About the Authors

PAMELA J. CARTER is a registered nurse and an award-winning instructor. After receiving her bachelor's degree in nursing from the University of Alabama in Huntsville, Pamela immediately began a career as a perioperative nurse. Over the course of her nursing career, she also worked in a physician's office and as a staff nurse in an intensive care unit.

Pamela started teaching informally while serving as an officer in the United States Air Force Nurse Corps. She formally entered the field of health care education by accepting a position at the Athens Area Technical Institute in Athens, Georgia, where she taught surgical technology. After obtaining a master's degree in adult vocational education from the University of Georgia, Pamela moved to Florida and took a position teaching nursing assisting students. She continued teaching nursing assisting after accepting a position at Davis Applied Technology College in Kaysville, Utah. During her first year at Davis Applied Technology College, Pamela piloted a new "open-entry/open-exit" method of curriculum delivery for the nursing assistant program at the college and was awarded the Superintendent's Award for Outstanding Faculty for her work. She then opened a surgical technology program at the college and has obtained national accreditation from the Commission on Accreditation of Allied Health Education Programs (CAAHEP) for delivery of this program using the "open-entry/open-exit" method. In 2002, Pamela received a National Merit Award for having her program rank in the top 10% in the nation for students passing their national certification exam.

Pamela's writing style reflects her love of teaching, and of nursing. She is grateful for the opportunity teaching and writing have afforded her to share her experience and knowledge with those just entering the health care profession, and to help those who are new to the profession to see how they can have a profound effect on the lives of others.

SUSAN LEWSEN holds a bachelor's degree in nursing from George Mason University, Fairfax, Virginia, and a master's degree in health administration from Webster University, Aurora, Colorado. She is currently the Certification Coordinator with the Utah Health Technology Certification Center in Kaysville, Utah, which administers the nurse aide registry for the state of Utah. Before coming to the registry, she served in the Army Nurse Corps for 21 years. While in the Army, Susan served as a staff nurse, charge nurse, supervisor, head nurse, and nurse educator, receiving numerous commendations and awards. Most recently, before she retired from the Army, Susan was training medics and practical nurses. Susan also has extensive experience in the area of home health. Throughout her nursing career she has remained an active volunteer with the American Red Cross, from which she received the Clara Barton award for her more than 30 years of volunteerism.

v

Lippincott's
Textbook *for* Nursing Assistants

Lippincott's
Textbook
for Nursing
Assistants

A Humanistic Approach to Caregiving

Pamela J. Carter, RN, BSN, M.Ed., CNOR
Program Coordinator/Instructor
School of Health Professions
Davis Applied Technology College
Kaysville, Utah

Susan Lewsen, MA, BSN, RN, LNC
Certification Coordinator
Utah Health Technology Certification Center
Kaysville, Utah

With Contributions By

LORRI POTTER NACEY, RN, BSN, MBA
Community Nursing Services
Salt Lake City, Utah

PAULA SICILIANO, APRN, MS, GNP
Assistant Professor
University of Utah—College of Nursing
Salt Lake City, Utah

SUSAN WRIGHT
Special Needs Coordinator
Davis County School District
Kaysville, Utah

LIPPINCOTT WILLIAMS & WILKINS
A **Wolters Kluwer** Company
Philadelphia • Baltimore • New York • London
Buenos Aires • Hong Kong • Sydney • Tokyo

Acquisitions Editor: Elizabeth Nieginski
Developmental Editor: Melanie Cann
Editorial Assistant: Josh Levandoski
Senior Production Editor: Tom Gibbons
Director of Nursing Production: Helen Ewan
Managing Editor/Production: Erika Kors
Art Director: Carolyn O'Brien
Senior Manufacturing Manager: William Alberti
Indexer: Kathy Pitcoff
Compositor: TechBooks
Printer: R.R. Donnelley—Willard

9 8 7 6 5 4 3 2 1

Library of Congress Cataloging-in-Publication Data

Carter, Pamela J.
   Lippincott's textbook for nursing assistants : a humanistic approach to caregiving / Pamela J. Carter, Susan Lewsen ; with contributions by Lorri Potter Nacey, Paula Siciliano, and Susan Wright.—1st ed.
      p. ; cm.
   Includes index
   ISBN 0-7817-3981-0 (hardcover : alk. paper)
      1. Nurses' aides.   2. Nursing.   I. Title: Textbook for nursing assistants.   II. Lewsen, Susan. III. Title.
      [DNLM: 1. Nurses' Aides.   2. Nursing Care. WY 193 C324L 2005]
RT84.C375 2005
610.73'06'98—dc22   2004012218

Care has been taken to confirm the accuracy of the information presented and to describe generally accepted practices. However, the authors, editors, and publisher are not responsible for errors or omissions or for any consequences from application of the information in this book and make no warranty, express or implied, with respect to the content of the publication.

The authors, editors, and publisher have exerted every effort to ensure that drug selection and dosage set forth in this text are in accordance with the current recommendations and practice at the time of publication. However, in view of ongoing research, changes in government regulations, and the constant flow of information relating to drug therapy and drug reactions, the reader is urged to check the package insert for each drug for any change in indications and dosage and for added warnings and precautions. This is particularly important when the recommended agent is a new or infrequently employed drug.

Some drugs and medical devices presented in this publication have Food and Drug Administration (FDA) clearance for limited use in restricted research settings. It is the responsibility of the health care provider to ascertain the FDA status of each drug or device planned for use in his or her clinical practice.

LWW.com

*To those who know me most deeply—my family. Mom and Dad quietly encouraged me to reach for higher ground. My sister Donna, although not quiet, kept me grounded and solid. My children, Jessi and Michael, gave up their mother to a stack of books and a computer screen for many evenings and weekends. Scott offered me a strong shoulder and Wednesday night dinners to keep me sane. I love you all so much! And also to all of my students. You truly have taught me as much as I ever taught you. —**P.J.***

*To my family, who always asked how things were going: my supportive husband Bob; Mom, who ran the house and did the cooking; and to our children—Michael, Patrick, and Kelly, for all their support. To all of my friends, for their moral and inspirational support —"Be wealthy in your friends" (William Shakespeare). To Lisa, who is the perfect role model for a CNA and will make an even better nurse. And to Miss Jasiecki, who gave me the desire to become a nurse and educator. I treasure our forty-plus years of friendship. She will always be my inspiration. —**S.L.***

Preface

The face of nursing assistant education is changing. Indeed, it must change if we are to keep pace with the needs of the health care industry. Today, the numbers of nursing assistants employed by hospitals, acute and extended-care facilities, hospice agencies, and home health care agencies are growing rapidly. In addition, the composition of the long-term care population (the population most frequently cared for by nursing assistants) is changing. Shorter hospital stays and advances in medicine and technology mean that today's long-term care resident tends to be older, sicker, and in need of more assistance with activities of daily living than the resident of 15 years ago. As educators, we must seek to provide our students with the skills and knowledge that they will need to meet the changing needs of their patients, residents, and clients, and to advance in their own careers.

In the past, the focus of nursing assistant education was on skill competency. However, that focus is shifting now toward graduating nursing assistants who not only possess the technical skills they need to provide competent care, but also the compassion and the communication and critical thinking skills they need to function effectively in the health care setting. It is no longer enough for nursing assistants to be competent at changing bed linens and measuring vital signs. Today's nursing assistants must also be able to recognize the person within the patient, resident, or client, and to understand that each person they are responsible for providing care for is unique and special, with individual needs that are very different from those of the person in the next bed. This textbook, *Lippincott's Textbook for Nursing Assistants,* has been written not only to help students develop the skills they need to become nursing assistants, but also to introduce them to a very humanistic approach to caregiving.

THEMES AND FEATURES

Three key beliefs guided us as we wrote this textbook:

1. Students need a textbook that captures their interest and increases their desire to learn.
2. Graduates of nursing assistant training programs must be able to provide competent, skilled care in a compassionate way.
3. The nursing assistant is a vital member of the health care team.

These beliefs form the basis for the textbook you hold in your hands.

LIPPINCOTT'S TEXTBOOK FOR NURSING ASSISTANTS IS WRITTEN WITH THE STUDENT IN MIND

One of our primary goals in writing this textbook was to make the information it contains interesting and accessible to the student. With that goal in mind, we have taken great care to present the student with a textbook that is easy and enjoyable to read, with a well-developed art program and proven learning aids.

A Student-Focused Writing Style

Educators know that a student can easily understand complex information if it is explained in a way that the student can understand. We have worked hard to develop a conversational, yet professional, writing style that respects the student's intelligence. Concepts are presented in a straightforward, accessible way, and the text is enlivened through the frequent use of examples and anecdotes from our own experience with patients and residents. Recognizing that many students entering nursing assistant training programs speak English as a second language or are resource students, we have had each chapter thoroughly reviewed by a special needs consultant to ensure an appropriate reading level.

An Art Program Developed Alongside the Text

The purpose of an art program is to reinforce and expand on concepts discussed in the text. To do this effectively, the art must be planned and developed alongside the manuscript. Numerous photographs, both alone and in combination with line art that has been created specifically for this textbook, help students to visualize and remember important concepts.

Proven Learning Aids in Every Chapter

Learning and remembering new information is challenging for many students. To help them meet the challenge of mastering the information in the textbook, we have developed features to assist students with studying and internalizing information:

- **What Will You Learn?** Each chapter begins with a *What Will You Learn?* section, which previews the chapter and helps to focus the student's reading. Each *What Will You Learn?* section begins with a paragraph that introduces the topic of the chapter to the student and explains why the topic is important. This introductory paragraph is then followed by a list of learning objectives and vocabulary words.
- **Summary.** Each chapter ends with a summary in a unique narrative outline format. This summary helps students to review the key, "take home" concepts of the chapter.
- **What Did You Learn?** Multiple-choice and matching exercises at the end of each chapter provide students with the opportunity to evaluate their understanding of the material they have just studied. Answers to these exercises are given in Appendix A.

LIPPINCOTT'S TEXTBOOK FOR NURSING ASSISTANTS IS DESIGNED TO PREPARE STUDENTS FOR CLINICAL PRACTICE

It is our desire to help prepare students to enter the health care profession with the knowledge, skills, and confidence that education and training can provide. Several of the textbook's features were designed specifically to help prepare the student for clinical practice:

- **Procedures.** Certainly, a major objective of any nursing assistant training course is to ensure that graduates are able to provide care in a safe and correct manner. Eighty-two core procedures are presented in this text. The procedures for each chapter are grouped at the end of the chapter, to avoid breaking up the text with lengthy boxes. *"Getting Ready"* and *"Finishing Up"* steps are reviewed at the beginning of each set of procedures and accompanied by icons to help students remember these very important pre- and post-procedure actions. The steps of the procedure are given using clear and concise language, and photographs and illustrations are provided as necessary. The concepts of privacy, safety, infection control, comfort, and communication are emphasized consistently in every procedure.

PROCEDURE 11-11
Transferring a Person from a Wheelchair to a Bed

Getting Ready   WGKIEPS

1. Complete the "Getting Ready" steps a through g.

Supplies
- transfer belt

Procedure

2. Make sure that the bed is lowered to its lowest position and that the wheels are locked. Raise the head of the bed, fanfold the top linens to the foot of the bed, and raise the opposite side rail.

3. Position the wheelchair close to the side of the bed, so that the person's strong side is next to the bed. Lock the wheelchair wheels, and either remove the footrests or swing them to the side.

4. Remove the person's lap blanket (if one was used) and release the wheelchair safety belt, if in use. Apply a transfer belt.

STEP 7 Help the person to stand.

5. Stand facing the person, with your feet spread about 12 inches apart and with your knees slightly bent to protect your back. With your back straight, slide the person to the front of the wheelchair seat.

6. Grasp the transfer belt (or pass your arms under the person's arms, placing your hands on her upper back). Position your feet along-

side the person's feet, flexing your knees. Place your shins against the person's shins to block the person's feet and keep her knees from buckling as she stands up.

7. Have the person rest her hands on your arms, and assist her to stand by pulling on the transfer belt as you straighten your knees. (If you are not using a transfer belt, assist the person into a standing position by gently pulling her up and forward as you straighten your knees.) Remember to keep your back straight. Alternatively, a person who requires less assistance can place her hands on the wheelchair arms for support and "push off" while you offer support.

8. Slowly help the person to turn toward the bed by pivoting on her strong leg. Help the person to sit on the edge of the bed.

9. Remove the person's robe and slippers, if appropriate.

STEP 8 Help the person to sit on the edge of the bed.

10. Move the wheelchair out of the way.

11. Place one of your arms around the person's shoulders and one arm under her legs. Swing the person's legs onto the bed.

- **Guidelines Boxes.** These boxes summarize general guidelines for various aspects of the nursing assistant's job. The unique "What You Do/Why You Do It" format helps students to understand why things are done a certain way. Rather than just presenting students with an endless list of guidelines to memorize, we have provided them with a tool for remembering why these guidelines are important to follow.

GUIDELINES BOX 9-1
GUIDELINES FOR PROTECTING YOURSELF FROM PHYSICAL INJURY

What you do	Why you do it
Make a habit of practicing good posture.	Keeping the body in proper alignment, regardless of the activity, reduces stress and fatigue to the muscles and joints.
Create a solid base of support by moving your feet apart, either by widening your stance or by placing one foot in front of the other.	A solid base of support improves your balance, reducing the chance that you will injure yourself during the maneuver.
Allow the weight of your own body to assist in pulling or pushing heavy objects.	Using coordinated body movement to move something minimizes the stress on your body while making the task you are trying to accomplish easier.
When moving or lifting people or objects, place your body as close as possible to the object being moved.	Bringing your body's center of gravity closer to the object improves your balance and allows the strong muscles of the shoulders and upper arms to assist in the move.
Squat, do not lean over, to lower your center of gravity when lifting.	Lowering your center of gravity improves your balance. However, this lowering should be accomplished by squatting, rather than leaning over. Squatting allows you to use the strong muscles of your lower body to move yourself, and the weight, upward. Leaning over while lifting weight strains the back joints and muscles.
Use the large, strong muscles of the hips, buttocks, and thighs to do the lifting.	Using the strong muscles of the legs to move yourself upward is preferable to placing strain on the muscles of the back, which are not meant to be used to lift substantial amounts of weight.
Do not lift heavy objects from a position higher than your head. Use a step stool or a short safety ladder to raise your entire body closer to the desired level.	Attempting to lift a heavy object from an awkward position (for example, with your arms raised above your head) interferes with your ability to balance and places you at risk for injury.
If an object is very heavy, do not attempt to lift it. Instead, pull, push, or roll the object.	Pushing, pulling, or rolling a heavy object places less strain on your body because you can use your body weight to help you accomplish the task. In other words, you can use the principle of coordinated movement.
Use assistive devices whenever possible to make the job easier.	Hand carts and dollies permit the easy movement of objects by placing them on wheels. Gait belts, draw sheets, and mechanical lifts (discussed in detail in Chapter 11) help make moving people easier.
Ask for help when lifting or moving heavy people or objects. You should also get help when you need to move a person who cannot offer any assistance, or is combative.	Heavy or awkward loads increase your risk of injury (and, if you are attempting to lift a person, increase that person's risk of injury as well.) A person who is "dead weight" or uncooperative is both heavy and awkward.
Keep your body in good physical condition by exercising regularly, eating nutritious foods, and getting enough rest.	Your body can be compared to an automobile. It must be properly maintained in order to provide you with years of solid performance.

- **Tell the Nurse! Notes.** A recurrent theme throughout the book is the important role the nursing assistant plays in making observations about a patient's or resident's condition and reporting these observations to the nurse. The *Tell the Nurse!* notes highlight and summarize signs and symptoms that a nursing assistant may observe that should be reported to the nurse.
- **Stop and Think! Scenarios.** Each chapter concludes with one or more *Stop and Think!* scenarios. These scenarios, which are excellent tools for initiating classroom discussion, encourage students to think

---

Tell the Nurse!

While providing hand and foot care, always be aware of potential signs and symptoms of illness or infection. Tell the nurse if you observe any of the following:

➤ Nailbeds that are either very pale or blue, or bruised

➤ Nails that are unusually yellow or white

➤ Nails that are unusually thick

➤ Nails that are broken or have been cut too short (especially if there is also bleeding or tenderness)

➤ Nails that are ingrown

➤ Cuticles that are torn, red, or swollen

➤ Skin that is blistered, red, or tender (especially on the feet)

➤ Any unusual rashes or odors

---

critically to solve problems, and help them to see that many situations they will encounter in the workplace do not have cut-and-dried answers.

Stop and think!

➤ Mr. Lovell, one of the residents with dementia at the long-term care facility where you work, has become very agitated. He is prone to falling, and should not get up without help. However, today he is refusing to stay in his bed or his wheelchair. You get him situated, and then as soon as you leave the room, he tries to get up again. This has happened twice, and you are only in the first hour of your shift. You are very concerned that Mr. Lovell will fall and hurt himself, but you cannot stay with him all day because you have other residents to attend to. Describe some things that you could do to help protect Mr. Lovell.

LIPPINCOTT'S TEXTBOOK FOR NURSING ASSISTANTS SEEKS TO INSTILL IN STUDENTS PRIDE IN THEMSELVES AND THEIR CHOSEN PROFESSION

Finally, it is our utmost desire to impress upon students entering the health care profession that no one is "just" a nursing assistant. Nursing assistants are often the members of the health care team with the most day-to-day contact with patients, residents, and clients. As such, they bear a large part of the responsibility for the well-being of those in their care. To highlight the contributions that nursing assistants make, each unit in the textbook concludes with a patient's, resident's, client's, or family member's first-person account of how a nursing assistant had a positive impact on their lives or the lives of their loved ones. The goal of these *Nursing Assistants Make A Difference!* stories is to help students to see that nursing assistants are vital members of the health care team. Nursing assistants who feel that they can and do make a difference in the lives of others will go the "extra mile" to ensure that the care they provide is holistic.

AN OVERVIEW OF *LIPPINCOTT'S TEXTBOOK FOR NURSING ASSISTANTS*

Lippincott's Textbook for Nursing Assistants is a comprehensive textbook, designed to prepare students to work as nursing assistants in any health care setting, as well as to open their eyes to the many career opportunities that exist within the health care field and to entice them to further their learning. We are in the midst of a health care crisis—profound demographic changes have led to an ever-widening gap between the number of people who need care and the number of people who are qualified to provide that care. As educators of future health care professionals, we are charged with providing the community with competent, dedicated, compassionate caregivers. In recognition of this need we have designed this textbook to be in accordance with standards for curriculum development established by organizations such as the National Consortium on Health Science and Technology Education (NCHSTE) and Health Occupations Students of America (HOSA). The eleven national health care skill standards, as put forth by NCHSTE, represent the basic skills and knowledge that a student needs to pursue a full range of career opportunities within the health care field.

A lifelong interest in learning new information is an important quality for any health care professional to have, as the body of information related to medicine and health care is constantly evolving. A lifelong interest in learning benefits the recipients of the care provided by our graduates, as well as our graduates themselves. Awareness of career pathways allows those just entering the health care profession to set goals for career advancement and reach them, over time receiving higher levels of compensation for higher levels of experience, skills, and responsibilities.

This textbook consists of eight units. The following is a brief survey of these units and the information they contain.

UNIT 1: INTRODUCTION TO HEALTH CARE

The six chapters that make up Unit 1 provide the student with basic background knowledge. Chapter 1 begins with an overview of how health care has evolved, and continues to evolve, in the United States. It then provides the student with a basic understanding of how the governmental regulations that control health care standards and payment came into existence. Chapter 1 also provides an overview of the many different types of health care facilities, and introduces the idea of holistic care and the "health care team." Chapter 2 focuses on the nursing assistant's roles and responsibilities as a member of the health care team, and on the concept of delegation. Professionalism, job-seeking skills, and the concept of work ethic are thoroughly discussed in Chapter 3, introducing students to the idea that a professional attitude promotes respect and is necessary for career advancement. Legal and ethical issues, including patient and resident rights and the Health Insurance Portability and Accountability Act (HIPAA), are covered in Chapter 4. Communication, one of the most essential responsibilities of the nursing assistant, is discussed in Chapter 5. We conclude this unit with Chapter 6, which focuses on the central member of the health care team—the patient, resident, or client. This final chapter introduces the concept of human needs and explains how the person being cared for in a health care setting has many needs other than those specifically associated with illness or disability.

UNIT 2: SAFETY

The six chapters that compose Unit 2 are concerned with the measures taken to ensure safety. Chapters 7 and 8 cover communicable disease, and how the spread of communicable disease is prevented in the health care setting. Chapter 9 deals with workplace safety, and includes an extensive discussion about the importance of using proper body mechanics to prevent work-related injuries. Chapter 10 explores some of the conditions that put patients, residents, or clients at risk for injury, followed by a discussion about methods used to prevent accidents from occurring. In Chapter 11, we cover the techniques used to safely assist patients, residents, and clients with repositioning and transferring. We conclude this unit with Chapter 12, which contains information related to recognizing emergencies and responding to them.

UNIT 3: BASIC PATIENT AND RESIDENT CARE

The eight chapters in this unit focus on the skills and equipment used to provide basic daily care to patients, residents, and clients. Chapters 13 and 14 introduce the student to the health care environment and explain the processes for admitting, transferring, or discharging patients, residents, and clients. Chapter 15 covers bedmaking. Chapter 16 covers vital signs, with an emphasis on exactly what function of the body is being measured and situations that may alter these measurements. We have also included practical hints and tips to take the mystery out of taking vital sign measurements, procedures that many students find intimidating and difficult to master at first. Chapters 17 and 18 cover bathing and grooming, with a focus on empathizing with the person receiving the care. In Chapter 19, we present information about basic nutrition in a factual, useful manner without undue emphasis on specific diets, as these continue to change as research dictates. We conclude Unit 3 with Chapter 20, a discussion about assisting with elimination. Again, much emphasis is placed on empathizing with the patient, resident, or client who requires assistance with this most intimate of activities.

UNIT 4: DEATH AND DYING

This unit has been written as two separate chapters to emphasize the fact that a person may cope with a terminal illness and the stages of grief for a long period of time before the actual physical process of dying takes place. Chapter 21 introduces the student to the stages of grief within the context of a discussion about terminal illness. Important concepts such as advance directives, wills, and palliative care are also introduced in this chapter. Chapter 22 focuses on the care a nursing assistant provides to the dying person and his or her family members in the hours immediately leading up to, and following, death. Both chapters in this unit include discussions about the grief a nursing assistant can expect to feel when a patient, resident, or client dies or receives a diagnosis of a terminal illness.

UNIT 5: STRUCTURE AND FUNCTION OF THE HUMAN BODY

Having a basic understanding of how each of the body's organ systems functions in health is essential to understanding how failure of an organ system to work properly leads to disease and disability. This unit begins with Chapter 23, which provides an overview of the body's organization and introduces the student to rehabilitation and restorative care as methods used to restore function when function has been changed or lost. The next 10 chapters (Chapters 24 through 33) each cover one of the organ systems. A basic explanation of the normal structure and function of the organ system is given, with an emphasis on homeostasis. Next, the normal effects of aging are discussed and differentiated from the effects of disease and disability. We then discuss key disorders specific to that particular body system. Diagnostic tests and treatments are covered next, along with rehabilitation and restorative care measures specific to the organ system under discussion. Throughout these chapters, the nursing assistant's role in recognizing problems and providing care is emphasized.

UNIT 6: SPECIAL CARE CONCERNS

This unit, which consists of five chapters, introduces the student to the special needs of certain groups of people. In Chapter 34, we review some of the major types of developmental disabilities. Chapter 35 is dedicated to a discussion about mental illness, including the importance of recognizing depression in elderly patients, residents, and clients. In Chapter 36, the student is introduced to the idea of dementia, and provided with specific information about how to communicate with, and care for, people suffering from this devastating condition. Chapter 37 discusses the diagnosis and treatment of cancer, as well as the special needs of people with cancer. The final chapter in this unit, Chapter 38, discusses the special needs of the person who is HIV-positive or has AIDS.

UNIT 7: ACUTE CARE

Nursing assistants provide care in many different types of health care settings. Many work in hospitals and clinics and assist nurses in caring for patients with acute conditions. The focus of the three chapters in Unit 7 is on special populations of patients that the nursing assistant may encounter in the acute care setting. Chapter 39 is dedicated to the surgical patient, Chapter 40 to obstetrical patients and newborns, and Chapter 41 to the pediatric patient.

UNIT 8: HOME HEALTH CARE

The two chapters in this final unit introduce the student to the home health care setting. Building on the basic knowledge and skills presented in previous units, this unit explores some of the concerns and issues that are unique to the home health care setting. Chapter 42 provides the student with an overview of what home health care is, who might require it, and how it is paid for, and explores some of the qualities that a person must have to succeed as a home health care aide. Chapter 43 covers specific issues related to safety and infection control within the home.

APPENDICES AND GLOSSARY

The textbook concludes with three appendices and a comprehensive glossary. Appendix A contains the answers to the *What Did You Learn?* exercises that appear at the end of each chapter. Appendix B summarizes the educational requirements for becoming a nursing assistant in each state. Appendix C introduces the student to the

language of health care. We chose to include this discussion about medical terminology as an appendix so that it could be introduced at any point during the training course, and referred to frequently. The tables containing common roots, prefixes, suffixes, and abbreviations are in close physical proximity to the glossary for easy and quick reference.

The glossary is the most comprehensive found in any nursing assistant textbook. A precise definition of each vocabulary word is given. The number in parentheses at the end of each entry indicates the chapter where the term is introduced as a vocabulary word. Extensive cross-references remind students of synonyms and antonyms, and help them to differentiate related words. All of the terms in the glossary are included on the audio glossary found on the CD included with the book, enabling students to hear the words pronounced, defined, and used in a sentence.

A COMPREHENSIVE PACKAGE FOR TEACHING AND LEARNING

To further facilitate teaching and learning, a carefully designed ancillary package is available. In addition to the usual print resources, we are pleased to present multimedia tools that have been developed in conjunction with the text.

RESOURCES FOR STUDENTS

- **Interactive back-of-book CD-ROM.** Packaged with the textbook at no additional charge, this CD contains an illustrated audio glossary and additional *Nursing Assistants Make A Difference!* stories read aloud.
- **Workbook to Accompany *Lippincott's Textbook for Nursing Assistants*.** Developed by an instructional design team, this four-color workbook provides the student with a fun and engaging way of reviewing important concepts and vocabulary. Multiple-choice questions, matching exercises, true-false exercises, word finds, crossword puzzles, coloring and labeling exercises, and other types of active-learning tools are provided to appeal to many different learn-

ing styles. The workbook also contains procedure checklists for each procedure in the textbook.

RESOURCES FOR INSTRUCTORS

- **Instructor's Resource Manual to Accompany *Lippincott's Textbook for Nursing Assistants.*** Authored by Pamela Carter and Lori Strong of Davis Applied Technology College, the instructor's manual contains four parts. Part 1 provides information about classroom management that many beginning instructors may find helpful. This part also introduces the reader to the "open-entry, open-exit" approach to structuring training programs. Part 2 reviews cognitive learning styles and includes a quiz that can be used to determine a student's learning style, as well as tips for appealing to each type of learner. Tips for making information accessible to resource and special needs students are also included in this part of the instructor's manual. Part 3 provides chapter-by-chapter teaching objectives, lecture outlines, teaching strategies, ideas for classroom activities and assignments, and points for discussion related to the *Stop and Think!* scenarios found in the textbook. The final part, Part 4, contains two 100-question multiple-choice exams that can be photocopied and given as practice exams to students at the conclusion of the course. Answer keys for these exams are also included in Part 4 of the Instructor's Manual.
- **Test Generator on CD-ROM.** Approximately 650 multiple-choice questions and the Diploma test generator are included on the *Instructor's Resource CD.* With the Diploma test generator, instructors can add their own questions, modify existing questions, and create chapter quizzes, unit quizzes, or comprehensive exams at the push of a button.
- **PowerPoint™ Lectures on CD-ROM.** A slide presentation to accompany each chapter in the book is available on the *Instructor's Resource CD.*
- **Image Bank on CD-ROM.** All of the illustrations in the text, as well as many of the photographs, are available on the *Instructor's Resource CD* in formats suitable for hard-copy printouts or incorporation into PowerPoint™ presentations or websites.

ADDITIONAL RESOURCES

- ***Lippincott's Video Series for Nursing Assistants.*** Procedure-based modules provide step-by-step demonstrations of the core skills that form the basis of the daily care the nursing assistant provides. *Getting Ready* and *Finishing Up* actions are reviewed on every procedure-based module, and the theme of communication is emphasized throughout. Four non-procedure–based modules, on the topics of preparing for entry into the workforce, caring for people with dementia, death and dying, and patient and resident rights, are also available.
- **Copper Ridge *Dementia Care Modules.*** Developed by the esteemed Copper Ridge Institute in affiliation with Johns Hopkins University School of Medicine, this two-CD set consists of nine interactive modules designed to teach students how to care for people with dementia. The causes and types of dementia are reviewed, along with dementia-related behaviors and the best way to manage them. Communication and compassion are emphasized throughout. Learning is enhanced through video clips, interactive exercises, and short multiple-choice quizzes at the conclusion of each module.

It is with great pleasure that we introduce these resources—the textbook, the ancillary package, the videos, and the Copper Ridge modules—to you. One of our primary goals in creating these resources has been to share with those just entering the health care field our sense of excitement about the health care profession, and our commitment to the idea that being a nursing assistant involves much more than just "bedpans and blood pressures." We hope we have succeeded in that goal, and we welcome feedback from our readers.

Pamela J. Carter
Susan Lewsen

To the Student

Welcome! By enrolling in this nursing assistant training course, you have taken a big first step. You may be taking this course for any number of different reasons. For example, you may be taking this course to "test the waters"—to see if working in health care is something you really want to do. Or, you may already know that you want to work in health care, and you are taking this course because it is the first step toward reaching your goal.

Health care is an exciting, yet demanding, field. During your training course, you will be expected to learn and apply a lot of new information. You will even have to learn a new language, the language of health care! My name is Pam Carter, and I am the lead author of the book you hold in your hands. It is my pleasure and my honor to assist you on your journey toward becoming a health care professional.

HOW TO USE THE BOOK TO PREPARE FOR CLASS AND STUDY

Learning is an active process. You need to read, make notes, and ask questions about anything you are having trouble understanding. Most students who are successful learners take a three-step approach to learning:

PREVIEW

During the *preview* stage of learning, you focus on preparing yourself for class. Most likely, your instructor will give you reading assignments that must be completed before each class. The course *syllabus* that you will receive at the beginning of the course will tell you when each reading assignment must be completed. The reading

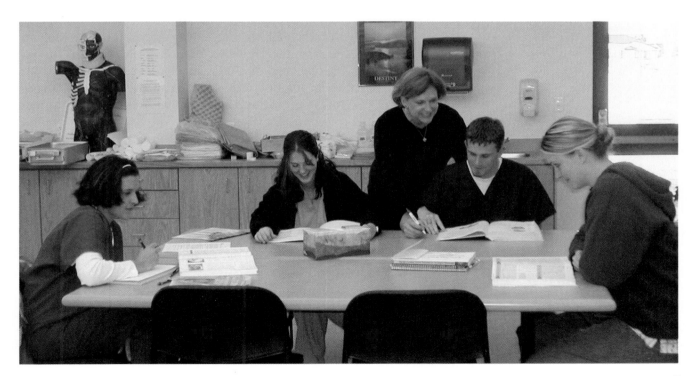

assignments give you the chance to get a general idea of what is going to be discussed in the next class.

To prepare for class, just read the assignment as if you were reading a novel or a newspaper for enjoyment. During the preview, you do not need to take notes or try to memorize facts—just read through the material to get the "big picture" of the information you are about to learn. Some people find it helpful to read the chapter out loud to themselves (or into a tape recorder, so that they can listen to the chapter again later). Others like to highlight parts of the chapter using a highlighting pen, or make notes in the margin. Learning becomes much easier when you discover what methods work best for you.

To assist you with previewing, we begin each chapter in the book with a *What Will You Learn?* section. This section contains a list of specific goals for the chapter, called *learning objectives*. Learning objectives tell you what you will be expected to know or be able to do to demonstrate complete understanding of the material in the chapter. During the preview stage, the learning objectives can be very useful in giving you an overview of the key goals of the chapter.

What will you learn?

There are many types of personal care routines. In the previous chapter, you learned how to help people with the most basic aspects of personal care, those activities related to keeping the body clean and healthy. **Grooming,** or activities related to maintaining a neat and attractive appearance, goes beyond basic personal hygiene. The routine care of the hands and feet (including the nails), shampooing and styling of the hair, the application of make-up, and shaving are all grooming practices that, while not necessarily *essential* for health, certainly play a role in maintaining both physical and emotional health. Imagine that you are a patient or a resident, and you are unable to complete your regular grooming activities. Your hair is uncombed, you have not applied make-up (if you are a woman) or shaved (if you are a man), and you are not dressed for visitors, yet company arrives anyway. How would you feel? Would you be able to fully enjoy your guests, or would you be worried about your appearance? Helping your patients and residents with "putting their best face forward," the subject of this chapter, is part of providing holistic care. When you are finished with this chapter, you will be able to:

1. Discuss how grooming differs from hygiene.
2. Describe factors that influence a person's grooming habits.
3. Explain the effect that illness or disability may have on a person's grooming habits.
4. List changes that occur in a person's feet as a result of aging or illness.
5. Understand the importance of proper hand and foot care.
6. Demonstrate proper technique for assisting with hand and foot care.
7. Discuss the various dressing needs that a patient or resident may have.
8. Demonstrate different methods of helping a person to dress and undress.
9. Discuss disorders a nursing assistant may observe when assisting with hair care.
10. Describe the different methods used to assist a person with shampooing his or her hair.
11. Describe methods used to style a person's hair.
12. Demonstrate proper technique for shampooing a bedridden person's hair and combing a person's hair.
13. Describe the tools and supplies used for shaving.
14. Demonstrate how to safely shave a man's face.
15. Explain how the use of make-up can affect a person's sense of well being.

Vocabulary

Use the CD in the back of your book to hear these terms pronounced, defined, and used in a sentence:

Grooming	Podiatrist	Seborrheic dermatitis	Pediculosis capitis
Hangnail	Dandruff	(cradle cap)	Nits
Tinea pedis	Tinea capitis	Alopecia	

The *What Will You Learn?* section also contains a list of the new vocabulary words you will

need to learn. The vocabulary words, which appear in **bold type** throughout the chapter, are listed in the order that they appear. You can use the CD in the back of your book to hear the words in each vocabulary list pronounced, defined, and used in a sentence. This is an effective and fun way to preview vocabulary words! Or you can look each word up in the glossary at the back of the book to find a complete definition. Familiarizing yourself with the chapter's vocabulary words before class puts you one step ahead, because when you hear those words in class, they will not sound strange to you, and you may already know what they mean.

VIEW

The *viewing* stage is when you get down to business and really work to understand the material. During the classroom lecture or discussion, highlight important points and take notes as you need to. Ask questions about any of the material that you do not fully understand. Remember, there are no "stupid" questions! If you do not fully understand something, you need to speak up so that the instructor can help you. This is your instructor's job.

REVIEW

After class, go back over the notes you took in class, and re-read the chapter in your book. Some students like to read the entire chapter over again. Others just skim the chapter, paying close attention to the topics they still have questions about. Read the chapter summary, which repeats and summarizes the key concepts of the chapter.

When you feel comfortable with your understanding of the material, test yourself! Go back to the learning objectives in the *What Will You Learn?* section at the beginning of the chapter and pretend they are questions. Try to answer them. If you have trouble answering them, then you know that you need to review certain parts of the chapter again. You can also test yourself using the *What Did You Learn?* section, at the end of each chapter. The answers to the questions in the *What Did You Learn?* section are in Appendix A in the back of the book so that you can see how well

SUMMARY

▶ Caring for the hands and feet (especially the fingernails and toenails), selecting an outfit to wear, shampooing and styling the hair, shaving, and applying make-up are grooming practices that people may engage in to make themselves feel more attractive and confident.

■ Grooming practices differ from hygiene practices in that grooming practices are performed mainly for the sake of appearance. Therefore, good grooming is more essential for emotional health than for physical health. However, grooming practices do benefit physical health as well.

■ Personal grooming practices are highly variable and are influenced by many factors, including culture, religion, upbringing, level of income, current fashion, and a person's feelings about his or her own sexuality. Respecting your patient's or resident's personal preferences is an important part of providing holistic care. Remembering this is very important when assisting with grooming.

▶ Care of the hands and feet focuses on keeping the skin and nails clean and healthy.

■ Assisting with hand and foot care gives the nursing assistant the chance to observe for potential health problems, including poor blood flow and fungal infections.

■ Poor blood flow to the feet is associated with many health problems, including decreased sensation and an increased risk for a

What did you learn?

Multiple Choice

Select the single best answer for each of the following questions.

1. You are a nursing assistant in a long-term care facility. Which one of the following procedures may be beyond your scope of practice?
   a. Assisting a resident with bathing
   b. Polishing a female resident's fingernails
   c. Trimming the toenails of a resident with diabetes
   d. Assisting a resident with oral hygiene

2. When helping a person to dress, which item of clothing would you put on first?
   a. Underpants
   b. Socks
   c. Slacks
   d. Sweater

3. Mrs. Dinksley, one of your residents, had a stroke that caused her left side to become weak. You are helping Mrs. Dinksley put on a cardigan sweater. Which arm should you put in the sleeve first?
   a. The left arm
   b. The right arm
   c. Either arm; it makes no difference
   d. Neither arm; Mrs. Dinksley should not be wearing a cardigan sweater

4. Mr. Bush has just been admitted to the long-term care facility where you work. You are telling him about the facility's policies. One of these policies is that residents are bathed on Monday, Wednesday, and Friday mornings. Mr. Bush looks worried, and says that he always bathes and shaves before he goes to bed, and he likes to do this every night. How do you react to this?
   a. You tell Mr. Bush that you're sorry, but he has to follow facility policy.
   b. You tell Mr. Bush "OK" but then schedule him for a bath every Monday, Wednesday, and Friday morning, just like everyone else.
   c. You respect Mr. Bush's choice and schedule him for a bath and a shave as part of evening care, every evening.
   d. You report Mr. Bush to the nurse because he is being difficult.

5. Brushing the hair is important to:
   a. Make it grow faster
   b. Make it soft and shiny and prevent tangles
   c. Keep it clean
   d. Keep it free from lice

6. When shaving a man's face with a safety razor and shaving cream, you should:
   a. Soften the beard with warm water before applying the shaving cream
   b. Apply aftershave lotion after the shave is complete, if the man requests it
   c. Give the man a mirror so that he can check his appearance when you are finished
   d. All of the above

7. When shaving a man's face, you should:
   a. Apply shaving cream sparingly
   b. Use upward strokes when shaving the cheeks
   c. Apply an antiseptic to any cuts or nicks
   d. Use downward strokes to shave the chin

8. Which one of the following statements about nail care is true?
   a. Scissors are used to trim the nails.
   b. Elderly people do not need nail care because their nails do not grow as fast.
   c. Providing nail care allows you to examine the hands and feet for signs of health and disease.
   d. Nail care is an activity that can be skipped if there is not enough time.

9. Which one of the following benefits does a patient or resident enjoy when you shampoo his or her hair?
   a. Improved circulation (blood flow) to the scalp
   b. A clean, neat appearance
   c. Increased feelings of well-being
   d. All of the above

10. Which one of the following statements about helping a resident to dress is true?
   a. Residents like staff members to decide what they are going to wear.
   b. Residents are used to being dressed in front of others.
   c. Residents care about how they look.
   d. Residents who are disabled do not need to dress in street clothes.

you understood the material you just studied. Again, if you have trouble answering these questions, then you will know that your studying is not quite finished! You may need to read certain parts of the chapter again, or ask your instructor for help.

Try to set aside short periods of time for studying each day. For example, you might study for 30 to 45 minutes, take a break to attend to other activities or chores, and then come back and study for another 30 to 45 minutes. After 30 to 45 minutes of studying, most people become tired and lose their ability to concentrate. Studying in short bursts will help keep you focused on the material you are trying to learn.

HOW TO PREPARE FOR TESTS

Did you learn the material or not? This is what instructors want to know when they give tests, quizzes, and exams. Not doing well on a test does not mean that you are a failure. It just means that you need to figure out what went wrong, and make an effort to improve the next time. Perhaps you did not study as well as you could have for the test. Or maybe you got so nervous, you forgot everything you learned when it came time to take the test!

The course syllabus will tell you when a test is scheduled to be given, and what material it will cover. Mark these dates on your calendar, so you are not surprised! Preparing for a test should not be a major event. If you use the preview–view–review approach and study each day, when it comes time to prepare for the test, you will be very well prepared. In the days leading up to the test, all you will need to do is review the material that will be covered on the test one more time, by skimming the chapters in the book and reviewing the notes you took in class.

When it comes time to actually take the test, remember the following tips:

- Relax! You have prepared for this test, and you know the answers to these questions!
- Take a deep breath and make sure you read the directions carefully. The directions will tell you whether there is only one correct answer for each question, or whether it is possible for a question to have more than one correct answer.
- Read each question completely and carefully. Many students answer questions incorrectly simply because they are in a hurry and miss important words, like "except" or "not."
- If the question is a multiple-choice question, try to state the answer in your head before looking at the answer choices. Then read each answer choice before choosing the one that best matches the answer you have in your head. This will increase your confidence that the answer you have selected is the correct one.
- After selecting an answer, avoid second-guessing yourself. Research has shown that your first choice is most likely to be correct, if you studied the material well. Sometimes, however, you will come across a question later in the test that makes you realize that you answered an earlier question incorrectly. In this case, when you are sure that you have made a mistake, it is all right to go back and change your answer. But if you do not have a clear idea of what the correct answer is, doubting your first choice will most likely result in changing a correct answer to an incorrect one!
- If you cannot answer a question, go on to the next. Often, another question on the test will jog your memory and help you to remember the answer to the question you skipped earlier. Just remember to go back over your answer sheet before you hand in your test to make sure you have answered all of the questions.

Many people think that the goal of studying is to pass a test. It is true that as you work through your training course, you will have to pass many tests. And most states require people who want to be nursing assistants to pass a certification exam at the end of the training course. But passing the test is a short-term goal. It is more important for you to be able to remember and use the information that you learned during your training course long after you complete the course and pass the certification exam. The people you will be caring for are depending on you to be knowledgeable and good at what you do. They are trusting you with their health and well-being. Study hard, ask questions, and remember that each and every person you care for throughout your career deserves the same type of competent, compassionate care that you would expect to be given to your own mother, father, spouse, sibling, or child. As a nursing assistant, you will have the chance to have a positive effect on the lives of many people.

Caring for those in need is very important work. Let me be among the first to thank you for your interest in pursuing a career in health care, and to wish you luck on your journey.

Sincerely,
Pam

Reviewers

We express our thanks to the many nursing assistant instructors who read the manuscript during its various stages of development and provided us with valuable suggestions for improving it:

Zaydie F. Abucejo
Southwestern College
Chula Vista, California

Katrina Allen
Faulkner State Community College
Bay Minette, Alabama

Deana Allison
Dawson Community College
Glendive, Montana

Judith A. Alter
Richmond Community College
Hamlet, North Carolina

Linda Amondson-Muller
Lower Columbia College
Longview, Washington

Linda Bacion
El Paso Community College
El Paso, Texas

Carol Bauck
Allen County Community College
Garnett, Kansas

Mary Anne Blackburn
Bolton Manor Nursing and Rehabilitation Center
Marlboro, Massachusetts

Rebecca J. Blanton
Manhattan Area Technical College
Manhattan, Kansas

Sue Boedeker
Gateway Technical College—Kenosha Campus
Kenosha, Wisconsin

DeLyna Bohnenblust
Labette Community College
Altamont, Kansas

Gail Breese
Spoon River College
Canton, Illinois

Betty Brock
Northeast Texas Community College
Mount Pleasant, Texas

Victoria Brown
Jefferson College
Hillsboro, Missouri

Claudia Campbell
Brevard Community College
Cocoa, Florida

Diane Cardamone
Wake Technical Community College
Raleigh, North Carolina

Anne Cassens
Normandale Community College
Bloomington, Minnesota

Linda Cater
Gadsden State Community College
Gadsden, Alabama

Kim Chacon
Trinidad State Junior College
Trinidad, Colorado

Lydia R. Chavana
South Texas Vocational Technical Institute
McAllen, Texas

Judith Conlin
Florida Department of Education
Tallahassee, Florida

Jean Cook
Templeton Developmental Center
Gardner, Massachusetts

Patricia DeiTos
Northern Virginia Community College
Fairfax, Virginia

Janetta DeOnna
Pennsylvania State University
University Park, Pennsylvania

Elaine Dinsel
Samaritan Health Services
Corvallis, Oregon

Patricia T. Doherty
Berks Heim—Berks County Home
Leesport, Pennsylvania

Julie Drake
Edmonds School District
Edmonds, Washington

Betty Earp
Mesa Community College
Mesa, Arizona

Toni Erickson
Pinellas Technical Education Center
Clearwater, Florida

Marie Etienne
Miami Dade College
Miami, Florida

Joan Fantozzi
Wilbur Wright College
Chicago, Illinois

Rhonda Ferrell
James Sprunt Community College
Kenansville, North Carolina

Sharon Franklin
Grayson County College
Denison, Texas

Mike Freel
Nebraska Methodist College
Omaha, Nebraska

Shirley Gaddis
Haywood Community College
Clyde, North Carolina

Mary Garcia
City Colleges of Chicago
Chicago, Illinois

Kimberly Gibson
Tennessee Technical Center at Athens
Athens, Tennessee

Candace Gioia
Pinellas Technical Education Center
Clearwater, Florida

Nathalie Grant
Health Careers Institute
West Palm Beach, Florida

Irmgard Grundner
Waubonsee Community College
Sugar Grove, Illinois

Barbara J. Gunderson
Carl Sandburg College
Galesburg, Illinois

Stephanie J. Guy
Southeast Arkansas College
Pine Bluff, Arkansas

Stacy Harper
Sunnyside Retirement Communities
Harrisonburg, Virginia

Terry Harper
Southwest Georgia Technical College
Thomasville, Georgia

Dalia Harrelson
Sam Houston State University
Huntsville, Texas

Lisa Hartwell
College of Medical Training
Lakewood, Washington

Ann Hess
Johnson County Community College Area
    Vocational School
Overland Park, Kansas

Pamela Hinckley
Redlands Adult School
Redlands, California

Sharon T. Hinton
Rural Nurse Resource Training Center
Floydada, Texas

Delores Holland
Wilbur Wright College
Chicago, Illinois

Judy A. Holton
Los Angeles Valley College
Los Angeles, California

Tim Inverso
The Center for Professional Personnel Development
    at The Pennsylvania State University
Teaching the Educator Program
State College, Pennsylvania
Nazareth Hospital
Philadelphia, Pennsylvania

Mary Jarmulowicz
Technical College of the Lowcountry
Beaufort, South Carolina

Judith Ann Johle
Kingwood College
Kingwood, Texas

Leslie Johnson
Lake Washington Technical College
Kirkland, Washington

Gail Joseph
Madison Area Technical College
Prairie du Sac, Wisconsin

Cheryl Jost
Lake Superior College
Duluth, Minnesota

Mary Krieg
Kennedy Western University
Cheyenne, Wyoming

Merlin A. Krull
Anderson County Career & Technical Center
Clinton, Tennessee

Charlene Kubic
Morton College
Downes Grove, Illinois

Debora Lemon
Walla Walla Community College
Clarkston, Washington

Bernice Lewis
Brunswick Community College
Supply, North Carolina

Doris Littlefield
Brevard Community College
Titusville, Florida

Gene Livingston
Texarkana College
Texarkana, Texas

Laura Logan
Angelina College
Lufkin, Texas

Marilyn Loptien
Arapahoe Community College
Littleton, Colorado

Cassie D. Matheson
Tennessee Technical Center
Harriman, Tennessee

Penelope McConley
Fayetteville Technical Community College
Fayetteville, North Carolina

Karen McConnell
Southeastern Illinois College
Harrisburg, Illinois

Betty McDonnell
John Wood Community College
Sterling, Illinois

Angela B. McDuffie
Southeastern Community College
Whiteville, North Carolina

Geraldine McGrann
Minuteman Regional School
Lexington, Massachusetts

Jeanne McKean
Lake Washington Technical College
Kirkland, Washington

Fawn Mefferd
Des Moines Area Community College
Des Moines, Iowa

Barbara Meinke
McHenry County College
Crystal Lake, Illinois

Joanne Moats
Seminole Community College
Winter Springs, Florida

Sherry Nantroup
Pierce College
Woodland Hills, California

Laura Noland
Country View Estates Care Home
Seneca, Kansas

Tanna Parker
Lake Superior College
Superior, Wisconsin

Elizabeth Ann Pelham
Our Lady of the Lake College
Baton Rouge, Louisiana

Gladys Petersen
Hawkeye Community College
Waterloo, Iowa

Beverly K. Pheifer
EHOVE Ghrist Adult Career Center
Milan, Ohio

Jewel Rankin
Walters State Community College
Morristown, Tennessee

Lyn Reardon
Washington County Technical College
Calais, Maine

Judith Rex
Northampton Community College
Bethlehem, Pennsylvania

Susan Richmond
McHenry County College
Crystal Lake, Illinois

Judy Ridinger
Memorial Medical Center
Springfield, Illinois

JoAnn Runewicz
LaSalle University
Philadelphia, Pennsylvania

Dianne Rush
University of Arkansas Community College
Batesville, Arkansas

Sheila Sarver
Lee County High Tech Center Central
Fort Myers, Florida

Jessica Sauld
Madison Area Technical College
Montello, Wisconsin

Tracy Schaetzl
Madison Area Technical College
Montello, Wisconsin

Dianna Scherlin
New Hampshire Community Technical College
Berlin, New Hampshire

Sally Scofield
Ohlone College
Fremont, California

Heidi Shinbargar
Itasca Community College
Grand Rapids, Minnesota

Linda Shows
Jones County Junior College
Ellisville, Mississippi

Cinda Siekbert
Great Oaks School of Practical Nursing
Georgetown, Ohio

Susan S. Simpkins
South Florida Community College
Avon Park, Florida

Mary Sirmons
Indian River Community College
Fort Pierce, Florida

Julie A. Slack
Mohave Community College
Colorado City, Arizona

Dana Spenger-Trantor
Quincy Area Vocational Technical Center
Quincy, Illinois

Linda C. Sullivan
Kansas City Kansas Community College
Kansas City, Kansas

Loretta Tacke
Montana State University
Bozeman, Montana

Acknowledgments

Certainly, the development and writing of a new textbook is a daunting task, even for an experienced author. For first-time authors, it is even more daunting! Writing a textbook requires many hours of research, planning, and just sitting in front of a blank computer screen waiting for one's fingers to make words appear. There are many people who have contributed to the making of this textbook, and each shares an incredible responsibility for what you will find between these covers.

We would especially like to thank all of the people at Lippincott Williams & Wilkins. Your vision has now become reality. Leigh Wells, National Manager Career Education Sales, was the first to have that vision, and became our lead cheerleader and attitude adjuster throughout this project. Although this book was conceived from our hearts and souls, it was Melanie Cann, Senior Development Editor, who truly gave it life. Melanie corrected our errors, gave us direction, and took our words and gave them magic. We would also like to thank everyone who assisted us with the art and design of the text: Elizabeth Morales, Art Development Editor; Nancy Lubars, Photo Researcher; Rick Brady, Photographer; and Carolyn O'Brien and Brett MacNaughton, Art Directors.

We also would like to thank the residents and staff at Highland Care Center in Salt Lake City, who appear in many of the photographs in this book:

Residents and Family Members

Lena Anderson
Mary Baker
Kenna Bancroft
Elsie Barrus
Shirley Barton
Shirley Beckstead
Maggie Beers
Heber Bishop
Josephine Bornhisel
Esther Bowen
Louis Bowen
Marjorie Call
Morris Cannegieter
Alice Cassell
Helen Christensen
Mary Jane Coleman
Mary Conklin
Becky Deppe

Russell Devitt
David Dunn
Betty Durham
Toby Ehrlich
Lila Erickson
Zina Feil
Blanche Fillmore
Venetta Flowers
Alice Fox
Marjorie Giles
Mary Gillespie
Marci Green
Tehya Green
Alberta Guyman
Marion Hardy
Dorothy Harkness
Alice Henze
Vivia Hopkins
Elizabeth Hunter
Eva Ingelby

Kathy Johnson
Lois Johnson
Viola Johnson
Frank Kearns
Elaine Leseuer
Bernice Littlefield
Arva Lovell
Rachel Lunt
Annis Mansfield
Grant Marcus
Lloyd Martin
May McGhie
Anna McKean
Bea Mickelson
Selma Miller
Esther Morris
Angela Nelson
Ruth Orlando
Easton Parratt
Fae Petersen

Maureen Poulson
Shirley Quist
Rosabelle Rodriguez
Norma Rolfsen
Ruth Ross
Dorothy Ruff
Marie Saterlie
Dorothy Shelton
Joellen Shumway
Virginia Smith
Afton Soderberg
Inez Steed
Carol Swalberg
Pinomi Taloa
Lottie Taylor
William Thompson
Paul Tingey
Mildred Tueller
Courtney Vander Veur
Kathleen Vander Veur
Arba Vanhouton
Nancy Watanabe
Ivan Watts
Betty Whetsel
Lovell Yamasaki

Staff

Jennifer Africano
Patricia Almeida
Maria Alvirez
Mary Angelo
Sharilyn Archuleta
Heather Baldwin
Troy Barnes
Krieg Benally
Melissa Benally
Doug Benson
Greg Bilbo
Valoree Bland
Alison Boehner
Andrew Bracken
Mallory Braithwaite
Carla Briggs
Misti Bunker
Rebecca Burns
Krista Burrow

Jason Button
Nicole Button
Lisa Bytheway
Martha Cabriales
Bonita Calvin
Eddie Calvin
Victor Campos
Melissa Chapman
Wendy Childs
Daiane Dacosta
Mark Dunn
JoAnn Eder
Jennifer Forster
April Galvin
Gerardo Garcia
Ignacio Garcia
Susan Geertsen
James Glines
Philip Greene
Tina Grimes
Valerie Halsey
Juan Hands
Matt Harmer
Jodie Hemmert
Javier Hernandez
Halley Hettich
Lisa Hettich
Bobbi Hollaway
Celeste Jones
Rose Jones
Mary Kelsey
Joy King
Kathy Knight
Franco Lampropoulos
Martha Langlois
Irven Larsen
Tracy Latturner
Joan Lewis
Dolores Lopez
Laura Lopez
Blanca Correa
Helena Maciel
Maria Magallanes
Lyn Marshall
Kathleen Martinez
Kathleen Metthea

Sinn Keno Mays
Tammi McCall
Jose Mendez
Isaiah Moore
Clelia Moreria
Stephanie Morgan
Dennis Munoz
Drew Naylor
Melanie Naylor
James O'Brien
Sandra Penuelas
Senovia Penuelas
Terry Petersen
Tammy Phomsouvanh
Shelly Pittman
Amy Pond
Brandi Rich
Tracy Rich
Liz Robies
Juana Rodriguez
Carly Rule
Anuar Sanchez
Carlos Sanchez
Renee Sanchez
Goarik Sekepyan
Angel Selis
Amanda Sequaptewa
Shadon Simmons
Gina Smith
Kaye Smith
Heather Stevens
Nicole Stewart
Teresa Sulsev
Sala Taloa
Glenda Trovenen
Merab Vargas
Orpha Vargas
Oscar Vazquez
Martha Velasquez
Yesenia Velasquez
Cherie Ward
Linda Whitaker
Connie Winkel
Jackie Winkel
Kim Wright
Mark Zwanziger

Finally, we would like to thank our colleagues at Davis Applied Technology College, the Utah State Office of Education, the Utah Department of Health, and Community Nursing Services for their support, advice, and confidence in our abilities.

Contents

UNIT **3**

BASIC PATIENT AND RESIDENT CARE   239

CHAPTER **17**

Cleanliness and Hygiene 323

CHAPTER **18**

Grooming 355

CHAPTER **19**

Basic Nutrition 378

CHAPTER **25**

The Musculoskeletal System   514

CHAPTER **26**

The Respiratory System   549

CHAPTER **27**

The Cardiovascular System   574

CHAPTER **28**

The Nervous System   594

CHAPTER **29**

The Sensory System   610

CHAPTER **30**

The Endocrine System   634

CHAPTER **31**

The Digestive System   649

CHAPTER 32

The Urinary System   664

CHAPTER 33

The Reproductive System   677

UNIT 6

SPECIAL CARE CONCERNS   695

CHAPTER 34

Caring for People With Developmental Disabilities   697

CHAPTER 35

Caring for People With Mental Illness   708

Introduction to Health Care

Welcome to the health care field! Today in the United States, the health care field is one of the largest fields, providing jobs for more than 11 million people in more than 469,000 health care organizations. In 2000, nearly 2 million of those employed by the health care industry were nursing assistants, with the number of job openings for nursing assistants expected to grow by 21% to 35% between 2000 and 2010.* The health care field is the focus of Unit 1.

*Occupational Outlook Handbook 2002–3 edition, published by the United States Bureau of Labor Statistics.
Photo: Welcome to the health care field! Nursing assistants are key members of the health care team.

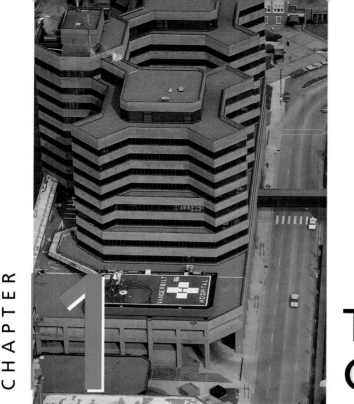

CHAPTER 1

The Health Care System

What will you learn?

As a health care professional, you will be part of the health care system. In this chapter, you will learn about the many different types of organizations that make up the health care system. You will also learn about some of the government regulations that affect the health care system. Finally, we will discuss some of the ways that health care is paid for in the United States. When you are finished with this chapter, you will be able to:

1. Identify changes that have occurred in how health care is delivered.
2. Describe the different types of health care organizations.
3. Briefly explain the structure of a health care organization.
4. Explain two important government regulations that affect the health care system.
5. Discuss how health care is paid for.

Vocabulary

Use the CD in the back of your book to hear these terms pronounced, defined, and used in a sentence:

Holistic
Mission
Hospital
Patient
Subacute care unit
  (skilled nursing unit,
  skilled nursing facility)
Long-term care facility
  (nursing home)

Resident
Assisted-living facility
Home health care agency
Client
Hospice organization
Health care team
Omnibus Budget
  Reconciliation Act
  (OBRA)

Occupational Safety and
  Health Administration
  (OSHA)
Group insurance
Precertification
  (preapproval) process
Managed care system
Preferred Provider
  Organization (PPO)

Health Maintenance
  Organization
  (HMO)
Medicare
Minimum Data Set
  (MDS)
Diagnosis-related
  groups (DRGs)
Medicaid

Photo: A hospital is just one of the many ways health care is delivered in the United States today.
(Photo Researchers, Inc.)

HEALTH CARE DELIVERY, PAST AND PRESENT

In the United States during the 18th, 19th, and early part of the 20th centuries, health care delivery focused mainly around the home and family. In many cases, the health care provider was trained, but as a generalist, rather than a specialist. He would deliver the babies, attend to wounds and broken bones, and provide comfort to both the dying person and the family (Fig. 1-1).

Until the early 1800s, the quality of health care in the United States was variable. Charlatans, people with no training or knowledge of medicine, traveled from town to town, offering worthless ("snake oil") cures in an effort to make a quick dollar. Hospitals typically caused more illness than they helped (Fig. 1-2). Patients were at the mercy of the "family doctor," and there was little they could do if the care they received was poor.

Present-day delivery of health care has changed dramatically. More intensive educational preparation for health care providers has become the standard and, in the United States, is required for those who want to care for those in need. Large facilities dedicated to providing on-site patient care have been established, replacing the home as the primary site for patient care. Due to advances in technology, a family doctor would no longer be able to carry the tools of his trade in the familiar black medical bag. A

FIGURE 1-1

In the past, health care was delivered in the home, usually by a "family doctor." *(Hafton/Archive by Getty Images.)*

FIGURE 1-2

Modern ideas about hospital cleanliness and patient care did not exist in the 1800s.

variety of medications and other treatments allow us to treat and cure many diseases that in the past would have been fatal, increasing the average person's life span by decades. The family doctor who attended a person from birth to death is now called a "general practitioner" or "family physician," and in many cases, he or she is supported by a team of specialists.

Although in the recent past, the trend was to *replace* the family doctor with a team of specialists, today we are seeing a return to a more holistic approach to health care. A **holistic** approach focuses on the care of the whole person, physically and emotionally. The best aspect of the care provided by the old-fashioned "family doctor"—the doctor's familiarity with the person as an individual—is combined with modern-day availability of specialized care when needed.

HEALTH CARE ORGANIZATIONS

As the health care system has developed and changed over the years, we have seen more and more variety in the organizations that provide health care to people in need. As a nursing assistant, you will be employed by a health care organization. All health care organizations have

a purpose, or **mission.** Some health care organizations, such as university hospitals, are associated directly with schools. The primary mission of a university hospital may be to train people in the field of health care. Other health care organizations are associated with a religious group. Some health care organizations are owned by corporations and use the health care industry as a financial investment in order to turn a profit. Although some health care organizations have very specific missions, others combine many of the following:

- To prevent disease by providing immunizations, teaching people how to control chronic health problems, and identifying factors that could place a person at risk for a disease
- To detect and treat disease
- To promote health by teaching people about ways to achieve and maintain both physical and mental fitness
- To offer rehabilitation (restorative care) services in order to help people return to their highest possible level of physical or emotional function
- To educate health care professionals by providing work-based training for medical students, student nurses, and many other types of students training for a career in the health care field

TYPES OF HEALTH CARE ORGANIZATIONS

There are many different types of health care organizations. Depending on where you live, you may be able to work as a nursing assistant in all of these organizations, or just some. For example, in some states, nursing assistants are only employed in long-term care facilities (nursing homes), but in others, nursing assistants can work in hospitals.

Hospitals

Probably the best known type of health care organization is the **hospital.** The services provided by a hospital differ according to the hospital's mission and location. Some hospitals, such as children's hospitals, women's centers, cancer centers, or orthopedic hospitals, have very specific missions, either in terms of the type of people they serve or the services that they offer. Other hospitals, sometimes called "general hospitals," provide a variety of services, such as:

- Delivering babies
- Diagnosing diseases
- Treating diseases with drugs, surgery, or both
- Providing emergency and intensive care services
- Providing mental health services
- Providing rehabilitation and physical therapy

People who receive the services of a hospital are typically referred to as **patients.** A hospital may admit a patient for care (have the patient stay for one or more nights). This is called inpatient care. Or a hospital may provide its services on an outpatient basis (the patient goes home the same day). For example, a patient with cancer who returns to the hospital every day for a period of time to receive radiation therapy would be receiving outpatient care.

Sub-acute Care Units (Skilled Nursing Units)

The care provided in a hospital is costly, and the number of beds in the hospital is limited. Therefore, once a patient has recovered enough to be out of danger, he or she is usually moved from the medical–surgical unit. Often, these patients still need some care from a skilled health care professional. This care may be provided in a **sub-acute care unit** (also called a **skilled nursing unit** or a **skilled nursing facility**). A sub-acute care unit may be a unit within a hospital or a long-term care facility, or it may be a separate facility.

Patients in sub-acute care units may require intravenous drugs, physical therapy, respiratory care or ventilator services, or wound management. The care given in these units focuses on rehabilitation and helping the patient to move from hospital care to home care (Fig. 1-3). Some patients in sub-acute care units recover fully, but others may need to move to a long-term care facility or arrange for continued care from home health-care services after they return home.

FIGURE 1-3

The care provided in sub-acute care units, also called skilled nursing units or skilled nursing facilities, often focuses on rehabilitation. Here, a physical therapist teaches a patient how to use a walker.

FIGURE 1-4

Residents of long-term care facilities (nursing homes) are unable to care for themselves at home, yet do not need to be hospitalized. (© *Will & Deni McIntyre/Photo Researchers, Inc.*)

Long-Term Care Facilities (Nursing Homes)

A **long-term care facility (nursing home)** is for people who are unable to care for themselves at home, yet do not need to be hospitalized (Fig. 1-4). Because the long-term care facility becomes the person's home, either temporarily or permanently, people being cared for in long-term care facilities are referred to as **residents,** rather than patients. Some residents will stay in the facility for a short period of time, until they are well enough to return home. Others will remain in the long-term care facility for the rest of their lives.

There are many reasons why a person would need to move to a long-term care facility. Many residents are elderly, but younger adults and children with conditions resulting from accidents or birth defects may also live in long-term care facilities. As with hospitals, long-term care facilities may provide care to residents with a wide variety of needs, or they may specialize. For example, some long-term care facilities provide skilled nursing care for residents who are unable to provide any of their own daily care. Others specialize in caring for residents with Alzheimer's disease. Still others help residents who have had a stroke or suffered a head injury to regain function.

Assisted-Living Facilities

An **assisted-living facility** is a type of long-term care facility. People who live in an assisted-living facility are able to provide most of their own care, but they may need some limited help with medications, transportation, meals, and housekeeping. The residents of an assisted-living facility usually live in private apartments and can feel safe and secure knowing that if they need help, someone is nearby to provide it, 24 hours a day (Fig. 1-5). Many retirement communities offer both assisted-living services and long-term care services. If the resident's needs change, he or she can move to the long-term care facility to receive more advanced care.

FIGURE 1-5

Residents of assisted-living communities often live in individual apartments. These residents are able to provide most of their own care but need help with certain things, such as medications, transportation, meals, or housekeeping. (*Courtesy of Country Pines Retirement Community, Clinton, UT.*)

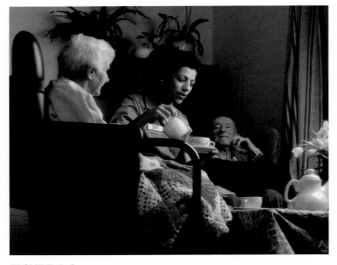

FIGURE 1-6

Nursing assistants who work for home health care agencies provide health care to people in their homes. A home health care aide's responsibilities might also include preparing and serving light meals and light housekeeping, depending on the client's needs and agency policy. (*SPL/CL Photo Researchers, Inc.*)

Home Health Care Agencies

Home health care agencies provide skilled care in a person's home (Fig. 1-6). In the home health care setting, people who receive care are typically called **clients,** rather than patients or residents. Home health care services are available for people of all ages with any number of different medical needs. For example, a new mother and her baby may need home care, especially if the baby was born too early. A person recovering from an accident, a stroke, or surgery may also need home care.

Hospice Organizations

Hospice organizations provide care for people who are dying and their families. People are able to receive the services of a hospice organization when they know that they have only 3 to 6 months to live. The focus of hospice care is on relieving pain and providing emotional and spiritual support for both the dying person and the family. Hospice care can be provided in the home, hospital, or long-term care facility, or in a facility devoted exclusively to providing care to the dying.

STRUCTURE OF HEALTH CARE ORGANIZATIONS

Most health care organizations are set up in a way similar to that shown in Figure 1-7. Most are governed by a board of trustees (also called a

board of directors), and most have divisions (groups in charge of certain aspects of the organization's function). An administrator or chief executive officer (CEO) usually manages the organization and is the link between the board and the organization.

The board is made up of community members. The board sets policies to ensure that the care offered by the organization is safe and of good quality. The board also makes sure that the organization meets the needs of the community. For example, think about a rural community where there is only one hospital. This hospital does not provide obstetric services, which means that pregnant women must travel out of the area to deliver their babies. The hospital's board surveys the people in the town and determines that the hospital needs to offer obstetric services in order to meet the community's need. The board then develops a plan to get funding to build a maternity ward, and to find qualified people to staff it.

Each division within a health care organization is responsible for one key aspect of the organization's function. Each division is managed by a division director or division manager. The medical services division is led by a medical director, and is responsible for the doctors on staff. Nursing services is headed by a director of nursing

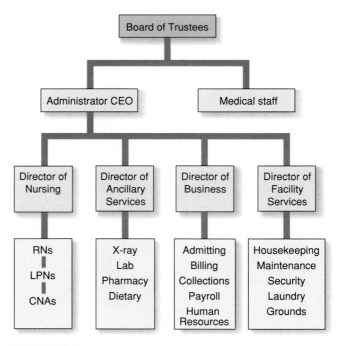

FIGURE 1-7

Most health care organizations are organized in similar ways. Each division within a health care organization is responsible for one key aspect of the organization's function.

(DON) or chief nursing officer (CNO), and is responsible for all aspects of the organization that have to do with patient or resident care. Business services is led by a business director, and usually oversees admissions, billing, and payroll. The business division may also oversee maintenance and housekeeping. The ancillary services division typically contains the departments in the organization that provide patient or resident services, such as social services and dietary services.

Within each facility, care of patients or residents is provided by a **health care team,** made up of many people with different types of knowledge and skill levels (Fig. 1-8). The patient or resident is always the focus of the health care team's efforts. The goal of the health care team is to provide holistic care (care of the whole person, physically and emotionally). Each member of the health care team's job is as important as any other member's. Think of the members of the health care team as links in the chain of care provided for the patient or resident. Because a chain is only as strong as its weakest link, each member of the health care team must provide care to the best of his or her ability. For example, the maintenance staff keeps the facility running smoothly by keeping equipment in good working order. The housekeeping staff keeps the facility clean. The people who work in the lab must be precise when performing laboratory studies and writing reports. In short, everyone must provide competent care in order for the health care team to function properly.

FIGURE 1-8

Care is provided by the health care team. The patient or resident is the primary focus of the health care team's efforts. Because a chain is only as strong as its weakest link, each member of the health care team must provide care to the best of his or her ability.

GOVERNMENT REGULATION OF THE HEALTH CARE SYSTEM

Government regulations protect the entire community by making sure that:

- Providers of health care are properly trained and competent
- Health care facilities meet standards of cleanliness and quality
- Quality health care is available to everyone

Government agencies monitor the activity of health care organizations and make sure that organizations do, in fact, provide the type of care they say they provide. The government inspects health care organizations regularly to make sure that the standards are being followed. Any problems are addressed and, if the problems are serious, the organization faces being fined or closed.

Two laws with far-reaching effects on the health care system were passed in the United States during the last half of the 20th century. One, the **Omnibus Budget Reconciliation Act (OBRA) of 1987,** was passed with the goal of improving conditions for people in long-term care facilities. Before OBRA, the quality of care in many long-term care facilities was poor. During the 1960s and 1970s, many long-term care facilities were run by people who were more interested in making money than in caring for the elderly and disabled. Neglect and abuse were common. Finally, in response to complaints from people who had family members in long-term care facilities, the Department of Health and Human Services (DHHS) began an in-depth investigation of long-term care facilities in the United States. This investigation led to OBRA in 1987.

OBRA improves the quality of life for people who live in long-term care facilities by making sure that residents receive a certain standard of care. This care must take into account the resident's physical, emotional, spiritual, and social needs. In addition, OBRA sets standards for the training and evaluation of nursing assistants who work in long-term care facilities. OBRA legislation is reviewed and passed by Congress each year. As you read this book, look for the OBRA icon, which highlights key information related to this law.

The other key piece of legislation, the Occupational Safety and Health Act of 1970, was passed in response to public concern over increasing numbers of on-the-job injuries and deaths. This legislation established safety and health standards for the workplace and led to the development of the **Occupational Safety and Health Administration (OSHA),** an agency within the Department of Labor. OSHA standards, which you will see referenced frequently throughout this text, protect you while you care for others.

PAYING FOR HEALTH CARE

As you surely know if you have ever received a bill for health care in the United States, health care can be expensive. Insurance can help to lessen these costs to the individual. As a nursing assistant, you should know a little bit about how health care is paid for in the United States.

PRIVATE AND GROUP INSURANCE

Although people can pay for health insurance privately, using their own funds, most people are covered by **group insurance** (insurance that is purchased at group rates by an employer or corporation). The employee may be covered in full as a benefit of employment, or he may pay a certain percentage of his coverage. The insurance company then pays for health care according to the individual policy.

Due to the increasing costs of medical care, the insurance industry has taken measures to control costs. Some insurance companies have a **precertification (preapproval) process.** This means that in order to be paid, the health care provider must prove that a person's medical condition meets certain criteria and obtain the insurance company's go-ahead for the proposed treatment before starting treatment.

Other insurance companies use a **managed care system.** Managed care systems assist in delivering health care to people who need it by arranging contacts with various health care providers (doctors' offices, hospitals, ambulance services, pharmacies). In addition, they help to reduce unnecessary costs associated with medical and surgical procedures by authorizing treatments before they are carried out. One form of managed care system is the **preferred provider organization (PPO).** In a PPO, health care

MINIMUM DATA SET (MDS) — *VERSION 2.0*
FOR NURSING HOME RESIDENT ASSESSMENT AND CARE SCREENING
FULL ASSESSMENT FORM
(Status in last 7 days, unless other time frame indicated)

SECTION A. IDENTIFICATION AND BACKGROUND INFORMATION

1. RESIDENT NAME
a. (First)   b. (Middle Initial)   c. (Last)   d. (Jr/Sr)

2. ROOM NUMBER

3. ASSESSMENT REFERENCE DATE
a. Last day of MDS observation period
☐☐ — ☐☐ — ☐☐☐☐
Month   Day   Year
b. Original (0) or corrected copy of form (enter number of correction)

4a. DATE OF REENTRY
Date of reentry from most recent temporary discharge to a hospital in last 90 days (or since last assessment or admission if less than 90 days)
☐☐ — ☐☐ — ☐☐☐☐
Month   Day   Year

5. MARITAL STATUS
1. Never married   3. Widowed   5. Divorced
2. Married   4. Separated

6. MEDICAL RECORD NO.

7. CURRENT PAYMENT SOURCES FOR N.H. STAY
(Billing Office to indicate; *check all that apply in last 30 days*)
Medicaid per diem	a.	VA per diem	f.
Medicare per diem	b.	Self or family pays for full per diem	g.
Medicare ancillary part A	c.	Medicaid resident liability or Medicare co-payment	h.
Medicare ancillary part B	d.	Private insurance per diem (including co-payment)	i.
CHAMPUS per diem	e.	Other per diem	j.

8. REASONS FOR ASSESSMENT
[Note—If this is a discharge or reentry assessment, only a limited subset of MDS items need be completed]
a. Primary reason for assessment
1. Admission assessment (required by day 14)
2. Annual assessment
3. Significant change in status assessment
4. Significant correction of prior full assessment
5. Quarterly review assessment
6. Discharged—return not anticipated
7. Discharged—return anticipated
8. Discharged prior to completing initial assessment
9. Reentry
10. Significant correction of prior quarterly assessment
0. NONE OF ABOVE
b. *Codes for assessments required for Medicare PPS or the State*
1. Medicare 5 day assessment
2. Medicare 30 day assessment
3. Medicare 60 day assessment
4. Medicare 90 day assessment
5. Medicare readmission/return assessment
6. Other state required assessment
7. Medicare 14 day assessment
8. Other Medicare required assessment

9. RESPONSIBILITY/ LEGAL GUARDIAN
(*Check all that apply*)
Legal guardian	a.	Durable power attorney/financial	d.
Other legal oversight	b.	Family member responsible	e.
Durable power of attorney/health care	c.	Patient responsible for self	f.
		NONE OF ABOVE	g.

10. ADVANCED DIRECTIVES
(*For those items with supporting documentation in the medical record, check all that apply*)
Living will	a.	Feeding restrictions	f.
Do not resuscitate	b.	Medication restrictions	g.
Do not hospitalize	c.	Other treatment restrictions	h.
Organ donation	d.	NONE OF ABOVE	i.
Autopsy request	e.		

SECTION B. COGNITIVE PATTERNS

1. COMATOSE
(*Persistent vegetative state/no discernible consciousness*)
0. No   1. Yes   (If yes, skip to Section G)

2. MEMORY
(*Recall of what was learned or known*)
a. Short-term memory OK—seems/appears to recall after 5 minutes
0. Memory OK   1. Memory problem
b. Long-term memory OK—seems/appears to recall long past
0. Memory OK   1. Memory problem

3. MEMORY/ RECALL ABILITY
(Check all that resident was **normally able to recall during** *last 7 days*)
Current season	a.	That he/she is in a nursing home	d.
Location of own room	b.		
Staff names/faces	c.	NONE OF ABOVE are recalled	e.

4. COGNITIVE SKILLS FOR DAILY DECISION-MAKING
(*Made decisions regarding tasks of daily life*)
0. INDEPENDENT—decisions consistent/reasonable
1. MODIFIED INDEPENDENCE—some difficulty in new situations only
2. MODERATELY IMPAIRED—decisions poor; cues/supervision required
3. SEVERELY IMPAIRED—never/rarely made decisions

5. INDICATORS OF DELIRIUM— PERIODIC DISORDERED THINKING/ AWARENESS
(*Code for behavior in the last 7 days.*) [*Note: Accurate assessment requires conversations with staff and family who have direct knowledge of resident's behavior over this time*].
0. Behavior not present
1. Behavior present, not of recent onset
2. Behavior present, over last 7 days appears different from resident's usual functioning (e.g., new onset or worsening)
a. EASILY DISTRACTED—(e.g., difficulty paying attention; gets sidetracked)
b. PERIODS OF ALTERED PERCEPTION OR AWARENESS OF SURROUNDINGS—(e.g., moves lips or talks to someone not present; believes he/she is somewhere else; confuses night and day)
c. EPISODES OF DISORGANIZED SPEECH—(e.g., speech is incoherent, nonsensical, irrelevant, or rambling from subject to subject; loses train of thought)
d. PERIODS OF RESTLESSNESS—(e.g., fidgeting or picking at skin, clothing, napkins, etc; frequent position changes; repetitive physical movements or calling out)
e. PERIODS OF LETHARGY—(e.g., sluggishness; staring into space; difficult to arouse; little body movement)
f. MENTAL FUNCTION VARIES OVER THE COURSE OF THE DAY—(e.g., sometimes better, sometimes worse; behaviors sometimes present, sometimes not)

6. CHANGE IN COGNITIVE STATUS
Resident's cognitive status, skills, or abilities have changed as compared to status of **90 days ago** (or since last assessment if less than 90 days)
0. No change   1. Improved   2. Deteriorated

SECTION C. COMMUNICATION/HEARING PATTERNS

1. HEARING
(*With hearing appliance, if used*)
0. HEARS ADEQUATELY—normal talk, TV, phone
1. MINIMAL DIFFICULTY when not in quiet setting
2. HEARS IN SPECIAL SITUATIONS ONLY—speaker has to adjust tonal quality and speak distinctly
3. HIGHLY IMPAIRED/absence of useful hearing

2. COMMUNICATION DEVICES/ TECHNIQUES
(*Check all that apply* during last 7 days)
Hearing aid, present and used	a.
Hearing aid, present and not used regularly	b.
Other receptive comm. techniques used (e.g., lip reading)	c.
NONE OF ABOVE	d.

3. MODES OF EXPRESSION
(*Check all used* by resident to make needs known)
Speech	a.	Signs/gestures/sounds	d.
Writing messages to express or clarify needs	b.	Communication board	e.
American sign language or Braille	c.	Other	f.
		NONE OF ABOVE	g.

4. MAKING SELF UNDERSTOOD
(*Expressing information content—however able*)
0. UNDERSTOOD
1. USUALLY UNDERSTOOD—difficulty finding words or finishing thoughts
2. SOMETIMES UNDERSTOOD—ability is limited to making concrete requests
3. RARELY/NEVER UNDERSTOOD

5. SPEECH CLARITY
(*Code for speech in the last 7 days*)
0. CLEAR SPEECH—distinct, intelligible words
1. UNCLEAR SPEECH—slurred, mumbled words
2. NO SPEECH—absence of spoken words

6. ABILITY TO UNDERSTAND OTHERS
(*Understanding verbal information content—however able*)
0. UNDERSTANDS
1. USUALLY UNDERSTANDS—may miss some part/intent of message
2. SOMETIMES UNDERSTANDS—responds adequately to simple, direct communication
3. RARELY/NEVER UNDERSTANDS

7. CHANGE IN COMMUNICATION/ HEARING
Resident's ability to express, understand, or hear information has changed as compared to status of **90 days ago** (or since last assessment if less than 90 days)
0. No change   1. Improved   2. Deteriorated

☐ = When box blank, must enter number or letter   [a.] = When letter in box, check if condition applies

MDS 2.0 September, 2000

FIGURE 1-9

Nurses in long-term care facilities that receive Medicare funding must complete a Minimum Data Set (MDS) report for each resident in their care. This report is used to assess the degree of assistance that each resident needs. A 9-page form is used when the resident is first admitted to the facility; a shorter, 3-page

Resident _____   Numeric Identifier _____

SECTION D. VISION PATTERNS

1.	VISION	*(Ability to see in adequate light and with glasses if used)* 0. *ADEQUATE*—sees fine detail, including regular print in newspapers/books 1. *IMPAIRED*—sees large print, but not regular print in newspapers/books 2. *MODERATELY IMPAIRED*—limited vision; not able to see newspaper headlines, but can identify objects 3. *HIGHLY IMPAIRED*—object identification in question, but eyes appear to follow objects 4. *SEVERELY IMPAIRED*—no vision or sees only light, colors, or shapes; eyes do not appear to follow objects
2.	VISUAL LIMITATIONS/ DIFFICULTIES	Side vision problems—decreased peripheral vision (e.g., leaves food on one side of tray, difficulty traveling, bumps into people and objects, misjudges placement of chair when seating self) a. Experiences any of following: sees halos or rings around lights; sees flashes of light; sees "curtains" over eyes b. *NONE OF ABOVE* c.
3.	VISUAL APPLIANCES	Glasses; contact lenses; magnifying glass 0. No 1. Yes

SECTION E. MOOD AND BEHAVIOR PATTERNS

1.	INDICATORS OF DEPRES- SION, ANXIETY, SAD MOOD	*(Code for indicators observed in last 30 days, irrespective of the assumed cause)* 0. Indicator not exhibited in last 30 days 1. Indicator of this type exhibited up to five days a week 2. Indicator of this type exhibited daily or almost daily (6, 7 days a week)

VERBAL EXPRESSIONS OF DISTRESS

a. Resident made negative statements—e.g., *"Nothing matters; Would rather be dead; What's the use; Regrets having lived so long; Let me die"*

b. Repetitive questions—e.g., *"Where do I go; What do I do?"*

c. Repetitive verbalizations—e.g., calling out for help, ("God help me")

d. Persistent anger with self or others—e.g., easily annoyed, anger at placement in nursing home; anger at care received

e. Self deprecation—e.g., "*I am nothing; I am of no use to anyone*"

f. Expressions of what appear to be unrealistic fears—e.g., fear of being abandoned, left alone, being with others

g. Recurrent statements that something terrible is about to happen—e.g., believes he or she is about to die, have a heart attack

h. Repetitive health complaints—e.g., persistently seeks medical attention, obsessive concern with body functions

i. Repetitive anxious complaints/concerns (non-health related) e.g., persistently seeks attention/reassurance regarding schedules, meals, laundry, clothing, relationship issues

SLEEP-CYCLE ISSUES

j. Unpleasant mood in morning

k. Insomnia/change in usual sleep pattern

SAD, APATHETIC, ANXIOUS APPEARANCE

l. Sad, pained, worried facial expressions—e.g., furrowed brows

m. Crying, tearfulness

n. Repetitive physical movements—e.g., pacing, hand wringing, restlessness, fidgeting, picking

LOSS OF INTEREST

o. Withdrawal from activities of interest—e.g., no interest in long standing activities or being with family/friends

p. Reduced social interaction

2.	MOOD PERSIS- TENCE	One or more **indicators** of depressed, sad or anxious mood **were not easily altered** by attempts to "cheer up", console, or reassure the resident over last 7 days 0. No mood indicators 1. Indicators present, easily altered 2. Indicators present, not easily altered
3.	CHANGE IN MOOD	Resident's mood status has changed as compared to status of **90 days ago** (or since last assessment if less than 90 days) 0. No change 1. Improved 2. Deteriorated
4.	BEHAVIORAL SYMPTOMS	**(A)** *Behavioral symptom frequency in last 7 days* 0. Behavior not exhibited in last 7 days 1. Behavior of this type occurred 1 to 3 days in last 7 days 2. Behavior of this type occurred 4 to 6 days, but less than daily 3. Behavior of this type occurred daily **(B)** *Behavioral symptom alterability in last 7 days* 0. Behavior not present OR behavior was easily altered 1. Behavior was not easily altered (A) (B)

a. WANDERING (moved with no rational purpose, seemingly oblivious to needs or safety)

b. VERBALLY ABUSIVE BEHAVIORAL SYMPTOMS (others were threatened, screamed at, cursed at)

c. PHYSICALLY ABUSIVE BEHAVIORAL SYMPTOMS (others were hit, shoved, scratched, sexually abused)

d. SOCIALLY INAPPROPRIATE/DISRUPTIVE BEHAVIORAL SYMPTOMS (made disruptive sounds, noisiness, screaming, self-abusive acts, sexual behavior or disrobing in public, smeared/threw food/feces, hoarding, rummaged through others' belongings)

e. RESISTS CARE (resisted taking medications/ injections, ADL assistance, or eating)

5.	CHANGE IN BEHAVIORAL SYMPTOMS	Resident's behavior status has changed as compared to **status of 90 days ago** (or since last assessment if less than 90 days) 0. No change 1. Improved 2. Deteriorated

SECTION F. PSYCHOSOCIAL WELL-BEING

1.	SENSE OF INITIATIVE/ INVOLVE- MENT	At ease interacting with others	a.
		At ease doing planned or structured activities	b.
		At ease doing self-initiated activities	c.
		Establishes own goals	d.
		Pursues involvement in life of facility (e.g., makes/keeps friends; involved in group activities; responds positively to new activities; assists at religious services)	e.
		Accepts invitations into most group activities	f.
		NONE OF ABOVE	g.
2.	UNSETTLED RELATION- SHIPS	Covert/open conflict with or repeated criticism of staff	a.
		Unhappy with roommate	b.
		Unhappy with residents other than roommate	c.
		Openly expresses conflict/anger with family/friends	d.
		Absence of personal contact with family/friends	e.
		Recent loss of close family member/friend	f.
		Does not adjust easily to change in routines	g.
		NONE OF ABOVE	h.
3.	PAST ROLES	Strong identification with past roles and life status	a.
		Expresses sadness/anger/empty feeling over lost roles/status	b.
		Resident perceives that daily routine (customary routine, activities) is very different from prior pattern in the community	c.
		NONE OF ABOVE	d.

SECTION G. PHYSICAL FUNCTIONING AND STRUCTURAL PROBLEMS

1.	**(A)** ADL SELF-PERFORMANCE—*(Code for resident's PERFORMANCE OVER ALL SHIFTS during last 7 days—Not including setup)*	

0. *INDEPENDENT*—No help or oversight —OR— Help/oversight provided only 1 or 2 times during last 7 days

1. *SUPERVISION*—Oversight, encouragement or cueing provided 3 or more times during last 7 days —OR— Supervision (3 or more times) plus physical assistance provided only 1 or 2 times during last 7 days

2. *LIMITED ASSISTANCE*—Resident highly involved in activity; received physical help in guided maneuvering of limbs or other nonweight bearing assistance 3 or more times — OR—More help provided only 1 or 2 times during last 7 days

3. *EXTENSIVE ASSISTANCE*—While resident performed part of activity, over last 7-day period, help of following type(s) provided 3 or more times:
—Weight-bearing support
—Full staff performance during part (but not all) of last 7 days

4. *TOTAL DEPENDENCE*—Full staff performance of activity during entire 7 days

8. *ACTIVITY DID NOT OCCUR* during entire 7 days

(B) ADL SUPPORT PROVIDED—*(Code for MOST SUPPORT PROVIDED OVER ALL SHIFTS during last 7 days; code regardless of resident's self-performance classification)*
0. No setup or physical help from staff
1. Setup help only
2. One person physical assist
3. Two+ persons physical assist   8. ADL activity itself did not occur during entire 7 days

			(A)	(B)
			SELF-PERF	SUPPORT
a.	BED MOBILITY	How resident moves to and from lying position, turns side to side, and positions body while in bed		
b.	TRANSFER	How resident moves between surfaces—to/from: bed, chair, wheelchair, standing position (EXCLUDE to/from bath/toilet)		
c.	WALK IN ROOM	How resident walks between locations in his/her room		
d.	WALK IN CORRIDOR	How resident walks in corridor on unit		
e.	LOCOMO- TION ON UNIT	How resident moves between locations in his/her room and adjacent corridor on same floor. If in wheelchair, self-sufficiency once in chair		
f.	LOCOMO- TION OFF UNIT	How resident moves to and returns from off unit locations (e.g., areas set aside for dining, activities, or treatments). **If facility has only one floor**, how resident moves to and from distant areas on the floor. If in wheelchair, self-sufficiency once in chair		
g.	DRESSING	How resident puts on, fastens, and takes off all items of **street clothing**, including donning/removing prosthesis		
h.	EATING	How resident eats and drinks (regardless of skill). Includes intake of nourishment by other means (e.g., tube feeding, total parenteral nutrition)		
i.	TOILET USE	How resident uses the toilet room (or commode, bedpan, urinal); transfer on/off toilet, cleanses, changes pad, manages ostomy or catheter, adjusts clothes		
j.	PERSONAL HYGIENE	How resident maintains personal hygiene, including combing hair, brushing teeth, shaving, applying makeup, washing/drying face, hands, and perineum (EXCLUDE baths and showers)		

MDS 2.0 September, 2000

FIGURE 1-9 (*Continued*)

version is completed after 30 days, 60 days, and 90 days. The MDS report helps to ensure that the resident receives quality care that is directed toward his or her specific needs by requiring the nursing staff to evaluate these needs at regular intervals.

providers contract with an insurance company to accept a standard payment as total payment for services rendered. In return for seeking care only from health care providers who are part of the PPO network, the insured person usually receives that care at a reduced cost. A **health mainte- nance organization (HMO)** is another type of managed care system. Like PPOs, HMOs contract with health care providers to provide health care services for a prepaid fee, and people seeking care agree to see only health care providers who are part of the HMO network. An underlying principle of HMOs is that it costs less to keep a person healthy than it does to treat an illness. Therefore, these organizations typically promote regular physical examinations and screening to detect and prevent illnesses.

MEDICARE

Medicare is a type of insurance plan that is fed- erally funded by Social Security, under the ad- ministration of the Center for Medicare and Medicaid Services (CMMS). People who are 65 years or older are eligible for Medicare, regard- less of their financial situation. Some younger people who are disabled also qualify for Medicare. The submission of fraudulent (fake) Medicare claims by health care facilities in the past has led to changes in the way the program is admin- istered. Health care facilities that are eligible to receive Medicare reimbursements must follow strict rules and guidelines to receive payment. For example, to receive Medicare reimburse- ments, long-term care facilities must complete a **Minimum Data Set (MDS)** report for each resi- dent in their care (Fig. 1-9). This report focuses on the degree of assistance or skilled care that the resident needs. Information, such as the person's weight, bowel and bladder habits, and ability to care for herself, is recorded regularly as part of the MDS report. Changes in these ar- eas could indicate that a higher level of care is needed, or that the person is not receiving the necessary care and as a result, her condition is getting worse.

Like insurance companies that insure the general public, the Medicare program is faced with the problem of controlling ever-increasing health care costs. In an effort to control these costs, Medicare has started a reimbursement program based on **diagnosis-related groups (DRGs).** Under this system, payment for hospital- ization, surgery, or other treatment is specified according to the diagnosis. Lengths of hospital stays are also determined by the diagnosis, and are typically short. Since being introduced by Medicare, the DRG system has been adopted by insurance companies in the private and group sectors as well, resulting in industry-wide changes. As a result of the DRG system, patients are discharged sooner and sicker, a situation that has created an increased need for extended care and home health care.

MEDICAID

Medicaid is a federally funded and state-regu- lated plan designed to help people with low in- comes to pay for health care. Elderly people, as well as those who are disabled, may also be eligi- ble, especially if they have limited incomes. To receive Medicaid reimbursement, a facility must be approved by the state agency. Not all facilities or health care providers choose to participate in the Medicaid plan.

SUMMARY

▶ Society has always sought to care for the sick and injured.
  ■ In the United States during the 1700s, 1800s, and early part of the 1900s, most people who needed health care received it in their homes. Most care was provided by family members and a "family doctor."
  ■ Today, health care is delivered in the home through home health care agencies and hospice organizations. In addition, people can go to health care facilities such as hos- pitals, sub-acute care units, long-term care facilities ("nursing homes"), and assisted- living facilities to receive health care.
▶ Today, we take a holistic approach to health care. That is, we take into consideration the person's emotional, as well as his or her phys- ical, needs.
  ■ Health care is provided by a team of people, each with different areas of expertise and job responsibilities.

- As a nursing assistant, you are a critical part of the health care team.
▶ In modern American society, various aspects of the health care system are regulated by the government.
  - The Omnibus Budget Reconciliation Act (OBRA) ensures that people in long-term care facilities receive a certain standard of care.
  - The Occupational Safety and Health Act was passed with the goal of reducing the number of on-the-job injuries that occur each year. The Occupational Safety and Health Administration (OSHA) was formed as a result of this act.
▶ As the health care system has become more complex, the cost of health care has increased, and the way health care is paid for has changed.

- Private and group insurance policies are one way that individuals pay for health care.
- Medicare is insurance that is funded by the United States government.
  - People who are 65 years or older are eligible for Medicare, regardless of their financial situation.
  - Health care facilities must meet government regulations in order to receive Medicare reimbursement for services provided. For example, long-term care facilities must complete a Minimum Data Set (MDS) report for each person in their care.
- Medicaid is also funded by the United States government, and is designed to help people with low incomes pay for health care.

What did you learn?

Matching

Match each numbered item with its appropriate lettered description.

_____ 1. Assisted-living facility

_____ 2. Medicaid

_____ 3. Long-term care facility (nursing home)

_____ 4. Holistic

_____ 5. Health maintenance organization (HMO)

_____ 6. Hospice

_____ 7. Diagnosis-related groups (DRGs)

_____ 8. Home health care agency

_____ 9. Preferred provider organization (PPO)

_____ 10. Minimum data set (MDS)

_____ 11. Omnibus Budget Reconciliation Act (OBRA)

_____ 12. Sub-acute care unit (skilled nursing unit, skilled nursing facility)

a. Type of insurance that promotes regular screening to prevent illnesses

b. Federally funded and state-regulated plan to help people with low income

c. Report that focuses on the degree of assistance or care a resident requires

d. Used to regulate the length of a hospital stay

e. Place where people who can provide for most of their own care but who need limited assistance can live

f. Provides skilled care in a person's home

g. Type of insurance that requires the insured person to seek care only from providers who are part of the network

h. Care of the whole person, physically and emotionally

i. Established standards for training and evaluation of nursing assistants

j. Provides care for people who cannot care for themselves, yet are not ill enough to be hospitalized

k. Care devoted exclusively to the dying

l. Provides care that is focused on rehabilitation; assists patients in making the transition from hospital care to home care

---

? Stop and think!

▶ Think about what health care was like in the United States 100 years ago. How has health care delivery changed in the United States since the early 1900s? What aspects of the "old-fashioned" way of delivering health care were good? Not so good? What aspects of modern health care delivery are good? Not so good?

The Nursing Assistant

What will you learn?

In the previous chapter, you were introduced to the idea of a "health care team," a group of employees with varying types of knowledge and skill levels who provide holistic care to a patient or resident. If you think of the members of the health care team as "links" in the chain of care, then as a nursing assistant, you are a very critical "link." What contributions does the nursing assistant make to the health care team, and what education is needed to become a nursing assistant? In this chapter we will answer those questions, as well as describe the various ways in which nursing care can be delivered. We will also discuss how the nursing assistant and nurse interact to achieve the goal of safe, efficient patient or resident care. When you are finished with this chapter, you will be able to:

1. Discuss the Omnibus Budget Reconciliation Act (OBRA) requirements for nursing assistant training.
2. Describe the contents of the registry.
3. Discuss the responsibilities of the nursing assistant.
4. List the members of the nursing team, and describe the role of each team member.
5. Discuss the delegation process as it relates to the nursing assistant.
6. List the five rights of delegation.

Photo: Nurses and nursing assistants work together to provide patient or resident care.

Vocabulary

Use the CD in the back of your book to hear these terms pronounced, defined, and used in a sentence:

Competency evaluation
Reciprocity
Registry
Licensed practical nurse
   (LPN) or licensed
   vocational nurse (LVN)

Registered nurse
   (RN)
Charge nurse
Head nurse
Director of nursing
   (DON)

Primary nursing
Functional (modular)
   nursing
Team nursing
Delegate
Scope of practice

Five rights of
   delegation

NURSING, PAST AND PRESENT

Very simply stated, the field of nursing involves caring for others. People who enter the field of nursing, such as nurses and nursing assistants, provide physical and emotional care for people who are sick, disabled, or injured. Many nurses also work to keep people healthy, by teaching them about ways to maintain health and prevent illness.

Perhaps you have heard of Florence Nightingale. Florence Nightingale (1820–1910) was a British nurse who is credited with making nursing into the profession that it is today (Fig. 2-1). Ms. Nightingale started training programs for nurses and set up practices for hospital cleanliness and patient care that are followed to this day. By establishing educational standards for nursing professionals, Ms. Nightingale improved conditions for both the people receiving health care and those providing it. For the first time, those in the nursing field were regarded as professionals in their own right, with specialized knowledge, skills, and responsibilities.

The knowledge, skills, and responsibilities of the nursing assistant have grown over the years too. Early nursing assistants, often referred to as "aides" or "orderlies," were employed in long-term care facilities and hospitals to help the nurses care for residents and patients. These aides usually did not have training in the health care field, which led to poor care in many cases. Today's nursing assistants, however, are well-trained members of the health care team with many important responsibilities (Box 2-1).

EDUCATION OF THE NURSING ASSISTANT

OBRA REQUIREMENTS FOR CERTIFICATION

As you learned in Chapter 1, a major objective of the Omnibus Budget Reconciliation Act (OBRA) was to improve the quality of care given to residents of long-term care facilities. To ensure that nursing assistants have the necessary knowledge and skills to give care, OBRA requires all nursing assistants who want to be employed in long-term care facilities to complete a training program and to pass a test that evaluates their knowledge and skills.

Training is offered in vocational schools and community colleges. In addition, many long-term care facilities have their own nursing assistant

---

BOX 2-1 The Nursing Assistant's Prayer

As I enter into my place of calling,
I ask for strength as I help those in needing.
Hide my tears for the sick and aging,
And let my smile be the hope they're seeking.
Guide my hands as they do for them the things
   they cannot do,
And we take for granted.
Allow my eyes to see those things that make
   my stay with them a blessing.
Provide the words I need to speak
To let them know I love them so.
As I do my work throughout the day
It is for my residents that I stay,
And for my residents that I pray.

Created by Steve and Shari Allen 11/23/97

rights, basic nursing skills, personal care skills, feeding techniques, and skin care. You will also learn how to help patients and residents move from place to place, change positions, dress, and perform range-of-motion exercises. In addition, you will learn the signs and symptoms of common diseases, and how to care for people who have problems with thinking and memory. During the practical experience portion of the course, you will practice performing nursing care procedures on real people.

The training ends with a **competency evaluation,** which involves a written test (consisting of approximately 75 multiple-choice questions) and a skills test (during which you will be asked to perform selected nursing skills learned in the training program). The actual number of test questions that you must answer and skills that you must demonstrate is determined by the state. You will have three opportunities to complete the evaluation successfully. This is mandated by OBRA. The pass rate (or score that you must attain in order to pass the evaluation) varies from state to state.

Some states allow a person who has on-the-job experience as a health care worker or one who has been trained in a related field to take the competency evaluation without completing the training course. However, the person must pass both the written and skills portions of the test on the first try. If he does not, then he must complete the course before taking the competency evaluation again.

FIGURE 2-1

Florence Nightingale was a British nurse who established educational standards for nursing professionals. (© *National Library of Medicine/Photo Researchers, Inc.*)

training programs. A minimum of 75 hours of training is required. This training must include classroom lectures and hands-on practice of skills, as well as supervised experience in an actual health care setting (Fig. 2-2). As you complete your nursing assistant training program, you will study communication skills, infection control, safety and emergency procedures, residents'

FIGURE 2-2

Part of a nursing assistant's training involves working with patients or residents in an actual health care setting.

When you complete your training program and pass the competency evaluation, you will be certified to work as a nursing assistant in the state where you completed your training and passed your competency evaluation. Requirements for training vary from state to state. Some states accept the OBRA minimum of 75 hours of training whereas others require more hours—see Appendix B: State Hourly Training Requirements and Registry Information. The principle of **reciprocity** means, however, that in many cases, your certificate will be valid in states other than where you originally trained. If you want to work in a state that requires more hours of training than you have, additional training can be obtained.

REGISTRY

OBRA requires every state to maintain a **registry,** an official record of the people who have successfully completed the nursing assistant training program. The registry contains the following information about each nursing assistant:

- Full name, including maiden name and any married names
- Last known home address
- Social Security number
- Date of birth
- Date the competency evaluation was passed
- Reported incidents of resident abuse or neglect, or theft of resident property

Registry information can be requested by any long-term care facility needing the information. Information about performance concerns, such as resident abuse, must remain in the registry for at least 5 years.

CONTINUING EDUCATION

Regular in-service education and performance reviews are also mandated by OBRA. Long-term care facilities must provide a minimum of 12 hours of in-service training per year to nursing assistants. During in-service training, new skills may be taught or existing skills reviewed, depending on the needs of the facility. OBRA also requires nursing assistants who have not worked for 2 consecutive years to undergo retraining and pass a competency evaluation.

RESPONSIBILITIES OF THE NURSING ASSISTANT

The duties of the nursing assistant vary according to the setting, but all nursing assistants assist nurses in giving care to patients or residents by performing simple, basic nursing functions. As a nursing assistant, most of your responsibilities will relate to meeting the basic physical needs of patients and residents, which include hygiene, safety, comfort, nutrition, exercise, and elimination (Fig. 2-3). In addition to taking care of patients' or residents' physical needs, you will play an important role in meeting patients' or residents' emotional needs. A kind word, a gentle touch, and a willingness to listen let your residents or patients know that they are important to you and that you care for them as individuals. Finally, you will play an important role as "observer and communicator." As the member of the health care team with the most opportunity to interact with the patients or residents, you will be in a unique position to observe changes in the patient's or resident's physical or mental status, and report these observations to the nurse.

THE NURSING TEAM

The nursing team, a subset of the health care team, is responsible for providing care to the patient or resident (Table 2-1). At minimum, the nursing team consists of a nurse and a nursing assistant. The nurse is either a **licensed practical nurse,** or **LPN** (referred to in some states as a **licensed vocational nurse,** or **LVN**), or a **registered nurse (RN).** The nurse carries out the doctor's orders, and the nursing assistant helps the nurse. Other members of the nursing team may include a **charge nurse,** an RN or LPN/LVN who supervises the other nurses for a particular shift, and a **head nurse,** an RN who is in charge of a department or section. Each health care organization has an RN who directs all of the nursing care within that facility. This person is the **director of nursing (DON).**

The way in which the members of the nursing team work together varies, depending on the setting. For example, in the home health care setting, the case manager (an RN) develops a care

---

**HIGHLAND CARE CENTER
JOB DESCRIPTION**

CERTIFIED NURSING ASSISTANT
(CNA)

SUPERVISOR : CHARGE NURSE/DIRECTOR OF NURSING

GENERAL QUALIFICATIONS

I. SKILL LEVEL AND EXPERIENCE:

   A   Must be a Certified Nursing Assistant as required by state and federal law.
   B   If applicant is an Aide in Training, certification must be obtained within 4 months of hire.
   C. Must complete orientation required by company policy.
   D. Must complete health screening and TB test (if required) within 2 weeks of employment.
   E. Must complete a mandatory drug test within 90 days of hire.
   F.   Must be free of criminal activity proven by a criminal background check.
   G. Must become familiar with and comply to all local, state, and federal regulations relating to the job.
   H. Must obtain a current Food Handler's Permit within 14 days of hire.
   I.   Must show within 3 days of hire satisfactory evidence of identity and eligibility for employment.
   J.   Previous experience as a CNA and experience in working with geriatric residents is preferred and may be required.

II. COMMUNICATION AND DECISION-MAKING SKILLS:

   A. Must possess the ability to work well and communicate effectively with other employees, residents, family member, visitors, government agencies, the general public, etc.
   B. Must be able to read, write, speak, and understand English sufficiently to perform required duties.
   C. Must be perceptive, with good judgment and decision-making/problem-solving skills.
   D. Must be able to understand and implement the plan of care and assess resident needs.
   E. Must be able to follow verbal and written instructions.

III. PERSONAL CHARACTERISTICS:

   A. Must show courtesy and respect to other employees, residents, family members, visitors, government agencies, the general public, etc.
   B. Must maintain good personal hygiene and dress and groom appropriately.
   C. Must not be a habitual abuser of drugs (prescription or non-prescription) or alcohol.

IV. WORKING CONDITIONS & ENVIRONMENTAL PARAMETERS:

   A. Must be very flexible and willing to cover shifts for other employees who are on vacation, sick, etc. Shift work will be required.
   B. Must be willing to work holidays and weekends.
   C. Must possess the ability to work in a wet or humid environment.
   D. Must be able and willing to work with body fluids, excretions, extreme odors, etc., while using universal precautions.
   E. Is subject to exposure to infectious waste, diseases, conditions, etc., including the AIDS and Hepatitis B viruses.
   F.   Must be able to relate to and work with the ill, disabled, elderly, emotionally upset, and, at times, hostile people within the facility.

V. PHYSICAL ABILITIES:

   A. Must be able to sit, walk, run, lift and carry in excess of 75 pounds, bend, climb, kneel, squat, stoop, push, pull, grasp, reach arms above head, and have hand and finger dexterity.
   B. Must be able to rapidly assist in the evacuation of all residents from the building in case of emergency.
   C. Must be able to cope with the mental and emotional stress of working daily with geriatric residents and dealing with emergency situations.

FIGURE 2-3

It is always a good idea to be very familiar with your formal job description at each facility where you work. Here is an example of a typical job description for a nursing assistant. (*Courtesy of Highland Care Center, Salt Lake City, Utah.*)

D.   Must be able to see, hear, and smell sufficiently to ensure the personal comfort, dignity, health, and safety of the residents, and to assure that the requirements of this position can be fully met.
E.   Must be in good general heath and be emotionally stable.
F.   Must be able to perform the essential job functions without posing a direct threat to residents, self, or others.

VI.   EQUIPMENT TO BE USED:

Must be able to operate the following equipment: fire extinguisher, blood pressure cuff, stethoscope, weight chair, mechanical lift, thermometer, restraints, whirlpool bath, gait belt, hair dryer, rollers, curling iron, and other equipment as required to do the job.

ESSENTIAL JOB FUNCTIONS

I.   POLICIES:

A.   Report on time as scheduled and follow all company policies and procedures.
B.   Attend staff meetings and in-service sessions and complete 12 hours per year continuing education.
C.   Become thoroughly familiar with emergency procedures and all applicable nursing procedures currently in use.
D.   Must be able to perform duties in a timely fashion, and within the prescribed sequences and schedules.
E.   Must be able to perform assigned tasks with a minimum of supervision and develop an awareness for and a willingness to perform other tasks, as needed, without constant supervision.
F.   Must possess the ability to seek out new methods and principles and be willing to incorporate them into existing practices.
G.   Must respect all resident rights, including the confidentiality of resident care information.
H.   Follow all established safety precautions when operating equipment, and report hazardous and defective equipment or conditions to your supervisor.
I.   Must be cooperative with other departments and be courteous and respectful in dealing with them at all times.
J.   Report immediately to the Charge Nurse, to the Administrator, and to the proper legal authorities if you have reason to believe a resident has been physically, emotionally, or sexually abused, or been a victim of theft of their personal property.
K.   Participate in and respond professionally to surveys (inspections) conducted by government agencies.
L.   Create and maintain an atmosphere of warmth, cheerfulness, enthusiasm, and love, giving the resident the quality of service you would want to receive personally.

II.   PATIENT CARE:

A.   The primary purpose of your position is to provide your assigned residents with routine daily nursing care in accordance with current regulations, established nursing care procedures, and as may be directed by your supervisors, and to provide quality patient care on a consistent basis.
B.   Assume the authority, responsibility, and accountability necessary to carry out the assigned duties.
C.   Assist residents as needed with activities of daily living. This includes bathing, hair care, nail care, oral care, shaving, dressing, eating, pericare, restraining (if ordered), assisting to and from bed, toileting, turning, transferring, lifting, changing when needed, etc.
D.   Bathe each resident according to schedule. Change bed linens completely on bath days, more often as needed. Clean showers and tub rooms thoroughly before and after each use.
E.   Make rounds regularly on each shift and assist each resident as needed, making sure they are safe, clean, and comfortable.
F.   Always respect resident privacy and confidentiality including all details of resident care. Refer all questions regarding patient's status to the Charge Nurse and all questions regarding operation of care center to the Administrator.
G.   Safeguard and use appropriately all resident belongings and appliances: hearing aids, eyeglasses, dentures, clothing, personal property, etc.
H.   Escort residents to scheduled activities (recreational, religious, etc.) according to care plan.
I.   Bring residents to the dining area, serve trays, feed residents as needed, and provide assistance to those not totally independent. Pick up trays and replace in kitchen cart for depository. Document meal intake percentage.
J.   Fill resident water pitchers with ice water at least once a shift.
K.   Perform restorative and rehabilitative nursing tasks as ordered. This includes turning and massaging bedfast residents every 2 hours, giving exercises as ordered, ambulating, checking and releasing restraints every 2 hours for 15 minutes, toileting every 2 hours or as ordered or as needed.
L.   Inform the Charge Nurse of any observed change in resident's condition. This includes decrease in level of response, alteration in bowel function, skin lesions, changes in skin color or temperature, bruises, rashes, falls or other accidents, altered behavior, etc.
M.   Accurately document all duties performed on the appropriate records. This includes flow sheets, charts, notes, accident reports, intake and output records, record of restraints, etc.

(Continued)

III.   LAUNDRY & CLEANING

A.   Make sure all resident clothing is properly marked and returned to the owner after being laundered.
B.   Take or send soiled linen and clothing to the laundry in properly secured laundry bags as soon as the bag is full and at the end of each shift, whether the bag is full or not. Linens soiled with feces, vomitus, blood, or any other bodily waste products must be thoroughly rinsed in the hopper room before being sent to the laundry.
C.   Keep resident rooms clean and orderly. (This includes nightstands, dressers, over-bed tables and closets.)Mop up spills and clean messes made by residents as needed.
D.   Help maintain cleanliness of work areas, break areas, and linen closets. Make sure that equipment and supplies are properly stored before leaving for breaks and at the end of each shift.
E.   If a resident has been discharged, have the cleaning staff completely clean and disinfect the area and get resident room ready for reoccupancy.

OTHER DUTIES

Perform other duties as may be assigned by the Charge Nurse or the Director of Nursing within the scope of CNA certification.

Check one

_____   I have read the above job description and can perform all duties as outlined.

_____   I have read the above job description and cannot perform the duties listed below and would like to discuss reasonable accommodation:

_____

_____

_____

_____   _____
          Signature   Date

---

plan along with the client and his family, and the nursing assistant follows this plan when she visits the client. Often, in this situation, the nursing assistant is the only health care provider who sees the client daily. The nurse may see the client only when she visits the home in a supervisory capacity (for example, every few weeks).

In the hospital or other settings where all of the members of the nursing team are "on-site," several different models for organizing the team's efforts have been developed.

- In **primary nursing,** one nurse (an RN or LPN/LVN) is assigned several patients or residents, and is responsible for planning and carrying out all aspects of care for those people. The nurse performs all of the nursing duties for his or her patients, from feeding and bathing to giving medications and other treatments. Other nurses and nursing assistants are responsible for the primary nurse's patients or residents when the primary nurse is not on duty, but all nursing efforts on behalf of those patients or residents are directed and coordinated by the primary nurse.

- In **functional (modular) nursing,** each member of the nursing team carries out the same assigned task for all patients or residents. For example, for a particular group or unit of patients or residents, one nurse may administer all medications while another nurse does assessments and special treatments. One nursing assistant may be assigned to take vital signs and

TABLE 2-1 ■ The Nursing Team

Team Member	Requirements to Practice	Contribution to Team
Registered nurse (RN)	A baccalaureate degree from a liberal arts college or university (4 years) OR An associate degree from a junior or community college (2 years) PLUS A license obtained by passing a state board examination	Develops nursing care plans and coordinates all aspects of patient or resident care Provides nursing care to patients or residents Delegates selected aspects of patient or resident care to other team members, and supervises these team members as they carry out the delegated tasks
Licensed practical nurse (LPN) OR Licensed vocational nurse (LVN)	A certificate from a 12- to 18-month training program offered by a vocational school, community college, or hospital PLUS A license obtained by passing a state board examination	Under the supervision of a registered nurse (RN), provides nursing care to patients or residents Delegates selected aspects of patient or resident care to other team members, and supervises these team members as they carry out the delegated tasks
Nursing assistant OR Patient care attendant Patient care technician (PCT) Nursing technician Nurse's aide Home health aide	A certificate from a 75- to 200-hour training program offered by a vocational school, community college, or health care facility, obtained by completing the training and passing a state-administered competency evaluation	Assists the RN or LPN with providing nursing care to patients or residents; responsibilities include basic nursing tasks related to meeting hygiene, safety, comfort, nutrition, exercise, and elimination needs

assist with meals, while another is assigned bathing and bedmaking.

- In **team nursing,** a team leader (an RN) determines all of the nursing needs for the patients or residents assigned to the team, and assigns tasks according to each team member's skills and level of responsibility. For example, the nurse may assist the nursing assistant with bathing a patient or resident, and then give that person his or her medication. Or two nursing assistants may work together to complete the tasks usually handled by nursing assistants, such as bathing and bedmaking.

DELEGATION

To **delegate** a task means to give another person permission to perform that task on your behalf. State nurse practice acts give RNs and LPNs the responsibility of performing nursing tasks and the authority necessary to fulfill this responsibility. In order to ensure that the nursing team functions efficiently, a nurse has the authority to delegate selected tasks to a nursing assistant, but the nurse is still responsible for the quality of the care. For example, if a nurse delegates a task to a nursing assistant that the assistant is not qualified to perform, and the nurse fails to adequately supervise the assistant as she carries out the task, then the nurse is liable for any harm to the patient or resident. However, if the nurse delegates a task to an assistant that is within the assistant's **scope of practice** (the range of tasks the assistant is legally permitted to do), and the assistant fails to perform the task properly, then the assistant is responsible for any injury to the patient or resident that occurs.

Typically, the nurse will delegate nursing tasks related to routine care (hygiene, comfort, exercise) to nursing assistants. An RN can also delegate certain nursing tasks, such as data collection and documentation, to a nursing assistant. However, nursing tasks that require professional judgment, such as assessment, planning, or evaluating, cannot be delegated to a nursing assistant. For example, a nursing assistant can take a person's vital signs and record this information on the person's chart, but the assistant is not qualified to interpret the data.

Understanding how a nurse decides which tasks to delegate will help you to understand why you may be asked to do certain tasks but not

TABLE 2-2 ■ Five Rights of Delegation

	Questions the Nurse Must Consider	Questions the Nursing Assistant Must Consider
The right task	Is this a task that can be delegated? Does the nurse practice act allow me to delegate the task? Is the task in the job description for the nursing assistant?	Does the state allow me to perform this task? Have I been trained to do this task? Do I have experience performing this task? Is this task in my job description?
The right circumstance	What is the patient's or resident's condition? Is he or she stable? What are the needs of the patient or resident at this time?	Can I perform this task safely, given the patient's or resident's condition?
The right person	Does the nursing assistant have the right training and experience to safely complete the task?	Am I confident that I can perform this task safely? Do I have any reservations about performing this task, and if so, what are they?
The right direction	Am I able to give the nursing assistant clear direction regarding how to perform this task? Am I able to explain to the nursing student what is expected?	Did the nurse give me clear instructions? Do I understand what the nurse expects?
The right supervision	Will I be available to supervise and answer questions?	Will the nurse be available to supervise and answer questions?

others. When delegating a task, the nurse must know the abilities and qualifications of the nursing assistant, and she or another licensed nurse must be available to provide supervision. In addition, she must consider the patient's or resident's individual needs. In order to enable nurses to make good decisions about which tasks to delegate and to whom, the National Council of State Boards of Nursing (NCSBN) has developed guidelines called the **five rights of delegation:**

1. **The right task.** Is this a task that can be delegated? Does the nurse practice act allow the nurse to delegate the task? Is the task in the job description for the nursing assistant?
2. **The right circumstance.** What is the patient's or resident's condition? Is he or she stable? What are the needs of the patient or resident at this time?
3. **The right person.** Does the nursing assistant have the right training and experience to safely complete the task?
4. **The right direction.** Will the nurse be able to give the nursing assistant clear direction regarding how to perform the task? Will he be able to convey to the nursing assistant what is expected?
5. **The right supervision.** Will the nurse be available to supervise or to answer questions?

You and the nurse share the responsibility for making sure that delegated tasks are carried out without causing harm to the patient or resident. The nurse is responsible for making good decisions about which tasks to delegate, and for providing adequate supervision. You are responsible for recognizing which delegated tasks are within your scope of practice and range of abilities, and using this knowledge as the basis for either accepting or refusing the assignment. Just as a nurse uses the five rights of delegation to decide which tasks to delegate and to whom, you can use the five rights of delegation to help you decide whether to accept or decline a delegated task (Table 2-2). When you agree to perform a task, you accept responsibility for your actions. You must ask for help when you have questions or are unsure about how to proceed, and you must communicate with the nurse by reporting what you have done and what you observed.

You should never refuse an assignment simply because you do not want to do it. You must have a good reason for refusing to carry out an assignment, or you could lose your job. Valid reasons for refusing an assignment include the following:

- The task is not in your job description. Box 2-2 summarizes tasks that are generally outside of the scope of practice of a nursing assistant.
- Carrying out the task could result in harm to the patient or resident.
- The task is illegal or unethical.
- The nurse is not available to supervise your efforts.

BOX 2-2 Tasks That Are Generally Beyond the Nursing Assistant's Scope of Practice

Administering medications (including oxygen). Some states allow nursing assistants to administer medications to residents in assisted-living facilities, if the nursing assistant has undergone specialized training to do so. Generally, only a licensed nurse (RN or LPN) or doctor is allowed to give medications. Nursing assistants may assist patients in taking medication by bringing water or helping to open the medicine bottle.

Receiving verbal orders (in person or over the telephone) from doctors. Licensed nurses (RNs or LPNs) are the only personnel authorized to receive doctors' orders.

Diagnosing illness and prescribing medications. Only doctors can diagnose illness and prescribe medical or surgical treatment.

Supervising other nursing assistants. Licensed nurses (RNs or LPNs) are responsible for supervising nursing assistants.

Performing procedures that require sterile technique. Nursing assistants are permitted to assist a nurse in performing a sterile procedure, but they are not trained to do these procedures themselves.

Inserting or removing tubes from a patient's body (bladder, esophagus, trachea, nose, ears). Nursing assistants generally are not trained in procedures that involve inserting or removing tubes from a patient's or resident's body. Exceptions may be made if the nursing assistant has had the opportunity to practice a procedure under an instructor's supervision.

- You do not have the proper equipment.
- The directions are not clear.
- You are not able to perform the task safely.
- You have not received adequate training about the task or the equipment used.

If you do make the decision to decline a task that you have been assigned to do, it is your responsibility to state clearly that you are not going to do the task and your reason why. Failure to communicate your refusal to complete a task to the person requesting your help can jeopardize the care or safety of the patient or resident. The person requesting your help assumes that you are doing the task, unless he or she hears otherwise.

GUIDELINES BOX 2-1
GUIDELINES FOR ACCEPTING OR DECLINING AN ASSIGNMENT

What you do	Why you do it
Always ask the nurse for clarification if there is something you do not understand.	It is your responsibility to make sure you know what is to be done and how it is to be done before going to the patient or resident.
Never perform a task that you have not been taught to do, or that you feel uncomfortable doing, unless you are supervised by a nurse.	The nurse is ultimately responsible for ensuring the patient's or resident's safety. This means that it is the nurse's responsibility to ensure that whoever is performing the task on her behalf is qualified to do so, and capable. It is irresponsible for you to misrepresent your abilities, or to proceed unsupervised with a task that you are not fully capable of doing well.
Never ignore an assignment because you do not know how to perform the task or the task is beyond your scope of practice.	The patient's or resident's needs must be attended to, either by you or by someone else. If you feel that you cannot perform the task that you are being asked to do, explain your concerns to the nurse so that she can either help you with the task or reassign it.

Declining a task is a discussion that you should have privately with the person requesting the task of you. Do not discuss the issue in front of the resident, patient, or visitors.

General guidelines for accepting or declining an assignment are given in Guidelines Box 2-1. A good general rule to keep in mind is that you should not perform any task that is not listed in your job description. Because a nursing assistant's duties can vary from state to state, and also from facility to facility, you must be familiar with your formal job description. Ask your supervisor about anything you do not understand. This is important to protect yourself, as well as your patients or residents.

SUMMARY

▶ No matter what the setting, nursing assistants are an integral part of the nursing team, a subset of the health care team.

- Like all of the members of the nursing team, nursing assistants undergo training that authorizes them to perform certain tasks.
- Nursing assistants assist the nurse by performing basic nursing functions, such as those related to hygiene, safety, comfort, nutrition, exercise, and elimination.

▶ In order to ensure that the nursing team operates smoothly and efficiently, a "chain of command" exists. This means that licensed nurses (RNs or LPNs) are able to assign (delegate) certain tasks to nursing assistants.

- The delegation of tasks cannot be taken lightly by either the delegator (the licensed nurse) or the delegatee (the nursing assistant). Both share the responsibility of ensuring that the procedure is carried out without harm to the patient or resident.
- The nursing assistant must know which tasks are within his or her scope of practice, and which tasks are not.

What did you learn?

Multiple Choice

Select the single best answer for each of the following questions.

1. Nursing assistants who work in the long-term care setting must complete a course of training and undergo a competency evaluation. These requirements are set by the:
   a. Centers for Disease Control (CDC)
   b. Food and Drug Administration (FDA)
   c. Omnibus Budget Reconciliation Act (OBRA)
   d. Occupational Safety and Health Administration (OSHA)

2. As a nursing assistant, it is your responsibility to:
   a. Plan the patient's or resident's care
   b. Perform the tasks your supervisor assigns to you
   c. Do the best you can without asking for help
   d. Compare assignments with your coworkers

3. If you do not know how to do an assigned task, you should:
   a. Call another nursing assistant for help
   b. Ask the patient or resident how he prefers to have it done
   c. Call the charge nurse and ask for help
   d. Follow the instructions in the procedure manual

4. Nursing assistants work under the supervision of:
   a. A doctor
   b. A registered nurse (RN) or licensed practical nurse (LPN)
   c. Other nursing assistants
   d. The long-term care facility administrator

5. To "delegate" means to:
   a. Do what you are told to do
   b. Give another person permission to perform a task on your behalf
   c. Transfer your duties to another assistant
   d. Have the charge nurse take your assignment

6. What information is included in the registry?
   a. The nursing assistant's full name
   b. The nursing assistant's Social Security Number
   c. Any reported incidents of abuse or theft
   d. All of the above

? Stop and think!

▶ You have just received your assignment for the shift. Another assistant does not like her assignment and asks to switch residents with you. This makes you uncomfortable because you have just started at the facility and do not know if switching assignments is permitted. What should you do?

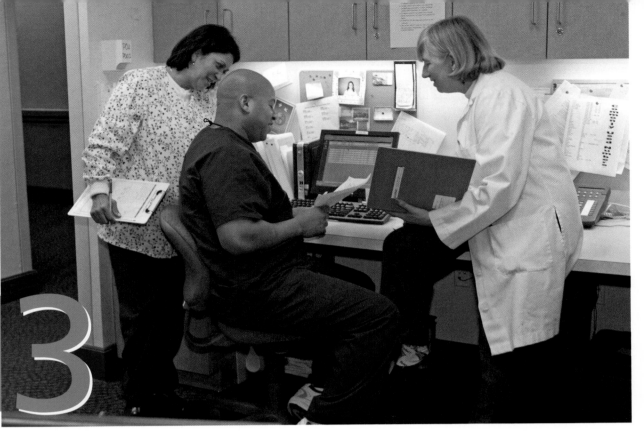

3

Professionalism and Job-Seeking Skills

What will you learn?

In the two previous chapters, you learned about the health care system in general, and the duties of a nursing assistant in particular. You learned about skills a nursing assistant must have in order to care for people in need, as well as about the duties and responsibilities of a nursing assistant. While having the knowledge and ability to perform your duties well is essential, showing professionalism and a strong work ethic are important too. In this chapter, we will explore the qualities of professionalism and a strong work ethic, and how possessing these qualities can help you to get a job, and excel at it. In addition, we will provide an overview of the process of applying and interviewing for a job. When you are finished with this chapter, you will be able to:

1. Define the terms *professional* and *professionalism*.
2. Discuss characteristics that health care workers demonstrate that promote professionalism.
3. List several sources of employment information for jobs in the health care industry.
4. Describe considerations one must explore when seeking employment.
5. Discuss the application process necessary for obtaining employment.
6. Define the term *work ethic* and describe how good work habits promote professionalism.
7. Understand the importance of personal health and hygiene for the health care worker.

Photo: The health care industry relies on all types of professionals to provide quality care to patients and residents.

Vocabulary

Use the CD in the back of your book to hear these terms pronounced, defined, and used in a sentence:

Professional	Equal Employment	Reference list	Interview
Professionalism	Opportunity	Human resources (HR)	Work ethic
Attitude	Commission	department	Hygiene
Résumé	(EEOC)	(personnel)	

WHAT IS A PROFESSIONAL?

What exactly is a professional? And how is professionalism measured? One definition of a professional is "a person with much experience and great skill in a specified role" who is "engaged in a specific occupation for pay or as a means of livelihood." Another definition relates the word "professional" to a "profession," or a sacred vow. The relationship between the word "profession" (in the sense of a sacred vow) and the word "professional" (in the sense of one who takes a sacred vow) is especially applicable to those of us who consider ourselves "health care professionals," for we do practice that "sacred vow" of providing care for those in need.

The health care industry gives the title of **professional** to those who have credentials, obtained through education and training, that enable them to become licensed or certified to practice a certain profession. This industry certainly relies on all types of professionals, such as physicians, nurses, and nursing assistants, to provide quality care to patients and residents. However, many people who are considered professionals do not need a license or a certificate to perform their jobs, and they may not even need a specific educational background. Being a professional also means having a professional attitude, or exhibiting **professionalism**.

An **attitude** is the side of ourselves that we display to the world, communicating outwardly how we feel about things. A person's attitude is apparent from things he says (and the way he says them), the way he behaves, and the way he looks. You may have heard it said about a person that he or she "has an attitude," meaning that the person's outward behavior is unpleasant. Well, an attitude is something we all possess and it can be positive instead of negative.

Possessing a positive attitude in the workplace means that you are caring and compassionate toward your patients or residents, and that you demonstrate a commitment to doing your job to the best of your ability at all times. This commitment to doing your best is the attitude that defines professionalism, the attitude of being a professional. While your job as a nursing assistant will allow you to earn a paycheck, a true professional views her work as a reflection of the role she plays in society. Income is important, but so is the sense of pride you will feel as a result of setting high standards for your performance and obtaining satisfaction from the work you do, in knowing that you are helping others. Regardless of the level of education, certification, or experience a health care professional has, professionalism is all about exhibiting the right attitude, to coworkers, patients or residents, and visitors. Professionalism is a choice you make and requires effort. What attitude will you chose to show?

JOB-SEEKING SKILLS

You are currently in the process of training to become a nursing assistant. You may have chosen to take this training for any number of reasons. You may have an interest in the health care profession and are taking this course to explore that interest. You may be entering the workforce after spending years raising a family, or you may find yourself in need of work due to a change in your financial situation. Some students are applying to nursing school and require the nursing assistant training to meet admission criteria. Regardless of your reason or reasons for entering the health care field, you will find many opportunities to put your training to use. The health care field is one of the most rapidly growing areas in industry, and the trend is expected to continue. Long-term care facilities, home health care agencies, hospice organizations, hospitals, doctor's offices, dialysis centers, rehabilitation centers, and many other types of health care organizations employ nursing assistants. Perhaps you already know what type of health care organization you would like to work in, or perhaps you will have to try a few different things before you find your special place.

GET READY!

So, you're ready to get a job. Before you begin the process of responding to notices about job opportunities, completing applications, and going on interviews, it is important that you take time to explore what you really want from your employment and what you will be able to offer to your employer (Fig. 3-1). Some questions to consider are:

- **What type of facility do you want to work at?** Do you like working with elderly people? If so, you might like working in a long-term care facility. Maybe you have always wanted to work with disabled children, or find the idea of caring for people in their homes appealing. Maybe you would thrive as part of the team working in the fast-paced environment of an acute care setting. Focusing on your interests, likes, and dislikes will help you to narrow the search, increasing the chance that you will find a job you will enjoy.

- **Are there limitations on the hours or shifts you are available to work?** If you are a parent with small children, you may be limited to working certain shifts depending on your childcare arrangements. Do not lead an employer to believe that you are available for any shift if you can realistically work only evenings.

- **Do you have reliable transportation to get to work?** Your employer will rely on you to come to work as scheduled and on time. If you rely on public transportation, apply for work at facilities serviced by that particular transportation method.

- **What are some of your personality strengths?** Are you self-motivated and independent, or do you like more supervision and guidance? A nursing assistant who

works well independently would be an asset for a home health care agency whereas one who prefers more supervision would probably be better suited for working in a facility.

Once you have some specific goals in mind, where do you start your search? There are many places to search for job openings. Certainly the classified ads in the local newspaper are a great place to start. Telephone directories list facilities and agencies that hire nursing assistants. You could try calling these organizations directly, or checking the Internet to see if the organizations you are interested in post job openings on their websites. In addition, you can use the Internet to check sites dedicated to helping people find jobs. The school that you are attending may offer a job placement service, where you can check job listings and obtain help with writing a résumé. You could also check for job postings on the bulletin board in the facility where you are receiving clinical training. Last but not least, friends and colleagues may know of openings. Start a list of positions that you hear of that interest you, so that you will have the information readily available.

Before actually making application for a particular job, you must prepare a **résumé**, a brief document that gives a possible employer general information about you and your education and work experience. Résumés should be typed or printed using a computer on white or off-white paper. With résumés, "plain" is best—no fancy lettering or designs are necessary! A résumé contains only facts and should be kept to one page, if at all possible (Fig. 3-2). Your résumé should include:

- Your full name, address, telephone number and, if you have one, your e-mail address
- A short objective, or career goal
- A history of your education (list the schools you attended most recently first, and for each school, include the dates you attended the school and the degree you graduated with)
- An employment history (list each of your previous employers, and for each employer, include the dates that you worked there, your job title, and your primary job duties)

Listing volunteer work on your résumé is appropriate, but only if it relates to the job you are applying for. There is some information that should never be included on a résumé, including your age, marital status, weight, religion, sexual preference, and whether or not you have children

FIGURE 3-1

The first step to finding a job is thinking about what sort of situation best fits your personality, lifestyle, and interests.

SUZIE SMITH
123 NORTH AVENUE
ANYWHERE, US 12345
(123) 456-7890

Career Objective:

To obtain a position as a Certified Nursing Assistant in a rehabilitation-centered healthcare facility that will allow me to utilize my skills to assist those in need.

Education:

Anywhere Vocational Center Anywhere, US	May–July 2002 Nursing Assisting Course CNA Certification: August 2002
State Jr. College Anywhere, US	August–December 2001 General Studies
Anywhere High School Anywhere, US	Graduated: June 2001 High School Diploma

Certifications:

Certified Nursing Assistant CPR Certification	August 2002 (Current) July 2002 (Current)

Employment History:

Sunshine Assisted Living   August 2002–Present
Anywhere, US

CNA, Rehabilitation Unit. Provided assistance with activities of daily living for residents, with an emphasis on rehabilitation. Worked closely with physical therapists to carry out therapy plan with meals and ambulation.

Quality Printing   July 2001–July 2002
Anywhere, US

Cashier/Customer Service. Worked part-time while attending college. Responsible for assisting customers with print orders and making end-of-day bank deposits.

Volunteer History:

Hospice   June 2000–July 2002
Anywhere, US

Respite Volunteer. Provided respite relief for families receiving hospice care. Sat with patients and read to them.

FIGURE 3-2

A résumé is a short, precise document with information about you, your work experience, and your education.

(or are planning to have them). This information should not matter to an employer who is considering you as an employee. In fact, according to the **Equal Employment Opportunity Commission (EEOC)**, it is against the law for an employer to ask a candidate questions related to these subjects at any time during the hiring process.

You may also want to prepare a cover letter to send out with your résumé. A cover letter is written as a way of introducing yourself to a potential employer. Your résumé contains information about your education, training, and experience, but a cover letter goes beyond the straight facts. A cover letter says, "Hello, this is why I want to work for your organization, and this is why I am the best person for the job" (Fig. 3-3). Your cover letter should be fairly short and typed or printed using a computer on white or off-white paper. Pay special attention to your grammar and spelling.

Suzie Smith
123 North Avenue
Anywhere, US 12345
February 1, 2004

Sandra Jones, Director of Human Resources
Sunny Hills Rehabilitation Center
1234 South Avenue
Anywhere, US 12345

Dear Ms. Jones,

  I would like to express my interest in the certified nursing assistant position at Sunny Hills Rehabilitation Center that was listed in the local want ads. In July, 2002, I completed my nursing assistant training at Anywhere Vocational Center. Since that time, I have been employed at Sunshine Assisted Living as a CNA in their rehabilitation unit.

  I am a hard worker and I learn new skills easily. I love working with the elderly and have heard that your facility is a very enjoyable place to work.

  Thank you for taking the time to review and consider my application. I am available for an interview at your convenience and look forward to meeting with you soon.

Sincerely,

Suzie Smith

Suzie Smith, CNA

FIGURE 3-3

A cover letter is a letter that you write to go along with your résumé. Your cover letter allows you to explain more fully why you want to work for a particular organization, and what qualities you have that make you the ideal person for the job opening in question.

The last document you should prepare before applying for a job is a reference list. A **reference list** is a list of three or four people who would be willing to talk to a potential employer about your abilities. When considering people to include on your reference list, think about people who know you well and have worked with you in a professional capacity, such as your teachers, coworkers, or previous supervisors. Before listing a person as a reference, make sure you have his or her permission to do so. Some people may hesitate to act as a reference. For example, they may not want their contact information given out, they may be too busy, or they may not think you did as good a job for them as you thought you did. After a person has agreed to be your reference, make sure you have accurate contact information for that person, including his or her full name and title (if any), a current and complete address, and a telephone number. Type your reference list on a sheet of paper that matches your résumé. Some employers will ask for a list of references at the time you turn in an application; others will want you to write your references on the actual application form. Either way, you will be prepared with correct and current information. How efficient and organized you will appear at that first meeting!

GET SET!

Now that you have thought about your ideal work situation, prepared a list of job opportunities to pursue, written your résumé and cover letter, and gathered your references, you are ready to place applications. Although it is acceptable and common practice to just stop by organizations where you are interested in working and ask to complete an application, you may want to call ahead to ask if there are any positions open for nursing assistants. Even if there are not any immediate openings, most facilities will keep applications on file for approximately 6 months, so ask if you may place an application to be kept on file.

In some facilities, the director of nursing (DON) handles the hiring of nursing assistants. In others, hiring is handled through the **human resources (HR) department (personnel)**. Usually, when you go to an organization to complete

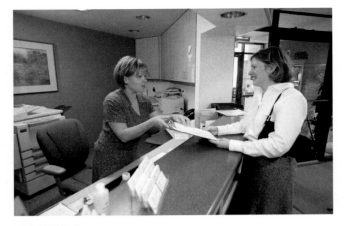

FIGURE 3-4

When you go to complete your application form, take your résumé, cover letter, and references with you, and dress neatly.

a job application, the receptionist at the main desk will give you the application to complete (Fig. 3-4). When you go to complete your application, take your résumé and references with you and dress appropriately, even though you expect only to complete the application and leave. Some facilities may choose to interview you at that time, especially if there is an opening. Appropriate dress means "clean and neat." Make sure your clothes are pressed and clean and your shoes are polished. Hair should be neatly arranged and out of your face. Jewelry should be simple and minimal, and if you wear perfume or cologne, the fragrance should be light. Women should make sure that their make-up is tastefully applied. Even if you do not interview, this will be the first impression you make on a possible employer. You can be sure that the people who do the hiring for the organization will do some preliminary screening by asking the receptionist whether you appeared neat and well-organized, and what your attitude was like.

A job application is a standardized form used to obtain basic pertinent information, such as which position you are applying for, how you can be reached, and what shifts you can work (Fig. 3-5). Remember the time you spent earlier thinking about practical factors that needed to be taken into consideration, such as childcare arrangements and transportation? Now you will be able to easily answer the questions on the application about your availability for work. The application form will also require you to provide information about your education, your work history, and the reasons you left your previous job. There are many legitimate reasons why a person would leave a place of employment:

- "I left to take a position that is closer to home."
- "I left because I was offered better hours/a pay increase."
- "I left to have children."
- "I left to go to school."
- "I left because we moved to a new city or town."
- "I left because I was laid off."

The reason for leaving a job could be that you were fired. If so, be honest. Your chances of finding new employment are much better if a potential employer hears the truth from you, instead of finding it out by calling your references. When giving a reason for leaving a job, avoid speaking negatively about your previous employer, even if the situation was not ideal. Doing so reflects poorly on you as a potential employee.

Some facilities will allow you to take the application home to be filled out and returned at a later date. Others will require you to complete the application while you are there. Most facilities will also request a copy of your résumé and reference list, along with the completed application. Be prepared to complete the application form in the facility. Have notes available with details that you will need to complete the application. Use blue or black ink and write clearly. The application form is a legal document, and your signature at the bottom states that all the information is true and accurate. An employer who finds out that you lied about any information on the application form has grounds to fire you without notice.

Ask for an appointment for an interview when you submit your cover letter, résumé, reference list, and completed application. Some facilities will make the appointment at this time. Others may want to review your résumé and application and call you for an appointment at a later date. If you have not heard from a potential employer in 1 week's time, it is appropriate to call and ask about the status of your application. A follow-up call shows a potential employer that you have initiative and are interested in the job.

GO!

You have an appointment for that interview! An **interview** is the chance for a potential employer to meet you personally and learn more about you

HIGHLAND CARE CENTER
APPLICATION FOR EMPLOYMENT

Highland Care Center is an equal opportunity employer, dedicated to a policy of non-discrimination in employment on any basis, including race, color, age, sex, religion, national origin or disability. Highland supports hiring people who have disabilities and meets all ADA requirements to provide reasonable accommodations for people with disabilities who are qualified to do the job. A mandatory drug test will be performed within 90 days of hire. Criminal background checks will be made on all new employees.

PERSONAL INFORMATION

Name:_____   Date:_____

        Please list any other names you have been known by or employed under:_____

Phone Number:_____   Social Security Number:_____

Position Desired:_____   Salary Desired:_____

Present Address:_____
                          Street   City   State   Zip Code

Permanent Address (if different from above):_____
                          Street   City   State   Zip Code

Have you ever applied for employment with Highland before?   Yes _____   No _____   If yes, when?_____

Have you ever worked for Highland before?   Yes _____   No _____   If yes, when?_____

Available for: Full Time _____   Part Time _____   On Call _____   Shifts available for: Morning ____   Afternoon ____   Night ____

If hired, when would you be available to begin work? _____

Are you eligible for employment in the United States?   Yes _____   No _____

How did you learn about Highland Care Center? _____

Have you ever been convicted of a felony or misdeamor?   Yes _____   No _____   Do you smoke? Yes _____   No _____

Upon hire a criminal background check will be conducted.

EDUCATION	Name and Location of School	Graduate?
High School		
College		
Business/Trade/Tech.		

List Other Job-Related Skills: _____

_____

Special Skills or Qualifications: _____

_____

FIGURE 3-5

A job application is a standardized form used to obtain basic information about each person who applies for a job with the organization. It is a legal document, and your signature at the bottom states that all of the information you have provided is true and accurate.

Please list your previous work experience below beginning with your present or most recent employer for the past five years or your last three employers, whichever you feel will provide us with the most helpful information about you.

Dates of Employment Must list month and year	Name, Address, Phone Number of Employer Name of Supervisor	Ending Wage	Ending Position	Reason for Leaving
Begin Date _____ End Date _____				
Begin Date _____ End Date _____				
Begin Date _____ End Date _____				

If a previous employer is not to be contacted, designate which

one: _____

Are there any comments you would like to share ? _____

_____

The information provided in this Application for Employment is true, correct and complete. If employed, any misstatement or omission of fact on this application may result in my dismissal. I understand that acceptance of an offer of employment does not create a contractual obligation upon Highland Care Center to continue to employ me in the future. Daywest HealthCare Services, Inc. Is a drug & alcohol free workplace. As a condition of employment all employees must successfully pass a drug test which will be administered some time during their orientation period. Criminal background checks will be made on all new employees.

Signature: _____   Date: _____

FOR HIGHLAND USE ONLY

Interviewed by: _____   Date: _____

References:

Person Contacted, Place and Date: _____

Person Contacted, Place and Date: _____

Person Contacted, Place and Date: _____

Remarks: _____

_____

_____

**HIGHLAND CARE CENTER
RELEASE OF INFORMATION**

Applicant Name: _____

Social Security #: _____   Date: _____

I authorize Highland Care Center to seek and obtain information from employers, supervisors and colleagues regarding the following as well as any other job-related information which will enable the facility to evaluate my suitability for employment.

____ work habits   ____ technical skills

____ performance record   ____ vaccination records

____ ability to form effective working relationships with co-workers

____ other: _____

I authorize those contacted to release this information to Highland Care Center.

By initialing below, I authorize Highland Care Center to obtain information from:

        ____ All former employers and current employer

        ____ Former employers only

Signature: _____   Date: _____

FIGURE 3-5

(continued)

in an effort to determine if you are the right person for the job. Equally as important, the interview is a chance for *you* to learn more about the employer and the position, in an effort to determine if they are right for you. Being properly prepared for the interview will allow you to gather as much information about the organization and the job as possible during the interview, so that you can make an informed decision about the job if it is offered to you. In addition, being properly prepared can make all the difference in how a potential employer views your potential! Your résumé and application contain all of the "hard" facts about your education and experience, but you are the one responsible for persuading the interviewer of your interest in the job, dedication to your profession, and abilities.

Before going to the interview, make a list of questions you would like answers to, and refer to this list during the interview. This shows that you are interested in the position and are taking the opportunity to interview seriously. Some questions you might want to ask include:

- "What are the major responsibilities or duties of the position? May I have a copy of the job description?"

- "Do you have to replace nursing assistants often, here? If so, why?"
- "May I see the unit where I will be working and meet the person who will be supervising me?"
- "What do you think nursing assistants like best about working here? Least?"
- "How many nursing assistants staff each unit?"
- "When would I be eligible for a performance evaluation, and what are the standards I will be evaluated against?"
- "What qualities are you looking for in a nursing assistant?"
- "What opportunities exist for career growth and furthering my education?"

Your dress for the interview should be neat and professional (Fig. 3-6). Men should wear slacks (not jeans), a button-down shirt or a polo shirt and a belt, and possibly a sport jacket if the weather is cool. A tie is optional. Your hair should be clean and neat. You should be freshly shaved, or, if you have a beard or a moustache, it should be neatly trimmed. Make sure your shoes are clean and polished, and wear socks. Your hands and nails should be clean and well cared

FIGURE 3-6

Dress like the professional that you are when you go for your interview! Clean, neat hair and nails and polished shoes are appropriate for both men and women. *(A)* An appropriate outfit for a man would be slacks, a button-down shirt or a polo shirt, and a belt. A tie is optional. *(B)* For a woman, an appropriate outfit would be a skirt and a blouse with stockings. Make-up and jewelry should be kept to a minimum.

A   B

for. Limit jewelry to functional items such as a watch and simple ring. Excessive jewelry, such as necklaces, and visible body piercings are not appropriate for either the interview or this career setting.

Women should wear a skirt (or dress slacks) and a blouse, or a simple dress. Stockings should be worn and the hem length of your skirt or dress should be modest. Your shoes should be clean and polished. Make sure your make-up is tasteful and professional. Avoid wearing too much make-up, or make-up that is too bright or dark. Limit the jewelry you wear to a few key accessories, and avoid clanking bracelets and long, dangling earrings, which can be distracting during an interview. If you wear cologne or perfume, it should be of a light fragrance. Nails should be trimmed and neat, and your hair should be neatly styled. If you have long hair, pin it back from your face with an attractive barrette or clip.

Make sure your clothing is pressed and all repairs, such as missing buttons or loose seams, have been taken care of before the interview. Carrying a small notebook containing the questions you want to ask during the interview and a copy of your résumé, reference list, and your certified nursing assistant certification or registration looks very professional. Do not chew gum during the interview, and make sure your cellular phone is turned off. You only have one chance to make a first impression, so make it a good one!

Give yourself adequate time to get to the interview. Ideally, you will arrive a few minutes early. After being introduced to the interviewer, shake his or her hand and take a seat when you are invited to do so. Do not address the interviewer by his or her first name, unless the interviewer specifically asks you to. Thank the person for the opportunity to interview at the beginning of the interview.

During the interview process, sit up straight and try not to fidget. You might be nervous and that is certainly understandable, but try to appear as confident and comfortable as you can under the circumstances. Maintain good eye contact during the interview and speak clearly. Common questions an interviewer might ask a candidate are listed in Box 3-1. Most interviewers will ask a potential employee about his or her strengths and weaknesses. Think about this ahead of time, and be honest. We all have some

---

BOX 3-1 Common Interview Questions

"Tell me about yourself. Why did you become a nursing assistant?"

"What part of your last job did you like the most? The least?"

"Why are you leaving your current job?" (or, "Why did you leave your last job?")

"What are you looking for in a manager?"

"How do you describe your work habits?"

"How do you set priorities?"

"How do you handle yourself under stress?"

"How do you handle problems with patients or coworkers?"

"Tell me about a specific situation that interfered with your ability to do your job, and how you handled it."

"What is the most satisfying workday you have had this year? Why?"

"Do you have a mentor? What have you learned from this person?"

"Who in your life would you consider to be 'successful'? Why?"

"What do you consider to be your greatest strength? Your greatest weakness?"

"Where do you want to go with your career? What steps have you taken to achieve your goal?"

"What is it about our organization that appeals to you?"

---

terrific strengths and we also have our weaknesses. Remember that a person who is aware of a weakness is capable of working to improve it. Try to answer questions concisely yet completely; it is best if you can strike a balance between listening and talking. If you do not know the answer to a question, simply say that you do not know—most interviewers are quick to recognize bluffing.

At the end of the interview, the interviewer will usually give you an opportunity to ask any questions that you may have. Now is the time to refer to your list! Asking questions of your own indicates that you have an active interest in making sure that you are a good fit for the job and the organization. The interviewer may have discussed salary and benefits (medical benefits, dental benefits, retirement plans, holiday and sick time, schedule for pay increases) during the course of the interview, but if he or she did not, it is best not to ask about these things now. The

February 6, 2004

Dear Ms. Jones,

I would like to thank you for the opportunity to interview for the nursing assistant position at Sunny Hills Rehabilitation Center. I was impressed by the quality of your facility and the competence of your staff and would like very much to become a member of your health care team. I look forward to hearing from you in the near future.

Thank you,

Suzie Smith

FIGURE 3-7

After your interview, send a thank-you note to the person who interviewed you, thanking her for her time and restating your interest in the position and the organization.

proper time to discuss pay and benefits is when a job offer is made. When the interview is over, thank the interviewer again for his or her time, and for considering you for the position. If the interviewer did not mention when you can expect to hear from him or her regarding the position, ask. Then leave! The interview is over, and there is nothing left to do but write a thank-you note.

You should write a short thank-you note within 1 day of interviewing for the position, thanking the interviewer for considering you for the position and briefly explaining why you are excited about the possibility of working for his or her organization (Fig. 3-7). Everyone wants to be complimented on his or her organization, and your interest in being a part of that organization is a compliment. You may hand-write your thank-you note on a plain notecard, or type it.

THE FINISH LINE!

As with dropping off the application, if you do not hear from the organization you interviewed with within the amount of time specified at the close of the interview, it is appropriate to follow up with a telephone call. When a representative

of the organization calls to offer you a job, you can take this opportunity to ask any questions that may have occurred to you since the interview, or that were not appropriate to ask during the interview. If you need time to think about the offer, it is acceptable to ask the person who has offered you the job if you can call him or her back with an answer within the next day or so.

Applying and interviewing for jobs can be a time-consuming process that requires a lot of effort. By taking the time to prepare, you increase your chances of finding a situation where you will be happy and satisfied with your work. However, landing the perfect job is just the beginning—in the next few sections, we will explore ways to ensure that you thrive in your new position.

WHAT IS A WORK ETHIC?

Interestingly enough, when nursing assistant instructors are called by potential employers to give a reference for a student, they are most often asked not how smart the student is, or what sort of grades the student made. Instead, they are most often asked about that student's **work ethic**. A work ethic can be described in many ways and measured by any number of standards, but simply put, it relates specifically to your attitude toward your work. We spoke earlier in this chapter about having a professional attitude and taking pride in doing your work to the best of your ability. Professionalism and a strong work ethic go hand-in-hand.

A strong work ethic is what separates an average employee from a great employee (Fig. 3-8). Two nursing assistants can have solid skills and be very good at getting their work done on time, but the nursing assistant with the strongest work ethic will be the one who enjoys the greatest professional success. A good work ethic not only allows a person to grow in her career (because her employer will be satisfied with the quality of her work), it allows her to experience the emotional rewards of knowing that she has made her best effort. What qualities does a person with a strong work ethic possess, and how can one go about developing these qualities?

FIGURE 3-8
Professionalism and a strong work ethic go hand-in-hand. Many qualities contribute to a strong work ethic.

FIGURE 3-9
Being punctual means that you are on time or a little early. It is important to come to work on time because many people are relying on you!

PUNCTUALITY

Being punctual means that you are on time, or a little bit early. Arriving to work on time prepared to start your duties is vital in the health care industry (Fig. 3-9). Many people are relying on you! The staff working the shift before yours is anxious for you to relieve them so that they can go home to their families and other responsibilities. If you work a morning shift, patients and residents will need your assistance in getting out of bed and preparing for breakfast, diagnostic tests, or surgery.

Organization is necessary to achieve punctuality. If you work a morning shift, plan ahead the evening before by packing your lunch and making sure your uniform is clean and pressed. If you have children, pack their lunches, lay out their clothes for the next day, and make sure any papers they need for school are completed. Setting the alarm 15 minutes earlier will not significantly affect the amount of sleep you get, but it will allow you that extra time you need to have breakfast before work, or tend to any small last-minute crises.

RELIABILITY

Reliability is an essential characteristic for a nursing assistant. Reliability means that others can count on you to come to work every day, as scheduled, and to remain there during your entire shift (in other words, that your attendance is consistent). Everyone certainly has to miss a day of work occasionally for sickness or emergencies, but frequent absences are a very poor reflection on your work ethic. Have alternative plans for transportation and childcare in place before the need arises, and try to keep yourself healthy to decrease your need to take sick days. Poor attendance and chronic lateness are primary reasons employers take corrective action against nursing assistants.

Reliability also means that others can count on you to do your job conscientiously and well, with minimal supervision. Your supervisor should not feel the need to look over your shoulder or "check up" on you to make sure your work has been finished.

ACCOUNTABILITY

Accountability is also an essential characteristic for a nursing assistant. An accountable person accepts responsibility for his or her actions, and the results of those actions. Being accountable means that you can accept criticism that is intended to help you improve, admit a mistake, and work to correct the situation. Although it can be difficult to admit that you have made a mistake, trying to conceal a mistake or blame it on someone else will only make matters worse. By acknowledging a mistake and taking measures to correct it, you are not only acting in the best interest of your patient or resident, you are letting your supervisors and colleagues know that you can be trusted to do your job to the best of your ability at all times, and that you are interested in learning how to prevent similar mistakes from happening in the future.

CONSCIENTIOUSNESS

Conscientious nursing assistants take their assignments seriously and make sure they follow directions carefully. They demonstrate responsibility by asking for additional explanation or clarification when necessary, seeking help with difficult tasks, and admitting that they may not know how to perform a particular task. If you have not been shown how to do a procedure that you have been asked to do, show that you are interested in learning how. A conscientious nursing assistant attends to details and goes the extra mile to complete a task with care. When you act conscientiously, you leave your patients or residents feeling like they are special and have received the "royal treatment."

COURTESY AND RESPECTFULNESS

Always treat other people with respect, both your patients or residents and your coworkers. The phrases *please, thank you,* and *excuse me* can improve the quality of almost any interaction. Avoid using "baby talk" or "talking down" to patients or residents. Address people as they prefer to be addressed. If in doubt, err on the side of formality ("Dr. Smith," "Mrs. Jones," "Mr. Davis," "Miss Thomson"). In some parts of the United States, such as the deep South, elderly people prefer to be addressed by their first names, preceded by "Miss" or "Mr." ("Miss Katharine"), and "ma'am" and "sir" are always used. Being polite and having good manners are correct in any situation. Considering another person's feelings and beliefs shows that you truly care about the person.

Show respect for your fellow workers and supervisors by not saying anything negative about them to your patients or residents, or other coworkers. Do not speak poorly about your place of employment to others, even if there are things that you are not happy with. People who hear you say negative things about your place of employment will begin to wonder about you and why you continue to work there if the situation is so bad. If the person you are speaking to is a patient or resident (or a family member of a patient or resident), he or she may begin to question the quality of care that is being given.

HONESTY

Honesty is a critical quality for health care workers to have. You are expected to accurately record vital signs and other information about the condition of the people you care for. You will have access to people's valuables, especially in the long-term care and home health care settings. You will be trusted with information of a very private nature regarding people's care and medical condition. Patients and residents will come to trust you and confide in you. If you act in a way that gives your patients or residents reason to lose confidence in their ability to trust you, it will be very difficult to reestablish your relationship.

COOPERATIVENESS

Being able to cooperate, or work as part of a team, is essential in the health care industry. Professionals with many different levels of education and areas of training work together to benefit the people they care for. Remember how important your part of the chain of care is and what an essential role you play in providing for the care and comfort of your patients or residents, and use this as a driving force. Making an effort to get along with your coworkers will make your work easier and will ease the burden on your coworkers as well. A good nursing assistant does not wait for a coworker to ask for help; he or she sees a need and offers a helping hand. You will undoubtedly have to work with people you may not especially like, but a professional is able to put his or her personal feelings aside for the benefit of the patient or resident.

EMPATHY

Empathy means that you are able to try and imagine what it would feel like to be in another person's situation. There are times when coworkers, patients or residents, or the family members of patients or residents will really try your patience, but if you think of how you would feel if you were in a similar situation, you may find that you are able to understand the offending behavior better. Empathy gives us another perspective and helps us to be kinder and more tolerant. Treating people with kindness is a better reflection of professionalism than, for example, displaying superior intellect.

There are many more qualities that are associated with a strong work ethic, such as cheerfulness and enthusiasm, a willingness to volunteer for new assignments, and a desire to learn new skills. Primarily, a nursing assistant with a strong work ethic is someone you can depend on and trust, someone who treats others with kindness, respect, and compassion. People with strong work ethics know how to do their jobs well, they like their jobs, and they continue to learn and improve. Last but not least, they smile a lot!

PERSONAL HEALTH AND HYGIENE

To care for your patients or residents to the best of your ability, you must first care for yourself. By taking proper care of yourself, you demonstrate that you are a professional who takes her responsibilities seriously.

MAINTAINING YOUR PHYSICAL HEALTH

The duties of a nursing assistant require much physical effort. You will be constantly lifting, bending, walking, and reaching as you perform your daily tasks at work. As you will learn in later chapters, there are many risks to your health and physical condition in the health care profession. Your employer, your coworkers, your family, and especially your patients or residents rely on you to be able to do your duties. In addition to giving you more energy, staying physically fit keeps your body strong and allows you to avoid many types of job-related injuries (Fig. 3-10). To keep your body in good physical condition:

- **Get enough sleep.** Most people need an average of 6 to 8 hours of sleep to function properly. Not only does rest relax the muscles, it also relaxes the mind and allows you to think clearly. Too little rest can weaken your immune system, making you more likely to get infections, such as cold and flu viruses.
- **Eat well-balanced meals.** A working body needs good nutrition, a subject you will learn more about in Chapter 19. You need fuel for your muscles and for your brain. Avoid fad diets because they often are responsible for the loss of muscle mass and strength.
- **Exercise regularly.** Regular physical exercise gives you more strength and energy, and keeps your heart and lungs healthy. In addition, regular exercise helps reduce the mental stress that sometimes goes along with intensely emotional jobs, such as those in the health care field.
- **Do not smoke.** Smoking causes the blood vessels in the body to narrow, reducing the flow of oxygen-carrying blood to the body's cells. It is well known that smoking is associated with lung cancer, emphysema, and heart disease. Infertility, impotence, and an increased risk of miscarriage are other negative effects of smoking. In addition to being a health risk, smoking makes your clothes and breath smell bad.
- **Do not take recreational drugs and limit your alcohol intake.** Recreational

FIGURE 3-10

There are many things you can do to keep your body in good physical condition. *(A)* Get enough sleep. *(B)* Eat well-balanced meals. *(C)* Exercise regularly. *(D)* Avoid smoking, excessive alcohol consumption, and the use of recreational drugs. *(E)* Get routine physical examinations to detect health problems early.

drugs are associated with many health problems. Many employers now perform drug screening of potential employees. Although many people feel that there is nothing wrong with occasionally having a drink if this is something you enjoy, drinking too much or too frequently can negatively impact your health and leave you unable to perform your job to the best of your ability. The health care profession needs workers who are clear-headed and able to make good decisions on behalf of others. Do not report to work while under the influence of recreational drugs or alcohol, or use these substances while on duty—doing so is dangerous for you, as well as for your patients or residents.

- **Have a routine physical examination.** Many chronic illnesses, such as high blood pressure and diabetes, go undetected until they have caused permanent damage to your body. Many types of cancers can be cured if detected early enough. Uncorrected vision and hearing problems can lead to errors when taking vital signs or reading medication labels. Routine physical examinations can help you to detect problems early, so that actions can be taken to correct them.

MAINTAINING YOUR EMOTIONAL HEALTH

Caring for others is an emotionally demanding job, as well as a physically demanding one, for many reasons:

- Due to the shortage of health care workers, as well as a need to cut costs, many facilities are understaffed, which means that employees are often overworked.
- Not all patients or residents are happy, or grateful for the care they are receiving. Many people in need of care do not feel well and, as a result, may be difficult or hard to manage. Sometimes a person who is ill or worried will become angry or very critical and he or she will take these feelings out on you, even though you have done nothing wrong.
- As a health care worker, you will have to face the death of some of your patients or residents. This can be difficult, especially in situations where you have had a chance to develop a relationship with the patient or resident and his or her family members.

Fortunately, there are actions you can take to help keep your emotions in check while you are on the job, and prevent emotional "burn-out":

- Maintain your physical health. It is proven that physical activity relieves mental and emotional stress.

FIGURE 3-11

Talking with a counselor can help you to manage work-related stress.

- Be sure to schedule time for yourself. Most of us are not just caregivers in the workplace; we are caregivers at home as well. It is important to make time for yourself, to do what you like to do, in order to avoid feeling overwhelmed by your responsibilities at home and at work.
- Take advantage of counseling services offered by your employer, or confide in a clergy member. Talking to a professional can help you to manage work-related stress and define your feelings and beliefs about difficult subjects, such as death and dying (Fig. 3-11)
- When a situation becomes particularly "heated" at work, take a physical and emotional break. Have someone relieve you (or make sure your patients are safe), and take a walk outside to calm down.
- Ask to be assigned to different work areas, or to different patients or residents, occasionally.

PERSONAL HYGIENE AND APPEARANCE

Personal **hygiene,** or cleanliness, addresses several issues. First, it promotes a professional image. If you care enough about yourself to keep yourself clean and neat, the people you care for will feel that you will do the same for them. Would you want to be cared for by someone with breath or body odors, or dirty hair? Second, good personal hygiene helps to prevent the spread of infection, both to your patients or residents and to you and your family. In a health care setting, the potential to come into contact with all types of "germs" is increased, and practicing good personal hygiene is necessary. To practice good personal hygiene:

- Bathe daily and use a deodorant.
- Shampoo your hair regularly and treat dandruff or other scalp conditions.
- Keep your nails short and clean.
- Brush and floss your teeth, and use mouthwash. Visit a dentist regularly. Poor dental health can cause breath odors and gum infections.
- Men should shave daily, or keep facial hair neatly groomed and trimmed.
- Wear a clean, pressed uniform each day.
- Wash your hands often.

Practicing good personal hygiene is essential to presenting a professional image. When you picture a health care professional, what does she look like? Is she wearing a wrinkled, stained uniform? Is her hair unkempt? Are her shoes dirty? Of course not! The health care worker you picture in your mind is clean and neat, with an unwrinkled uniform and clean shoes (Fig. 3-12). Her hair is neatly styled and held back off the face. Keeping your hair controlled and away from your face is important in order to keep it away from equipment, out of your eyes, and out of your work. Most people unconsciously reach up to move hair out of their eyes. If your hair is not secured back, when you move your hair out of your eyes, any dirt on your hands will be transferred to your hair and face.

FIGURE 3-12

In the health care field, many of the traits we have come to associate with a professional image are related to maintaining safety and health.

Accessories must be kept to a minimum. A watch with a second hand is an essential part of a nursing assistant's uniform, but bracelets, necklaces, rings, and dangling earrings not only look unprofessional, they can be dangerous. A child or confused person might pull the earrings through your earlobes. Necklaces and bracelets get in the way, and can get caught in equipment and broken. If you wear rings, germs can become trapped underneath them, which makes handwashing less effective. Rings can also scratch a person's skin when you are providing care. Long, polished nails are attractive, but in the health care setting they are not appropriate. Germs can "hide" under the tips of long nails. Long nails can also scratch a person's skin. Frequent handwashing can cause acrylic and false nails to lift, allowing water to become trapped underneath and leading to a fungal infection in the nailbed. In the health care field, many of the traits we have come to associate with a professional image are related to maintaining safety and health.

SUMMARY

▶ The health care industry relies on all types of professionals to provide quality care to patients and residents.
  - Professionals, such as doctors, nurses, and nursing assistants, have certain credentials that are obtained through education and training.
  - Being a professional also means having a professional attitude.
▶ Job-seeking skills are useful for finding an employment situation that matches your individual needs.

- Advance planning about the type of employment you want helps to give your job search direction.
- Résumés provide potential employers with information about your education and skills. Job applications are legal documents that provide pertinent information about your employment history.
- A job interview is an opportunity for the potential employer to evaluate you, and for you to evaluate the potential employer.
▶ After becoming employed, you must exhibit a strong work ethic in order to be successful and grow professionally.
  - A nursing assistant with a strong work ethic possesses qualities that make her both pleasant to work with and dependable.
  - A nursing assistant with a strong work ethic demonstrates compassion and respect for his patients or residents.
▶ In order to care for your patients or residents to the best of your ability, you must first care for yourself.
  - Taking care of the body's physical needs helps keep your body strong, healthy, and able to handle the physical demands of being a nursing assistant.
  - Taking steps to maintain your emotional health helps to prevent emotional "burn-out" and helps you to keep your emotions in check, both at work and at home.
  - Good personal hygiene helps to prevent the spread of infection and promotes a professional appearance.

What did you learn?

Multiple Choice

Select the single best answer for each of the following questions.

1. A person with much experience and great skill in a specified role is referred to as a(n):
   a. Apprentice
   b. Professional
   c. Graduate
   d. Novice

2. In many states, nursing assistants can be employed at all of the following except:
   a. Hospitals
   b. Long-term care facilities
   c. Research centers
   d. Rehabilitation centers

3. A short, precise document with information about you, your work experience, and your education is called a:
   a. Minimum Data Set (MDS)
   b. Résumé
   c. Reference
   d. Cover letter

4. All of the following information should be included on your résumé, except for your:
   a. Name
   b. Address
   c. Employment history
   d. Religion

5. An organization's human resources (HR) department is also known as:
   a. Personnel
   b. Dietary
   c. Administration
   d. Education

6. Which one of the following is a standardized form that is also a legal document used when applying for a job?
   a. Résumé
   b. Cover letter
   c. Reference list
   d. Application

7. The chance for a potential employer to meet you personally occurs during the:
   a. Application process
   b. Interview process
   c. Job posting process
   d. Reference checking process

8. A nursing assistant can promote his or her own physical health by doing all of the following except:
   a. Eating well-balanced meals
   b. Getting plenty of rest
   c. Smoking and drinking socially
   d. Attending aerobics classes

9. A nursing assistant's personal cleanliness is referred to as:
   a. Grooming
   b. Neatness
   c. Hygiene
   d. Fashion

10. Qualities that characterize a good work ethic include all of the following except:
    a. Reliability
    b. Punctuality
    c. Honesty
    d. Tardiness

11. What type of a nursing assistant accepts responsibility for his or her actions?
    a. An accountable nursing assistant
    b. A respectful nursing assistant
    c. A courteous nursing assistant
    d. A punctual nursing assistant

12. What type of a nursing assistant is able to imagine what it would feel like to be in another person's situation?
    a. A creative nursing assistant
    b. An empathetic nursing assistant
    c. An experienced nursing assistant
    d. An honest nursing assistant

13. What type of a nursing assistant can be counted on to come to work everyday?
    a. A punctual nursing assistant
    b. A nursing assistant with access to public transportation
    c. A reliable nursing assistant
    d. An ethical nursing assistant

Stop and think!

▶ Imagine that you have just completed your nursing assistant training and taken the state test. While you are waiting for your test results, you decide to begin reading job postings to see what opportunities are available. At this point, you are considering several options. You are excited about beginning your career in the health care field, and you are anxious to get into the workforce and put your new skills to use. However, you think that you might also want to continue your education, and become either a licensed practical nurse (LPN) or a registered nurse (RN) someday. What sorts of organizations may be looking for nursing assistants in your community? How could working as a nursing assistant now help you to further define your career goals?

▶ Your best friend Martha is also a nursing assistant at the long-term care facility where you work. She has a very difficult time managing her personal life and her professional life. Many times, Martha has asked you to clock her in when you get to work so that your supervisors will not see that she is late. This makes you uncomfortable, but you do not want to lose Martha's friendship. What should you do?

▶ One of your coworkers, Robert, has returned to work after completing a drug abuse rehabilitation program. For awhile, things seemed to be going smoothly, but lately, you have noticed that Robert is spending a lot of time hanging around the nurse's station and the drug cart. Furthermore, you know from something one of the nurses said that the drug counts on the cart have been incorrect on several occasions. You think Robert might be stealing drugs, especially since you have noticed that on a few occasions, his speech has been slurred and he seems somewhat "out of it." What should you do?

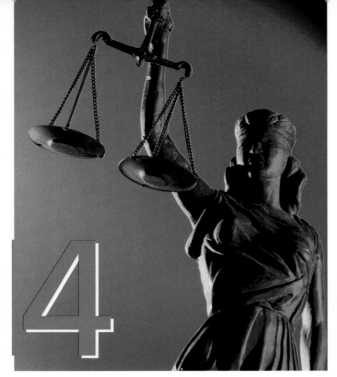

Legal and Ethical Issues

What will you learn?

As members of society, we make decisions every day about how to behave. Some of these decisions are dictated by society's laws, or rules established by the governing authority, and we act a certain way because we know that failing to obey these rules can result in punishment. Other decisions are dictated by our own personal ethical code, or moral sense of what is right and wrong. Many factors influence an individual's ethical code, including spiritual beliefs and values instilled by the person's family. Generally, when we act according to our ethical code, we act a certain way because we believe it is the right way to act, not because we risk punishment if we do not behave in that way. Obeying society's laws and upholding our own personal ethical standards allow us to function as members of society. Just as laws and ethics guide our behavior in society, laws and ethics guide our behavior in the workplace, as health care providers. (Recall the discussion in Chapter 3 about the importance of having a "work ethic.") This chapter explores some of the legal issues that can affect you, as a nursing assistant, and describes general ethical principles that should guide your behavior in the workplace. When you are finished with this chapter, you will be able to:

1. List and discuss patients' and residents' rights, as set forth by the American Hospital Association (AHA) and the Omnibus Budget Reconciliation Act (OBRA), respectively.
2. Discuss the legal aspects of health care delivery.
3. List common legal violations that are related to the provision of health care.
4. Display the awareness that health care workers must have in order to avoid legal dilemmas.
5. Define the types of abuse and describe signs that indicate abuse.
6. Discuss the health care worker's obligations in the reporting of suspected abuse.
7. Explain the difference between legal and ethical issues.
8. Describe the ethical standards that govern the nursing profession in particular, and the health care profession in general.

Photo: Lady Justice symbolizes the fair and equal administration of the law.
(© Comstock IMAGES.)

Vocabulary

Use the CD in the back of your book to hear these terms pronounced, defined, and used in a sentence:

Laws	Defamation	Health Insurance	Elder abuse
Civil laws	Slander	Portability and	Ethics
Criminal laws	Libel	Accountability Act	Beneficence
Litigation	Assault	(HIPAA)	Nonmaleficence
Liability	Battery	Larceny	Justice
Tort	Informed consent	Abuse	Fidelity
Unintentional tort	Fraud	Physical abuse	Autonomy
Negligent	False imprisonment	Psychological	Value
Malpractice	Invasion of privacy	(emotional) abuse	
Intentional tort	Confidentiality	Sexual abuse	

PATIENTS' AND RESIDENTS' RIGHTS

PATIENTS' RIGHTS

Guidelines have been established to protect patients who receive our care, and to create an atmosphere of open communication among everyone who is involved in the patient's care: the patient (and the patient's family), the health care workers who are providing the care, and the administrators of the health care organization from which the patient is receiving care. In 1973, the American Hospital Association (AHA) first adopted a series of statements called *A Patient's Bill of Rights*. Since 1973, the health care industry has changed dramatically, and *A Patient's Bill of Rights* has been revised to reflect those changes. For example, rather than being regarded as passive recipients of health care, patients are now authorized to become informed and cooperative participants when it comes to making decisions related to their health care. Also, health care workers are expected to provide care with sensitivity to a person's culture, race, language, religious beliefs, age, and gender. In brief, the twelve points describing patient rights in the *Patient's Bill of Rights* are as follows:

1. The patient has the right to considerate and respectful care.
2. The patient has the right to information about her diagnosis, treatment, and prognosis.
3. The patient has the right to make decisions about her plan of care, and to refuse a recommended treatment.
4. The patient has the right to specify her wishes regarding her health care in advance in case the time comes when she can no longer make her wishes known herself. (Methods of doing this, such as advance directives and durable powers of attorney, are discussed in detail in Chapter 21.)
5. The patient has the right to privacy.
6. The patient has the right to expect that all communication (written and oral) pertaining to her care will be treated with confidentiality.
7. The patient has the right to review the records related to her medical care, and to have the information they contain explained or interpreted as necessary.
8. The patient has the right to suggest alternatives to her planned care, or to transfer to another facility if she so desires.
9. The patient has the right to be informed of any business relationships between parties that influence the care she receives (the hospital and an insurance provider; the hospital and a university).
10. The patient has the right to participate in, or decline to participate in, experimental studies.
11. The patient has the right to be informed of her options for care when she is discharged from the hospital.

12. The patient has the right to know how the hospital settles disputes, what the hospital charges for its services, and what options for payment are available.

In addition to having rights, the patient has responsibilities. Patients are responsible for:

1. Cooperating with health care providers
2. Respecting the property, comfort, environment, and privacy of other patients
3. Making an effort to understand, and follow, instructions concerning treatment
4. Providing accurate and complete information about their health status by answering questions as truthfully and completely as possible
5. Ensuring payment for services received (including providing insurance information in a cooperative and timely manner)
6. Informing the health care staff of any medications brought from home
7. Accepting responsibility for the consequences of refused treatment or disregarded instructions

RESIDENTS' RIGHTS

Similar guidelines concerning the rights of residents of long-term care facilities are ordered by the federal government and must be followed if a facility receives any federal payments from Medicare. These guidelines are called the *Resident Rights* and are included as part of the Omnibus Budget Reconciliation Act (OBRA). In brief, the twelve major points of the *Resident Rights* portion of OBRA are as follows:

1. The resident has the right to make decisions regarding his care, including choosing his own physician, participating in planning and implementing his own care, having his individual needs and preferences accommodated, and voicing grievances about care.
2. The resident has the right to privacy, including privacy while receiving treatments and nursing care, making and receiving telephone calls, sending and receiving mail, and receiving visitors. The resident has the right to confidentiality of personal and medical records.
3. The resident has the right to be free from physical or psychological abuse, including the improper use of restraints.
4. The resident has the right to receive visitors, and to share a room with a spouse if both partners are residents in the same facility.
5. The resident has the right to use personal possessions.
6. The resident has the right to control his own finances.
7. The resident has the right to information about eligibility for Medicare or Medicaid funds, and to be protected against Medicaid discrimination.
8. The resident has the right to information about the facility's compliance with regulations, planned changes in living arrangements, and available services (and the fees for these services).
9. The resident has the right to remain in the facility unless transfer or discharge is required by a change in the resident's health, an inability of the resident to pay for the services he is receiving, or the facility is closed.
10. The resident has the right to organize and participate in groups organized by other residents, or the families of residents. For example, residents or their families may organize groups dedicated to improving life for residents, by suggesting changes that could be made at the facility or by planning group outings and activities. The resident also has the right to participate in social, religious, and community activities of his choosing.
11. The resident has the right to information about advocacy groups.
12. The resident has the right to choose to work at the facility, either as a volunteer or a paid employee. For many people, working or helping others gives them a sense of purpose. However, under no circumstances is a resident obligated to work (for example, in exchange for services).

The AHA's *Patient's Bill of Rights* and the *Resident Rights* portion of OBRA were written to guide the way patients and residents, health care providers, and the administrators of health care organizations interact with one another. In respecting the rights of patients and residents, health care workers behave according to legal standards; they also behave according to ethical standards.

LAWS: A WAY OF PRESERVING PATIENTS' AND RESIDENTS' RIGHTS

On July 4, 1776, the representatives of the 13 North American colonies declared the colonies' independence from England. The document recording that historic event, the Declaration of Independence, states that " . . . all men are created equal, that they are endowed by their Creator with certain unalienable Rights, that among these are Life, Liberty, and the pursuit of Happiness. That to secure these rights, Governments are instituted among Men, deriving their powers from the consent of the governed...." In other words, all people are entitled to certain basic human rights, and the government, which is put in place by the people, plays a role in making sure that these rights are honored.

One way the government works to preserve its citizens' basic human rights is by making and enforcing **laws.** Laws are rules that are made by a controlling authority, such as the state or federal government. By formally establishing principles to guide behavior, laws give society a way of settling disputes in a civilized, orderly way. Laws enacted by the federal and state governments serve to protect basic human rights for all people, regardless of race, religion, gender, or income.

There are two types of laws: **civil laws** and **criminal laws.** Civil laws are concerned with relationships between individuals. Criminal laws are concerned with the relationship between the individual and society as a whole. People found guilty of violating civil laws usually must pay a fine or make a financial settlement to the party that was wronged. Those who violate criminal laws are often sentenced to prison. **Litigation** is the lawsuit, or legal action, taken against a person who is accused of breaking a law. The responsibility of an individual to act within the confines of the law is called **liability.** Each individual is considered responsible, and held accountable, for her own actions in accordance with the law.

VIOLATIONS OF CIVIL LAW

When a patient or resident is admitted to a health care facility, he signs a form giving the facility permission to provide medical care. A health care worker employed by that facility likewise agrees to provide that care to the patient or resident. This arrangement is, basically, a contractual agreement. Contracts, such as the contract that exists between a nursing assistant and the person she cares for, fall under the jurisdiction of civil law. When this civil law is violated, a **tort**, or wrong, is committed. An **unintentional tort** occurs when someone causes harm or injury to another person or that person's property without the intent to cause harm. A person who commits an unintentional tort is considered **negligent** for failing to do what a "careful and reasonable" person would do (Fig. 4-1). For example, in each of the following scenarios, the nursing assistant would be considered negligent:

- A nursing assistant becomes distracted by another resident's needs and forgets to lock the wheels on the wheelchair she has just placed by the resident's bed. As the resident moves from the bed to the wheelchair, the wheelchair rolls, causing the resident to fall.
- While changing a patient's bed, a new nursing assistant forgets to check the linens for personal objects. As a result, the patient's dentures are sent to the laundry with the soiled linens, and the dentures are damaged when they go through the washing machine.
- A nursing assistant who is caring for a resident with a reputation for complaining fails to report the resident's complaints of pain to the nurse. It turns out that this time the resident's complaints were valid.

Negligence committed by people who hold licenses to practice their profession, such as doctors, nurses, lawyers, dentists, and pharmacists, is considered **malpractice.** Nursing assistants

FIGURE 4-1

The nursing assistant who was responsible for this patient has committed an unintentional tort and would be considered negligent for failing to lock the wheels on the wheelchair, an action that would have prevented the patient from falling out of bed.

(who receive certification, but not licensure) are not charged with malpractice.

A violation of civil law committed by a person with the intent to do harm is considered an **intentional tort.** Intentional torts that nursing assistants are particularly at risk for committing in the workplace include defamation, assault, battery, fraud, false imprisonment, invasion of privacy, and larceny.

Defamation

Defamation is making untrue statements that hurt another person's reputation. Statements in oral form are called **slander,** whereas statements in written form are called **libel.** It is best to avoid saying negative things or spreading rumors about a coworker, supervisor, doctor, patient, or resident (Fig. 4-2). Although it is easy to become hurt, angry, or defensive when you feel that someone has treated you unfairly, making untrue

FIGURE 4-2

Never say negative things or spread rumors about coworkers, patients, or residents. Doing so is unprofessional, and it could get you in trouble with the law!

FIGURE 4-3

Try to avoid letting your emotions get out of check. Making angry gestures toward another is considered assault.

remarks about that person is not the professional way to handle these feelings.

Assault

Assault is threatening or attempting to touch a person without his consent, causing that person to fear bodily harm (Fig. 4-3). A person can be found guilty of committing assault on the basis of an angry statement ("If you get up out of that wheelchair once more without calling for help, I'll tie you down!") or an angry gesture (shaking a fist in someone's face or acting as if you are going to slap her). Even Biblical Job would have his patience tried by some situations that face nursing assistants! In order to avoid doing something you will regret later, "take a break" (physically and emotionally) when you feel your emotions get on edge.

Battery

Battery is touching a person without her consent. For example, a health care worker could be accused of battery for physically restraining a person who is trying to leave the room, or for performing a procedure that the person or the person's family has not consented to. In order to avoid being charged with battery, health care

providers must obtain **informed consent** from patients and residents before starting a treatment or procedure. Informed consent, which is discussed in detail in Chapter 39, implies that the person has been informed of the need for a procedure or treatment, and that he has given his permission to the health care provider to perform the procedure or administer the treatment. Even if a person initially consents to a treatment or procedure, he is able to withdraw that consent and refuse the treatment or procedure at any time.

Fraud

Fraud is deception that could cause harm to another person. A health care worker who misrepresents his or her professional qualifications (for example, by telling a patient or resident that she is a nurse or a doctor, when in fact, she is not, or lying about previous training or employment on a job application) is committing fraud.

False Imprisonment

False imprisonment is confining another person against his or her will. In the health care setting, it is sometimes necessary to confine a person to a chair, a bed, or a room in order to maintain that person's safety (or the safety of others). However, the use of restraints can be considered false imprisonment if the restraints are not justified for the safety of the patient, the resident, or the staff (see Chapter 10).

Invasion of Privacy

Invasion of privacy is violating another person's right to keep certain information and aspects of himself away from the examination of others. In the health care setting, discussing a patient's or resident's physical condition, diagnosis, prognosis, or behavior in a public area (such as an elevator, hallway, or cafeteria) violates that person's right to confidentiality, and can be considered an invasion of privacy if someone overhears your discussion (Fig. 4-4). **Confidentiality** means keeping personal information that someone shares with you to yourself. Confidentiality applies not only to spoken and observed information, but also to written information. Always make sure that charts, medical records, or computer screens with patient or resident information are

FIGURE 4-4

It is fine to chat with coworkers in public areas about topics that are not related to work, but never discuss your patients or residents, or their care, in a place where you could be overheard by others.

not left where others can read them. The only time it is acceptable to discuss a patient or resident is when it is necessary to exchange information about that person's care with someone else who is directly involved in caring for that person. Failure to maintain a person's physical privacy (e.g., by leaving a door or curtain open during a procedure, or exposing a person's entire body when it is only necessary to expose a certain part) is also considered an invasion of privacy.

The **Health Insurance Portability and Accountability Act (HIPAA)** originated in 1996. HIPAA is a federal privacy regulation that helps to keep personal information about patients and residents private. HIPAA:

- Regulates who has the right to view a person's medical records, data, or other private information
- Sets standards on how a person's medical information is to be stored and transmitted from one place to another
- Requires that health care organizations set policies that allow a patient or resident to have access to his or her medical records

Larceny

Larceny is simply the act of stealing another person's property. In the health care setting, especially in the long-term care and home health care settings, but also in the hospital setting, health care workers have access to patients' or residents' personal belongings. It is never acceptable

to take something belonging to another person, even if the item is not of great monetary value or if the person does not seem to "need" it. People who are elderly or ill are particularly vulnerable to theft, and not just at the hands of health care workers—family members, neighbors, or fellow residents may also commit larceny. As a nursing assistant, it is important for you to be aware of others who may steal from one of your patients or residents, and to report any suspicions according to your facility's or agency's policy.

VIOLATIONS OF CRIMINAL LAW—ABUSE

Abuse, the repetitive and deliberate infliction of injury on another person, is a criminal act, and is punishable by a court of law. A person can commit abuse by *actively doing something to* another person, or by *failing to do something for* another person, such as provide adequate care or attention. Abuse takes many forms. The injury that results from the abuse may be physical or emotional.

Forms of Abuse

Physical abuse results in injury to the abused person's body. Striking, biting, slapping, shaking, and handling another person roughly are all actions that make up physical abuse. In a situation where one person depends on another for care, the caregiver can commit physical abuse by failing to provide for the basic physical human needs (adequate food and drink and physical cleanliness) of the person in his or her care. In the health care setting, failure to reposition a person frequently can lead to pressure ulcers and is also considered a form of physical abuse.

Psychological (emotional) abuse can be inflicted in many ways. Making another person fearful by threatening him with physical harm or abandonment is one form of psychological abuse, as is teasing a person in a cruel way. Isolating a person by preventing him from interacting with others (an act called *involuntary seclusion*) is another form of psychological abuse. Involuntary seclusion can involve keeping a person in a room alone with the door closed. In extreme cases, it may involve locking a person in a closet or attic for years.

Sexual abuse is forcing another person to engage in sexual activity. Making inappropriate, sexually aggressive comments or threats is also a form of sexual abuse.

Risk Factors for Abuse

Anyone can become the victim of abuse, but those who depend on others for their care (the very young, the disabled, and the elderly) are particularly at risk. The greater the extent of disability, the more at risk the person is for abuse or neglect.

Elder abuse is the abuse of an older person. It is estimated that there are 700,000 to 1 million cases of elder abuse in the United States each year. It is hard to tell exactly how many cases occur each year because only 1 of every 14 cases is reported to the authorities. Among elderly people who depend on others for their care, 1 in 10 is abused or neglected by family members or other care providers. Elder abuse takes many forms:

- Infliction of physical pain or injury
- Failure to provide food, water, care, and medications
- Involuntary confinement or seclusion
- Withholding of Social Security checks and other sources of income (or intentional mismanagement of funds)
- Sexual abuse

Perpetrators of Abuse

There are many reasons why a person may become abusive toward another. Sometimes, abuse is rooted in the desire of one person to overpower and dominate another. Many abusers were victims of abuse themselves. Other times, in a situation where a person requires a great deal of care, the primary caregiver may become overly tired, frustrated, and overwhelmed by the responsibility of providing care, leading to abuse and neglect. This is often the case with an adult child who finds herself in the situation of caring for an ill and demanding elderly parent, without the proper training or support system.

Even people who are trained to administer care may become overwhelmed by their responsibilities or a particular situation. A health care worker is particularly at risk for becoming abusive when the patient or resident is "difficult" or hard to manage, and the relationship is long-term, rather than short-term. As described in Chapter 3, many facilities have counseling serv-ices to help employees deal with the emotional stress that caring for others can create.

Regardless of the reason abuse occurs, abuse is never an acceptable form of behavior! Be very careful not to place yourself in the position of potentially abusing a patient or resident. Being found guilty of abuse could destroy your potential for future employment in the health care field.

Role of the Nursing Assistant in Reporting Abuse

As a nursing assistant, you may find yourself in a situation where you suspect that one of your patients or residents is being abused (Box 4-1). Laws require that any health care worker who suspects the abuse of a child or elderly person must report his or her suspicions to the proper authorities. Your facility or agency will have specific policies regarding the chain of reporting. Some organizations will require that you report to your supervisor or nurse, whereas others require reporting to a risk management representative. It is not your responsibility to investigate whether or not abuse

---

BOX 4-1 Signs of Abuse

- Poor personal hygiene, as evidenced by an unclean body, clothes, or both; an unshaven face or uncombed hair; skin irritation (from wearing urine-soaked undergarments for long periods of time); dried stool on buttocks; or a lack of oral hygiene
- Loss of weight or dehydration (see Chapter 19 for signs and symptoms of dehydration)
- Unexplained bruises or bruises in various stages of healing; explanations of injuries that are not consistent with the location of the injury
- Patches of missing hair
- Burn marks from cigarettes or abrasions from ropes or other bindings
- Unclean or unsafe living conditions, as evidenced by rotting food, unchanged sheets, or a lack of heat or water services
- An anxious, fearful or withdrawn demeanor, especially in the presence of the abuser
- Uncontrolled medical conditions (possibly the result of a lack of prescribed medication or treatment)

FIGURE 4-5

In order to stay within the legal limits of your job, know your scope of practice (as defined by the state and your job description), familiarize yourself with your employer's "policies and procedures" manual, and always seek clarification from your supervisor if there is something you do not understand.

has actually occurred, or who has caused it. The state agencies that handle abuse reports will proceed through the proper channels. Your responsibility is to simply report your suspicions.

During your career, you will be exposed to a variety of circumstances and situations. Always bear in mind the legal responsibilities and obligations that you have as a caregiver. There may be many times when you wonder whether a situation poses legal liability issues for you or your employer. Make sure that you are familiar with your employer's policies, and with your duties and obligations as listed in your job description. Do not perform duties that are not described in your job description, and always ask your supervisor any questions you may have regarding legal issues. Be aware of the limits of practice for nursing assistants in your state; these limits are set by each state's certification agency and may differ from state to state. Keeping yourself informed is critical to ensure that the care you give is within the legal limits of your job (Fig. 4-5).

ETHICS: GUIDELINES FOR BEHAVIOR

As you have learned, laws serve to preserve basic human rights. As such, laws generally deal with issues that are either "black" or "white": An ac-

tion is either within the law, or outside of it. But what about situations that are not so easily defined? The dramatic changes in health care that have been brought about by advances in technology and research have greatly impacted legal and ethical issues surrounding the medical profession, and have created some unique moral dilemmas. Consider the following questions:

- What should be done with human embryos that have been frozen for future use, if the parents decide they do not want to have any more children?
- How does one decide who receives a donor organ, when there are so many people in need but few organs available?
- When does human life begin?
- Should doctors be allowed to end a person's life, at that person's request?

Clearly, these are difficult questions to answer because the answers to these questions depend on the individual's values and beliefs. When definitive answers to questions are not available, we rely on ethical standards to decide what to do. **Ethics** are moral principles or standards that govern conduct. The word "ethics" is derived from the Greek word *ethos*, which means "beliefs that guide life." Ethical standards, which are less prescriptive than laws, help us to determine the difference between right and wrong in areas where the law fears to tread.

PROFESSIONAL ETHICS

Each profession has a code of ethics, or guidelines pertaining to standards of conduct and practice, for that profession. The code of ethics for nursing assistants falls within the American Nurses Association (ANA) code of ethics for nursing (Box 4-2). In addition, there are some general ethical principles that guide all health care workers:

- **Beneficence.** Do good for those in your care by preventing harm and promoting the health and welfare of the person above all else.
- **Nonmaleficence.** Avoid harming those in your care. Use kindness and gentleness when administering care.
- **Justice.** Treat people fairly and equally, regardless of race, religion, culture, disability, or ability to pay.
- **Fidelity.** Act with integrity to earn others' trust.

Box 4-2 Code of Ethics for Nursing Assistants

- Treat patients and residents with respect for their individual needs and values.
- Respect the patient's or resident's right to choice in regard to the individual's right to control his or her own care.
- Hold confidential all information about patients and residents learned in the health care setting.
- Be guided by consideration for the dignity of patients and residents.
- Fulfill the obligation to provide competent care to patients and residents.

- **Autonomy.** Respect a person's rights and personal preferences.
- **Confidentiality.** Maintain a person's privacy by allowing the person to discuss sensitive issues with the knowledge that the information will be kept secret.

PERSONAL ETHICS

Many factors influence a person's ethics, which are derived from a person's values. A **value** is simply a cherished belief or principle. Factors that influence a person's values include his or her religious or spiritual beliefs, level and type of education, culture and heritage, and life experiences. Each person's value system is unique, and as a nursing assistant, you need to think about how you feel about certain moral and ethical issues. Only then will you be able to understand that although another person's values may differ from yours, that person's values are as important to her as yours are to you. Respect for the individual is one of the principles that forms the basis of the code of ethics for nursing (Fig. 4-6).

Ethical dilemmas arise when we attempt to judge other people by our own ethical standards. Satisfactory resolutions to ethical dilemmas in the health care field can be solved only by allowing the patient or resident to become an informed, active participant in his or her care, and by following ethical standards when administering care.

FIGURE 4-6

Values, which are derived from religious and spiritual beliefs, culture and heritage, and a person's family, are the basis of ethics. Not everyone has the same values. It is important to recognize and respect your patients' or residents' values, even if they are not the same as yours.

SUMMARY

▶ A professional acts in a way that is legally and ethically appropriate.
▶ The American Hospital Association's *Patient's Bill of Rights* and the *Resident Rights* portion of the Omnibus Budget Reconciliation Act protect the people who receive our care and create an atmosphere of open communication among everyone involved in that care.
▶ Laws are rules that are made by a controlling authority, such as the state or federal government, that serve to protect basic human rights.
   ■ Civil laws are concerned with relationships between individuals. Criminal laws are concerned with the relationship between an individual and society as a whole.

- An unintentional tort occurs when someone causes harm or injury to another person or that person's property without the intent to cause harm. A person who commits an unintentional tort is considered negligent for failing to do what a careful and reasonable person would do.
- A violation of civil law committed by a person with the intent to do harm is called an intentional tort. Examples of intentional torts that may be committed by nursing assistants in the workplace are defamation, assault, battery, fraud, false imprisonment, invasion of privacy, and larceny.

▶ Abuse, the repetitive and deliberate infliction of injury on another person, is a criminal act and is punishable by a court of law.

- Abuse can be committed by either actively doing something to another person, or by failing to do something for another person.
- Abuse can be physical or emotional.
- People who depend on others for their care, such as the very young, the disabled, and the elderly, are particularly at risk for abuse.
- Laws require that any health care worker who suspects the abuse of a child or elderly person must report his or her suspicions to the proper authorities.

▶ Ethics are moral principles or standards that govern conduct. Ethical dilemmas in the health care field can be solved only by allowing the patient or resident to become an informed, active participant in his or her care, and by following ethical standards when providing care.

What did you learn?

Multiple Choice

Select the single best answer for each of the following questions.

1. All of the following are legal terms that relate to making false statements that injure another person's reputation except:
   a. Defamation
   b. Gossip
   c. Slander
   d. Libel

2. If a registered nurse (RN) fails to raise the side rails on the bed of a confused patient, and the patient falls out of bed and is injured, the nurse may be charged with:
   a. Malpractice
   b. Negligence
   c. An intentional tort
   d. Assault

3. *Resident Rights* are a part of which legislation?
   a. American Medical Association (AMA)
   b. Omnibus Budget Reconciliation Act (OBRA)
   c. Federal Emergency Management Agency (FEMA)
   d. Social Security Act

4. Which ethical principle relates to the concepts of informed consent and a person's right to refuse treatment?
   a. Beneficence
   b. Autonomy
   c. Fidelity
   d. Justice

5. Confidentiality means:
   a. Only sharing information with those directly involved in a patient's or resident's care
   b. Respecting a patient's or resident's right to privacy
   c. Never sharing information with anyone
   d. Both "a" and "b"

6. All residents have basic rights. Which of the following is a basic right of residents?
   a. Right to choice
   b. Right to privacy and confidentiality
   c. Right to be free from verbal abuse, or any other abuse
   d. All of the above

7. You are a nursing assistant working in a home health care setting. You suspect that one of your clients is being emotionally and physically abused by her husband. What should you do first?
   a. Call the police
   b. Keep your suspicions to yourself but continue to observe the situation
   c. Immediately report your suspicions to the case manager
   d. Tell another nursing assistant at the agency

8. One of your fellow nursing assistants has been having a very hard time with one of her residents. The resident is confused and, as a result, is being uncooperative. In a moment of complete frustration, your coworker says to the resident, "If you don't shut up and behave yourself right now, I'm going to slap you!" What kind of an intentional tort has this nursing assistant committed?
   a. Assault
   b. Battery
   c. Negligence
   d. Malpractice

9. A nursing assistant answers the telephone at the nursing station. The doctor who is calling wants to give a verbal order, and the nursing assistant tells the doctor that she is a nurse and can take the order. What intentional tort has the nursing assistant committed?
   a. Slander
   b. Fraud
   c. Libel
   d. Informed consent

10. What does the Health Insurance Portability and Accountability Act (HIPAA) protect?
    a. The patient's or resident's right to privacy
    b. The patient's or resident's right to sue negligent health care workers
    c. The patient's or resident's right to be free from abuse
    d. The patient's or resident's right to choose who will provide his or her care

Matching

Match each numbered item with its appropriate lettered description.

_____ **1.** Civil laws

_____ **2.** Liability

_____ **3.** Fraud

_____ **4.** Ethics

_____ **5.** Beneficence

a. The responsibility of an individual to act within the confines of the law

b. A system of moral principles or standards used to govern conduct

c. Protecting a patient or resident from harm

d. Deception that could cause harm to another person

e. Laws that deal with relationships between individuals

? *Stop and think!*

► A licensed practical nurse (LPN) who works with you in a long-term care facility stops in Mrs. Taylor's room to give Mrs. Taylor her daily medications. Mrs. Taylor is in the bathroom and you are changing the linens on her bed. The nurse hands you the medication cup, which contains three pills, and asks you to have Mrs. Taylor take the pills as soon as she comes out of the bathroom. You are aware that in your state, nursing assistants who work in long-term care facilities are not allowed to give medications. When you mention your concern about giving Mrs. Taylor her medication to the nurse, she says, "It's okay; the other nursing assistants do this for me all of the time." What should you do?

Communication Skills

What will you learn?

Being able to effectively communicate, or participate in the exchange of information, is a critical skill for all people in the health care field to possess. Every day, you will need to communicate with your patients or residents, and with other members of the health care team. If just one link in the chain of communication is broken, the quality of care given to the patient or resident can be seriously jeopardized. In this chapter, we will describe techniques for, as well as obstacles to, effective communication. In addition, we will review some of the tools that are commonly used by members of the health care team to ensure that information is readily available to all who are involved with the care of a patient or resident. When you are finished with this chapter, you will be able to:

1. Define communication.
2. Describe the two major forms of communication, and give examples of each.
3. Discuss techniques that promote effective communication.
4. Describe blocks to effective communication and discuss methods used to avoid them.
5. Identify causes of conflict, and discuss ways of resolving conflicts.
6. Demonstrate proper telephone communication skills.
7. Discuss the methods of reporting and recording information in a health care setting.
8. Explain how the patient's or resident's medical record makes communication easier among members of the health care team.
9. Describe communication technologies that are being used in the health care field today.
10. Explain why the nursing assistant is a vital link in the communication chain, and describe how the nursing assistant communicates information to other members of the health care team.
11. List the steps of the nursing process, and describe how the nursing team uses the nursing process to plan the patient's or resident's care.
12. Understand the role of effective communication in the provision of quality health care.

Photo: A nursing assistant checks a resident's medical record. The medical record is one way members of the health care team share information with each other.

Vocabulary

Use the CD in the back of your book to hear these terms pronounced, defined, and used in a sentence:

Communication	Observation	Reporting	Nursing process
Verbal communication	Objective data	Recording	Nursing diagnosis
Nonverbal communication	Signs	Medical record	Interventions
	Subjective data	Kardex	Goals
Conflict	Symptoms	Nursing care plan	

WHAT IS COMMUNICATION?

Communication is simply defined as an exchange of information. The key to understanding what communication truly is lies within the word "exchange." If you exchange gifts with another person, you give that person a gift, and in return, you receive one back. In the exchange of information that defines communication, there is a constant back-and-forth flow of information. Communicating is not just about telling someone something (giving information). It is also about listening and observing (receiving information).

In order for effective communication to occur, all of the people who are involved must actively participate in the exchange of information. Communication involves at least two people, a *sender* and a *receiver*. The sender is the person with information to share, and the receiver is the person for whom the information is intended. The sender

delivers the information in the form of a *message,* which the receiver may or may not understand. Through *feedback,* or a return message, the receiver lets the sender know whether the message was received and understood (Fig. 5-1). Note that as information is transmitted back and forth, the sender and the receiver switch roles.

There are two major forms of communication, verbal and nonverbal. **Verbal communication** involves the use of language, either spoken or written. Sign language, a system of hand gestures used to make letters of the alphabet and words, is also considered a form of verbal communication. Verbal communication tends to be deliberate—when we use language to express a thought, it is usually with the intent of giving specific information to another person. **Nonverbal communication,** on the other hand, tends to be more subtle. In nonverbal communication, a person gives information through the use of facial expressions, gestures, and body language. For example,

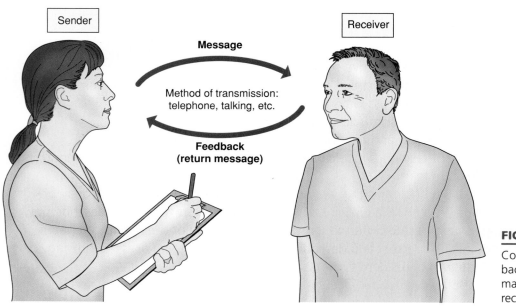

Sender

Message

Method of transmission: telephone, talking, etc.

Feedback (return message)

Receiver

FIGURE 5-1

Communication involves the back-and-forth flow of information between a sender and a receiver.

consider a resident with disabling arthritis. Not wanting to seem a "burden" to the health care staff, the resident may tell you that she feels fine when you ask. However, you note that she makes a face when she tries to get out of her chair, an observation that would indicate that she is not being entirely truthful with you about how she is feeling. Of the two forms of communication, nonverbal communication is perhaps the most reliable method of "reading" another person, especially in the health care field. For various reasons, such as embarrassment, shyness, or a fear of being perceived as foolish, people may not say what they really mean. Being observant and aware of others' nonverbal cues will give you a greater understanding of what your patients or residents are feeling and thinking.

COMMUNICATING EFFECTIVELY

As a nursing assistant, you must be a successful communicator, both as a sender and a receiver of information, with both those you care for and your coworkers. For example, you will use communication skills to comfort, reassure, and teach your patients or residents. Because nursing assistants typically spend more time with patients and residents, and get to know them better, than any other member of the health care team, you will become one of the strongest links between the patient or resident and the other health care team members. As you form relationships with your patients or residents, they will talk to you, confide in you, listen to you, and trust you. In addition, by carefully watching your patients or residents for nonverbal communication cues, you may be the first member of the health care team to notice that Mr. Jones' color is not quite right, or that Mrs. Smith is having abdominal pain after eating, even though she is not complaining verbally.

In addition to communicating well with patients or residents, communicating well with your coworkers is also essential. Supervisors will delegate tasks to you, and you must be sure that you understand what they are asking you to do and how you are to go about doing it. Additionally, you will be the "eyes and ears" of the nurses, physical therapists, dietitians, social workers, and other members of the health care team.

Relaying vital information about your patient's or resident's condition to the nurse is an essential part of your duties. As a nursing assistant, you are not trained to diagnose and treat medical problems. However, your knowledge of your patient or resident will allow you to gather important information that, when communicated to the nurse, will alert the health care team members to changes in that person's condition and influence the care he or she receives. Your responsibility as a communication link between the patient or resident and the rest of the health care team is very important (Fig. 5-2)!

Clearly, it is important for a nursing assistant to learn good communication skills. There are many ways that communication can fail. Remember that good communication is a "two-way street" and involves the *exchange* of information. In order to see where problems in communication can occur, let's look at each part of the process of exchanging information:

1. **The sender creates a message.** Information needs to be organized and relevant to the person who will be receiving it. Your message, whether it is spoken or written, should convey the relevant facts, organized in an easily accessible manner. Use language that the receiver understands— this could mean getting help from an interpreter, if the receiver does not speak the same language you do, or using

FIGURE 5-2

As a nursing assistant, you are an important link between the patient or resident and the other members of the health care team.

simple, common words in place of more complex, medical words. Speak clearly and loudly enough for the receiver to hear you without straining. Written messages should be legible and organized so that the information is complete and concise.

2. **The sender delivers the message.** Information can be transmitted from one person to another in many different ways. Speaking directly to another person, or "face-to-face," permits nonverbal communication to take place. Other methods of transmission, such as letters, memos, e-mails, telephone calls, and intercom conversations are primarily methods of verbal communication. Nonverbal communication is impossible with these methods of transmission because the sender and the receiver are physically separated. When relying on a written form of transmission, be sure your handwriting is neat and your spelling is accurate. With oral methods of transmission, such as telephone calls and intercom conversations, it is important to ensure that background noise or static does not interfere with the receiver's ability to hear your message.

3. **The receiver receives the message.** In order for successful communication to occur, the receiver must be physically able to receive the message and mentally engaged in the communication exchange. For example, a person with a hearing loss could not physically receive a spoken message. A person who cannot read would not be able to understand a message sent in written form. A person who has had a stroke may be able to hear your words perfectly, but may not be able to understand their meaning. Sign language or communicating through nonverbal means (e.g., nodding your head "yes" to a person's question) would not be effective if the person is blind. These are all examples of physical problems that can interfere with a person's ability to receive a message. Communication can also fail when a receiver is mentally distracted, or not really paying attention to the sender.

4. **The receiver provides feedback.** Have you ever spoken to someone and had him ignore you? Did you wonder whether or not the person even heard you? You did not receive feedback from that person. Feedback, like the other parts of communication, can be verbal (spoken or written) or nonverbal. During an exchange of information, it is important for the receiver to provide feedback to the sender, and it is important for the sender to listen and watch for this feedback. If the receiver does not provide feedback, the sender should make an effort to get a response of some sort. When feedback does not occur, or indicates that the message the sender sent was not interpreted correctly, other methods of enhancing communication may be necessary.

TACTICS THAT ENHANCE COMMUNICATION

Good communication skills will serve you well, both in your professional life and your personal life. There are many ways you can enhance communication with others.

When You Are the Receiver, Be a Good Listener

Listening is perhaps the most useful communication skill, especially in the health care setting. Active listening requires focusing your attention on the speaker. Sit down or assume a relaxed posture so you do not appear rushed or in a hurry to move on, and make eye contact with the person (Fig. 5-3).

FIGURE 5-3

Being a good listener is essential to being a good communicator.

Do not interrupt or try to finish the person's sentence for her. Interrupting a person may make her forget what she was trying to tell you in the first place. Let the person finish what she was saying before you ask another question or make a comment, and focus on the person and the information she is trying to give you—try not to think about what *you* intend to do or say next. After the person has finished speaking, you should ask questions to help clarify any information that you do not understand. Your comments and questions will let the speaker know whether you understood her message, or whether she needs to provide additional information.

When You Are the Sender, Make Sure Your Message Is Clear

Speak clearly and use words that the person you are speaking to understands. A nurse or a fellow nursing assistant will understand medical terminology, and using medical terminology is appropriate when you are communicating with one of your coworkers. However, a patient, resident, or family member may not be familiar with medical terminology. To make sure the patient or family member understands your message, try to use common words instead of technical words whenever it is appropriate to do so. For example, you could say, "Miss Lewis, we're going to go for a walk down the hall now, to get you up and moving" instead of "Miss Lewis, I'm going to ambulate you now."

Sometimes, it is necessary to communicate with someone who does not speak the same language as you do, or who has a physical problem that makes certain forms of communication less effective than others. In order to meet the regulation that requires patients and residents to give informed consent for treatments and procedures, health care facilities must provide interpreters for patients or residents who speak languages other than English. By definition, a person cannot give informed consent unless he understands what he is consenting to! A hearing-impaired person may need a sign language interpreter to assist with communication, or you could try writing out important questions for the person to read and respond to. A picture board, a tool that allows a person to point to a picture of what he or she is trying to say, is often useful when trying to communicate on a basic level with someone who speaks a different language or is hearing impaired (Fig. 5-4). More information about communicating with patients and residents with special needs can be found in Chapters 28 and 29.

Learn Techniques for Encouraging People to Talk

When you need to get information from someone, try asking the person an open-ended question. Questions that can be answered with a simple "yes" or "no" usually get just that response, and the conversation grinds to a halt. In contrast, open-ended questions encourage the person to talk. Another question that can cause a conversation to end is "Why?" If a patient complains that he does not like his dinner or choice of

FIGURE 5-4

A picture board can be used to communicate when illustrations are more effective than words.

snack, instead of asking "Why?" (which can be intimidating), you could ask the person to tell you what his favorite food or snack is. For example, consider the following two conversations:

Conversation 1

Nursing assistant: "Good morning, Mr. Hopkins. Did you have breakfast this morning?"

Mr. Hopkins: "No."

Nursing assistant: "Why not?"

Mr. Hopkins: "I don't know...I just wasn't hungry, I guess."

Conversation 2

Nursing assistant: "Good morning, Mr. Hopkins. What did you have for breakfast this morning?"

Mr. Hopkins: "Not much. They sent up scrambled eggs. I've never liked scrambled eggs—not since I was a child—so I just had some buttered toast and coffee."

Nursing assistant: "I didn't know you didn't like scrambled eggs! Let me see what I can do about that. Do you dislike eggs in general, or just scrambled eggs? In the meantime, are you hungry?"

In the second conversation, the nursing assistant achieved two key goals: She engaged Mr. Hopkins in the conversation, and in the process, she made him feel as though she really cared about him as an individual.

Rephrasing what someone says to you is another way to encourage someone to talk. For example, if one of your residents tells you that she feels sad and lonely, instead of asking "Why?" try repeating the person's statement back to her as a question: "You are feeling sad and lonely?" By rephrasing and asking an open-ended question, you will invite the person to say more. In addition, encouraging the person to talk more about what she is feeling shows the person that you are, in fact, actively listening to what she is saying to you.

Provide and Seek Feedback

Providing and seeking feedback is a critical communication skill that will come into play with both your coworkers and your patients or residents. Consider two conversations, one between you and the nurse, and the other between you

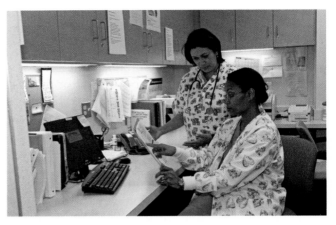

FIGURE 5-5

By indicating to the nurse that she understands what she is being asked to do, this nursing assistant is providing good feedback.

and one of your patients or residents. In the first, you are the "receiver"—the nurse is asking you to do a task. After the nurse has finished speaking, you could say, "Let me make sure I understand this correctly," and repeat the information back to her. What awesome feedback! The nurse now knows that you were listening, and that you understand what is being asked of you (Fig. 5-5). The *exchange* of information has occurred. You are communicating effectively.

In the second conversation, you are the "sender" and one of your residents is the "receiver"—you are trying to give instructions to the resident about how to use the call light control system in the room, and you want to make sure that he understands how the system works. You might say, "Now repeat that information back to me so I can make sure you've got it," but asking for feedback in this way could be intimidating to the resident. A more gracious way of finding out whether the resident understood your message would be to say, "Now, if you could just repeat these instructions back to me so I can make sure I didn't leave anything out...." This approach makes the resident feel that he is helping you by repeating the information, and in the process, you are able to tell whether or not he understands your instructions clearly.

Be Mindful of Your Body Language

Use appropriate body language when listening or talking to other people. Negative body language, such as crossing your arms across your chest, tapping your feet or fingers, rolling your eyes, or

FIGURE 5-6

If you were a patient or resident, what message would this nursing assistant be sending to you?

FIGURE 5-7

Putting yourself at eye level with a patient or resident indicates to the person that you are interested in what he or she has to say, and that you have time to listen.

constantly looking at your watch or toward the door sends the very clear message that you are bored or uninterested (Fig. 5-6). In contrast, displaying positive body language, such as facing the person, nodding as he speaks, smiling or looking serious as appropriate, and making occasional vocal sounds, such as "uh huh" or "hmm," indicates to the person that you are interested in what he is saying. Positioning your body so that you are at eye level with the speaker also shows interest (Fig. 5-7). Children are especially responsive to the adult who comes "down to their level" to listen to what they have to say.

Remember the Value of Silence and a Comforting Touch

There will be many times throughout your career as a nursing assistant when words will not be enough to communicate your care and concern to a patient or resident, or to a family member of one or your patients or residents. Silence and a comforting touch will say more than words can (Fig. 5-8). Touch is perhaps the most universal of all languages, but remember to be sensitive to the individual's comfort level. Many patients and residents appreciate affection and will enjoy a hug or sitting and holding your hands as you talk. Other people may not be as comfortable with affection, and will be satisfied with a light pat on the shoulder or top of the hand as you greet them or say good-bye.

In addition to allowing us to communicate when words are not enough, touch is comforting and establishes a bond. So much has been

FIGURE 5-8

Of the many techniques for enhancing communication, nothing says "I care about you and I want to help you" more effectively than a simple touch on a person's hand or shoulder.

written about the "healing powers of touch"—for example, consider the role of therapeutic massage in the treatment of physical ailments. Research has also shown that babies, even when given adequate food and physical care, fail to grow and thrive without human touch and attention.

BLOCKS TO EFFECTIVE COMMUNICATION

Some behaviors and attitudes can block effective communication. Perhaps the most common obstacle to effective communication is not listening carefully to what another person is saying. You must be especially careful not to "tune out" your patients or residents, despite the fact that you will be busy, and many of the people you will care for could be easily labeled "complainers." Imagine the consequences if you ignore a patient's or resident's complaint, and it turns out to be valid.

Being judgmental of others will also block communication. If a person feels that you do not believe or respect what he is trying to tell you, he will most likely stop talking and will probably refuse to answer any questions you may pose later. A judgmental attitude, indicating that you do not really care to hear what the person is trying to tell you, can be revealed through negative body language or comments you may make.

Communication blocks can occur when you assume that someone else knows what you are thinking. Your patient should know that she should not adjust the flow rate on her intravenous (IV) line, shouldn't she? Your coworkers should know without bothering you that Mrs. Jones has already been up to the bathroom, shouldn't they? Your husband should know why you are mad at him, shouldn't he? The assumption that other people know what you know, think the way you think, and feel the way you feel presents a major block to effective communication and can lead to conflict and confusion. To avoid this communication pitfall, be proactive in your interactions with others, and keep them informed. For example, give instructions and gentle reminders to patients or residents, tell your coworkers what has already been accomplished and what still needs to be done before you go on break, and ask your husband to take out the trash instead of getting angry because he did not think of it himself!

CONFLICT RESOLUTION

Conflict, or discord resulting from differences between people, can occur when one person is unable to understand or accept another's ideas or beliefs. Conflict can also arise when one person's expectations for another differ from that person's expectations for himself. Other times, conflict arises because one person misunderstands another person's words or intentions. How many times have you been angry with a friend because you thought she said or meant one thing, only to find out after talking with her that what you thought she said or meant is not what she said or meant at all? Conflict can occur when another person's needs or wants conflict with our own needs and wants.

Some degree of conflict in our lives is inevitable, by virtue of the fact that we are each individuals with unique personalities, feelings, and beliefs. Conflict is a fairly common occurrence in the health care field, because health care is a people-oriented business. It is also a very emotional business. Patients and residents are sick, hurting, confused, and frightened. Family members feel helpless and sad. Nursing assistants and other health care workers are often stressed by the emotional and physical demands of their work. As a result, conflicts may arise between a member of the health care team and a patient or resident, between two patients or residents, or between two members of the health care team (Fig. 5-9). Getting along with other people, while a very important part of your job, can sometimes be the hardest part of your job.

FIGURE 5-9

Conflict can occur between a member of the health care team and a patient, resident, or visitor for a number of reasons. Poor communication is one of the most common!

Conflict makes the people directly involved, as well as those around them, uncomfortable. This discomfort can affect a patient's or resident's ability to recover or a staff member's quality of work. Good communication is essential to preventing conflict, as well as helping to resolve it. If you find yourself involved in a conflict, remember what it means to be a professional, and take the time to talk calmly with the person you are upset with. It is important to address areas of conflict early, before they have time to get worse and involve more people. Approaches for resolving conflict include the following.

- Ask to speak privately with the person you have a conflict with. Because the two of you may be able to resolve your disagreement on your own, try this approach before asking a supervisor to mediate, if at all possible. Remain polite and professional and thank the person for her time.
- During your conversation, focus on the specific area of conflict. Do not focus on how you feel about the other person, or how you think she should have acted under the circumstances.
- Be specific about what you understand the problem to be, and express why you are upset in terms of "I," rather than the more accusatory "you." For example, instead of saying, "You really hurt my feelings by what you said the other day," say, "I am bothered by what you said the other day." In this manner, you take responsibility for the emotion and allow the other person to explain her side of the story.
- Be prepared to hear how the other person may feel toward you or the problem, even if it is not pleasant. Perhaps you were the one who was initially misunderstood.
- Be gracious enough to apologize for misunderstanding the other person, or for being the one who was misunderstood.
- Ask the other person for insight into solutions for resolving the conflict. Her suggestions may surprise you!
- Sometimes it is necessary to "agree to disagree." People with differing opinions and beliefs can focus on the things they have in common, such as caring about the patient's or resident's well-being, and still disagree on certain issues (Fig. 5-10).

FIGURE 5-10
Sometimes, the best solution to a conflict is to simply "agree to disagree." Instead of focusing on your differences, focus on your similarities. In the professional setting, for example, even if you and a resident's family member cannot agree about what is "best" for the resident, you can certainly respect the fact that both of you care deeply about the resident and want to do what is best for him.

Learning to respect others' beliefs is an important part of being professional.
- If you are unable to resolve a conflict with a coworker, a patient or resident, or a patient's or resident's family member on your own, seek the advice of your supervisor. A conflict that affects the quality of the care you provide must not be allowed to continue!

TELEPHONE COMMUNICATION

The telephone was first presented to the American public at the Centennial Exposition, held in Philadelphia in 1876, and we have never looked back. Although initially available only to certain professionals (such as doctors) and wealthy families, the technology soon became available to everyone, and we have used the telephone as a primary means of communication ever since. In fact, use of the telephone to communicate with others is probably increasing now that cellular phones are common.

Today, the telephone remains a primary tool of communication in the health care field. Other departments will call to verify an order or request, doctors will call to ask about a patient or resident or to give orders, and family members will call to get an update on the condition of a loved one. The

FIGURE 5-11

Developing a good phone manner is important, because you will find yourself using the telephone to communicate frequently!

telephone at the nursing station is in use constantly...it is almost as if a teenager lives there! As a nursing assistant, you will usually be required to answer the telephone, either at the nursing station or in a patient's or resident's room (Fig. 5-11). Much has been written about telephone etiquette and methods of communicating on the telephone (Box 5-1).

When you answer the telephone, make sure your voice is pleasant and unhurried. Believe it or not, a caller can "hear a smile" in your voice. This can be very comforting to an anxious family member who is calling to check on a sick loved one. You must remember to be as professional on the telephone as you are in person. There will be times when a caller may be impatient or angry; resist the urge to respond in a similar manner. You do not know the cause of the caller's impatience or anger, and you certainly do not want to add to it. The way you handle yourself on the telephone reflects directly on your facility. If callers perceive you as kind and professional when they speak to you on the phone, they will feel that the people you are caring for are receiving the same kind, professional care.

Confidentiality is of concern when the telephone is used as a means of communication. When you are discussing a person's care over the telephone, be sure that other patients, residents, or visitors cannot overhear your conversation. Know your facility's policy regarding what information can be provided over the telephone. For example, some facilities, such as those that provide mental health care or substance abuse rehabilitation, protect their patients' and residents' right to privacy through policies that prohibit staff from confirming or denying that a person is even

BOX 5-1 Telephone Etiquette

- Answer the telephone promptly, within the first three rings.
- Answer with a pleasant greeting, such as "Good morning" or "Good afternoon."
- Identify yourself by name and title and by your unit or floor according to facility policy: "3 West; Mary Smith, CNA, speaking."
- Because the caller obviously needs something (otherwise, he would not be calling), ask "How may I help you?"
- Know how to perform basic functions using your facility's telephone system, such as how to transfer a call or place a caller on hold.
- If you must place a caller on hold, ask her permission first ("May I put you on hold for a minute?"). Be aware of the length of time a caller has been on hold; if the time becomes excessive (more than 5 minutes), ask the caller if she wants to continue to hold, leave a message, or call back later.
- If the person the caller wants to speak to is unavailable, offer to take a message. When

  taking a telephone message, be sure to write down the date and time of the call, the name of the caller, a telephone number where the caller can be reached, and your name. Write clearly, and ask the caller to spell his or her name if you are not sure how to spell it. Be sure to deliver the message to the person for whom it was intended.
- A nursing assistant is not to take doctor's orders, receive or give results of diagnostic tests, or release patient or resident information to anyone, even family members. Calls of this nature should be handled by a nurse.
- Do not use the telephone at the nurse's station to make or receive personal calls. Personal calls should be made from a pay phone or your own cellular phone, while you are on break or at lunch. Never tie up a telephone used for health care communication by using it for personal business.

receiving treatment at the facility. To give out such information could result in litigation against the facility, and ultimately cost you your job. The Health Insurance Portability and Accountability Act (HIPAA), discussed in Chapter 4, specifically regulates who may be given information about a person in a health care facility.

COMMUNICATION AMONG MEMBERS OF THE HEALTH CARE TEAM

So far, you have learned about the skills that allow people to communicate effectively, and some of the common obstacles to effective communication. You have also been introduced to one of the primary tools health care team members use to communicate with each other and the outside world, the telephone. Next, we will explore recording and reporting, two methods of communication used by health care team members to make sure that everyone who is responsible for the care of a patient or resident has the same information about that person's status and care.

As you have already learned, the nursing assistant plays a very important role in gathering and sharing information about patients and residents with other members of the health care team. As you interact with your patients or residents, you will have the opportunity to make **observations.** An observation is something that you notice about the patient or resident, typically related to a change in the person's physical or mental condition. The amount of time you will spend with your patients or residents, combined with the type of duties you are responsible for performing daily (e.g., bathing, feeding, ambulating, toileting), will give you a chance to observe things that other health care team members may overlook.

Two types of data can lead to observations, objective data and subjective data. **Objective data** are information that you obtain directly, through measurements or by using one of your five senses. In the professional setting, the senses you will use most often are sight, hearing, touch, and smell. For example, certain indicators of a person's health, called vital signs, can be objectively measured. (The vital signs are temperature, pulse, respiratory rate, and blood pressure.) You

FIGURE 5-12

When you make an objective observation, you obtain information using one of your five senses. Here, the nursing assistant is feeling the resident's forehead to assess whether or not the skin is hot and dry or cool and clammy.

can see the color of a person's skin, and feel that it is cool and clammy (Fig. 5-12). You can see the color of a person's urine, smell any foul odor, and measure the amount that was voided. You can hear wheezing or gurgling as a person breathes. You can see bruises, swelling, or rashes on the skin when you help a person bathe. You can see how much breakfast the person ate and measure how much juice she drank. These are all objective observations. Objective observations, such as an elevated temperature, a rash, or a low urine output, are called **signs. Subjective data,** on the other hand, are information that cannot be objectively measured or assessed. The basis for a subjective observation is usually a person's complaint, or **symptom.** For example, a patient or resident may tell you that he has a headache or stomachache. You cannot see, feel, measure, or hear his pain, but he can describe it to you (Fig. 5-13).

When you are communicating subjective observations to the other health care team members, it is useful to quote the patient directly, whether you are relaying the complaint verbally (reporting) or writing the information in the patient's medical record (recording). It is also useful to support subjective observations with objective ones. For instance, Mrs. White tells you that she feels dizzy when she stands up (a subjective observation). To gather more information, you ask Mrs. White if she has gotten dizzy before, and

FIGURE 5-13

A subjective observation is information that is derived "second-hand." This nursing assistant knows that her resident is experiencing stomach pain because the resident is describing it to her, not because she detected the resident's pain using one of her five senses.

whether or not her dizziness is accompanied by a headache or nausea. Her answers to these questions would also be subjective observations. Next, you observe Mrs. White's skin for paleness or redness; touch her skin to see if it is warm, or cool and clammy; measure her blood pressure; and take her pulse. All of these objective observations give you still more information. By gathering objective facts to add to Mrs. White's subjective statements, and then organizing this information in a logical way and relaying it to the nurse, you are truly communicating! Not only have you told the nurse about Mrs. White's symptoms, you have given her objective data that may help her determine what is causing those symptoms.

Once you have made an observation, you must decide on the most effective method of communicating that observation to the nurse. Nursing assistants use two methods of communicating observations about their patients or residents and documenting the care provided so that other health care team members are kept "in-the-know." These methods are reporting and recording. Some observations need to be reported to the nurse immediately, such as a patient's or resident's complaint of pain or a change in her vital signs. Other observations only need to be recorded in the person's medical record. Throughout this text, observations that need to be reported to the nurse immediately are highlighted as "Tell the Nurse!" notes.

REPORTING

Reporting is the spoken exchange of information between health care team members. Reporting is used throughout the shift to communicate changes about a patient's or resident's status to other health care team members (Fig. 5-14). Nursing assistants use reporting to communicate the following information to the nurse:

- Observations that suggest a change in the patient's or resident's condition
- Observations regarding the patient's or resident's response to a new treatment or therapy
- A patient's or resident's complaints of pain or discomfort
- A patient's or resident's refusal of treatment
- A patient's or resident's request for clergy

When reporting information, follow the guidelines that help promote effective communication. Make sure the information that you are reporting is accurate—refer to the patient or resident by name and room number, and if you are reporting measurements, such as vital signs, write the numbers down so that you do not forget them or report them incorrectly. Report your observations in an orderly, concise manner. Avoid adding information that is not relevant to what you are trying to communicate. Use correct terminology when reporting, and make sure the person you are reporting to gives you feedback so that you know he received the information and will act on it.

Reporting is also routinely used when shifts change to keep the staff members who are

FIGURE 5-14

This nursing assistant is reporting a change in one of her resident's vital signs to the nurse.

reporting for work aware of all the information that is necessary to ensure a smooth continuation of care for the patient or resident. For example, the end-of-shift report is when oncoming staff members would be informed of new patients or residents and their care requirements, changes in the care plan for established patients or residents (such as new orders or treatments), and changes in a patient's or resident's status (such as rest or appetite changes).

RECORDING

Recording, sometimes referred to as "charting," is communicating information about a patient or resident to other health care team members in written form. Tools associated with recording include the medical record (chart) and the Kardex.

Medical Record (Chart)

A person's **medical record (chart)** is a legal document where information about the person's current condition, the measures that have been taken by the medical and nursing staff to diagnose and treat the condition, and the person's response to the treatment and care provided is recorded. Because the medical record, a legal document, is a formal accounting of the care the person received from the health care facility, it can be retrieved at any time and used in a court of law as evidence in a litigation claim.

The medical record is usually organized in sections with specific forms contained in each section. Some of these forms provide general information about the patient or resident. Others are specific to a particular health care department. The forms used may vary depending on the type of facility or health care agency. Typically, however, a medical record contains the following forms:

- **Admission sheet.** The admission sheet provides standard information about the person, including the person's name, address, date of birth and age, Social Security number, gender, insurance and employment information, emergency notification information, and advance directive information.
- **Medical history.** Usually, the medical record contains a dictated and typed medical history from the person's doctor.

The medical history contains information about the person's previous surgeries and medical conditions, current medications, allergies, and current medical diagnosis.

- **Nursing history.** The nursing history is completed by the nurse at the time of the person's admission to the facility. The nursing history provides information related to the person's care needs, such as information about physical disabilities or limitations, bowel and bladder habits, dietary preferences, and use of ambulation aids. An example of a nursing history is given in Chapter 14, Figure 14-4.
- **Physician's order sheet.** The physician's order sheet is used by the doctor to communicate to the other members of the health care team what should be done for the patient or resident. For example, the doctor may use the physician's order sheet to order treatments (such as medications), specify dietary orders or activity status, or order diagnostic tests.
- **Medication sheet.** The medications ordered for the patient or resident are listed here, along with the dosage and the time at which they are to be administered. This form is also used to record when medications are given, and by whom. Some long-term care and assisted-living facilities provide additional training to allow nursing assistants to give medications. If giving medications is within your scope of practice, then you will record your activities on the medication sheet.
- **Physician's progress notes.** The doctor uses this form to record his notes and observations about the person's progress and response to treatment.
- **Narrative nurse's notes.** The nurse uses this form to document the person's complaints (symptoms) and the actions taken by the nursing staff in response to them (Fig. 5-15). Some facilities allow nursing assistants to make notations in the narrative nurse's notes, and some do not.
- **Graphic sheet.** This is where information that is gathered routinely—such as vital signs, the frequency of urination and bowel movements, and food and fluid intake —is documented (Fig. 5-16). Some long-term care facilities use a type of graphic sheet to

Date	Time	Department (Nursing, P. T., ect.)	Prob. No.	◄ Progress Note ◄ Signature/Title	
12/02	1410	N		P. Abdish.CNA	Resident c/o pain in Rt. arm. BP 142/86,
					P. 92, R. 18, T. 99.2(0). RN notified.
12/02	1415	N		S. Carter, RN	Demerol 50mg, p.o. administered. Rt. arm elevated on
					pillow. Fingers warm and pink.
12/02	1500	N		S. Carter, RN	Resident states "My arm feels much
					better now."

Patient's Name (Last, First, MI)	Attending Physician	Room Number	Patient Number
Hayes, Ethel J	Sanders	302	1301

FIGURE 5-15

The care provided by the nursing staff, and the patient's or resident's response to this care, is documented in the narrative nurse's notes.

record a resident's activities of daily living (ADLs) and exercise therapy. The graphic sheet is the form used by nursing assistants most often to document the care that they provide.

- **Miscellaneous documents.** Laboratory reports, radiology reports, and reports related to other diagnostic tests or therapeutic treatments are usually included in specific sections of the person's medical record.

The information recorded on these various forms allows the members of the health care team to communicate with each other efficiently. For example, consider the following scenario:

Three days ago, Mrs. Wilson was admitted to 2 North for abdominal pain. Yesterday, when Mrs. Wilson's doctor reviewed the graphic sheet in Mrs. Wilson's chart, she saw that Mrs. Wilson had developed a fever. The doctor recorded her observations and impressions on the physician's progress notes form, and then ordered an antibiotic for Mrs. Wilson using the physician's order sheet. The ward clerk read the physician's order sheet and notified the pharmacy about the antibiotic. After giving the antibiotic to Mrs. Wilson, the nurse recorded when the antibiotic was given on the medication sheet. Throughout the rest of that day and night, the nursing assistants who were caring for Mrs. Wilson measured and recorded Mrs. Wilson's temperature at regular intervals on the graphic sheet. When the doctor made her rounds the next day, she was able to see that the antibiotic had been given as ordered and could tell by the temperature recordings that Mrs. Wilson was responding to the medication.

By using the medical chart properly, the health care team members were able to commu-

UNIVERSITY MEDICAL CENTER	GRAPHIC SHEET	PATIENT, TEST ACCT# 111111111111 MR# 222222222 DOB: 1/01/1940 AGE: 55 YRS ADM DT: 7/03/02 9228 GNS DR: REYNOLDS, VERNON

TODAY'S WEIGHT: 132	YESTERDAY'S INTAKE: 2550	
YESTERDAY'S WEIGHT: 132.5	YESTERDAY'S OUTPUT: 2350	YESTERDAY TEMP MAX: 99.4

DATE:	7/5/02
TIME:	8 15⁰ 18¹⁰ 22¹⁵
INITIALS:	AB CD CD EF

A = Axillary
R = Rectal

(temperature graph grid with markings at 105°, 104°, 103°, 102°, 101°, 100°, 99° (normal), 98°, 97°, 96°)

Circle pulse if apical (below)   96°

PULSE	84	92		78
RESPIRATIONS	16	20		16
SYST. BLOOD PRESSURE	120	132		124
DIAST BLOOD PRESSURE	84	80		86
L=LIE, S=SIT, T=STAND	L	L		L
O² SATURATION				

SIGNATURE	Alice Boyd, RN	AB	SIGNATURE	
SIGNATURE	Carol Davis, RN	CD	SIGNATURE	
SIGNATURE	Ellen Fisk, RN	EF	SIGNATURE	

FIGURE 5-16

The graphic sheet is used to record information that is more easily and accurately expressed visually, as opposed to verbally. For example, here you can see how the patient's temperature has fluctuated throughout the day.

UNIVERSITY MEDICAL CENTER
DATE: 7/5/02

I & O SHEET

PATIENT, TEST   ADM: 7/03/02
ACCT# 111111111111   MR# 222222222
DOB: 1/01/1940   AGE: 55 YRS
DR: REYNOLDS, VERNON   9228   GNS

Legend:
- T = Tubing Change
- ▲ = Dressing Change
- D = Diuretic
- + = Positive Blood
- − = Negative Blood

D5½NS ↓30K | Meds | PO
Column headers (output): urine | JP#1 | JP#2 | BM

TIME	INIT	SITE✓	D5½NS ↓30K	Meds	PO	INTAKE			INTAKE OR OUTPUT		urine	JP#1	JP#2	BM
0700														
0800	AB	✓	249/60		400						200			
0900														T
1000	AB	✓	180/60	50	100									
1100														
1200	AB	✓	120/60		400									
1300											400			
1400	AB	✓	60/60	50								15	25	
			240	100	900						600	15	25	
Shift Cumulative Total						1240				Shift Cumulative Total	640			
1500				T										
1600	CD	✓	1000/60								400			
1700														
1800	CD	✓	930/70	100 T	240									
1900														
2000	CD	✓	880/50		100									
2100											500			
2200	CD	✓	820/60	50								15	30	
			240	150	340						900	15	30	
Shift Cumulative Total						730				Shift Cumulative Total	945			
2300											400			
2400	EF	✓	770/60	50										
0100														
0200	EF	✓	705/65											
0300														
0400	EF	✓	650/55											
0500														
0600	EF	✓	580/80									10	25	
			240	50							400	10	25	
Shift Cumulative Total						290				Shift Cumulative Total	440			

CUMULATIVE 24° TOTAL	INTAKE	2260		OUTPUT	2030
SIGNATURE			SIGNATURE		
SIGNATURE			SIGNATURE		
SIGNATURE			SIGNATURE		

FIGURE 5-16

(continued)

nicate with each other in an organized, efficient way. The doctor did not need to find the nurse or nursing assistant to ask whether Mrs. Wilson was receiving the antibiotic, or to find out whether her fever had gone away.

Each facility or agency has specific policies about whether or not a nursing assistant is allowed to record information in the medical record. In some agencies or facilities, you may be able to record information on the graphic sheet, but not on the narrative nurse's notes. In others, you will be required to make entries in the narrative nurse's notes as documentation of the care you provide and the observations you make. Whenever you enter information on a person's medical record, date and time your entry correctly. Most medical facilities and agencies use the 24-hour time clock, also called "military time," for recording the time in a patient's medical record (Fig. 5-17). Guidelines for recording are given in Guidelines Box 5-1.

The way information is organized and entered into a medical record, and the policies dictating who is permitted to enter information into the record, differ from facility to facility. However, two policies regarding the handling of medical records are always the same, no matter where you work:

- The information contained in a person's medical record is considered confidential and is only to be read by members of the health care team who are directly involved in the care of that person and need access to the information in the record to provide that care. For example, although a custodial worker is part of the health care team, he does not need access to the information in the medical record in order to perform his duties. Therefore, custodial workers generally do not have access to patients' or residents' charts.
- To keep patients and residents safe, each form in the medical record must be stamped or printed with the patient's or resident's identification information. Accidentally placing a physician's order sheet meant for one person in another person's medical record could cause someone to receive a treatment or medication in error. A miscommunication of this nature could have serious, possibly even fatal, consequences.

FIGURE 5-17

Most medical facilities and agencies use the 24-hour time clock, also referred to as "military time," for recording the time in a patient's medical record. The 24-hour time clock eliminates the need to differentiate between morning (A.M.) and night (P.M.), thus reducing errors in recording. On the 24-hour time clock, the morning hours are the same as on the conventional clock. To indicate a time in the afternoon, add "12" to the time on the conventional clock. When time is stated according to the 24-hour time clock, the first two numbers indicate the hour and the last two numbers indicate the minute (for example, 8:24 P.M. conventional time = 2024 military time). Conventional time = *blue;* morning hours = *yellow;* afternoon hours = *green.*

Conventional time	24-hour time
1:00 A.M.	0100
2:00 A.M.	0200
3:00 A.M.	0300
4:00 A.M.	0400
5:00 A.M.	0500
6:00 A.M.	0600
7:00 A.M.	0700
8:00 A.M.	0800
9:00 A.M.	0900
10:00 A.M.	1000
11:00 A.M.	1100
12:00 P.M. (noon)	1200
1:00 P.M.	1300
2:00 P.M.	1400
3:00 P.M.	1500
4:00 P.M.	1600
5:00 P.M.	1700
6:00 P.M.	1800
7:00 P.M.	1900
8:00 P.M.	2000
9:00 P.M.	2100
10:00 P.M.	2200
11:00 P.M.	2300
12:00 A.M. (midnight)	2400

GUIDELINES BOX 5-1
GUIDELINES FOR RECORDING

What you do	Why you do it
Write legibly, using blue or black ink. Your facility may have specific policies regarding the color of ink used.	It is important to write legibly to avoid miscommunication. A pen is used instead of a pencil because pencil can be erased, enabling someone to change the person's medical record. Blue and black ink reproduce best when a document is photocopied.
Always sign or initial your entry, according to facility policy.	By signing or initialing your entry, you indicate that you are the person who needs to be consulted if further clarification of the information you have entered is necessary. Additionally, signing or initialing your entry indicates that you accept legal responsibility for what you have written.
Only record observations that you have made, or care that you have given. Do not make entries for another person.	By making an entry in a medical record, you accept legal responsibility for that entry. Therefore, it is best to record only information that you, personally, can vouch for.
Date and time your entries correctly (see Fig. 5-17).	The date and time that actions occurred or observations were made are extremely important elements of the medical record, which is a legal account of care provided.
Check the patient's or resident's name on the medical record and on the form where you are recording.	By verifying the patient's or resident's identification information, you will ensure that you are recording the person's information in the correct medical record.
Use appropriate medical terminology and facility-approved abbreviations when recording.	Using correct terminology and abbreviations will prevent others from having to second-guess your meaning.
Do not record care as given or procedures as performed before you have provided the care or performed the procedure. Only document after the fact.	You may become distracted or involved in another situation that prevents you from carrying out the duties you have already charted. If you record duties as "completed" in the medical record, but then do not actually complete these duties, you will have committed fraud.
Record information in a timely manner. If you must wait to record something, keep notes about your observations and care so that the information you record in the medical record will be accurate.	If you wait until the end of your shift to record, you may forget important information.
If you make an error, do not erase, use correction fluid to cover, or scribble through the mistaken entry. Simply draw a line through the mistake and initial it according to facility policy.	Striking through an error is the only legal way to indicate a change in the medical record. Erasing or using correction fluid to correct an error could be seen as an attempt to hide or change existing information.
Remember that in a liability situation, care not recorded was care not provided.	Proper and conscientious recording of patient or resident information protects the patient or resident, your employer, and you.

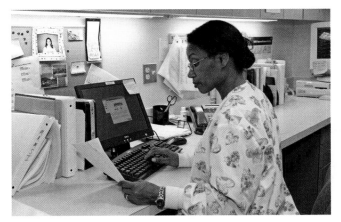

FIGURE 5-18

Computerized charting is becoming more widespread.

As the use of computers becomes more wide-spread, computerized charting is replacing paper charting in some facilities and agencies (Fig. 5-18). In computerized charting, the person's medical record is maintained by entering data into a computer in response to the computer's prompts, rather than by filling in a paper form. Medical records created in this way tend to be more accurate and legible because they are typed rather than handwritten. Using a computer to maintain and access a patient's or resident's medical record does not require advanced computer training. If your facility or agency uses computerized charting, your employer will provide training in the use of the computer as part of your new employee orientation. During this training, you will learn how to enter data about your patients or residents, as well as how to quickly retrieve information that you need about a patient or resident in order to provide his or her care.

Although computerized charting offers many advantages over paper charting, patient and resident confidentiality is a primary concern when the computer is used to store patient data. To promote patient or resident confidentiality, each user of the computer is assigned a password, which permits the user to have access to certain patients' or residents' medical records. Never give anyone else your password or leave the computer active after you have used it. If you fail to log off after using the computer, the information on the screen may be visible or accessible to people who are not authorized to have access to it. Additionally, if you fail to log off when you are finished with the computer, someone else could enter information under your password, and it will appear that you have entered it. Computer monitors

should be positioned so that the screen is not visible to the public when you are working. Your facility or agency will have specific policies (mandated by HIPAA) regarding computer use and confidentiality. Make sure you are familiar with these policies, and follow them carefully.

Kardex

The **Kardex** is a card file, containing condensed versions of each patient's or resident's medical record. The Kardex card contains a summary of the person's current diagnosis, the diagnostic tests and treatments ordered by the doctor, and information about routine care measures, such as the person's diet, level of ambulation, and bathing schedule (Fig 5-19). The Kardex card is updated as the person's condition or doctor's orders change. By providing a one-page summary of the patient's or resident's medical record, the Kardex card keeps health care team members from having to search through the entire record every time they need information about the person's status and care plan.

THE NURSING PROCESS

Although the doctor is responsible for diagnosing a person's medical problems and ordering medication or other therapies to correct those problems, the nursing team is responsible for carrying out the doctor's orders and providing holistic care to the patient or resident. To achieve its goals, the nursing team develops a specific plan of care, called the **nursing care plan,** for each patient or resident. The communication method that is used to develop the nursing care plan is called the **nursing process.** The nursing process allows members of the nursing team to communicate with each other regarding the patient's or resident's specific needs (in regard to nursing care), what steps will be taken to meet those needs, and whether or not the steps were effective in meeting the person's needs. The nursing care plan, which is derived from the nursing process, makes sure that all members of the nursing team are "on the same page." The nurse who is acting as the nursing team leader is responsible for developing the nursing care plan. She does this with the help of other health care team members, including the patient or resident, the nursing assistant, and members of specific departments, such as dietitians, social workers, and physical therapists.

ADVANCED DIRECTIVES

- X Living will
- ___ Autopsy request
- ___ Do not resuscitate
- ___ Feeding restrictions
- ___ Do not hospitalize
- ___ Medication restrictions
- X Organ donation
- ___ Other treatment restrictions
- ___
- ___ NONE OF THE ABOVE

Allergies: **Sulfa**

(Write in red or highlight)

Nutritional/Oral

Diet _Regular_

Supplements: _n/a_

Meal Location: Breakfast _Dining room_

Lunch _Dining room_

Dinner _Dining room_

- ___ Swallowing Difficulty
- ___ Thicken Liquids
- ___ Tube Feeding
- ___ NPO
- ___ I-O
- ___ Fluid Restriction
- ___ TPN

Elimination   QOL program(s) _n/a_

Bladder:

- X Continent
- ___ Incontinent
- ___ Catheter

Bowel:

- X Continent
- ___ Incontinent
- ___ Ostomy

Cognition

- ___ Short term memory problem
- ___ Decision-making difficulty
- ___ Difficulty expressing self

Oriented to:

- X Person
- X Place
- X Time
- X Situation

Behavior   QOL program _n/a_

- ___ Verbally Abusive
- ___ Physically Abusive
- ___ Socially Inappropriate
- ___ Resistant to Care
- ___ Wandering/Exit Seeking   QOL program _n/a_

Communication

Primary Language:

- X English   ___ Other: _____
- ___ Alternative methods used:
- ___ Communication board   ___ Writing
- ___ Sign language   ___ Gestures
- ___ Other _____

Appliances

- ___ Hearing Aide   ___ R   ___ L
- X Glasses   ___ Contacts
- X Dentures   ___ Upper   ___ Lower   X Partial
- ___ Anti-embolism hose
- X Prosthesis/Splint/Brace (description) _Cast-Rt_
  Forearm

Respiratory

- ___ Pulse Oximetry
- ___ Tracheostomy   ___ Oxygen
- ___ Ventilator   ___ Suctioning

Skin Management   QOL program _____

- ___ Turn & Position   ___ Other _____
- ___ Mattress   _____

Additional Quality of Life Program(s) or Medical Specialty Treatment Program(s)

Physical Therapy rt. arm

_____

_____

ADL's		Self-Performance	Support (# of Persons)
Bathing	_____	I S (L) E T	(1) 2
Dressing	_____	I S (L) E T	(1) 2
Toileting	_____	(I) S L E T	1 2
Eating	_____	I S (L) E T	(1) 2
Transferring	_____	(I) S L E T	1 2
Walking	_____	I S (L) E T	(1) 2

I - Independent   E - Extensive
S - Supervised   T - Total
L - Limited

Mobility: Weight bearing status _Good_

- ___ Mechanical lift   ___ W/chair
- ___ ROM   ___ Walker
- X AROM   X Cane
- ___ PROM   ___ Other: _____
- ___ Bedfast/chairbound

Weight schedule X mo ___ why ___ other
QOL program _____
Restraint: Type: _____   When: _____
QOL Program _____

Resident Preferences:	Bathing type:	Bathing Day/time:
	___ Shower	
Name: _Miss (Ethel)_	X Tub	M (T) W (Th)
Time to arise _7 am_	___ Other:	F (Sa) Su
Time to rest: _1 pm_		
Time to retire _10 pm_		AM (PM)
Likes/dislikes: ___		

Special Precautions:
Please assist at mealtime by opening milk and cutting food into small pieces

Diagnoses:
Primary: _____
Secondary: _FX Rt. radius & ulna_

RESIDENT NAME	ADMISSION DATE	PHYSICIAN	DOB	AGE	Medical Record Number
Ethel Hayes	_12/01/01_	_Sanders_	_03/06/1929_	_72_	_1301_

FIGURE 5-19

The Kardex card, kept in a Kardex file, summarizes the most up-to-date information about a patient's or resident's condition and care needs.

The nursing process is organized into a series of steps:

1. **Assessment.** During this step, information specific to the patient or resident is gathered. Sources of this information are the person's medical history, the nursing history, family members, and most importantly, the person himself. As part of the assessment process, the nurse examines the patient or resident and asks questions about his abilities, level of discomfort, eating and toileting habits, and specific needs.

2. **Diagnosis.** Using the information gathered during the assessment step, the nurse then develops a **nursing diagnosis,** or a statement that describes a problem the person is having, as well as the cause of the problem. Unlike a medical diagnosis, which identifies a medical problem that must be identified and managed by a doctor, a nursing diagnosis identifies a problem that the nursing staff can identify and treat independently. For example, consider a person who has a broken arm. The medical diagnosis for this person might be "fractured radius and ulna." The nursing diagnosis might be "impaired nutritional status due to inability to feed self because of dominant hand being in a cast."

3. **Planning.** The next step in the nursing process involves making a plan for the person's care. Using information obtained from the nursing diagnosis, the nurse develops **interventions** (actions that will be taken to help the person) and **goals** (descriptions of what the interventions are meant to achieve). For example, in order

to achieve the goal of improved nutritional status for the person with the cast on his arm, the intervention may be to cut the person's food into bite-sized pieces to make it easier for him to eat. The interventions and goals that have been set for the patient or resident are written down in a formal way. This document (the nursing care plan) becomes part of the patient's or resident's medical record and may be included on the Kardex.

4. **Implementation.** During the implementation step, the interventions that were detailed in the nursing care plan are carried out. (The nursing care plan specifies the team members who are responsible for doing each intervention.)

5. **Evaluation.** During the evaluation step, the nursing team checks the effectiveness of the nursing care plan and revises it as necessary. Is the care plan working? Are the goals being met? What needs to be improved or changed to meet the goals? Has the patient's or resident's status changed? Is the existing nursing care plan still appropriate for the patient or resident? If certain interventions are not working, or if the goals have been met, the nursing care plan will change.

The nursing process is ongoing. The nursing staff continually assesses the patient or resident and adjusts the nursing care plan as the person's needs change. As a nursing assistant, you will participate in the nursing process by carrying out interventions and communicating observations to the nurse. When you communicate observations to the nurse, you help him or her with the assessment and evaluation steps of the nursing process. Your observations and communications to the nurse and other health care team members will ensure that the patient or resident remains the focus of quality, compassionate care that is carefully planned, implemented, and evaluated.

SUMMARY

▶ Communication is the exchange of information.
  ■ For good communication to occur, a sender must send a clear message directly to a receiver who can understand the message. The receiver must provide feedback that lets the sender know that the message was heard "loud and clear."
  ■ Effective communication among health care team members is essential to ensure that patients or residents receive top-quality, safe care. It is important for nursing assistants to have good communication skills because the exchange of information with patients, residents, and coworkers is a key part of the nursing assistant's job.
  ■ Nursing assistants are an important link between the patient or resident and other members of the health care team. The nursing assistant is often the first member of the health care team to become aware of a change in a patient's or resident's condition that could be a sign of something serious.

▶ There are many ways to improve communication with others.
  ■ Listening is one of the most important communication skills, especially in the health care field.
  ■ Speaking clearly, asking open-ended questions, and using appropriate body language when talking with other people are other ways to improve communication.

▶ Reporting and recording are two methods of communication used by the health care team to make sure that everyone involved in the care of a patient or resident has current, reliable information about that person. Observations about a patient's or resident's condition are reported, recorded, or both. Observations may be subjective or objective.
  ■ Reporting is the spoken exchange of information between members of the health care team. Observations about a change in a patient's or resident's condition must be reported to the nurse immediately.
  ■ Recording is the written exchange of information between members of the health care team. Recording is done in the person's medical record or chart.

▶ The nursing process is a communication method that allows members of the nursing team to meet a patient's or resident's specific care needs. The nursing assistant plays a role in the nursing process by carrying out interventions and communicating observations to the nurse.

What did you learn?

Multiple Choice

Select the single best answer for each of the following questions.

1. Which one of the following is an open-ended question?
   a. "Are you Mrs. Brown?"
   b. "Mr. Jones, when you were growing up, what was your favorite meal?"
   c. "Are you feeling okay, Mrs. Smith?"
   d. "It's beautiful outside today, Mrs. Murphy! Do you want to go for a walk?"

2. Which one of the following is an example of positive body language?
   a. Nodding encouragingly as someone speaks
   b. Crossing your arms across your chest
   c. Tapping your feet or fingers
   d. Rolling your eyes

3. An example of an action that blocks effective communication is:
   a. Interrupting
   b. Not listening carefully
   c. Being judgmental
   d. All of the above

4. Which one of the following is an objective observation?
   a. "Mr. Wohl says that his back hurts when he coughs."
   b. "Ms. O'Connell's urine is cloudy, and has a strong odor."
   c. "Mr. McAndrews is complaining of a headache."
   d. "The resident in room 201B is complaining of a stomachache."

5. Which one of the following is an example of nonverbal communication?
   a. Using sign language to communicate with a deaf person
   b. Recording vital sign measurements in a patient's or resident's chart
   c. Gently touching a patient or resident on the shoulder to reassure her
   d. Making a telephone call

6. What usually forms the basis for a subjective observation?
   a. A symptom, or patient complaint
   b. A measurement
   c. A doctor's order
   d. All of the above

7. Which step of the nursing process involves gathering information about a patient or resident?
   a. Implementation
   b. Assessment
   c. Planning
   d. Evaluation

8. With regard to telephone communication, nursing assistants are responsible for all of the following except:
   a. Writing down the caller's name and telephone number if the person the caller wants to speak to is not available, and delivering this message to the intended recipient
   b. Answering the telephone promptly, with a pleasant greeting
   c. Taking down doctor's orders if the nurse is not available and a doctor calls
   d. Identifying themselves to the caller by name and title, per facility policy

9. When recording information in a person's medical chart, what should you remember to do?
   a. Use pencil so that errors can be corrected neatly
   b. Sign or initial and date and time your entry, per facility policy
   c. Update all of your patients' or residents' charts at one time at the end of each shift
   d. All of the above

10. What is it called when people have differences and they are unable to come to an agreement?
    a. Communication
    b. Conflict
    c. Culture
    d. Personality difference

Matching

Match each numbered item with its appropriate lettered description.

_____ **1.** Admission sheet

_____ **2.** Narrative nurse's notes

_____ **3.** Medical history

_____ **4.** Physician's order sheet

_____ **5.** Graphic sheet

a. Used to record patient complaints and the actions that were taken by the nursing team to provide relief

b. Used to record routine data, such as vital signs, frequency of urination and bowel movements, and food and fluid intake

c. Used to order diagnostic tests and treatments, and to specify dietary orders or activity status

d. Typed or dictated document that lists a patient's previous surgeries and medical conditions, current medications, allergies, and current medical diagnosis

e. Document that contains essential information about the patient, including his or her name and address, birth date, insurance information, advance directives information, and emergency contact information

Stop and think!

▶ Juanita is assigned to care for Mr. Thompson today. Juanita has taken care of Mr. Thompson before, and he is not one of her favorite residents. It seems like he is always unhappy about something. As expected, the moment Juanita walks into his room, Mr. Thompson begins to complain—his children have left him here to die! His grandchildren expect him to remember their birthdays (and send money), but they never remember his! The food in this place is terrible! Juanita is focused on getting Mr. Thompson out of bed, washed, and ready for breakfast. While Juanita is busy getting the bathroom ready and collecting linens, Mr. Thompson starts to complain that his chest feels "tight," and he "can hardly breathe." Assuming that this is just another item in Mr. Thompson's long list of complaints, Juanita continues with what she was doing. If you were Juanita, would you have handled this situation differently? If so, how? If not, why not? What blocks to effective communication do you see here?

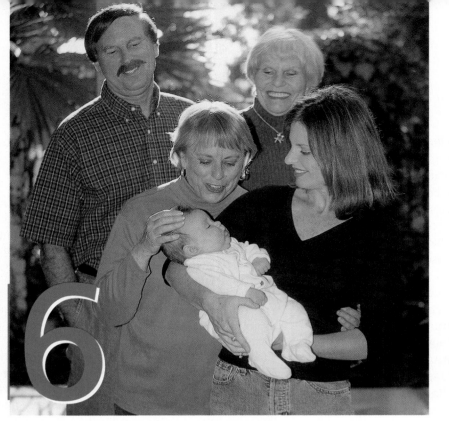

6

Those We Care For

What will you learn?

As we start on the final chapter in this introductory unit, you are probably beginning to realize that there is much more to being a nursing assistant than blood pressures and bedpans. A health care worker can go to the most well-known schools, receive the most intense training, and graduate at the top of his class, but if he is not able to connect on a human level with his patients or residents, he will fail. In this chapter, we will explore the qualities that we, as humans, share, as well as the ones that make us unique individuals. When you are finished with this chapter, you will be able to:

1. Recognize that health care is a people-focused service.
2. Discuss why people need health care intervention.
3. Differentiate between acute, chronic, and terminal conditions, and give an example of each.
4. Describe how the health care industry classifies people, and list the types of people you might have the opportunity to work with.
5. List and briefly describe the stages of human growth and development.
6. Understand that developmental changes are common throughout the life span of a person.
7. Draw Maslow's hierarchy of basic human needs, and explain each level.
8. Describe ways that a nursing assistant helps patients and residents to meet their needs.
9. Understand the difference between sex and sexuality and discuss how a person's sexuality can be affected by illness.
10. Explain the concept of diversity, and why it is important for health care workers to recognize their patients' and residents' diversity.

Photo: Throughout the course of our lives, we pass through a series of stages. Here, members from the same family represent the stages of infancy, young adulthood, middle adulthood, and later adulthood. (©Grantpix/Photo Researchers, Inc.)

Vocabulary

Use the CD in the back of your book to hear these terms pronounced, defined, and used in a sentence:

Acute illness	Puberty	Sex	Masturbation
Chronic illness	Menarche	Heterosexual	Culture
Terminal illness	Nocturnal emissions	Homosexual	Race
Growth	Menopause	Bisexual	Religion
Development	Need	Transsexual	
Tasks	Sexuality	Transvestite	
Neonate	Intimacy	Coitus	

PATIENTS, RESIDENTS, AND CLIENTS

If someone asked you "As a nursing assistant, who do you care for?" you might answer (depending on where you work) "I care for patients," or "I care for residents," or "I care for clients." (As you will recall from Chapter 1, a patient is a person who is receiving health care in a hospital, clinic, or extended-care facility. A resident is a person who is living in a long-term care facility or an assisted-living facility, and a client is a person who is receiving care in his or her own home, from a home health care agency.) These are all terms for people who, because they are sick, injured, or unable to care for themselves, need the services that the health care industry offers. At the most basic level, patients, residents, and clients are "those we care for."

There are three general types of illnesses or conditions that can cause a person to need health care services. An **acute illness** is a condition characterized by a rapid onset and a relatively short recovery time. Because the onset is rapid, acute illnesses are usually unexpected. Conditions such as pneumonia, appendicitis, a broken bone, or labor and delivery would be considered acute conditions. In contrast, a **chronic illness** is a condition that is ongoing. A person with a chronic illness generally needs continuous medication or treatment to control the condition. Occasionally, acute flare-ups of the chronic condition lead to hospitalization. Examples of chronic illnesses include diabetes, asthma, arthritis, and high blood pressure (hypertension). Finally, a **terminal illness** is an illness or condition from which recovery is not expected. People who have a terminal illness will die as a result of their illness, usually within a short period of time. Examples of terminal illnesses include some types of cancer, end-stage emphysema, and some heart conditions.

In order to make providing care more efficient, the health care industry groups people according to their ages, illnesses or medical conditions, or special health care needs (Fig. 6-1). For example, it would not make sense to have adults and small children on the same ward, or a critically ill person rooming with a woman who is merely recovering from delivering a baby. In some cases, specialized training is needed in order to care for a certain type of patient, so it would make sense to group all of the patients requiring that type of specialized care together. Examples of terms that are often used to describe people, based on the person's age, illness, or special health care needs, include the following.

- **Surgical patients** have illnesses or conditions that are treated by surgery, such as appendicitis or certain types of tumors. Surgical patients are admitted to the hospital for surgery and the recovery period afterwards. Many surgical procedures are performed on an outpatient basis, which means that the patient is admitted to the hospital for surgery, but then sent home to recover. The care of surgical patients is discussed in Chapter 39.
- **Medical patients** have an illness or condition that is treated with interventions other than surgery, such as medication, physical therapy, or radiation. Examples of medical conditions include pneumonia, myocardial infarction ("heart attack"), stroke, and some stomach disorders (such as ulcers).

A

B

C

D

E

F

G

FIGURE 6-1

Examples of the many ways in which people are grouped by the health care industry. (*A*) Surgical patient. (*B*) Medical patient. (*C*) Obstetrical patient. (*D*) Pediatric patient. (*E*) Geriatric patient. (*F*) Rehabilitation patient. (*G*) Intensive care patient. (*A, ©Pete Saloutos/CORBIS; B, © Richard T. Nowitz/CORBIS; C, ©Viviane Moos/CORBIS; D, © Tom Stewart/CORBIS; E, ©LWA-Dann Tardif/CORBIS; F, ©LWA-Stephen Welstead/CORBIS; G, ©Grafton Marshall Smith/CORBIS.*)

- **Obstetrical patients** are those who are pregnant or have just given birth. Obstetrical care extends throughout the pregnancy and labor and delivery, and then continues for about 8 weeks after delivery. Although most obstetrical patients are admitted to the hospital for the actual labor and delivery, and remain hospitalized for a brief time afterward, most of the care before and after the delivery is provided on an outpatient basis (unless the mother or baby experiences complications.) The care of obstetrical patients is discussed in Chapter 40.

- **Pediatric patients** are children and adolescents. Pediatrics has become a specialty because children and teenagers are at risk for some diseases that adults are not. In addition, sometimes special considerations must be taken into account when providing treatments and care for younger patients because a child's body does not function in exactly the same way an adult's does. Sometimes an entire facility is dedicated to the care of the pediatric patient. Other times, a special unit within the hospital or long-term care facility is designated as the pediatrics unit.

The care of pediatric patients is discussed in Chapter 41.

- **Geriatric patients** are adults 75 years and older. Health care workers who specialize in geriatrics are trained to recognize the physical and mental effects of the normal aging process and help older adults adjust to these changes. They are also trained to care for people with diseases that are particularly common among this age group.

- **Psychiatric patients** are people with impaired mental health. Psychiatric patients are often treated on an outpatient basis, using a combination of counseling and medication. However, mentally ill people who are deemed a danger to themselves or others may be admitted to a health care facility for treatment.

- **Rehabilitation patients** are those who are undergoing therapy to restore their highest level of physical, emotional or mental, or vocational functioning. People born with physical disabilities or deformities may require physical rehabilitation. So might people who have had a stroke or are recovering from surgery or an injury. Emotional or mental rehabilitation may be necessary for people with substance abuse problems. Vocational rehabilitation focuses on providing the person with special training after an injury or surgery so that he or she can return to a particular type of work. Rehabilitation facilities or units provide services both on an inpatient and outpatient basis.

- **Subacute or extended-care patients** are usually recovering from an acute illness or condition. They do not need the total care provided by a hospital, but are not quite ready to return home. They may continue to have a need for intravenously administered medications, physical therapy, or other treatments that cannot be provided by untrained caretakers.

- **Intensive care patients.** Patients needing very specialized, or intensive, care are usually admitted to an intensive care unit or a special care unit. After heart or brain surgery, or after suffering from a heart attack or stroke, a patient will stay in the special care unit until her condition improves. She will then be moved to a regular hospital unit.

As you can see, the people we care for can be classified in many different ways. However, those in need of health care services are not merely defined by their illnesses and disabilities. First and foremost, patients, residents, and clients are human beings. In the rest of this chapter, we will take a closer look at some of the things that all people have in common, as well as some of the things that make us different.

GROWTH AND DEVELOPMENT

Throughout the course of our lives, we all pass through a series of stages. We are constantly changing, from conception until the time of death. Changes that occur physically are known as **growth.** Changes that occur psychologically or socially are known as **development.** Growth is demonstrated by changes in height and weight and by physical maturation of the body's organ systems. Development is evidenced by changes in a person's behavior and way of thinking. Both growth and development occur in an orderly fashion and progress from the simple to the complex. Physically, a baby must develop the muscle strength and coordination that will enable him to sit, then stand, and finally to walk. Developmentally, that baby will smile at his mother, then coo, say his first word, and soon speak in complete sentences.

The process of growth and development is divided into stages of normal progression (Fig. 6-2). Although all people progress through the stages of growth and development in a series of expected steps, they do not progress through the stages at the same rate. For example, one child may walk at 8 months and speak his first word at 10 months. His sister, on the other hand, may talk relatively early at 7 months, but not walk until the age of 14 months. Although the stages of growth and development can be generalized by age, it is important to note that each person, like the brother and sister described here, progresses through the stages at his or her own pace. A person cannot progress to the next stage without successfully completing the **tasks,** or growth and development milestones, associated with the stage she is currently in. With young children and teenagers, it is quite common

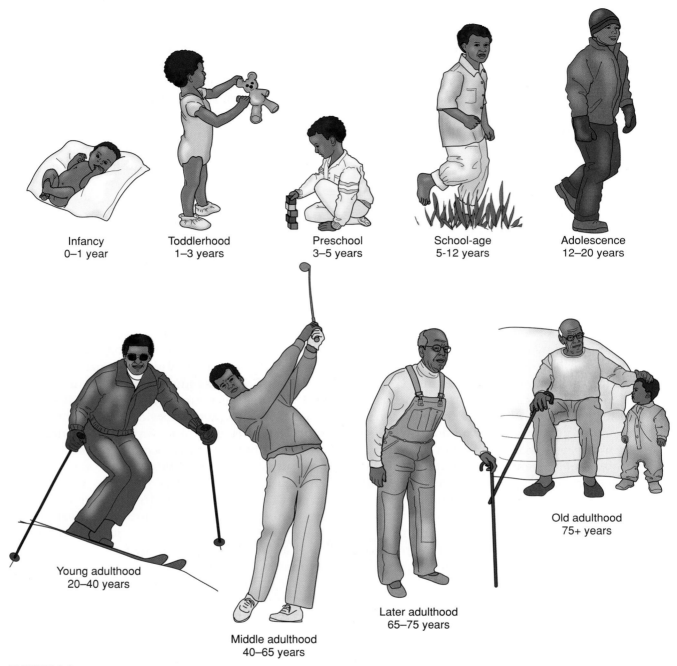

Infancy
0–1 year

Toddlerhood
1–3 years

Preschool
3–5 years

School-age
5-12 years

Adolescence
12–20 years

Young adulthood
20–40 years

Middle adulthood
40–65 years

Later adulthood
65–75 years

Old adulthood
75+ years

FIGURE 6-2

Everyone passes through the same stages of growth and development.

to see some overlap in the stages. This is because growth and development occurs unevenly, or in spurts, with one part occurring faster that the other. A 5-year-old may have matured quickly emotionally and prefer the company of older children, but lack certain motor skills that would allow him to ride a bike or play baseball. This can be quite frustrating for the child until he has physi-

cally grown enough to keep up. Another child may reach physical maturity quickly, but will then need to "catch up" emotionally. The basic principles of growth and development are highlighted in Box 6-1.

Psychologists are people who study the mind and behavior. Many psychologists have developed theories about human development throughout

BOX 6-1 Principles of Growth and Development

- Growth and development occurs continuously throughout a person's life span, from conception until death.
- Growth and development occurs step by step and in an orderly progression. Each stage has specific characteristics and tasks that must be accomplished before the person can progress to the next stage.
- Growth and development tasks progress from the simple to the complex.
- Growth and development tasks progress from head to toe, and from the center of the body outward.
- Growth and development occurs at variable rates for each individual, and may occur unevenly or in spurts.

the life span. Depending on which psychologist's work you study, you may find that the growth and development stages are defined slightly differently, in terms of age ranges and tasks. Additionally, the age at which a person begins or ends a certain stage of development varies slightly according to the individual. Figure 6-2 and the descriptions of the various stages in the sections

that follow are generalizations, obtained from the large amount of research that has been done on the subject of human growth and development. Throughout your career as a nursing assistant, you may have the opportunity to care for people of all different ages, from premature newborns to those who have lived for more than a century. As a person grows and ages, the physical and psychological changes that occur affect the type of care the person needs, and the way in which we communicate with him or her. Becoming familiar with the various stages of growth and development, and the tasks commonly associated with these stages, will help you to become a more able caregiver.

INFANCY (BIRTH TO 1 YEAR)

Infancy is the stage during which physical and psychological changes occur most rapidly. By his first birthday, an infant will typically weigh three times what he did when he was born, and he will have progressed from a totally helpless **neonate** (a newborn infant, 28 days or younger) to a child learning how to walk (Fig. 6-3). During this stage, new tasks are accomplished on a weekly and monthly basis. The infant begins to smile and laugh, recognize parents and siblings, play

A

B

FIGURE 6-3

During the infancy stage, growth and development tasks are accomplished in leaps and bounds. Within the space of a year, an infant goes from being totally helpless (A) to being able to move around independently (B).

peek-a-boo, and say simple words. He progresses from drinking only mother's milk or formula to feeding himself solid foods. What a year!

TODDLERHOOD (1 TO 3 YEARS)

Physical growth slows down during toddlerhood, but development of the muscular and nervous systems allows the toddler to become quite active. The toddler can walk, run, climb, jump, and peddle a tricycle easily (Fig. 6-4). Suddenly, parents and caretakers must work hard to remove unsafe objects and curb the natural curiosity of the toddler! In addition to permitting increased mobility, development of the muscular and nervous systems permits greater control of the bladder and bowels, so this is when toilet training begins.

Developmentally, the toddler learns the words to express emotions, such as "sad" or "scared," and is able to express herself in short, complete sentences. Toddlers become quite independent and sometimes have trouble following rules of behavior. The toddler's world revolves around the toddler! Toddlers will engage actively in play, but usually play alone or alongside another child without many interactions. Toddlers do not separate from a parent or familiar caregiver easily. Therefore, medical procedures that require separation of the child and the caregiver can be very frightening for a toddler.

PRESCHOOL (3 TO 5 YEARS)

The preschooler is an adventure waiting to happen! The preschooler's physical coordination improves a great deal, and he learns to dress himself and tie his own shoes. Toileting becomes more independent. Preschoolers become involved in playing with other children, and will use their active imaginations to create detailed play stories and scenes (Fig. 6-5). During this stage, children become aware of gender differences and roles and are very curious about the differences between boys and girls. They ask questions all the time and love to have stories told or read to them. As the preschooler begins to know the difference between right and wrong behavior, he begins to develop a conscience and is able to more easily follow rules.

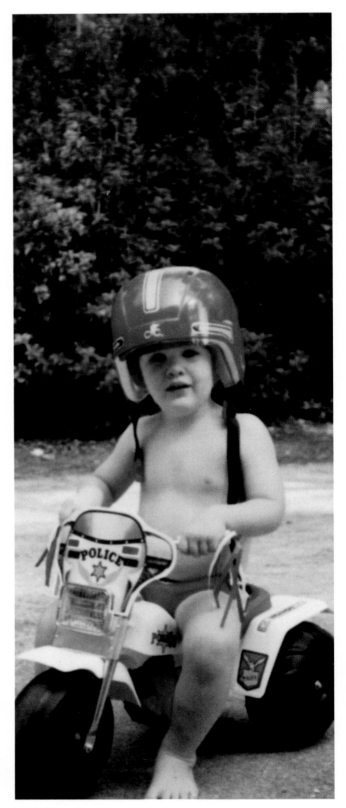

FIGURE 6-4

During the toddler stage, development of the nervous and muscular systems leads to increased mobility.

FIGURE 6-5

Preschoolers enjoy interacting with others and playing "make-believe." (© *Joseph Sohm; Chromo Sohm, Inc./CORBIS.*)

Physical growth and development during adolescence is considerable. In girls, the development of breasts and the growth of hair in the pubic and armpit (axillary) regions occurs before the onset of menstruation, or **menarche.** Throughout adolescence, a girl's breasts continue to develop and her hips broaden, leading to the curves that characterize the female shape. In boys, the genitals increase in size. Pubic, axillary, and facial hair develops, and the voice deepens. Ejaculation, or the release of semen, signals the onset of puberty; adolescent boys often experience **nocturnal emissions** (commonly known as "wet dreams") while sleeping. A growth spurt occurs, and the adolescent boy may gain more than a foot in height over the course of a few months. His shoulders broaden and his muscles become more developed.

SCHOOL-AGE (5 TO 12 YEARS)

The school-aged child experiences several major physical growth spurts, which lead to increases in both height and weight. As her fine motor skills develop, the child's ability to write and draw improves. Play usually involves groups of same-sex friends. Popular activities, such as belonging to a scout troop, help with developing gender identity (Fig. 6-6). With school attendance comes an increased ability to follow society's rules. Children in this age group actively seek approval from authority figures and peers. They develop logical thinking patterns and learn to incorporate other people's perspectives into their own thinking. Morals develop and school-aged children may feel very strongly about issues being either right or wrong, with no gray area. Spirituality and religious beliefs, as well as a concern for other living things, also take root during this developmental stage.

ADOLESCENCE (12 TO 20 YEARS)

The ages of children in this developmental stage vary considerably. Adolescence begins at the onset of **puberty,** when the secondary sex characteristics appear and the reproductive organs begin to function. In girls, the onset of puberty usually occurs between the ages of 10 and 14 years, and in boys, it occurs between the ages of 12 and 16 years.

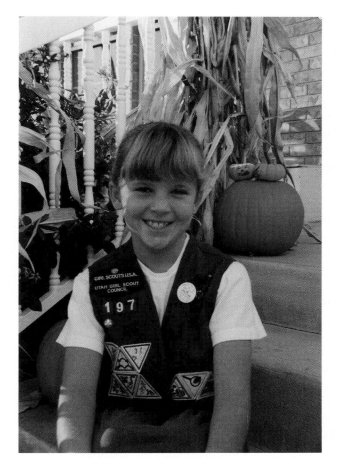

FIGURE 6-6

School-age children like activities that allow them to interact with members of the same sex.

FIGURE 6-7

Adolescence can be a difficult yet exciting time. (© *Comstock IMAGES.*)

FIGURE 6-8

Many young adults choose to get married and begin families of their own.

Psychologically, the period of adolescence is stormy. Adolescents may be self-conscious about their changing bodies and increased awareness of their own sexuality (Fig. 6-7). They are torn between wanting to be treated as grown-ups and being afraid to make their own decisions. Adolescents experiment with new styles of dress and hair, and follow very closely with their friends. They begin to date and to question the moral teachings of authority figures and parents. As a result, experimentation with alcohol, drugs, and sex may occur during this stage. As a reflection of their increasing emotional maturity, adolescents take jobs to make extra cash, learn to drive, and begin to make plans for their future education or the beginning of a career.

YOUNG ADULTHOOD (20 TO 40 YEARS)

After the turmoil of adolescence, young adulthood comes as a relief. Young adults typically enjoy stable, supporting friendships and good health. The primary tasks of this stage center on completing one's education, starting on a career, and, possibly, finding a partner and marrying. The young adult learns to be successful on his or her own, and if he or she marries, adjusts to living with a partner. Many young adults choose to start families (Fig. 6-8). For many women, the most significant physical change that will occur during young adulthood is pregnancy. Otherwise, the physical changes that occur in young adults are generally minor. The adult height is achieved during adolescence.

MIDDLE ADULTHOOD (40 TO 65 YEARS)

Middle adulthood frequently finds people at the height of their careers and productivity. Many middle adults find themselves in the role of caretaker to their children as well as to their aging parents. As the children grow up and become less reliant, many middle adults find that they have more time to travel or participate in leisure activities (Fig. 6-9). During middle adulthood, many people become grandparents. Physically, the middle adult begins to show signs of aging, such as wrinkles or a few gray hairs. Women typically experience **menopause** (i.e., cessation of menstruation and fertility) in their early 50s. Although good health is usually still enjoyed, some chronic illnesses, such as hypertension and diabetes, become apparent during this stage.

LATER ADULTHOOD (65 TO 75 YEARS)

During this stage, the physical signs of aging and the development of chronic illnesses become more prevalent. Strength diminishes, as do many senses, such as hearing and sight. Retirement may place the older adult on a fixed income, but

FIGURE 6-9

Many middle adults have raised their families and now have more time to reconnect as a couple and pursue their own interests and hobbies. (© *Chuck Savage/CORBIS*.)

FIGURE 6-11

Many older adults feel that they have lived a good life. (© *Bill Binzen/CORBIS*.)

OLDER ADULTHOOD (75 YEARS AND BEYOND)

During this stage, a primary task is preparing for one's own death. Although some older adults continue to be relatively healthy and independent, many must adjust to failing health and a growing dependency on others. Even if their health or physical abilities prevent them from being totally independent, many older adults continue to feel fulfilled and needed until death, and enjoy sharing the wisdom of their years with younger people (Fig. 6-11).

BASIC HUMAN NEEDS

Clearly, all patients and residents are not alike. The people you will care for will be in different growth and development stages, and as such, they will have different needs. The primary mission of health care is to administer to the physical and emotional needs of those we care for. But what exactly are needs?

MASLOW'S HIERARCHY OF HUMAN NEEDS

A **need** can be defined as something that is essential for a person's physical and mental health. Abraham Maslow (1908–1970), a famous American psychologist, defined what he thought

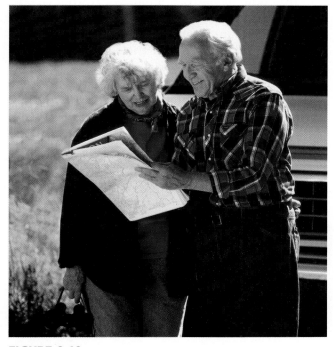

FIGURE 6-10

During late adulthood, many people retire from their careers and begin to enjoy the results of a lifetime of hard work, such as grandchildren and travel.

those who have planned wisely are able to travel and pursue hobbies that they did not have time for when they were employed (Fig. 6-10). During this stage, many people must cope with the loss of friends or a spouse due to death.

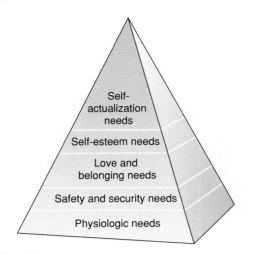

FIGURE 6-12

Maslow's hierarchy of human needs. A "hierarchy" shows the relationship of one idea to another. By arranging the basic human needs in a pyramid shape, Maslow created a visual representation of the idea that basic needs must be fulfilled before more complex ones.

to be the basic human needs, and then arranged them in a pyramid to show that certain needs are more basic than other needs (Fig. 6-12). Maslow's pyramid, called *Maslow's hierarchy of human needs,* reflects Maslow's belief that the more basic, lower-level needs must be met, at least to some degree, before the higher-level needs can be met. Many people can meet their needs with little or no outside help. But people who are ill, injured, or disabled must rely on the help of the health care team to make sure that their needs are met.

Physiologic Needs

The most basic level in Maslow's hierarchy of needs is the physiologic (physical) needs, such as oxygen, water, food, shelter, elimination, rest and sleep, physical activity, and sexuality. Meeting the physiologic needs is essential for survival. Therefore, meeting these needs is of the highest priority. A person must have enough oxygen or he will die within minutes. Water and food are essential for life, as is the ability of the body to eliminate waste products, such as carbon dioxide, urine, and feces. Shelter protects a person from the elements and extremes in temperature. Rest and sleep are essential for preventing physical exhaustion, which can lead to

disability and illness. Physical activity keeps the nervous, skeletal, and muscular systems functioning and prevents wasting. Sexuality involves both the individual's need to have a sexual identity, as well as the need to engage in sexual activity, which allows for a species to reproduce and avoid extinction. Nursing assistants perform many duties that assist patients in meeting their physiologic needs: Assisting with meals, toileting, and ambulating and providing a relaxing environment in which to sleep are just some of the many ways you will help people to meet their most basic needs (Fig. 6-13).

Safety and Security Needs

Safety and security needs are both physical and emotional. Not only must we *be* safe, we must also *feel* safe. For example, parents of young children take measures, such as covering electrical outlets, padding sharp surfaces, and keeping household cleaners and medications in a locked cabinet, to make sure that their children remain physically safe from harm. Nursing assistants follow policies and procedures that are designed to ensure their own safety, as well as that of their patients or residents. For example, to prevent the spread of infection, a nursing assistant follows the procedure for handwashing. In order to protect a resident who is at risk for falling, the

FIGURE 6-13

The nursing assistant shown here is helping her resident to meet her need for nutrition, one of the most basic human needs.

nursing assistant always makes sure that the resident has his walker close at hand. In the next unit, Unit 2, you will learn about the many ways in which nursing assistants work to ensure their own safety, as well as that of the people they care for.

The emotional part of safety and security involves trusting others and being free of fear of harm. For example, parents help their children feel safe and secure by tucking them into bed at night, establishing routines, and letting them know that "mommy and daddy will always be there." A nursing assistant can help a patient or resident feel safe by remembering that the entire experience of being in an unfamiliar place and having unfamiliar tests and treatments done is very frightening for many people. By explaining procedures and having questions answered promptly, the nursing assistant can help to relieve much of this anxiety (Fig. 6-14).

Love and Belonging Needs

All people need to feel loved, accepted, and appreciated by others. People meet this need for one another by showing affection and forming close (intimate) relationships. Family life helps us to meet our love and belonging needs. We need to feel that we are part of an accepting group. When this need is unmet, feelings of loneliness and isolation develop. Babies and children fail to grow, and older people can actually "die of loneliness." Being a patient or a resident in a health care facility can cause a person to feel isolated, unlovable, and unappreciated. Patients and residents often feel that they have become a medical condition, instead of a person. By taking an interest in the person and showing respect for the person's specific likes and dislikes, nursing assistants can help to meet that person's need to feel loved, accepted, and appreciated by others. A smile, a kind word, or a gentle touch can go a long way toward making someone feel loved, appreciated, and like she "belongs" (Fig. 6-15).

Self-Esteem Needs

Self-esteem is influenced by how a person perceives herself, and how she thinks others perceive her. Everyone wants to be respected and thought well of by others. Being hospitalized or moving to a long-term care facility can affect a person's self-esteem in many ways. Many things can affect the self-esteem of a person who is receiving health care, such as:

- Having to wear a hospital gown
- Having surgery that might cause the person's physical appearance to change
- Having to depend on others for something one used to be able to do for oneself

Nursing assistants help to preserve their patients' and residents' self-esteem by providing for

FIGURE 6-14

Understanding how the bed-positioning controls work can make a nervous patient or resident feel more secure in her unfamiliar environment.

FIGURE 6-15

All human beings need to feel that they are loved and needed by others.

FIGURE 6-16
By helping this resident to look her best, this nursing assistant is helping to foster the resident's self-esteem.

FIGURE 6-17
Helping patients and residents to set small, realistic goals helps them to meet their need for self-actualization.

privacy when it is necessary to expose someone's body, by allowing people to wear their own clothing (as opposed to a hospital gown) whenever possible, and by assisting people with basic grooming (Fig. 6-16).

Self-Actualization Needs

The highest level on the hierarchy of needs is self-actualization. In order to achieve self-actualization, a person must reach his or her fullest potential. Most of us try throughout life to meet this need, because we are constantly setting new goals for ourselves. As a health care worker, you will have the unique opportunity to help the people you care for achieve self-actualization, by helping them to set small, realistic goals for a positive outcome (Fig. 6-17). Examples of goals that patients or residents may have include taking one step (for a person who has had a stroke), delivering a healthy baby (for a pregnant woman), or returning home (for a person who has broken a hip).

The needs of the people you care for will change as their conditions improve or decline. By helping people to meet their most essential needs first, you will enable them to meet their higher-level needs. For example, it is difficult to work on a person's self-esteem if he is struggling to breathe! Recognizing needs that people have difficulty meeting on their own, and helping them to meet these needs, is one of the most valuable contributions you will make as a nursing assistant.

HUMAN SEXUALITY AND INTIMACY

All human beings are sexual beings. **Sexuality** is an integral part of our personalities; it is how a person perceives his or her maleness or femaleness. Sexuality differs from **intimacy,** which is a feeling of emotional closeness to another, and **sex,** which is the physical activity one engages in to obtain sexual pleasure and reproduce. A person's sexuality can be influenced by many factors, including the person's culture and religious beliefs. From birth, we are surrounded by symbols of our sexuality—little boys receive baseball mitts and miniature toolboxes "just like Dad's"; little girls receive dolls and tea sets (Fig. 6-18). We grow up being taught by our parents and peers what is appropriate behavior for a "little girl" or for a "big boy."

As we progress through the developmental stages of life, we develop personal ideas and beliefs about our own sexuality. Many women like to express their sexuality by dressing in a feminine manner and wearing make-up, whereas others may prefer a more casual, natural look. Men also have preferences in their dress. For example, some feel most masculine in suits and ties, others in jeans and boots. People also develop preferences for the types of people they are sexually attracted to. For example, **heterosexuals** are attracted to members of the opposite sex, whereas **homosexuals** are attracted to members of the

FIGURE 6-18

Society influences our ideas about our sexuality from an early age.

same sex. **Bisexuals** are attracted to members of both sexes.

Sometimes, a person's feelings about his or her sexuality do not correspond with the person's physical body. These people, called **transsexuals,** believe that they should be members of the opposite sex. Some transsexuals have a surgical procedure (a "sex change operation") to physically become a member of the opposite sex, after receiving psychiatric counseling to ensure that they are good candidates for the surgery. In other cases, the way a person chooses to express his or her sexuality does not match what society has defined as typically "male" or "female." For example, a **transvestite** is a person who becomes sexually excited by dressing as a member of the opposite sex. Most transvestites are men who prefer to dress like women. A person with transvestite tendencies is not necessarily a transsexual or a homosexual—in fact, most transvestites are heterosexual men.

As a nursing assistant, you will meet people whose feelings about their sexuality, and the ways in which they express these feelings, might be very different from your feelings about your sexuality and the way you express those feelings. You must avoid being judgmental or critical of how another person chooses to express his or her sexuality. Acceptance of another person's views does not mean that you approve of that person's beliefs and practices. It only means that you respect that person's right to make his or her own decisions.

Because society so often associates youth and beauty with sexuality, we often do not consider the sexual needs of aging people. Sexuality (or the need to perceive oneself as a sexual being) and intimacy (the need to share emotional closeness with another) are basic human needs, common to all people, young and old (Fig. 6-19). Many elderly people in long-term care facilities have lost their sexual partners, either as a result of death or divorce. Quite often, they have the chance to find happiness again in their golden years with someone they meet in a nursing facility.

There are many ways that, as a nursing assistant, you can help patients and residents to fulfill their need to be thought of as sexual beings, and to engage in intimate relationships with others:

- Avoid being judgmental.
- Help your patients and residents with rituals that make them feel either feminine or masculine, such as dressing and applying make-up, perfume, or aftershave lotion.
- Allow for privacy. If the person is in a private room, close the door and use a "do not disturb" sign as the person requests. If the person has a roommate, suggest to the roommate that the two of you take a walk or participate in another activity, outside of the room. Privacy is necessary for people in

FIGURE 6-19

Although sexual activity is a part of some intimate relationships, it is not necessarily a part of all. Many people share intimacy by just cuddling or caressing. Sometimes illness or physical disabilities make coitus (sexual intercourse) difficult or impossible, but there are other ways in which two people can love each other. (*©CORBIS.*)

intimate relationships, whether or not they involve **coitus** (sexual intercourse). It is also necessary for people who want to engage in **masturbation** (stimulation of the genitals for sexual pleasure or release, by a means other than sexual intercourse).

- If a person is masturbating in a public room (some confused patients or residents will do this), take the person to his or her room and provide for safety and privacy.
- Always knock before entering a person's room. If you do interrupt a sexual encounter, excuse yourself quietly and say you will return later.

Some people become sexually aggressive and will behave in an unpleasant or unwelcome way toward you or another patient or resident. It is important for you to be able to recognize situations that could be considered sexual abuse or assault. However, before you get upset and report the person's inappropriate behavior to a supervisor, stop and think about a few things. Although a patient or resident, especially if he or she is elderly, may seem unattractive to you, think about what that person sees when he or she looks at you. You may be young and very attractive. You may remind the patient or resident of his or her spouse, when that person was young. The patient or resident may have poor eyesight and mistake you for someone else, or he or she may be confused or disoriented as a result of a disease process. Although it is totally inappropriate for you to attend to the sexual needs of your patients or residents, it is important to avoid being unkind or hateful in your response. Depending on the situation, tell the patient or resident kindly, yet firmly, that you are not going to do what he or she is asking you to do, or that he or she must not touch you in that manner. Avoid giggling or teasing the patient or resident in a flirtatious manner. This will only serve to reinforce the inappropriate behavior. If the behavior does not stop, or if the behavior is directed at another patient or resident, you should discuss the matter with your supervisor.

CULTURE AND RELIGION

You can see that there are many things that, as human beings, we all have in common. For example, everyone has the same basic needs, although some needs may be more pressing than others at any given time for any one individual. Similarly, we all pass through the same stages of growth and development, although not at the same time or at the same rate. Culture, the subject of this section, is another thing that makes human beings human. All people have a culture, although everyone's culture is not the same. **Culture** is made up of the beliefs (including religious or spiritual beliefs), values, and traditions that are customary to a group of people. It is a view of the world that is handed down from generation to generation. A culture can be shared by people of the same race or ethnicity, by people who live within the same geographic area or speak the same language, or by a combination of these two (Fig. 6-20). While racial identity is often mixed with a person's culture, **race** is a general characterization that describes skin color, body stature, facial features, and hair texture.

One of the most unique things about the United States is the diversity of cultures that are represented here. Diversity has enriched this country, yet problems can arise when people are not sensitive to, or respectful of, the cultural uniqueness of each individual. As a health care worker, it is important for you to learn as much as possible about the characteristics of other cultural or ethnic groups of people, because your patients or residents will have cultural differences

FIGURE 6-20

This African-American family is celebrating Kwanzaa, a holiday celebrated by Africans and people of African descent throughout the world. Kwanzaa, a celebration of African history and culture, with a special emphasis on family life, occurs from December 26 through January 1. Kwanzaa is a cultural holiday, not a religious one. Celebrants are united by their African heritage, not their religion. (©*Lawrence Migdale*.)

that may affect their preferences regarding health care. Additionally, a primary goal of the nursing team is to provide for the comfort of those we care for. A person who feels that his culture is not understood or respected by the people who are caring for him will feel uncomfortable.

There are many ways in which a health care worker can accidentally be disrespectful of a patient's or resident's culture, which can lead to conflict. Sometimes, misunderstandings occur simply because a health care worker is not aware of how a certain person's culture influences her behavior. Although it is difficult to make generalizations about culture—not everyone from the same geographic region, or with the same skin tone, necessarily has the same beliefs or value system—being aware of what a patient or resident is telling you can help you to know when cultural differences need to be taken into account. Areas where culture and health care often intersect include beliefs and practices associated with food and meals; religious beliefs and practices; and attitudes toward health, sickness, and death.

Liking certain types of food, or food prepared a specific way, is very cultural. For example, a person from the southern United States may prefer "grits" (cornmeal) to oatmeal. Sometimes, a patient or resident may request or refuse a certain food or combination of foods in order to follow religious beliefs or practices. For example, a person of the Catholic faith may not want to eat meat on Fridays during Lent, and a person of the Jewish faith may follow the practice of not drinking milk with a meal that contains meat. In some cultures, it is believed that certain combinations of foods can aid or inhibit healing. For example, according to Taoism (a philosophy that originated in Asia), illness occurs when the body is out of balance. To restore balance, certain foods may be chosen over others. If one of your patients or residents requests or denies a certain food or combination of foods for religious or other reasons, be sure to tell the nurse. She will work with the dietary department to meet the person's request.

A person's spiritual beliefs, or **religion,** are often very closely linked with his or her culture. Members of some cultural groups have certain rituals that they feel will bring them good luck or aid in healing. For example, you may encounter a person from Turkey who believes

hanging an "evil eye" talisman will ward off bad spirits, or a person from Panama who believes that wearing strings on the wrist will relieve pain. A person might want to light candles while praying to a specific saint. Many people are very spiritual and find comfort and solace in prayer, reading scriptures or spiritual books, singing, and praying. If a patient or resident asks to see a spiritual leader or clergy member, communicate the request promptly and according to your facility's policy, and allow for privacy during the visit. Other persons' religious beliefs may be very different from yours, but you can be certain that their beliefs are as important to them as yours are to you. You do not have to believe in a person's religion to offer the kind of care that reading their scriptures to them when they cannot will show (Fig. 6-21).

There are other examples of cultural practices that we must be respectful of, even if we think they are wrong. Remember, your culture gave you your value system, and your patient's or resident's culture gave her hers. Respecting another person's values does not mean that you have to agree with that person, or her values. For example, some cultures do not allow women certain freedoms that we take for granted in this country. Imagine that you are a male nursing assistant, caring for a Middle Eastern woman. In some Middle Eastern cultures, a woman is not allowed to be questioned or examined by a male health care provider unless her husband is present. Your patient's husband has not yet

FIGURE 6-21

A nursing assistant can help people to obtain comfort from their religious beliefs, even if he or she does not share those same beliefs.

arrived at the hospital, and you need to perform a procedure for this patient. Although it would be tempting to go ahead with the procedure without the husband present, you know that your patient would not be comfortable if you were to put her in a difficult situation. You would be devaluing her belief system by trying to overrule it.

Throughout your career, you may be lucky enough to care for people from many different cultural and religious backgrounds. You will most likely encounter situations, practices, and beliefs that no book could have prepared you for! Take time to listen to your patients or residents, and to learn from them. Exposure to cultures other than your own is enriching, both professionally and personally.

RESPECTING THE INDIVIDUAL

As a health care professional, you are trained to care for a person's physical needs. Treating illness and promoting good health are two primary goals of all health care providers. However, sometimes we are so focused on treating a patient's or resident's problems, we forget to consider the desires of the individual. A holistic approach to health care, as you have learned, takes into consideration a person's emotional needs as well as his or her physical ones. Making an effort to accommodate a person's cultural beliefs and practices is one way that health care workers provide holistic care. Another way is by allowing patients and residents to make decisions related to their own quality of life.

As a nursing assistant, you will learn that a person who has diabetes must control her diet carefully. You will learn that a person with heart disease should eat fewer foods high in cholesterol and stop smoking. But, what if your patient or resident does not comply with the recommendations of the health care team? Is the woman with diabetes a bad person if she truly loves sweets and does not want to give them up? Is the man with heart disease a bad person if he cannot bear to give up his daily breakfast of eggs and bacon at the diner? What if a person refuses a treatment or surgery that may prolong his or her life? Should the health care profession simply write that per-

son off and focus only on those willing to follow medical advice?

If a health care worker gives a person the proper information about his illness or condition, and educates him about the steps that can be taken to treat or resolve the condition, then the health care worker has provided the person with the information he needs to make a conscientious decision concerning his own health. The person must make these decisions according to his own personal values and sense of what is best for himself, as an individual. This is where the idea of *quality of life* comes into play. Quality of life has to do with getting satisfaction and comfort from the way we are living. The idea of what quality of life means differs for each person and may vary as a person's situation changes. For example, during your career as a health care worker, you will care for terminally ill people who want every treatment available to help them fight for life, even if the procedures are dangerous or painful. You will also care for terminally ill people who decline painful or risky treatments because they feel that their ability to enjoy life and derive pleasure from living will be too compromised by the treatments. Each of your patients and residents must be allowed to make decisions concerning his or her quality of life. In order to provide holistic care for your patients or residents, you must respect their decisions related to maintaining their quality of life.

WHAT IS IT LIKE TO BE A PATIENT OR RESIDENT?

Focus for a moment on why people need health care and what it is like to be a patient or resident. Being sick, injured, or unable to care for oneself creates a state where a person will need the services the health care industry offers. People do not choose illness or infirmity, and most very desperately want to "get better" quickly.

What is it like to be a patient? Patients feel scared and lonely. They feel sick. They are unsure about their health, now and in the future. Some patients worry about whether they will be able to return to work, and they are concerned about how their illness will affect the financial future of their families. Others worry about how they will look after surgery (e.g., a woman who has had a mastectomy to treat breast cancer may worry that her husband will no longer find her attractive). Some medical treatments can also cause a change in a person's physical appearance (e.g., loss of hair as a result of chemotherapy). Patients worry about spouses, children, and pets at home, and whether they are being cared for properly. They worry about the emotional effects of their illness on their family members. The hospital environment itself can be frightening and uncomfortable, full of strange noises and smells. If you were in this circumstance, how would you feel and how might this affect your behavior?

Similarly, what is it like to be a resident? Imagine what it would be like to have to move from a home you loved to a long-term care facility. You have lived a long, full life. You have worked hard and raised a family. You really liked your little house with your cat and the shady back porch where you could sit on hot summer evenings. Now, you are not managing as well as you once did—you have fallen twice, and left the teakettle on numerous times and forgotten about it. Even though, logically, you know it makes sense to move to a place where there is always someone around to "take care of you," when you gave up your home, you gave up a certain amount of your independence along with it. You cannot take all of your furniture, and you must find a new home for your beloved pet cat. You have a roommate (at your age!) and you have to eat the meals that are prepared for you, when they are served to you. Gone are the lazy summer evenings eating peaches on the porch for dinner and relaxing in the bathtub with a glass of wine. How would you feel about this loss of independence, and how might this affect your behavior?

People who find themselves as patients and residents often feel that they are at the mercy of the health care industry. While some patients and residents are cheerful, compliant, and grateful, others may be depressed, angry, anxious, or just downright mean. When you must care for a patient or resident who makes you wish you had never chosen to be a nursing assistant (and you can be certain you *will* encounter patients or residents like this), stop and think for a moment about the reasons that person may be acting out of sorts. When you look beyond the illness or condition,

past the technical duties and procedures, and into that person's eyes, you will find your reason for choosing to be a nursing assistant...a person who needs you very much.

SUMMARY

▶ Patients, residents, and clients are people who need the services of the health care industry because they are sick, injured, or unable to care for themselves.
  ■ Acute, chronic, or terminal illnesses can cause a person to need health care services.
  ■ People in health care settings are grouped according to their ages, illnesses or medical conditions, or special health care needs.
▶ People in health care settings have many different physical and emotional needs.
  ■ Basic needs must be met before higher-level needs can be met.
  ■ Maslow's hierarchy of human needs includes physiologic needs, safety and security needs, love and belonging needs, self-esteem needs, and self-actualization needs.
  ■ Sexuality is how a person perceives his or her maleness or femaleness. Sexuality differs from intimacy (the need to feel emotionally close to another person) and from sex (a physical act engaged in for pleasure and reproduction). Sexuality and intimacy are basic human needs.
  ■ Patients and residents who are not able to meet their needs on their own rely on the health care team to recognize and help meet these needs for them.
▶ The people you will care for are individuals, with unique feelings, memories, goals, and personalities.
  ■ You will care for people in varying stages of growth and development.
  ■ You will care for people from different cultural and religious backgrounds.
  ■ Recognizing and respecting the differences in the people you care for will allow you to provide holistic care. When you provide holistic care, you make a difference in the lives of your patients or residents and their family members.

What did you learn?

Multiple Choice

Select the single best answer for each of the following questions.

1. Sally is caring for Mrs. Norville, who lives in a long-term care facility. Sally encourages Mrs. Norville to make her own decisions about what to do each day. She helps her with dressing and grooming, but lets her do as much as she can for herself. These activities help fulfill Mrs. Norville's need for:
   a. Security
   b. Shelter
   c. Spirituality
   d. Self-esteem

2. When caring for people from different cultures, you should try to:
   a. Understand and respect their special needs
   b. Encourage them to change their beliefs while in your facility
   c. Pretend that the cultural differences do not exist
   d. Avoid talking to them

3. Which one of the following is an example of an acute condition?
   a. Appendicitis
   b. Emphysema
   c. Diabetes
   d. High blood pressure (hypertension)

4. A resident's religion forbids him from eating pork. Pork chops are being served for dinner. What should you do?
   a. Tell the resident that religious restrictions on diet do not count in times of illness
   b. Ask the nurse to call the dietary department
   c. Insist that the resident eat the pork, because it contains protein, an essential nutrient
   d. Reassure the resident by telling him that the doctor ordered this diet

5. A resident in a long-term care facility may show her sexuality by doing all of the following except:
   a. Desiring sexual intercourse
   b. Engaging in public fondling
   c. Giving her granddaughter a doll for her birthday
   d. Applying make-up and scented powder before receiving a male visitor

6. Which one of the following is not a basic human need?
   a. Fear
   b. Self-actualization
   c. Self-esteem
   d. Water

7. Which one of the following is a basic social need?
   a. Food
   b. Water
   c. Air
   d. Love

8. What is a person who becomes sexually excited by dressing as a member of the opposite sex called?
   a. A transsexual
   b. A transvestite
   c. A bisexual
   d. A homosexual

Matching

Match each numbered item with its appropriate lettered description.

1. Infancy
2. Toddlerhood
3. Preschool
4. School-age
5. Adolescence
6. Middle adulthood
7. Older adulthood

_____ **a.** A 16-year-old girl going to the junior prom

_____ **b.** A 42-year-old executive running his own company

_____ **c.** A 2-year-old boy starting toilet training

_____ **d.** A 6-month-old girl learning to sit up

_____ **e.** A 92-year-old great-grand-mother moving to a long-term care facility

_____ **f.** A 4-year-old boy learning to tie his shoes

_____ **g.** An 11-year-old Boy Scout participating in his troop's annual canned food drive

? Stop and think!

▶ You are caring for Mr. Spencer, whose wife passed away several years ago. When you enter his room, after knocking to announce yourself, you find Mr. Spencer being fondled by Miss Rich, another resident. You are embarrassed, as well as somewhat disgusted—you were raised to believe that sex is something that only married people engage in. What should you do?

Nursing Assistants Make a Difference!

"I have spent more than 20 years working as an operating room nurse. A few years ago, I took a job working in an outpatient surgical department, where I cared for many elderly patients who were having cataract surgery. Many of these elderly patients were very healthy, and excited about having surgery to restore their vision.

One day, we were scheduled to perform cataract surgery on a resident from a local nursing home, Mrs. Lindgren. I was somewhat surprised to meet my patient! Mrs. Lindgren had Alzheimer's disease and was quite confused. She also hadn't walked for more than a year, and spent her days in a wheelchair. Susan, a nursing assistant who had cared for Mrs. Lindgren regularly for about 3 years, came with her to the surgery. Needless to say, I questioned the wisdom of putting Mrs. Lindgren through surgery, which would most certainly be a frightening experience for her. What was the surgeon thinking?

When I expressed my concerns to Susan, she told me a little bit about Mrs. Lindgren. Susan told me that before Mrs. Lindgren's Alzheimer's disease had progressed to the point where she was no longer able to care for herself, she had loved to sit in her garden and watch the birds gather around the many bird feeders that she kept filled. Knowing this, Susan began to take Mrs. Lindgren into the garden at the nursing home so that she could enjoy the birds there. However, over the course of the last 3 years, Mrs. Lindgren's cataracts had gotten so bad that now, all she could do was sit and listen to the birds. Susan noticed that the birds still gave Mrs. Lindgren great pleasure, and when she mentioned this fact to Mrs. Lindgren's family, they began to think about how they could help Mrs. Lindgren to see the birds again. The hope was that restoring Mrs. Lindgren's eyesight would bring some light and enjoyment into a life that had gone dark in more ways than one.

On hearing Susan's explanation, I felt ashamed that I had questioned the necessity of the eye surgery for Mrs. Lindgren. Susan's ability to focus on her resident and her specific needs was certainly a lesson this nurse needed to relearn. Now, as I teach other health care professionals, I always remember Susan and Mrs. Lindgren and I try to share the lesson that compassionate nursing assistant taught me."

You can listen to more stories about how nursing assistants make a difference on the CD in the back of your book.

Safety

As you have learned, being a nursing assistant is physically demanding work that places you in close contact with people. Many of the people you will care for will be ill, injured, frail, or a combination of the three. Not only must you know how to protect yourself in the workplace (from communicable disease and from physical injury), but you must also know how to protect those entrusted to your care. Maintaining safety is the focus of Unit 2.

Photo: A nursing assistant helps a resident to walk safely.

107

Communicable Disease and Infection Control

What will you learn?

Communicable diseases are diseases that can be spread from one person to another. There are many factors that come together in the health care setting to make it easy for communicable diseases to spread. In this chapter, you will learn how to minimize these factors, so that you can protect yourself, your family members, and your patients or residents from catching a communicable disease. You will also learn about the causes of communicable disease, and the ways communicable diseases are spread from one person to another. After all, it is hard to protect yourself and others from communicable disease if you do not know what causes it or how it is spread! When you are finished with this chapter, you will be able to:

1. List the different types of "germs" (microbes) that cause disease and discuss the conditions that are essential for their survival and growth.
2. Define the terms *normal flora* and *pathogen*.
3. Define the term *infection* and describe the chain of events required for infection to occur.
4. Explain the defense mechanisms the body uses to fight infection.
5. Discuss factors that affect the proper functioning of the immune system.
6. Define the term *nosocomial* and discuss ways a person could get an infection within the health care system.
7. Discuss the techniques of medical asepsis and infection control.

(continued)

Photo: Escherichia coli, *a microbe that can cause disease. Color was added to this photograph, which was taken with a special microscope.*
(©Howard Sochurek/CORBIS.)

8. Describe methods used in the health care setting to destroy microbes.
9. State how personal protective equipment (PPE) is used in infection control.
10. Explain how isolation (transmission-based) precautions are used to help prevent the spread of infection.
11. Demonstrate proper handwashing, gloving, masking, gowning, and double-bagging technique.

Vocabulary

Use the CD in the back of your book to hear these terms pronounced, defined, and used in a sentence:

Communicable disease	Methicillin-resistant *Staphylococcus aureus* (MRSA)	Vector	Personal protective equipment (PPE)
Microbe (microorganism)		Virulence	Isolation (transmission-based) precautions
Normal (resident) flora	Vancomycin-resistant enterococcus (VRE)	Nosocomial	
Pathogens		Infection control	Airborne precautions
Opportunistic microbes	Infection	Medical asepsis	Droplet precautions
Colonies	Chain of infection	Sanitization	Contact precautions
Aerobic	Contaminated	Antisepsis	
Anaerobic	Fomite	Disinfection	
Antibodies		Sterilization	
		Transient flora	

WHAT IS A MICROBE?

You may recall from one of your science classes that all plants and animals are made up of cells, the basic unit of life. You may have even looked at one of your own cells (from the inside of your cheek) or the cell of an onion plant under a microscope, a tool used to see structures that are not visible to the naked eye. Maybe you even studied the structures of a typical animal or plant cell, such as the nucleus and cell wall.

A **microbe,** also called a **microorganism,** is a living thing that cannot be seen with the naked eye. Many (but not all) microbes consist of just one cell. (To give you an idea of how small a cell is, consider that it is estimated that the adult human body is composed of approximately 50 million *million* cells!) Microbes are found in the air, in the soil, in water, in food, and in and on the bodies of plants and animals, including humans.

Most microbes cause no harm and are actually essential for healthy living. For example, some of the microbes that live in the human digestive tract help us to get certain vitamins from the foods that we eat. Others help to maintain an environment that is unfriendly to harmful microbes. The harmless microbes that help the human body to function properly are called **normal (resident) flora.**

Some microbes, however, can cause illness and are known as **pathogens.** Sometimes microbes can be considered normal flora in one part of the body and pathogens in another. For example, *Escherichia coli* is a microbe that normally lives in our large intestines, where it is harmless. However, when *E. coli* finds its way out of the intestine and into another part of the body where it is not normal flora, such as the bladder, it can cause an infection. These types of microbes are called **opportunistic microbes.** Given the chance, opportunistic microbes can change from harmless to pathogenic.

There are many different types of microbes that live and prosper among us. Microbes can generally be classified as bacteria, viruses, fungi, or parasites (Table 7-1).

BACTERIA

Bacteria cause many of the infections you will encounter in the health care setting. Many scientists believe that bacteria lived on Earth long

TABLE 7-1 ■ Types of Microbes

	Type	Examples of Commonly Caused Infections
	Bacteria	"Strep throat," urinary tract infections, abscesses, tuberculosis (TB), bacterial meningitis, Lyme disease, Rocky Mountain spotted fever, syphilis
	Viruses	HIV/AIDS, hepatitis, fever blisters, common cold
	Fungi	Ringworm, "athlete's foot," vaginal yeast infections (candidiasis), oral yeast infections (thrush)
	Parasites	
	Insects	Scabies, pediculosis (lice)
	Helminths (worms)	Pinworm infestation
	Protozoa	Malaria, amebic dysentery

Top to bottom: *Lester V. Bergman/CORBIS. ©Ron Boardman; Frank Lane Picture Agency/CORBIS. ©Lester V. Bergman/CORBIS. ©Mike Buxton; Papilio/CORBIS. ©Lloyd Birmingham/Custom Medical Stock Photo.©Lester V. Bergman/CORBIS.*

before any other life forms. Bacteria have been found in polar ice caps, as well as in deep cracks in the ocean floor. The ability of bacteria to adapt to all sorts of environments is proof of this life form's ability to survive.

Most bacteria consist of only one cell, and reproduce by dividing in half. Although bacteria usually consist of only one cell, they often group together to form **colonies.** Scientists classify and name bacteria in many different ways:

- By their shape
- By the way they arrange themselves in a colony
- By the way they stain (how they react to the dye scientists use to make microbes more visible under a microscope)

For example, round bacteria are called *cocci,* rod-shaped bacteria are called *bacilli,* and spiral-shaped or curved bacteria are called *spirilla* (Fig. 7-1). Bacterial colonies may consist of pairs of bacteria (indicated by the prefix *diplo-*), chains of bacteria (indicated by the prefix *strepto-*), or grape-like clusters of bacteria (indicated by the prefix *staphylo-*). So, what would you know if you saw the word *Staphylococcus aureus* on a person's medical record? You would know that this person had an infection caused by a round bacterium (*-coccus*) that arranges itself in clusters (*Staphylo-*)! There are thousands of types of bacteria and not all of them are named using this method. However, this example illustrates how you can learn the meaning of a word that might be unfamiliar to you by taking it apart. In Appendix C, "Introduction to the Language of Health Care," you can learn about many more prefixes, suffixes, and roots that are used to form words commonly used in the health care setting.

Bacteria, like all other living things, have certain basic requirements for survival. These requirements vary, according to the type of bacteria. For example, some bacteria, called **aerobic** bacteria, need oxygen to live. Others, called **anaerobic** bacteria, die if oxygen is present. Most bacteria that can cause illness need a warm, moist, dark environment and a source of nutrition in order to grow—requirements the inside of the human body meets perfectly! Some types of bacteria can surround themselves with a hard shell, called an *endospore,* and enter a state of inactivity. If the inactive bacterium's best growing conditions become available, the bacterium will become active again. Because of their protective endospores, these types of bacteria are very difficult to kill using the standard techniques described later in this chapter. Examples of illnesses caused by bacteria that form endospores include tetanus (lockjaw) and botulism (food poisoning).

Bacteria are the most common cause of infection in the health care setting. Some common illnesses caused by bacteria include "strep throat" (caused by *Streptococcus pyogenes*), some bladder infections (such as those caused by *E. coli*), and some skin infections (such as those caused by *S. aureus*). Several types of small, rod-shaped bacteria are transmitted by ticks and fleas and cause diseases such as Rocky Mountain spotted fever and typhus. Bacteria are also responsible for some types of pneumonia and some infections of the reproductive and urinary systems.

VIRUSES

Viruses, the smallest of all microbes, can only be seen using a special kind of microscope, called an electron microscope. Viruses are not even complete cells—they are just small bundles of protein. Because viruses are not complete cells, they cannot carry out normal cellular activities, such as reproduction, by themselves. Instead, they must take over a host cell, usually a plant or animal cell. Once inside the host cell, the virus uses the host cell's "machinery" to make copies of itself. Eventually, the virus and all of its copies (called *progeny*) break through the host cell's wall, killing the host cell and freeing the viruses to infect other, neighboring host cells. Many illnesses are caused by viruses, including the common cold, fever blisters (caused by herpes simplex virus), chickenpox (caused by varicella zoster virus), hepatitis, and acquired immunodeficiency syndrome (AIDS, caused by human immunodeficiency virus, or HIV).

A. Cocci (spheres)   B. Bacilli (rods)   C. Spirilla (spirals)

FIGURE 7-1

Bacteria can be spherical, rod-shaped, or spiral-shaped.

FUNGI

Fungi are a group of plant-like organisms that scientists have classified together because of certain characteristics, including the make-up of their cell walls. Not all fungi are microscopic—for example, mushrooms are a type of fungus! Other types of fungi you may be familiar with include yeasts (such as the yeast that is used to make bread rise and beer foamy) and molds (such as the mildew that grows inside a shower stall or the growths that appear on bread and cheese if left too long). Many fungi help us (or, at least, do not harm us). However, some fungi are capable of causing illness. If you have ever had ringworm (caused by *Tinea corporis*), athlete's foot (caused by *Tinea pedis*), thrush (a yeast infection in the mouth), or candidiasis (a vaginal yeast infection), then you have been the victim of a fungus!

PARASITES

Parasites live in or on a host, such as a plant or animal, and use that host for food and protection. Some parasites can be transmitted from one person to another through physical contact. For example, scabies, an itchy skin condition, is caused by a mite that burrows under the skin. Pediculosis (lice) is caused by wingless insects that live on the scalp or body and feed on the host's blood. Both scabies and lice are often seen in the health care setting. Other parasites are transferred from one person to another through feces or blood.

Helminths, a type of parasite, are worm-like organisms that live in the human body (as well as the bodies of other animals). Examples of helminths include pinworms, tapeworms, and roundworms. Although the way these organisms are transmitted from one host to another varies, transmission usually involves eating or inhaling the worm eggs, which then grow in the host's digestive tract. The mature worms produce eggs or larvae of their own, which are then passed out of the host's body with the feces. Once the eggs reach the outside world again, they are free to be eaten or inhaled by another host, and the life cycle of the helminth continues.

Protozoa, another type of parasite, are said to be "animal-like" because they can take in food. Protozoa cause illnesses such as malaria (transmitted by the bite of a mosquito) and amebic dysentery (a type of diarrhea caused by drinking water contaminated with protozoa).

DEFENSES AGAINST COMMUNICABLE DISEASE

THE IMMUNE SYSTEM

Many, many microbes share the Earth with us. If microbes are everywhere, and some of them can make us sick, then why aren't we all always sick? The answer to this question lies in the body's immune system, the wonderful defense system that protects us from infection. Some of the body's defenses are nonspecific, which means that they help to protect us from all pathogens. Other defenses are specific, which means that they help to protect us only from certain pathogens.

Nonspecific Defense Mechanisms

Our main nonspecific defense mechanism is healthy, intact skin and mucous membranes. Skin that is without cuts, scrapes, or wounds physically prevents pathogens from entering the body. In addition, the natural lubricants on our skin contain substances that help to prevent the growth of pathogens. Mucous membranes line all of the organ systems that come in contact with the outside world (namely, the respiratory, digestive, urinary, and reproductive systems). The special cells of the mucous membranes secrete mucus, a sticky substance that creates a physical barrier by trapping and destroying pathogens. Keeping the skin clean helps to reduce the number of pathogens on the skin. Good oral hygiene and drinking plenty of fluids helps to keep mucous membranes functioning properly. These are important measures to take for yourself, as well as for your patients or residents. Stomach acid (which kills many of the microbes contained in the food that we eat), tears (which contain a substance that kills microbes), and the acts of coughing and sneezing (which remove inhaled microbes) are also nonspecific defense mechanisms that prevent microbes from "setting up shop" in our bodies.

If a pathogen manages to get past these first lines of defense and an infection results, the body

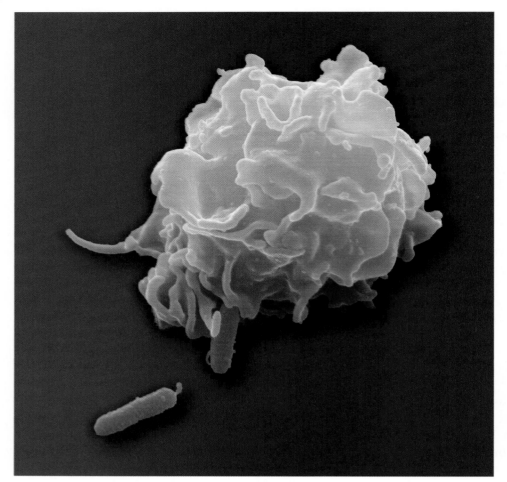

FIGURE 7-2

In this photograph, a white blood cell (*white*) is killing a pathogen (*red*) by eating it. This is a process called phagocytosis (*phago-* means "eat" and *cyt-* means "cell"). (*SPL/Photo Researchers, Inc.*)

activates a general immune response that helps to fight off the infection. Blood vessels around the site of the infection dilate (widen), allowing more blood flow to the area. The increased blood flow brings more oxygen and nutrients to the tissues, along with large numbers of white blood cells (leukocytes). White blood cells destroy pathogens that invade the body, either by ingesting them (Fig. 7-2) or by secreting substances that cause them to die. The increased blood flow causes the infected area to become red, warm, swollen, and painful (Fig. 7-3). A person who is fighting off an infection may have a high body temperature (fever). If you remember, most pathogens prefer a nice, normal body temperature. The fever helps to destroy the pathogens and is a normal response for many infections.

As a nursing assistant, it is important for you to watch for signs of infection in your patients or residents. Many patients or residents may not be able to communicate that they do not feel well or that they have pain. Some infections, if not treated at an early stage, can be very dangerous

for people. If one of your patients or residents has signs or symptoms of an infection, the doctor may order a diagnostic test, called a *culture and sensitivity*, to find out which microbe is causing the infection and which medication is best suited to

FIGURE 7-3

The site of infection is typically hot, red, swollen, and painful. This means the body's general immune response is at work! (*Custom Medical Stock Photo.*)

fight it. The culture and sensitivity may be performed on urine, wound drainage, or other body fluids or substances.

 ## Tell the Nurse!

Possible signs of infection that should be reported to the nurse immediately include:

- An increase in body temperature
- A rapid pulse, a rapid respiratory rate, or changes in blood pressure
- Pain or difficulty breathing
- Redness, swelling, or pain
- Foul-smelling or cloudy urine
- Pain or difficulty urinating
- Diarrhea or foul-smelling feces
- Nausea or vomiting
- Lack of appetite
- Skin rashes
- Fatigue
- Increased confusion or disorientation
- Any unusual discharge or drainage from the body

Specific Defense Mechanisms

The body's nonspecific defense mechanisms, including physical barriers and the general immune response, are one way our immune systems help us to prevent and fight off infections. The immune system also has the ability to develop specialized proteins called **antibodies,** which help our bodies to fight off specific microbes. A person develops antibodies following exposure to the microbe. This exposure may come from a previous infection with the microbe, or through a vaccination (shot). For example, the antibodies that build up in the body following an episode of measles or chickenpox are the reason most of us only get these "childhood diseases" once. Similarly, when you get your annual "flu shot," what you are getting is a dose of the virus strains that cause the flu. The viruses have been killed, so that you do not actually get sick, but the exposure is enough to cause your immune system to begin producing antibodies against those particular strains of the virus. That way, if you are exposed later, you will be immune.

ANTIBIOTICS

Many times, our immune systems can fight off invading pathogens on their own. Other times, however, some outside help is required. An *antibiotic* is a drug that is able to kill bacteria or make it difficult for them to reproduce and grow. The first antibiotic, penicillin, came into widespread use during World War II, and completely changed how we treat infectious disease. Today, there are many types of antibiotics, used to treat many different types of bacterial infections. Antimicrobial agents (used to treat fungal and parasitic infections) and antiviral agents (used to treat some viral infections) are other drugs that we use to treat infection.

The story of the war between humans and pathogens, however, does not end with the invention of antibiotics and associated drugs. Bacteria, as you will recall, are very adaptable organisms that have been around since the beginning of time. As such, some bacteria have used their ability to change to develop resistance to the antibiotics used to fight them. This means that the antibiotics that used to work against these bacteria no longer work. Two types of bacteria, **methicillin-resistant *Staphylococcus aureus* (MRSA)** and **vancomycin-resistant enterococcus (VRE),** have become resistant to two of the most powerful antibiotics we have invented to date (methicillin and vancomycin).

S. aureus and enterococci are common microbes. *S. aureus* is often found on a person's skin and is transmitted easily through person-to-person contact. Enterococci are commonly found in a person's digestive tract and are transmitted through contact with feces. In a health care setting, these pathogens can be very dangerous because many patients and residents do not have healthy immune systems and, therefore, are less able to fight off infection. If infection occurs, it is difficult to treat because these microbes have become resistant to the drugs used to treat them in the past. MRSA and VRE are well-known examples of bacteria that have developed resistance to antibiotics. It is reasonable to expect that in the future, other bacteria will become resistant to antibiotics as well.

Although antibiotics have given us more options for treating infectious disease than we had in the past, they do not work against all pathogens all of the time. The best policy is clearly to avoid infection in the first place. You can keep your immune system strong and healthy through proper nutrition, adequate rest, and regular exercise. You can also take steps to limit your exposure to pathogens. In the next few sections, we will look at how pathogens are spread from one person to another, and what you can do to help control their spread.

COMMUNICABLE DISEASE AND THE CHAIN OF INFECTION

An **infection** is an illness caused by a pathogen (a microbe that can cause illness). Infections can be local (affecting a small, defined area of the body), generalized (affecting a general area or an organ), or systemic (affecting the entire body). Many, but not all, infections are communicable, which means that they can be transmitted from one person to another, either directly or indirectly. Sometimes the terms *communicable* and *contagious* are used to mean the same thing, but the two terms are not truly synonymous. *Contagious* is more accurately used to describe an infection that can be easily transmitted from one person to another through casual contact, such as a common cold. For example, you can get a cold just by touching a button in an elevator after someone who has a cold has touched it, or by sitting next to someone with a cold on a crowded bus. Therefore, a common cold is not only communicable, it is contagious. On the other hand, infections such as AIDS and hepatitis, while still communicable, are not referred to as *contagious* because they are not transmitted through casual contact.

For a person to get a communicable infection, six key conditions must be met. These six key elements are known as the **chain of infection** (Fig. 7-4).

1. A *pathogen* must be present.
2. A *reservoir* must be present. A reservoir is a place where something is stored. In this particular context, a reservoir is a place that is suitable for the pathogen's survival. Pathogens collect in the reservoir, and sometimes, they multiply there as well. Possible reservoirs of pathogens include humans and other animals, food, water, milk, and objects that come in contact with an infected person's secretions or body fluids.

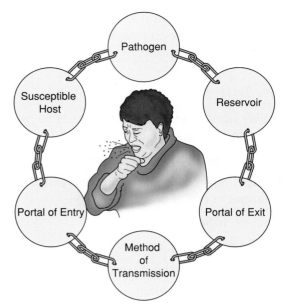

FIGURE 7-4

The chain of infection. For a person to get an infection, all six links in the chain must be present.

3. A *portal of exit* must be available. The portal of exit is the way the pathogen leaves the reservoir. (The word *portal* means "door.") The way a pathogen leaves its reservoir varies, depending on the type of pathogen and the reservoir. For example, when the reservoir is a human being, common portals of exit for pathogens include the digestive tract (through feces, saliva, or vomitus), the respiratory tract (through mucus), the genitourinary tract (through urine, semen, or vaginal secretions), and the skin (through blood, pus, or other drainage from wounds).
4. A *method of transmission* must be available. After the pathogen leaves its reservoir via the portal of exit, it must have a way of physically getting from one person to another. This is called the pathogen's method of transmission, and it may be direct or indirect. Direct transmission requires close contact between an infected and a noninfected person. Pathogens can be directly transmitted when a noninfected person makes physical contact with an infected person, or inhales or ingests droplets exhaled by the infected person (for example, when that person coughs,

FIGURE 7-5
Pathogens can live on objects such as linens, bedpans, and drinking glasses. When an uninfected person touches or uses these items, he might pick up some of the pathogens on them and become sick. Non-living objects that are capable of transmitting disease are called fomites.

talks, or sneezes). Indirect transmission occurs when a noninfected person comes into contact with a non-living object that has been **contaminated** (soiled) by pathogens. These objects are called **fomites.** For example, a water glass or a bed sheet can become a fomite if it becomes contaminated by pathogens from a person with an infection, because if a noninfected person uses the contaminated water glass or sleeps on the contaminated bed linens, he could become infected (Fig. 7-5). Other pathogens, such as the protozoan that causes malaria, are transmitted by way of a **vector,** or a living creature (in the case of malaria, a mosquito). Some pathogens can be transmitted by more than just one method.

5. A *portal of entry* must be available. Now that the pathogen has left its reservoir and been successfully transmitted to another person, it must have a way of entering the new person's body. The respiratory, urinary, digestive, and reproductive systems are common portals of entry. So are breaks in the skin. A pathogen can leave one person's body and be transmitted to another person, but if the pathogen is not able to enter the new person's body, infection will not occur.

6. A *susceptible host* must be available. Microbes that can cause infection enter the human body continuously. The defense systems of the body, both those we are born with and those we acquire (such as vaccines), can fight off most of these pathogens. However, many factors

can place us at risk for infection. This is when the pathogen "makes its move." Risk factors that make a person more likely to get an infection include:

- **Very young or very old age.** The very young and the very old are more likely to get an infection. The young have not had time to develop an effective defense mechanism for fighting infections, and the elderly lose their defenses as they age.
- **Poor general health.** A person who is sick or debilitated ("worn down") is more at risk for infection because the body's defenses are already weakened by illness. Therefore, the person is not able to fight off the pathogen as easily. Additionally, certain medical treatments, such as chemotherapy or radiation therapy, can affect the functioning of the body's immune system and put a person more at risk for infection.
- **Stress and fatigue.** Lack of rest and emotional stress can affect the body's ability to defend itself from pathogens.
- **Indwelling medical devices.** Medical devices, such as catheters, feeding tubes, and intravenous (IV) lines, increase a person's risk of infection by increasing the availability of a portal of entry for a pathogen.

Many of the people you will care for as a nursing assistant have risk factors for infection. Your patients or residents will be sick, recovering from surgery, elderly, or have a chronic illness or conditions that will increase their risk of getting an infectious disease. A major part of your responsibility in caring for other people involves protecting them from infection.

The chain of infection can be broken by taking away just one of the six required elements (Fig. 7-6). For example, taking the right antibiotic for a bacterial infection quickly turns a person's body into an unfriendly reservoir for bacteria. Covering an infected wound with a dressing eliminates a pathogen's portal of exit by containing the pathogen within the dressing. Washing your hands and making sure that linens, utensils, glassware, and other possible fomites are properly cleansed eliminates a method of transmission. Wearing gloves and keeping your skin healthy and intact removes one potential portal of entry available to pathogens. Receiving required

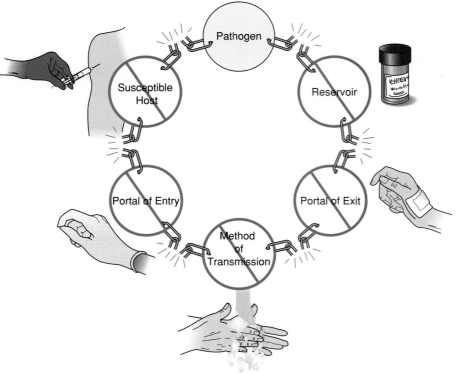

FIGURE 7-6

The chain of infection can be broken by removing just one of the six elements that must be present for infection to occur.

immunizations and maintaining general good health make you a less susceptible host. All of these actions break a link in the chain of infection, stopping the infection from being transmitted. Other factors that determine whether or not an infection will be transmitted are the **virulence** (strength or disease-producing potential) of the pathogen and the actual number of pathogens that enter the body.

INFECTION CONTROL IN THE HEALTH CARE SETTING

What do you think of when you think of a health care facility? Health care professionals in clean, fresh uniforms, a smell of antiseptic in the air, and miles of shiny tile floors? Most of us think of health care facilities as clean, possibly even sterile, environments. Maintaining cleanliness in health care facilities is essential, because exposure to pathogens is increased in these settings. Additionally, most of the people in health care facilities are there because they are not in good overall health. Therefore, their potential to become infected is increased. The chance of getting an infection while in

a health care facility is so great, there is even a word for it: nosocomial. A **nosocomial** infection is an infection gotten while in a hospital or other health care setting. Interestingly, the most common method of transmission for nosocomial infections, including the very dangerous VRE, is on the hands of health care workers!

All health care facilities follow basic practices that are designed to decrease the chance that an infection will be spread from one person to another. These practices are called **infection control.** There are four major methods of infection control—medical asepsis, surgical asepsis, barrier methods, and isolation (transmission-based) precautions.

MEDICAL ASEPSIS

Medical asepsis involves physically removing or killing pathogens, and is primarily achieved through processes involving soap, water, antiseptics, disinfectants, or heat. The goal of medical asepsis is to remove pathogenic microbes from surfaces, equipment, and the hands of health care workers. There are four techniques that make up the practice of medical asepsis:

A. Sanitization

C. Disinfection

B. Antisepsis

D. Sterilization

FIGURE 7-7

There are many approaches to medical asepsis, a general term used to describe techniques used to remove or kill microbes. (*A*) Sanitization is physically removing microbes from surfaces. Here, a home health aide washes dishes. (*B*) Antisepsis involves the use of agents that kill microbes or slow down their growth, such as iodine (Betadine) or rubbing alcohol. Here, a nurse cleans a patient's skin with a Betadine swab. (*C*) Disinfection also involves the use of agents that kill microbes. Because disinfectants are strong chemicals, disinfection is used only to clean non-living objects. This nursing assistant is using a disinfectant to clean an over-bed table. (*D*) Sterilization involves the use of pressurized steam heat or very strong chemicals to kill microbes. This technician is opening a steam autoclave, a device used to sterilize instruments and equipment. (*D*, *©Wedgwood/Custom Medical Stock Photo.*)

sanitization, antisepsis, disinfection, and sterilization (Fig. 7-7):

- **Sanitization** is the word we use to describe practices associated with basic cleanliness, such as handwashing, cleansing of eating utensils and other surfaces with soap and water, and providing clean linens and clothing. Sanitization practices physically remove pathogens, thereby preventing their spread. General guidelines for maintaining a sanitary environment in a health care setting or home are given in Guidelines Box 7-1.

- **Antisepsis** takes sanitization one step further, by actually killing microbes or stopping them from growing. An antiseptic is a chemical that is capable of killing a pathogen, or preventing it from growing. Antiseptics can be used on the skin or other surfaces to kill pathogens. Rubbing alcohol and iodine are common antiseptics used on the skin to prevent infection. Many soaps used in the health care setting now contain an antiseptic agent as well.

- **Disinfection** involves the use of stronger chemicals to kill pathogens. The chemicals

GUIDELINES BOX 7-1
GUIDELINES FOR MAINTAINING A SANITARY ENVIRONMENT

What you do	Why you do it
Wash your hands after contact with any body fluid or substance, whether it is your own or another person's. Examples of body fluids and substances include blood, saliva, vomitus, urine, feces, vaginal discharge, semen, wound drainage, pus, mucus, and respiratory secretions.	Pathogens often leave the body through the gastrointestinal tract, genitourinary tract, respiratory tract, or breaks in the skin. In addition, some pathogens are transmitted in blood and other body secretions, such as breast milk.
Wash your hands frequently, especially after using the bathroom; before handling food, drink, or eating utensils; and before and after any contact with a patient or resident.	Frequent handwashing eliminates a method of transmission for microbes.
Cover your mouth or nose with a tissue when you cough or sneeze, and teach your patients and residents to do the same. Dispose of tissues properly by placing them in a waste container.	Some microbes are transmitted in particles of saliva or sputum. Covering your nose or mouth with a tissue contains these particles and helps to prevent the spread of infection.
Provide each patient or resident with individual personal care items, such as toothbrushes, drinking glasses, towels, washcloths, and soap.	If not properly cleaned after use, these items can act as fomites. Therefore, it is better to limit their use to one person.
Keep contaminated or dirty items, such as soiled linens, away from your uniform.	Microbes can be transferred from the dirty item to your uniform, which can then act as a fomite.
When cleaning, take care not to stir up dust. For example, wiping dusty surfaces with a damp cloth or mop helps prevent the movement of dust and lint into the air. Do not shake linens when making beds.	Dust can act as a fomite and carry microbes from one area to another.
Dispose of trash properly. Follow established procedures for preparing dirty linens and clothing for the laundry.	If not disposed of properly, trash can provide an ideal environment for microbial growth, especially if the trash contains food or other materials susceptible to rotting. Soiled items and clothing act as fomites and must be handled in a way that will lessen the chance of someone else coming in contact with the contaminated item.
Maintain good personal hygiene, and help your patients or residents to do the same. Bathing, washing hair, brushing teeth, and wearing clean clothing are all grooming practices that help prevent the spread of infection.	Personal grooming practices help to reduce the number of microbes present on the skin.

used for disinfection are too strong to be used on the skin. Instead, disinfectants are used to clean non-living objects that come in contact with body fluids or substances, such as bedpans, urinals, and tray tables.

- **Sterilization** is the most thorough method of killing microbes. Sterilization is used on objects that must be completely free of any microbe, such as surgical instruments, hypodermic needles, or intravenous (IV) catheters. These objects must be sterilized because they are placed in the patient's or resident's body. Therefore, they can act as portals of entry for microbes. Equipment is sterilized either by placing items in an autoclave (a machine that uses pressurized steam heat to kill microbes) or by soaking the items in chemicals that destroy all microbes. Although covering items in boiling water will kill most microbes, boiling is not an effective method of sterilization.

Before disinfecting or sterilizing an object, the object must be cleaned first using basic sanitation methods. The chemicals used to disinfect or sterilize an object cannot work properly unless the surface to be disinfected or sterilized is clean and free of any organic material (material from a living organism, such as blood, urine, or feces). Organic materials contain fats and proteins that coat the surface of the object, much like an egg yolk coats the surface of a plate. If the plate is not washed with detergent and warm water before the egg yolk dries, the hardened yolk becomes very difficult to remove. The same principle applies to dirty bedpans, urinals, and other pieces of equipment—if the piece of equipment is not washed first using soap and water, any organic material that is present can harden, making it difficult for the disinfectant or sterilization agent to kill the microbes underneath the dried material. Therefore, equipment must be properly cleaned using basic sanitation methods before moving on to disinfection or sterilization.

Handwashing

As a nursing assistant, the technique of medical asepsis that you will use most frequently is handwashing. According to the Centers for Disease Control (CDC), *handwashing is the single most important method of preventing the spread of infection.* This is true in the "real world," as well as in the health care setting. However, in the health care setting, handwashing takes on a special importance because the chance of picking up a pathogen and passing it on to someone else is greater than in normal, everyday life. In addition, many of the people who are in health care facilities are less able to handle an infection, should they get one. The easiest way to protect yourself and your patients or residents is to be conscientious about washing your hands!

Before you move from one person's room to another in a health care facility, you must always wash your hands. In the process of taking care of your patients or residents, you will collect a variety of microbes on your hands. These microbes could then be easily transferred to the next patient or resident you care for, yourself, or one of your family members. Failing to wash your hands

before giving care to a patient or resident could even be considered abuse.

There are two main types of microbes found on a person's hands. Earlier in this chapter, you learned about the first type, normal (resident) flora. These are the microbes that normally live on a person's skin and usually do not cause infections. Normal flora lives deep in the pores of the skin and cannot be totally removed. The other type of microbe typically found on a person's hands is called **transient flora.** Transient flora is picked up from touching contaminated objects or people who have an infectious disease. Most nosocomial infections are caused by transient flora—the hands of the health care worker serve as the method of transmission from one person to another. Transient flora lives on the surface of the skin and is easily removed by proper handwashing.

There are differences in opinion about handwashing techniques, such as the time required, the type of cleaning agents that should be used, and the frequency with which handwashing should occur. Certain situations may require specific handwashing techniques. For example, health care workers who work in the operating room, intensive care unit, neonatal unit, or labor and delivery units may be required to use an antiseptic cleaning agent, a scrub brush, or both because patients in these settings have higher infection risks (Fig. 7-8). Antiseptic cleaning agents remove the transient flora from the surface of the skin. They also slow down the growth of the normal flora, which can be helpful in certain areas of

FIGURE 7-8

This person is performing a surgical scrub in preparation for entering an operating room.

health care. Procedure 7-1 describes the basic handwashing procedure. Although the specifics of how handwashing is performed vary from setting to setting, one aspect of handwashing always remains the same—it must be performed thoroughly, properly, and consistently. At the minimum, wash your hands:

- When you first arrive at your facility
- Before entering a patient's or resident's room
- Before entering a "clean" supply room
- Before obtaining clean linen from a linen cart
- Before handling a patient's or resident's meal tray
- Before you go on break and before you leave your shift
- Before and after drinking, eating, or smoking
- Before and after inserting contact lenses
- After using the bathroom
- After coughing, sneezing, or blowing your nose
- After touching anything that may be considered dirty—especially objects contaminated with blood or other body fluids or substances
- After picking an object up from the floor
- After removing disposable gloves, including those times when you are replacing a torn glove
- After handling your hair or applying make-up or lip gloss

When washing your hands, make sure you clean those areas that microbes love to hide, under and around the fingernails and between the fingers. As you learned in Chapter 3, long, glamorous fingernails and jewelry do not really have a place in the nursing assistant's professional life. Long fingernails trap microbes underneath them and therefore are harder to clean. Nail polish cracks and peels, providing many places for transient microbes to hide. False nails, acrylics, and wraps often lift, creating an excellent breeding ground for microbes. For the same reason, it is not a good idea to wear rings and bracelets while on the job. Many health care workers think that by removing their jewelry before washing their hands, they can remove any microbes trapped underneath the jewelry. But, think about this: even if you remove your jewelry before you wash your hands, the jewelry itself is still dirty, so you will be putting dirty jewelry back onto your clean

hands. For the sake of efficiency and cleanliness, it is best to keep your fingernails short and unpolished, and to leave your jewelry at home when performing your duties as a nursing assistant.

A good lather of soap and the physical motion of rubbing your hands together removes skin oils and lotions, which can harbor microbes. Rinsing thoroughly removes microbes, along with the dirt and lather. Because frequent handwashing can cause the skin to become excessively dry, leading to cracking, applying a lotion or hand cream after washing is recommended. Remember, your own intact skin is important to help protect you from infection too.

While nothing can replace the effectiveness of good handwashing to remove visible dirt, blood, or other body fluids or substances, the CDC issued guidelines in October, 2002, recommending the use of alcohol-based hand rubs for routine hand decontamination. Alcohol-based hand rubs have several advantages:

- Using an alcohol-based hand rub is quicker than washing your hands at the sink, which means that during duties that require frequent handwashing, using an alcohol-based hand rub can save time.
- Alcohol-based hand rubs are gentler on the skin than soap and water.
- Alcohol-based hand rubs are used without water, so they can be used anywhere. In many facilities, alcohol-based hand rubs can be dispensed at the patient's or resident's bedside, saving many trips back and forth to the sink. Many even come in containers small enough to be carried in your uniform pocket.

It is very simple to use an alcohol-based hand rub. The label on the product will tell you how much product to use. Apply this amount to one of your palms and rub your hands together, covering your hands and fingers (front and back) with the product. Continue rubbing your hands together until your skin is dry. That's all there is to it!

Remember, if your hands are visibly soiled with dirt, blood, or other body fluids or substances, you must wash them at the sink, using soap and water. However, if your hands are not visibly soiled, than it is acceptable to use an alcohol-based hand rub to decontaminate your hands, instead of handwashing.

SURGICAL ASEPSIS

Surgical asepsis is used for procedures that involve entering a person's body. Examples of procedures that require surgical asepsis include surgical procedures, injections, the insertion of intravenous (IV) catheters, and the insertion of urinary catheters. Because these procedures disrupt the body's natural protective barriers, all instruments and equipment used must be sterile, or totally free from microbes. In most states, performing procedures that require surgical asepsis is not within a nursing assistant's scope of practice. However, some facilities will provide extra training in this area if performing procedures that require surgical asepsis is part of your job description.

BARRIER METHODS

In addition to medical asepsis and surgical asepsis, barrier methods are used to control infection in the health care setting. A *barrier* is an object that physically prevents microbes from reaching a health care provider's skin or mucous membranes. Examples of barriers used in infection control, called **personal protective equipment (PPE),** include disposable gloves, gowns, masks, and protective eyewear. While in use, the barrier becomes contaminated with microbes and must be removed in a way that prevents transmission of the microbes onto the skin of the health care worker.

Gloves

Gloves are the most commonly used barrier method. Gloves are worn in the following situations:

- When there is a possibility that you will come in contact with body fluids or substances
- When you are performing or assisting with perineal care (cleaning of the area between the legs)
- When you have a cut or abrasion on your hands
- When you are shaving a patient or resident
- When you are performing care on a patient or resident who has an open wound or other break in the skin

To effectively prevent contamination of your hands, gloves must be intact (without holes or tears), and they must fit properly. Gloves that are too tight are uncomfortable. Gloves that are too loose will not stay on your hands. Many people are allergic or sensitive to latex, the material that is most commonly used to make disposable gloves. If you or someone you are caring for is sensitive to latex, then you should use gloves made from another synthetic material, such as vinyl. Health care facilities must provide non-latex barrier methods for people who are sensitive to latex.

The most common error made by people who wear gloves for barrier protection is becoming too comfortable with the fact that they are protecting themselves, and forgetting to protect others! If you are wearing gloves and you touch a surface that is contaminated, then your gloves become contaminated. If you then touch another surface, such as the side rail, light switch, or doorknob, with your contaminated gloves, the pathogens will be transferred from your gloves to that surface. The next person who touches the surface could then pick up the microbes you deposited there with your dirty gloves (Fig. 7-9). Gloves that become contaminated with material that may contain pathogens should be removed before touching any other surface. You may need to change gloves several times during one procedure to prevent the transfer of microbes from dirty areas to clean areas (for example, when cleaning feces from a person who has soiled himself, or

FIGURE 7-9

Do not make this mistake! By touching the light switch with her gloved hands, this nursing assistant has transferred whatever microbes were on her gloves onto the light switch, where they could be easily transferred onto the hands of the next person who turns on the light.

changing soiled sheets). And always wash your hands after removing your gloves. Procedure 7-2 describes the proper way to remove gloves.

Gowns

A gown (fabric or paper) should be used when it is likely that your uniform will be soiled with body fluids or substances. The use of the gown prevents contamination of your uniform. Each gown is worn only once. Any gown, fabric or paper, is considered contaminated if it becomes wet. Procedures 7-3 and 7-4 describe how to put on and take off a gown, respectively.

Masks

Masks prevent you from breathing in microbes through your nose or mouth, and are worn when there is a chance that you will be exposed to pathogens that are transmitted through the air or in droplets of saliva. For example, the virus that causes measles and the bacterium that causes tuberculosis (TB) are airborne pathogens, and the microbes that cause diseases such as pneumonia, strep throat, and meningitis are transmitted in droplets of saliva. You could be exposed to these pathogens when a person with one of these diseases talks, coughs, or sneezes.

Surgical masks are most commonly used, but if you are caring for a person with TB, you may be required to wear a special high-filtration mask (Fig. 7-10). Surgical masks are "one size fits all,"

but high-filtration masks are available in various sizes and you must be fitted for them in advance. All masks are used only once. You must discard and replace your mask if it becomes wet or soiled. Procedure 7-5 explains how to put on and take off a mask.

Protective Eyewear

Goggles, face shields, and other types of protective eyewear are used to protect your eyes from substances that may splash (Fig. 7-11). Blood and other body fluids, as well as the fluid used to clean wounds, may contain pathogens, which can enter your body through your eyes. Goggles fit close to your face and can be worn over prescription eyeglasses. Face shields may be attached to a mask, or to an elastic band that fits around the head. Your employer is required to provide you with appropriate protective eyewear.

In many situations, you may need to wear more than one article of PPE. The best sequence for putting these items on is as follows: mask, gown, protective eyewear, gloves. The order is reversed when it is time to get out of the PPE. Procedure 7-6 describes how to remove PPE when more than one article is being used. After use, PPE is considered contaminated. Removal of PPE in the correct sequence helps to protect you from infection. For instance, you would not want to remove your mask first, because this would mean that you would have to touch your face with your contaminated gloves.

FIGURE 7-10

Masks cover your nose and mouth and protect you from inhaling pathogens transmitted in the air or in saliva. (*Left*) A surgical mask. (*Right*) A high-filtration respirator mask, worn when caring for people with tuberculosis (TB).

FIGURE 7-11

Face shields (*left*) and goggles (*right*) are used to protect your eyes from substances that may splash.

ISOLATION (TRANSMISSION-BASED) PRECAUTIONS

The last major method of controlling the spread of infection throughout a health care facility is by using isolation (transmission-based) precautions. **Isolation (transmission-based) precautions** are guidelines, based on a pathogen's method of transmission, that we follow to contain the pathogen and limit others' exposure to it as much as possible. There are two "levels" of isolation precautions. The first level, called standard precautions, is a set of precautions used to protect against pathogens that are transmitted in blood. Standard precautions, which you will learn more about in Chapter 8, are taken with every patient or resident. The second "level" of isolation precautions includes precautions that are used when a person is known to have a disease that is transmitted a certain way, for example, via the air, in droplets, or by direct contact.

Airborne precautions are used when caring for people infected with pathogens that can be transmitted through the air, and are described in detail in Chapter 8. Airborne pathogens enter the respiratory tract of people breathing the same air as the infected person. Therefore, airborne precautions include placing the patient or resident in a private room with the door closed, wearing a mask when caring for the person, and minimizing the amount of time the person spends out of his private room. When it is necessary for the infected person to leave his room, he wears a mask. Diseases caused by pathogens that can be transmitted in the air include TB, chickenpox, and measles.

Droplet precautions are used when caring for people with diseases caused by pathogens that are transmitted by direct exposure to droplets released from the mouth or nose (for example, when the person coughs, sneezes, or talks). Droplet precautions must also be taken when performing procedures that involve contact with an infected person's mouth or nose. Diseases caused by pathogens that can be transmitted in droplets include mumps, influenza, whooping cough, strep throat, scarlet fever, rubella, meningitis, pneumonia, diphtheria, and epiglottitis. Droplet precautions are the same as airborne precautions, except that it is usually only necessary to wear a mask when you are within 3 feet of the infected person.

Contact precautions are used when caring for people with diseases caused by pathogens that are transmitted directly (by touching the person) or indirectly (by touching fomites). Diseases that can be transmitted by contact include skin and wound infections, digestive tract infections, and some respiratory tract infections. Contact precautions involve using barrier methods whenever you must touch the infected person or items contaminated with wound drainage or body substances. Contaminated linen and waste materials must be contained and disposed of properly. Procedure 7-7 describes how to transfer contaminated items out of a person's room when contact precautions are being followed.

When caring for a person with a communicable disease, it is very important to remember the person. We work hard to follow all of the procedures that help to prevent the spread of infection, and this is a very important part of providing care. However, sometimes it is easy to forget about how the person with the infection might feel. A person with a communicable disease often feels dirty or unwanted. Think about it—how would you feel if a health care worker had to wear gloves or a mask every time he or she came near you? When airborne or droplet precautions are in effect, the person with the communicable disease may feel isolated and lonely, and desperately miss the company of other people. Friends and family members may avoid visiting the person. When you are caring for a patient or resident with a communicable disease, checking on the person frequently and taking the time to talk with the person when you are providing care can help to make the person feel better.

SUMMARY

▶ A huge variety of microbes share our planet.
- Major types of microbes include bacteria, viruses, fungi, and parasites.
- Some cause disease, and are called pathogens, while others are harmless. Harmless microbes that live in and on our bodies are called normal flora.

▶ Our immune systems help us to fight off infections.
- The human immune system's nonspecific defense mechanisms include the physical

barriers provided by the skin and mucous membranes, and the general immune response.

- The human immune system's specific defense mechanisms include antibodies.

▶ Health care facilities provide the perfect environment for the spread of infection.

- The chain of infection describes the elements that must be present in order for infection to occur. The six elements of the chain of infection are pathogen, reservoir, portal of exit, method of transmission, portal of entry, and susceptible host.

- Breaking just one link in the chain of infection stops the spread of infection from one person to another.

▶ Some of the people you will care for will be receiving health care because they have a serious communicable disease. Others may have a serious communicable disease and not even know it. In addition, many of the people you will care for will be more at risk for catching a communicable disease because they are not entirely healthy to begin with. Therefore, infection control is very important in the health care setting.

- Health care workers take many approaches to infection control. As a nursing assistant, it is your ethical and legal responsibility to protect your patients or residents from infectious disease. You must also protect yourself and your family members. The techniques used to help control the spread of infection are effective only if performed properly and consistently.

- Medical asepsis involves physically removing or killing pathogens.
  - Methods of medical asepsis include sanitization, antisepsis, disinfection, and sterilization.
  - Handwashing, a form of medical asepsis, is the single most important method of controlling the spread of infection.

- Surgical asepsis is required for procedures that involve entering a person's body.

- Barrier methods prevent a pathogen from gaining access to a health care worker's body. Commonly used barrier methods include gloves, gowns, masks, and protective eyewear.

- Isolation (transmission-based) precautions are based on a pathogen's mode of transmission (blood, air, droplet, direct contact).

Chapter 7 Procedures

1. Gather needed supplies, if not present at the handwashing area: *soap or the cleansing agent specified by your facility, hand lotion* (optional), *paper towels, a waste container, a nailbrush* (optional), *an orange stick* (optional).

2. Stand away from the sink, so that your uniform does not touch the sink. Push your sleeves up your arms 4 to 5 inches; if you are wearing a watch, push it up too.

STEP 3 Use a clean paper towel to turn on the faucet.

3. Use a clean paper towel to turn on the faucet, adjusting the water temperature until it is warm. Dispose of the paper towel in a facility-approved waste container.

STEP 7 Interlace your fingers.

4. Wet your hands, keeping your fingers pointed down. This will cause the water to run off your fingertips and into the sink. Do not allow water to run up your forearms.

5. Press the hand pump or step on the foot pedal to dispense the cleaning agent into one cupped hand.

6. Lather well, keeping your fingers pointed down at all times. Make sure the lather extends at least 1 inch past your wrists.

7. Rub your hands together in a circular motion, washing the palms and backs of your hands. Interlace your fingers to clean the spaces between your fingers. Continue for 10–15 seconds.

8. Rub the fingernails of one hand against the palm of the opposite hand to force soap underneath the tips of the fingernails, *or* clean underneath the tips of the fingernails with the blunt edge of an orange stick or a nailbrush.

STEP 8 Clean under your fingernails.

9. Rinse your hands, keeping your fingers pointed down at all times.

10. Dry your hands thoroughly with a clean paper towel. Dispose of the paper towel in a facility-approved waste container, being careful not to touch the container.

(continued)

PROCEDURE 7-1 (Continued)

Handwashing

11. With a new paper towel, turn off the faucet. Carefully dispose of the paper towel.

STEP 9 Always point your fingertips down.

12. As you leave the handwashing area, if there is a doorknob, open the door by covering the doorknob with a clean paper towel. If there is no doorknob, push the door open with your hip and shoulder to avoid contaminating your clean hands.

13. After leaving the handwashing area, apply a small amount of hand lotion to keep your skin supple and moist.

PROCEDURE 7-2

Removing Gloves

1. With one gloved hand, grasp the other glove at the palm and pull the glove off your hand. Keep the glove you have removed in your gloved hand. (Think, "glove to glove.")

STEP 1 "Glove to glove."

2. Slip two fingers from the ungloved hand underneath the cuff of the remaining glove, at the wrist. Remove that glove from your hand, turning it inside-out as you pull it off. (Think, "skin to skin.")

STEP 2 "Skin to skin."

3. Dispose of the soiled gloves in a facility-approved waste container.

4. Wash your hands.

PROCEDURE 7-3
Putting on a Gown

1. Gather needed supplies: *a gown, gloves.*

2. Remove your watch and place it on a clean paper towel. (If you are wearing jewelry, remove that as well.) Roll up the sleeves of your uniform so that they are about 4–5 inches above your wrists.

3. Wash your hands.

STEP 4 Slip your arms into the sleeves.

4. Put on the gown by slipping your arms into the sleeves.

5. Secure the gown around your neck by tying the ties in a simple bow or by fastening the Velcro™ strips.

STEP 6 Overlap and tie.

6. Reach behind yourself and overlap the edges of the gown so that your uniform is completely covered. Secure the gown at your waist by tying the ties in a simple bow or by fastening the Velcro™ strips.

7. Put on the gloves. The cuffs of the gloves should extend over the cuffs of the gown.

PROCEDURE 7-4
Removing a Gown

1. Untie the waist ties (or undo the Velcro™ strips at the waist).

2. Remove and dispose of your gloves as described in Procedure 7-2.

3. Untie the neck ties (or undo the Velcro™ strips at the neck). Be careful not to touch your neck or the outside of the gown.

4. Grasping the gown at the neck ties, loosen it at the neck.

5. Slip the fingers of your dominant hand under the cuff of the gown on the opposite sleeve, and pull the sleeve over your hand. Be careful not to touch the outside of the gown with either hand.

STEP 5 Be careful not to touch the outside of the gown.

6. Use your gown-covered hand to pull the sleeve over your other hand, and then pull the gown off both arms.

STEP 6 Use your gown-covered hand to pull the sleeve over your other hand.

7. Holding the gown away from your body, roll it downward, turning it inside out as you go. Take care to touch only the non-contaminated side of the gown.

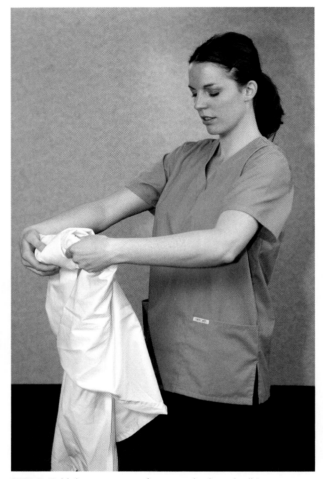

STEP 7 Hold the gown away from your body and roll it downward, turning it inside out.

8. After the gown is rolled up, contaminated side inward, dispose of it in a facility-approved container.

9. Wash your hands.

PROCEDURE 7-5
Putting on and Removing a Mask

Putting on a Mask

1. Gather needed supplies: *a mask.*
2. Wash your hands.

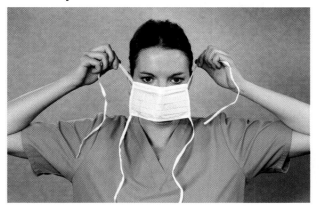

STEP 3 Be careful not to touch your face with your hands.

3. Place the mask over your nose and mouth, being careful not to touch your face with your hands.

STEP 4 Tie the top strings securely.

4. Tie the top strings of the mask securely behind your head.

STEP 5 Tie the bottom strings securely.

5. Tie the bottom strings of the mask securely behind your neck. Make sure that the mask fits snugly around your face. You want to breathe through the mask, not around it.

Removing a Mask

1. Wash your hands. (You do not want to touch your face with dirty hands.)
2. Untie the bottom strings first, and then untie the top strings.
3. Remove the mask by holding the top strings. Dispose of the mask, holding it by its ties only, in the facility-approved container located inside the patient's or resident's room.
4. Wash your hands.

PROCEDURE 7-6
Removing More Than One Article of Personal Protective Equipment (PPE)

1. Untie the gown's waist ties (or undo the hook-and-fastener strips at the waist).
2. Remove and dispose of your gloves as described in Procedure 7-2.
3. Wash your hands.
4. Remove and dispose of the mask as described in Procedure 7-5.

5. Untie the gown's neck ties (or undo the hook-and-fastener strips at the neck), and loosen the gown at the neck. Remove and dispose of the gown as described in Procedure 7-4.
6. Remove your protective eyewear.
7. Wash your hands.

PROCEDURE 7-7
Double-Bagging (Two Assistants)

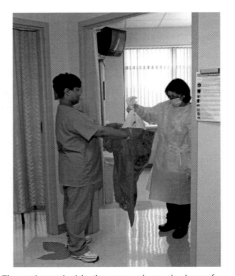

1. The nursing assistant inside the person's room places the contaminated items into an isolation bag (usually a color-coded plastic bag), and secures the bag with a tie.

2. Another nursing assistant, referred to as the "clean" nursing assistant, stands outside of the person's room, holding a plastic bag cuffed over her hands. The cuff at the top of the bag protects the "clean" nursing assistant's hands.

3. The nursing assistant inside the isolation unit deposits the bag of contaminated items into the bag held by the "clean" nursing assistant.

4. The "clean" nursing assistant secures the top of the plastic bag tightly and disposes of the double-bagged items according to facility policy.

STEP 3 The assistant inside the room places the bag of contaminated items in the bag held by the nursing assistant outside of the room.

What did you learn?

Multiple Choice

Select the single best answer for each of the following questions.

1. When you wash your hands, you should:
   a. Use the hottest water possible
   b. Scrub with a brush for 3 minutes
   c. Rinse with your fingers pointed up
   d. Rinse with your fingers pointed down

2. When should you wash your hands?
   a. When you wake up in the morning and before you go to bed at night
   b. Before and after contact with a patient or resident
   c. When the charge nurse tells you to
   d. When you notice that they look or feel dirty

3. You have been told to follow contact precautions with one of your residents. Therefore, this resident's soiled linen should be:
   a. Thrown away
   b. Bagged prior to removing it from the room
   c. Taken directly to the laundry
   d. Placed in the linen hamper

4. Which of the following procedures best destroys all bacteria?
   a. Sterilizing
   b. Washing with bleach
   c. Soaking in alcohol
   d. All of the above

5. Bacteria may enter the body through:
   a. The mouth
   b. The nose
   c. Cuts in the skin
   d. All of the above

6. Which statement about the handwashing procedure is correct?
   a. As long as soap is used, the temperature of the water does not matter
   b. The faucet is clean and may be touched during handwashing
   c. Wash at least one inch above the wrist
   d. All of the above

7. Microbes can be spread by:
   a. Looking at a person with a communicable disease
   b. Coughing or sneezing
   c. Touching a person with a communicable disease
   d. Both "b" and "c"

8. Which one of the following statements about protective gowns is true?
   a. The outside is considered the "clean" side
   b. The gown opens in the front
   c. A gown may be used more than once
   d. A gown is considered contaminated when wet

9. Which one of the following could be a fomite?
   a. A water glass that has been used
   b. A mosquito
   c. Linens that have just come back from the laundry
   d. A cut in the skin

10. Which one of the following must be present in order for infection to spread?
    a. A nursing assistant
    b. An indwelling medical device
    c. A susceptible host
    d. A patient or resident who looks ill

Matching

Match each numbered item with its appropriate lettered description.

_____ 1. Communicable disease

_____ 2. Pathogen

_____ 3. Leukocyte

_____ 4. Opportunistic microbe

_____ 5. Fomite

_____ 6. Aerobic

_____ 7. Nosocomial

_____ 8. Vector

_____ 9. Anaerobic

_____ 10. Antibody

a. Describes bacteria that need oxygen to survive

b. Special proteins that help fight specific pathogens

c. Can be transferred from one person to another

d. Microbe that can cause illness

e. Non-living object that is contaminated

f. White blood cell

g. Can change from harmless to pathogenic, given a chance

h. Infection gotten in the health care setting

i. A living creature that transmits disease

j. Describes bacteria that die if oxygen is present

Stop and think!

▶ You have just received your shift report and will be caring for Mrs. Grande, who is recovering from a stroke, and her roommate, Miss Murphy, who is receiving intravenous antibiotic therapy for a foot infection caused by methicillin-resistant *Staphylococcus aureus* (MRSA). What do you need to be concerned about when caring for Mrs. Grande and Miss Murphy? What suggestions would you have for minimizing Mrs. Grande's risk of infection?

8

Bloodborne and Airborne Pathogens

What will you learn?

As a nursing assistant, you will have close contact with patients and residents, some of whom will have life-threatening communicable diseases. Although your risk of getting these diseases is real, there are things you can do to minimize that risk. Additionally, the Occupational Safety and Health Administration (OSHA) has developed standards for employers to make sure that you have the equipment and training you need to maintain your safety at work. In this chapter, you will learn about some of the communicable diseases that pose the most risk to health care workers, and how these diseases are transmitted. You will learn what you can do to minimize your risk of getting one of these infections. And you will also learn about the standards that have been developed by OSHA with the goal of protecting you at work while you provide quality care for your patients or residents. When you are finished with this chapter, you will be able to:

1. Describe the types of bloodborne pathogens and the risks they pose to the health care worker.
2. State the OSHA standards for bloodborne pathogens.
3. Identify body fluids that can contain bloodborne pathogens.
4. Define the term *standard precautions.*
5. Identify the requirements for an exposure control plan.
6. Explain how engineering and work practice controls help to protect the nursing assistant (and others) from exposure to bloodborne and airborne diseases.
7. Explain the various methods used to protect against tuberculosis (TB) exposure.

Photo: Following standard precautions, such as wearing personal protective equipment (PPE) whenever contact with blood or other body fluids is likely, helps to protect you from bloodborne pathogens.

Vocabulary

Use the CD in the back of your book to hear these terms pronounced, defined, and used in a sentence:

Bloodborne pathogen
Body fluids
Hepatitis
Hepatitis A virus (HAV)
Oral–fecal route
Hepatitis B virus (HBV)
Carrier

Centers for Disease
  Control and
  Prevention (CDC)
Hepatitis C virus
  (HCV)
Hepatitis D virus
  (HDV)

Hepatitis E virus (HEV)
Human
  immunodeficiency
  virus (HIV)
Acquired
  immunodeficiency
  syndrome (AIDS)

T cell
Standard precautions
Exposure control
  plan
Airborne pathogen
Tuberculosis (TB)

BLOODBORNE PATHOGENS

A **bloodborne pathogen** is a disease-producing microbe that is transmitted to another person through blood or other body fluids. **Body fluids** are liquid or semi-liquid substances produced by the body, such as blood, urine, feces, vomitus, saliva, drainage from wounds, sweat, semen, vaginal secretions, tears, cerebrospinal fluid, amniotic fluid, and breast milk. For a bloodborne pathogen to be transmitted from one person to another, blood or body fluids from an infected person must enter the bloodstream of a person who is not infected. There are several ways this could occur in the workplace:

- Needlesticks (puncture wounds caused by dirty hypodermic needles)
- Cuts from contaminated, broken glass (such as that from a broken blood tube)
- Direct contact between infected blood and broken skin, mucous membranes, or the eyes

Additionally, bloodborne pathogens can be transmitted via sexual intercourse, or through blood transfusions.

Several diseases are caused by bloodborne pathogens. The most common are:

- Hepatitis B, C, and D
- Human immunodeficiency virus (HIV), which causes acquired immunodeficiency syndrome (AIDS)
- Malaria
- Syphilis
- Ebola

Of these, hepatitis and HIV pose the greatest occupational risk to the health care worker.

HEPATITIS

Hepatitis is inflammation of the liver, the organ that removes toxic substances from the bloodstream (Fig. 8-1). Hepatitis is most commonly caused by a viral infection, but it may also be caused by chemicals, drugs, or drinking alcohol. Some infections with a hepatitis virus are mild, producing no lasting effects on the liver. Others are chronic and affect the liver's ability to function over time. If the liver failure is severe, the person will die unless she receives a liver transplant. Currently, five types of hepatitis virus have been identified: the hepatitis A, B, C, D, and E viruses.

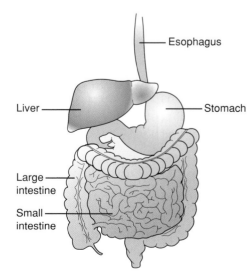

Esophagus

Liver

Stomach

Large
intestine

Small
intestine

FIGURE 8-1

Hepatitis is inflammation of the liver, the organ that removes toxic substances from the blood.

Hepatitis A Virus (HAV)

Hepatitis A virus (HAV) is not a bloodborne pathogen. This virus is transmitted through the **oral–fecal route,** which means that the virus lives in the digestive tract of an infected person and leaves the person's body through the feces. The feces can contaminate food or water. Then, when a person eats or drinks the contaminated food or water, he becomes infected. (*Oral* means mouth. In this case, the infection is transmitted by taking contaminated food or water into the mouth.) For example, HAV can be passed on when a food service worker who has the virus uses the restroom but fails to wash her hands properly before returning to work and handling a customer's food (Fig. 8-2). Hepatitis A outbreaks are also found in areas where raw sewage comes into contact with bodies of water where shellfish, such as oysters, live. The virus infects the shellfish and is then passed on to unsuspecting people who eat the contaminated shellfish raw. Fortunately, the illness caused by HAV (commonly referred to as *infectious hepatitis*) is usually acute and the person usually recovers fully. An effective vaccine against this virus is available and recommended for the general public.

Hepatitis B Virus (HBV)

Hepatitis B virus (HBV), a bloodborne pathogen, is a serious threat for the health care worker. The virus is found in blood, as well as in other body fluids, such as semen and vaginal secretions. This means that HBV can be transmitted through transfusion of infected blood or blood products, across the placenta from mother to infant, and through unprotected sexual intercourse (both heterosexual and homosexual). Health care workers are at risk for getting HBV through:

- Needlestick injuries
- Cuts from contaminated objects
- Exposure of broken skin or mucous membranes to contaminated blood or other body fluids (Fig. 8-3)

In addition to blood, semen, and vaginal secretions, body fluids known to carry high amounts of HBV include wound drainage and cultures, cerebrospinal fluid, amniotic fluid, and breast milk. Other body secretions do not typically have high viral counts unless there is visible blood present.

Infection with HBV causes an acute illness in most people, but some people can be infected by the virus and never develop symptoms. These people are considered **carriers.** Carriers do not have

FIGURE 8-2

Hepatitis A virus (HAV) is transmitted via the oral–fecal route. The virus lives in an infected person's digestive tract and leaves the body in the feces. If the person's hands become contaminated with feces and then the person handles food, the infection could be passed on to the person who eats the contaminated food.

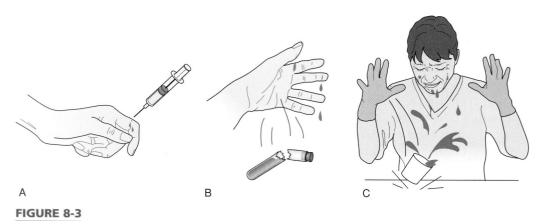

FIGURE 8-3

In the workplace, hepatitis B virus (HBV) can be transmitted by (*A*) a needlestick injury, (*B*) cuts from contaminated glass, or (*C*) direct contact with blood, for example, through a blood splash to the face.

symptoms of the disease and therefore may be unaware that they have it. However, the virus lives in their bodies and can be transmitted to another person. Between 5% and 10% of HBV infections become chronic. People with chronic infections may never have symptoms and become carriers. Or, they may have flare-ups of symptoms every so often, resulting in months of disability. An effective vaccination against HBV is available and is recommended by OSHA for health care workers, as well as the general public (Fig. 8-4).

Health care workers who have any direct contact with patients or residents can be exposed to body fluids that contain HBV. Although the virus is not known to be transmitted in saliva, the gums of people with periodontal (gum) disease may

FIGURE 8-4

A vaccine against hepatitis B virus (HBV) is available. The Occupational Safety and Health Administration (OSHA) requires employers to make the vaccine available to nursing assistants free of charge.

bleed during oral care and tooth brushing, exposing the health care worker to potentially contaminated blood. There is always the risk of nicking a patient or resident with the razor during shaving, and patients or residents may fall and injure themselves, resulting in wounds that bleed. A used hypodermic needle could be lost in the bed linens or accidentally tossed in the trash, placing an unsuspecting health care worker at risk for a puncture injury. Because of these occupational risks, the **Centers for Disease Control and Prevention (CDC)** recommends that all health care workers who have even the slightest potential for being exposed to blood or contaminated body fluids should receive the hepatitis B vaccination, which provides immunity to the virus. OSHA requires employers to offer this vaccine to employees free of charge.

Hepatitis C Virus (HCV)

Hepatitis C virus (HCV) is also a bloodborne pathogen. The most common mode of transmission is through contaminated blood transfusions, although some needlestick exposures have caused infection. Although the mode of HCV transmission is mainly bloodborne, in more than 40% of people who are diagnosed with HCV, no obvious route of transmission is found. The illness that results from infection with HCV tends to be more chronic and serious than that resulting from infection with HBV. As many as 85% of people with hepatitis C develop chronic disease, and of these, 20% go on to develop end-stage cirrhosis (a fatal liver disease), liver failure, or liver cancer. Hepatitis C is the leading cause for liver transplantation in the United States. Currently, no vaccine against HCV is available.

Hepatitis D Virus (HDV)

Hepatitis D virus (HDV), also a bloodborne pathogen, is found only in people who are already infected with HBV. Vaccination against HBV protects against HDV.

Hepatitis E Virus (HEV)

Hepatitis E virus (HEV) is not a bloodborne type of hepatitis. Like HAV, HEV is spread through the oral–fecal route of transmission. HEV infection is most common in countries with poor sanitation controls. There is no vaccination for this virus.

HIV AND AIDS

Human immunodeficiency virus (HIV) is the virus that causes **acquired immunodeficiency syndrome (AIDS).** HIV is a bloodborne pathogen, and is transmitted in the same way as HBV. Its effect on the body, however, is very different.

As described in Chapter 7, the human immune system recognizes and destroys pathogens (microbes that can enter the body and cause illness). One way the immune system does its job is through **T cells,** special white blood cells (leukocytes) that play a role in the immune response to invading pathogens. There are two main types of T cells. One type of T cell recognizes cells that are foreign to the body, such as those infected by viruses, and kills them by producing substances that cause the foreign cells to burst. The other type of T cell produces substances that help other cells in the immune system to defend the body against pathogens.

T cells are the main target of HIV (Fig. 8-5). The virus invades the T cell. But, instead of killing the T cell immediately, it uses the T cell to make copies of itself and increase its numbers. Eventually, the virus kills the T cell, and then the virus (and all of its copies) move on to repeat the process in other T cells. This process, over a period of time, results in an increase in the virus count and a decrease in the T cell count.

In addition to invading and killing T cells, HIV invades the cells that form new T cells. This causes the body to produce T cells that cannot

FIGURE 8-5

This photograph was taken by a special microscope, and color was added to enhance it. It shows a T cell (*green*) that is infected with the human immunodeficiency virus (HIV), shown in *red*. Infection with HIV can lead to the development of acquired immunodeficiency syndrome (AIDS), a fatal disease. (*NIBSC/Photo Researchers, Inc.*)

TABLE 8-1 ■ **Comparison of Hepatitis B Virus (HBV) and Human Immunodeficiency Virus (HIV)**

	Hepatitis B Virus (HBV)	Human Immunodeficiency Virus (HIV)
Virus's ability to live outside of the body	HBV can live on a dry surface in the form of dried blood or body fluid for as long as **7 days.**	HIV can live for up to **24 hours** on a dry surface.
Virus content per cc/mL of blood*	**1,000,000,000 (1 billion)** virus particles per cc/mL of blood	**1,000 (1 thousand)** virus particles per cc/mL of blood
Risk of getting virus from a needlestick injury	**6%–30%**	**Less than 0.1%**[†]
Modes of transmission	Not transmitted by casual contact. Outside of the health care profession, HBV can be transmitted by having unprotected sexual intercourse or sharing needles used to inject drugs. It can also be transmitted to a fetus across the placenta or following exposure to the mother's blood during birth.	Not transmitted by casual contact. Outside of the health care profession, HIV can be transmitted by having unprotected sexual intercourse or sharing needles used to inject drugs. It can also be transmitted to a fetus across the placenta or following exposure to the mother's blood during birth.
Associated annual death rate among health care workers	Approximately 250 health care workers die each year from HBV	Statistic not available

* One cc/mL of blood is equal to approximately one large drop of blood. Therefore, even minor cuts can be significant in terms of their ability to expose the health care worker to bloodborne pathogens.
† 97.7% of occupational exposures do not result in HIV infection.

recognize pathogens. The body then becomes unable to recognize and fight off infections, leading to the condition known as AIDS. People with AIDS do not die from the virus itself. They die from infections that the body is no longer able to fight. To date, there is no cure for AIDS and no vaccine for HIV.

STANDARD PRECAUTIONS

Clearly, bloodborne pathogens, such as HIV and HBV, pose an occupational risk to the health care worker (Table 8-1). Because of the type of work you do, you will come in contact with substances that carry these viruses. Additionally, in many cases, you will not be able to easily identify patients or residents who have these diseases. For example, HIV can be present in the blood of an infected person for a very long time without causing symptoms or being detected using the diagnostic tests that are currently available. Similarly, recall that the virus that causes hepatitis B can live in a person's body without causing signs or symptoms. For these reasons, we in the health care field *must* treat each patient or resident we have contact with as if he may be infected with a bloodborne pathogen—thus, the

term **standard precautions.** These precautions are taken with each patient. Standard precautions involve the use of barrier methods, as well as certain environmental control methods, to protect the health care worker (Box 8-1). *For these methods to be effective, they must be used consistently!*

OSHA BLOODBORNE PATHOGENS STANDARD

Your safety in the workplace is a shared responsibility. You are responsible for following the standard precautions. Your employer is responsible for making sure that you have the equipment and training you need to maintain your safety in the workplace. To help employers to meet their responsibilities toward their employees, OSHA has created certain standards that all employers must follow.

According to the OSHA Bloodborne Pathogens Standard:

1. People working in an area where exposure to bloodborne pathogens is possible must receive training on the risks associated with bloodborne pathogens and on the methods they can use to safeguard themselves. Proof

BOX 8-1 Standard Precautions

1. Gloves must be worn if the *possibility* exists that the hands could come in contact with blood or other body fluids. Gloves must also be worn when touching any surface or linen that could be contaminated with infected materials. Remember that you cannot see a virus with the naked eye.

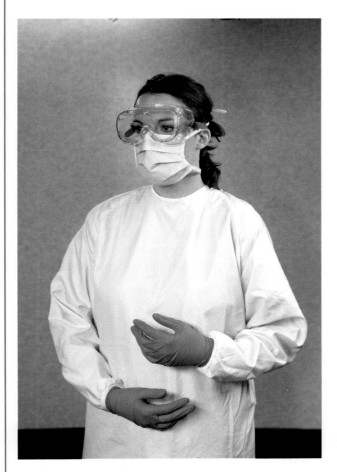

4. Sharps, such as used needles, razors, or broken glass, must be disposed of properly in labeled, OSHA-approved containers. Contaminated, broken glass items should not be handled, even with gloved hands. They should be swept or vacuumed up for disposal.
5. Spills of blood or other body fluids must be cleaned up promptly with an approved viricidal cleaning agent or a solution of 1 part household bleach to 10 parts water. Personal protective equipment (PPE), such as gloves and a gown, should be worn while cleaning up spills.

2. A waterproof (impervious) gown must be worn if the *possibility* exists that your clothes could become soiled with blood or other body fluids.
3. A mask, face shield, and eye goggles must be worn if the *possibility* exists that blood or other body fluids could splash or spray.

6. ***Handwashing is the single most important method of preventing the spread of infection!*** Hands must be washed when you remove your gloves. If accidental exposure to blood or other body substances occurs, hands must be washed thoroughly and immediately.

of initial training (at orientation) is to be on file in the employee's records and training must be updated annually.
2. Employers must make the hepatitis B vaccine available to workers who are at

risk, free of charge. If an employee refuses the vaccination, a disclaimer signed by the employee must be kept on file. If the employee decides to accept the vaccine at a later date, the employer must provide it.

3. The employer must provide adequate personal protective equipment (PPE), as required by the employee's duties. This includes gloves (non-latex, if the employee has allergies), face and eye protection, gowns and aprons, and scrub attire. It is the employee's responsibility to use the PPE consistently and conscientiously.

4. Environmental control methods must be used to protect both the employees and the patients or residents. Environmental control methods include special ventilation systems to keep the air clean, procedures for the disposal of liquid waste, the availability of sharps disposal containers, and procedures for handling contaminated linen and trash. Housekeeping and cleaning methods must also meet OSHA's standards.

5. Each health care facility must have an **exposure control plan** in place, in case an employee is exposed to blood or other body fluids from a patient or resident. This plan must be up-to-date, available in written form, and available to all employees. It is the employee's responsibility to report any exposure incidents so that the employer can arrange for appropriate medical tests and treatment.

Any health care facility that does not follow the OSHA standards for bloodborne pathogens may risk heavy fines and serious penalties, such as closure of the facility. For health care workers who do not follow standard precautions, the penalty can be even greater—a deadly illness. Additionally, if you have an exposure accident and are not following the recommended precautions, you may not be covered by worker's compensation if you become sick as a result of the exposure. The consequences of not following proper procedures in the workplace are not worth the risk.

It is important to remember that although those who choose to work in the health care field place themselves at risk for exposure to substances that can cause disease, the risk of encountering these substances outside of the workplace also exists. In fact, your behavior outside of the workplace could put you at much higher risk for getting one of these diseases. For example, having unprotected sexual intercourse is the most common way of getting HBV and HIV, and the rate of new hepatitis B and AIDS cases is growing fastest among young, heterosexual men and women. Your job exposes you to risks, such as needlesticks, that people in other professions do not need to worry about. But, if you follow the standard precautions, your risk of getting a bloodborne disease in the workplace will probably be lower than your risk of getting a bloodborne disease outside of it!

AIRBORNE PATHOGENS

Airborne pathogens are disease-producing microbes that are transmitted through the air. When an infected person coughs or sneezes, the microbes leave the body through particles of saliva or sputum (Fig. 8-6). As these particles spray through the air, they dry out and remain in the air for a long time (much like particles of dust caught in a shaft of sunlight). Like dust, the dried-out droplets containing microbes are in the air we breathe and on the surfaces we touch. Infection spreads when a person breathes the air containing the suspended pathogens. Infections that are transmitted in this way include measles, chickenpox, and tuberculosis (TB). Although vaccines are available to prevent measles and chickenpox, there is currently no vaccine against TB.

TUBERCULOSIS (TB)

Tuberculosis (TB) is an infection caused by a bacterium that usually infects the lungs, but may also infect the kidneys or bones. The bacteria are

FIGURE 8-6

Airborne pathogens are transmitted through the air when a person sneezes, coughs, laughs, sings, or speaks. (*Jonathan Watts/Photo Researchers, Inc.*)

present in the sputum of an infected person and are spread by airborne droplets when the person coughs, sneezes, speaks, or sings. People who have close, frequent contact with a person who has TB are most likely to get the disease. A person infected with TB may have the disease for years before she shows any symptoms. TB is usually diagnosed following a routine skin test (used to screen for the disease) or chest x-ray (Fig. 8-7). Health care facilities and agencies routinely screen new employees for existing infections and regularly re-screen employees according to their potential for exposure.

In the early 1900s, TB caused many deaths. It was often called "consumption" because the disease progressed slowly and caused a wasting effect on the person. (In other words, the person grew very thin, and appeared to be eaten, or "consumed," by the disease). During this time, people with TB were usually sent to special hospitals called *sanatoriums,* which offered treatment and also served as a way of limiting the spread of the disease, by keeping people with TB away from others. In the early 1950s, the development of antibiotics that worked against the bacterium that causes TB resulted in a decrease in the number of people with the disease. However, since the mid-1980s, there has been an increase in the number of new cases of TB.

Many factors seem responsible for these new cases:

- Strains of the bacterium that cause TB have become resistant to the antibiotics used to treat the infection, making the antibiotics less effective.
- People with immunodeficiency syndromes, such as AIDS, are more at risk for infections such as TB, and the number of people with immunodeficiency syndromes has increased.
- More people are traveling to developing nations, where TB is still common.
- People who are poor or who live in crowded urban areas (e.g., homeless people, illegal immigrants) are at increased risk for TB.

A

B

FIGURE 8-7

Health care facilities and agencies routinely screen employees for tuberculosis (TB). (*A*) A simple skin test is used to screen for exposure to TB. A small amount of test material, called tuberculin, is placed under the skin on the arm using a needle or tines. In a few days, the area is checked. A person who has been exposed to the bacterium that causes TB will develop redness and swelling in the area (*shown here*). A person who has not been exposed will not have any reaction to the tuberculin. (*B*) TB causes changes in the lungs that can be seen on a chest x-ray. The chest x-ray of a person with a TB infection in the upper part of the lungs is shown here. (*A, Dr. P. Marazzi, Photo Researchers, Inc.; B, B. Bates M.D./Custom Medical Stock Photo.*)

BOX 8-2 Airborne Precautions

1. Patients or residents known or suspected to be infected with an airborne pathogen are to be placed in private rooms with special ventilation systems.
2. Health care workers should wear masks when caring for patients or residents with known or suspected tuberculosis (TB). If the health care worker has not been exposed to measles or chickenpox (and is therefore not immune), then he is at risk for these diseases, and a mask should be worn when caring for patients or residents with measles or chickenpox. If the health care worker is immune to measles or chickenpox, a mask is not necessary.
3. A surgical mask should be placed over the patient's or resident's face if she must be transported from one location to another. Transport of the patient or resident should be kept to a minimum.
4. All precautions for preventing transmission of TB should be implemented if the patient or resident is known or suspected to have TB.

People who get TB need to be treated for a long time, with many different antibiotics. Unfortunately, the people who are most likely to get the disease are least likely to complete the course of treatment for it because they lack money, a stable home, or both.

AIRBORNE PRECAUTIONS

Because the number of new TB cases is increasing, and because the disease may go undiagnosed, a very real potential for exposure to TB in the workplace exists. For this reason, isolation (transmission-based) precautions should be followed, as described in Chapter 7. Additionally, if a patient or resident is known or suspected to have an infection that is caused by an airborne pathogen, such as TB, chickenpox, or measles, the airborne precautions in Box 8-2 should be taken as well.

SUMMARY

► Hepatitis B virus (HBV), hepatitis C virus (HCV), hepatitis D virus (HDV), and human immunodeficiency virus (HIV) are bloodborne pathogens that a health care worker may be exposed to. These viruses cause serious, possibly even life-threatening, diseases.
  ■ For a bloodborne pathogen to be transmitted from one person to another, blood or body fluids from an infected person must enter the bloodstream of a noninfected person.
    ● Needlesticks, cuts from contaminated glass, and splashes and sprays of contaminated blood can put a health care worker at risk for a bloodborne disease.
    ● Bloodborne diseases can also be transmitted through sexual intercourse and through blood transfusions.
    ● A person who is infected with a bloodborne pathogen may not appear to be ill.
  ■ You and your employer share the responsibility for maintaining your safety in the workplace.
    ● Employers must follow the standards outlined by the Occupational Safety and Health Administration (OSHA) to ensure that the work environment is safe (the OSHA Bloodborne Pathogens Standard).
    ● Employees must follow the recommended precautions for preventing the spread of disease (standard precautions). Following the recommended standard precautions, at all times, is the single most important thing you can do to ensure your own safety.

- A vaccine against HBV is available, and offers protection against HDV as well. Currently, there is no vaccine available for HCV or HIV.
- ► Tuberculosis (TB) is caused by an airborne pathogen. The pathogen that causes TB is spread when an infected person coughs, sneezes, speaks, or sings.
  - The number of TB cases is on the rise. A person with TB may not appear to be ill.
  - Although antibiotics are available to treat TB, treatment is difficult, time-consuming, and expensive. There is currently no vaccine available for TB.
- ► You will face exposure to many infections, some life-threatening, while caring for others. Learning about these infections and how they are transmitted, as well as staying well-informed about new developments and treatments for these diseases, will allow you to provide quality care to those you are responsible for.

What did you learn?

Multiple Choice

Select the single best answer for each of the following questions.

1. Hepatitis B virus (HBV), a bloodborne pathogen, can be found in all of the following body fluids except:
   a. Blood
   b. Semen
   c. Wound drainage
   d. Sweat

2. When are goggles a necessary part of personal protective equipment (PPE)?
   a. Whenever blood is present
   b. Whenever blood may splash or spray
   c. Whenever you are taking care of a person with tuberculosis (TB)
   d. Goggles are not really a necessary part of PPE

3. Human immunodeficiency virus (HIV) can be transmitted through all of the following means except:
   a. Blood splash to mucous membrane
   b. Sexual intercourse
   c. Sharing needles
   d. A mosquito bite

4. A vaccination against which one of the following bloodborne diseases is available?
   a. Lyme disease
   b. AIDS
   c. Hepatitis C
   d. Hepatitis B

5. Hepatitis B is a viral disease of the:
   a. Spleen
   b. Liver
   c. Blood
   d. Heart

6. For health care workers, which of the following is the most important method of preventing the spread of infection?
   a. Standard precautions
   b. Handwashing
   c. Wearing gloves
   d. Wearing gowns and goggles

7. Personal protective equipment (PPE) refers to:
   a. Sterilization and disinfection
   b. Security personnel
   c. Disposable gloves, face masks, and gowns
   d. Isolation precautions

? Stop and think!

► You are providing care to Mr. Torres, who has hepatitis B. This morning, while you are helping Mr. Torres to brush his teeth, he coughs, spraying your uniform and arms with bloody mucus. You are wearing gloves, but no gown or mask. Is it possible that you have been exposed to an infectious disease? What should you do?

9

Workplace Safety

What will you learn?

As you have learned in Chapters 7 and 8, the risk of infectious disease is a work-related hazard faced by all people in the health care system—patients and residents, family members and visitors, and health care workers. Although minimizing the spread of infectious disease is a major safety concern for health care workers, it is not the only one. In this chapter, we will explore other threats to the safety of people who work or live in a health care facility, and the measures you can take to minimize these threats. When you are finished with this chapter, you will be able to:

1. Describe hazards present in the workplace that can affect the safety of the nursing assistant.
2. Define the term *body mechanics* and demonstrate actions that make the body more effective when working.
3. Demonstrate the use of good body mechanics when lifting.
4. Describe ways to prevent back injury.
5. Describe hazards that increase the risk of falls in the health care setting.
6. Demonstrate how to assist a person who is falling.
7. Discuss electrical hazards found in the health care setting and ways to avoid them.
8. Describe chemical hazards found in the health care setting.
9. List the elements necessary for a fire to start and continue to burn.
10. Describe the RACE fire response plan.
11. Demonstrate how to use a fire extinguisher.
12. List disaster situations that may affect a health care facility, and describe the focus of a disaster preparedness plan in a hospital versus in a long-term care facility.

Photo: A competitive weightlifter uses good body mechanics to complete the lift safely. (Pascal Rondeau / Getty Images.)

Vocabulary

Use the CD in the back of your book to hear these terms pronounced, defined, and used in a sentence:

Body mechanics
Alignment
Balance
Coordinated
  movement
Grounded

Materials Safety
  Data Sheet
  (MSDS)
RACE fire response
  plan
Disaster

FIGURE 9-1

When the body is held in proper alignment, the back is in a "neutral" position, with the curve of the lower spine intact. Holding the body in proper alignment prevents strain on the joints and muscles.

PROTECTING YOUR BODY

Performing the same action over and over again places stress on the body—for example, think of the stress on a baseball catcher's knees as he squats, then stands, then squats again hundreds of times throughout a single game. In addition, moving a large, awkward, or heavy object also places undue strain on the body and can lead to injury. As a nursing assistant, you will place stress on your body as you lift, push, pull, stoop, and bend repeatedly on a daily basis. In addition, in many cases, you will need to move a person or piece of equipment that is larger and heavier than you are. There is no doubt about it—being a nursing assistant is extremely physically demanding! Fortunately, by practicing good body mechanics and learning proper lifting techniques, you can minimize your risk for physical injury.

THE "ABCs" OF GOOD BODY MECHANICS

The efficient movement and use of the wonderful machine we call the body is accomplished through good **body mechanics.** The basic components (the "ABCs") of good body mechanics are **A**lignment, **B**alance, and **C**oordinated movement.

Alignment is simply good posture. For the body to work most efficiently, proper alignment is necessary to ensure that no excess strain is placed on the joints and muscles. The back is held in a "neutral" position, with the natural curvature of the lower back intact. Imagine that you are looking at a person who is holding her body in proper alignment (Fig. 9-1). On the side view, you

would be able to draw a straight line connecting the person's ear, shoulder, hip, knee, and ankle. From the front view, you would be able to draw a straight line that connected the nose, the sternum (breastbone), and the navel, and then continued between the legs, dividing that space equally in half.

Balance involves holding your center of gravity, or area of largest mass, close to your base of support. For example, when you are standing, your base of support is your feet (which are placed squarely on the floor), and your center of gravity is your torso, the heaviest part of your body. The larger your base of support, and the closer the heaviest part of your body is to that base of support, the more balanced you will be. How, then, can you stabilize your body and maximize your ability to remain balanced? There are two ways:

- You can increase your base of support by spreading your feet further apart.
- You can bring your center of gravity closer to your base of support by bending at the knees and hips, so that your torso is closer to your feet.

Imagine that you are standing with your legs together and your ankles touching. If someone pushed you, you might lose your balance and fall. Now imagine that you are standing with your feet about shoulder-width apart. The same shove

A   **B**

FIGURE 9-2

Maintaining balance. (*A*) The distance between this person's feet (his base of support) is small, and the heaviest part of his body (his center of gravity) is far away from his base of support, making him more prone to lose his balance. (*B*) By increasing the distance between his feet and lowering his body toward the ground, the person has increased his ability to maintain his balance.

FIGURE 9-3

Coordinated body movement involves using the weight of your body to help with movement. Pulling a heavy cart up a hill is much easier than pushing it, because of coordinated body movement.

might not cause you to lose your balance. And if you were then to lower your body into a squat, it would be even harder to push you over! Increasing your base of support by standing with your feet apart, and positioning yourself so that your center of gravity (your torso) is close to your base of support (your feet) improves your balance and is a very important part of practicing good body mechanics (Fig. 9-2).

Coordinated body movement involves using the weight of your body to help with movement. For example, imagine that you must pull a heavy cart up a hill. You would stand facing the cart, holding the cart handle in your hands. Then you would take a step backward, bending at the knees and hips. With each backward step, the weight of your body would shift from the foot closest to the cart to the back foot, and the cart would roll forward. In this way, your body movement makes the task of moving the cart up the hill easier (Fig. 9-3). In Chapter 11, which focuses on repositioning and lifting people who cannot get out of bed, you will see other examples of how coordinated body movement can make a task easier. For example, when moving a person up in bed, you stand facing the bed, with your feet apart. As you step sideways to move the person's head and shoulders up, you trans-

fer your weight from one foot to the other and the momentum helps you to move the person.

LIFTING AND BACK SAFETY

Practicing good body mechanics is very important, especially when you must lift heavy equipment or move people who have trouble moving on their own. Lifting is a required task for nursing assistants who provide direct care to patients or residents. Therefore, it is important to learn proper technique. Failure to use good body mechanics when lifting something or someone can result in back injuries. Back injuries are the most common work-related injury in the nursing field. Injuries of the back range from muscle strains and soreness to ruptured vertebral discs (a condition that may require surgery and a long recovery period). Back injuries are painful and costly (in terms of medical care and missed work), and can be serious enough to end your career and prevent you from participating in other activities that you enjoy (Fig. 9-4). If you do not take precautions to prevent back injuries, you could find yourself in the position of being the patient instead of the care provider!

If you have ever watched the weightlifting event in the Olympics, you know that competitive weightlifters can lift more than 500 pounds. The weightlifter's lifting technique is an excellent example of good body mechanics being used. The athlete squats low to the ground, using his arms and shoulders to pull the weight close to his body at chest level. He then uses his hips and legs to

FIGURE 9-4

Back injuries are the most common work-related injury in the nursing field.

stand up with the weight. After becoming upright, he widens his base of support by moving one foot ahead of the other. These maneuvers allow the large, strong muscles of the body to do the work of lifting and also protect the back from injury.

The muscles of the arms and legs are attached to the long bones in our limbs. The muscle contracts by pulling against the bone it is attached to. This allows us to move and to lift weight. In contrast, the muscles of the back are flat and fan-like, and are not designed to lift weight. When the competitive weightlifter lifts his weights, he uses his leg muscles, not his back muscles. As he raises himself out of the squat, he uses the powerful muscles in his buttocks, hips, and thighs to move himself, and the weight, upward. Although you will not be required to practice competitive weightlifting at work, you should try to imitate the professionals with your technique! For example, if

you had to move a patient or resident from the bed to a chair, you would bend your knees and hold the person close to the center of your body. Then, you would use the muscles in your thighs and hips to lift and move the person from the bed to the chair. Proper lifting technique is summarized in Fig. 9-5.

Many health care facilities and agencies require employees who must lift to wear back supports. If your facility requires you to wear a back support when lifting, make sure you have been properly trained in its correct use. Use the support correctly. Improper or prolonged use of a back support can actually weaken the back muscles. But, when used correctly, the back support will remind you to hold your body in proper alignment when lifting. Bending at the waist with a tight back support around you is very uncomfortable (Fig. 9-6).

Guidelines for protecting yourself from injury as a result of the physical nature of your job are summarized in Guidelines Box 9-1. To protect your health, remember the principles of good body mechanics and apply them consistently, both at work and at home.

PREVENTING FALLS

In Chapter 10, you will learn about situations that increase a patient's or resident's risk for falling, such as poor vision, a limited ability to move, or confusion. But what about factors that increase a nursing assistant's chances of falling?

Nursing assistants work very hard and have many duties that must be completed during a shift. Being in too much of a hurry can increase your risk of falling. Even in an emergency situation, when you need to move quickly, be aware of your surroundings and move only as fast as you are safely able. You are not a help in an emergency if you fall and hurt yourself!

Wet floors also increase your risk of falling. Helping patients and residents with showers and baths often results in wet feet for you and water on the floor. A resident who is incontinent (unable to control her bladder) can leave a puddle of urine in the hallway that you could slip in, especially if you are in a hurry. If you see water or other fluids or substances on the floor, you should immediately stop what you are doing and dry the area (Fig. 9-7). Failure to do so puts you, your patients

Plan your lift.

Ask for help.

Widen your base of support.

Bend your knees

FIGURE 9-5

Proper lifting technique.

Tighten your stomach muscles.

Lift with your leg muscles.

Keep your load close.

Keep your back straight.

or residents, visitors, and coworkers at risk for falling.

Helping a very weak, unsteady, or uncooperative person to walk or transfer from one place to another without help can cause both of you to fall. You may not want to ask a busy coworker for help, but resist the temptation to "go it alone." If the patient or resident you are attempting to help falls, she will take you with her, potentially resulting in serious injury to you both. Attempting to prevent a patient or resident from falling can also result in a back injury for you. Please ask for help whenever you feel you need it in order to safely continue. If you are assisting a person who begins to fall, follow the steps in Box 9-1 to minimize the risk of injury for everyone involved.

PREVENTING CHEMICAL INJURIES

Health care facilities use many chemicals on a daily basis—for example, cleaning solutions and disinfectants, sterilizing agents, and chemothera-

peutic drugs. Many of these chemicals can be harmful if they are inhaled, swallowed, absorbed through the skin, or splashed in the eyes. Some chemicals are relatively harmless alone but can become dangerous if accidentally mixed with another product.

The Occupational Safety and Health Administration (OSHA) requires all employers to maintain a list of the chemicals that are used in the facility, from household cleaners to highly toxic solutions, and to inform and educate all workers about the chemicals that are in use in their workplace. One way of communicating information about chemicals to employees is through a **Materials Safety Data Sheet (MSDS),** which the manufacturer of the chemical is required to supply (Fig. 9-8). The MSDS for each chemical in use must be kept on file and be readily available in each unit of the health care facility. The MSDS summarizes key information about the chemical, such as what it is made from, which exposures may be dangerous, what to do if an exposure occurs, and how to clean up spills. Container labels also provide information about the chemicals in the container,

FIGURE 9-6

A back support can help to hold your body in proper alignment when lifting.

FIGURE 9-7

Mopping up spills is an important safety measure. Failing to do so can lead to falls.

and all containers must be clearly labeled. As a nursing assistant, it is your responsibility to be familiar with the chemicals that you may come in contact with in your facility, and to know the proper, safe way to handle each chemical in use.

PREVENTING ELECTRICAL SHOCKS

There are many electrical appliances used in the health care setting, from complex monitoring devices to the common hair dryer. Knowing how to safely operate and maintain electrical equipment in the workplace will help create a safe working environment for you and a safe living environment for your patients or residents.

Precautions, such as using grounded appliances and power strips, help to minimize the risk of electrical shock. Most electrical equipment used in the health care setting is **grounded.** This means that it has a way of returning stray electrical current to the outlet so that the risk of electrical shock is reduced. Grounding may be achieved through a three-prong plug (Fig. 9-9*A*) or a safety outlet with a ground-fault breaker (Fig. 9-9*B*). The use of extension cords is not recommended and outlets should not be overloaded. If more than two items must be plugged into an outlet, a facility-approved power strip should be used (Fig. 9-9*C*).

As a nursing assistant, you must be alert for electrical items that pose potential shock or fire hazards. Residents of long-term care facilities often bring small electrical items with them to furnish their rooms, such as radios, televisions, and table lamps. Most facilities require items like these to be inspected by the maintenance department before the resident can use them. However, if you should notice anything unsafe about an electrical appliance that is being used, such as frayed wires or loose plugs, you should remove the appliance from use immediately. This is true of facility-owned equipment as well, such as electrically controlled hospital beds and call light controls. Most health care facilities have a system for tagging a defective item and sending it for repair (Fig. 9-10). Follow your facility's policy. Failure to properly tag a defective electrical device could result in injury or even death to the next person who uses it.

GUIDELINES BOX 9-1
GUIDELINES FOR PROTECTING YOURSELF FROM PHYSICAL INJURY

What you do	*Why you do it*
Make a habit of practicing good posture.	Keeping the body in proper alignment, regardless of the activity, reduces stress and fatigue to the muscles and joints.
Create a solid base of support by moving your feet apart, either by widening your stance or by placing one foot in front of the other.	A solid base of support improves your balance, reducing the chance that you will injure yourself during the maneuver.
Allow the weight of your own body to assist in pulling or pushing heavy objects.	Using coordinated body movement to move something minimizes the stress on your body while making the task you are trying to accomplish easier.
When moving or lifting people or objects, place your body as close as possible to the object being moved.	Bringing your body's center of gravity closer to the object improves your balance and allows the strong muscles of the shoulders and upper arms to assist in the move.
Squat, do not lean over, to lower your center of gravity when lifting.	Lowering your center of gravity improves your balance. However, this lowering should be accomplished by squatting, rather than leaning over. Squatting allows you to use the strong muscles of your lower body to move yourself, and the weight, upward. Leaning over while lifting weight strains the back joints and muscles.
Use the large, strong muscles of the hips, buttocks, and thighs to do the lifting.	Using the strong muscles of the legs to move yourself upward is preferable to placing strain on the muscles of the back, which are not meant to be used to lift substantial amounts of weight.
Do not lift heavy objects from a position higher than your head. Use a step stool or a short safety ladder to raise your entire body closer to the desired level.	Attempting to lift a heavy object from an awkward position (for example, with your arms raised above your head) interferes with your ability to balance and places you at risk for injury.
If an object is very heavy, do not attempt to lift it. Instead, pull, push, or roll the object.	Pushing, pulling, or rolling a heavy object places less strain on your body because you can use your body weight to help you accomplish the task. In other words, you can use the principle of coordinated movement.
Use assistive devices whenever possible to make the job easier.	Hand carts and dollies permit the easy movement of objects by placing them on wheels. Gait belts, draw sheets, and mechanical lifts (discussed in detail in Chapter 11) help make moving people easier.
Ask for help when lifting or moving heavy people or objects. You should also get help when you need to move a person who cannot offer any assistance, or is combative.	Heavy or awkward loads increase your risk of injury (and, if you are attempting to lift a person, increase that person's risk of injury as well.) A person who is "dead weight" or uncooperative is both heavy and awkward.
Keep your body in good physical condition by exercising regularly, eating nutritious foods, and getting enough rest.	Your body can be compared to an automobile. It must be properly maintained in order to provide you with years of solid performance.

BOX 9-1 Minimizing the Risk of Injury as a Result of a Fall

1. If the person complains of dizziness or seems unsteady, help him to sit in a chair. If a chair is not close by, help the person to sit on the floor. Stay with the person and call for assistance. This action can prevent a fall completely.

2. If a fall cannot be avoided, place your body behind the person and place your arms around his torso, pulling him close to your body. Do not grab the person's arm in an attempt to prevent the fall, because doing so may actually cause more extensive injuries in some people (such as elderly people, who may have brittle bones, and people with weaknesses on one side of the body).

3. With the person's body pulled close to yours, widen your base of support by placing one foot behind the other, and allow the person to slide down your body toward the floor.

4. As the person slides down, squat while still supporting his body and gently lower him to the floor. Lower yourself to the floor and assume a sitting position with the person's head in your lap.

5. Stay with the person and call for assistance.

When using electrical equipment, be aware of the safety hazard posed by operating an electrical appliance around water. Do not operate hair dryers, electric razors, curling irons, radios, or other electrical appliances around showers and bathtubs. The risk of electrical shock or electrocution must be taken seriously.

FIRE SAFETY

In a health care facility, a fire that gets out of control can have tragic consequences. Not only is the facility either a permanent or temporary home to hundreds of people, many of these

----
   5. ENVIRONMENTAL INFORMATION   (continued)

RECOMMENDED DISPOSAL:
  Discharge spent solutions and small quantities (less than 5 gal.(19
  L)) to a wastewater treatment system. Flush spent solutions and
  small quantities (less than 5 gal.(19 L)) to a wastewater treatment
  system. Reduce discharge rate if foaming occurs. Incinerate in a
  permitted hazardous waste incinerator in the presence of a
  combustible material.

  Empty container may be sanitary landfilled.

ENVIRONMENTAL DATA:
  Not determined.

REGULATORY INFORMATION:
  Volatile Organic Compounds: ca. 4.00 gms/liter.
  VOC Less H2O & Exempt Solvents: N/D.

  Since regulations vary, consult applicable regulations or authorities
  before disposal. U.S. EPA Hazardous Waste Number = D002 (Corrosive)

EPCRA HAZARD CLASS:
 FIRE HAZARD: Yes PRESSURE: No REACTIVITY: No ACUTE: Yes   CHRONIC: Yes

----
   6. SUGGESTED FIRST AID

EYE CONTACT:
  Immediately flush eyes with large amounts of water for at least 15
  minutes. Get immediate medical attention.

SKIN CONTACT:
  Immediately flush skin with large amounts of water for at least 15
  minutes in a chemical safety shower while removing contaminated
  clothing and shoes. Get immediate medical attention. Wash
  contaminated clothing before reuse.

INHALATION:
  If signs/symptoms occur, remove person to fresh air. If
  signs/symptoms continue, call a physician.

IF SWALLOWED:
  If swallowed, do NOT induce vomiting. Give victim two glasses of
  water. Call a physician immediately. Never give anything by mouth to
  an unconscious person.

  Note to physician: Probable mucosal damage may contraindicate the use
  of gastric lavage.

Abbreviations: N/D - Not Determined N/A - Not Applicable CA - Approximately

FIGURE 9-8

Part of a Materials Safety Data Sheet (MSDS). The MSDS provides important information about each chemical in use in the workplace.

A   **B**   **C**

FIGURE 9-9

(A) Three-prong plugs, (B) outlets with ground-fault breakers, and (C) power strips help to reduce the risk of electrical shock and fire.

people are relatively unable to help themselves in the event of an emergency. As a health care worker, you must know how to prevent fires in the workplace, and what to do in the event that a fire does occur.

PREVENTING FIRES

For a fire to occur, three elements must be present: fuel (something to burn), heat (something to ignite the fuel), and oxygen (Fig. 9-11).

Common sources of fuel in the health care setting include:

- Cloth, such as bed linens, mattresses, and clothing
- Paper
- Substances that easily catch fire and burn quickly, such as cooking oil, gasoline, and nail polish remover
- The building itself

Heat can be provided by:

- An electrical spark (such as may occur with a frayed electrical cord, a "short" in a piece of electrical equipment, or even a lightning strike)
- Lighted smoking materials (such as cigarettes, cigars, or matches)
- Lighted candles

- Heating elements (such as radiators or furnaces)
- Stoves

Oxygen is found in the air around us, and generally the better the air supply, the better a fire will burn. Remember that in a health care facility, many patients and residents receive oxygen therapy, which increases the content of the oxygen in the air in the immediate area. Safety precautions that are used to prevent fires (Guidelines Box 9-2) are extremely important

FIGURE 9-10

If you notice that a piece of electrical equipment is malfunctioning or presents a safety hazard, follow your facility's policy for removing it from use and getting it repaired.

FUEL
- Cloth
- Paper
- Building materials
- Cooking oil or grease
- Flammable substances (e.g., nail polish remover)

HEAT
- Electrical spark
- Lighted smoking materials
- Lighted candles

OXYGEN
- Normal air
- Oxygen tank

FIGURE 9-11

Three things must be present for a fire to occur: fuel, heat, and oxygen.

when oxygen therapy is in use. The patient or resident and any visitors should be made aware of the added risks (Fig. 9-12).

REACTING TO A FIRE EMERGENCY

Sometimes, despite taking precautions, a fire will occur. In some cases, the fire will be small and can be dealt with rather easily if the situation is

FIGURE 9-12

Oxygen therapy is common in health care facilities. "Oxygen In Use" signs are posted to warn patients or residents and their visitors that extra precautions are needed when oxygen therapy is in use.

addressed promptly and correctly. For example, imagine a fire that begins in a resident's room because a visitor drops a half-lit cigarette in a wastebasket full of paper, or a stovetop fire that begins in the hospital kitchen. In both of these situations, an alert person who knew what to do could control the fire and it is possible that others outside of the immediate area would not even be aware of the disturbance. However, sometimes a fire can begin on a much larger scale, for example, as a result of faulty electrical wiring in the walls of the building, a gas leak, or even a terrorist attack. In situations like these, a large-scale evacuation (removal) of those in the facility will most likely be necessary.

The general actions that are taken in the event of a fire emergency are known as the **RACE fire response plan** (Fig. 9-13):

Remove any patients or residents who are in immediate danger to safety. Escort people who can walk. Use wheelchairs for unsteady people. To prevent a confused or disoriented person from accidentally wandering back into the fire area, assign another, alert patient or resident or a visitor to attend to the person. People who cannot get out of bed should be moved in their beds, if possible. If the bed cannot be moved out of the room, or if stairs must be used, the patient or resident can be pulled to safety using the linens from the bed (Box 9-2). Some facilities will train you in special techniques that are used to carry a person to safety.

Activate the alarm, if the alarm has not been sounded. Follow your facility's policy for reporting a fire. For example, you may be required to pull the fire alarm, or use the intercom or telephone system.

Contain the fire by closing doors and windows. This action helps to slow the spread of the fire.

Extinguish the fire if possible, or, if the fire is large or spreading quickly,

Evacuate the building.

Extinguishing Fires

As you know, there are three elements that must be present for a fire to continue burning—fuel, heat, and oxygen. If you remove just one of these elements, you can put out (extinguish) the fire. Not all fires are alike. Fires are classified as either "A" type, "B" type, or "C" type fires (Table 9-1).

GUIDELINES BOX 9-2
GUIDELINES FOR PREVENTING FIRES

What you do	Why you do it
Supervise patients or residents who are disoriented or who may fall asleep while smoking, any time that they smoke.	A sleepy or disoriented person is not paying close attention to the lighted smoking material, which increases the chance that a fire will start.
Do not allow any patient or resident to smoke in bed, especially if the person is receiving oxygen therapy.*	A person who smokes in bed is bringing all three elements necessary for a fire together (fuel = bed linens; heat = lighted smoking material; oxygen = surrounding air). Smoking in bed is especially dangerous because the person is more likely to fall asleep and forget about the lighted smoking material. In addition, the use of oxygen therapy increases the oxygen content of linens and bedding in the immediate area. If burning ashes from a cigarette should happen to drop on the bed, a fire would be more likely to start and would burn much faster as a result of the added oxygen.
If smoking is permitted in the facility, make sure that all smoking occurs only in designated smoking areas.	Designated smoking areas have ashtrays for properly extinguishing lit smoking materials. They are also located in a part of the building where oxygen therapy is not in use.
Keep smoking materials, lighters, and matches in a place where children and confused patients or residents cannot reach them.	Children do not understand that playing with these materials can be dangerous. A confused person is not able to use these materials responsibly on his or her own, and should be supervised.
Keep all electrical equipment in good working order.	A spark from a frayed wire, an improperly grounded plug, or an electrical "short" can start an electrical fire.
Handle flammable substances safely and clean up any spills immediately. Do not use flammable substances near a heat source such as a hair dryer or heater, or while smoking.	Flammable substances ignite easily and burn quickly. Therefore, if they come in contact with a heat source, a fire is likely to start.
Report any malfunctioning smoke detectors immediately.	A smoke detector is the best early fire detection device available, but only if it is functioning properly.
Investigate smoke or smells of anything burning promptly. Be aware of the location of fire alarms and fire extinguishers and know how to activate and use them.	Early investigation and quick action can help to contain a fire before it gets out of control.
Be familiar with your facility's fire safety policies and know the location of all exits.	If a fire does occur, you may need to evacuate patients or residents. You will be much more effective in your duties if you are able to remain calm, and your calmness will also help to calm others.

*Although health care facilities prohibit smoking in patient or resident rooms, some people may forget or disregard the rules.

Remove

Activate

Contain

Extinguish or Evacuate

FIGURE 9-13

The RACE fire response plan.

This classification determines the best way to put them out.

A commonly used tool for putting out fires is a fire extinguisher (Fig. 9-14). There are fire extinguishers that are specific for each type of fire, but the most common type of fire extinguisher, an ABC extinguisher, can be used for all types of fires. ABC fire extinguishers use carbon dioxide to remove the oxygen from the fire. This smothers

---

BOX 9-2 Using Bed Linens to Evacuate a Bedridden Person

1. Loosen the bottom sheet from the foot of the person's bed.
2. Make sure that the bed is lowered to its lowest position and that the wheels are locked.
3. Clasp the top of the bottom sheet near the person's shoulders and lower the person's upper body slowly to the floor, allowing the person's lower body to follow naturally. Be sure to use good body mechanics during this maneuver.
4. Pull the sheet, with the person cradled in it, toward the nearest exit.
5. If it is necessary to move the person down stairs, support the person's upper body by pulling up on the sheet and proceed down the steps backward, pulling the person behind you head-first. (In other words, allow the person's feet to bump against each step, not his or her head!)

---

the fire, putting it out. All health care facilities must have easily accessible fire extinguishers, in case a fire should occur. You are responsible for knowing where fire extinguishers are kept in your facility. During your orientation, you will be trained in the use of your facility's fire extinguishers, and these instructions will be reviewed with you each year. In the event of a small fire, you should be able to use a fire extinguisher to put the fire out safely and effectively. When using a fire extinguisher, remember the word **PASS:**

Pull the safety pin out.

Aim the hose toward the base of the fire.

Squeeze the handle.

Spray the contents of the fire extinguisher at the base of the fire.

Evacuating the Building

If a large, uncontrollable fire breaks out, you will need to know how to get your patients or residents and yourself to safety. Health care facilities must regularly practice and evaluate fire safety plans. You should take these fire drill exercises seriously so that if a fire emergency should occur, your actions will be almost second nature. By knowing what to do and acting calmly, you will increase the efficiency of the evacuation and help to calm those around you.

TABLE 9-1 ■ Types of Fires

Type	Description	Method of Extinguishing
A	Fueled by ordinary material such as wood, paper, cloth, leaves, and grass	Water effectively extinguishes a Type A fire by removing the heat.
B	Fueled by a petroleum product (e.g., gasoline, automotive oil), cooking oil, or grease	Do not try to put these fires out with water! Instead, smother the fire by sprinkling powder (such as baking soda) on it or by using a fire extinguisher made for a Type B fire. A stovetop fire that starts in a pan can be extinguished by covering the pan and removing it from the heat source.
C	An electrical fire	Attempting to put an electrical fire out with water can result in shock or electrocution. Use a fire extinguisher that is specific to an electrical fire instead.

DISASTER PREPAREDNESS

A **disaster** is a sudden, unexpected event that causes injury to many people, major damage to property, or both. Disasters can be caused by acts of nature (such as tornadoes, earthquakes, hurricanes, floods, blizzards, or ice storms), or they may be the result of explosions, accidents, or acts of war or terrorism. Your facility or agency will have a disaster preparedness plan that will direct the actions of the health care team in the event of such an occurrence. If you work for a hospital, your facility's disaster plan may focus on preparing staff to handle the simultaneous admission and treatment of multiple people with injuries. If you work in a nursing facility, the focus of your facility's disaster plan may be more on how to provide safe care for your residents in the event of a power failure. In the event of a disaster, you may have to help evacuate residents and patients to safer quarters. Know the particular duties that will be required of you in the event of a disaster and remain calm.

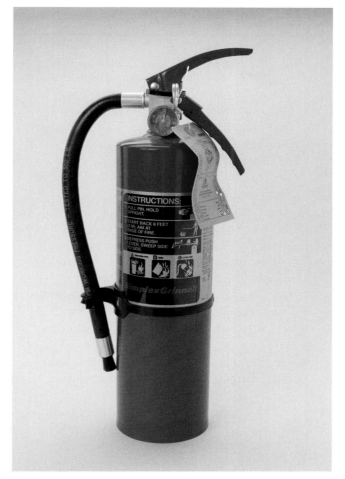

FIGURE 9-14

An ABC fire extinguisher is effective against all types of fires.

SUMMARY

▶ There are many factors that contribute to workplace safety and there are many people that the safety of the workplace affects.

■ It is your responsibility to help make your workplace safe, both for yourself and others, by following the guidelines for safety and by reporting any unsafe conditions to the appropriate person.

■ The Occupational Safety and Health Administration (OSHA) oversees safety regulations in all types of workplaces and addresses everything from safe lifting techniques to the control of hazardous materials.

● OSHA mandates that employers inform workers of all safety risks that are present in their workplace.

● OSHA requires employers to provide regular training about the safety risks in the work environment, and how injury is to be avoided. Your employer must keep records of any training you have received that meets OSHA regulations.

▶ Practicing good body mechanics allows you to use your body effectively when lifting and moving patients and equipment, and helps to protect you from injury as you perform your daily duties.

■ The "ABCs" of good body mechanics are alignment, balance, and coordinated movement.

■ Learning proper lifting technique is especially critical to preventing back injuries.

▶ Falling poses a risk to both the health care worker and the patient or resident. Asking for assistance and knowing how to properly assist a person who is falling can help to prevent injuries to everyone involved.

▶ Most health care facilities use many chemicals in their daily operation. Information about how to respond to a chemical exposure is found on the Materials Safety Data Sheet (MSDS), which each chemical manufacturer must supply, and on the labeled container.

▶ Malfunctioning electrical appliances, or electrical appliances that are used improperly, can lead to electric shock, electrocution, and electrical fires.

▶ A fire in a health care facility can have tragic consequences because many of the people who are housed in health care facilities are unable to move independently or quickly in the event of a fire.

■ Three elements are necessary to start a fire and keep it burning: fuel, heat, and oxygen.

■ The RACE fire response plan describes the general actions that are to be taken in the event of a fire emergency: **R**emove people in the immediate area, **A**ctivate the alarm, **C**ontain the fire, and **E**xtinguish or **E**vacuate as indicated by the situation.

▶ In the event of a disaster, follow your facility's disaster preparedness plan.

What did you learn?

Multiple Choice

Select the single best answer for each of the following questions.

1. In the event of a fire in a resident's room, your first action should be to:
   a. Remove the resident to a safe place
   b. Get the fire extinguisher
   c. Sound the fire alarm
   d. Notify the head nurse

2. When lifting, remember to use the large muscles of your:
   a. Chest
   b. Hips, buttocks, and thighs
   c. Back
   d. Shoulders

3. You accidentally knock over a water pitcher, spilling water on the floor of a patient's room. What should you do?
   a. Call housekeeping
   b. Continue with your assignment and make a mental note to wipe up the spill later
   c. Throw a towel over the spill to absorb the liquid and alert others to be careful
   d. Wipe the spill up immediately

4. While you are walking with Mrs. Davis in the hallway, she complains of chest pains and dizziness. Your first response should be to:
   a. Assist her to the floor and call for help
   b. Assist her to the floor and go get help
   c. Ask Mrs. Davis to breathe deeply and reassure her that everything will be fine
   d. Encourage Mrs. Davis to continue walking because she needs the exercise

5. As you come around the corner on your unit, you hear Mrs. Petersen shouting in alarm, and you see smoke and flames coming from the wastebasket in her room. You should:
   a. Run to the telephone and call the fire department

   b. Take Mrs. Petersen's cigarettes away
   c. Assist Mrs. Petersen out of the room and close the door
   d. Throw water on the flames

6. Using good body mechanics to lift an object off the floor means that you would:
   a. Use a mechanical lift
   b. Kneel down to get the broadest base of support and lift up
   c. Squat and lift with your legs
   d. Lean over at the waist, keeping your back flat

7. Unsafe conditions in a health care facility can be caused by:
   a. Health care workers who allow patients or residents to get out of bed
   b. Health care workers who stop doing an assigned task to clean up a spill
   c. Overloaded outlets and extension cords
   d. Patients and residents who smoke in "smoking only" areas

8. All of the following actions could cause a fire except:
   a. Using a three-prong plug
   b. Emptying an ashtray into a wastebasket
   c. Smoking in a room where a person is receiving oxygen therapy
   d. Placing a stack of linens on a heating unit to warm them

9. Where should you direct the foam when using a fire extinguisher to put out a fire?
   a. At the base of the fire
   b. In a circle around the fire, to prevent the fire from spreading
   c. At the top of the fire
   d. Anywhere in the general area of the fire

10. What are the "ABCs" of good body mechanics?
    a. Assess, Balance, Complete
    b. Assign, Begin, Complete
    c. Alignment, Balance, Coordinated movement
    d. Attempt, Brace, Change

11. You are a new nursing assistant and have been assigned to clean the room of a resident who has just been discharged. The nurse shows you the cleaning closet, which contains towels, rags, and containers holding liquids and powders of various colors and odors. How can you find out what cleaning products are appropriate for your assigned task?

a. Read the nursing care plan

b. Read the Material Safety Data Sheet (MSDS)

c. Use your senses—smell the contents of each container and use whichever has the most pleasant smell

d. There is no need to find out which product is most appropriate—the cleaning closet contains only products used for cleaning

? Stop and think!

▶ You work on the second floor of a large long-term care facility. As you are on your way from the nurses' station to answer a resident's call light, you see smoke coming from another resident's room. You know that the occupant of that room, Miss Verna, is a committed smoker. Although Miss Verna knows she is not supposed to smoke, she often tries to "sneak" a cigarette. She has emphysema, a terminal lung disease caused by smoking, and is receiving oxygen therapy. Much to your horror, when you enter the room, you see that Miss Verna has dozed off, dropping a lit cigarette onto her bed linens. The sheets have begun to smolder and catch on fire. What should you do first—sound the fire alarm? Turn off the flow of oxygen? Wake Miss Verna up and assist her to safety? Explain the logic behind your answer.

10

Patient and Resident Safety and Restraints

What will you learn?

Life has taught us many lessons in safety. When you were a child, your parents constantly reminded you to look both ways before crossing the street. As a teen learning to drive, you were cautioned to wear your seatbelt and to observe the rules of the road. As an adult, you remember to lock the door at night and turn off the coffeepot before you leave home. As you remember from Chapter 6, safety is a basic human need. If we feel safe, we can relax and rest and we feel secure and comfortable. The previous chapters have explained principles and procedures designed to help keep you safe while you perform your duties as a nursing assistant. In this chapter, we will focus on principles and procedures that help to keep those you care for safe. When you are finished with this chapter, you will be able to:

1. Identify risk factors that may put people in a health care facility at higher risk for accidents and injury.
2. Describe basic safety methods designed to prevent accidents in a health care facility.
3. Understand the importance of reporting and recording occurrences.
4. List the different types of restraints.
5. Describe methods used to reduce the need for restraints.
6. Identify safety concerns of restraint use.
7. Demonstrate the proper application of a vest restraint, a wrist or ankle restraint, and a lap or waist (belt) restraint.

Photo: As a nursing assistant, you will play an important role in keeping your patients or residents safe. Here, a nursing assistant helps a resident to get out of bed safely.

Vocabulary

Use the CD in the back of your book to hear these terms pronounced, defined, and used in a sentence:

Paraplegia	Comatose	Physical restraint	Procedures
Quadriplegia	Incident (occurrence)	Chemical restraint	Pre-procedure actions
Hemiplegia	report	Restraint alternatives	Post-procedure actions

ACCIDENTS

RISK FACTORS

For many reasons, certain groups of people are more at risk than others to have an accident (Fig. 10-1). Recognizing the factors that can increase a person's chances of having an accident will help you to minimize the chance that an accident will occur.

Age

Infants and young children are at high risk for accidents. Infants are helpless. As a result, they are prone to accidental suffocation and falls. Young children are not helpless, but they lack knowledge about things that are dangerous. As a result, young children are at risk for injuries such as falls, burns, poisoning, and drowning. You can find out more about safety issues related to children in Chapter 41.

The elderly are at high risk for accidents also. Although an elderly person can recognize a dangerous situation, some of the physical and mental effects of the aging process can affect his or her ability to be safe.

Medication

The effects of medications, especially pain medications, can affect the ability of a person to be safe, regardless of age or other factors. For example, under the influence of a pain medication (which has a sedative effect), a person who normally smokes a cigarette while watching the evening news could fall asleep in front of the television while smoking, causing a fire. Driving and operating machinery are dangerous under the influence of some medications. Medications that affect blood pressure can cause a person to become dizzy if he or she stands up quickly, leading to a fall. Some medications cause confusion in the elderly, especially if they are not taken properly.

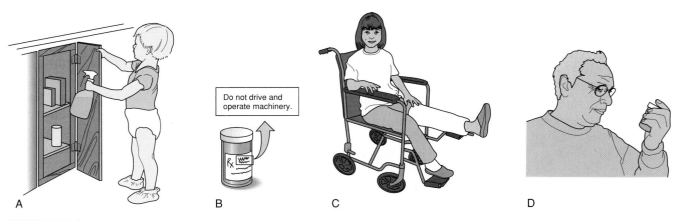

A   B   Do not drive and operate machinery.   C   D

FIGURE 10-1

Some predisposing factors that place people at risk for accidents: (*A*) very young or very old age; (*B*) medication effects;. (*C*) impaired mobility (an inability to move easily); (*D*) sensory impairment (an inability to see, hear, smell, taste, or detect pain or changes in temperature).

Paralysis

Paralysis (an inability to move or to feel) can be caused by a spinal cord injury or a stroke ("brain attack"). Depending on where a spinal cord injury occurs, a person can be paralyzed from the waist down, or from the neck down. Paralysis from the waist down is known as **paraplegia.** Paralysis from the neck down is known as **quadriplegia.** A quadriplegic or paraplegic person's abilities vary, according to the exact level of the spinal injury. A stroke can cause **hemiplegia,** or paralysis on one side of the body. Not only is a person with paraplegia, quadriplegia, or hemiplegia unable to move the affected areas of his body, he is usually unable to sense pain, heat, or cold in these areas. The inability to move properly increases the person's risk for falling. The lack of sensation increases the person's risk for other injuries, such as burns.

Poor Mobility

An inability to move easily can put a person at risk for falling. Pain and stiffness from arthritis can make it difficult for a person to get around easily. A stroke can sometimes cause a person to shuffle his feet when he walks. This can make a person more likely to trip over carpeted areas and uneven outside surfaces. Although elderly people tend to have more trouble with mobility than younger people, this is a risk factor that can affect all age groups. For example, a person recovering from knee surgery or a broken leg will be more likely to fall because of difficulty with mobility.

Sensory Impairment

We rely on our five senses (vision, hearing, touch, smell, and taste) to give us information about our environment and to keep us safe. Perhaps the sense we rely on the most is sight—not being able to see clearly can put anyone at risk for accidents. Poor vision increases the risk of falls, especially on stairs or over objects left on the floor. A person who wears bifocals may misjudge distance when stepping on or off curbs and steps, leading to falls. Additionally, poor vision can increase the chances of accidental poisoning from medications, if the person is not able to clearly read the directions on the medication label.

Our sense of hearing also plays a large role in keeping us safe. A person with hearing difficulties may not be able to hear signs of danger approaching, such as the sound of an oncoming car. She may also miss warning alarms, such as the sound made by a smoke or carbon monoxide detector. When being given instructions or directions (for example, regarding how to take a medication), a hearing-impaired person may be able to hear part of what is being said, but not enough to understand completely.

Touch and smell play a role in informing us about our environment as well. Certain conditions, such as diabetes, can decrease a person's sense of touch. People with an impaired sense of touch may not be able to tell that their bath water is too hot, leading to increased risk for burns. Because their ability to feel pain is lessened, they may be unaware that a favorite pair of shoes is causing blisters, leading to infection. Similarly, a decreased ability to smell (such as often occurs as part of the normal aging process) can leave a person unable to detect spoiled food, a natural gas leak in the home, or smoke.

Limited Awareness of Surroundings

There are many reasons a person may not be aware of his surroundings. Confusion and disorientation can be caused by reactions to medication, head injuries, dementia, and other medical conditions. It can also be caused by something as simple as a change in environment or forgetting to put one's glasses on. Confusion can cause a person in a health care facility to forget to call for help when he needs to get up. A person who is unconscious or **comatose** is totally unable to respond to his environment and will also need your assistance to remain safe.

As you can see, there are many factors that can affect a person's ability to avoid accidents. When several of these factors are combined, complex safety issues can result. As a nursing assistant, you must evaluate each person and situation individually so that you can provide a safe environment for those you care for.

AVOIDING ACCIDENTS

Many accidents that occur in health care facilities could have been prevented. Most safety measures do require an extra step or two, meaning more work for an already overworked staff of health care workers. However, remember your obligation to provide the same quality of care for your patients or residents that you would want for a member of your own family. Take that extra step to help ensure the safety of those you care for.

Preventing Falls

Falls are the leading cause of accidental death among elderly people. Falls are also the most common type of accident that occurs in the health care setting. In Chapter 9, you learned how to assist a person who is falling. However, preventing a fall is always the best policy.

Many health care facilities, especially hospitals and long-term care facilities, evaluate each new patient or resident for risk factors that increase the person's risk for falls (Fig. 10-2). Measures that can be taken to prevent falls are then included in the person's nursing care plan. Guidelines for preventing falls are given in Guidelines Box 10-1.

Preventing Burns

As you learned earlier, people who have a reduced sense of touch (reduced sensation) may be at risk for burns. A burn can be life-threatening to a patient or resident. Measures for preventing burns include the following:

- If a person will be taking a tub bath or shower, always check the water temperature first using a bath thermometer. The water temperature should be between 105°F (40.5°C) and 115°F (46°C). If the person is elderly, the water temperature should be at the lower end of this range. Many long-term care facilities have whirlpool tubs that allow you to set the water temperature before filling the tub.
- If you will be giving a person a bed bath, you should measure the temperature of the water in the basin. The water in the basin can be hotter than the water in a bathtub or shower because it cools off quickly and the person will not be immersed in it. The temperature range for a bed bath is between 110°F (43.3°C) and 115°F (46°C).
- Teach patients or residents who will be bathing themselves to check the water temperature with a thermometer or a hand or wrist before getting into the bathtub or shower.
- Use extreme care with heat applications (discussed in detail in Chapter 25).

FIGURE 10-2

Many health care facilities use a form like this one to assess a new patient's or resident's risk of falling. Once the risk factors are known, precautions can be taken to decrease the person's risk of falling. (Modified with permission from Hollinger, L. & Patterson, R. [1992]. A fall prevention program for the acute care setting. In S.G. Funk, E.M. Tomquist, M.T. Champagene, and R.A. Wiese [Eds.], *Key aspects of elder care: Managing falls, incontinence, and cognitive impairment.* New York: Springer.)

FALL RISK ASSESSMENT TOOL

Client Factors	Date	Initial Score	Date	Reassessed Score
History of falls		15		15
Confusion		5		5
Age (greater than 65 years)		5		5
Impaired judgment		5		5
Sensory deficit		5		5
Unable to ambulate independently		5		5
Decreased level of cooperation		5		5
Increased anxiety/emotional lability	5			5
Incontinence/urgency		5		5
Cardiovascular/respiratory disease affecting perfusion and oxygenation		5		5
Medications affecting blood pressure or level of consciousness		5		5
Postural hypotension with dizziness		5		5
Environmental Factors				
First week on unit (e.g., lack of familiarity with facility, services)			5	
Attached equipment (e.g., intravenous pole, chest tubes, appliances, oxygen, tubing)		5		5

Total points:_____
Implement fall precautions for a total score of 15 or greater.

GUIDELINES BOX 10-1
GUIDELINES FOR PREVENTING FALLS

What you do	Why you do it
Check the person's clothing and shoes. Clothing should fit properly. Shoes should provide good foot support and have nonskid soles.	Long or loose clothing (such as a robe) or shoes that provide inadequate foot support or have slippery soles could lead to tripping.
Encourage the person to use rails along hallways and stairways while walking.	The additional support offered by rails may be all that is needed to allow a person to move about safely and independently.
Observe the person for signs of unsteadiness and offer physical assistance as needed.	Offering assistance as needed allows the person to remain as independent as possible, while minimizing the risk of falls.
Observe the person's ability to use walking aids, such as canes and walkers, and correct incorrect use.	Using a piece of equipment improperly can be just as hazardous as not using it at all.
Check equipment, such as walkers and wheelchairs, to ensure that it is in good condition. Non-skid tips should be intact on walkers. Wheelchair wheel locks should function properly.	Malfunctioning or broken equipment increases a person's risk for accidents.
Make sure a patient or resident who needs glasses is wearing them when he or she is out of bed.	A person who cannot see clearly is more at risk for falls.
Remove any clutter or obstacles from walkways and provide adequate lighting.	Proper lighting enhances the ability to see. Removal of obstructions is an easy way to minimize falls.
Keep beds in the lowest position. Keep bed wheels locked.	Keeping the bed in the lowest position minimizes the distance from the bed to the floor, should the person fall out of bed. Keeping the wheels on the bed locked prevents the bed from rolling. A rolling bed could result in injury to the nursing assistant, the patient or resident, or both.
Keep side rails up or down, according to the care plan for that particular person.	Side rails can prevent a person from falling out of bed. Because side rails are considered a form of restraint, they should always be lowered, unless the person's medical condition is such that he or she needs the protection that is offered by having the side rails raised.
Always make sure the call light control is within easy reach of the person. Answer call lights promptly, and offer to help the person with toileting frequently.	Many falls are the result of a person trying to make it to the bathroom without assistance.
Wipe up any spills immediately.	Wet surfaces may not be obvious (especially to people with some degree of visual impairment) and greatly increase the risk of slipping.
Keep people who are at risk for falling and disoriented close to the nursing station. Offer frequent assistance with walking.	Keeping a person who is disoriented and at risk for falling close to the nursing station allows staff to "keep an eye" on the person, and also minimizes the chance that a person who feels lonely will attempt to get up to look for company. A person who is offered help with walking on a fairly regular basis is less likely to attempt to get up on his or her own, thereby minimizing the chance of a fall.
Orient a newly admitted patient or resident to the unit and his or her room.	Falls and other accidents often occur when a person is unfamiliar with his or her surroundings.

- Warn people that a food or beverage is hot before giving it to them. Many burns occur when hot liquids (such as soup, coffee, or tea) spill. Some people may need a cup with a lid for their coffee or tea if weakness or unsteadiness puts them at risk for spilling.
- Follow the guidelines for using electrical appliances that are given in Chapter 9. Electrical burns can occur if an appliance malfunctions or is used near water.

Preventing Accidental Poisonings

Many people think of accidental poisonings as a problem that affects only children, but elderly people are at risk for accidental poisonings too. Poor eyesight, confusion, or a decreased sense of taste or smell can cause an elderly person to eat or drink something that will cause her harm. Accidental poisonings can also occur if a person takes too much, or the wrong, medication. An elderly person might not be able to read the medication label, or he might forget that he has already taken his medication that day, and take it again. To minimize the risk of accidental poisonings:

- Never store household cleaners or other chemicals in containers meant for food or beverages.
- Keep household cleaners and chemicals in a locked cabinet.
- Make sure the contents of all containers are clearly marked on the outside.
- Provide help with reading labels as necessary.

REPORTING ACCIDENTS

Accidents will happen despite the precautions taken by even the most conscientious of health care workers. Some accidents occur as a result of faulty equipment or from unfamiliarity with new equipment. Other accidents are the result of carelessness on the part of a health care worker or family member of the patient or resident involved. When accidents do occur, you must know exactly how to report the accident at your particular facility or organization.

All accidents are to be verbally reported immediately to the nurse. In addition, most facilities require the accident to be reported in written form as well. This written report is called an **incident (occurrence) report.** It generally takes the form of a preprinted document that must be completed (Fig. 10-3). Information about the accident should be provided in a straightforward and factual manner, without opinion or blame.

The completed incident (occurrence) report is used by the quality assurance department and is very important for follow-up. For example, consider a situation where an accident has occurred because a wheelchair's brakes did not hold properly. Following the completion of the proper forms by the nursing assistant, the quality assurance department might find that several similar accidents have occurred with wheelchairs of the same type, or after repairs from the same shop, or on the same shift of work scheduling. This would show a trend that could help prevent accidents like this from happening in the future.

Some health care workers hesitate to report an accident because they feel responsible for the accident or are afraid they will be blamed for the accident. Other times, they know that a coworker will be blamed for carelessness and do not want to report the coworker's error to a supervisor. As described in Chapter 3, the nursing assistant must be honest and dependable in carrying out her duties. Reporting accidents promptly helps to protect your patients, your facility, and yourself.

RESTRAINTS

Restraints, referred to as "reminder devices" in some facilities, are sometimes necessary to help keep a person safe. Restraints are used to restrict a person's freedom of movement, or to prevent a person from reaching parts of his body. For example, a restraint might be used for an agitated, disoriented patient who continually tries to remove an intravenous (IV) line from her arm.

Restraints can be either physical or chemical. A **physical restraint** is a device that is attached to or near a person's body to limit a person's freedom of movement or access to her body (Fig. 10-4). Physical restraints confine a person to a bed or a chair or prevent movement of a specific body part and cannot be easily removed by the restrained person. Physical restraints can be applied to parts of the body,

COMMUNITY NURSING SERVICE
INCIDENT REPORT

EMPLOYEE INVOLVED:

Name: _____

Address: _____

Phone: _____

Employee: _____
              (RN, PT, Aide, etc.)

PATIENT INVOLVED:

Name: _____

Address: _____

Phone: _____

FID #: _____

OTHERS INVOLVED: Name: _____ Phone: _____

Address: _____ Relationship: _____

- -

Date of Incident: _____ Time of Incident: _____

Location of Incident: _____

Incident Reported to: _____ Time: _____ Date: _____

DESCRIPTION OF INCIDENT: (Complete Workers Comp. form if on-job injury)

_____
                                                    Employee Signature

FOLLOW-UP

Family aware of incident: _____

Physician aware of incident: _____

Action Taken:

Follow-up / Supervisor's Comments:

FIGURE 10-3

An incident (occurrence) report like this one must be completed if an accident occurs. The report provides information that might help to prevent a similar accident from happening again.

A. Vest restraint

D. Mitt restraint

B. Jacket restraint

E. Lap restraint

C. Wrist restraint

F. Lap buddy

G. Chair with a tray table

FIGURE 10-4

Physical restraints are attached on or near a person's body. They limit freedom of movement. Some examples of physical restraints are shown here. (*A*) A vest restraint. (*B*) A jacket restraint. (*C*) A wrist restraint. (*D*) A mitt restraint. (*E*) A lap restraint. (*F*) A lap buddy and (*G*) a chair with a tray table are considered restraints if the person cannot remove the lap buddy or tray table independently.

such as the wrists, ankles, chest, waist, or elbows. Additionally, some types of chairs or attachments to chairs can act as restraints. So can the side rails of beds or tightly tucked sheets. Not permitting a person free access to other rooms or parts of the facility is also considered a form of physical restraint.

A **chemical restraint** is any medication that alters a person's mood or behavior, such as a sedative or tranquilizer. There is a fine line between using medications to help calm an anxious, combative (physically aggressive), or agitated (very upset) person and using medications for staff convenience. These medications should assist in the control of anxiety, combative behavior, or agitation. They should not be used in so high a dose as to make the person sleepy or unable to function in a normal fashion.

USE OF RESTRAINTS

Restraints are never used as punishment or for the staff's convenience. They are used to provide postural support, to protect the patient or resident from harm, and/or to protect the staff from harm (in the case of a combative or violent patient). Restraints are to be used only if all other methods have failed (see "Restraint Alternatives," below) and the person is considered to be a danger to herself or others if restraints are not applied. Examples of situations where the use of restraints may be appropriate (Fig. 10-5) include, but are not limited to:

- A person who is at risk for falling but cannot remember to call for help before attempting to get up
- A person who is at risk for wandering away from a facility, because of dementia
- A person who attempts to remove or pull out tubing necessary for medical treatment (this is particularly common among small children, confused patients or residents, and patients or residents who are intubated and uncomfortable)
- A person who has overdosed on alcohol or medications and is demonstrating combative behavior (due to withdrawal symptoms) or is on suicide precautions

The use of restraints is clearly defined in guidelines issued by the Omnibus Budget Reconciliation Act (OBRA), the Joint Commission on Accreditation of Healthcare Organizations (JCAHO), and the Food and Drug Administration (FDA).

A

B   C   D

FIGURE 10-5

Restraints are to be used only with a doctor's order and only if the person is considered to be a danger to himself or others if restraints are not applied. The use of restraints is a last resort. However, in some situations, the use of a restraint may be appropriate. (*A*) A person who is at risk for falling but will not stay in his bed or a chair and will not call for help may need to be restrained. (*B*) A person who may wander away from the facility may need to be restrained. (*C*) A person who tries to remove tubing needed for medical treatment may need to be restrained. (*D*) A person who is combative (physically aggressive) may need to be restrained.

The *Resident Rights* portion of OBRA addresses a person's right to be free from physical and chemical restraints. According to OBRA, the improper use of restraints can be considered holding a person against his or her will, or false imprisonment. Current standards of care set forth by JCAHO and the Centers for Medicare and Medicaid Services (CMS) require that health care facilities minimize their use of restraints. Today, many health care facilities, especially long-term care facilities, are almost restraint-free.

Each health care facility has policies and procedures detailing the use of restraints for patients and residents. As a nursing assistant, you must understand your facility's policies, and your responsibilities, regarding the use of restraints. Failure to follow these policies can result in a situation that is dangerous for your patient or resident. Additionally, failure to follow these policies can leave you and your facility open for litigation. Guidelines for the use of restraints are given in Guidelines Box 10-2.

COMPLICATIONS ASSOCIATED WITH RESTRAINT USE

There are many complications and dangers that can result from the use of restraints. Restraints are dangerous even when used properly, but doubly so if they are not. A person who is restrained is eight times more likely to die than a person who is not restrained. Consider the following:

- Strangulation, which can lead to death, can occur if a vest restraint is improperly applied or if the restraint gets tangled in a piece of furniture.
- Bruises, nerve damage, and skin abrasions can result if a restrained person pulls at the restraint.
- Permanent tissue damage as a result of impaired blood flow can occur if a restraint is placed incorrectly or too tightly. All of the tissues of the body require oxygen to live, and oxygen is carried to the tissues in the blood. If something stops blood from flowing to a certain part of the body, the affected tissues can be permanently damaged from lack of oxygen. In some cases, amputation (removal of a limb) may even be necessary.

- Broken bones and other serious injuries can occur if a restrained person tries to get out of the restraints. For example, a person restrained in a chair may still attempt to get up, which could result in serious injury if the chair overturns. Similarly, a person who is improperly restrained in a bed could slide between the bed and the side rails, or attempt to climb over the side rails, actions that could lead to injury or death if the restraint gets caught in the side rails.
- Pneumonia, pressure ulcers, and blood clots (complications of immobility) can occur if a person is left in a restraint for too long.
- Incontinence (an inability to control one's bowel, bladder, or both) can occur if a person is not taken to the bathroom regularly.
- The mental effects associated with the use of restraints can be serious and include agitation, increased confusion, humiliation, and embarrassment.

Physically and emotionally, restraints have a very negative impact on a person's quality of life.

RESTRAINT ALTERNATIVES

Although the use of physical or chemical restraints is not forbidden by any regulating agency, measures must be taken to avoid their use. In other words, **restraint alternatives** must be sought and used. The measures taken to avoid the use of restraints on a person must be documented before resorting to the use of restraints to protect that person's safety. There are many good actions that a nursing assistant can take that may eliminate or reduce the need for restraints. They all require planning and effort on the part of the caregiving staff, but the effort is considered part of the quality, individualized care that should be given to each person. Some alternatives to using chemical or physical restraints are shown in Figure 10-6. For example, a nursing assistant can:

- Provide an environment in which the person feels safe and secure. Placing a confused person close to the nurses' station, where he can be observed and the person can, in turn, watch others and not feel left alone, is often helpful.

GUIDELINES BOX 10-2
GUIDELINES FOR USING RESTRAINTS

What you do	Why you do it
Do not use a restraint without a written doctor's order that states the reason for the restraint.	OBRA and state laws protect patients and residents from being unnecessarily restrained.
Never use a restraint to "punish" a patient or resident, or for your own convenience.	Physically and emotionally, the use of restraints has a very negative impact on the person's quality of life. Therefore, restraints are only used when absolutely necessary, after all other methods of ensuring the person's safety have failed.
Use the least restrictive restraint for the least amount of time.	Minimizing the use of restraints is important to preserve the person's quality of life.
Follow the manufacturer's instructions, nurse's direction, and facility policy for applying restraints.	Improper application of restraints can lead to serious medical complications, injury, or even death.
Use a restraint that is the correct size and in good condition.	If the restraint is too large, the person may be able to remove it, either completely or partially. This puts the person at risk for falling and strangulation. If the restraint is too small, complications such as restriction of blood supply to areas beyond the restraint can result. If the restraint is in poor condition, it may not properly restrain the person, or the person may be injured when the restraint is applied.
Use commercial restraints. Do not use makeshift restraints, such as bed sheets or locks.	Using anything other than a commercial restraint to restrain a person is unprofessional and dangerous.
Restraints are always applied over clothing, pajamas, or a gown.	Clothing offers a layer of protection between the restraint and the person's skin.
Restraints are to be tied in simple, easy-to-release knots placed out of reach of the patient's or resident's hands.	Easy-to-release knots must be used in case a person needs to be released from the restraint quickly due to an emergency (for example, choking).
Ensure that you have enough help when applying a restraint.	Attempting to apply a restraint to an uncooperative, combative person can lead to injury of the person, you, or both.
Check on the restrained person every 15 minutes to make sure that feeling and blood flow are normal in any restrained extremity (arm or leg).	A restraint that is applied too tightly can lead to poor blood flow, which in turn can lead to permanent tissue or nerve damage. In addition, checking on the person regularly helps to prevent him or her from feeling abandoned.
Completely remove the restraint every 2 hours, for a total of 10 minutes.	Releasing the restraint allows you to reposition the person. All patients and residents should be repositioned at least every 2 hours, whether they are restrained or not.
Record any care given to a restrained person promptly and according to your facility's policy.	In a litigation situation, any action not recorded is considered not done. You can provide the best care possible, but if you do not record it, your effort will not protect you or your facility if legal action is taken.
Use restraints only if you have been properly trained in their use.	**Incorrect use of restraints can result in death!**

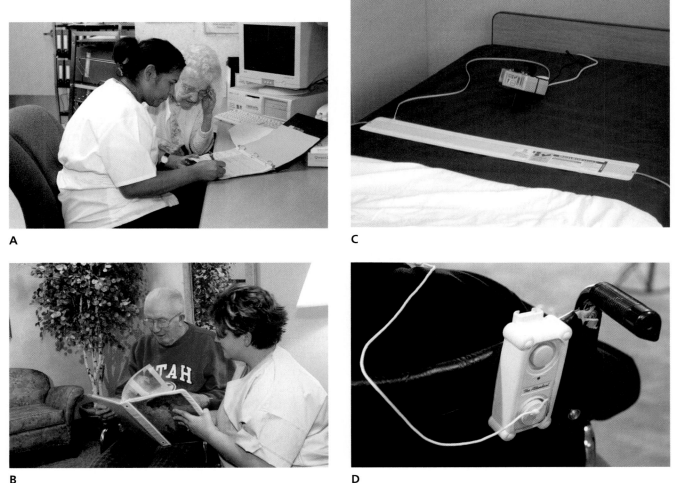

FIGURE 10-6

Alternatives to physical and chemical restraints should always be tried first. (*A*) Moving the person to a place, such as the nurses' station, can help ease feelings of loneliness. Sometimes all people want is company or to be where the action is. (*B*) Volunteers, other residents, or family members can be called on to provide company to a person too. (*C*) A pressure-sensitive bed monitoring system is shown here. The pressure-sensing mat is secured across the mattress (under the sheet), located where the person's buttocks will be. The monitor, shown here next to the mat, is then usually hung from the headboard, out of the person's reach and sight. If the person tries to get out of bed, an alarm will sound, alerting the staff that the person needs help. Systems like this are helpful for patients or residents who are likely to fall if they try to get up unassisted. Similar systems are available for chair or wheelchair seats as well. (*D*) A wanderer monitoring system is a sensor that is attached to the person's wheelchair or worn around the wrist or ankle. If the person tries to leave the facility through a doorway that leads to an unsafe area, an alarm will sound, alerting the staff so that someone can guide the person back to safety. Systems like this are useful for patients or residents who are likely to stray away from the facility, such as those with dementia. (*C courtesy of Bed-Check® Corp., Tulsa, Oklahoma.*)

Taking time to speak to the person often or sitting beside him while you complete paperwork offers the person company and companionship. Soft music, television, or other methods of entertainment can be calming.

• Provide frequent attention to the person's physical needs. Take the person to the bathroom and offer a drink or snack regularly, per facility policy or more frequently if necessary. Assist the person with walking or change her position frequently, to help maintain comfort. Answer call lights promptly and make sure that the call light control is within easy reach of the person.

- Explain procedures and reassure the person. Being in a situation or having a condition that requires the use of restraints can be confusing and embarrassing.
- Get help from family members, volunteers, or other residents of the facility. Providing companionship can be an effective alternative to the use of restraints. Additionally, this approach improves the quality of a person's life.
- Use restraint methods that are less restrictive. For example, pressure-sensitive alarm systems are placed on a person's wheelchair seat or bed. If the person tries to get up without help, the alarm will sound, alerting the staff. Sometimes the alarm will remind the person to call for help when he needs to get up. Another type of alarm system, called a wanderer monitoring system, involves a small sensor that is worn around the wrist or ankle, or placed on the person's wheelchair. If the person tries to leave the facility, an alarm will sound, alerting the staff so that the person can be gently and safely led back inside. These sensors work the same way as anti-shoplifting devices in shopping malls work.

APPLYING RESTRAINTS

In some situations, restraint alternatives will not be enough to keep the patient or resident safe, and it will be necessary to apply a physical restraint. Only a doctor can order a restraint for a patient or resident. If a doctor orders a restraint for one of your patients or residents, always follow your facility's policies regarding the application and use of restraints in order to protect yourself, your facility, and, most important, your patient or resident.

Most facilities require either a registered nurse (RN) or a licensed practical nurse (LPN) to apply the restraint, but as a nursing assistant, you will be responsible for providing care for the person while he is restrained. For example, you must check on the person every 15 minutes and help him with repositioning, range-of-motion exercises, and meeting nutritional and toileting needs. The restraint must be removed every 2 hours. Be sure to consider how frightening and humiliating it can be for a person to be restrained. Do not forget to provide the care necessary to meet the person's emotional, as well as his physical, needs. All care that you give to a restrained person must be recorded promptly.

In addition to providing and recording care, you will also be responsible for observing the person's response to the restraint and reporting any signs of trouble to the nurse immediately. Any restraint that is tied should be tied with a "quick-release" knot (Fig. 10-7). A quick-release knot, or slip knot, will hold tightly if the restrained person pulls against it, but can be undone quickly by pulling on its "tails." The use of a quick-release knot will allow you to free a person from a restraint quickly in the event of an emergency.

FIGURE 10-7

To make a quick-release knot, make a regular overhand knot, but slip a loop (instead of the end of the strap) through the first loop.

⫸ *Tell the Nurse!*

Each time you attend to a person who is wearing a restraint, you should be alert to signs and symptoms related to the use of the restraint. Tell the nurse immediately if:

⫸ The restrained person complains of, or exhibits any signs of, shortness of breath or difficulty breathing

⫸ The hand or foot beyond the restraint is pale, blue, or cold

⫸ The restrained person complains of pain, numbness, or tingling at or below a restrained body part

⫸ The restrained person has become more confused, disoriented, or agitated

To ensure that the care you provide is safe and correct, **procedures,** or lists of routine steps or actions, have been developed for the application of the various types of restraints. The procedures for applying restraints are the first of many procedures that you will find in this book that will be performed on or for the person you are caring for. Following the recommended steps of a procedure helps to protect the person you are caring for, and it protects you. Certain steps, called **pre-procedure actions,** are followed before performing any procedure on a patient or resident. In this book, we call these actions "Getting Ready" actions (Box 10-1). Similarly, there is a group of actions that are routinely performed at the end of each procedure, called **post-procedure actions.** In this book, we call these actions "Finishing Up" actions (Box 10-2). As you review the procedure boxes throughout this book, you will see references to these "Getting Ready" and "Finishing Up" actions in each of them. You must learn these steps and perform them before and after every procedure.

Applying a Vest Restraint

A vest restraint is applied to a person's chest to protect the person from falling out of bed or a chair. The person's arms are placed through the armholes of the vest, and the flaps of the vest are crossed over each other, across the person's chest. A vest restraint should never be put on backwards (that is, with the back of the vest on the person's chest and the flaps crossed across her back). Putting the vest on backwards can

BOX 10-1   Getting Ready (Pre-procedure Actions)

a. **W**ash your hands. Apply gloves and follow standard precautions if contact with blood or body fluids is possible.

b. **G**ather needed supplies.

c. **K**nock on the door and identify yourself by name and title to the person.

d. **I**dentify the person, and greet him or her by name. Methods of identifying patients and residents will vary depending on where you work. Common methods of identifying people in health care facilities include wrist bands and photographs.

e. **E**xplain the procedure and encourage the person to participate as appropriate. Show any visitors where they may wait, if necessary, until you have completed the procedure.

f. **P**rovide privacy by closing the door and the curtain. Drape the person for modesty as appropriate.

g. **S**ee to safety. Take safety precautions by following standards of body mechanics, equipment use, and infection control. In procedures that involve getting a person out of bed, you will be instructed to lower the bed to its lowest position. This is to decrease the distance between the bed and the floor, should the person fall. In procedures that involve providing care while the person remains in bed, you will be instructed to raise the bed to a comfortable working height. This is to protect your back.

cause the person to strangle if she slides down against the improperly placed restraint, because the back of the restraint is higher than the front. The procedure for applying a vest restraint is given in Procedure 10-1.

A jacket restraint is similar to a vest restraint, in that it is applied to the chest, but a jacket restraint has sleeves and closes in the back.

BOX 10-2 Finishing Up (Post-procedure Actions)

a. **C**onfirm that the person is comfortable and in good body alignment.

b. **L**eave the call light control, telephone, and fresh water within easy reach of the person.

c. **S**ee to safety. Return the bed to the lowest position, lock the wheels, and raise the side rails (if side rails are in use).

d. **O**pen the curtain and door if desired by the patient or resident, and inform visitors that they may return to the room.

e. **W**ash your hands. If gloved, remove and discard the gloves following facility policy, and then wash your hands.

f. **R**eport and record actions as required by your facility.

Applying Wrist or Ankle Restraints

In some cases, wrist or ankle restraints are applied to keep a person from moving his arms, legs, or both. When keeping a person in bed is the goal, the doctor may specify the number of extremities that are to be restrained. For example, a two-point restraint would involve two extremities (e.g., both wrists), a three-point restraint would involve three extremities, and a four-point restraint would involve all four extremities.

Although wrist restraints are sometimes used to confine a person to bed, a more common use is to prevent a person from removing tubes and catheters. When preventing a person from removing a tube or catheter is the purpose of the wrist restraint, a mitt restraint may be used instead. This mitten-like variation of a wrist restraint restricts finger movement. A mitt restraint prevents the person from grasping tubes or catheters, but allows for more freedom of arm movement.

The procedure for applying wrist or ankle restraints is given in Procedure 10-2.

Applying Lap or Waist (Belt) Restraints

Lap restraints are used to prevent a person from sliding out of a chair. Waist (belt) restraints can be used to secure a person in a chair or in a bed. The procedure for applying a lap or waist (belt) restraint is given in Procedure 10-3.

SUMMARY

▶ Safety is a basic human need.
  ■ If we feel safe, we can relax and rest because we feel secure and comfortable.
  ■ Nursing assistants are responsible for helping to ensure the safety of those they care for.
▶ There are many factors that can put a person at increased risk for an accident, including age, impaired mobility, use of certain medications, and sensory impairment.
▶ Most accidents that occur in a health care facility are avoidable.
  ■ Providing for the safety of those we care for is a never-ending process.
  ■ A nursing assistant must be continuously aware, observing patients and residents and their environment for safety risks. Nursing assistants must also perform their duties in accordance with specified policies and procedures that have been established for safety.
  ■ If an accident does occur, it should be reported immediately and an incident (occurrence) report should be completed promptly. Proper reporting and recording of accidents helps to protect your patients and residents, your facility, and yourself.
▶ Restraints are sometimes necessary to help ensure a person's safety. Because the use of restraints can be associated with complications (and possibly even death), restraints are used only when all other measures to ensure a person's safety have failed.
  ■ Restraints are never used to punish a person, or for the convenience of the staff.
  ■ Physically and emotionally, restraints have a very negative impact on a person's quality of life. The use of restraints requires extra care on the part of the nursing assistant to protect the patient's or resident's safety and dignity.

Chapter 10 Procedures

Getting Ready Steps

a. **W**ash your hands and observe standard precautions as necessary.

b. **G**ather needed supplies.

c. **K**nock and introduce yourself.

d. **I**dentify the person and greet him or her by name.

e. **E**xplain the procedure.

f. **P**rovide privacy.

g. **S**ee to safety.

Finishing Up Steps

a. **C**onfirm comfort and good body alignment.

b. **L**eave the call light control within easy reach.

c. **S**ee to safety.

d. **O**pen the curtain and door.

e. **W**ash your hands.

f. **R**eport and record.

PROCEDURE 10-1

Applying a Vest Restraint

Getting Ready WGKIEPS

1. Complete the "Getting Ready" steps **a** through **g**.

Supplies

• vest restraint in proper size

Procedure

2. Get help from another nursing assistant, if necessary.

3. Assist the person to a sitting position by locking arms with him or her.

4. Support the person's back and shoulders with one arm, while slipping the person's arms through the armholes of the vest using your other hand. Apply the restraint according to the manufacturer's instructions. The vest should cross in the front, across the person's chest.

5. Make sure there are no wrinkles across the front or back of the restraint.

6. Bring the ties through the slots.

7. Help the person to lie or sit down.

8. Make sure the person is comfortable and in good body alignment.

STEP 4 Support the person's back and shoulders while slipping her arms through the armholes of the vest.

STEP 9 Attach the straps to the bed frame, never the side rails.

(continued)

PROCEDURE 10-1 (Continued)

Applying a Vest Restraint

9. If the person is in a chair, thread the straps *between* the seat and the armrest or *between* the back of the seat and the back of the chair, according to the manufacturer's directions. If the person is in bed, attach the straps to the bed frame, never the side rails. Always use the quick-release knot approved by your facility.

STEP 10 Check to make sure the restraint is not too tight.

10. Make sure the restraint is not too tight. You should be able to slide a flat hand between the restraint and the person. Adjust the straps if necessary.

Finishing Up CLSOWR

11. Complete the "Finishing Up" steps **a** through **f**.
12. Check on the restrained person every 15 minutes.
13. Release the restraint every 2 hours and:
    a. Reposition the person.
    b. Meet the person's needs for food, fluids, and elimination.
    c. Give skin care and perform range-of-motion exercises.
14. Reapply the restraint.
15. Report and record the procedure, noting the type of restraint used, the time the restraint was applied, and the person's response to the restraint. Include any other relevant observations and sign the chart. Be sure to include your title as well as your name.

PROCEDURE 10-2

Applying Wrist or Ankle Restraints

Getting Ready WGKIEpS

1. Complete the "Getting Ready" steps **a** through **g**.

Supplies

- appropriate number of wrist restraints, ankle restraints, or both

Procedure

2. Get help from another nursing assistant, if necessary.

STEP 4 You should be able to slip two fingers between the person's wrist and the restraint.

3. Apply the wrist or ankle restraint following the manufacturer's instructions. Place the soft part of the restraint against the skin.
4. Secure the restraint so that it is snug, but not tight. You should be able to slide two fingers under the restraint.
5. Attach the straps to the bed frame. Always use the quick-release knot approved by your facility.
6. If applying two-point, three-point, or four-point restraints, repeat steps 9 through 11.

Finishing Up CLSOWR

7. Complete the "Finishing Up" steps **a** through **f**.
8. Check on the restrained person every 15 minutes.
9. Release the restraint every 2 hours and:
    a. Reposition the person.

(continued)

PROCEDURE 10-2 (Continued)

Applying Wrist or Ankle Restraints

b. Meet the person's needs for food, fluids, and elimination.

c. Give skin care and perform range-of-motion exercises.

10. Reapply the restraint.

11. Report and record the procedure, noting the type of restraint used, the time the restraint was applied, and the person's response to the restraint. Include any other relevant observations and sign the chart. Be sure to include your title as well as your name.

PROCEDURE 10-3

Applying Lap or Waist (Belt) Restraints

Getting Ready

1. Complete the "Getting Ready" steps **a** through **g**.

Supplies

• lap or waist restraint in proper size

Procedure

2. Get help from another nursing assistant, if necessary.

3. If the person is in a chair, assist him or her to a proper sitting position, making sure that the person's hips are as far back against the back of the chair as possible. (If the person is in a wheelchair, make sure the brakes are locked first, and position the footrests to support the person's feet.)

4. Wrap the restraint around the person's abdomen, crossing the straps behind the person's back.

5. Bring the ties through the loops at the sides of the restraint, according to the manufacturer's directions.

6. Make sure the person is comfortable and in good body alignment.

7. Thread the straps between the chair arm and the chair back before securing the straps out of the person's reach, at the back of the chair. Always use the quick-release knot approved by your facility.

8. Secure the restraint, making sure it is not too tight. You should be able to slide a flat hand between the restraint and the person.

Finishing Up

9. Complete the "Finishing Up" steps **a** through **f**.

10. Check on the restrained person every 15 minutes.

11. Release the restraint every 2 hours and:

a. Reposition the person.

b. Meet the person's needs for food, fluids, and elimination.

c. Give skin care and perform range-of-motion exercises.

12. Reapply the restraint.

13. Report and record the procedure, noting the type of restraint used, the time the restraint was applied, and the person's response to the restraint. Include any other relevant observations and sign the chart. Be sure to include your title as well as your name.

What did you learn?

Multiple Choice

Select the single best answer for each of the following questions.

1. After applying a restraint to a patient or resident:
   a. Try to ignore the person's complaints; he or she just wants attention
   b. Check the restraint every 6 hours
   c. Change the restraint once a day
   d. Remove the restraint at least every 2 hours

2. Vest restraints are applied so that the flaps:
   a. Cross in the back
   b. Cross in the front
   c. Are left open
   d. Are wrapped tightly around the person's chest

3. Which one of the following should not be done when applying a restraint to a patient or resident?
   a. Explain the procedure to the patient or resident
   b. Introduce yourself by name and title
   c. Make sure the patient or resident is asleep
   d. Make sure you have a written doctor's order for the restraint

4. A person with quadriplegia is paralyzed:
   a. From the waist down
   b. From the neck down
   c. On the left side
   d. On the right side

5. What is the leading cause of accidental death among elderly people?
   a. Burns
   b. Falls
   c. Poisonings
   d. Drowning

6. Mary is helping Mr. Watkins to get out of bed when he becomes dizzy, loses his balance, and falls. How should Mary report this accident?
   a. She should tell the nurse about it
   b. She should fill out an incident (occurrence) report
   c. She should tell the nurse about it and fill out an incident (occurrence) report
   d. She should tell the doctor about it

7. Why is a restraint used?
   a. To make caregiving easier for the staff
   b. To punish residents or patients who refuse to follow the rules
   c. To protect a person from harming himself or others, when all other methods of keeping the person safe have failed
   d. All of the above

8. You work in the pediatrics unit of a hospital. One of your small patients has a nasogastric feeding tube that is causing her discomfort, and she keeps trying to pull it out. What should you do to prevent the child from removing the feeding tube?
   a. Apply a mitt restraint
   b. Report your observations to the nurse
   c. Explain to the child that she has to leave the tube alone
   d. Use a sensor alarm

? Stop and think!

▶ Mr. Lovell, one of the residents with dementia at the long-term care facility where you work, has become very agitated. He is prone to falling, and should not get up without help. However, today he is refusing to stay in his bed or his wheelchair. You get him situated, and then as soon as you leave the room, he tries to get up again. This has happened twice, and you are only in the first hour of your shift. You are very concerned that Mr. Lovell will fall and hurt himself, but you cannot stay with him all day because you have other residents to attend to. Describe some things that you could do to help protect Mr. Lovell.

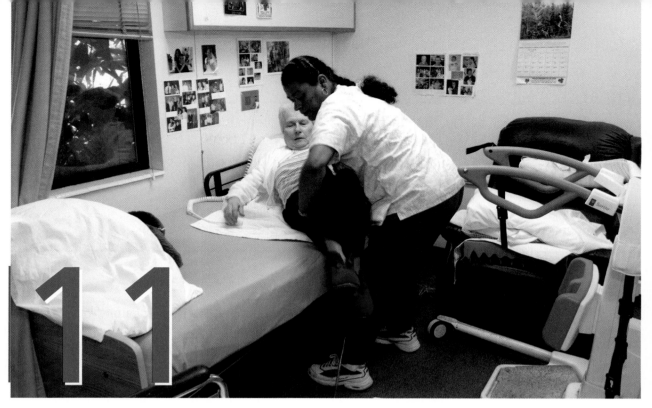

11

Positioning, Lifting, and Transferring Patients and Residents

What will you learn?

At one time or another, all of us have been awakened from sleep because the position we were in was uncomfortable. Surely, when this has happened to you, you have rolled over, found a more comfortable position, and gone back to sleep. Can you imagine what it would be like to be unable to change positions, especially if the position you were in was uncomfortable? Most of the people you will care for as a nursing assistant will be able to move with little or no help. But others will need help to reposition themselves or get out of their bed or chair.

Repositioning, lifting, and transferring people is a major part of the nursing assistant's daily routine. You will do this several times a day. By following the guidelines for body mechanics and back safety that you learned in Chapter 9, you can protect yourself from fatigue and injury. In this chapter, you will learn how to keep your patients or residents safe while assisting them with movement. When you are finished with this chapter, you will be able to:

1. Explain the complications of immobility.
2. Describe the concept of proper body alignment.
3. Identify the different body positions and explain the purpose of regular, frequent repositioning.
4. Discuss safety measures related to lifting and transferring people.
5. Demonstrate techniques of safe lifting and transfer.

Photo: A nursing assistant helps a resident to transfer out of bed.

Vocabulary

Use the CD in the back of your book to hear these terms pronounced, defined, and used in a sentence:

Pressure ulcers	Fowler's position	Prone position	Transfer belt
Contractures	Semi-Fowler's	Sims' position	(gait belt)
Body alignment	(low Fowler's)	Shearing	Weight bearing
Supportive devices	position	Friction	
Supine (dorsal	High Fowler's position	Logrolling	
recumbent) position	Lateral position	Transfer	

POSITIONING PATIENTS AND RESIDENTS

Changing position frequently helps us to stay comfortable while we are sitting or lying down. It also prevents complications that can result from spending long periods of time in the same position. Additionally, in a health care setting, a person may need to get into a certain position to have a procedure done, or to recover from one. Although many of your patients or residents will be able to reposition themselves, some will need your help. For these reasons, helping people who must stay in bed or a wheelchair to reposition themselves is an important responsibility of the nursing assistant.

There are many reasons why a person may not be able to shift positions without help. For example, the person could be recovering from surgery, wearing a body cast, or in traction. He or she may be totally or partially paralyzed, unconscious or in a coma, or very weak from a disease or illness. For these people, the inability to change positions regularly can lead to discomfort and, potentially, serious complications. For example, consider a person with limited mobility who has been positioned in a sitting position in bed. With time, this person will begin to slide down in the bed, leading to discomfort and an inability to breathe easily (Fig. 11-1).

In addition to discomfort, a person who cannot reposition herself is at risk for developing serious complications (Fig. 11-2). Some of the most serious complications affect the skin, bones and muscles, lungs, and heart:

- **Integumentary system (skin).** The most common complication of immobility is pressure ulcers. **Pressure ulcers,** also known as *decubitus ulcers* or *bed sores*, form when

bony areas press against the mattress. The pressure slows down blood flow to the tissues that are pressed between the bone and the mattress. This results in a sore, which can be very difficult to heal and might even be fatal. Pressure ulcers are discussed in detail in Chapter 24.

FIGURE 11-1

Gravity causes a person who is sitting in bed to slide down over time, leading to discomfort and interfering with the person's ability to breathe.

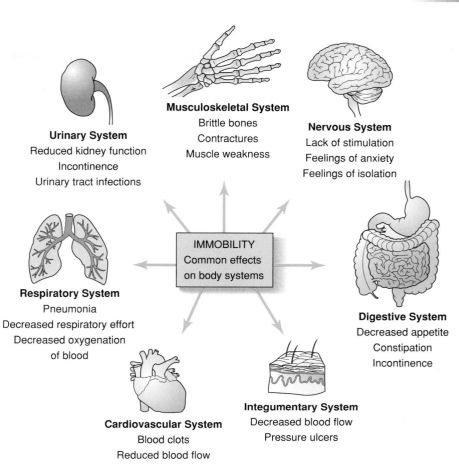

Urinary System
Reduced kidney function
Incontinence
Urinary tract infections

Musculoskeletal System
Brittle bones
Contractures
Muscle weakness

Nervous System
Lack of stimulation
Feelings of anxiety
Feelings of isolation

IMMOBILITY
Common effects
on body systems

Respiratory System
Pneumonia
Decreased respiratory effort
Decreased oxygenation
of blood

Digestive System
Decreased appetite
Constipation
Incontinence

Cardiovascular System
Blood clots
Reduced blood flow

Integumentary System
Decreased blood flow
Pressure ulcers

FIGURE 11-2

Immobility can cause complications in almost every body system.

- **Musculoskeletal system (bones and muscles). Contractures,** discussed in detail in Chapter 25, occur when a joint is held in the same position for too long a time. Contractures cause stiffness and shortening of the tendons, leading to loss of motion of the joint that may be permanent. Long-term immobility can also cause loss of muscle mass and strength. Finally, immobility can cause the loss of calcium from the bones, causing the bones to become brittle.

- **Respiratory system (lungs).** Lying in one position for a long period of time can prevent the lungs from completely filling with air when the person breathes. This causes the small air sacs in the lungs, called *alveoli,* to close. As a result, the person's ability to get oxygen into his or her bloodstream is decreased. In addition, decreased filling of the lungs with air allows fluids and mucus to collect in the lungs. This fluid and mucus creates an environment that is favorable for the types of bacteria that cause pneumonia.

- **Cardiovascular system (heart).** When we walk, the large muscles in our legs contract. Contraction of the leg muscles squeezes the veins, helping to move blood from the legs back up to the heart. People who must stay in bed are not using their leg muscles. Therefore, the blood flow from the legs back up to the heart becomes slow. This situation can lead to the formation of blood clots in the lower legs.

BASIC POSITIONS

Proper positioning is necessary for good **body alignment** and may help relieve some of the discomfort associated with a person's medical condition. A person in proper body alignment is positioned so that his spine is not twisted or crooked. To check for alignment, imagine a line that connects the person's nose, breastbone (sternum), and pubic bone, and then continues between the person's knees and ankles. This imaginary line should be straight whether the

A

B

C

FIGURE 11-3

When a person is in proper body alignment, an imaginary straight line can be drawn connecting the person's nose, breastbone (sternum), and pubic bone. (*A*) Proper body alignment for a person who is lying on her back in bed (supine). (*B*) Proper body alignment for a person who is lying on her side in bed (lateral). (*C*) Proper body alignment for a person who is lying on her stomach in bed (prone).

FIGURE 11-4

Some people require extra support to maintain proper body alignment. This support can be achieved by using pillows; a rolled-up towel, sheet, or blanket; or a supportive device made especially for this purpose.

person is lying on his back, side, or abdomen (Fig. 11-3). If the person's legs are spread apart, each leg should be the same distance from the imaginary line. When helping to position one of your patients or residents, imagine yourself in that particular position and remember how your body is most comfortable.

Proper body alignment is most comfortable for the patient or resident. It relieves strain on muscles and joints, promotes good heart and lung function, and helps prevent contractures and pressure ulcers. Sometimes **supportive devices,** such as pillows; rolled sheets, towels, or blankets; and devices designed specifically for the purpose of offering support (Fig. 11-4), are needed to keep the person in proper body alignment. Learning to

position these supports correctly is essential. Proper use of supportive devices helps to keep your patients or residents both safe and comfortable. Make sure you ask the nurse or physical therapist about the proper use of any supportive devices for your patients or residents.

There are several basic positions that are used when a person must stay in bed or seated for long periods of time (Fig. 11-5). As you work as a nursing assistant, you may see variations on these positions for reasons specific for your patient or resident. A doctor may order restrictions on positions for a person after some surgeries or diagnostic procedures. Refer to the person's care plan or ask the nurse if there are any limitations or special positioning needs that the person may have.

Supine (Dorsal Recumbent) Position

When a person is in the **supine (dorsal recumbent) position,** she is simply lying on her back. The bed is flat and the person's head is supported by a pillow. Sometimes, pillows are placed to support the arms and hands as well. Some people may be more comfortable with a pillow under their knees and lower legs to take strain off the lower back. Others may ask for a small pillow under their lower back.

Fowler's Position

A variation of the supine position is **Fowler's position,** in which the head of the bed is elevated to

FIGURE 11-5

There are several basic positions that are used when a person must remain in bed or seated for a long period of time. (*A*) Supine position. (*B*) Fowler's position. (*C*) Lateral position. (*D*) Prone position. (*E*) Sims' position. (*F*) Sitting position.

A Supine (dorsal recumbent) position

B Fowler's position

C Lateral position

D Prone position

E Sims' position

F Sitting position

between 45 and 60 degrees. In **semi-Fowler's (low Fowler's) position,** the head of the bed is elevated approximately 30 to 45 degrees. In **high Fowler's position,** the head of the bed is elevated approximately 60 to 90 degrees (Fig. 11-6). The knee-gatch area of the bed may be bent or a pillow may be placed under the person's knees and calves. Pillows may also support the arms and hands.

The semi-Fowler's position is comfortable for people who are resting in bed and want to read, watch television, or talk with visitors. It is also the most comfortable position for a person who has trouble breathing when lying flat. Some medical conditions, such as hiatal hernia with reflux, and some situations, such as tube feedings, require the person to be positioned in the semi-Fowler's position. High Fowler's position is useful when a person is eating a meal in bed, and during grooming procedures.

Lateral Position

A person who is in the **lateral position** is lying on his side. When documenting the lateral position, the side of the person that is on the bed is used as the descriptor. For example, a person lying with his left side down on the mattress is in "left lateral position." The person's lower leg is straight and his upper leg is bent at the knee, so that the knees are not pressed together. Pillows are placed under the person's head and neck, between the legs, and under the upper arm to keep the spine in alignment. A small pillow or rolled sheet may be placed close against the back to keep the person from rolling backward.

A variation of the lateral position may be used to keep pressure off the side of the hip. In the semi–side-lying position, pillows are placed either against the person's back and hip or along the front of her body. The pillows cause the person to lie either a little more forward or a little more toward the back. When the pillows are placed along the person's back and hip, she will lie a little more on her back, leaning toward the pillows. When the pillows are placed along the person's front, she will lie a little more on her abdomen.

The lateral position is often used for people with back pain, to relieve pressure on the spine, and for those in a body cast. Also, the lateral position is part of the cycle of positions for people who are unable to reposition themselves—the person is moved from the supine position to the lateral position, then back to the supine position,

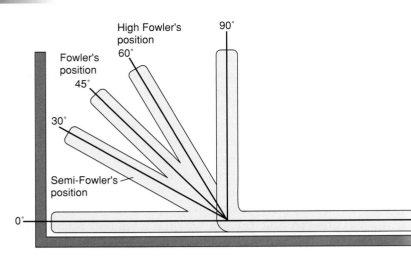

FIGURE 11-6

In Fowler's position, the head of the bed is elevated. Variations of Fowler's position include semi-Fowler's (low Fowler's) position and high Fowler's position.

and then to the lateral position on the other side every 2 hours, routinely.

Prone Position

A person who is in the **prone position** is lying on his abdomen with his head turned to one side. A small pillow is placed under the person's head. Another small pillow is placed under the lower abdomen and pelvis to allow room for the chest to expand when the person breathes. (Alternatively, a rolled towel can be placed under each of the person's shoulders to reduce pressure on the chest.) A pillow is also placed under the person's shins to keep the feet in proper position. The person's arms are bent at the elbows and his hands are placed on either side of the head, palms facing down. Many people, especially elderly people, are not comfortable in the prone position. Make sure you check with the nurse before placing a person in this position.

Sims' Position

Sims' position is an extreme side-lying position that is almost prone. The person's head is turned to one side and her knee on that side is bent sharply and supported by a pillow. The corresponding arm is bent at the elbow with the hand in front of the face, palm down, resting on a pillow. The lower leg is straight and the lower arm extends out from the side with the hand down near the hips and the palm turned upward. Sims' position is used for people who are receiving enemas, and to relieve pressure on areas that may be prone to developing pressure ulcers, such as the coccyx (the "tailbone") and the greater trochanter of the femur (the "hip bone").

Sitting Position

Positioning and body alignment are important for everyone, not just people who must stay in bed. Proper sitting position holds a person's body in correct alignment while she is sitting in a chair. The person's feet should rest flat on the floor or on the footrests of the wheelchair. Her knees are bent at approximately 90 degrees and the calves of her legs do not touch the chair. The person's buttocks and back rest against the back of the chair. Paralyzed arms should be supported on pillows. A person who cannot hold her body upright for long periods of time may need postural supports to assist in good body alignment.

REPOSITIONING A PERSON

Some people will have conditions that require repositioning as frequently as every hour, but most people will require repositioning every 2 hours. Each time you reposition a person, you should be alert to signs and symptoms of complications related to immobility.

▶ Tell the Nurse!

Possible signs and symptoms of complications related to immobility that should be reported to the nurse immediately include:

▸ Reddened skin, especially over bony areas, that does not return to its normal color after gentle massage of the surrounding tissue

▸ Pale, white, or shiny skin over a bony area

▸ Tears, scrapes, or skin that looks burned

⟶ Hot, reddened, painful areas in the lower legs (do not rub these areas because doing this could dislodge a blood clot, which could then move to a vital organ such as the heart, lungs, or brain)

⟶ New occurrence of urinary or bowel incontinence

⟶ New complaints of pain on movement

⟶ Any disconnected or heavily draining tubes or drains

To assist a person who is in bed into a new position, you will need to know how to lift and turn the person without causing injury to yourself or the person you are trying to move. People who are being moved in bed are particularly at risk for shearing and friction injuries if they are not moved properly. Perhaps you remember sliding across a vinyl car seat or down a metal sliding board while wearing shorts, and feeling pain as you moved and your skin "stuck to" the vinyl or metal. That pain is similar to the pain caused by shearing and friction. **Shearing** is caused by pulling a person across a sheet or other surface that offers resistance. When a person is pulled against a surface that offers resistance, the skin is dragged in a direction opposite that of the underlying tissues and muscles, injuring the blood vessels and connective tissue under the skin and starting the process of skin breakdown. **Friction** occurs when two surfaces, such as a sheet and the person's skin, rub against each other. The rubbing action can injure the skin and contribute to skin breakdown. The risk of shearing and friction can be minimized by rolling or lifting, instead of pulling or dragging, a person who needs to be moved. Guidelines for repositioning a person are given in Guidelines Box 11-1.

Moving a Person to the Side of the Bed

There are many reasons why you may need to reposition a person so that he is lying on one side of the bed or the other. For example, if you want to turn a person, you would first want to move the person to the side of the bed so that when the turn is completed, he is in the middle of the bed (not on one side). You might also need to move a person to the side of the bed before performing a personal care procedure, so that the person is closer to you

during the procedure. Depending on the situation, you may be able to move the person to the side of the bed by yourself (Procedure 11-1), or you may need help (Procedure 11-2). Generally speaking, you should get help from a coworker if the patient or resident is large, seriously ill or injured, or uncooperative.

Helping a Person to Move Up in Bed

As mentioned earlier, people who are sitting up in bed tend to slide down, toward the foot of the bed, over time. To keep a person who is sitting in bed comfortable and in proper body alignment, you must help him with moving up in the bed periodically. Again, depending on the situation, you may be able to do this by yourself (Procedure 11-3), or you may need assistance (Procedure 11-4).

Raising a Person's Head and Shoulders

Often, you will need to lift a person's head and shoulders away from the bed. For example, you may need to do this to help a person with drinking or to rearrange the pillow. Procedure 11-5 explains how to lift a person's head and shoulders away from the bed safely.

Turning a Person Onto His or Her Side

Helping a person to roll over in bed helps to keep the person comfortable. It also helps to prevent many of the complications associated with remaining in a single position for a long period of time. The person may be turned away from you (Procedure 11-6) or toward you, depending on the situation.

Logrolling a Person

Logrolling is performed whenever it is necessary to move a person who has had back surgery or an injury to the spine. In turning, the person's body is moved in segments (first the upper body is turned and then the lower body, or vice versa). In logrolling, the person is rolled in one fluid motion so that the head, torso, and legs move as one unit and the body (the "log") is kept in alignment. Two or three assistants, plus a lift sheet, are usually necessary to logroll a person. Procedure 11-7 explains how to logroll a person safely.

GUIDELINES BOX 11-1
GUIDELINES FOR REPOSITIONING A PERSON

What you do	Why you do it
Before attempting to reposition a person, plan how you will go about it and get help from others if necessary.	Depending on the person's medical condition or size, extra equipment or people may be necessary. Planning ahead helps to ensure that the procedure will be carried out efficiently, and with the most consideration for the person's safety and comfort.
Make sure you are aware of any limitations or restrictions concerning the movement or positioning of a person. Know the specific positioning guidelines for each person in your care.	Failure to take a person's limitations into consideration can cause you to injure the person while moving him.
Explain the procedure to the person, even if he is unconscious.	People who cannot move on their own may feel helpless and frightened at the thought of being lifted or moved by someone else. Understanding how the procedure is performed builds trust and lets the person feel like an active participant. Although it may seem that an unconscious person would be unaware of being moved, imagine how frightening it would be to sense that someone is attempting to move you without telling you what she is doing!
Make sure that you allow the person to assist in the repositioning to the full extent of her ability.	Being able to assist with one's own repositioning promotes feelings of independence and lessens the embarrassment some people may feel over having to rely on someone else for assistance.
Provide for the person's modesty by keeping his body covered.	Keeping the person's body covered preserves his dignity.
Take care to protect any tubes or drains from being pulled out while the person is being moved.	Dislodging tubes or drains is painful for the person. In addition, if tubes or drains become dislodged, it is necessary to reinsert them, which can cause additional discomfort.
Follow safety precautions and use good body mechanics when helping to reposition a person.	Using good body mechanics will protect you, as well as the patient or resident, from injury.
Use a gentle touch to avoid injury to delicate skin and fragile bones. Use a lift sheet to reposition the person whenever possible. (A lift sheet, also called a draw sheet, is a small sheet that is placed over the bottom sheet so that it extends from the person's shoulders to below her buttocks. Lift and draw sheets are discussed in detail in Chapter 15.)	A lift sheet allows you to lift the person (instead of dragging her across the sheets). This helps to prevent shearing and friction injuries.
Avoid moving or lifting someone by holding onto his arm or leg.	People who are weak or paralyzed do not have the muscle strength necessary to keep an extremity from being pulled out of its socket, or a joint from being stretched beyond its range of motion.

(continued)

GUIDELINES BOX 11-1 (Continued)
GUIDELINES FOR REPOSITIONING A PERSON

What you do	Why you do it
After repositioning a person, make sure that the bed linens are free of wrinkles, and that the person's clothing is not twisted or wrinkled up underneath the person.	Lying on wrinkled bed linens or clothing can lead to skin breakdown. Skin breakdown increases the person's risk of getting a pressure ulcer.
Gently move the person's clothing aside to check the person's skin, especially on the part of the body the person was just lying on.	Reddened or pale skin can be a sign that a pressure ulcer is starting.

TRANSFERRING PATIENTS AND RESIDENTS

To **transfer** means to move from one place to another. As a nursing assistant, you will help people with transfers many times each day. For example, people transfer from the bed to a chair and back again, or from a wheelchair to a dining chair or commode and back again. Many people are able to transfer from one place to another with little or no help, whereas others require a lot of help. The assistance you offer will vary from just providing a steadying hand to totally lifting a person from one place to another.

A person's ability to assist with her own transfers may be affected by the person's ability to bear weight. **Weight bearing** refers to a person's ability to stand on one or both legs. A limited ability to bear weight could be caused by surgery that affects the legs, injury to one or both legs, or paralysis. Some people with paraplegia have learned to transfer themselves by using their arms to support the weight of their body as they move from one surface to another.

A **transfer belt** is a webbed or woven belt with a buckle that is used to assist a weak or unsteady person with standing, walking, or transferring. (When used to help a person walk, a transfer belt becomes a **gait belt**.) The belt is approximately 1.5 to 2 inches wide, and it is 54 to 60 inches long. Many health care facilities require nursing assistants to use a transfer belt when helping people to stand, walk, or transfer. The transfer belt is applied around the person's waist (Procedure 11-8), giving the nursing assistant a place to grasp and support the person (other than by the person's arms or ribcage). When using a transfer belt, remember:

- Some patients or residents may have medical conditions that make it dangerous to use a transfer belt on them. For example, a transfer belt should not be applied to a person who is recovering from abdominal surgery. Transfer belts are also not used with people with certain heart disorders. If you are in doubt about using a transfer belt on a patient or resident, check the nursing care plan or ask the nurse for specific directions.
- A transfer belt is only an assist device and should never be used to "lift" a person who is unable to bear weight. A person who is unable to bear weight should be moved with a mechanical lift device.

Before beginning a transfer, advance planning is always necessary. Ask the nurse or physical therapist about any specific limitations the patient or resident has and what the recommended method of transfer is. Many nursing care plans will also have this information. Gather any needed equipment (e.g., a mechanical lift or wheelchair) and make sure the equipment is in good working condition. If necessary, move the furniture in the room to make space for a safe transfer. Finally, ask others for help as necessary.

Remember that a person who needs your assistance during a transfer may feel weak and shaky. The person may be frightened, or embarrassed about having to rely on others to help her do something that always seemed so easy before. Always explain the transfer procedure to the person, and make certain she understands how she is expected to help. Allow the person to assist as much as possible. Encouragement and reassurance from you, along with firm, steady assistance, will help your patient or resident gain confidence in her own abilities and learn to trust that you will be there to offer help as necessary.

It is important that you learn safe transfer techniques to protect yourself and your patients or residents. Accidents are common during the act of transferring, for both the nursing assistant and the person being transferred. Regardless of the particular type of transfer, the safety measures summarized in Guidelines Box 11-2 should always be followed. Specific procedures for various types of transfers are described in the sections that follow.

TRANSFERRING A PERSON TO AND FROM A WHEELCHAIR OR CHAIR

Wheelchairs have been used for many years to provide people who have difficulty walking with a way of getting around. Advances in technology, combined with an awareness for the individual needs of the person, have led to the availability of wheelchairs with a wide variety of features. For example, some wheelchairs are motorized to provide an even greater degree of independence.

GUIDELINES BOX 11-2
GUIDELINES FOR ASSISTING A PERSON WITH TRANSFERRING

What you do	*Why you do it*
Before attempting to transfer a person, plan how you will go about it and get help from others if necessary.	Depending on the person's medical condition or size, extra equipment or people may be necessary. Planning ahead helps to ensure that the procedure will be carried out efficiently, and with most consideration for the person's safety and comfort.
Use correct body mechanics. Keep your body close to the person and bend at the knees. Use a transfer belt.	Using good body mechanics will protect you, as well as the patient or resident, from injury.
Make sure that beds are lowered to their lowest position and wheels are locked on beds, stretchers, and wheelchairs.	Lowering the bed to the lowest position makes it easier and safer for the person to transfer, because the lowest position allows the person to put his feet on the floor. Locking the wheels on equipment prevents the equipment from moving out from under the person as he transfers.
Check the person's clothing and shoes. Clothing should fit. Shoes should provide good foot support and have nonskid soles.	Long or loose clothing (e.g., a robe) and shoes that do not provide enough support or have slippery soles could lead to tripping.
Plan the transfer so that the person is leading with her strongest side, if possible.	Doing so allows the person to bear weight in the direction she is going.
Do not allow a person to hold onto you around your neck. Instead, have an unsteady person grasp the arm of the chair or your arm for support.	If the person stumbles or falls while grasping you around the neck, you could be injured seriously.
Do not place your hands under a person's arms to help support him.	If the person stumbles or falls, he may be injured when you lift up as he is falling down.

Wheelchair use, although a common practice, presents some specific safety issues. Wheelchairs, like any other piece of equipment, need to be checked before use to ensure safety. Check to make sure that there are no broken or missing parts, that the wheels turn smoothly, that any safety straps are secure, and that the brakes hold well. Trying to transfer a person into or out of a wheelchair with unlocked or poorly locked wheels is a common cause of accidents. Procedure 11-9 describes how to transfer a person into a wheelchair or chair by yourself. Procedure 11-10 describes how to transfer a person into a wheelchair or chair with assistance. Procedure 11-11 explains how to transfer a person from a wheelchair or chair to a bed.

TRANSFERRING A PERSON TO AND FROM A STRETCHER

Stretchers are used to transport people to other parts of the facility for surgery or diagnostic testing. Critically ill and comatose people are also transported on stretchers. Procedure 11-12 describes how to transfer a person from a bed to a stretcher. Procedure 11-13 describes how to transfer a person from a stretcher to bed.

TRANSFERRING A PERSON USING A MECHANICAL LIFT

A mechanical lift is used to move people who are helpless or very heavy (Fig. 11-7). Before using a mechanical lift, always make sure the person you need to transfer weighs less than the weight limit specified on the lift. Some facilities require two staff members to operate the mechanical lift. Make sure you know your facility's policy. Procedure 11-14 describes one method of transferring a person using a mechanical lift. Because lifts from different manufacturers may vary greatly in their procedures for use, do not use a mechanical lift until you have been taught specifically how to use that lift.

ASSISTING A PERSON WITH WALKING (AMBULATING)

Some patients and residents may be able to transfer without using a wheelchair or stretcher, if they are offered assistance with walking. In

FIGURE 11-7

A mechanical lift is used to move a person who is very heavy, completely unable to assist with the move, or both. There are many different types of mechanical lifts in use. You should be trained how to operate the lift at the facility where you work before using it. Most lifts have similar parts, however, as diagrammed here.

addition, it is important to encourage people who are able to walk (either with or without assistance) to walk on a regular basis. Frequent ambulation helps to preserve mobility, improves heart and lung function, and promotes digestion. In addition, walking helps the person to remain as independent as possible for as long as possible. A person who feels weak or unsteady benefits, both physically and emotionally, from being encouraged to walk with assistance.

Sitting on the edge of the bed, also called "dangling," is the first step for someone who is going to get out of bed and walk. Procedure 11-15 explains how to help a person to sit on the edge of the bed. When a person has been resting in bed, especially for a long time, sitting up and then standing causes blood to flow to the legs and away from the head. This can lead to dizziness and fainting. Dangling allows time for the heart and blood vessels to make up for the change in position. Blood flow is sent to the head. This reduces the person's risk of falling due to dizziness or loss of consciousness.

There are many different devices people use to help them walk (Fig. 11-8). These devices are specially fitted to the individual and, therefore, should not be shared.

A. Walker

C. Crutches

B. Cane

FIGURE 11-8

Many people use assistive devices when walking. (*A*) A walker. (*B*) A cane. (*C*) Aluminum crutches.

- **A walker** is a lightweight frame (usually made of aluminum) with four rubber-tipped legs or two legs and two front wheels. The person uses the walker by grasping the top of the frame and lifting up while moving one leg forward, then resting the walker squarely on the ground before repeating the process to move the other leg forward. The walker is placed 10 to 18 inches in front of the body with each step, and the person leans on the top of the frame for support between steps.
- **Canes** are used by people whose bodies are weak on one side. Some canes have a single tip, and some have three or four tips. (A four-tipped cane is called a **quad cane**). The person holds the cane on his strong side, placing it in front of his body and using it to support his weight while moving. The weaker leg is moved forward first, followed by the stronger leg. The handle of the cane should be even with the person's hip.
- **Crutches** are made of either wood or aluminum. Aluminum crutches are lighter than wooden ones. The person supports

his weight on the handgrips to reduce the amount of body weight that he must bear on either one or both legs.

Procedure 11-16 describes how to assist a person with walking. Be alert to potential problems and be sure to report these to the nurse. Safety guidelines for assisting a person with walking are summarized in Guidelines Box 11-3.

▶ *Tell the Nurse!*

Each time you assist a person with a transfer, tell the nurse immediately if:

➤ The person complains of dizziness, shortness of breath, chest pain, a rapid heart beat (palpitations), or sudden head pain

➤ The person complains of pain when he tries to bear weight, and this is new

➤ You observe any changes in the person's usual grip, strength, or ability

➤ A usually cooperative person refuses to participate ("I just don't feel like it today")

➤ The equipment is not working properly or is broken

GUIDELINES BOX 11-3
GUIDELINES FOR ASSISTING A PERSON WITH WALKING (AMBULATION)

What you do	*Why you do it*
Use correct body mechanics.	Using good body mechanics will protect you, as well as the patient or resident, from injury.
Watch the person for fatigue or discomfort.	A person who is tired or uncomfortable is at greater risk for tripping or fainting.
Check the person's clothing and shoes. Clothing should fit. Shoes should provide good foot support and have nonskid soles.	Long or loose clothing (e.g., a robe) and shoes that do not provide enough support or have slippery soles could lead to tripping.
Check ambulation devices to ensure that they are in good condition. Tips on canes and walkers should not be cracked, worn, or missing.	The tips on canes and walkers provide traction. If they are cracked or worn, they can slip, causing the person to fall.
If the person is using a walker, make sure that she is not placing the walker too far ahead of her body, or walking too far into the frame of the walker.	If the person places the walker too far ahead of herself, she is too far from her base of support and she could fall. Similarly, if she places the walker too close to herself, she could trip over it.
If the person is using a walker, a cane, or crutches, make sure he is placing the tip or tips flat on the floor. If the person is using a three- or four-tipped cane, all of the tips must be placed flat on the ground at the same time.	Placing the tips of a walker, cane, or crutches squarely and evenly on the ground reduces the person's risk of slipping and falling.

SUMMARY

▶ For many different reasons, people in a health care setting may be unable to reposition themselves without assistance.

- The resulting immobility can cause serious complications, including pressure ulcers, contractures, pneumonia, and the formation of blood clots in the legs.
- Preventing the complications of immobility, through frequent repositioning and transferring, is a major responsibility of the nursing assistant.
  - Some people will have conditions that require frequent, regular repositioning, as often as every hour, but at least every 2 hours.
  - There are several basic positions that are used when a person must remain in bed for extended periods of time: the supine (dorsal recumbent), Fowler's, lateral, prone, and Sims' positions. Proper positioning helps to ensure proper body alignment, which relieves strain on the muscles and joints, promotes good heart and lung function, and helps to prevent contractures and pressure ulcers. It is essential for comfort.
  - When repositioning a person, it is important to take care to prevent shearing and friction injuries to the skin.

▶ Nursing assistants also help people to transfer from one place to another many times throughout the day.

- Advance planning and proper technique help to ensure a safe transfer.
- Some patients and residents may be able to walk on their own, with help. Encouraging and assisting patients and residents to walk enhances their quality of life by providing both physical and emotional benefits.

Chapter 11 Procedures

Getting Ready Steps

a. **W**ash your hands and observe standard precautions as necessary.

b. **G**ather needed supplies.

c. **K**nock and introduce yourself.

d. **I**dentify the person, and greet him or her by name.

e. **E**xplain the procedure.

f. **P**rovide privacy.

g. **S**ee to safety.

Finishing Up Steps

a. **C**onfirm comfort and good body alignment.

b. **L**eave the call light control within easy reach.

c. **S**ee to safety.

d. **O**pen the curtain and door.

e. **W**ash your hands.

f. **R**eport and record.

PROCEDURE 11-1

Moving a Person to the Side of the Bed (One Assistant)

Getting Ready WGKIEPS

1. Complete the "Getting Ready" steps **a** through **g**.

Procedure

2. Make sure that the bed is positioned at a comfortable working height (to promote good body mechanics) and that the wheels are locked.

3. Place the pillow at the head of the bed, on its edge against the headboard. This gets the pillow out of the way. It also pads the headboard in case you move the person up a little too much or too fast!

4. If the side rails are in use, lower the side rail on the working side of the bed. The side rail on the opposite side of the bed should remain up. Lower the head of the bed so that the bed is flat (as tolerated). Fanfold the top linens to the foot of the bed.

5. Stand at the side of the bed, with your feet spread about 12 inches apart and with your knees slightly bent to protect your back.

6. Gently slide your hands under the person's head and shoulders and move the person's upper body toward you.

7. Gently slide your hands under the person's torso and move the person's torso toward you.

8. Gently slide your hands under the person's hips and legs and move the person's lower body toward you.

9. Now, position the person as planned (e.g., in the prone or lateral position).

10. Reposition the pillow under the person's head and straighten the bottom linens. Draw the top linens over the person. Raise the head of the bed as the person requests.

11. Make sure that the bed is lowered to its lowest position and that the wheels are locked. If the side rails are in use, return them to the raised position.

Finishing Up CLSOWR

12. Complete the "Finishing Up" steps **a** through **f**.

PROCEDURE 11-2

Moving a Person to the Side of the Bed (Two Assistants)

Getting Ready

1. Complete the "Getting Ready" steps **a** through **g**.

Supplies

• lift sheet (if one is not already on the bed)

Procedure

2. Make sure that the bed is positioned at a comfortable working height (to promote good body mechanics) and that the wheels are locked.

3. Place the pillow at the head of the bed, on its edge against the headboard. This gets the pillow out of the way. It also pads the headboard in case you move the person up a little too much or too fast!

4. If the side rails are in use, lower the side rails. Lower the head of the bed so that the bed is flat (as tolerated). Fanfold the top linens to the foot of the bed.

5. If the lift sheet is already on the bed, make sure that it is positioned so that it is under the person's shoulders and hips. (If a lift sheet is not already on the bed, position one under the person's shoulders and hips—see Procedure 15-2.)

STEP 6 Stand opposite your co-worker.

6. Stand at the side of the bed, opposite your coworker, with your feet spread about 12 inches apart and with your knees slightly bent to protect your back.

7. Grasp the edge of the lift sheet and roll it over as close to the person's body as possible. This will provide for a better grip. (Your coworker does the same.)

STEP 8 Grasp the rolled lift sheet with both hands, palms and fingers facing down.

8. Grasp the rolled edge of the lift sheet with both hands, palms and fingers facing down. One hand should be level with the person's shoulders and the other should be level with his or her hips.

9. On the count of "three," slowly and carefully lift up on the lift sheet in unison and move the person to the side of the bed.

10. Now, position the person as planned (e.g., in the prone or lateral position).

11. Reposition the pillow under the person's head and straighten the bottom linens. Draw the top linens over the person.

12. Make sure that the bed is lowered to its lowest position and that the wheels are locked. If the side rails are in use, return them to the raised position.

Finishing Up

13. Complete the "Finishing Up" steps **a** through **f**.

PROCEDURE 11-3
Moving a Person up in Bed (One Assistant)

Getting Ready

1. Complete the "Getting Ready" steps **a** through **g**.

Procedure

2. Make sure that the bed is positioned at a comfortable working height (to promote good body mechanics) and that the wheels are locked.

3. If the side rails are in use, lower the side rail on the working side of the bed. The side rail on the opposite side of the bed should remain up. Fanfold the top linens to the foot of the bed.

4. **Method "A":**

   a. Remove the pillow. Lower the head of the bed so that the bed is flat (as tolerated).

   b. Face the head of the bed. Position your outside foot (i.e., the foot that is farthest away from the edge of the bed) 12 inches in front of the other foot, and bend your knees slightly to protect your back.

STEP 4 Position your outside foot 12 inches in front of your inside foot.

   c. Place your arm that is nearest the head of the bed under the person's head and shoulders. Lock your other arm with the person's arm that is closest to you.

   d. Have the person bend her knees.

   e. Tell the person that on the count of "three," she is to lift her buttocks and press her heels into the mattress as you lift her shoulders. On the count of "three," help the person move smoothly toward the head of the bed.

5. **Method "B":**

   a. Place the pillow at the head of the bed, on its edge against the headboard. This gets the pillow out of the way. It also pads the headboard in case you move the person up a little too much or too fast!

   b. Have the person grasp the head of the bed or a trapeze, if there is one.

   c. Face the head of the bed. Position your outside foot (i.e., the foot that is farthest away from the edge of the bed) 12 inches in front of the other foot, and bend your knees slightly to protect your back.

   d. Place your hands under the person's back and buttocks.

   e. Have the person bend his knees.

   f. Tell the person that on the count of "three," he is to lift his buttocks and press his heels into the mattress. On the count of "three," help the person move smoothly toward the head of the bed.

6. Reposition the pillow under the person's head and straighten the bottom linens. Draw the top linens over the person. Raise the head of the bed as the person requests.

7. Make sure that the bed is lowered to its lowest position and that the wheels are locked. If the side rails are in use, return them to the raised position.

Finishing Up

8. Complete the "Finishing Up" steps **a** through **f**.

PROCEDURE 11-4
Moving a Person up in Bed (Two Assistants)

Getting Ready WORKTEPS

1. Complete the "Getting Ready" steps **a** through **g**.

Supplies

• lift sheet (if one is not already on the bed)

Procedure

2. Make sure that the bed is positioned at a comfortable working height (to promote good body mechanics) and that the wheels are locked.

3. Place the pillow at the head of the bed, on its edge against the headboard. This gets the pillow out of the way. It also pads the headboard in case you move the person up a little too much or too fast!

4. If the side rails are in use, lower the side rails. Lower the head of the bed so that the bed is flat (as tolerated). Fanfold the top linens to the foot of the bed.

5. If the lift sheet is already on the bed, make sure that it is positioned so that it is under the person's shoulders and hips. (If a lift sheet is not already on the bed, position one under the person's shoulders and hips—see Procedure 15-2.)

6. Stand at the side of the bed, opposite your coworker, with your feet spread about 12 inches apart and with your knees slightly bent to protect your back.

7. Grasp the edge of the lift sheet and roll it over as close to the person's body as possible. This will provide for a better grip. (Your coworker does the same.)

8. Grasp the rolled edge of the lift sheet with both hands, palms and fingers facing down. One hand should be level with the person's shoulders and the other should be level with his or her hips.

9. On the count of "three," slowly and carefully lift up on the lift sheet in unison and move the person toward the head of the bed. Avoid dragging the person across the bottom linens.

10. Reposition the pillow under the person's head and straighten the bottom linens. Draw the top linens over the person. Raise the head of the bed as the person requests.

11. Make sure that the bed is lowered to its lowest position and that the wheels are locked. If the side rails are in use, return them to the raised position.

Finishing Up CLSOWR

12. Complete the "Finishing Up" steps **a** through **f**.

PROCEDURE 11-5
Raising a Person's Head and Shoulders

Getting Ready WORKTEPS

1. Complete the "Getting Ready" steps **a** through **g**.

Procedure

2. Make sure that the bed is positioned at a comfortable working height (to promote good body mechanics) and that the wheels are locked.

3. Place the pillow at the head of the bed, on its edge against the headboard. This gets the pillow out of the way. It also pads the headboard in case you move the person up a little too much or too fast!

4. If the side rails are in use, lower the side rail on the working side of the bed. The side rail on the opposite side of the bed should remain up. Fanfold the top linens to the foot of the bed.

5. Face the head of the bed. Position your outside foot (i.e., the foot that is farthest away from the edge of the bed) 12 inches in front of the other foot, and bend your knees slightly to protect your back.

6. Slide one hand under the person's shoulder that is nearest to you.

(continued)

PROCEDURE 11-5 (Continued)

Raising a Person's Head and Shoulders

7. Slide the other hand under the person's upper back.

8. On the count of "three," slowly and carefully lift the person's head and shoulders.

9. Reposition the pillow under the person's head and straighten the bottom linens. Draw the top linens over the person. Raise the head of the bed as the person requests.

10. Make sure that the bed is lowered to its lowest position and that the wheels are locked. If the side rails are in use, return them to the raised position.

Finishing Up CLSOWR

11. Complete the "Finishing Up" steps **a** through **f**.

PROCEDURE 11-6

Turning a Person onto His or Her Side

Getting Ready WCKIEPS

1. Complete the "Getting Ready" steps **a** through **g**.

Supplies

- additional pillows (if not already in the room).

Procedure

2. Make sure that the bed is positioned at a comfortable working height (to promote good body mechanics) and that the wheels are locked.

3. Place the pillow at the head of the bed, on its edge against the headboard. This gets the pillow out of the way. It also pads the headboard in case you move the person up a little too much or too fast!

4. If the side rails are in use, lower the side rail on the working side of the bed. The side rail on the opposite side of the bed should remain up. Lower the head of the bed so that the bed is flat (as tolerated). Fanfold the top linens to the foot of the bed.

5. Stand at the side of the bed with your feet spread about 12 inches apart and with your knees slightly bent to protect your back.

6. Move the person to the side of the bed nearest you, using the method described in either Procedure 11-1 or Procedure 11-2.

7. Stand by the side of the bed nearest the person, with your feet spread about 12 inches apart and with your knees slightly bent to protect your back.

8. Cross the person's arm that is nearest you over the person's chest.

9. Bend the person's leg that is nearest you, placing the foot on the bed. (Or, cross the person's leg that is nearest to you over his or her other leg.)

STEP 9 Bend the person's leg that is nearest you, placing the foot on the bed.

10. Place one of your hands on the person's shoulder that is nearest you, and place your other hand on the person's hip that is nearest you.

11. Gently roll the person away from you, toward the opposite side of the bed.

12. Reposition the pillow under the person's head and straighten the bottom linens. Support the person by placing a pillow lengthwise between the person's legs. The person's lower leg

(continued)

PROCEDURE 11-6 (Continued)

Turning a Person onto His or Her Side

should be bent slightly at the knee, and the upper leg should be kept straight on top of the pillow. Place additional pillows under the person's upper arm, and behind his or her back. Draw the top linens over the person.

13. Make sure that the bed is lowered to its lowest position and that the wheels are locked. If the side rails are in use, return them to the raised position.

Finishing Up CLSOWR

14. Complete the "Finishing Up" steps **a** through **f**.

PROCEDURE 11-7

Logrolling a Person (Two Assistants)

Getting Ready WGKIEPS

1. Complete the "Getting Ready" steps **a** through **g**.

Supplies

• lift sheet (if one is not already on the bed)

Procedure

2. Make sure that the bed is positioned at a comfortable working height (to promote good body mechanics) and that the wheels are locked.

3. Place the pillow at the head of the bed, on its edge against the headboard. This gets the pillow out of the way. It also pads the headboard in case you move the person up a little too much or too fast!

4. If the side rails are in use, lower the side rail on the working side of the bed. The side rail on the opposite side of the bed should remain up. Lower the head of the bed so that the bed is flat (as tolerated). Fanfold the top linens to the foot of the bed.

5. Stand with the other assistant on the side of the bed with the lowered side rail. Stand facing the bed, with your feet spread about 12 inches apart and with your knees slightly bent to protect your back. One assistant is aligned with the person's head and shoulders; the other is aligned with the person's hips.

6. Place your hands under the person's head and shoulders, while your coworker places her hands under the person's hips and legs (or vice versa). Lifting in unison, gently move the person toward the side of the bed closest to you.

7. Place a pillow lengthwise between the person's legs, and fold the person's arm so that it will be on top of his chest when he is turned.

8. Raise the side rail and make sure that it is secure.

9. Go to the opposite side of the bed and lower the side rail.

10. Working with the other assistant, turn the person onto his side.

   a. If a lift sheet is being used, turn the person by reaching over him and grasping the lift sheet. One assistant should place one hand on the lift sheet at the level of the person's shoulder and the other hand at the level of the person's hip; the other assistant should place one hand on the lift-sheet at the level of the person's hip and the other at the level of the person's calves.

STEP 10a Reach over the person and grasp the lift sheet.

(continued)

PROCEDURE 11-7 (Continued)

Logrolling a Person (Two Assistants)

b. If a lift sheet is not being used, one assistant should position her hands on the person's shoulders and hips, and the other assistant should place her hands on the person's thigh and calves.

11. On the count of "three," roll the person toward the side on which you are standing in a single movement, being sure to keep the person's head, spine, and legs aligned.

STEP 11 On the count of "three," roll the person in one fluid movement.

12. Reposition the pillow under the person's head and straighten the bottom linens. Support the person by bolstering his back with pillows. If the person's condition allows, a small pillow or folded towel may be used to support his head and neck. The pillow between the person's legs should remain in place, and additional pillows or folded towels should be used to support the person's arms. Draw the top linens over the person.

13. Make sure that the bed is lowered to its lowest position and that the wheels are locked. If the side rails are in use, return them to the raised position.

Finishing Up CLSOWR

14 Complete the "Finishing Up" steps **a** through **f**.

PROCEDURE 11-8

Applying a Transfer (Gait) Belt

Getting Ready WCKIEDS

1. Complete the "Getting Ready" steps **a** through **g**.

Supplies

• transfer belt

Procedure

2. If the person is in bed, make sure that the bed is lowered to its lowest position and that the wheels are locked. If the side rails are in use, lower the side rail on the working side of the bed. The side rail on the opposite side of the bed should remain up. Fanfold the top linens to the foot of the bed. Assist the person to sit on the edge of the bed (see Procedure 11-15).

3. Apply the belt around the person's waist, over his or her clothing. Buckle the belt in the front by threading the tongue of the belt through the side of the buckle that has "teeth" first, and then placing the tongue of the belt through the other side of the buckle.

STEP 3 Thread the tongue of the belt through the side of the buckle that has "teeth" first.

(continued)

PROCEDURE 11-8 (Continued)

Applying a Transfer (Gait) Belt

4. Before tightening the belt, turn it so that the buckle is off-center in the front, or to the side.

STEP 6 Use an underhand grasp to hold the belt.

5. Tighten the belt and check for fit. The belt should be snug, but you should be able to slip your fingers between the belt and the person's waist. When applying a transfer belt to a woman, make sure that her breasts are not trapped underneath the belt.

6. Use an underhand grasp when holding the belt to provide greater safety.

Finishing Up   CLSOWR

7. When the person has finished transferring and is ready to return to bed, reverse the procedure.

8. Complete the "Finishing Up" steps **a** through **f**.

PROCEDURE 11-9

Transferring a Person from a Bed to a Wheelchair (One Assistant)

Getting Ready   WGKIEPS

1. Complete the "Getting Ready" steps **a** through **g**.

Supplies
- wheelchair
- lap blanket (optional)
- person's robe
- person's slippers or shoes
- transfer belt

Procedure

2. Determine the person's strongest side, and then place the wheelchair alongside the bed. Position the wheelchair so that the person will move toward the chair "strong side first." Whenever possible, position the wheelchair so that it is against a wall or a solid piece of furniture so that it will not slide backward during the transfer.

3. Lock the wheelchair wheels, and either remove the footrests or swing them to the side.

4. Fanfold the top linens to the foot of the bed.

5. Make sure that the bed is lowered to its lowest position and that the wheels are locked. Raise the head of the bed as tolerated.

6. Help the person to move toward the side of the bed where the wheelchair is located (see Procedure 11-1).

STEP 7 Have the person roll onto her side, facing the side of the bed where the wheelchair is located.

7. Have the person roll over onto her side, facing the side of the bed where the wheelchair is located (e.g., if the wheelchair is on the right side of the bed, then the person will roll over so that the right side of her body is against the mattress). Have the person flex her knees and bend the arm she is lying on

(continued)

PROCEDURE 11-9 (Continued)

Transferring a Person from a Bed to a Wheelchair (One Assistant)

in preparation for using it to prop her upper body up. Have the person bend her top arm so that her hand is in a position that will enable her to push off the bed.

8. Instruct the person to rise to a sitting position by using the elbow of her bottom arm to raise her upper body while pushing against the mattress with her other hand. Advise the person to allow her legs to swing over the edge of the bed while you help to guide her into an upright position.

9. Allow the person to rest on the edge of the bed. The person should be sitting squarely on both buttocks, with her knees apart and both feet flat on the floor (to offer a broad base of support). The person's arms should rest alongside her thighs. Watch for signs of dizziness or fainting. Position yourself in front of the person so that you can offer assistance in case she loses balance.

10. Help the person put her shoes or slippers on, and help her get into a robe. Apply a transfer belt.

11. Help the person to stand.

    a. Stand facing the person.

b. Have the person put her hands on the edge of the bed, alongside each thigh.

c. Make sure the person's feet are flat on the floor.

d. Have the person lean forward.

e. Grasp the transfer belt at each side, using an underhand grasp. (If you are not using a transfer belt, pass your arms under the person's arms and rest your hands on her shoulder blades.)

f. Position your feet alongside the person's feet, flexing your knees. Place your shins against the person's shins to block the person's feet and keep her knees from buckling as she stands up.

g. Have the person push down on the bed with her hands and stand on the count of "three." Assist the person into a standing position by pulling on the transfer belt as you straighten your knees. (If you are not using a transfer belt, assist the person into a standing position by gently pulling her up and forward as you straighten your knees.) Remember to keep your back straight.

STEP 11 Help the person to stand. Brace the person's knees with your knees, and the person's feet with your feet.

STEP 12 Support the person in the standing position.

(continued)

PROCEDURE 11-9 (Continued)

Transferring a Person from a Bed to a Wheelchair (One Assistant)

12. Support the person in the standing position by holding the transfer belt or by keeping your hands on her shoulder blades. Continue to block the person's feet and knees with your feet and knees.

STEP 13 Help the person to turn so that she can grasp the arms of the wheelchair and sit down.

13. Help the person to turn by pivoting on the stronger leg toward the chair. This will allow

the person to grasp the far arm of the wheelchair. The backs of the person's legs should touch the edge of the chair.

14. Continue to assist the person with turning until she is able to grasp the other armrest.

15. Lower the person into the wheelchair by bending your hips and knees.

16. Make sure the person's buttocks are at the back of the chair. Make sure the person is comfortable and in good body alignment.

17. Remove the transfer belt.

18. Position the person's feet on the footrests of the wheelchair. Buckle the wheelchair safety belt (if ordered), and cover the person's lap and legs with a lap blanket, if desired. Make sure that the lap blanket does not drag on the floor.

Finishing Up   CLSOWR

19. Position the wheelchair according to the person's preference.

20. Complete the "Finishing Up" steps **a** through **f**.

PROCEDURE 11-10

Transferring a Person from a Bed to a Wheelchair (Two Assistants)

OBRA ✓

Getting Ready   WGKIEpS

1. Complete the "Getting Ready" steps **a** through **g**.

Supplies

- wheelchair
- lap blanket (optional)
- person's robe
- person's slippers or shoes

Procedure

2. Place the wheelchair alongside the bed, facing the foot of the bed. Whenever possible, position the wheelchair so that it is against a wall or a solid piece of furniture so that it will not slide backward during the transfer.

3. Lock the wheelchair wheels, and either remove the footrests or swing them to the side.

4. Fanfold the top linens to the foot of the bed.

5. Make sure that the bed is positioned at a comfortable working height (to promote good body mechanics) and that the wheels are locked. Raise the head of the bed as tolerated.

6. Help the person to move toward the side of the bed where the wheelchair is located (see Procedure 11-2).

7. Help the person put his shoes or slippers on, and help him get into a robe.

8. Stand by the side of the bed, behind the wheelchair. Standing behind the person, pass your arms under the person's arms and grasp his forearms. The other assistant grasps the person's thighs and calves.

9. Working in unison with the other assistant, lift the person from the bed and bring him toward the wheelchair on the count of "three." Lower the person into the wheelchair.

(continued)

PROCEDURE 11-10 (Continued)

Transferring a Person from a Bed to a Wheelchair (Two Assistants)

10. Make sure the person's buttocks are at the back of the chair. Make sure the person is comfortable and in good body alignment.

11. Position the person's feet on the footrests of the wheelchair. Buckle the wheelchair safety belt (if ordered), and cover the person's lap and legs with a lap blanket, if desired. Make sure that the lap blanket does not drag on the floor.

Finishing Up CLSOWR

12. Position the wheelchair according to the person's preference.

13. Complete the "Finishing Up" steps **a** through **f**.

PROCEDURE 11-11

Transferring a Person from a Wheelchair to a Bed

Getting Ready WCKIEPS

1. Complete the "Getting Ready" steps **a** through **g**.

Supplies

• transfer belt

Procedure

2. Make sure that the bed is lowered to its lowest position and that the wheels are locked. Raise the head of the bed, fanfold the top linens to the foot of the bed, and raise the opposite side rail.

3. Position the wheelchair close to the side of the bed, so that the person's strong side is next to the bed. Lock the wheelchair wheels, and either remove the footrests or swing them to the side.

4. Remove the person's lap blanket (if one was used) and release the wheelchair safety belt, if in use. Apply a transfer belt.

5. Stand facing the person, with your feet spread about 12 inches apart and with your knees slightly bent to protect your back. With your back straight, slide the person to the front of the wheelchair seat.

6. Grasp the transfer belt (or pass your arms under the person's arms, placing your hands on her upper back). Position your feet alongside the person's feet, flexing your knees. Place your shins against the person's shins to block the person's feet and keep her knees from buckling as she stands up.

7. Have the person rest her hands on your arms, and assist her to stand by pulling on the transfer belt as you straighten your knees. (If you are not using a transfer belt, assist the person into a standing position by gently pulling her up and forward as you straighten your knees.) Remember to keep your back straight. Alternatively, a person who requires less assistance can place her hands on the wheelchair arms for support and "push off" while you offer support.

STEP 7 Help the person to stand.

8. Slowly help the person to turn toward the bed by pivoting on her strong leg. Help the person to sit on the edge of the bed.

9. Remove the person's robe and slippers, if appropriate.

(continued)

PROCEDURE 11-11 (Continued)

Transferring a Person from a Wheelchair to a Bed

STEP 8 Help the person to sit on the edge of the bed.

10. Move the wheelchair out of the way.

11. Place one of your arms around the person's shoulders and one arm under her legs. Swing the person's legs onto the bed.

12. Help the person to move to the center of the bed and position her comfortably.

13. Straighten the bottom linens and make sure the person is comfortable and in good body alignment. Draw the top linens over the person.

14. If the side rails are in use, return them to the raised position.

Finishing Up CLSOWR

15. Complete the "Finishing Up" steps **a** through **f**.

PROCEDURE 11-12

Transferring a Person from a Bed to a Stretcher (Four Assistants)

Getting Ready WGKIEPS

1. Complete the "Getting Ready" steps **a** through **g**.

Supplies

- stretcher
- lift sheet (if one is not already on the bed)
- blanket

Procedure

2. Position the stretcher alongside the bed. Lock the stretcher wheels and move the stretcher safety belts out of the way.

3. Raise the bed to its highest level. (The stretcher should be slightly lower than the bed.) Lower the head of the bed so that the bed is flat. Make sure that the bed wheels are locked.

Lower the side rails. Fanfold the top linens to the side of the bed opposite the stretcher.

STEP 5 Stand at the side of the bed facing your co-worker, who is positioned along the outside edge of the stretcher. Another pair of assistants does the same.

(continued)

PROCEDURE 11-12 (Continued)

Transferring a Person from a Bed to a Stretcher (Four Assistants)

4. If the lift sheet is already on the bed, make sure that it is positioned so that it is under the person's shoulders and hips. (If a lift sheet is not already on the bed, position one under the person's shoulders and hips—see Procedure 15-2.)

5. Two assistants stand at the side of the bed facing their coworkers, who are positioned along the outside edge of the stretcher.

6. Grasp the edge of the lift sheet and roll it over as close to the person's body as possible. This will provide for a better grip. (Your coworkers do the same.)

7. On the count of "three," all four assistants slowly and carefully lift up on the lift sheet in unison and move the person to the side of the bed.

8. On the count of "three," all four assistants slowly and carefully lift up on the transfer sheet in unison and move the person to the side of the stretcher.

9. Position the person on the stretcher and make sure he or she is in good body alignment. Reposition the pillow under the person's head and cover the person with a blanket for modesty and warmth. Buckle the stretcher safety belts across the person and raise the side rails on the stretcher. Raise the head of the stretcher as the person requests.

Finishing Up CLSOWR

10. Transport the person to the appropriate site. A person on a stretcher should always be transported "feet first." Remain with the person; never leave someone alone on a stretcher.

11. Complete the "Finishing Up" steps **a** through **f**.

PROCEDURE 11-13

Transferring a Person from a Stretcher to a Bed (Four Assistants)

Getting Ready WCKIEps

1. Complete the "Getting Ready" steps **a** through **g**.

Supplies

• lift sheet (if one is not already on the stretcher)

Procedure

2. Position the stretcher against the bed and lock the stretcher wheels.

3. Raise or lower the bed so that it is slightly lower than the stretcher. Lower the head of the bed so that the bed is flat. Make sure that the bed wheels are locked. Lower the side rails. Fanfold the top linens to the side of the bed opposite the stretcher.

4. Unbuckle the stretcher safety belts and lower the side rails on the stretcher.

5. Two assistants stand at the far side of the bed facing their coworkers, who are positioned along the outside edge of the stretcher. (Some facilities allow the assistants on the far side of the bed to kneel on the bed to complete the transfer; follow your facility's policy.)

STEP 5 Stand at the side of the bed facing your co-worker, who is positioned along the outside edge of the stretcher. Another pair of assistants does the same.

6. If the lift sheet is already on the stretcher, make sure that it is positioned so that it is

(continued)

PROCEDURE 11-13 (Continued)

Transferring a Person from a Stretcher to a Bed
(Four Assistants)

under the person's shoulders and hips. (If a lift sheet is not already on the stretcher, position one under the person's shoulders and hips—see Procedure 15-2.)

7. Grasp the edge of the lift sheet and roll it over as close to the person's body as possible. This will provide for a better grip. (Your coworkers do the same.)

8. On the count of "three," all four assistants slowly and carefully lift up on the lift sheet in unison and move the person to the bed.

9. Help the person to move to the center of the bed and, if desired, remove the lift sheet by turning the person first to one side, then the other. Position the person comfortably.

10. Straighten the bottom linens and make sure the person is comfortable and in good body alignment. Draw the top linens over the person.

11. Make sure the bed is lowered to its lowest position and that the wheels are locked. If the side rails are in use, return them to the raised position.

Finishing Up CLOSURE

12. Complete the "Finishing Up" steps **a** through **f**.

PROCEDURE 11-14

Transferring a Person Using a Mechanical Lift (Two Assistants)

Getting Ready WCKIEPS

1. Complete the "Getting Ready" steps **a** through **g**.

Supplies

- wheelchair
- mechanical lift
- sling in proper size
- lap blanket (optional)
- lap restraint (if ordered)

Procedure

2. Make sure that the bed is positioned at a comfortable working height (to promote good body mechanics) and that the wheels are locked.

3. If the side rails are in use, lower the side rails.

4. Fanfold the top linens to the foot of the bed.

5. Center the sling under the person. (To get the sling under the person, move the person as if you were making an occupied bed—see Procedure 15-2.) The lower edge of the sling should be positioned underneath the person's knees.

6. Raise the head of the bed as tolerated.

7. Move the release valve on the lift to the closed position.

8. Raise the lift so that it can be positioned over the person.

9. Spread the legs of the lift to provide a solid base of support. The legs must be locked in this position, or the lift could tip over, injuring you, the person you are trying to transfer, or both.

STEP 5 Center the sling under the person.

STEP 10 Move the lift into position over the person.

(continued)

PROCEDURE 11-14 (Continued)

Transferring a Person Using a Mechanical Lift (Two Assistants)

10. Move the lift into position over the person.

11. Fasten the sling to the straps or chains of the lift. Make sure the hooks face away from the person.

STEP 11 Fasten the sling to the lift according to the manufacturer's instructions.

12. Attach the sling to the swivel bar with the short side attached to the top of the sling and the long side attached to the bottom of the sling.

13. Cross the person's arms across her chest. The person may hold onto the straps, but do not let her hold onto the swivel bar.

14. Lower the head of the bed.

15. Raise the lift until the person and the sling are clear of the bed.

STEP 15 Raise the lift until the person and the sling are clear of the bed.

16. Place the wheelchair alongside the bed, facing the foot of the bed. Lock the wheelchair wheels.

17. Have your coworker support the person's legs as you move the lift into position over the wheelchair.

STEP 17 A co-worker supports the person's legs as you move her into position over the wheelchair.

18. Turn the person so that she is facing the mast of the lift and is centered over the base. (The person's back should be facing the wheelchair.)

19. Move the lift so that the person is over the seat of the wheelchair.

20. Slowly open the release valve on the lift. Gently lower the person into the wheelchair. Make sure the person's buttocks are at the back of the chair.

STEP 20 Gently lower the person into the wheelchair.

21. Lower the swivel bar so that you can unhook the sling. Leave the sling under the person.

22. Make sure the person's buttocks are at the back of the chair. Make sure the person is comfortable and in good body alignment.

23. Position the person's feet on the footrests of the wheelchair. Buckle the wheelchair safety belt (or place a lap restraint, if ordered). Cover the person's lap and legs with a lap blanket, if desired. Make sure that the lap blanket does not drag on the floor.

(continued)

PROCEDURE 11-14 (Continued)

Transferring a Person Using a Mechanical Lift (Two Assistants)

Finishing Up CLSOWR

24. Position the wheelchair according to the person's preference.

25. Follow the "Finishing Up" steps **a** through **f**.

26. When the person is ready to return to bed, reverse the procedure.

PROCEDURE 11-15

Assisting a Person with Sitting on the Edge of the Bed ("Dangling")

Getting Ready WGKIEpS

1. Complete the "Getting Ready" steps **a** through **g**.

Procedure

2. Make sure that the bed is lowered to its lowest position and that the wheels are locked.

3. If the side rails are in use, lower the side rail on the working side of the bed. The side rail on the opposite side of the bed should remain up. Raise the head of the bed as tolerated. Fanfold the top linens to the foot of the bed.

4. Stand at the side of the bed with your feet spread about 12 inches apart and with your knees slightly bent to protect your back.

5. Have the person bend his knees and plant his feet on the bed.

6. Gently slide one arm behind the person's upper back. Slide the other arm under his knees and rest your hand on the side of the person's thigh.

STEP 6 Slide one arm behind the person's upper back. Slide the other arm under her knees.

7. With a single smooth movement, slide the person's legs over the side of the bed while moving his head and shoulders upward, so that the person is sitting on the edge of the bed.

STEP 7 Help the person to sit on the edge of the bed.

8. Have the person put his hands on the edge of the bed, alongside each thigh, for support. Watch for signs of dizziness or fainting. If the person feels faint, help the person to lie down and call for the nurse.

9. Allow the person to "dangle" his legs over the side of the bed for the specified period of time, and then either take the person's vital signs (if indicated), help the person to lie back down, or assist him to a standing position. Stay with the person during the entire time.

Finishing Up CLSOWR

10. Complete the "Finishing Up" steps **a** through **f**.

PROCEDURE 11-16
Assisting a Person with Ambulating

Getting Ready WGKIEPS

1. Complete the "Getting Ready" steps **a** through **g**.

Supplies

- transfer belt
- cane or walker (if indicated)
- person's robe
- person's slippers or shoes (nonskid soles)

Procedure

2. If the person is in bed, make sure that the bed is lowered to its lowest position and that the wheels are locked.

3. Assist the person to "dangle" (see Procedure 11-15). Check the person's pulse; a weak pulse could lead to lightheadedness. If the person's pulse is weak, stay with the person and alert the nurse before attempting ambulation.

4. Help the person put her shoes or slippers on, and help her into a robe. Apply a transfer belt.

5. Help the person to stand.

   a. Stand facing the person.

   b. Have the person put her hands on the edge of the bed, alongside each thigh.

   c. Make sure the person's feet are flat on the floor.

   d. Have the person lean forward.

   e. Grasp the transfer belt at each side, using an underhand grasp. (If you are not using a transfer belt, pass your arms under the person's arms and rest your hands on her shoulder blades.)

   f. Position your feet alongside the person's feet, flexing your knees. Place your shins against the person's shins to block the person's feet and keep her knees from buckling as she stands up.

   g. Have the person push down on the bed with her hands and stand on the count of "three." Assist the person into a standing position by pulling on the transfer belt as you straighten your knees. (If you are not using a transfer belt, assist the person into a standing position by gently pulling her up

and forward as you straighten your knees.) Remember to keep your back straight.

6. Have the person grasp the cane or walker, if she is using one, in order to maintain balance. The person should hold the cane on her strong side.

STEP 13 Grasp the transfer (gait) belt with an underhand grip from the back.

7. Help the person to walk. Stand slightly behind the person on her weaker side. Grasp the transfer belt with an underhand grip from the back. If the person is using an ambulation device, make sure she is using it correctly.

8. After returning to the person's room, help her back into bed or a chair.

Finishing Up CLSOWR

9. Complete the "Finishing Up" steps **a** through **f**.

What did you learn?

Multiple Choice

Select the single best answer for each of the following questions.

1. Which of the following describes good standing posture when helping to reposition or transfer a person?
   a. Feet 12 inches apart
   b. Abdominal muscles relaxed
   c. Arms out straight
   d. Feet close together

2. When assisting a person to move to the head of the bed, you should:
   a. Face the head of the bed
   b. Unlock the bed wheels
   c. Place a pillow under the person's head
   d. Place the foot that is farthest away from the bed edge behind the other foot

3. Which person is likely to need help moving and turning in bed?
   a. A person who is ambulatory
   b. A person who has Alzheimer's disease
   c. A sleeping person
   d. An unconscious person

4. To transfer a person correctly from a bed to a stretcher, you must:
   a. Use a mechanical lift
   b. Get help from at least five coworkers
   c. Use good body mechanics
   d. Raise the far side rail of the stretcher first

5. When moving and positioning people, you should:
   a. Avoid friction and shearing
   b. Use good body mechanics
   c. Use pillows and rolled towels to maintain the position
   d. All of the above

6. Sitting a person on the side of the bed is called:
   a. Semi-sitting
   b. Proning
   c. Supining
   d. Dangling

7. When transferring a person from one place to another, you should:
   a. Use a transfer belt (unless the person has a condition that prevents the use of a transfer belt)
   b. Adjust the bed to the lowest possible height
   c. Lock the brakes of the bed, wheelchair, or stretcher
   d. All of the above

8. A person in the prone position is lying on his:
   a. Right side
   b. Left side
   c. Abdomen
   d. Back

9. When moving a person by yourself and the person is wearing a transfer belt:
   a. Lift from the side
   b. Use an underhand grasp
   c. Use an overhand grasp
   d. Stand behind the person

10. A nurse asks you to place a patient in the semi-Fowler's position while his tube feeding is running. You know the head of the bed should be elevated:
    a. 90 degrees
    b. 60 degrees
    c. 30 degrees
    d. 15 degrees

11. A mechanical lift can be used to:
    a. Move a patient or resident who is very heavy
    b. Move a patient or resident who is very weak
    c. Help a nursing assistant carry out her duties without injuring herself
    d. All of the above

12. When transferring a person from a bed to a stretcher, you should position the bed:
    a. At its lowest level
    b. At its highest level
    c. In the high Fowler's position
    d. In the supine position

13. A person who cannot reposition himself independently is at risk for developing:
    a. Pressure ulcers
    b. Blood clots
    c. Pneumonia
    d. All of the above

14. What is it called when a joint is held in one position for too long, and the tendons shorten?
    a. A pressure ulcer
    b. A bed sore
    c. A contracture
    d. A shearing injury

15. Why is it important to ensure that your patients or residents are in good body alignment every time you reposition them?
    a. Good body alignment is most comfortable for the patient or resident
    b. Good body alignment helps prevent complications, such as pressure ulcers and contractures
    c. Good body alignment helps the person to breathe easier and improves blood flow to tissues
    d. All of the above

16. What technique would you use to move Rosemary, a 15-year-old patient who has just had spinal surgery?
    a. Logrolling
    b. A mechanical lift
    c. Dangling
    d. Turning

? Stop and think!

▶ Cynthia, a new nursing assistant, has been assigned to take care of Mrs. Adkins. Mrs. Adkins weighs more than 250 pounds and has had a stroke, so she is paralyzed completely on her left side. Cynthia has to transfer Mrs. Adkins from her bed to a wheelchair so she can go to the shower room. If you were Cynthia, what would be the first step you would take?

▶ You have been assigned to the north hall and have five residents you must awaken and dress for breakfast. You walk into Mr. Clark's room and announce cheerfully that it is time to get up for breakfast. Mr. Clark is a very large man, with many medical problems. Although he can sit up and get out of bed, he tends to be unsteady on his feet. How would you go about getting Mr. Clark up and dressed?

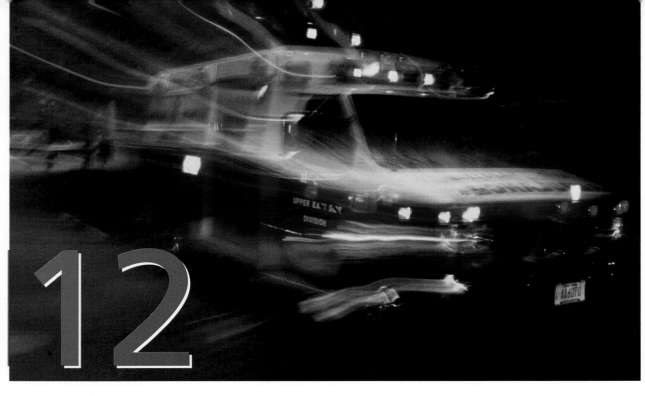

CHAPTER

12

Basic First Aid and Emergency Care

What will you learn?

An emergency can occur as a result of an accident, or as a result of a medical condition (such as a heart attack or a stroke). Most emergencies that are not caused by a medical condition are caused by an accident that could have been prevented. This is why safety and accident prevention are emphasized so heavily. Accidental injuries (such as trauma from falls or automobile accidents, drownings, poisonings, burns, and electrocutions) are the leading cause of death among young people. However, as you will recall from Chapter 10, both young and elderly people are at risk for accidental injuries—the very young because they lack judgment and experience, and the very old because of the physical and mental effects of the aging process. In addition to being at risk for accidental injury, people who are elderly, disabled, or in otherwise poor health are at high risk for developing an unexpected medical condition, such as a heart attack, diabetic reaction, stroke, medication reaction, or seizure disorder. As a nursing assistant, you must be prepared to provide safe, compassionate care for a person in an emergency situation. When you are finished with this chapter, you will be able to:

1. Define the term *emergency* and give examples of emergency situations.
2. Define terms used to describe a person's condition in an emergency situation.
3. List some of the organizations that offer approved training in first aid and basic life support (BLS) measures.
4. Discuss your role in an emergency situation.

(continued)

Photo: An ambulance speeds through the city streets to aid a person in need. (T. McCarthy/Custom Medical Stock Photo.)

5. List and discuss the steps of basic life support (BLS).
6. List the signs and symptoms of a "heart attack" and describe the actions that a nursing assistant would take to assist a person with these signs and symptoms.
7. List the signs and symptoms of a stroke.
8. Describe how you would assist a person who complains of feeling faint, or who has fainted.
9. Describe how you would assist a person who is having a seizure.
10. Describe how you would assist a person who is bleeding uncontrollably (hemorrhaging).
11. Describe some of the types and causes of shock, and describe how you would assist a person who is in shock.
12. Demonstrate how to clear the airway of a choking adult or child older than 1 year by using the Heimlich maneuver.
13. Demonstrate the method used to clear the airway of a choking infant.
14. Describe the steps of the chain of survival.

Vocabulary

Use the CD in the back of your book to hear these terms pronounced, defined, and used in a sentence:

Emergency	Rescue breathing	Emergency medical	Shock
Respiratory arrest	Cardiopulmonary	services (EMS) system	Cardiogenic shock
Cardiac arrest	resuscitation	Pulse points	Hemorrhagic shock
Clinical death	(CPR)	Syncope	Septic shock
Biological death	Oriented to person,	Grand mal seizure	Anaphylactic shock
First aid	place, and time	Petit mal (absence)	Aspiration
Basic life support	Disoriented	seizure	Heimlich maneuver
(BLS)	Unresponsive	Hemorrhage	Chain of survival

WHAT IS AN EMERGENCY?

An **emergency** is a condition that requires immediate medical or surgical evaluation or treatment in order to prevent the person from dying or having a permanent disability. Often, when a person requires immediate care, it is because something has occurred that affects one or both of the processes necessary for life, breathing and circulation. As you learned in Chapter 7, the human body is made up of millions of cells. Each of these cells requires oxygen to live. When we inhale, we take air, which contains oxygen, into our lungs. Once in the lungs, the oxygen in the air passes from the tiny air sacs of the lungs (called the alveoli) into the blood in the blood vessels that surround the alveoli. Each time the heart beats, the oxygen-rich blood is sent to all of the cells in the body.

Any process that affects our ability to take air into our lungs, or to send oxygen-rich blood to the cells and tissues of the body, is an emergency. Without oxygen, the cells of the body begin to die. Human beings can live for days without food and water, but only for a few minutes without oxygen.

Respiratory arrest means that breathing has stopped (*arrest* means "stop"). If a person cannot breathe well for whatever reason, the oxygen content of the blood decreases, and there is not enough oxygen for the cells of the body to function properly. Eventually, key organs such as the brain and the heart stop functioning. A person who is in respiratory arrest may have a heartbeat initially, but if breathing is not started again soon, his heart will stop beating. This condition is called **cardiac arrest.** A person who has no pulse or is not breathing is said to be *clinically dead.* **Clinical death** can sometimes be reversed with prompt emergency treatment that restarts the heart and breathing. However, if clinical death is not promptly reversed, allowing oxygen-rich blood to reach the tissues of the brain and heart, **biological death** soon follows. Biological death is not reversible.

There are several ways that breathing and circulation can be hindered, leading to respiratory arrest, cardiac arrest, or both (in short, an emergency situation). For example:

- When a person chokes, the airway becomes blocked, and oxygen-containing air cannot reach the lungs. Remember that oxygen passes from the lungs into the bloodstream for distribution to the cells of the body, so if oxygen is not reaching the lungs, then it is not reaching the bloodstream, or the body's cells, either.
- A person who is hemorrhaging is losing large amounts of blood in a short period of time, and as a result, there is not enough blood to carry oxygen to the all of the cells in the body.
- During a "heart attack," the muscular heart is not able to contract normally, which means that oxygen-rich blood is not circulated throughout the body efficiently.

As you can see, there are many different mechanisms that can lead to impaired breathing or circulation, and thus to an emergency situation.

RESPONDING TO AN EMERGENCY

TRAINING PROGRAMS

There are many types of training programs that teach people, both health care workers and those who work in fields other than health care, how to react in case of an emergency. General training programs cover principles of **first aid,** the care given to an injured or sick person while waiting for more advanced help to arrive, and **basic life support (BLS),** or basic emergency care. Techniques, such as **rescue breathing** and **cardiopulmonary resuscitation (CPR),** used to sustain breathing and circulation for a person who has gone into respiratory or cardiac arrest, are also taught. Some training programs may focus on only one aspect of first aid or BLS, such as how to perform CPR, or they may focus on more advanced lifesaving techniques, such as giving

supportive medications. First aid courses are offered through organizations such as the American Red Cross (ARC), the National Safety Council (NSC), and the American Heart Association (AHA). The programs offered by these organizations are taught by certified instructors, using approved teaching methods (Fig. 12-1).

Your facility or organization may require first aid and CPR training as a requirement for employment. In some states, first aid and CPR training are provided as part of the nursing assistant training course. As the result of ongoing research, improvements are periodically made in the way some of these techniques, such as CPR, are taught. Therefore, we have not provided specific instructions for all first aid and BLS techniques in this text. You are, however, encouraged to get training in first aid and BLS techniques from a reputable program, such as one offered by the ARC, the NSC,

FIGURE 12-1

A student practices cardiopulmonary resuscitation (CPR) on a mannequin during a CPR training course. (*Stewart Cohen/ Index Stock Imagery, Inc.*)

or the AHA. The additional training, whether required by your employer or not, will allow you to be better prepared for emergency situations that may arise in your workplace, home, or community.

THE ROLE OF THE NURSING ASSISTANT IN AN EMERGENCY

As you learned in Chapter 5, the nature of your daily duties will bring you in close and frequent contact with your patients or residents. This unique relationship gives you insight that others might not have. Through your interactions with your patients or residents, you become aware of their individual qualities, personalities, and habits. For example, you know that Mrs. Smith typically has an above-average blood pressure reading, even though she is taking medication. You know that Mr. Martin complains about his arthritis, especially in the morning. You know that Mr. Allen always says that he is starving after eating a full meal. You know which of your patients or residents are "morning people," and which are grumpy and slow until after they have had their first cup of coffee. Your familiarity with your patients or residents makes you more likely to notice signs and symptoms that could alert the health care team to the fact that an emergency situation is lurking.

For example, the first sign of a stroke is often just a slight slurring of speech or a small change in a person's personality. Heart attacks may be signaled by complaints of fatigue or indigestion. Other emergency situations are recognized by changes in vital functions (such as respiratory rate, heart rate, and blood pressure) or behavior. The people you care for will have varying levels of ability and awareness, and you will come to learn what is normal for each person. A change in a person's usual abilities or level of awareness can be a sign that a problem is brewing beneath the surface. A person who is usually alert and **oriented to person** (able to tell you who he is and who you are), **place** (able to tell you where he is), and **time** (able to tell you the year, the day of the week, and the time of day) can suddenly become **disoriented,** or unable to answer those basic questions. A person is said to be **unresponsive** if she is unconscious and cannot be aroused, or conscious but not responsive when spoken to or touched. Either of these conditions should be

FIGURE 12-2

Being able to recognize an impending emergency is a life-saving skill.

reported to the nurse immediately. By conscientiously reporting signs or symptoms that seem unusual or give you cause for alarm to the nurse, you may prevent an emergency situation from developing (Fig. 12-2).

If an emergency situation does occur, your responsibilities as a nursing assistant are clear-cut. You should:

1. **Recognize that an emergency exists.** Use your observation skills and familiarity with the patient or resident to detect changes in behavior or physical condition.

2. **Decide to act.** Stay calm now and organize your thoughts. Check the scene to make sure that you are not entering a situation that is potentially dangerous for you, or for other members of the health care team. For example, a person who has been electrocuted may still be tangled in live electrical wires, which could shock you. Or, you could be entering an area that is contaminated with hazardous materials or gases. Acting hastily can make the problem worse in some situations. For example, someone who has fallen from a ladder may have injuries to the spinal column that would be made worse if the person were moved.

3. **Check for consciousness.** If it is safe to do so, gently shake the person and call to him. The person may have just fainted ("passed out"), in which case you will need to call the nurse for help. Keep the person lying down until the nurse arrives. The nurse will make sure that no other injuries

are present and work to find out why the person fainted. If the person does not respond when you gently shake his arm and call to him, then you will need to...

4. **Activate the emergency medical services (EMS) system.** An **EMS system** is a network of resources (including people, equipment, and facilities) that is organized to respond to an emergency. Hospitals typically have a code or procedure for calling EMS assistance from within the facility. Home health care agencies, assisted-living facilities, and long-term care facilities may require you to dial "911" or some other emergency telephone number. Know your facility's or agency's policy so that you can get help quickly. Early activation of the EMS system allows a person in an emergency situation to get advanced medical care as soon as possible. This greatly increases the person's chances of survival. When you call, be prepared to give accurate information about your location and the condition of your patient or resident. If you work in a long-term care facility, an assisted-living facility, or for a home health care agency, the people who respond to your call may be emergency medical technicians (EMTs) or paramedics. In an acute-care facility, such as a hospital, the people who respond will be a specially trained group of nurses, doctors, and other health care workers.

5. **Provide appropriate care until the EMS personnel arrive.** Start first aid or BLS measures according to the situation and your level of training. (As in any situation, you should perform only those procedures that you have been trained to do and that are within your scope of practice.) Speak gently and calmly to the person, and reassure him that more help is on the way.

BASIC LIFE SUPPORT (BLS) MEASURES

BLS measures are taken to help a person who is at risk for, or is already in, respiratory arrest, cardiac arrest, or both. When you use certain BLS measures, such as rescue breathing and CPR, you are essentially performing the vital functions of breathing and circulation for someone who is unable to perform these functions on her own. If you find one of your patients or residents in a state of respiratory or cardiac arrest, be sure you know the person's wishes for resuscitation before undertaking any BLS measures. For example, a person who is terminally ill may not want to be resuscitated if she goes into respiratory or cardiac arrest. In this case, the person's chart would carry a no-code or do not resuscitate (DNR) order. (See also Chapter 21, where the subject of advance directives is covered more fully.) If a person is on DNR status, follow your facility's or agency's policy accordingly.

The goal of BLS is to prevent respiratory arrest, cardiac arrest, or both. If the person is already in respiratory or cardiac arrest, BLS is used to keep the person alive until advanced medical assistance arrives. The steps of BLS are:

1. **"A" is for "airway."** Open the person's airway by tilting his head back and lifting his chin (Fig. 12-3). A person who has fainted can stop breathing if the tongue relaxes and falls backward against the back of the throat. Remember that respiratory arrest will lead to cardiac arrest if not quickly corrected.

2. **"B" is for "breathing."** Check to see if the person is breathing by leaning close and placing your ear over his mouth and nose. Listen for the sounds of breathing, feel the person's breath moving against your cheek, and look for the rise and fall of his chest (Fig. 12-4). The person is not breathing unless there is air movement as well as chest movement! For example, a person who has suddenly died will exhale when you open his airway, but he will not

FIGURE 12-3

"A" is for "airway." Tilting the head back and lifting the chin helps to maintain an open airway.

continue to breathe in and out. A person with an obstructed airway may make efforts to breathe that will cause his chest to rise and fall, but you will not be able to feel air moving from his mouth or nose. If the person is breathing, keep his airway open or position him in the recovery position (the lateral position). Continue to monitor the person's condition closely while waiting for assistance. If the person is not breathing, start rescue breathing according to your training. Remember that if an airway is not established and oxygen is not sent to the person's lungs, the person will not survive the incident, no matter what additional measures are taken.

3. **"C" is for "circulation."** Check the person's pulse. You can feel an adult's or child's pulse by placing your fingers on either side of the Adam's apple, over the carotid artery in the neck. An infant's pulse is felt over the brachial artery, in the upper arm. A person in an emergency situation may have a rapid, weak, erratic (irregular), or very slow pulse. A person with no pulse is in cardiac arrest and needs immediate CPR (Fig. 12-5).

4. **Check for bleeding.** Severe bleeding (hemorrhage) must be controlled. This can be accomplished by applying pressure directly to the wound to slow or stop the bleeding. If direct pressure does not work and the source of the blood is a wound on the person's arm or leg, you can elevate the extremity and apply pressure to a pulse point between the wound and the heart. **Pulse points** are the points where the large arteries run close enough to the surface of the skin to be felt as a pulse (see Chapter 16, Fig. 16-8). At these points, the artery can be pressed against a bone by applying direct pressure, helping to slow blood loss from a wound. A tourniquet is a device that is placed tightly around an arm or a leg to cut off nearly all blood supply. A tourniquet is only used as a last resort to control bleeding, and should always be applied by a specially trained emergency responder.

FIGURE 12-4

"B" is for "breathing." To make sure that a person is breathing, you should listen for the sound of his breath, feel for his breath against your cheek, and look for the rise and fall of his chest.

EMERGENCY SITUATIONS

Many different emergency situations can occur, both in the home and community and in the health care setting. In this section, we will review some of

FIGURE 12-5

"C" is for "circulation." In cardiopulmonary resuscitation (CPR), which is used for a person in cardiac arrest, oxygenated blood is circulated throughout the person's body by manually compressing his heart. (A) This is a cross-sectional view of the human body when a person is lying down. The sternum (breastbone) covers the heart. (B) When CPR is given, pressure is applied to the sternum with the hands to compress the heart, causing blood to flow throughout the body.

Breastbone (sternum)
Heart
Lung
Lung
Esophagus
Vertebra

A.

B.

the most common emergency situations, as well as what you should do if you find yourself in a position to help a person in one of these situations.

"HEART ATTACKS" AND STROKES

Both heart attacks and strokes can occur suddenly. These are life-threatening situations that require emergency care. Perhaps the classic emergency situation is that of a "heart attack," or myocardial infarction (MI). The myocardium is the muscular wall of the heart. An infarction occurs when blood flow to a part of the body is blocked, depriving the cells of oxygen and causing them to die. So when a person has a myocardial infarction (MI), blood flow to the muscular wall of the heart is blocked, and part of the heart muscle dies. The crippled heart muscle is unable to pump blood effectively throughout the body, creating an emergency situation. If the damaged area of the heart is large enough, cardiac arrest can occur.

The signs and symptoms of a heart attack can vary greatly from one person to the next. The most typical symptom is pain or tightness in the chest, which may or may not extend to the neck or arm. In addition, the person's skin may become pale or grayish and the person may sweat excessively. He may have trouble breathing, and may complain of nausea or heartburn-like pain. If you observe that a person is having signs or symptoms of a heart attack, have the person lie down. Raise the person's head to help make breathing easier, and call the nurse or activate the EMS system immediately. Prompt medical intervention can help to minimize damage to the heart muscle. If the person goes into respiratory or cardiac arrest, you will need to begin BLS.

Strokes, also known as "brain attacks" or cerebrovascular accidents (CVAs), are also caused by blocked blood flow to a body part. In the case of a stroke, the affected body part is the brain, rather than the heart. Like a heart attack, a stroke can cause different signs and symptoms in different people. For example, a stroke might cause only mild physical changes in some people. In others, it might cause loss of consciousness or a coma. Signs of a stroke could include any of the following:
- A change in a person's level of orientation or consciousness
- Slurred speech
- Muscle weakness or paralysis
- Drooping of the eyelid or a corner of the mouth
- Severe headache

If you think that a person is having or has had a stroke, report your observations to the nurse and activate the EMS system. Keep the person lying down and watch for signs of respiratory arrest until advanced care arrives. New advances in the treatment of stroke have resulted in improved outcomes for some patients, when treatment is started early.

FAINTING (SYNCOPE)

Fainting occurs when the blood supply to the brain suddenly decreases, resulting in a loss of consciousness. Although fainting may be an early sign of a serious medical condition, such as a heart problem, it can also be the result of hunger ("low blood sugar"), pain, extreme emotion, fatigue, medication side effects, a "stuffy" room (poor ventilation), excessive heat, or standing for a long time. Fainting is not life-threatening in and of itself, but because a person who faints is at risk for injury from falling, it is important to act quickly if you believe a person is about to faint. A person who is about to faint may complain of dizziness or a temporary loss of vision. His skin may be pale and clammy from excessive sweating. He may breathe shallowly, and his pulse may be weak.

If you think that a person is about to faint, have the person lie down in the supine position and elevate his legs 12 inches, or ask him to sit down and bend forward, placing his head between his knees (Fig. 12-6). These actions will increase blood flow to the brain, which may prevent the person from losing consciousness. Loosen any restraints or tight clothing (such as a belt or necktie), and have the person remain in the supine or sitting position (with his head between his knees) for at least 5 minutes. Do not leave the person unattended during this time. If necessary, use the call light control to call the nurse.

If a person you are assisting does faint, lower him to the floor or other flat surface, remembering to use good body mechanics (see Chapter 9, Box 9-1). Position the person on his back with his head turned to the side, in case he vomits. If you are sure that the person does not have any injuries to the head, neck, or spinal cord, raise his legs 12 inches, and loosen any tight clothing or restraints.

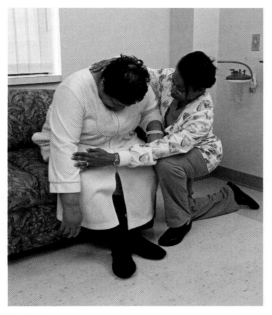

FIGURE 12-6
Having a person sit with her head between her knees increases blood flow to the brain and may prevent a fainting episode.

Make sure the person is breathing, and call for help. Then check the person's vital signs. Even if the person recovers from the episode quickly, have him continue to lie down until the nurse arrives.

 ### Tell the Nurse!

Because fainting may be a sign of a serious medical condition, it is important to note the following for the nurse:

⮕ What time the person fainted

⮕ Whether there was a change in the person's level of consciousness, and if so, how long this change lasted

⮕ Whether the person vomited

⮕ The person's appearance at the time of the incident (for example: overheated, pale, sweaty)

⮕ Whether the person complained of anything before the incident (for example: loss of vision, dizziness, nausea)

⮕ The actions you took to assist the person

SEIZURES

Seizures, also known as *convulsions*, occur when brain activity is interrupted. Seizures can result from head injuries (either recent or past), strokes,

infections, high fevers, poisonings, brain tumors, and epilepsy. When most of us think of the seizures associated with epilepsy, we think of **grand mal seizures,** which are characterized by generalized and violent contraction and relaxation of the body's muscles. However, not all seizures are characterized by violent contraction and relaxation of the muscles. A person who is having a **petit mal (absence) seizure** may show no signs other than appearing to be momentarily absent from the present situation. The person may stare into space or stop speaking in mid-sentence, only to "come back" a few moments later.

Although petit mal seizures are not an emergency situation, grand mal seizures usually are. Grand mal seizures cause a loss of consciousness and, because of the violent jerking of the muscles, place the person who is having the seizure at risk for injuring herself. If a person is standing or sitting in a chair when a seizure begins, she could be injured when she falls as the result of losing consciousness. A person who is having a seizure is also at risk for injuring herself by striking nearby objects or by severely biting her own tongue and lips. A grand mal seizure may last for just a few seconds, or it may go on for as long as 5 to 10 minutes.

First aid for a person having a grand mal seizure involves protecting the person until the seizure is over, and keeping the airway open during the period of unconsciousness afterwards. If a person is standing or sitting when a seizure begins, gently help the person to the floor and move furniture or other objects that might cause injury out of the way. Protect the person's head by placing a pillow or folded towel underneath it and call for help while allowing the seizure to run its course. Although in the past, it was common practice to insert a tongue blade into the person's mouth to prevent the person from biting her own tongue, you should not do this. Never attempt to place anything in the person's mouth or between the teeth. You may hurt the person or get bitten. It is common for a person who is having a seizure to lose control of her bladder or bowels. Because the gag reflex may also be temporarily lost, saliva may pool in the mouth. After the seizure is over, turn the person to her side (place her in the recovery position) and allow any secretions to drain from her mouth to prevent choking. Provide warmth and a quiet environment (Fig. 12-7). A person who has just had a seizure may be very disoriented, tired, or both, and she may have no memory of the episode at all.

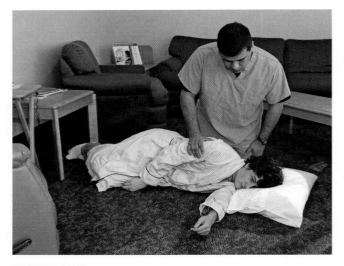

FIGURE 12-7

After the seizure has passed, place the person in the recovery position and allow secretions to drain from the mouth.

HEMORRHAGE

Hemorrhage (severe, uncontrolled bleeding) can be caused by trauma to a blood vessel or by certain illnesses, such as gastric ulcers. Ordinarily, when a blood vessel wall is injured, a blood clot forms to prevent the loss of blood. However, if the trauma to the blood vessel wall is major, or if the person lacks the clotting factors needed to form blood clots, the bleeding will not stop. It should be noted that people who are taking medications to prevent blood clotting are at high risk for hemorrhage as well, because the medication decreases the body's normal clotting response.

Hemorrhage can be either external (plainly visible) or internal (occurring within the body). Internal hemorrhage may be very well hidden unless the person vomits blood or passes blood through the rectum. Hemorrhage can be either venous or arterial, depending on the type of blood vessel that is injured. Venous hemorrhage flows steadily. Arterial hemorrhage spurts or pulses with the heartbeat. If hemorrhage is not controlled quickly, death will result.

If a person is hemorrhaging, call for help and make sure the person is lying down. Take standard precautions to protect yourself from exposure to bloodborne pathogens. Apply firm, steady pressure directly to the wound using a sterile dressing, a clean towel, or whatever else is clean and available for use as a compress. Continue to apply pressure to the wound until more advanced medical help comes. If the direct pressure does not stop or slow the flow of blood, raise the affected body part (if it is an arm or leg) and apply pressure to a pulse point above the wound (see Chapter 16, Fig. 16-8).

SHOCK

Shock results when the organs and tissues of the body do not receive enough oxygen-rich blood. There are many different causes and types of shock. For example:

- **Cardiogenic shock** can occur when the heart is unable to pump enough blood throughout the body to meet the tissues' need for oxygen.
- **Hemorrhagic shock** results from massive blood loss, which means that there is not enough blood in the vessels to supply the tissues of the body.
- **Septic shock** is caused by severe bacterial infections that involve the entire body. The toxins produced by the bacteria cause the blood vessels to dilate (widen), leading to pooling of blood away from the heart and poor circulation.
- **Anaphylactic shock** is caused by a severe allergic reaction (for example, to medications, bee stings, or certain foods, such as nuts). As in septic shock, widening of the blood vessels occurs, causing the blood to pool away from the heart. In addition, the tiniest tubes in the lungs (called bronchioles) close off, preventing the oxygen in the air from passing into the lungs and reaching the blood.

To treat shock, the underlying cause of the shock must be addressed. For example, if a person is in shock because of hemorrhage, the bleeding must be stopped and the fluid replaced intravenously to prevent death. If the pumping action of the heart is too weak or erratic to circulate blood to the organs and tissues, the heart's ability to pump must be restored through medications or other measures, such as the implantation of a pacemaker.

A person entering a state of shock will have low blood pressure that continues to decrease. His pulse will be rapid and weak. His skin will be cool, clammy, and pale. He will be confused

FIGURE 12-8

The EpiPen Auto-Injector, a self-injectable cartridge of epinephrine, is used to treat anaphylactic shock. The yellow EpiPen is for adults. The white one is for children. (*Photo courtesy of L.P. Dey.*)

or disoriented. He will breathe rapidly, and if he is conscious, he may complain of thirst. Make sure that advanced emergency medical care has been called and keep the person warm and calm. The treatment for anaphylactic shock is the immediate administration of a medication called epinephrine (adrenaline). People who know that they are allergic to something that could cause them to go into anaphylactic shock (for example, bee stings) often carry this medication with them (Fig. 12-8). If a person who is in anaphylactic shock is unable to give himself this medication, someone else will need to do this for him.

AIRWAY OBSTRUCTIONS ("CHOKING")

As you now know, the organs and tissues of the body need oxygen to function. Occasionally, foreign material, such as food or vomitus, becomes lodged in the airway ("windpipe"), blocking the flow of air to the lungs. The accidental inhalation of foreign material into the airway is called **aspiration.** Airway obstructions are most often caused by aspirated pieces of food—people often do not chew their food properly, and, usually, they are distracted from the process of chewing and swallowing because they are interacting with others at the table. Aspiration can occur when a person takes a breath to laugh or speak, and a piece of food is sucked into the airway. If the piece of food is large enough or goes down the airway far enough, the person may not be able to cough it up. People with poorly fitting dentures or who are missing teeth are at increased risk for aspiration, because they cannot chew their food properly.

Children are at particularly high risk for airway obstruction, for several reasons. First of all, children cannot or do not always chew their food well,

and they can choke on very small pieces of food. Foods that ordinarily would not cause a problem for adults, such as hard candies, hotdogs, popcorn, apples, grapes, carrots, and nuts, can be choking hazards for children. Second, children may attempt to continue eating while running, playing, laughing, or crying. Last, children tend to place small toys and other foreign objects in their mouths.

People who are not conscious or who have weak coughing or swallowing reflexes as a result of paralysis or the effects of a medication (for example, some pain medications) are also at an increased risk for aspiration. Most people who are vomiting can keep their airway clean and will choke and gag easily, but people with an impaired gag reflex may aspirate vomitus. This is why, when you are assisting a person who is vomiting or at risk for vomiting, you turn the person's head to the side to help keep the airway clear.

An airway obstruction can be either partial or complete. In a partial airway obstruction, the object is not totally blocking the airway and some air can pass through. A person who is coughing strongly and has good skin color most likely has a partial airway obstruction with good air exchange (that is, an adequate ability to breathe). Stay with the person and allow him to continue to cough. If the person is not already in an upright position, assist him into one to make breathing easier. If the person does not quickly cough up the object, call for help because advanced emergency medical assistance may be necessary to remove the item. Also, there is the risk that the item will move and totally obstruct the airway, in which case the person will need immediate assistance. A partial airway obstruction with poor air exchange (that is, an inadequate ability to breathe) is demonstrated by a weak, ineffective coughing effort; high-pitched, "crowing" sounds as the person tries to breathe; and a bluish skin color. A person with this type of airway obstruction needs immediate help.

A complete airway obstruction is one that totally blocks all airflow to the lungs. The person cannot cough, speak, or breathe and will lose consciousness quickly if the object that is blocking airflow is not removed. The person will be frightened, and may run to the bathroom if the obstruction occurs in a public place, such as in a restaurant or dining room. (If you suspect that someone who has left the table is choking, please follow him.) The person may grab his throat in what is considered the universal choking sign (Fig. 12-9).

FIGURE 12-9

Grasping the throat is the universal sign for "I'm choking!"

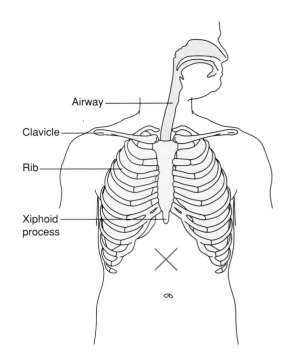

FIGURE 12-10

Applying pressure to the abdominal cavity (*red X*) forces the air out of the lungs, which in turn forces the object out of the person's airway.

Clearing the Airway in Adults and Children Older Than 1 Year

Abdominal thrusts, commonly called the **Heimlich maneuver,** are used to clear an obstructed airway in an adult or a child older than 1 year who is choking. The thoracic cavity, which contains the heart and lungs, is separated from the abdominal cavity, which contains the stomach and other organs, by the diaphragm, a flat muscle. During the Heimlich maneuver, the area beneath the diaphragm (the abdominal cavity) is compressed, forcing the air out of the lungs. This dislodges the object that is blocking the airway (Fig. 12-10). The procedure for performing the Heimlich maneuver on a person who is conscious is given in Procedure 12-1. The procedure for performing the Heimlich maneuver on a person who is unconscious is given in Procedure 12-2.

The Heimlich maneuver is done the same way in both children older than 1 year and adults, except that in children, less force is applied to the abdomen. This is to avoid injuring the child's ribs, sternum (breastbone), and internal organs. In very heavy people or pregnant women, the Heimlich maneuver is modified so that chest thrusts, rather than abdominal thrusts, are used. This is because in these situations, giving abdominal thrusts would be either impossible or dangerous. In the case of a very heavy person, it is too hard to get your arms around the person. In the case of a pregnant woman, applying pressure to the abdomen could harm the baby. Procedure 12-3 explains how to give chest thrusts to both conscious and unconscious people.

When a person is choking, the EMS system should be activated as soon as possible. While you wait for help, perform the Heimlich maneuver repeatedly, until the airway is open again and the person starts breathing on his own. If the person does not start breathing on his own, perform rescue breathing after the airway is cleared. You may need to start CPR if the person goes into cardiac arrest. However, you must understand that until the obstruction has been removed and air is sent to the lungs, CPR will not be effective.

Clearing the Airway in Infants

In children younger than 1 year, the Heimlich maneuver is not used because of the risk for damaging the baby's internal organs. Instead, a combination of back blows and chest thrusts is used. Clearing the airway in a conscious infant is described in Procedure 12-4. Clearing the airway in an unconscious infant is described in Procedure 12-5. You can give back blows and chest thrusts while standing or sitting. If the infant is large or your hands are small, you may prefer to sit.

THE CHAIN OF SURVIVAL

A person's ability to survive an emergency, and to survive it without any permanent damage, relies on a series of events called the **chain of survival:**

1. Someone must recognize that an emergency situation exists, and activate the EMS system.
2. First responder care (basic first aid, including BLS if applicable) must be given by able people at the scene of the emergency.
3. Medical intervention, such as that provided by an EMT, a paramedic, a nurse, or a doctor, must be provided as soon as possible.
4. After the immediate crisis passes, hospital care may be needed to help the person survive. As the person's condition improves, she may be transferred to a subacute care unit or return to a long-term care facility or private home for further recovery.
5. Rehabilitation, the final step in the chain of survival, focuses on improving the general health status of the person. One goal of rehabilitation may be to help the person to recover abilities that may have been lost as a result of the emergency. For example, a person who has suffered a stroke may need to relearn skills such as walking or speaking. Another goal of rehabilitation may be to help the person learn how to prevent further progression of a disease. For example, a person who has had a heart attack may be taught new diet management skills, and started on an exercise program.

As a nursing assistant, you can play a vital role in helping to see a person through the immediate crisis (steps 1 and 2). You may also find yourself caring for someone who is in the recovery phase (steps 4 and 5).

SUMMARY

▶ Breathing and circulation are processes that are essential to life. Disruption of either of these processes leads to an emergency situation. Common emergency situations include fainting, seizures, hemorrhaging, shock, and choking.
  ■ Fainting, seizures, and choking may interfere with breathing.
  ■ Hemorrhage and shock interfere with circulation.
▶ Basic life support (BLS) measures focus on preserving breathing and circulation for people who cannot perform these functions on their own, until more advanced medical care arrives. BLS involves maintaining the person's airway, making sure that the person is breathing, evaluating the person's pulse to make sure that the heart is beating and blood is circulating throughout the body, and controlling bleeding.
▶ Nursing assistants play a vital role in preventing, recognizing, and responding to emergency situations.
  ■ Your knowledge of your patient's or resident's usual condition, combined with keen observation skills, may allow you to recognize a potential emergency situation. By communicating what you have observed to the nurse, you may be able to prevent the emergency from occurring, or to minimize the effects if it does occur.
  ■ You may find yourself in the position of assisting someone who needs emergency care, either at work, at home, or in the community. Participation in first aid and BLS training programs will increase your skills and allow you to care for people in emergency situations confidently and safely.
▶ Receiving skilled first aid, along with early medical intervention, increases a person's chance of surviving an emergency and minimizes the person's chances of having permanent disabilities as a result of the incident.

Chapter 12 Procedures

PROCEDURE 12-1

Performing Abdominal Thrusts in Conscious Adults and Children Older Than 1 Year

1. Check the person's ability to breathe and speak by tapping him or her on the shoulder and saying, "Are you okay? Can you talk? I can help you." A person who cannot breathe or speak needs immediate help.

STEP 5 Place your fist just above the person's navel and below the sternum.

2. If the person starts to cough, wait and see if the coughing will dislodge the foreign body. If the person's cough is weak and ineffective, or if the person is in obvious distress, continue with step 3.

3. Stay with the person and call for help. Have the person who is helping you activate the emergency medical services (EMS) system.

4. Stand behind the person with the obstructed airway and wrap your arms around his or her waist.

5. Make a fist with one hand and place the thumb of the fist against the person's abdomen, just above the navel and below the sternum (breastbone). Grasp your fist with the other hand.

6. Being careful not to put pressure on the person's ribs or sternum with your forearms, press your fist inward and pull upward, using quick thrusting motions, until the foreign body is expelled, the person begins to cough forcefully, or the person loses consciousness.

   a. If the foreign body is expelled, stay with the person, and follow the nurse's directions.

   b. If the person begins to cough, wait and see if the coughing results in expulsion of the foreign body. If it does not, continue giving abdominal thrusts.

   c. If the person loses consciousness, lower the person to the floor and initiate Procedure 12-2, beginning with step 7.

7. The person should be evaluated by a doctor following the choking incident.

PROCEDURE 12-2

Performing Abdominal Thrusts in Unconscious Adults and Children Older Than 1 Year

1. Check the person's consciousness by tapping him or her on the shoulder and saying, "Are you okay? Can you talk? I can help you." An unresponsive person needs immediate help.

2. Stay with the person and call for help. Have the person who is helping you activate the emergency medical services (EMS) system.

3. **Head tilt/chin lift maneuver.** Position the person on his or her back on a hard, flat surface. Open the person's airway by tilting the head back and lifting the chin (see Fig. 12-3). Look, feel, and listen for signs of breathing.

STEP 4 Rescue breathing.

4. **Rescue breathing.** If the person is not breathing, keep his or her head tilted back and the chin lifted. Blow two slow breaths into the person's mouth through a ventilation barrier device, removing your mouth from the device and inhaling between each breath. If the air does not go in, repeat the head tilt/chin lift maneuver and attempt rescue breathing once again.

STEP 5 Foreign body check/finger sweep maneuver.

5. **Foreign body check/finger sweep maneuver.** If no air enters the person's lungs after the second attempt, perform a foreign body check followed by a finger sweep maneuver to try to dislodge and remove the foreign body. To do a foreign body check followed by a finger sweep maneuver:

   a. Kneel beside the person's head. With the person's head tilted back and the chin lifted, grasp the person's lower jaw and tongue with one hand, lifting the lower jaw upward.

   b. Look for the foreign body.

   c. Insert the index finger of the other hand into the person's mouth, placing it alongside the person's cheek. The tip of your finger should be at the base of the person's tongue.

   d. Using a "hooking" action, sweep your index finger across the inside of the person's mouth to try and dislodge and remove the foreign body. Be careful not to push the foreign body deeper into the person's throat.

6. Repeat the head lift/chin tilt maneuver. Blow two slow breaths into the person's mouth through a ventilation barrier device, removing your mouth from the device and inhaling between each breath. If the air does not go in, repeat the head lift/chin tilt maneuver and attempt rescue breathing once again.

STEP 7 Abdominal thrusts.

7. **Abdominal thrusts.** If no air enters the person's lungs after the second attempt, give five

(continued)

PROCEDURE 12-2 (Continued)

Performing Abdominal Thrusts in Unconscious Adults and
Children Older Than 1 Year

abdominal thrusts. To give abdominal
thrusts to an unconscious person:

    a. Straddle the person's thighs.

    b. Place the heel of one hand on the person's
abdomen, above the navel and well below
the sternum (breastbone). Your fingers
should be pointing toward the person's
head.

    c. Place your other hand on top of the first
and position your shoulders directly above
the person's abdomen.

    d. Press your hands inward and upward, us-
ing quick thrusting motions, five times.

8. Perform a foreign body check followed by a
finger sweep maneuver.

9. Repeat the head lift/chin tilt maneuver.
Blow two slow breaths into the person's
mouth through a ventilation barrier device,
removing your mouth from the device and
inhaling between each breath. If the air does
not go in, repeat the head lift/chin tilt maneuver and attempt rescue breathing once
again.

10. Repeat the abdominal thrust–foreign body
check/finger sweep–rescue breathing sequence until the foreign body is expelled, rescue breathing is successful, or other trained
personnel arrive and take over.

11. The person should be evaluated by a doctor
following the choking incident.

PROCEDURE 12-3

Performing Chest Thrusts in Adults and Children
Older than 1 Year

·If the Person Is Conscious

1. Stand behind the person and place your arms
under the person's armpits and around his or
her chest.

STEP 2 Place your fist over the person's sternum.

2. Make a fist with one hand and place the
thumb of the fist against the center of the person's sternum. Be sure that your thumb is
centered on the sternum, not on the lower tip
of the sternum (the xiphoid process) and not
on the ribs.

3. Give up to five quick chest thrusts by
grasping your fist with your other hand
and pressing inward five times. Each
thrust should compress the chest 1½ to
2 inches.

4. Continue to give chest thrusts until the
foreign body is expelled, the person begins to
cough forcefully, or the person loses
consciousness.

    a. If the foreign body is expelled, stay with the
person, and follow the nurse's directions.

    b. If the person begins to cough, wait and see
if the coughing results in expulsion of the
foreign body. If it does not, continue giving
chest thrusts in groups of five.

    c. If the person loses consciousness, lower the
person to the floor and initiate the procedure below.

(continued)

PROCEDURE 12-3 (Continued)

Performing Chest Thrusts in Adults and Children Older than 1 Year

5. The person should be evaluated by a doctor following the choking incident.

If the Person Is Unconscious

1. Kneel next to the person.

2. Place the heel of one hand on the center of the person's sternum, and place your other hand on top. Be sure that the heel of your hand is centered on the sternum, not on the lower tip of the sternum (the xiphoid process) and not on the ribs.

3. Give up to five quick chest thrusts by pressing straight down five times. Each thrust should compress the chest 1½ to 2 inches.

4. After giving five chest thrusts, perform a foreign body check followed by a finger sweep maneuver and initiate rescue breathing as described in Procedure 12-2.

5. Repeat the chest thrust–foreign body check/finger sweep–rescue breathing sequence until the foreign body is expelled, rescue breathing is successful, or other trained personnel arrive and take over.

6. The person should be evaluated by a doctor following the choking incident.

PROCEDURE 12-4

Clearing the Airway in a Conscious Infant

1. Check the infant's ability to breathe and cry. An infant who cannot breathe or cry needs immediate help.

2. Stay with the infant. Call for help and have the person who is helping you activate the emergency medical services (EMS) system.

STEP 3 Hold the infant on his back between your forearms.

3. Position the infant on his or her back on your forearm. Place your other arm on top of the infant, using your thumb and forefinger to hold the infant's jaw while sandwiching the infant between your forearms.

4. Rotate your arms, so that the infant is facing downward, still sandwiched between your forearms. Lower your arm onto your thigh so that the infant's head is lower than his or her chest.

5. Give five firm blows to the back (between the infant's shoulder blades), using the heel of your hand. Be sure that you continue to support the infant's head and neck by firmly holding the baby's jaw between your thumb and forefinger.

6. If the back blows do not dislodge the foreign body, you must turn the infant over in preparation for administering chest thrusts. Turn the infant over by placing your free hand and forearm along the infant's head and back so that the infant is sandwiched between your hands and forearms. Continue to support the infant's head between your thumb and forefinger from the front, while you cradle the back of the head with your other hand. Turn the infant onto his or her back. Lower your arm onto your thigh so that the infant's head is lower than his or her chest.

(continued)

PROCEDURE 12-4 (Continued)

Clearing the Airway in a Conscious Infant

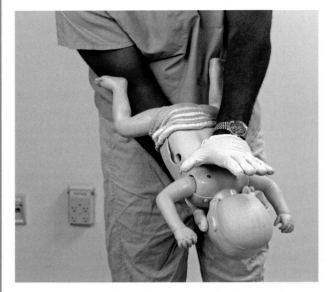

STEP 5 Use the heel of your hand to deliver back blows while supporting the infant's head and neck.

STEP 7 Place the pads of your first three fingers on the infant's sternum to give chest thrusts.

7. To locate the correct place to give chest thrusts, imagine a line running across the infant's chest between the nipples. Place the pads of your first three fingers on the infant's sternum (breastbone), even with this imaginary line. If you feel the notch at the end of the infant's sternum, move your fingers toward the infant's head so that your fingers are over the center of the sternum.

8. Lift your ring finger off the chest, and using the pads of the two remaining fingers, compress the sternum ½ to 1 inch, and then let the sternum return to its normal position. Give five chest thrusts.

9. Repeat the back blow–chest thrust sequence until the foreign body is expelled, the infant begins to cough forcefully, or the infant loses consciousness.

   a. If the foreign body is expelled, stay with the infant, and follow the nurse's directions.

   b. If the infant begins to cough, wait and see if the coughing results in expulsion of the object. If it does not, continue giving five back blows followed by five chest thrusts.

   c. If the infant loses consciousness, initiate the procedure described in Procedure 12-5, beginning with step 4.

10. The infant should be evaluated by a doctor following the choking incident.

PROCEDURE 12-5

Clearing the Airway in an Unconscious Infant

1. Check the infant's responsiveness by gently shaking the infant and speaking to him. An unresponsive infant needs immediate help.

2. Stay with the infant and call for help. Have the person who is helping you activate the emergency medical services (EMS) system.

3. **Head tilt/chin lift maneuver.** Position the infant on his or her back on a hard, flat surface. Open the infant's airway by tilting the head back slightly and lifting the chin until the infant's nose points toward the ceiling. Look, feel, and listen for signs of breathing.

4. **Rescue breathing.** If the infant is not breathing, keep his or her head tilted back and the chin lifted. Cover the infant's nose and mouth with your mouth or an airway device and blow two slow breaths into the infant's mouth, removing your mouth from the infant's nose and mouth and inhaling between each breath. If the air does not go in, repeat the head tilt/chin lift maneuver and attempt rescue breathing once again.

5. If no air enters the infant's lungs after the second attempt, assume that the infant's airway is blocked.

6. **Back blow/chest thrust sequence.** Give five back blows, followed by five chest thrusts, as described in Procedure 12-4.

7. **Foreign body check.** If the back blow–chest thrust sequence is not successful, perform a foreign body check. To do a foreign body check:

   a. Kneel beside the infant's head. Open the infant's mouth, using your hand that is

nearer the infant's feet. Put your thumb into the infant's mouth and your fingers underneath his or her lower jaw, and lift the jaw upward.

   b. Look for the foreign body. If you can see it, try to remove it by using your thumb and index finger in a "pincer"-type motion. If you cannot see the foreign body, skip ahead to step 8.

STEP 7 If you see the foreign body in the infant's mouth, try to remove it using a "pincer"-type motion.

8. Blow two slow breaths into the infant's nose and mouth, removing your nose and mouth from the infant's mouth and inhaling between each breath. If the air does not go in, repeat the head tilt/chin lift maneuver and attempt rescue breathing once again.

9. Repeat steps 6 through 8 until the foreign body is expelled, rescue breathing is successful, or other trained personnel arrive and take over.

10. The infant should be evaluated by a doctor following the choking incident.

What did you learn?

Multiple Choice

Select the single best answer for each of the following questions.

1. A person with an airway obstruction will usually:
   a. Have a seizure
   b. Vomit
   c. Be able to speak and breathe normally
   d. Clutch at his or her throat

2. The first step in the chain of survival is:
   a. Rehabilitation
   b. Recognizing that an emergency exists and calling for help
   c. Giving first aid
   d. Initiating basic life support (BLS) measures

3. In the ABCs of basic life support (BLS), the "C" stands for:
   a. Cardiac
   b. Consciousness
   c. Circulation
   d. Check for bleeding

4. You are helping to prepare a holiday dinner at your mother's house, when suddenly your sister misses the vegetable she is trying to slice and cuts deeply into her finger instead. Blood is spurting from the cut, which indicates to you that your sister:
   a. Is hemorrhaging internally
   b. Has cut a vein
   c. Has cut an artery
   d. Requires the application of a tourniquet

5. Where do you place your fist while clearing an obstructed airway in an unconscious adult?
   a. On the person's back
   b. Above the person's navel
   c. On the person's chest
   d. Below the person's navel

6. If a person is coughing but able to breathe, you should:
   a. Administer oxygen
   b. Use a finger sweep to remove the object that is obstructing the person's airway
   c. Perform the Heimlich maneuver
   d. Stay with the person and allow him or her to continue coughing

7. Which is a sign or symptom of shock?
   a. Low blood pressure
   b. A weak, rapid pulse
   c. Cool, clammy, pale skin
   d. All of the above

8. Which of the following actions should you take to assist a person who is having a grand mal seizure?
   a. Protect the person's head by placing a pillow underneath it
   b. Clear the area by moving furniture out of the way
   c. Avoid placing anything in the person's mouth
   d. All of the above

Matching

Match each numbered item with its appropriate lettered description.

_____ **1.** Emergency medical services (EMS) system

_____ **2.** First aid

_____ **3.** Basic life support (BLS)

_____ **4.** Clinically dead

_____ **5.** Respiratory arrest

_____ **6.** Cardiac arrest

_____ **7.** Grand mal seizure

_____ **8.** Petit mal (absence) seizure

_____ **9.** Anaphylactic shock

_____ **10.** Fainting (syncope)

a. Occurs when the blood supply to the brain suddenly decreases, resulting in a loss of consciousness

b. Condition of a person who has no pulse or is not breathing

c. Breathing has stopped

d. A potentially deadly allergic reaction (for example, to a bee sting or certain foods, such as nuts)

e. Heart has stopped

f. Care given to an injured person before more advanced medical assistance arrives

g. A network of resources, including people, equipment, and facilities, that is organized to respond to an emergency

h. The person stares off into space or stops speaking for a moment

i. Measures taken to help a person who is at risk for, or is already in, respiratory arrest, cardiac arrest, or both

j. Generalized and violent contraction and relaxation of the body's muscles

? Stop and think!

▶ You work as a nursing assistant in a nursing home. One of your responsibilities is to check on the residents while the nurses are attending the change-of-shift report. You enter Mrs. Oblonsky's room and find her on the floor. She has no roommate, so no one witnessed what happened. It does not appear that Mrs. Oblonsky fell out of bed. Her color is pale, and her lips are turning blue. What do you first?

▶ One of your responsibilities is to oversee the residents of the long-term care facility where you work while they are in the recreation room. Today, the residents are gathered and getting ready for an activity. Everyone is busy talking, selecting teams, and generally having fun. Everyone, that is, except for Mr. Grant. Normally outgoing and friendly, today Mr. Grant is just sitting in his wheelchair, staring into space without moving. You know that Mr. Grant has a history of seizures, but he has been taking his medications for months with no problems. In fact, recently, he has even put on some weight and you think the extra pounds suit him well. Everyone, staff members and residents alike, has been eating more lately, ever since the facility hired a new cook who makes exceptionally tasty food. You are getting ready to go across the room to see Mr. Grant when all of a sudden, he stiffens, thrusts his hands out in front of him, lifts his feet out of the footrests, falls out of his wheelchair, and begins convulsing! What should you do? What could have caused this sudden change in behavior?

Nursing Assistants Make a Difference!

"My name is Hal, and I have been a resident of the Sunnydale Nursing Facility for the past 6 years. I came to live here after a stroke partially paralyzed my right side and left me unable to walk. I am well cared for, and have grown to care for most of the people who work here like my own family. I've also made many new friends. It's funny—since coming to live here, I actually get to see more people and do more things than when I lived at home, alone. There are always planned activities—such as bingo games, poetry readings, jigsaw puzzle get-togethers, and card games—that allow us residents to get together and socialize. Perhaps my favorite social activity of all is dinner in the dining room. The dining room has large bay windows and French doors that look westward out over the mountains, giving us "front row seats" for the sunset. There is also a piano, and on most nights, Mitch, a volunteer from the community, comes and plays wonderful music on the piano as we eat.

"One night not too long ago, however, I had a horrible scare in the dining room. I was chewing a piece of chicken when I laughed at a joke one of my friends told. The chicken slid down my throat the wrong way, and got stuck in my windpipe. I couldn't breathe or speak....I was so frightened! I was convinced that after working so hard to survive my stroke, I would die from choking on a stupid piece of chicken! Fortunately for me, one of the nursing assistants, Paula, saw my terrified expression from across the room and rushed to my aid. She asked if I was choking and told me that she could help. As she positioned herself behind me, she called to another nursing assistant that I was choking, and asked him to call the nurse. In the meantime, Paula performed that maneuver—the Heimlich, I think they call it—and the piece of chicken flew right out of my mouth!

"After the excitement had died down, Paula stayed with me for a while just to make sure I was OK. I didn't want to admit how scared I was, but secretly, I was really glad to have her company. I actually slept well that night, knowing that angels disguised as nursing assistants like Paula were watching over me. Although I still love having dinner in the dining room with my friends, I now try to pay a little bit more attention to my food. I never want to experience the feeling of choking again!"

You can listen to more stories about how nursing assistants make a difference on the CD in the back of your book.

Basic Patient and Resident Care

You may have chosen to pursue a career as a nursing assistant for many reasons, but chances are good that at least one of those reasons had to do with a desire to help and care for others. As a nursing assistant, you will have the chance to fulfill this desire many times over! In Unit 3, we will explore the skills and responsibilities that form the basis for the daily care you will provide for your patients and residents.

Photo: Taking blood pressures is a skill you will use every day.

13

The Patient or Resident Environment

What will you learn?

Have you ever moved into a new house or apartment? If so, you probably remember how strange the place felt, until you managed to get some boxes unpacked and make it your own. After you had added your own personal touch, even if it was just to hang a picture, then the place probably felt more like "home." For a person who is entering a health care facility, whether just for a few nights' stay or for the rest of his or her life, the idea of "home" takes on a whole new meaning. Suddenly, "home" may only be one room, or even half of one room, and everything that the person has always associated with "home" is gone, except for perhaps a few select items. Items that were never part of the person's home environment before, such as special beds and medical equipment, may now be present. In this chapter, we will take a closer look at the physical environment in a health care facility, and how that environment can affect a person's well-being. We will also provide an overview of the standard equipment and furniture that is typically found in a patient's or resident's room. When you are finished with this chapter, you will be able to:

1. Describe the types of rooms that are commonly found in different health care settings.
2. Discuss the Omnibus Budget Reconciliation Act (OBRA) regulations relating to the physical environment in long-term care facilities.
3. Understand your role in helping to keep the patient's or resident's environment clean and comfortable.
4. Describe the standard equipment and furniture found in a person's room in a health care facility.
5. Discuss the importance of allowing a person to have and display personal items.

Photo: Residents of long-term care facilities are encouraged to make their rooms as "home-like" as possible.

Vocabulary

Use the CD in the back of your book to hear these terms pronounced, defined, and used in a sentence:

Unit
Ventilation system
General lighting
Task lighting
Gatches
Trendelenburg's
  position

Reverse
  Trendelenburg's
  position
Over-bed table
Call light system

THE PATIENT OR RESIDENT UNIT

In Chapter 1, you learned about the many different types of health care facilities, such as hospitals, long-term care facilities, and assisted-living facilities. You also learned that some people receive health care in their homes, from home health care agencies or hospice organizations. A patient's or resident's room, also referred to as a patient's or resident's **unit,** will vary in the way it is set up according to the type of facility and the needs of the person. However, no matter what form the person's room takes—whether it is a single room, a room shared with a roommate, or an apartment-like suite of rooms—the room is considered the person's home.

HOSPITALS

Several different types of rooms are usually found within a hospital (Fig. 13-1). Most patients who are recovering from an illness or surgery will stay in double-occupancy rooms (rooms that can accommodate two people). Patients who are very ill may have private rooms in the intensive care unit (ICU) or critical care unit (CCU). These rooms contain special equipment that helps the health care team monitor and care for very ill patients. On the maternity ward, new mothers and babies may receive care before, during, and after the birthing process in a room called a birthing suite. A birthing suite is typically very home-like, with curtains, attractive furniture, and attractive cabinets that contain monitoring equipment and an entertainment center. Other special accommodations include an attached room for waiting family members, a special bed designed to make the process of labor and delivery easier, and possibly even a whirlpool bath! Some hospitals have subacute care (skilled nursing) units for patients who are not quite well enough to go home, but not quite sick enough to be in a typical hospital room. The subacute care unit is usually designed to be more home-like, and may include a common (communal) dining room and activity rooms for the patients.

All patient rooms have with some form of bathroom. However, the set-up varies according to the type of room. Usually, the bathroom is attached to the patient's room and will include a shower or bathtub, a toilet, and a sink. Some attached bathrooms may contain only a sink and a toilet, with communal bathing facilities located down the hall. The bathrooms in health care facilities usually have special features, such as handrails and a toilet that is higher than a regular toilet, to help people who may be unsteady or have limited mobility. There may also be more "open space," to accommodate a wheelchair. Finally, there will be a call light or an intercom system to ensure that a person can obtain help if necessary (Fig. 13-2).

LONG-TERM CARE FACILITIES

As you will recall, long-term care facilities provide care for people who are not able to care for themselves independently. In most cases, a person moving into a long-term care facility is making a permanent move into what is truly a new home. For most people, moving into a long-term care facility represents a major change. For example, a person who once enjoyed an apartment or home with several rooms would now have to adjust to living in a single room, possibly with a roommate. To help ease the transition, people who are moving into a long-term care facility are usually allowed to furnish their rooms with one or two favorite pieces of furniture and various personal items (Fig. 13-3).

A. Typical hospital room

C. Birthing suite

B. Intensive care unit

D. Sub-acute care unit

FIGURE 13-1

Patient rooms in the hospital vary, depending on the needs of the patient. (*A*) A typical hospital room. (*B*) A room in the intensive care unit (ICU). (*C*) A birthing suite in the maternity ward. (*D*) A room in the sub-acute care unit. (*B, Custom Medical Stock Photo; D, Ron Gould/Custom Medical Stock Photo.*)

FIGURE 13-2

Most bathrooms in health care facilities have modifications for people who have trouble with mobility. For example, the bathroom usually has handrails, an elevated toilet, or both to make it easier for a person to get up and sit down. The bathroom also has a call light or intercom system, so that a person can call for help if necessary.

Each room in a long-term care facility may have a full private bath, consisting of a shower or tub, a toilet, and a sink. Or it may have a partial bath, consisting of a toilet and a sink, that is shared between two rooms. In this case, a communal bath area, designed to accommodate the bathing of several residents at the same time, is located down the hall. Like a bathroom in a patient room, a bathroom in a resident room will have special modifications, such as handrails and a means of calling for help.

In addition to resident rooms, long-term care facilities usually have common rooms where residents gather to socialize, such as the dining room, day (or activity) rooms, and a small chapel where religious services are held. Long-term care

FIGURE 13-3
People moving into a long-term care facility are often encouraged to bring one or two favorite pieces of furniture, as well as small decorative items, to furnish their new home.

FIGURE 13-4
Residents of assisted-living facilities may have an apartment with a kitchen. (*Catrina Genovese/Index Stock Imagery, Inc.*)

FIGURE 13-5
When a person is receiving health care at home from a home health care agency, the bedroom, living room, or dining room becomes the person's "unit."

facilities may also be designed with patios and gardens to allow the residents access to outdoor activities.

ASSISTED-LIVING FACILITIES

Assisted-living facilities are a type of long-term care facility. However, the residents of assisted-living facilities are usually still somewhat independent. In some assisted-living facilities, residents live in private apartments consisting of a common area, one (or maybe even two) bedrooms, a bathroom, and possibly even a small kitchen (Fig. 13-4). In other assisted-living facilities, residents live in suites consisting of a private bedroom and bath, with communal dining and activity rooms.

HOME HEALTH CARE

Some people receive health care services in their homes. Usually in this situation, the person's bedroom, living room, or dining room becomes the patient care unit (Fig. 13-5). The home health care setting is discussed in more detail in Unit 8.

ENSURING COMFORT

Environmental conditions, such as a room's cleanliness, temperature, noise level, and quality of light, affect how we feel. Imagine what it would be like if you were confined to bed in a dirty room, or one that smelled bad or was too hot or too noisy or too dark. To enhance the comfort and well-being of patients and residents, hospitals and long-term care facilities have policies designed to regulate the environment within the health care facility. In long-term care facilities, these policies are set by Omnibus Budget Reconciliation Act (OBRA) regulations. Facilities that receive federal funding from Medicare must follow these regulations. The following aspects of the resident's environment are regulated by OBRA:

- The size of the room
- The lighting that must be available
- The temperature at which the facility must be maintained
- The measures that must be taken to maintain air quality
- The measures that must be taken to control noise
- The types of furnishings and equipment that must be present
- The types of modifications to the room that must be present to ensure safety (such as handrails and a call light or intercom system in the bathroom)
- The minimal amount of personal space for storage of belongings that each resident is allowed to have

FIGURE 13-6

Keeping the facility neat and clean is the responsibility of each member of the health care team.

CLEANLINESS

A facility's cleanliness and overall appearance is something that people who are receiving health care at the facility, as well as their family members and other visitors, notice. The appearance of the facility is a reflection on the quality of service provided. To make a good impression, a facility does not need to be new or filled with state-of-the-art equipment—but it does need to be kept clean and neat. Not only is cleanliness essential for making a good impression, it is essential for controlling the spread of infection and odors.

Each member of the health care team is responsible for keeping the facility clean (Fig. 13-6). The housekeeping or custodial staff does major, routine cleaning of the facility (such as mopping floors, emptying waste containers, and cleaning bathrooms). However, each member of the health care team also has specific duties related to maintaining cleanliness. For example, nursing assistants are responsible for changing the bed linens according to facility policy and for helping patients and residents to keep their personal belongings neat and clean. In addition, if you notice something out of place, then it is your responsibility to correct the problem. For example, if you notice something spilled on the floor or a countertop, you should wipe it up.

If you see a stray piece of trash, you should pick it up and dispose of it properly. If you notice that there is an ongoing problem, such as wastebaskets not being emptied or bathrooms not being cleaned properly, you should report this observation to the nurse, so that she can follow up with the appropriate people.

ODOR CONTROL

In a health care setting, the potential for unpleasant smells to exist is greater than under normal circumstances. The odors from vomit (emesis), wound drainage, urine, or feces can make any environment unpleasant! However, there are things you can do to help minimize odors and maintain a pleasant environment:

- Follow your facility's policy regarding the handling of waste and soiled linens.
- Keep the lids on laundry and waste receptacles closed.
- Empty and clean emesis basins, urinals, bedside commodes, and bedpans promptly.
- Use a facility-approved air freshener when appropriate.
- Assist your patients and residents with routine personal care. Clean skin and good

oral hygiene are essential for controlling odors.

- Pay attention to your own personal hygiene, especially if you are a smoker. The odors from smoking can cling to your clothes and hair and are considered unpleasant by many people. Make sure you wash your hands after smoking and use a mint or breath freshener before continuing your patient or resident care duties.

VENTILATION

A **ventilation system** provides fresh air and keeps air circulating. A well-functioning ventilation system is essential for carrying away unpleasant odors, for keeping the air from seeming stale, and for preventing rooms from feeling stuffy. However, good ventilation systems can also create drafts (chilly currents of air), especially near the circulation vents. Infants, elderly people, and people who are ill may become easily chilled and may require an extra blanket, a sweater, or a lap robe to stay warm (Fig. 13-7). Also, be sure to position chairs and beds so that

FIGURE 13-7

Although good ventilation is essential for health and comfort, elderly people, infants, and people who are ill often "catch a chill." Provide additional layers as needed, and be sure to position people away from drafts created by the ventilation system.

your patient or resident is not in a drafty area. For example, avoid placing furniture and wheelchairs right underneath a circulation vent.

ROOM TEMPERATURE

Most people prefer a room temperature that is somewhere between 68° and 74°F. However, people who are ill, elderly, or relatively inactive may prefer a warmer room temperature. OBRA regulations require the temperature in a long-term care facility to be kept between 71° and 81°F. Although this temperature may seem quite warm to you, especially when you are moving around and busy with your daily duties, remember that the temperature regulations are intended to ensure the comfort of the people you care for.

LIGHTING

There are two major types of lighting used in the health care setting: general lighting and task lighting. Usually, both lighting types are used in a single room. **General lighting** provides overall illumination (light), allowing a person to see and move about safely. Sunlight is one common source of general lighting. Usually the general light provided by an uncovered window is supplemented by light from a ceiling fixture. Many people prefer to have the drapes or blinds covering the windows in a room opened during the day, to allow natural light in. Others may prefer a darkened room, or to illuminate the room with light from a ceiling fixture instead of sunlight. You should ask each of your patients or residents what he or she prefers, and act accordingly (Fig. 13-8).

Task lighting directs bright light toward a specific area. In a patient or resident room, task lighting is usually provided by a fixture mounted over the head of the bed. Some of these fixtures provide both general and task lighting with dual switches. The patient or resident may use task lighting for activities that require good light to prevent eyestrain, such as reading, needlework, or doing a crossword puzzle. You would use task lighting when providing patient or resident care, so that you could see clearly while carrying out the procedure. The focused illumination provided by task lighting also helps you to notice changes

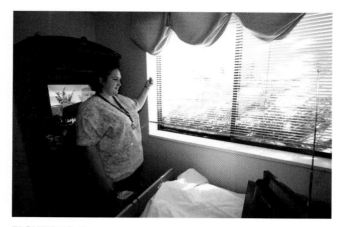

FIGURE 13-8

Some people prefer to have the blinds or drapes opened during the day to let in the sunlight. Others prefer a darkened room and will want to have the blinds or drapes drawn. Always ask the patient or resident about his or her preference.

that should be reported to the nurse. For example, you may notice a change in a person's skin tone or a strange new rash that might otherwise go unnoticed.

NOISE CONTROL

Health care facilities can be such busy, noisy places! Imagine that you are a patient on a typical floor in a hospital. It is about 11:30 in the morning, and there is a lot of activity. The telephone is ringing at the nurse's station. Here comes the man with the cart carrying the food trays up from the kitchen. You know he is coming because his cart has a squeaky wheel. A nurse and a nursing assistant are having a conversation in the hallway about what needs to be done that afternoon. A patient down the hall, who is a little bit hard of hearing, has the volume turned all the way up on his television set. He is watching a talk show, and every once in awhile, you can hear the audience clapping. Several visitors are going down the hallway to visit a friend who is recovering from surgery, and they are laughing and talking as they go. A radio is playing somewhere. You are not feeling very well, and you wonder if things will ever quiet down enough for you to get some rest!

Although a certain level of noise in a busy place is to be expected, too much noise can affect the level of comfort of patients and residents. Many hospitals and long-term care facilities are built with materials that help to contain and

minimize noise, such as noise-absorbing ceiling tiles and carpeting. In addition, members of the health care team must do their part to keep the noise level to a minimum. For example, answering phones promptly, reporting noisy equipment that needs to be oiled or adjusted, and being aware of the volume of your own voice are all things you can do to help control the noise level in the facility where you work. OBRA regulations require long-term facilities to take measures to control noise.

FURNITURE AND EQUIPMENT

The furniture and equipment that is considered "standard" for a patient's or resident's room will differ according to the facility and to the specific needs of the patient or resident. To ensure your own safety, as well as that of your patients or residents, you must make sure that you know how to operate and adjust any furniture and equipment that is considered standard in the facility where you work. The furniture and equipment described in this section would be considered standard for a typical room in a hospital or a long-term care facility. In a facility that offers specialized care (for example, a burn unit or rehabilitation center), items considered standard might vary from this list.

BEDS

An adjustable bed, commonly referred to as a *hospital bed,* is used in most health care settings (Fig. 13-9). The frame of an adjustable bed can be raised or lowered, moving the entire bed either further away from, or closer to, the floor. This helps health care workers maintain good body mechanics when performing care procedures. It also helps the patient or resident to get into or out of the bed. The mattress platform on an adjustable bed can also be positioned in a variety of ways to keep the patient or resident comfortable. Sometimes, the doctor will order a specific mattress position for a patient or resident.

The mattress platforms of most adjustable beds have joints at the hips and knees, which allow the mattress to "break." These joints are called **gatches,** after Willis Gatch, the surgeon who developed the first bed that was adjustable at the hips and knees. The hip gatch raises the person's upper

A. The bed can be moved up or down in terms of distance from the floor.

Trendelenburg's position

Reverse Trendelenburg's position

45°

Hip gatch

Knee gatch

Fowler's position

B. The mattress can be adjusted to assist with positioning of the patient or resident.

FIGURE 13-9

Most beds used in health care settings are adjustable, both in terms of (A) their height from the floor and (B) the position of the mattress.

body to a semi-sitting position (Fowler's position; see also Chapter 11). The knee gatch raises the person's knees to help prevent the person from sliding toward the end of the bed while in the Fowler's position. In addition to having hip and knee gatches, most adjustable beds permit the mattress to be "tilted" without bending the person at the waist. In **Trendelenburg's position,** the foot of the mattress is raised so that the person's head is lower than her feet. Trendelenburg's position is sometimes used for a person who has gone into shock and has a very low blood pressure, to encourage blood flow

to the heart. In the **reverse Trendelenburg's position,** the head of the mattress is raised so the person's head is higher than her feet. The reverse Trendelenburg's position is useful for people who are recovering from spinal cord injury or back surgery, or who are in traction.

Adjustable beds are adjusted either electrically, using control buttons located on or near the side rails, or manually, using a system of cranks located at the foot of the bed (Fig. 13-10). One advantage of electrically operated beds is that the control buttons are located in a place that is

Raises/lowers head of bed

Moves bed closer to\further away from floor

Raises/lowers foot of bed

A.

Raises/lowers head of bed

Moves bed closer to/further away from floor

Raises/lowers foot of bed

B.

FIGURE 13-10

Adjustable beds may be adjusted electrically (*A*) or by hand (*B*).

accessible to the patient or resident, as well as to members of the health care team. When using an electrically operated bed, remember that it is a piece of electrical equipment. Appropriate safety precautions should be taken when operating it to avoid electrical shock (see Chapter 9). When using a manually operated bed, remember to fold the cranks down and away under the bed after you are finished using them, so that people who are walking near the foot of the bed do not bump into them.

In addition to being adjustable, adjustable beds usually have two other features that regular beds do not—side rails and wheels (casters). The side rails on a bed are raised to help prevent a person from falling out of the bed. Always remember, however, that side rails can be considered a form of restraint, and should only be used according to your facility's policies and the person's individual care plan. Some of your patients or residents may want to have one of the side rails raised, so that they can use it as an assistive device for repositioning. The patient or resident can grab the side rail and use it to reposition himself in bed or to get up.

Wheels make the bed easier to move from place to place, which is sometimes necessary when a person needs to be moved from one part of the facility to another without leaving his or her bed. Wheels are also useful when it is necessary to move the bed to clean underneath it. The wheels have locking

devices that are used to keep the bed steady and prevent it from rolling. Always make sure the bed's wheels are locked, unless you are moving it (Fig. 13-11)! A person could be injured while getting into or out of the bed if the bed shifts out from

FIGURE 13-11

Wheel locks help to prevent unintentional movement of the bed. There are different types of wheel locks. In the type shown here, the red pedal locks the wheel, and the green pedal unlocks it.

underneath him. Additionally, you may be injured if the bed suddenly shifts away from you while you are providing care to a patient or resident.

In some cases, you may care for a person who is in a regular bed, instead of an adjustable bed. For example, some assisted-living and long-term care facilities allow people to bring their own beds from home, if they prefer. Also, a person who is being cared for in her home may not have an adjustable bed. When you are caring for a person in a regular bed, you can use blocks to elevate the head of the bed. Positioning devices, such as pillows shaped to support a person in a sitting position, are available to help achieve the other positions.

CHAIRS

A person's room should be furnished with one or two chairs that are comfortable for the person and will accommodate any visitors. Some people with disabilities require special chairs, such as geri-chairs, wheelchairs, or chairs with special lifting devices that help the person to get in and out of the chair easily. A person who is recovering from hip or spinal surgery may need a chair that has firm upholstery, a straight back, and no armrests. Many residents of long-term care facilities will bring a favorite chair or two from home. These chairs may recline or have a rocking action that the person finds very comfortable.

OVER-BED TABLES

Most health care facilities furnish patient and resident rooms with **over-bed tables,** which fit over the bed or a chair and can be raised or lowered as needed. You will use the over-bed table to hold basins and other articles when carrying out personal care for a patient or resident (Fig. 13-12). The patient or resident may use the over-bed table as a surface for writing a letter, or for eating a meal or snack. When kept in easy reach of the person, the over-bed table is an excellent place to keep a water pitcher or any other items the person may want close by. Because the over-bed table is considered a "clean" area, items placed there should be either sterile or clean. One way to help remember this is to consider the over-bed table the person's dining room table—you would never place dirty items, such as bedpans or soiled linens, there.

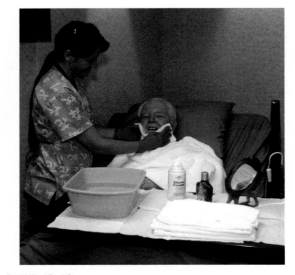

FIGURE 13-12

Over-bed tables are used when performing personal care. Here, the over-bed table holds shaving supplies.

STORAGE UNITS

Various types of bedside tables are used to furnish the patient's or resident's room. Many of these bedside tables have drawers or a combination of drawers and closed shelves that are used to store personal care items. The person's toothpaste and toothbrush, lotion, soap, deodorant, and other personal hygiene items are usually stored in the top drawer, whereas basins, bedpans, and other care equipment are stored neatly underneath in the lower drawers or shelves. The telephone, a flower arrangement, and other personal items may be placed on top of the bedside table (Fig. 13-13).

Additional storage for a person's personal items may be provided in the form of a closet, a wardrobe, or a chest of drawers. OBRA regulations require long-term care facilities to provide each resident with enough storage space for his or her clothing and other personal items. The resident must have free access to this storage space and the items it contains. Because the resident's closet, wardrobe, or chest of drawers is considered private, personal property, you must have the person's permission to remove items from it (Fig. 13-14).

Occasionally, you will need to inspect a resident's personal storage area. For example, you may suspect that a resident is keeping something in the storage area that is not permitted, such as food. Food can spoil and may attract insects and rodents. In this situation, you would be permitted to inspect the personal storage space, but first

FIGURE 13-13

Personal care items are usually stored in the bedside table.

FIGURE 13-14

The resident's closet is considered private, personal property.

you must inform the resident of your intent to do so, and the search must be conducted in the resident's presence. If you must carry out an inspection of a resident's personal storage space, it may be a good idea to have another staff member present during the inspection to verify that you acted appropriately and within the regulations.

CALL LIGHT AND INTERCOM SYSTEMS

Patients and residents must have a way of communicating with the health care staff at all times. Most health care facilities have a **call light system,** which patients or residents can use to alert a staff member that they need help. Many also have an intercom system, which allows staff members to speak to a patient or resident in his room from the nurses' station.

A call light system consists of a call light control (usually either a cord that is pulled or a hand-held button device), a light in the hall (over the doorway of the patient's or resident's room), and a panel of lights at the nurses' station or some other central location. When the person pulls the cord or pushes the button on the call light control, the light over the doorway blinks and the light on the panel at the nurses' station lights, alerting the staff that the person needs help. A staff member who is at the nurses' station

could then use the intercom system to communicate with the patient or resident before going to the person's room (Fig. 13-15).

The call light control must always be within a person's reach, whether the person is in the bed or in a chair. An unconscious or comatose person will be unable to call for help and should be checked on very frequently. It is also important to note that a person who is hearing impaired will have difficulty communicating with an intercom system. The person simply will not be able to understand what you are saying, so remember to respond in person to a hearing-impaired person's calls. Answer all requests for assistance promptly, even though it can be frustrating to respond to numerous, seemingly silly requests from any particular person, especially when you are very busy. Sometimes people who use the call light system excessively are feeling scared and lonely. What they are really seeking is reassurance that if a problem actually does occur, someone will come quickly to their aid. Part of helping to meet a person's safety and security needs is your quick response to a request for help.

PRIVACY CURTAINS AND ROOM DIVIDERS

Each patient or resident unit will have privacy curtains (which are usually hung from the ceiling) or room dividers. The privacy curtain should be

A. Call light control

C. Intercom system

B. Panel of lights at the nurses' station

FIGURE 13-15

Most health care facilities use a call light system along with an intercom system to allow communication between patients or residents and the members of the health care team. (*A*) The call light control may be a cord that is pulled or a hand-held button device. (*B*) Pulling the cord or pushing the button turns on a light in the hallway over the doorway to the person's room (not shown). It also turns on a light on the panel at the nurses' station. (*C*) A nurse or nursing assistant can use the intercom system at the nurses' station to communicate with the patient or resident before going to the room.

closed, or a room divider used, when you are providing care for your patients or residents. The door to the room should also be closed, as the privacy curtains do little to keep voices and other sounds private. OBRA regulations require long-term care facilities to use privacy curtains or room dividers to protect the privacy of each resident.

OTHER EQUIPMENT

Depending on the type of facility and the purpose of the room, other equipment may be present. For example, many rooms have hanging intravenous (IV) poles and outlets for oxygen and suction devices. The Occupational Safety and Health Administration (OSHA) requires personal protective equipment (PPE), such as gloves, and disposal equipment, such as sharps containers, to be kept in every patient or resident care area for your use. Therefore, the room may be equipped with a wall-mounted sharps disposal box and a wall-mounted box of disposable gloves.

PERSONAL ITEMS

When a person enters a health care facility, he may bring personal items along to add a "touch of home." Usually the number and type of personal items depends on whether the stay at the health care facility is temporary or permanent. For example, a person entering the hospital for a brief stay may just bring along a favorite photograph or a religious item. A person who is moving into a long-term care facility may bring along furniture and larger decorative items.

Many residents in long-term care facilities bring their own bedspreads or comforters to make up the standard facility bed. They may have their own clothing, jewelry, books, and favorite wall hangings. Some residents bring a television, a stereo, or even a personal computer to their new home, and many have a private telephone line installed in their rooms so that they can keep in touch with loved ones and friends. You may see plants, drawings from grandchildren, and maybe even a small pet, such as a bird or a fish, in your residents' rooms!

OBRA states that a resident's unit must be safe, clean, orderly, and free from obstacles where people must walk. You should help your residents to decorate their rooms according to their own individual taste and preference, while making sure that they stay within the safety standards established by OBRA and your facility. You must respect a person's personal items as if they belonged to you. Remember that even a small scrap of paper can be very precious to a resident, especially if it is a note from someone the person loves. While you may consider a resident's personal things quite a bit of clutter, especially if you have to help keep them neat, just remember that each one of those items represents a piece of that person's life. When you show respect for, and take an interest in, a patient's or resident's personal belongings, you are letting the person know that you truly care for him or her.

 ### Tell the Nurse!

You are responsible for making sure that the patient's or resident's room is home-like, clean, and safe. Report the following situations to a nurse immediately:

◉➡ You notice that a piece of equipment or furniture in the room is not working properly

◉➡ A patient or resident has been injured by a piece of equipment or furniture in the room

◉➡ You have been injured by a piece of equipment or furniture in the room

◉➡ You suspect that a patient or resident is storing unwrapped food in a drawer or closet area

◉➡ A patient or resident, or one of his family members, complains that personal items are missing from the room

◉➡ You accidentally break a personal item belonging to a patient or resident

◉➡ Bathroom fixtures and floors do not appear to be properly cleaned or wastebaskets are not emptied

◉➡ There is an odor in the room that cannot be eliminated

SUMMARY

▶ Patient or resident rooms in a health care facility will vary according to the purpose of the facility and the needs of the person being cared for in the room.
- A patient room in a hospital is a person's temporary home.
- A resident room in a long-term care or assisted-living facility usually becomes a person's permanent home.

▶ The physical environment of a health care facility contributes to a person's overall comfort, health, and well-being. Long-term care facilities that receive federal funding must follow Omnibus Budget Reconciliation Act (OBRA) regulations concerning the physical environment of the resident's room.
- Many people judge a facility according to its level of cleanliness. In addition, a clean environment is essential for odor and infection control.
  - Providing a clean and comfortable environment for patients and residents is a responsibility of all members of the health care team.
  - Nursing assistants are responsible for helping patients and residents keep their rooms neat and clean.
- Odor control is achieved by promptly removing and cleaning dirty emesis basins, urinals, bedpans, and linens. Assisting patients and residents with bathing and brushing their teeth also helps to prevent odors.
- Good ventilation helps carry away unpleasant odors and prevents stale air. However, it is important to protect your patients and

residents from becoming chilled as a result of the drafts created by the ventilation system.

■ The temperature of a patient's or resident's room should be maintained between 71° and 81°F.

■ Adequate light must be provided for all activities that take place in a person's room.
  • General lighting, such as that provided by sunlight or an overhead ceiling fixture, provides overall illumination.
  • Task lighting focuses bright light on one particular area.

■ Too much noise interferes with a person's ability to rest.

▶ Most patient and resident rooms contain the same basic furniture and equipment.

■ All patient or resident rooms contain a bed. In most cases, the bed will be an electrically or manually operated adjustable bed.

■ All patient or resident rooms contain at least one chair, to accommodate a visitor and to provide a "change of scenery" for the patient or resident. Many residents in long-term care facilities bring a favorite chair from home to furnish their rooms.

■ Over-bed tables fit over a person's bed to provide a work surface for both the patient or resident and the health care worker. The over-bed table is considered a "clean" area.

■ Personal care items, such as toiletries, are usually stored in the bedside table.

■ In long-term care facilities, a closet, wardrobe, or chest of drawers is used to provide private storage space for the resident's personal belongings.

■ Call light and intercom systems are used for communication.
  • The call light system allows patients or residents to signal that they need help.
  • The intercom system allows members of the health care team to communicate with patients or residents without leaving the nurses' station.

■ Privacy curtains or room dividers are used to help maintain a resident's or patient's privacy when care is being given.

▶ People entering a health care facility may want to bring personal items to add a "touch of home." Always show as much care for a person's personal items as you would for your own most treasured belongings.

What did you learn?

Multiple choice

Select the single best answer for each of the following questions.

1. How should a resident's room look?
   a. Functional and sparsely decorated
   b. Like a hospital room
   c. As home-like as possible
   d. Like a hotel room

2. You show respect to a patient or resident when you:
   a. Knock before entering his or her room
   b. Close the door and pull the privacy curtain when you are providing care
   c. Handle the person's personal belongings with care
   d. All of the above

3. The nurse tells you that Mr. Haskill's bedside table is looking a little bit disorderly, and asks you to clean it up a bit. You should:
   a. Search the shelves for hidden food and throw anything that you find away
   b. Remove the bedpan and washbasin, because these items do not belong there
   c. Straighten the items on the top of the table and on the shelves, removing any dirty items so that they can be cleaned and returned
   d. All of the above

4. Which regulations state that a resident's unit must be clean, safe, orderly, and free of obstacles in the pathway?
   a. Occupational Safety and Health Administration (OSHA) regulations
   b. Omnibus Budget Reconciliation Act (OBRA) regulations
   c. Medicare regulations
   d. Medicaid regulations

5. One of your patients has had back surgery, and the nurse asks you to position his bed so that the head of the bed is elevated. The patient's body needs to remain flat against the mattress. What position would the nurse tell you to put the patient in?
   a. Reverse Trendelenburg's position
   b. Fowler's position
   c. Prone position
   d. Trendelenburg's position

6. Each member of the health care team has specific duties related to maintaining a clean patient or resident environment. You have noticed that your residents' bathrooms have been less well-kept than usual lately. The sinks are not being cleaned thoroughly, and sometimes the wastebaskets are not emptied. Who has fallen down on the job?
   a. The residents—routine upkeep of the bathroom is their responsibility
   b. You—routine upkeep of the bathroom is your responsibility
   c. The housekeeping staff—routine upkeep of the bathroom is their responsibility
   d. The nurse—routine upkeep of the bathroom is her responsibility

7. How can you help to control unpleasant odors in the workplace?
   a. Empty emesis basins promptly
   b. Assist your patients or residents with skin care and oral hygiene
   c. Use facility-approved air fresheners as necessary
   d. All of the above

Matching

Match each numbered item with its appropriate lettered description.

_____ **1.** Side rails

_____ **2.** Patient or resident unit

_____ **3.** Over-bed table

a. The patient's or resident's pitcher and meal trays may be placed here

b. The space where a patient or resident lives in a health care facility

c. Used to prevent a person from falling out of bed, and as an assistive device; may also be considered a form of restraint

---

? Stop and think!

▶ You've been assigned to take care of Mr. Knutson, who is 101 years old. He is pretty independent, considering his age. When you enter Mr. Knutson's room to assist him with his morning routine, you notice that he has left his full bedpan on the bedside table next to his water glass and pitcher. What should you do? What would you say to Mr. Knutson?

▶ You have been assigned to straighten up Mr. Grant's room. Mr. Grant can be difficult, especially when he feels that his "personal space" is being invaded. You enter his room and explain to him that you are going to straighten up and dust. He immediately says, "Get out of here, and leave me alone. I don't need your help." What should you do?

14

Admissions, Transfers, and Discharges

What will you learn?

Checking people into and out of a health care facility is a routine, daily occurrence in many health care settings. Routine, that is, unless you are the person being admitted ("checked in"), discharged ("checked out"), or transferred (moved from one room in the facility to another, or moved to another facility altogether). All of these events cause a major change to the patient's or resident's daily routine and normal lifestyle. For many people, this is very upsetting. In this chapter, you will learn how admissions, transfers, and discharges are carried out. You will also learn about things you can do to help make these times of change easier for your patients or residents. When you are finished with this chapter, you will be able to:

1. Explain why admission to a health care facility may be emotionally difficult for a person and his or her family members.
2. Discuss how the nursing assistant can help to make a person's admission into a health care facility a more pleasant experience.
3. List the duties of the nursing assistant during the admission process.
4. Describe some of the reasons a person in a health care facility might need to be moved to another room, or to another facility.
5. Describe a nursing assistant's duties when assisting with the transfer of a patient or resident.
6. Discuss the purpose of discharge planning.
7. Describe a nursing assistant's duties during the discharge process.

Photo: A new resident arrives at a long-term care facility.

Vocabulary

Use the CD in the back of your book to hear these terms pronounced, defined, and used in a sentence:

Admission
Admission sheet
Nursing history
Resident inventory
　sheet

Transfer
Discharge
Against medical advice
　(AMA)
Discharge planning

ADMISSIONS

An **admission** is the official entry of a person into a health care setting. A person who needs health care must be formally admitted to the health care facility that will be providing the care, whether the length of the stay is:

- A few hours (for example, a person entering an outpatient surgical unit for same-day surgery)
- A few days or weeks (for example, a person entering a hospital to receive treatment for a complication of diabetes)
- A few months, or
- The rest of the person's life (for example, a person entering a long-term care facility because of advanced Alzheimer's disease)

In the case of a home health care agency, the health care setting is the client's home, but there may still be an admissions process. This is because admission is a time of orientation, for both the new patient, resident, or client and the health care team. During the admissions process, the patient, resident, or client is informed of her rights and the policies of the facility or agency, and introduced to the people who will be caring for her. At the same time, the members of the health care team are introduced to the person and her family, and the process of gathering the information that the health care team needs to care for the person properly begins.

Although the members of the health care team may regard the process of admitting a person to the facility as a normal, uneventful occurrence, to the person being admitted, the occurrence is very eventful. A person being admitted for health care services must take on a new role—that of a patient, resident, or client. Taking on this new role can be very traumatic because most people are used to thinking of themselves as independent, unique individuals, not as dependent people in need of the services of the health care industry. The person may feel a loss of identity, as the illness or condition takes "center stage," causing all of the other qualities that make the person unique to fade into the background. This is why the members of the health care team must always make an effort to treat each new patient or resident as if he is a guest in the facility. Make the person feel welcome, not like he is just another body to wash. Ask the person how he prefers to be addressed. This helps maintain the person's sense of identity and individuality. Never refer to a patient or resident as "the gallbladder in room 212." If you cannot remember the person's name, at least say "the person in room 212 who has gallbladder problems."

In addition to feeling stressed by the need to adjust to a new role, a person who is being admitted to a health care facility (and the person's family members) may also be feeling fear and anxiety about the future. For example, a person who is entering a long-term care facility may worry that she will not like her new home, and she may be sad about giving up her old one. In many cases, admission to a long-term care facility is as traumatic for family members as it is for the resident herself. A person who is being admitted to the hospital may worry that diagnostic tests will reveal bad news, or that a surgery will not be successful, and it is likely that his family members will share these worries. Even if the reason for the admission to a health care facility is joyous (for example, to deliver a baby), there may still be some lingering fear and anxiety (for example, about what labor and delivery will actually be like, or whether the baby will be healthy). The health care setting itself may be frightening. Imagine how you would feel if you were entering an environment filled with strangers asking personal questions about your life and poking and prodding your body with strange equipment. One way to help ease the fear and anxiety felt by patients, residents, and their family members is to include the family members in the admission process. Make sure that family members know that their presence is welcome, and their support of the patient or resident is beneficial (Fig. 14-1).

FIGURE 14-1

Being admitted to a health care facility is often stressful for the patient or resident, as well as his or her family members. Involving family members in the admissions process can help to put everyone at ease.

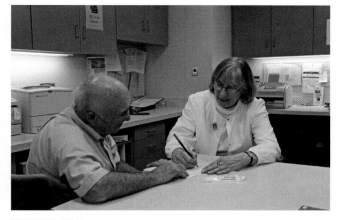

FIGURE 14-2

The admissions clerk or nurse helps the patient or resident to fill out the admissions sheet.

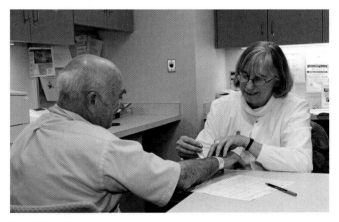

FIGURE 14-3

Each patient receives an identification bracelet in the admissions office.

THE ADMISSIONS PROCESS

Because the admission process is an emotional time for the patient or resident and his family members, you must focus on the person and his needs, as well as on the process and the paperwork. Most admissions follow a process established by the health care facility:

1. The admissions process usually begins in a doctor's office, unless the admission is caused by an emergency. In the case of an emergency, the person may arrive at the health care facility without seeing her doctor first. Normally, however, the admission process begins when a doctor writes orders regarding the specific needs of the person. These orders usually include the doctor's diagnosis of the person's condition, and specify dietary orders, activity status, medications, diagnostic tests, and the type of room required by the person.

2. On arrival at the health care facility, the person first goes to the admissions office, where she meets with an admission clerk or a nurse who is responsible for admissions. The health care team member who is handling the admission will help the person to complete an **admission sheet,** which gathers standard information about the person, such as her name, address, date of birth and age, social security number, gender, insurance and employment information, emergency

notification information, and advance directive information (Fig. 14-2). The admission clerk or nurse will also have the person sign a consent form giving the facility permission to treat the person's medical condition. When the admissions paperwork is completed, the admissions clerk or nurse will provide the patient or resident with a way of being identified. In a hospital, an identification bracelet will be issued (Fig. 14-3). In a long-term care facility, a photograph of the person will be taken for identification purposes.

3. After completing the admissions paperwork, the person will be escorted to her room by the admissions clerk or nurse, a volunteer, or a nursing assistant.

Depending on the situation, the person may be able to walk to her room, or she may be taken there in a wheelchair or on a stretcher.

4. A nursing assistant is usually responsible for helping the person to unpack and settle in, and for taking and recording the person's vital signs, height, and weight. If you work in a hospital, you may need to help the person change into a hospital gown or pajamas. Make sure that the person is comfortable by helping her into bed or a chair. Next, a nurse will come to the patient's or resident's room to complete the **nursing history.** As you will remember from Chapter 5, the nursing history is used to gather information about the person's preferences, abilities, disabilities, and habits (Fig. 14-4). The nurse completes this document by interviewing the patient or resident (or, in some cases, a family member of the patient or resident).

TACTICS FOR MAKING A NEW PATIENT OR RESIDENT FEEL WELCOME

When a new patient is being admitted to a hospital, the admissions staff will usually notify the nursing staff as soon as the person arrives in the admissions office. This gives the nursing team time to prepare for the person's arrival. When a person is being admitted to a long-term care facility, the nursing staff typically has a few days' advance notice of the new arrival. As a member of the nursing team, you will play a very important role in making sure that the person feels expected and welcomed when he arrives at the health care facility. A good first impression can go a long way toward easing a person's anxiety, especially if one of the things the person is anxious about is the quality of care that he will be receiving while staying at your facility. As a nursing assistant, you will use the following tactics to make sure that the admission goes as smoothly as possible.

Prepare the Person's Room in Advance of His or Her Arrival

Ask the nurse about any special requirements that your new patient or resident may have. Does the person use a walker or some other ambulation device, or will he be arriving in a wheelchair or on a stretcher? If so, you will want to check the placement of the furniture in the room and move it as necessary to ensure easy entry into the room. If necessary, adjust the lighting and temperature of the room. Open the blinds or drapes and prepare the bed by turning the sheets back, lowering the bed to the lowest position, and making sure the wheels are locked (see Chapter 15). If the person is arriving by stretcher, you would prepare the bed in a slightly different manner (also described in Chapter 15).

Gather the equipment you will need for taking and recording the person's vital signs (see Chapter 16). Make sure any other equipment needed by the incoming patient or resident, such as oxygen tubing, a suctioning device, or an intravenous (IV) pole, is in the room before the person arrives. If your facility provides them, obtain an admissions pack for the person. A typical admissions pack would consist of a basin, a water pitcher, a drinking cup, a package of tissues, and assorted personal care items (such as toothpaste, soap, and shampoo). Preparing the room in a thoughtful manner indicates to the new patient or resident that his arrival was anticipated and planned for (Fig. 14-5).

Greet the Person Warmly and Introduce Yourself

When you meet the person and his family members for the first time, be sure to introduce yourself. Give your title and explain how you will be involved in the care of the person. A warm, courteous, professional greeting helps to put people at ease and gives them confidence that they will be well taken care of by the health care team.

Help the Person Settle into His or Her New Home

Always take the time to give a new patient or resident a "tour" of the room (Fig. 14-6). Point out the location of the bathroom. Show the person how to use the call light control, how to adjust the bed, how to adjust the lights, and how to operate any other appliances or pieces of equipment in the room. For example, in a hospital setting, you may need to show the person how to get an outside line on the telephone, or how to turn the television on and off and adjust the volume.

Admission Database

CURRENT MEDICATIONS, SUPPLEMENTS, NON-PRESCRIPTION DRUGS:

NAME	DOSE/FREQUENCY	LAST DOSE
Aspirin	2 prn	1 month
Maalox	prn	this Am

☐ MEDICATION TO PHARMACY ☐ MEDICATION SENT HOME

ALLERGEN: (DRUGS, FOOD, TAPES, DYES, OTHERS)

ALLERGEN	SYMPTOMS
Penicillin	rash

DATE __1-16-00__ TIME __0900__

ADMISSION ☐ OBSERVATION

☒ AMBULATORY ☐ WHEELCHAIR ☐ STRETCHER
☐ CORRECT IDENTIFICATION BAND
ADMITTED FROM: ☒ HOME ☐ NURSING FACILITY
　　　　　 ☐ EMERGENCY ROOM ☐ OTHER_____
INFORMATION GIVEN BY: ☐ FAMILY MEMBER ☐ FRIEND ☒ PATIENT
　☐ UNABLE TO TAKE HISTORY · PATIENT UNRESPONSIVE/CONFUSED;
　　NOT ACCOMPANIED BY FAMILY OR FRIEND
　☐ PREVIOUS MEDICAL RECORD

ORIENTATION TO ROOM
☒ VISITING HOURS ☒ CALL LIGHT IN REACH: ☒ EXPLAINED
☒ OPERATION OF BED AND SIDE RAILS ☒ USE OF PHONE
☒ VALUABLES SENT HOME ☐ IN SAFE ☐ IN POSSESSION
　SPECIFY _____
☒ PATIENT HANDBOOK ☒ INTRODUCED TO ROOMMATE

LEGAL GUARDIAN (NAME/PHONE)_____
CONTACT PERSON (NAME/PHONE) __Mrs. Solle, 335-4001__
PHYSICIAN NOTIFIED __✓__ TIME __0830__
PRIMARY CARE PHYSICIAN __Dr. Wills__

MEDICAL HISTORY
ADMITTED MEDICAL DIAGNOSIS __Peptic Ulcer__

PAST HOSPITALIZATIONS AND/OR ILLNESS: (MEDICAL, SURGICAL, EMOTIONAL PROBLEMS) __1986 - Appendectomy__

WHAT IS REASON FOR ADMISSION? (PATIENT'S OWN WORDS)_____
"My doctor says I have An ulcer"

*SUBJECTIVE DATA:

1. HEALTH PERCEPTIONS/HEALTH MANAGEMENT PATTERN
GENERAL HEALTH __Excellent__
USE OF: ☐ TOBACCO: HOW MUCH/HOW LONG? __No__
　　　 ☐ ALCOHOL: HOW MUCH/HOW LONG? __No__
　　　 ☐ OTHER DRUGS TYPE(s) __None__

2. NUTRITIONAL/METABOLIC PATTERN
DIET/RESTRICTIONS/SUPPLEMENTS: __Regular diet__

☐ INSTRUCTED IN DIET PREVIOUSLY BY:_____
TIME OF LAST P.O. INTAKE: __0700__
FLUID INTAKE (AMOUNT/DAY) __5-6 glasses__
WEIGHT: ☐ NO PROBLEMS_____
☐ GAIN_____ ☒ LOSS/HOW MUCH/HOW LONG __10 lbs__ | __1 month__
☒ SKIN NORMAL ☐ HEALING PROBLEMS
　☐ COLOR CHANGE OF SKIN
　☐ SKIN LESIONS/RASH_____

3. RESPIRATION/CIRCULATION PATTERN
HISTORY OF: ☐ COUGH ☐ SPUTUM _____
☐ SHORTNESS OF BREATH ☐ WITHOUT EXERCISE ☐ WITH EXERCISE

HISTORY OF: ☐ PACEMAKER ☐ RATE_____
　　　 ☐ BLOOD CLOTS ☐ CHEST PAIN ☐ PEDAL EDEMA

☒ CHECK BOX IF DATA IS PERTINENT
*SEE NURSES NOTES FOR FURTHER NOTATIONS OR ANY CHANGES.

*OBJECTIVE DATA:

1. CLINICAL DATA
AGE __36__ HEIGHT __5'6"__
WEIGHT __122__ ☒ BEDSCALE ☐ STANDING APPROXIMATE_____
TEMP: __98.4__ PULSE: __118__ RESPIRATIONS __16__
BLOOD PRESSURE (RIGHT ARM) __120/68__ (LEFT ARM) __122/70__
　　　　　 ☒ SITTING ☐ LYING
N.T./N.A. INITIALS __O.B.__

2. NUTRITIONAL/METABOLIC PATTERN
ORAL MUCOSA: ☒ HEALTHY COLOR_____
　☐ MOIST ☐ DRY ☐ LESIONS_____
TEETH: ☒ NO PROBLEM CONDITION:_____
　☐ DENTURES ☐ UPPER ☐ LOWER ☐ PARTIAL
　☐ MISSING TEETH ☐ CAPS/CROWNS
☒ WELL NOURISHED ☐ OBESE ☐ EMACIATED
SKIN: ☒ TURGOR NORMAL ☐ OTHER_____
　☒ INTACT ☐ OTHER _____
　TEMP __warm__ COLOR __brown__ ☐ DIAPHORESIS
☐ TUBES _____

3. RESPIRATION/CIRCULATION PATTERN
BREATH SOUNDS __Clear__
LIP COLOR __pink__ ☐ USE OF ACCESSORY MUSCLES
COUGH: ☐ NON-PRODUCTIVE ☐ PRODUCTIVE SPUTUM COLOR_____
APICAL RATE __120__ RHYTHM: ☒ REGULAR ☐ IRREGULAR
ABNORMAL HEART SOUNDS NOTED __No__
NECK VEIN DISTENTION AT 45 DEGREES: ☐ PRESENT ☒ ABSENT
☐ EDEMA: LOCATION _____
RIGHT DORSALIS PEDAL PULSE: ☒ STRONG ☐ WEAK ☐ ABSENT
LEFT DORSALIS PEDAL PULSE: ☒ STRONG ☐ WEAK ☐ ABSENT
CALF TENDERNESS ☒ NO ☐ YES ☐ N/A
EXTREMITIES COLOR __brown__
　　　TEMP __warm__

4. ELIMINATION PATTERN
ABDOMEN: ☒ SOFT ☐ FIRM
　　　 ☐ NON-TENDER ☐ TENDER
　　　 ☐ NON-DISTENDED ☐ DISTENDED _____ Girth
☐ OSTOMIES/TUBES: TYPE _____
☐ NORMAL BOWEL SOUNDS ☐ HYPOACTIVE ☒ HYPERACTIVE ☐ ABSENT

(continued)

FIGURE 14-4

The nursing history is used to gather information about the person's preferences, abilities, disabilities, and habits. The nurse completes the nursing history. (*Courtesy of Southeast Missouri Hospital, Cape Girardeau, Missouri.*)

Admission Database *(continued)*

*SUBJECTIVE DATA (Cont'd) LBM_____

4. ELIMINATION PATTERN

BOWEL HABITS: STOOLS/DAY **2** COLOR **dk. brown** ☒ SOFT/FORMED

☐ CONSTIPATION: ☐ LAXATIVE ☐ ENEMA

☐ DIARRHEA ☐ INCONTINENCE

BLADDER HABITS: URINATES/DAY **5-6** ☒ NO PROBLEM ☐ SELF-CATH

☐ URGENCY ☐ FREQUENCY ☐ NOCTURIA

☐ DYSURIA ☐ HEMATURIA ☐ INCONTINENCE

5. SEXUALITY/REPRODUCTIVE PATTERN (IF APPROPRIATE)

LAST MENSTRUAL PERIOD **1-10-00** MENSTRUAL PROBLEMS ☐ YES ☒ N/A

BIRTH CONTROL MEASURES **None** # PREGNANCIES **2**

COMPLICATIONS OF PREGNANCIES **None**

HX VENEREAL DISEASE **No**

SEXUAL CONCERNS: **None**

6. ACTIVITY/EXERCISE PATTERN

ENERGY LEVEL: ☐ TIRES EASILY ☐ AVERAGE ☒ HIGH/ENERGY

ABLE TO: ☒ FEED SELF ☒ BATHE SELF

☐ BATHE/FEED SELF WITH ASSISTANCE

☒ AMBULATE ☒ CLIMB STAIRS !

☒ CAN DO HOUSEHOLD CHORES

AIDS: ☐ CANE ☐ WALKER ☐ WHEELCHAIR ☐ OTHER _____

GAIT: ☐ STEADY ☐ UNSTEADY ☐ LIMP ☐ UNABLE TO WALK

PROTHESIS _____

7. SLEEP/REST PATTERN

DO YOU FEEL RESTED AFTER SLEEP? ☒ YES ☐ NO ☐ NO PROBLEM

SLEEP PROBLEMS: ☐ TROUBLE FALLING ASLEEP ☐ EARLY AM WAKING

☐ OTHER _____

8. COGNITIVE/PERCEPTUAL PATTERN

HEARING: ☒ NORMAL ☐ IMPAIRED: ☐ LEFT EAR ☐ RIGHT EAR ☐ AID

VISION: ☐ NORMAL ☐ IMPAIRED ☒ GLASSES ☐ PROTHESIS

☐ FARSIGHTED ☐ NEARSIGHTED

OTHER PROBLEMS _____

COMMUNICATION: LANGUAGE SPOKEN **English**

UNDERSTANDS _____ UNABLE TO: ☐ READ ☐ WRITE

ABLE TO: ☒ READ ☒ WRITE ☐ LIP READ

COGNITION: ☒ NO PROBLEMS ☐ RECENT MEMORY CHANGE

☐ DIFFICULTY LEARNING

DISCOMFORT/PAIN: ☐ NO ☒ YES DESCRIBE **Epigastric**

HOW DO YOU MANAGE YOUR PAIN? **Bland food, Maalox**

9. COPING/STRESS TOLERANCE PATTERN

SPECIAL CONCERNS REGARDING HOSPITALIZATION? ☐ NO ☒ YES

Care of Children

10. SELF-PERCEPTION/SELF-CONCEPT PATTERN

CONCERNS ABOUT HOW YOUR ILLNESS AFFECTS YOU? ☐ NO ☒ YES

Concerned about health

11. ROLE/RELATIONSHIP PATTERN

MARITAL STATUS: ☐ MARRIED ☐ SINGLE ☐ WIDOWED ☒ DIVORCED

CHILDREN (#) **2** OTHER DEPENDENT(S) **0**

OCCUPATION **Secretary**

RESIDENCY (TYPE) **apartment**

WHO LIVES AT HOME WITH YOU? **Children**

SUPPORT SYSTEM (CLOSE FRIEND/FAMILY MEMBER) **Yes**

FAMILY CONCERNS ABOUT HOSPITALIZATION? **Yes**

12. VALUE/BELIEF PATTERN

RELIGIOUS AFFILIATION **Baptist**

RELIGIOUS RESTRICTIONS **0**

☐ WOULD LIKE CHAPLAIN TO VISIT (IF YES, NOTIFY CHAPLAIN)

☒ WOULD LIKE FAMILY MINISTER TO VISIT

NAME **Mr. Ame** PHONE **314-6000**

RELIGIOUS ACTIVITIES IMPORTANT TO YOU **Bible**

SUBJECTIVE DATA SIGNATURE **P. LeMone RN** _____ (Nurse)

6. ACTIVITY/EXERCISE PATTERN

ROM: ☒ FULL ☐ OTHER _____

BALANCE AND GAIT: ☒ STEADY ☐ UNSTEADY ☐ LIMP _____

HAND GRASPS: ☒ EQUAL ☒ STRONG

☐ WEAKNESS/PARALYSIS ☐ RIGHT ☐ LEFT

LEG MUSCLES: ☒ EQUAL ☒ STRONG

WEAKNESS/PARALYSIS ☐ RIGHT ☐ LEFT

8. COGNITIVE/PERCEPTUAL PATTERN

LEVEL OF CONSCIOUSNESS: ☒ ALERT ☒ RESPONDS TO PAIN

ORIENTED TO: ☒ TIME ☒ PLACE ☒ PERSON

MOOD: ☒ CALM ☐ SAD ☐ ANGRY

☐ WITHDRAWN ☐ OTHER _____

PUPILS: ☒ EQUAL ☒ REACTIVE ☐ OTHER _____

COGNITION: ☒ ABLE TO FOLLOW SIMPLE COMMANDS

☒ RESPONDS APPROPRIATELY TO QUESTIONS

☐ UNABLE TO FOLLOW COMMANDS

☐ OTHER _____

HEARING: ☒ NORMAL ☐ OTHER _____

VISION: ☒ NORMAL ☐ OTHER _____

MANIFESTATIONS OF PAIN _____

10. SELF-PERCEPTION/SELF-CONCEPT PATTERN

EYE CONTACT: ☒ APPROPRIATE ☐ DOWNCAST ☐ STARING

BODY POSTURE: ☒ RELAXED ☐ STOOPED ☐ RIGID

BEHAVIOR: 1 ②(2) 3 4 5 (CIRCLE)

RELAXED NERVOUS

OTHER _____

11. ROLE/RELATIONSHIP PATTERN

BEHAVIOR: ①(1) 2 3 4 5 (CIRCLE)

PASSIVE ASSERTIVE AGGRESSIVE

INTERACTION WITH FAMILY/SIGNIFICANT OTHER: ☐ N/A

☒ RELAXED ☐ TENSE ☐ ANGRY ☐ WITHDRAWN ☐ OTHER _____

COMMENTS: _____

Worried about effect of illness and possible surgery on care of children, job, and income. Has strong support of family.

SIGNATURE **P. LeMone, RN** _____ (Nurse)

FIGURE 14-4

(continued)

FIGURE 14-5

Turning the bed sheets down and opening the blinds or drapes to let the sunshine in says to a new patient or resident, "Welcome! We were expecting you!" Making sure the room is stocked with the necessary equipment and supplies, including personal toiletry items, also indicates to the new patient or resident that his or her arrival was planned for and expected.

FIGURE 14-6

A new patient or resident must be taught how to operate the equipment in the room. Here, a nursing assistant shows a new resident how to use the call light control.

You should also help the person to unpack and find appropriate places for her personal belongings (Fig. 14-7). If you work in a long-term care facility, you will need to complete a resident inventory sheet as part of the unpacking process. The **resident inventory sheet** is a document that lists and briefly describes all of the resident's personal belongings. When completing the resident inventory sheet, make sure that you describe each item objectively. For example, when describing a resident's ring, you would write, "yellow metal ring with two blue stones" instead of "gold ring with two sapphires" because you do not know for sure that the ring is

FIGURE 14-7

Helping the person to unpack and find suitable spots for personal items can make a new environment feel more "home-like" instantly.

Inventory of Personal Effects

Resident _____ Room No. _____

Description :

Bathrobe	Cane
Bed Jackets	Comb Brush
Belts	Crutches
Blouses	Dentures-Full Upper ( ) Lower ( )
Bras	Partial Upper ( ) Lower ( )
Coat	Furniture
Dresses	Glasses-Rimmed ( ) Rimless ( )
Girdles	Luggage
Hat	Other
Hose	Prosthesis
Nightgowns	Purse
Pajamas	Radio
Panties	Razors - Electric ( ) Safety ( )
Shirts	Rings
Shoes	Toothbrush
Skirts	Walker
Slips	Watch
Slippers	Wheelchair
Sweaters	
Ties	
Trousers	
Undershirts	
Undershorts	
Wallet	

I certify that the above is a correct list of my personal belongings.
I take full responsibility for retaining in my possession the articles listed above and any others brought to me while a resident in this facility.

ALL ITEMS BROUGHT FOR THE PERSONAL USE OF THE RESIDENT MUST BE PROPERLY MARKED AND LISTED AS ARE THE ABOVE. Please bring additional items to the Nurses' Station for proper handling.

Resident's washable clothing to be: _____ taken home for laundering _____ laundered here at the center.

I understand the Management will not be responsible for any valuables, money, or clothing left in the possession of the resident._____ Date_____

Signature of Resident (or Relative) _____ Date _____
Signature of Nurse _____ Date _____

Disposition on Discharge   *Upon Discharge, all personal items are sent with resident or picked up by responsible party. Upon transfer, all personal items are to be boxed and placed in designated storage area for safekeeping.

Signature of Nurse _____   Signature of Resident/Relative _____
Date _____   Date _____

FIGURE 14-8

A resident inventory sheet is completed when a person is admitted to a long-term care facility. This document is used to keep track of each person's belongings.

gold or the stones are sapphires. The resident inventory sheet is used to help make sure that a resident leaves the facility with all of her belongings, in the event of a transfer or discharge (Fig. 14-8). It is also used to assist with tracking if belongings are misplaced or borrowed. Some long-term care facilities require each resident to write her name inside of each article of clothing to help with laundry sorting. You may need to help the resident do this if it has not been done already.

If the person has brought personal items to decorate with, let the person know that you will be willing to assist in any way that you can. For example, a resident of a long-term care facility may need your help with hanging a favorite picture on the wall, or obtaining a bulletin board to display treasured cards and pieces of art.

Practice Good Communication Skills

While you are helping the person to get settled, talk to him! Involving the person in conversation will indicate to the person that you are interested in him, personally, and it will let you get to know the person a little bit better. You know your own duties better than anyone else, and questions that you ask the patient or resident will help you to plan each person's care. For example, you might ask the person when he likes to bathe, whether he likes to take a nap between lunch and dinner, or whether he would prefer to take meals in the dining room or in his room. Be sure to listen to what the person is saying to you, both on his own and in response to your questions. Is the person asking questions or expressing feelings that suggest that he is scared, worried, or upset? Answer questions about your specific responsibilities to the best of your ability. Questions the patient or resident may have about his medical care should be directed to the nurse. Report any concerns that you may have about the person's ability to adjust to the new environment to the nurse.

TRANSFERS

A **transfer** occurs whenever a patient or resident is moved within or between health care settings. A transfer can be:
- From one room to another (for example, from a semi-private to a private room)
- From one unit to another [for example, from the intensive care unit (ICU) to a standard care floor]

- From one health care facility to another (for example, from a long-term care facility to a hospital for the treatment of an acute illness)

Transfers can occur when a person's medical condition improves, or when it worsens. Transfers can also occur when a preferred room becomes available for a person on a waiting list, or when it is necessary to move people to resolve conflicts between roommates.

As is the case with admissions, transfers can be stressful for the patient or resident, as well as her family members. The reason for the transfer may cause anxiety, especially if the person's condition has worsened or if the person is being transferred from a hospital to a long-term care facility. These transfers may not be expected or desired by either the person or the person's family members. They are usually the result of necessity. Even if the transfer is expected and desirable (for example, a resident in a long-term care facility is moving from one room to another because the view is better), the person being transferred may still experience some stress as a result of the change.

The physical transfer can be carried out in a number of ways. The patient or resident may simply walk, or she may be transported in a wheelchair or on a stretcher. Sometimes, the person does not even need to get out of bed. The bed (with the person in it) is simply moved to another room or unit. An ambulance may be used when a person is being moved from one health care facility to another. However, many people are transferred from one facility to another by their regular means of transportation, such as a car or taxi.

Your duties related to assisting with transfers will vary according to the type of facility where you work. In a hospital or acute care setting, you will be responsible for gathering and packing the person's belongings. It is very important that you help to make sure that all of the person's belongings are packed and sent along with her, so that nothing gets lost. You may also need to assist the nurse in transporting the person to the new room or unit, or to the waiting ambulance, car, or taxi. The nurse is usually responsible for reporting information about the person's medical condition and medications or other treatments to the receiving nurse. If the transfer is taking place within the hospital, you may be asked to report information about the person's preferences and habits to the receiving nursing assistant.

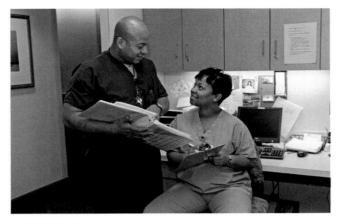

FIGURE 14-9

Two nursing assistants meet to discuss the personal care needs of a resident who is being transferred from one part of the facility to another.

In a long-term care facility, the assistance you provide will be more personal. Although the nurse will report medical information about the resident to the receiving nurse, you will be responsible for reporting personal care information about the resident to the receiving nursing assistant (Fig. 14-9). This is appropriate, because you are the caregiver who is most likely to know the most about your resident's personal preferences. For example, you would know that Mr. Vasquez does not like overcooked vegetables, that he requires minimal assistance in the bathroom, and that he likes to read the paper after breakfast. By providing the new nursing assistant with this information, you are helping to ensure that the transition from one caretaker to another is as seamless as possible for your resident.

DISCHARGES

A **discharge** is the official release of a patient or a resident from a health care facility to his or her home. A patient's or resident's discharge is ordered by the doctor. Occasionally, a person will insist on leaving a health care setting without a doctor's order, or **against medical advice (AMA).** A person who is mentally competent may choose to leave a facility if she wants to. However, that person must sign certain documents first. By signing these documents, the person states that she understands that leaving the facility without a doctor's order releases the doctor and the health care facility from any legal responsibility regarding her health status because she has refused to follow the recommendations for her care. If a person tells you that she is leaving the facility, you must report this to the nurse immediately. The nurse will follow the facility's policy for ensuring that a person who is leaving AMA is aware of the consequences of her actions.

Although some people initiate their own departure from a health care facility, most people wait to be officially discharged. Many times, the official discharge is a happy event, but sometimes, people have mixed emotions about leaving. As you will recall from Chapter 1, the ever-increasing costs of health care have created a situation where patients are being discharged from hospitals before they are fully recovered. Many patients are still acutely ill or need complicated treatment and care at the time of their discharge from the hospital. For these people and their family members, leaving behind the safe, professional care provided by the hospital staff can be a frightening experience.

To help ease the transition from a health care facility to home for patients and residents, preparations for discharge begin as soon as a person is admitted to the health care facility. **Discharge planning** is the process used by the members of the health care team to help prepare a patient or resident to leave the facility. Discharge planning helps to make sure that the person continues to receive quality care, either from a home health care agency or from family members, after the discharge. The purpose of discharge planning is to identify the needs that a person will have after his discharge and to make arrangements for meeting these needs after the person goes home. For example, as a result of discharge planning:

- A patient's family members may be taught how to change a wound dressing before the patient is sent home
- A resident and his family may receive help in planning a special diet before the resident is sent home
- Arrangements may be made to transfer a patient from the hospital to a long-term care facility for a short recovery period
- The services of a home health care agency may be obtained

The ultimate goal of discharge planning is to help the patient or resident achieve the best health

FIGURE 14-10

Nurses are responsible for discharge planning, a process that helps to ensure a continuation of care for people after they leave a health care facility. Here, a nurse is showing a patient's family member how to change a wound dressing.

status possible after he or she leaves the health care facility (Fig. 14-10).

When a patient or resident is discharged from a health care facility, the nurse is responsible for making sure that the person and his family members have been taught what they need to know about the person's condition and how to monitor or care for it. Your responsibilities when a person is discharged are related more to helping the person to gather and pack his belongings and say goodbye to friends and caretakers. Ask the nurse or the person about the estimated time of discharge so that you can have the person ready to leave on time, taking into account the time the person needs to pack and say his goodbyes. You may need to assist the person out of the facility or help to carry his belongings.

➡ *Tell the Nurse!*

The changes that accompany discharges, transfers, and admissions to health care facilities can be very stressful for a person and for his family members. Often, a lot of information is communicated in a very short period of time, and the patient or resident (as well as his family members) may have trouble absorbing and understanding everything. Make sure you observe and listen carefully to your patient or resident, and to his family members, during these transitions. Report any of the following to the nurse immediately:

➠ Any questions that have to do with a person's medical condition or transfer

➠ Any comments that would indicate that the person or a family member does not fully understand what she has been told by a doctor or nurse

➠ Any signs of anxiety, such as crying, confusion, agitation, or other unexplained behavior

➠ Any changes in the person's vital signs or mental status

➠ Any mention of leaving the facility against medical advice (AMA)

SUMMARY

▶ Admission to a health care facility is a time of orientation. The patient or resident must learn to accept his new environment and his new status as a "patient" or "resident," and the members of the health care team must learn about their new patient or resident.

■ Assuming the role of a patient or resident can be very traumatic for a person. Therefore, the person's physical and emotional needs must always remain the focus of the admissions process.

■ Newly admitted patients or residents should be welcomed as if they are guests in your facility.

■ A smooth admissions process helps to reduce a person's anxiety about entering the health care facility. Many of the nursing assistant's duties revolve around making the admissions process easier for the patient or resident and his family members.

● Nursing assistants are responsible for preparing the person's room, taking the person's vital signs and measuring his height and weight, helping the person to unpack, and teaching the person how to use the equipment in the room.

● By actively listening to the comments made by the person and his family members during the admissions process, the nursing assistant can notify the nurse of any specific concerns that may need to be addressed.

▶ Transfers occur when a patient or resident is moved, either within a health care setting or between health care settings.

■ Transfers can occur when a person's medical condition improves, or when it worsens.

■ When a person is transferred within a hospital or long-term care facility, the nursing assistant is responsible for passing vital information about the resident's care to the receiving nursing assistant.

▶ Although many people look forward to going home after being discharged from a health care facility, some might wonder whether they will be able to manage on their own, or with only the help of family members.

■ Discharge planning helps to ensure that a patient or resident continues to receive quality health care, even after being released from a health care facility. Discharge planning begins at the time of admission and is the responsibility of the nurse.

■ The nursing assistant is responsible for helping a person prepare for discharge by gathering and packing all of a person's personal items.

What did you learn?

Multiple Choice

Select the single best answer for each of the following questions.

1. One of your patients is being transferred to another unit in the hospital. What would you pack for him to take along with him?
   a. His bed linens
   b. His medical record
   c. His personal belongings
   d. All of the above

2. One of your patients, Mrs. Sarandis, mentions to you that she is leaving the hospital, and her son is coming to pick her up. Before Mrs. Sarandis can be permitted to leave the premises, she must have:
   a. A nurse's order for discharge
   b. A doctor's order for discharge
   c. An admissions sheet on record
   d. A completed resident inventory sheet

3. As a nursing assistant, one of your tasks during the admission process will be to:
   a. Take and record the new patient's or resident's vital signs
   b. Assess the new patient's or resident's medical condition
   c. Hurry the new patient or resident through the admissions process to keep things running smoothly
   d. Reassure the new patient or resident by telling him or her that everything will be fine

4. Who writes the orders on admission for a person's diet, medications, level of activity, and type of room?
   a. The admissions clerk
   b. The patient or resident, or one of his or her family members
   c. The Director of Nursing
   d. The person's doctor

5. Discharge planning begins:
   a. A couple of days before the patient or resident is scheduled to be discharged
   b. When the patient or resident is admitted to the health care facility
   c. The day the patient or resident is scheduled to be discharged
   d. Before the patient or resident is admitted to the health care facility

6. The ultimate goal of discharge planning is to:
   a. Make sure that the room is clean and ready for the next patient or resident
   b. Close out the nursing care plan
   c. Help the person who is being discharged achieve his or her best level of health
   d. Make sure that all of the patient's or resident's belongings are accounted for

7. Who is responsible for carrying out the actions prescribed by the discharge plan (for example, teaching a patient's family member how to change a dressing)?
   a. The doctor
   b. The hospital social worker
   c. The nurse
   d. The nursing assistant

8. Mr. Singer, one of your patients, tells you that he hates the food at the hospital and feels that being hospitalized is actually doing him more harm than good. He says that he has called his wife, and she is coming that afternoon to take him home. As far as you know, Mr. Singer's discharge has not been ordered. What should you do?
   a. Apply a restraint
   b. Help Mr. Singer pack; it is his right to leave if he wants to
   c. Tell the nurse immediately
   d. Remind Mr. Singer's roommate that the door to the room must be kept shut and locked at all times

9. Why should a newly admitted patient or resident be given a warm welcome?
   a. Because he represents more revenue for the facility
   b. Because he will be a good roommate for another lonely patient or resident
   c. Because he may be feeling scared and uncomfortable about entering a health care facility
   d. He should not be given a warm welcome; after all, admissions happen every day and a "business as usual" attitude is best to avoid upsetting the other patients or residents

10. One of your residents has just been discharged, and you assisted with the discharge. What should you report to the nurse?
    a. The resident left in a limousine!
    b. The resident was accompanied by a care-taker
    c. The resident was discharged at 1500
    d. All of the above

> **? Stop and think!**
>
> ▶ A new resident, Mrs. Becker, arrives at your facility in an ambulance. Mrs. Becker has been transferred to your facility from a local hospital's skilled nursing unit because she needs more physical therapy before she can go home. Mrs. Becker is slightly confused, and quiet. After the paramedics leave the room, Mrs. Becker's daughter starts complaining—she wants a single room for her mother, and she does not like the view. She immediately wants to see the administrator and have her mother transferred to another facility. Mrs. Becker's oldest daughter (not the daughter who accompanied Mrs. Becker to the facility) is Mrs. Becker's legal guardian, and she is not present. This means that the daughter who is present does not have the authority to have Mrs. Becker transferred to another facility. You have been assigned to be Mrs. Becker's nursing assistant. What can you do to make the admissions process more comfortable for Mrs. Becker, in spite of her demanding daughter?
>
> ▶ Mr. Gardner has been a resident in your facility for several months and he has reached his maximum potential in therapy. Medicare will no longer pay for his care. Mr. Gardner's son is transferring him to an assisted-living facility for monetary reasons. Mr. Gardner tells you that he is uncomfortable and scared about the new facility, since he does not know anyone there. How can you help Mr. Gardner?

15

Bedmaking

What will you learn?

For someone who is tired or ill, nothing is quite as comforting as clean, crisp linens on the bed. Clean linens are essential not only for your patient's or resident's comfort, but also for infection control and the prevention of skin breakdown and pressure ulcers. A neat, well-made bed is a sign that the facility provides capable, competent care to its patients or residents. When you are finished with this chapter, you will be able to:

1. Describe ways that a properly made bed can increase a person's comfort and well-being.
2. List the different types of linens and their uses.
3. Demonstrate the proper way to handle and care for linens.
4. Explain the infection control measures that are used during bedmaking.
5. Demonstrate techniques of proper bedmaking, including making a closed bed, opening a bed, preparing a surgical bed, and making an occupied bed.

Vocabulary

Use the CD in the back of your book to hear these terms pronounced, defined, and used in a sentence:

Draw sheet	Pressure-relieving	Footboard	Open bed
Lift sheet	mattress	Mitered corner	Surgical bed
Bed protector	Bed board	Closed bed	Occupied bed
Bath blanket	Bed cradle	Fanfolded	Toe pleat

Photo: A well-made bed is essential to a person's mental and physical well-being. Here, a nursing assistant tucks in a draw sheet.

LINENS AND OTHER SUPPLIES FOR BEDMAKING

LINENS

Many types of linens are used to make a bed. On your bed at home, you probably have a mattress pad, a bottom (or fitted) sheet, a top (or flat) sheet, a pillow covered in a pillowcase, and a bedspread or comforter. If you live in a cold climate, you may add a blanket to your bed during the winter months to provide extra warmth. In a health care facility, all of these basic linens are used, and some special ones may be added, depending on the needs of the patient or resident. Linens that you may see in use in a health care facility include the following.

Mattress Pads

A mattress pad is a thick layer of padding that is placed on the mattress to help make the bed more comfortable for the patient or resident, and to protect the mattress from moisture and soiling. The mattress pad may be "fitted." In this case, it will have elasticized sides that wrap around and underneath the mattress, holding the pad securely to the mattress. Or, the mattress pad may be "flat" (non-fitted).

Often, in health care facilities, the mattress has a rubber coating that helps to keep the mattress dry. When no mattress pad is used, and a bottom sheet is placed directly on the rubberized mattress, the person may become very warm and start to sweat because the rubber retains the person's body heat. The bottom sheet becomes damp and stays damp, because the rubberized mattress does not absorb the extra moisture. Lying on a damp sheet is uncomfortable for the patient or resident. In addition, lying on a damp sheet can cause the skin to become reddened and irritated, which can lead to skin breakdown and pressure ulcers. Therefore, when a rubberized mattress is in use, a mattress pad may be used to help pull moisture away from the person's skin.

In a home environment or a long-term care facility, the person may use a standard mattress on his own bed. In this situation, a waterproof mattress pad can be used to help protect the mattress, especially if the person is incontinent (unable to control his bladder or bowels).

Bottom and Top Sheets

The sheets used to make a bed may be white or colored, plain or print. Regardless of their other characteristics, however, sheets need to be clean and wrinkle-free. A bed is made with two sheets, a bottom sheet and a top sheet. Some facilities use flat, or non-fitted, sheets as bottom sheets, or the bottom sheet may be fitted. When you are using a flat sheet as the bottom sheet, it is important to tuck the sheet tightly so that movement does not cause the sheet to loosen and wrinkle underneath the person. Wrinkled sheets are uncomfortable and can create areas of pressure on a person's skin, which can lead to skin breakdown.

The top sheet is a flat sheet.

Draw Sheets

A **draw sheet** is a small, flat sheet that is placed over the middle of the bottom sheet, covering the area of the bed from above the person's shoulders to below his or her buttocks (Fig. 15-1). When a rubberized mattress is in use, a draw sheet may be used instead of a mattress pad to form a protective, moisture-absorbing barrier between the person's body and the rubberized mattress. Some facilities use rubberized or plastic draw sheets to protect the mattress from soiling. If a rubberized draw sheet is used, it is always covered with a cotton draw sheet to protect the person's skin from contact with the rubber. The sides of the draw sheet are tucked tightly under the mattress to prevent wrinkling.

FIGURE 15-1

A draw sheet is a small sheet that is placed over the middle of the bottom sheet to absorb extra moisture when a mattress pad is not used. Sometimes, draw sheets are used to assist with turning or lifting a person. When a draw sheet is used for this purpose, it is called a "lift sheet."

A **lift sheet** is simply a draw sheet that is used to help lift or reposition a person who needs assistance with moving in bed (see Chapter 11). A draw sheet or a lift sheet can be made easily by folding a flat sheet in half. If a folded flat sheet is being used as a lift sheet, the folded edge of the sheet is positioned above the person's shoulders and the loose ends are positioned below the buttocks. When a draw sheet is to be used as a lift sheet, the sides are usually allowed to hang free, although some facilities may require you to tuck the sides of the lift sheet under the mattress after lifting or repositioning the person, to reduce wrinkling.

Bed Protectors

A **bed protector** is a square of quilted absorbent fabric backed with waterproof material. The bed protector measures approximately 3 feet by 3 feet. Bed protectors may be disposable, or they may be laundered and reused. In addition to being used for people who are incontinent, bed protectors are often used for people with draining wounds. The urine, feces, or wound drainage is pulled away from the person's body by the absorbent layers of the bed protector, and the waterproof layer keeps the liquid from soiling the rest of the linens on the bed. Sometimes, only the bed protector needs to be changed, resulting in more efficient and economical care.

Blankets

Blankets provided by a facility are usually woven cotton and should be available as requested by a person for his or her comfort. Residents of long-term care facilities or home health care clients may use their own blankets, which may be wool, cotton, or synthetic, depending on the person's preference and the climate. Electric blankets should be checked for faulty wiring or plugs and may not be safe to use if the person is incontinent or unable to adjust the controls independently (for example, if the person is very old or very young). Electric blankets should only be used according to facility policy.

Bedspreads

A bedspread adds the finishing touch to a well-made bed and can add a decorative touch to a person's room. Hospitals and extended-care facilities may supply bedspreads for their patients to use. Other types of health care facilities or agencies may encourage their residents to use their own bed coverings. Allowing a person to use her bedspread from home is one way that long-term care facilities help to foster a sense of independence and individuality in residents.

Pillows and Pillowcases

Pillows are used for comfort and to aid in positioning. They may be available in many sizes and are made from a variety of materials. Some pillows are covered with waterproof material or treated with a waterproofing substance to protect them from moisture and to aid with cleaning. Pillows are always covered with clean pillowcases. Care for pillows that become wet or soiled will vary according to facility.

Bath Blankets

A **bath blanket** is a lightweight cotton blanket or flannel sheet that is used to provide modesty and warmth during a bed bath or a linen change. A flat sheet may also be used for this purpose if the facility does not provide a special bath blanket. The bath blanket is not made into the bed, but because it is used during bed baths and linen changes, it is gathered along with the other linens.

OTHER BEDMAKING SUPPLIES

Occasionally, other equipment or supplies are used on a person's bed, depending on the specific needs of the patient or resident. Some of the items used include the following.

- A **pressure-relieving mattress** may be placed on top of the regular mattress to help prevent skin breakdown in patients and residents who must stay in bed for long periods of time. Thin foam pads that resemble the inside of an egg carton, called "egg crate mattresses," were used in the past to help relieve pressure, but now are used only for comfort. Use of foam pads is decreasing because the foam is difficult to keep clean and dry, especially if the person is incontinent. Newer versions of pressure-relieving mattresses may be filled with air or water, and are made out of a material that is easily cleaned.

FIGURE 15-2

A bed cradle is used to keep the top sheet, the blanket, and the bedspread off the patient's or resident's feet. The linens are tucked in at the end of the bed and along the sides to keep the person from getting cold.

- A **bed board** is a piece of wood (usually plywood) that is placed under the mattress to provide extra support. The bed board keeps the mattress from sagging, helping to keep the person's body properly aligned. Bed boards are most commonly used in the home health care and long-term care settings.
- A **bed cradle** is a metal frame that is placed between the bottom and top sheets to keep the top sheet, the blanket, and the bedspread away from the person's feet (Fig. 15-2). Bed cradles are often used for people who are recovering from burns to prevent the top sheet from touching the burned skin, which would be very painful. They are also often used for people who are at risk for developing pressure ulcers on their feet.
- A **footboard** is a padded board that is placed upright at the foot of the bed (Fig. 15-3). The person's feet rest flat against the footboard, helping to keep the feet in proper alignment.

HANDLING OF LINENS

The types of linens used for bedmaking will vary, depending on the facility and the needs of the patient or resident. Some facilities will use fitted mattress pads and bottom sheets, whereas others will use non-fitted mattress pads and flat

FIGURE 15-3

A footboard is placed against the end of the bed to keep the person's feet in proper alignment. (*Courtesy of the Posey Company.*)

sheets for bottom sheets. Some facilities will use rubberized draw sheets to protect the bottom sheet and mattress, whereas others will use bed protectors. During your employee orientation, you will learn which linens to use to make the beds. Additional information specific to each patient or resident will be provided on the nursing care plan.

No matter which linens are used in your facility, you should always collect the linens in the order that they will be used—mattress pad, bottom sheet, draw sheet, top sheet, blanket, bedspread, pillowcases. Once you have collected your stack of linens, flip the stack over so that the item you will need first is on the top of the stack (Fig. 15-4). Collecting linens in the order that they will be put on the bed helps you to remember which linens you need to collect. In addition, because the linens will be arranged in order of use, you will be able to make the bed more efficiently, without searching through the stack for the proper item.

Always remember that linens can act as fomites, or objects capable of spreading infection. For this reason, you should always use infection control practices when handling linens. Always wash your hands before collecting clean linens, and avoid letting clean linens come into contact with dirty surfaces, such as your uniform or the floor. When removing used linens from the bed, wear gloves, and roll the linens toward the center of the bed (down from the top and up from the bottom) to confine any soiled areas on the inside (Fig. 15-5). You may be required to place the used linen in a plastic bag as it is removed from the bed to help prevent the spread of pathogens. The linen bag is then removed from the room and

A

B

FIGURE 15-4

Handling linens. (A) First, collect the linens in the order that they will be used. Here, the nursing assistant has gathered a mattress pad, a bottom sheet, a draw sheet, a top sheet, a blanket, a bedspread, and two pillowcases. The mattress pad is on the bottom of the stack and the pillowcases are on the top. Note that the nursing assistant is holding the linens away from his body. (B) Next, flip the stack of linens over so that the item you will need first is on top. Now the pillowcases are on the bottom of the stack and the mattress pad is on top, ready to be put on the bed.

taken to a designated area. If a linen bag is not used, then the used linens are placed in the linen hamper immediately, as per your facility's policy. Do not place dirty linens on the floor, or hold them against your uniform.

Guidelines Box 15-1 summarizes some general guidelines for the handling of linens. These guidelines apply no matter where you work.

FIGURE 15-5

Gloves are worn to remove linens from the bed, because the linens may be soiled with body fluids. The soiled area is rolled toward the center of the bed.

STANDARD BEDMAKING TECHNIQUES

Routine bedmaking is usually done in the morning, before visiting hours, while your patients or residents are bathing or dressing. How often the linens on a person's bed are changed will vary according to the type of health care facility and the person's needs. For example, in a hospital, the policy may be to change each person's linens completely on a daily basis. In a long-term care setting, the policy may call for less frequent linen changes. However, a person's bed must be remade each time any of the linens become soiled or excessively wrinkled, regardless of the time of day. Soiling of the sheets can occur as a result of spilled food or drink or as a result of excessive sweating, vomit, urine, feces, wound drainage, or leakage from a feeding tube. In each of these instances, a linen change would be required. Change as many of the bed linens as necessary to ensure a clean, dry, wrinkle-free bed for your patient or resident. General guidelines for bedmaking are given in Guidelines Box 15-2.

To make a bed, you will need to know how to make a **mitered corner** (Fig. 15-6). Mitering is a

GUIDELINES BOX 15-1
GUIDELINES FOR HANDLING LINENS

What you do	*Why you do it*
Always wash your hands before collecting clean linens.	Washing your hands prevents microbes on your hands from being transferred to the clean linens.
Do not hold linens, clean or dirty, against your uniform.	If you hold clean linens against your uniform, microbes on your uniform could be transferred to the linens. If you hold dirty linens against your uniform, then microbes from the dirty linens could be transferred to your uniform.
When collecting linens, collect only those that you will need for that person's bed. For example, if a draw sheet is not needed, do not collect one.	Extra linens brought into a person's room are considered soiled, and therefore must not be returned to the clean linen cart or used for another person. These linens must now be laundered, which costs the facility extra money and manpower and creates additional wear on the linens, shortening their lifetime of use.
Collect linens in the order that they will be used. Once you have collected your stack of linens, flip the stack over so that the item you will need first is on the top of the stack.	Collecting linens in the order that they will be put on the bed helps you to remember which linens you need to collect. In addition, because the linens will be arranged in order of use, you will be able to make the bed more efficiently, without searching through the stack for the proper item.
Place clean linens on a clean surface in the room, such as the over-bed table or a chair. Do not place clean linens on the floor.	Clean linens can become contaminated with microbes if you place them on a "dirty" surface, such as the floor.
Wear gloves when removing used linens from a bed. Roll the linens toward the center of the bed to confine the soiled area inside.	Any item contaminated with blood or other body substances is a potential source of exposure to pathogens for the health care worker. Following the standard precautions and wearing proper personal protective equipment (PPE) will help to minimize your exposure. Confining the soiled area to the inside of the linens helps to ensure that other people, such as the people in the laundry, do not come in contact with the potentially infectious material.
If body fluids or substances leak through the linens to the mattress or bed frame, the mattress or bed frame should be wiped with an appropriate cleaning solution before placing clean linens on the bed. Remove your gloves and wash your hands before handling the clean linens.	These infection control methods help to prevent the clean sheets from becoming contaminated.
After removing the dirty linens from the bed, place them in the linen hamper immediately. Your facility may require you to place dirty linens in a plastic bag or pillowcase before placing them in the linen hamper. Do not place dirty linens on the floor or on any other surface.	Placing the dirty linens in the linen hamper immediately helps to control the spread of infection.

GUIDELINES BOX 15-2
GUIDELINES FOR BEDMAKING

What you do	Why you do it
Always place linens on the bed so that the seams of the sheets face away from the person's skin.	The seams of the sheets can rub the person's skin, causing irritation and leading to skin breakdown.
Linens must be pulled tightly to avoid wrinkling. Layering should be kept to a minimum.	The wrinkles and extra layers of linens can cause skin breakdown and contribute to the formation of pressure ulcers.
Linens should be changed whenever they become soiled or wet, regardless of the time of day.	Besides causing discomfort, soiled or wet sheets can cause skin breakdown and contribute to the formation of pressure ulcers.
Do not shake linens when placing them on the bed.	Recall that dust is a transport mechanism for microbes. Shaking linens stirs up dust from the floor. The dust then settles on surfaces in the room and can be easily transferred onto eating utensils or into a wound, causing an infection.
When you need to change the linens on a person's bed with the person still in the bed, always be sure to explain what you are doing throughout the procedure. Close the door, pull the privacy curtain, and keep the person covered.	Having the bed linens changed while still in the bed can be a very frightening experience for a bedridden person, particularly if the person is unconscious. Even if the person is conscious, movement may cause pain, and incontinence (the involuntary loss of urine or feces) can be very embarrassing if it occurs. If the person is mentally impaired, he or she may become combative. Talk reassuringly to the person, even if the person is unconscious and you think that the person cannot hear you. Always provide for privacy and modesty by keeping the person covered at all times.
Check the bed linens for personal items before removing the linens from the bed.	Personal items, such as dentures, eyeglasses, or jewelry, may become lost in the bed linens. If these linens are removed from the bed, bundled up, and sent to the laundry, the mislaid personal items may not be discovered and they could be damaged in the wash cycle, or they may be lost altogether. Personal items may be expensive and inconvenient to replace. If they hold sentimental value, they may be irreplaceable. Therefore, you must take care not to mishandle personal items.

way of folding and tucking the sheet so that it lies flat and neat against the mattress. When a flat sheet is used as the bottom sheet, the mitered corners are made at the top of the bed to help secure the sheet to the mattress. Mitered corners are made at the foot of the bed to hold the top sheet, blanket, and bedspread in place.

CLOSED (UNOCCUPIED) BEDS

A **closed bed** is an empty bed (Fig. 15-7A). A bed that is unoccupied because the previous patient or resident has been discharged from the facility and a new patient or resident has yet to arrive is considered a closed bed. Similarly, a bed that is

FIGURE 15-6

How to make a mitered corner. Here, a mitered corner is being made on a top sheet. (*A*) The sheet is hanging over the side of the bed. (*B*) Grasp the edge of the sheet about 12″ from the foot of the bed and lift it up, forming a triangle. Lay the triangular fold on the top of the bed, and smooth the hanging portion of the sheet against the side of the mattress. (*C*) Tuck the hanging portion of the sheet underneath the mattress, while holding the triangular fold taut against the top of the bed. (*D*) Bring the triangular fold back down over the edge of the mattress, and tuck it underneath.

unoccupied because the patient or resident is simply not in it at the moment (and is not expected back any time soon) is also considered a closed bed. For example, many long-term care facilities make closed beds each day for residents who are not bedridden. Procedure 15-1 explains how to make a closed bed.

When the top sheet, blanket, and bedspread of a closed bed are turned back, or **fanfolded,** the closed bed becomes an **open bed,** or a bed ready to receive a patient or resident. For example, you would open a bed in preparation for a new admission, or after you have changed the linens while a patient or resident is bathing or out of the room for a diagnostic test. Because the patient or resident would be expected to return to the bed shortly, you would fanfold the linens back in anticipation of his return. Similarly, in some long-term care facilities, the linens on the beds of residents who are not bedridden are folded back in the evening, before the residents return to their rooms. To open a closed bed, you first grasp the bedspread, blanket, and top sheet and fold them back to the foot of the bed, creating a fanfold (Fig. 15-7B). Finish by making sure that the bed is in the lowest position and the bed wheels are locked. Place the call light control near the head of the bed, clipping it to the bottom sheet.

A **surgical bed** is a closed bed that has been opened to receive a patient or resident who will be arriving by stretcher. A surgical bed may be prepared for a patient who is returning to the room following surgery or a diagnostic procedure, or for one who is being transferred from another unit (such as the emergency room). When preparing a surgical bed, instead of folding the top sheet, blanket, and bedspread to the foot of the bed, you loosen these linens from the foot of the bed and fold them toward the side of the bed, leaving one side open and ready to receive the person (Fig. 15-7C). After folding the linens to the side, raise the bed so that the stretcher will be slightly higher than the bed. Make sure that the bed wheels are locked, and ensure a clear path by moving any furniture away from the bed.

OCCUPIED BEDS

"She went out of the room and came back with the old nurse of the early morning. Together they made the bed with me in it. That was new to me and an admirable proceeding."

—*A Farewell to Arms*, Ernest Hemingway

Some conditions make it difficult or impossible for a person to get out of bed for a linen change. When this is the case, it is necessary to change the linens while the person is still in the bed. This is

A

C

B

FIGURE 15-7

Types of beds. (*A*) A closed bed is an unoccupied bed. (*B*) When a closed bed is "opened," the top sheet, blanket, and bedspread are "fanfolded" to the foot of the bed. (*C*) A surgical bed is a closed bed that has been "opened" to receive a person on a stretcher. The top linens are fanfolded to the side of the bed.

called making an **occupied bed** (Procedure 15-2). In most facilities, this procedure is carried out on a routine basis after the person has been bathed. However, as always, if the linens become wet or soiled in between scheduled linen changes, then they must be changed. Because it can be frightening for a bedridden person to have the linens changed while he or she is still in the bed, remember to explain to the person what you are doing throughout this procedure. Keep the privacy curtain and the door closed during the procedure, to help maintain the person's modesty. If the linens you are removing from the bed are soiled with blood or other body substances, you must wear gloves. Remember to remove the soiled gloves and put on clean ones before handling the clean linens.

SUMMARY

▶ A well-made bed is essential to a person's mental and physical well-being.

■ Clean, dry, wrinkle-free linens help make a person who is ill feel cared for and more comfortable.

■ Clean, dry, wrinkle-free linens help to prevent complications, such as pressure ulcers. Dampness contributes to skin breakdown and wrinkled sheets can cause friction, both of which are factors in the development of pressure ulcers.

■ Clean, dry linens are important for odor and infection control.

▶ A variety of linens are used to make a bed. Facility policy and the patient's or resident's particular needs dictate which linens are used to make the bed.

▶ Special devices, such as pressure-relieving mattresses and bed cradles, are used to improve the patient's or resident's comfort and to prevent the development of complications related to spending long periods of time in bed, such as pressure ulcers.

▶ Because linens soiled with body fluids and substances can act as fomites, it is important to use good infection control practices when handling soiled linens.

- Never hold dirty linens against your uniform, or place them on the floor or other surface in the room. Dirty linens must be placed in the linen hamper or linen bag immediately.
- Always wash your hands before handling clean linens. Never hold clean linens against your uniform, or place them on the floor. Clean linens may be placed on a clean surface in the room, such as the over-bed table.
- Always wear gloves when it is possible you will be handling linens soiled with body fluids or other substances.

▶ A bed is either unoccupied ("closed") or occupied. A closed bed may be "opened" in anticipation of receiving a patient or resident by fanfolding the sheets to allow easier access.

Chapter 15 Procedures

Getting Ready Steps

a. **W**ash your hands and observe standard precautions as necessary.

b. **G**ather needed supplies.

c. **K**nock and introduce yourself.

d. **I**dentify the person, and greet him or her by name.

e. **E**xplain the procedure.

f. **P**rovide privacy.

g. **S**ee to safety.

Finishing Up Steps

a. **C**onfirm comfort and good body alignment.

b. **L**eave the call light control within easy reach.

c. **S**ee to safety.

d. **O**pen the curtain and door.

e. **W**ash your hands.

f. **R**eport and record.

PROCEDURE 15-1
Making an Unoccupied (Closed) Bed

OBRA ✓

Getting Ready WGKIEPS

1. Complete the "Getting Ready" steps **a** through **g**.

Supplies

- mattress pad
- bottom sheet
- draw sheet or bed protector (if necessary)
- top sheet
- blanket
- bedspread
- pillowcase

Procedure

2. Make sure that the bed is positioned at a comfortable working height (to promote good body mechanics) and that the wheels are locked.

3. Place the linens on a clean surface close to the bed (e.g., the over-bed table).

4. Lower the side rails and move the mattress to the head of the bed (it may have shifted to-ward the foot of the bed if the occupant of the bed had the head of the bed elevated).

Note: The mattress pad, bottom sheet, and draw sheet are positioned and tucked in on one side of the bed before moving to the other side to complete these actions. This is most efficient in terms of energy and time.

5. Place the mattress pad on the bed and unfold it, so that only one vertical crease remains. Make sure that this crease is centered on the mattress. If the mattress pad is fitted, carefully pull the corners of the near side over the corners of the mattress and smooth down the sides. If the mattress pad is not fitted, make sure the top of the pad is even with the head of the mattress. Open the mattress pad across the bed, taking care to keep it centered.

6. Place the bottom sheet on the bed. If the bottom sheet is fitted, carefully pull the corners of the near side over the corners of the mattress and smooth down the sides. If the bottom sheet is not fitted:

   a. Place the sheet so that when you unfold it, the wide hem will be at the head of the bed

(continued)

---

*It is assumed that the dirty linens have been removed from the bed, and the bed frame has been cleaned, as per facility policy, prior to beginning this procedure.

PROCEDURE 15-1 (Continued)

Making an Unoccupied (Closed) Bed

and the hem stitching will be against the mattress, away from the person who will be occupying the bed.

b. Unfold the sheet so that only one vertical crease remains. Make sure that this crease is vertically centered on the mattress.

STEP 6b Unfold the sheet so that only one vertical crease remains.

c. Open the sheet across the bed, taking care to keep it centered. The same length of sheet (approximately 12 to 18 inches) should hang over each side of the bed. Make sure that the lower edge of the sheet is even with the foot of the mattress.

STEP 6c Open the sheet across the bed, taking care to keep it centered.

d. Tuck the sheet under the mattress at the head of the bed and miter the corner (see Fig. 15-6).

e. Tuck the near side of the sheet underneath the mattress, working from the head of the bed toward the foot. As you tuck, make sure there are no wrinkles in the sheet and that the mattress pad remains smooth and in place.

7. Place the draw sheet on the bed so that the top of the sheet is approximately 12 inches from the head of the mattress (see Fig. 15-1). If you are using a plastic or rubberized draw sheet, place a cotton draw sheet on top of it. Smooth the draw sheet across the bed, and tuck the near side under the mattress.

STEP 6e After mitering the corner at the head of the bed, tuck the side of the sheet underneath the mattress.

8. Now, move to the other side of the bed and repeat the process of aligning the mattress pad, mitering the corner, and tucking in the bottom sheet and draw sheet.

9. Place the top sheet on the bed so that when you unfold it, the wide hem will be at the head of the bed and the hem stitching will be facing upward, away from the person who will be occupying the bed.

a. Unfold the sheet so that only one vertical crease remains. Make sure that this crease is centered vertically on the mattress.

b. Open the sheet across the bed, taking care to keep it centered. The same length of sheet (approximately 12 to 18 inches) should hang over each side of the bed. Make sure that the top edge of the sheet is even with the head of the mattress. Pull the bottom of the sheet over the foot of the bed, but do not tuck it in yet (it will be tucked in with the blanket and bedspread).

10. Place the blanket on the bed and unfold it in the same manner as the sheet, keeping the center crease in the center of the bed. The same length of blanket (approximately 12 to 18 inches) should hang over each side of the bed. Make sure that the top edge of

(continued)

PROCEDURE 15-1 (Continued)

Making an Unoccupied (Closed) Bed

the blanket is approximately 6 to 8 inches from the head of the mattress. Fold the top edge of the sheet back over the top edge of the blanket, creating a cuff. Pull the bottom edge of the blanket over the sheet at the foot of the bed, but do not tuck anything in yet.

11. Place the bedspread on the bed and unfold it in the same manner as the sheet, keeping the center crease in the center of the bed. The sides of the bedspread should be even and cover all of the other bed linens. Make sure that the top of the bedspread is even with the head of the mattress, unless the pillow is to be tucked under the bedspread (in which case you will need to allow more length at the top). Pull the bottom of the bedspread over the blanket and sheet at the foot of the bed.

12. Together, tuck the bedspread, the blanket, and the top sheet under the foot of the mattress. Make a mitered corner at the foot of the bed on both sides.

13. Fold the top of the bedspread back over the blanket to make a cuff.

14. Rest the pillow on the bed. Grasping the closed end of the pillowcase, turn the

pillowcase inside out over your hand and arm. Grasp the pillow through the pillowcase and pull the pillowcase down over the pillow. Make sure any tags or zippers are on the inside of the pillowcase.

STEP 14 Grasp the pillow through the pillowcase and pull the pillowcase down over the pillow.

15. Place the pillow on the bed with the open end of the pillowcase facing away from the door.

Finishing Up   CLSOWR

16. Complete the "Finishing Up" steps **a** through **f**.

PROCEDURE 15-2

Making an Occupied Bed

Getting Ready   WCKIEpS

1. Complete the "Getting Ready" steps **a** through **g**.

Supplies

- gloves
- bath blanket
- mattress pad
- bottom sheet
- draw sheet
- bed protector (if necessary)

- top sheet
- blanket
- bedspread
- pillowcase

Procedure

2. Make sure that the bed is positioned at a comfortable working height (to promote good body mechanics) and that the wheels are locked.

3. Place the linens on a clean surface close to the bed (e.g., the over-bed table).

4. Remove the call light control and check the bed for dentures or any other personal items.

5. Lower the head of the bed so that the bed is flat (as tolerated).

6. Put on the gloves (the linens may be wet or soiled).

7. Remove the bedspread and blanket from the bed. If they are to be reused, fold them and place them on a clean surface, such as a chair.

8. Loosen the top sheet at the foot of the bed, and spread a bath blanket over the top sheet (and the person).

(continued)

PROCEDURE 15-2 (Continued)

Making an Occupied Bed

9. If the person is able, have him or her hold the bath blanket. If not, tuck the corners under the person's shoulders. Remove the top sheet by pulling it out from underneath the bath blanket, being careful not to expose the person.

STEP 9 Remove the top sheet by pulling it out from underneath the bath blanket.

10. Place the top sheet in the linen hamper or linen bag.

11. If the side rails are in use, lower the side rail on the working side of the bed. The side rail on the opposite side of the bed should remain up. Turn the person onto his or her side, so that he or she is facing away from you (see Chapter 11, Procedure 11-6). Reposition the pillow under the person's head, and adjust the bath blanket to keep the person covered.

12. Loosen the draw sheet, bottom sheet, and (if necessary) the mattress pad.

13. Fanfold the bottom linens toward the person's back, tucking them slightly underneath the person.

STEP 13 Fanfold the bottom linens toward the person's back.

14. Straighten the mattress pad (if it is not being changed). If the mattress pad is being changed, place the clean mattress pad on the bed and unfold it, so that only one vertical crease remains. Make sure that this crease is centered vertically on the mattress. If the mattress pad is fitted, carefully pull the corners of the near side over the corners of the mattress and smooth down the sides. If the mattress pad is not fitted, make sure the top of the pad is even with the head of the mattress. Fanfold the opposite side of the mattress pad close to the patient or resident.

15. Place the clean bottom sheet on the bed. If the bottom sheet is fitted, carefully pull the corners over the corners of the mattress and smooth down the sides. If the bottom sheet is not fitted:

   a. Place the sheet so that when you unfold it, the wide hem will be at the head of the bed and the hem stitching will be against the mattress, away from the person who will be occupying the bed.

   b. Unfold the sheet so that only one vertical crease remains. Make sure that this crease is centered vertically on the mattress.

   c. Open the sheet across the bed, taking care to keep it centered. The same length of sheet (approximately 12 to 18 inches) should hang over each side of the bed. Make sure that the lower edge of the sheet is even with the foot of the mattress. Fanfold the opposite side of the sheet close to the patient or resident.

STEP 15c Open the sheet across the bed, taking care to keep it centered.

   d. Tuck the sheet under the mattress at the head of the bed and miter the corner (see Fig. 15-6).

(continued)

PROCEDURE 15-2 (Continued)

Making an Occupied Bed

e. Tuck the near side of the sheet underneath the mattress, working from the head of the bed toward the foot. As you tuck, make sure there are no wrinkles in the sheet and that the mattress pad remains smooth and in place.

16. Place the draw sheet on the bed so that the top of the sheet is approximately 12 inches from the head of the mattress (see Fig. 15-1). If you are using a plastic or rubberized draw sheet, place a cotton draw sheet on top of it. Fanfold the opposite side of the draw sheet close to the patient or resident. Smooth the draw sheet across the bed, and tuck the near side under the mattress.

17. Raise the side rail on the working side of the bed. Help the person to roll toward you, over the folded linens. Reposition the pillow under the person's head, and adjust the bath blanket to keep the person covered.

18. Move to the other side of the bed and lower the side rail.

19. Loosen and remove the soiled bottom linens, and place them in the linen hamper or linen bag. Change your gloves if they become soiled.

20. Now, repeat the process of aligning the mattress pad, mitering the corner, and tucking in the bottom sheet and draw sheet.

21. Help the person to move to the center of the bed and position him or her comfortably. Raise the side rail on the working side of the bed.

22. Change the pillowcase (see Procedure 15-1, step 20) and place the pillow under the person's head.

23. Place the clean top sheet over the person (who is still covered with the bath blanket), being careful not to cover the person's face. The sheet should be placed so that when you unfold it, the wide hem will be at the head of the bed and the hem stitching will be facing upward, away from the person who will be occupying the bed.

a. Unfold the sheet so that only one vertical crease remains. Make sure that this crease is centered vertically on the mattress.

b. Open the sheet across the bed, taking care to keep it centered. The same length of sheet (approximately 12 to 18 inches) should hang over each side of the bed.

c. If the person is able, have him or her hold the top sheet. If not, tuck the corners under the person's shoulders. Remove the bath blanket by pulling it out from underneath the top sheet, being careful not to expose the person. Place the bath blanket in the linen hamper or linen bag.

24. Place the blanket, and then the bedspread, over the top sheet. Together, tuck the bedspread, the blanket, and the top sheet under the foot of the mattress. Make a mitered corner at the foot of the bed on both sides.

25. Make a **toe pleat** by grasping the top sheet, the blanket, and the bedspread over the person's feet and pulling the linens straight up. The toe pleat allows the person to move his or her feet and helps to relieve pressure on the feet from tightly tucked linens.

STEP 25 Make a toe pleat by pulling straight up on the top linens.

26. Lower the bed to its lowest position and make sure that the wheels are locked. Raise the head of the bed as the person requests.

27. Remove your gloves and dispose of them in a facility-approved waste container.

Finishing Up CLSOWR

28. Complete "Finishing Up" steps **a** through **f**.

Multiple Choice

Select the single best answer for each of the following questions.

1. What is a draw sheet?
   a. A fitted bottom sheet
   b. A half-sized sheet that is placed over the middle of the bottom sheet and has varied uses, including protecting the mattress from soiling
   c. A half-sized sheet that is placed over the middle of the top sheet and used to make toe pleats
   d. A sheet used to add a decorative touch to the person's room

2. What is a bed that has a person in it called?
   a. An open bed
   b. A closed bed
   c. A surgical bed
   d. An occupied bed

3. A bed that has the top linens fanfolded to the side has been prepared for what type of patient?
   a. A patient who is paraplegic
   b. A patient who is incontinent
   c. A patient who will be arriving on a stretcher
   d. A patient who will be returning to bed in the evening

4. A sheet of wood that is placed under the mattress for extra support is called:
   a. A bed cradle
   b. A bed board
   c. A stretcher
   d. An egg crate mattress

5. When you are handling linens, always remember to:
   a. Shake the bedspread to remove dust
   b. Place the dirty linens on the floor, to get them out of your way
   c. Hold the linens away from your body
   d. All of the above

6. What do you call a metal frame that is placed between the bottom and top sheets to keep the bed linens from resting on the person's feet?
   a. A bed board
   b. A pressure-relieving mattress
   c. A bed cradle
   d. A footboard

7. What personal protective equipment (PPE) should be worn when removing used bed linens?
   a. Gloves
   b. A gown
   c. Eye goggles
   d. No PPE is necessary

8. When are bed linens changed?
   a. When they become wet or soiled
   b. According to facility policy
   c. When they become excessively wrinkled
   d. All of the above

9. Mrs. Owens is returning to her room following a diagnostic procedure. She will be arriving on a stretcher. What sort of bed should you make?
   a. An open bed
   b. A closed bed
   c. A surgical bed
   d. An occupied bed

? Stop and think!

▶ You are making an occupied bed. There is no linen hamper in the room and you have already removed the soiled linens from the bed. What should you do with the soiled linens until you can take them to the linen room or hallway hamper? Mrs. O'Shea, the resident, is lying on her side in the bed, covered with a bath blanket.

▶ Barbara is a nursing assistant on 3 West. She has already changed the bed linens twice during her shift for one of her patients, Mrs. Bridges. Mrs. Bridges is receiving chemotherapy for cancer and one of the side effects of the medication is uncontrollable diarrhea. It is getting close to the end of her shift and Barbara has her fingers crossed that she can make it to 4 P.M. without having to change Mrs. Bridges' linens again. Just then, the light over Mrs. Bridge's doorway lights up. With a sigh, Barbara grabs another assistant, Linda, to help her move Mrs. Bridges because she knows it will be much easier to change the bed with help. As the two assistants enter the room, Mrs. Bridges starts to cry and says, "I'm so sorry to bother you again, but I couldn't hold it any longer. I'm so, so sorry. I wish this stuff would stop." What could Barbara say to make Mrs. Bridges feel better? What should Barbara look for while she is cleaning up Mrs. Bridges and changing her bed linens?

16

Vital Signs, Height, and Weight

What will you learn?

The word "vital" means "necessary to life." This is why those in the health care field refer to certain key measurements that provide essential information about a person's health as **vital signs.** When we evaluate a person's vital signs, we look at the person's body temperature, heart beat (pulse), breathing (respirations), and blood pressure. One of the many important duties you will perform as a nursing assistant will be to routinely measure and record your patients' or residents' vital signs. A person's height and weight, although not technically vital signs, also provide insight into a person's overall health status. Therefore, you will also be responsible for obtaining and recording these measurements (although not as frequently as the vital sign measurements). Because a change in a person's normal vital sign measurements can be a sign of illness, your ability to detect a change and report this to the nurse promptly is essential to the well-being of your patients or residents. When you are finished with this chapter, you will be able to:

1. Define the term *vital signs* and discuss how the vital signs reflect changes in a person's medical condition.
2. Understand the importance of accurately measuring and recording vital signs, and of reporting any changes to the nurse.
3. Describe the factors affecting a person's body temperature.
4. Discuss various terms used to describe an abnormal body temperature.
5. List common sites used for measuring a person's body temperature, and the advantages and disadvantages associated with each site.

(continued)

Photo: A nursing assistant gets ready to take a resident's pulse.

6. Demonstrate the proper use of a glass thermometer, an electronic or digital thermometer, and a tympanic thermometer.
7. Define the term *pulse* and describe factors that may affect a person's pulse.
8. Describe the different qualities of the pulse that a nursing assistant should be aware of when taking a person's pulse.
9. List common sites used for taking a person's pulse.
10. Diagram the parts of the stethoscope and explain how this tool is used.
11. Demonstrate the proper way to measure and record a radial pulse and an apical pulse.
12. Describe the factors that may affect a person's respirations.
13. Explain the terms used to describe a person's respirations.
14. Demonstrate the proper way to measure and record a person's respirations.
15. Define the term *blood pressure* and describe factors that may affect a person's blood pressure.
16. Discuss various terms used to describe an abnormal blood pressure.
17. Discuss the various methods used to measure a person's blood pressure.
18. Explain how a sphygmomanometer works, and demonstrate how to use this tool to measure a person's blood pressure.
19. List and describe the Korotkoff sounds, which are heard while taking a person's blood pressure.
20. Discuss factors that can lead to a change in a person's weight.
21. Demonstrate the proper way to measure a person's height and weight using an upright scale.
22. Demonstrate the proper way to measure a person's weight using a chair scale.
23. Demonstrate the proper way to measure a person's height when the person is in bed.

Vocabulary

Use the CD in the back of your book to hear these terms pronounced, defined, and used in a sentence:

Vital signs	Stethoscope	Respiratory rate	Blood pressure
Body temperature	Diaphragm	Respiratory rhythm	Systolic pressure
Metabolism	Bell	Depth of	Diastolic pressure
Pyrexia	Pulse deficit	respiration	Pulse pressure
Febrile	Tachycardia	Eupnea	Sphygmomanometer
Pulse	Bradycardia	Tachypnea	Korotkoff sounds
Pulse rate	Ventilation	Bradypnea	Hypertension
Pulse rhythm	Inhalation (inspiration)	Dyspnea	Hypotension
Dysrhythmia	Exhalation	Hyperventilation	Orthostatic
Pulse amplitude	(expiration)	Hypoventilation	hypotension

WHAT DO VITAL SIGNS TELL US?

Vital signs reflect functions that are regulated automatically by the body, such as:
- How fast the heart beats
- The internal temperature of the body
- The rate at which a person breathes

Because the body is always trying to maintain a state of balance, "control centers" (located mostly in the brain) regulate what is going on inside the body and make adjustments as necessary to keep things within the range of normal. Therefore, a change in a vital sign may indicate that something has put the body out of balance, and the body is trying to get that balance back.

There are many factors that can cause changes in a person's vital sign measurements. A person's vital sign measurements may vary over the course of a day (for example, in response to emotional or physical stress or a change in position), while still staying within the range of "normal." However, a major or a long-lasting change in one or more of a person's vital sign measurements may indicate a response to illness or injury. As you read this chapter, pay attention to the ranges that are considered "normal" for each vital sign. Knowing these ranges will allow you to quickly recognize measurements that are not within the range of normal. Also remember that your definition of "normal" will vary according to the person, especially if you are lucky enough to care for a patient or resident for an extended period of time. For example, you may come to know that Ms. Goldblum's blood pressure tends to be at the low end of the normal range, whereas Mr. Hanson's tends to be a little bit higher than average. Your knowledge of your patient or resident will allow you to know whether the vital sign measurements you have obtained are normal readings for that person.

MEASURING AND RECORDING VITAL SIGNS

Vital signs are measured and compared with normal values (as well as the values that are considered normal for the individual) under many different circumstances. For example, it is routine for vital signs to be taken each time a person visits the doctor, and when a person is admitted to a hospital or long-term care facility. It may also be necessary to check a person's vital signs:

- Before and after certain medications are given
- Before, during, and after a surgical or diagnostic procedure
- In an emergency situation

Patients in a hospital may have their vital signs taken every shift or every few hours, whereas residents of a long-term care facility may have their vital signs taken only once daily or even weekly. A patient who is critically ill may be attached to machines that measure his vital signs continuously and display the results on a monitor. The nursing care plan, the doctor's order

sheet, or both will specify how often each of your patient's or resident's vital signs are to be measured and recorded. However, it is also within your scope of practice to take a person's vital signs if the person complains of dizziness, nausea, or pain, or if you notice that the person just is not looking or acting like he or she normally does. If a person has been participating in an activity that may affect her vital signs (e.g., walking, drinking, eating) you should give the person a few minutes to sit and relax before taking her vital signs.

Facilities and agencies will have different policies regarding how vital signs are recorded. Some facilities will record vital sign measurements on one flow sheet for the unit, which lists the names of all of the patients or residents on a particular unit. Other facilities will use one flow sheet per patient or resident. This flow sheet may be kept in the person's medical record, or at the person's bedside. If you take a person's vital signs and get a measurement that is abnormal (either higher or lower than normal for that particular person), you should take the measurement again for the sake of accuracy and then report your findings to the nurse immediately.

The skills you will use to measure a person's vital signs may seem difficult when you are first learning them, but practice will make you more comfortable with taking vital sign measurements. Measuring and recording vital sign measurements accurately is critical because many people rely on this information to make important decisions about the patient's or resident's care. In addition, a problem may go unnoticed if a vital sign measurement is measured or recorded inaccurately. Always ask for assistance, either from another nursing assistant or a nurse, if you are having difficulty when checking a person's vital signs. Asking for help when you need it is not a sign of failure or an inability to do your job—rather, it demonstrates that you are responsible and interested in seeing that your patient or resident receives the best possible care. Let's take a look now at the individual vital signs, starting with body temperature.

BODY TEMPERATURE

The **body temperature** is simply how hot the body is. When we measure someone's body temperature, what we are measuring is the difference between the heat produced by the person's body and the heat lost by the person's body. The human body produces heat as a normal process of **metabolism.** Metabolism is the word used to describe the physical and chemical changes that occur when the cells of the body change the food that we eat into energy. Muscle movement also produces heat. This is why we become hotter when we exercise, and why we shiver when we are cold (shivering moves the muscles, producing heat). Heat loss occurs normally through the skin, through the passing of urine and feces, and through the process of breathing, and is increased by bodily responses such as sweating. The body temperature is regulated by a "control center" that is located in the brain.

FACTORS AFFECTING THE BODY TEMPERATURE

Although a healthy person's body temperature is usually fairly constant, small changes may occur as a result of physical or emotional stress, the environmental temperature, or even the time of day. For example, it is typical for a person's body temperature to be lower in the morning and increase slightly throughout the day, probably from an increase in activity levels. Stress causes the release of hormones that increase metabolism and the heart rate, readying the body to respond to the source of the stress. This response, called the "fight or flight" response, is discussed in detail in Chapter 30. The increase in metabolism and heart rate can lead to an increase in body temperature as well. Finally, exposure to either very hot or very cold environmental temperatures can cause changes in a person's body temperature.

A person's age and gender also play a role in determining body temperature. Very young people and very old people tend to be more sensitive to environmental temperature changes. Infants often have immature control centers, which means that their bodies are slower to adjust to changes in temperature. In addition, infants usually lose body heat through their skin more easily. An elderly person's body may not produce as much heat as it did in younger years, due to muscle loss as a result of normal aging. Finally, a woman's body temperature tends to change more frequently than a man's, because of the hormonal changes that occur with the menstrual cycle and during pregnancy and menopause.

MEASURING THE BODY TEMPERATURE

The body temperature can be measured from several different areas of the body:

- The mouth (an *oral temperature*)
- The rectum (a *rectal temperature*)
- The armpit (an *axillary temperature*)
- The ear (an *aural temperature*)
- The forehead (a *temporal temperature*)

Where the body temperature is measured depends on facility policy and the needs of the patient or resident. Because the method used to measure the temperature affects the accuracy of the measurement, you should note which method was used when you record the temperature, as per your facility's policy. For example, many facilities use "O" for oral, "R" for rectal, "T" for tympanic, and "A" for axillary. The body temperature is measured in either degrees Fahrenheit (°F) or degrees Celsius (°C), using a clinical thermometer.

Types of Clinical Thermometers

There are many different types of clinical thermometers in use.

Glass Thermometers

When most of us think of a thermometer, we think of a glass thermometer (Fig. 16-1). Glass thermometers consist of a glass bulb attached to a thin glass tube that is marked with a temperature scale and filled with mercury (a metallic substance). The mercury inside the thermometer expands with heat and moves up the glass tube, showing the temperature on the scale. The Fahrenheit thermometer is scaled from 94°F to 108°F, whereas the Celsius thermometer is scaled from 34°C to 43°C (Fig. 16-2). Before you use a glass thermometer, the mercury must be "shaken down" to below the 94° mark on a Fahrenheit thermometer, or the 34° mark on a Celsius thermometer (Fig. 16-3).

In most facilities that use glass thermometers, each patient or resident has her own thermometer, which is kept in a case at the person's bedside. Because glass thermometers are not

FIGURE 16-1

Temperatures have traditionally been taken with glass thermometers. Glass thermometers are used less often in health care settings now that other types of thermometers are available. The glass thermometer on *top,* used for taking an oral or axillary temperature, has a long, narrow bulb. The glass thermometer on the *bottom,* used for taking a rectal temperature, has a short, round bulb.

disposable, they must be cleaned properly after each use, according to facility policy. Sometimes, a clear plastic cover called a *sheath* is used to cover the thermometer, and then the sheath is discarded. The thermometer is washed with warm water and soap (never hot water, which can cause the thermometer to shatter), rinsed with cool water, and placed in a disinfectant solution. The amount of time that the thermometer must soak in the disinfectant will vary, depending on the type of disinfectant solution used. If a glass thermometer breaks while you are cleaning it (or at any other time), avoid touching the mercury and the broken glass, and prevent others from doing so as well. Call the nurse immediately. Mercury is a hazardous material and must be cleaned up according to facility policy.

FIGURE 16-3

A glass thermometer is "shaken down" before use by holding the thermometer firmly by the stem and snapping your wrist downward.

Because of the dangers associated with breakage and spilled mercury, many facilities have stopped using glass thermometers. Some facilities still use glass thermometers, but have switched to using newer models, which contain a substance that behaves the same way as mercury but is less toxic.

Electronic and Digital Thermometers

Because glass thermometers can break, posing a danger to both the patient or resident and the health care worker, more and more facilities are using electronic or digital thermometers instead (Fig. 16-4). Electronic and digital thermometers are powered by batteries, and the temperature is displayed on a screen on the front of the instrument. A probe, covered with a disposable sheath, is placed in the patient's or resident's mouth, rectum, or armpit to measure the temperature. After an electronic or digital thermometer is used, the disposable sheath is discarded.

A. Fahrenheit (F°) thermometer

B. Celsius (C°) thermometer

FIGURE 16-2

(*A*) A Fahrenheit thermometer is scaled from 94°F to 108°F. Each long line indicates 1 degree, and each short line indicates ²/₁₀ (0.2) of a degree. (*B*) A Celsius thermometer is scaled from 34°C to 43°C. Each long line indicates 1 degree, and each short line indicates ¹/₁₀ (0.1) of a degree.

A

B

FIGURE 16-4

Battery-operated electronic and digital thermometers display the person's temperature on a screen. (A) A digital thermometer. The battery in a digital thermometer is usually not rechargeable. When the battery is depleted, the thermometer is thrown away. (B) An electronic thermometer. Electronic thermometers come with battery chargers, which keep the battery continuously charged. Always remember to return an electronic thermometer to its charger after each use. (*A Chris Priest/Photo Researchers, Inc.; B courtesy of Medline Industries, Inc.*)

Tympanic Thermometers

A tympanic thermometer (Fig. 16-5) is used to measure the body temperature in the ear. The probe of this battery-operated instrument is inserted into the ear canal, where it rests near the eardrum (tympanic membrane). The person's temperature is displayed on a screen after a few seconds. Tympanic thermometers are often used for children because they allow a temperature to be measured in a safe, quick, and relatively painless manner.

FIGURE 16-5

A tympanic thermometer is inserted into the ear canal. (*Samuel Ashfield/Photo Researchers, Inc.*)

Temporal Artery Thermometers

The temporal artery thermometer represents the latest development in thermometer technology (Fig. 16-6). Remember how your mother used to place her cool hand on your hot forehead to check for a fever? The temporal artery thermometer is simply a "high-tech" version of Mom's gesture. As the device is passed over a person's forehead, it detects the body temperature at numerous points. It then performs a series of calculations on the readings to arrive at the person's peak body temperature. The temporal artery thermometer is even more accurate than a tympanic thermometer, and it is considered the least invasive of all of the thermometers available (because it does not have to be inserted into any body opening).

Sites for Measuring Body Temperature

Mouth (Oral Temperature)

Measuring a person's body temperature by placing the thermometer in his or her mouth is simple and causes the person minimal discomfort. Because the thermometer is being placed in the mouth, which is not an entirely enclosed space, the temperature reading may not be as accurate as with some of the other methods. For example, measuring the temperature in the rectum or ear gives a more accurate reading, because the

FIGURE 16-6

A temporal artery thermometer. The scanner is placed in the middle of the person's forehead and swept toward the ear, stopping behind the ear. (*Courtesy of Exergen Corporation, 2004.*)

thermometer is placed into a tightly closed space. However, many times, the reading provided by placing the thermometer in the mouth is accurate enough. An oral temperature may be measured using a glass thermometer (Procedure 16-1) or an electronic or digital thermometer (Procedure 16-2).

If a person eats, drinks, smokes, or chews gum within 15 minutes of having his or her temperature taken orally, the temperature measurement may not be accurate. If one of your patients or residents has engaged in any of these activities shortly before you intend to take his temperature orally, then you must either use a different method or wait for a period of time as specified by

your facility's policy (usually 15 to 30 minutes). In certain situations, an oral temperature should not be taken. For example, an oral temperature should not be taken if the patient or resident:

- Is unconscious
- Is unable to keep his or her mouth closed (necessary in order to keep the thermometer in place)
- Is unable to breathe through his or her nose
- Is likely to bite the oral thermometer (for example, a child younger than 5 years, a disoriented person, or a person with a history of seizures)
- Is coughing or sneezing
- Has recently had mouth surgery or an injury to the mouth
- Is receiving oxygen by a face mask (because the oxygen may cause the temperature measurement to be inaccurate)

Rectum (Rectal Temperature)

Measuring a person's body temperature by placing the thermometer in the rectum provides a more accurate measurement of the person's body temperature because the thermometer is placed in an enclosed space. However, placing the thermometer rectally is also the most risky method of taking a temperature, and it can be uncomfortable and embarrassing for the patient or resident.

A rectal temperature may be obtained using a glass thermometer (Procedure 16-3) or an electronic or digital thermometer (Procedure 16-4). In facilities where the same type of glass thermometer is used for both oral and rectal temperatures, the thermometers for rectal use have a red dot on the end. Similarly, when an electronic thermometer is used, the red probe is used rectally and the blue probe is used orally. The thermometer must be lubricated and inserted carefully into the rectum, not more than one-half inch in a child or one inch in an adult.

When you are taking a temperature rectally, it is important that you stay with the patient or resident during the entire procedure, both to hold the thermometer in place and to make sure that the person is all right. The thermometer could stimulate the vagus nerve, an important nerve that begins in the brain and sends branches to the heart, lungs, stomach, and rectum. Stimulation of the vagus nerve may temporarily decrease the person's heart rate and blood pressure, which can be dangerous. A different method of measuring the temperature should be used if the person:

- Has hemorrhoids, rectal bleeding, or a disease involving the rectum
- Has diarrhea
- Has had rectal surgery
- Has certain heart conditions

Armpit (Axillary Temperature)

An axillary temperature is measured by placing the thermometer under the person's arm and then having the person hold his arm close to his body. The axillary method provides the least reliable measurement of body temperature, but if the oral and rectal methods are not safe, and a tympanic or temporal thermometer is not available, then the axillary method can be used. The axillary temperature may be taken using a glass thermometer (Procedure 16-5) or an electronic or digital thermometer (Procedure 16-6). If the person has just washed under his or her arms, or applied deodorant or antiperspirant, then you must wait for at least 15 minutes before taking the axillary temperature. Also, if the person has recently had chest or breast surgery, and it is necessary to take the person's temperature using the axillary method, then the thermometer should be placed on the unaffected side of the body.

Ear (Aural Temperature)

Because a tympanic thermometer measures the temperature of the blood in the small vessels in the eardrum, the temperature it gives is very accurate. The aural temperature is taken with a tympanic thermometer (see Fig. 16-5). Procedure 16-7 describes how to take a tympanic temperature.

Forehead (Temporal Temperature)

A temporal artery thermometer is swept across a person's forehead to obtain a body temperature measurement (see Fig. 16-6).

NORMAL AND ABNORMAL FINDINGS

The normal body temperature varies slightly from person to person. In fact, a person's normal body temperature may be anywhere from 0.5°F to 1°F higher or lower than the range generally considered normal. The normal range also varies

TABLE 16-1 ■ Normal Adult Temperature Ranges

Method Used to Obtain Temperature	Fahrenheit (°F)	Celsius (°C)
Oral	97.6 to 99.6	36.5 to 37.5
Rectal	98.6 to 100.6	37 to 38.1
Axillary	96.6 to 98.6	36 to 37
Aural	98.6	37
Temporal	98.6	37

according to what method is used to measure the body temperature (Table 16-1).

The state of having a body temperature that is much higher than normal is called **pyrexia** (*pyr-* means "fire"). A person who has an increased body temperature is said to have a fever, or be **febrile**. Pyrexia is a common finding with illness and is the body's normal response to infection. If you think that one of your patients or residents is febrile, you should take the person's temperature (using whichever method is most appropriate for your patient or resident) and report your findings to the nurse immediately. Early detection of illness allows for earlier treatment of the problem and a better outcome for the person. A person with a fever needs to be closely monitored to make sure that her temperature does not become too high. Sometimes the doctor will order medications, such as aspirin or acetaminophen, for a person with a fever to bring her temperature down. These medications are called *antipyretic* or *fever-reducing* drugs. A person with a very high fever may benefit from additional measures, such as a cool sponge bath.

PULSE

Each time the heart beats, it sends a wave, or **pulse,** of blood through the arteries. The arteries are the blood vessels that carry oxygen-containing blood away from the heart to all of the tissues of the body. The pulse, a throbbing sensation just underneath the skin, can be felt (palpated) by placing your fingers gently over an artery that runs close to the surface of the skin, such as the carotid artery in the neck or the radial artery in the wrist (Fig. 16-7). Although we can only feel the pulse in a few of the body's arteries (those

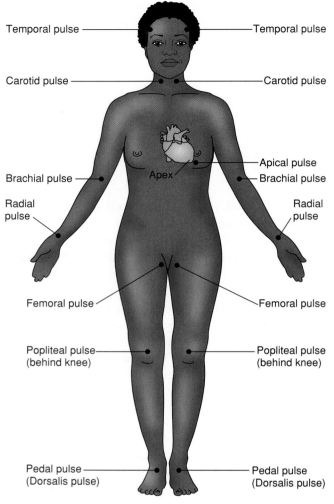

FIGURE 16-7

The pulse points are places where the arteries run close to the surface of the skin, allowing the pulse to be felt. When taking a person's pulse, it is common to place your fingers on the radial artery (in the wrist). An apical pulse can be taken by placing a stethoscope on the person's chest, over the apex of the heart.

that run closest to the surface of the skin), all of the arteries in the body have a pulse. The pulse tells us many things:

- By feeling for and counting the pulse, we are able to measure the **pulse rate,** or the number of pulsations that can be felt in 1 minute. The pulse rate tells us the heart rate, or how fast the heart is beating.
- In addition to measuring the pulse rate, we can detect the **pulse rhythm,** or the pattern of the pulsations and the pauses between them. Normally, the pulse rhythm is smooth and regular, with the same amount of time in between each pulsation. An irregular

pulse rhythm is called a **dysrhythmia** (*dys-* means "bad" or "difficult").

- Finally, we can evaluate the force or quality of the pulse, known as the **pulse amplitude** or the pulse character. Each pulsation should be strong, and easy to feel. Pulses that are difficult to feel may be described as "weak" or "thready." A weak or thready pulse usually means that the heart is having trouble circulating blood throughout the body.

FACTORS AFFECTING THE PULSE

The rate at which the heart beats is controlled automatically by the body's central nervous system. When the nervous system senses that the tissues need more oxygen and nutrients (for example, when a person is exercising), it increases the heart rate so that blood reaches the tissues faster. A person's heart rate will also increase during times of anger and anxiety, illness, pain, fever, and excitement, and when taking certain medications.

MEASURING THE PULSE

Radial Pulse

One common way of measuring the pulse rate is by placing the middle two or three fingers over the radial artery, which is located on the inside of the wrist (see Fig. 16-7), and counting the number of pulses that occur in either 30 seconds or 1 minute. The thumb is not used to palpate the artery because the thumb has its own pulse. Although the pulse may be taken at other pulse points, taking the pulse at the radial artery is easiest for the patient or resident. The carotid or femoral arteries may be used to assess the pulse during an emergency situation when cardiopulmonary resuscitation (CPR) is being administered. Procedure 16-8 describes how to take a radial pulse.

Apical Pulse

The apical pulse is measured by listening (auscultating) over the apex of the heart with a stethoscope. The apex of the heart (that is, the lower tip of the heart) is located approximately 2 inches below the level of the left nipple (see

Fig. 16-7). An apical pulse is taken when a person has a weak or irregular pulse that may be difficult to feel in the radial artery. An apical pulse may also be used to measure heart rate in infants and in people with known heart disease.

A **stethoscope,** a device that makes sound louder and transfers it to the listener's ears, is used to take an apical pulse. The stethoscope allows you to hear, rather than feel, each beat of the person's heart. The stethoscope has the following parts (Fig. 16-8):

- Earpieces, which are placed in your ears
- A brace and binaurals, which connect the earpieces to the rubber or plastic tubing that conducts the sound
- An amplifying device, which makes the sound louder

The amplifying device, which is the part of the stethoscope that is placed against the person's skin, is usually two-sided. One side, called the

diaphragm, is a large flat surface that is used to hear loud, harsh sounds like an apical pulse, blood rushing through the arteries, or respiratory sounds. The other side, called the **bell,** is a small rounded surface that is designed to pick up faint sounds like heart murmurs or difficult-to-hear blood pressures. The bell side is also commonly used to listen to apical pulses in infants and small children. The amplifying device rotates so that the sound comes from either the diaphragm or the bell, but not both at the same time.

Before using a stethoscope, clean both the earpieces and the diaphragm or bell by wiping them with alcohol wipes. Place the earpieces in each ear canal. You will know that the earpieces are placed correctly when they fit snugly, yet comfortably, and block out any outside sound. Next, tap lightly on the diaphragm. You should be able to hear the tapping. If you cannot hear the tapping, rotate the amplifying device and tap again. When you can hear the tapping, you are ready to go! Procedure 16-9 describes how to take an apical pulse using a stethoscope.

The apical pulse rate and the radial pulse rate should be the same in any single person. Occasionally, however, the heart does not pump strongly enough to send enough blood through the arteries with each beat. This means that while each beat of the heart may be heard over the apex of the heart using a stethoscope, it may not be felt in the wrist. This difference between the apical pulse rate and the radial pulse rate is known as the **pulse deficit.** The pulse deficit is measured by having one member of the nursing team take the person's apical pulse while another team member takes the person's radial pulse. The two counts are then compared to determine the pulse deficit. For example, if the apical pulse is 84 beats per minute and the radial pulse is 80 beats per minute, the difference between the apical pulse and the radial pulse (that is, the pulse deficit) is 4 beats per minute ($84 - 80 = 4$). The apical pulse rate will always be higher than the radial pulse rate, because it is easier to hear a heartbeat at the source than to feel it.

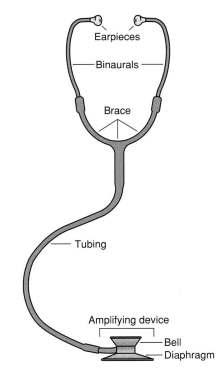

FIGURE 16-8

A stethoscope is used to listen to the heartbeat (when taking an apical pulse) or blood moving through the arteries (when taking a blood pressure). The sound is made louder by the amplifying device and transmitted by the rubber tubing to the earpieces, which fit snugly in the user's ear canals. The brace and binaurals, which are usually made of metal, connect the rubber or plastic tubing to the earpieces and prevent it from twisting or kinking, which could distort the sound. The rubber or plastic tubing may be single (as shown) or double.

NORMAL AND ABNORMAL FINDINGS

As with temperature, there is an accepted normal pulse rate. The pulse rate is faster in infants and small children and gradually slows as a person reaches adulthood. **Tachycardia** is a rapid heart rate, or a pulse rate of more than 100 beats per minute for an adult (*tachy-* means "fast" and *cardia* means "heart"). A heart rate that is slower than normal (that is, a pulse rate of less than 60 beats per minute) is called **bradycardia** (*brady-* means "slow"). Certain illnesses or conditions can cause bradycardia. Bradycardia may also be a normal finding in a young, athletic person who is very physically fit, because the person's physical conditioning allows the heart to pump stronger and more effectively, which slows the heart rate. Any change in pulse rate, rhythm, or amplitude should be reported to the nurse immediately.

RESPIRATION

Respiration is the exchange of gases between the body and the environment. As you know, in order to live, we must have oxygen, a gas that is essential for life. However, the intake of oxygen is only half of the story. We must also get rid of waste products that are created as a result of normal cellular function (metabolism). One of these waste products is carbon dioxide, a gas.

Respiration is accomplished through **ventilation,** or the mechanical process of moving air in and out of the lungs (breathing). The first phase of ventilation is **inhalation** (also called **inspiration**). When we inhale, we take oxygen-containing air into the body. Once in the lungs, the oxygen in the air passes across a thin membrane into the bloodstream, where it is carried by the red blood cells to all of the cells in the body by the action of the heart, which pumps the oxygen-rich blood throughout the body. As the body's cells use the oxygen and nutrients delivered to them by the blood, they give off carbon dioxide, which the blood takes back to the lungs. There, the carbon dioxide crosses the same thin membrane, moving from the blood into the air still remaining in the lungs. **Exhalation** (also called **expiration**) is the second phase of ventilation. When we exhale, we breathe out the carbon dioxide in the lungs. Therefore, you can see that the process of breathing performs two vital functions—it brings oxygen, a substance necessary for life, into the body, and it removes carbon dioxide, a waste product that is not necessary for life, from the body.

During the inhalation (inspiration) phase, the chest expands (rises) as air is brought into the lungs. During the exhalation (expiration) phase, the chest deflates (falls) as air moves out of the lungs. When we measure a person's respirations, what we are really looking at is the person's ventilation, or the mechanical process of breathing. We look at the person's:

- **Respiratory rate,** or the number of times a person breathes in 1 minute (one breath is both an inhalation and an exhalation)
- **Respiratory rhythm,** or the regularity with which a person breathes
- **Depth of respiration,** or the quality of each breath (for example, is it deep or shallow?)

FACTORS AFFECTING RESPIRATION

As with other vital functions, the process of breathing is controlled mainly by the central nervous system, in a part of the brain called the medulla. Control centers, called chemoreceptors, are located in the medulla and in some of the major arteries. These control centers monitor the carbon dioxide and oxygen content of the blood and adjust the rate and depth of breathing accordingly. For example, exercise increases the body's use of oxygen as well as its production of carbon dioxide and will increase both the rate and depth of a person's respirations. Other factors that may affect respiration rate, depth, and regularity include anxiety, pain, fear, fever, infections and diseases of the heart and lungs, stroke or head injury, and certain medications.

In addition to being controlled automatically by the nervous system, breathing can also be controlled to a certain extent by the individual (for example, when we "hold our breath" while swimming). In this respect, breathing is different from the other vital signs.

MEASURING RESPIRATION

Many tests are available to evaluate a person's respiratory function. The simplest approach involves no equipment, other than a watch. The respiratory rate is easily determined by watching the rise and fall of a person's chest and counting the number of breaths that occur in either 30 seconds or 1 minute. (Remember that one breath consists of both an inhalation and an exhalation.) Usually, the rise and fall of the chest can be easily observed by standing beside the person, or by watching his or her back. In some situations, you may need to stand slightly behind the person while she is seated and look down at the chest to detect the movement. Or, you can actually place your hand either near the collarbone or on the person's side to feel her breathing if it is not easily seen. Most small children and some older adults use their abdominal muscles to assist with breathing. In these people, breathing can be easily seen by watching the abdomen move instead of the chest.

Because a person can consciously control her respirations if she is aware that she is being observed, a more accurate measurement may be obtained if you measure the respiratory rate right after you take the person's pulse, with your fingers still on the person's wrist as if you were still counting the pulse. It is also easy to count a person's respirations while she sleeps, before you have awakened her to measure other vital signs. This is the one instance where it is acceptable to carry out a task without telling the patient or resident exactly what you are doing! Procedure 16-10 describes how to measure a person's respiratory rate.

NORMAL AND ABNORMAL FINDINGS

Under normal conditions, a healthy, resting adult will breathe about 16 to 20 times a minute, while infants and children may have a significantly higher respiratory rate. A normal respiratory rate is called **eupnea.** (The prefix *eu-* means "good" and the suffix *-pnea* means "breathing.") A respiratory rate that is higher than normal (greater than 24 breaths/min in an adult) is called **tachypnea,** whereas a respiratory rate that is lower than normal (less than 10 breaths/min) is called **bradypnea.** (Recall that *tachy-* means "fast," and *brady-* means "slow.") Any respiratory rate greater than 20 breaths/min or less than 12 breaths/min should be reported to the nurse.

Normally, the chest should rise and fall evenly, in a regular rhythm. Breathing should be quiet and easy. Labored or difficult respirations are termed **dyspnea** (recall that *dys-* means "bad" or "difficult"). Other notable respiratory patterns are **hyperventilation** (increased rate and depth of breathing) and **hypoventilation** (decreased rate and depth of breathing). Respirations that are shallow or labored should be reported to the nurse. If you notice that the person's chest does not rise equally on both sides, you should report that to the nurse as well.

BLOOD PRESSURE

The force that the blood exerts against the arterial walls is known as the **blood pressure.** There are two pressure levels that are measured when taking a person's blood pressure measurement. The first, known as the **systolic pressure,** is the pressure that is caused by the blood when the heart muscle contracts, sending a wave of blood through the artery. The second, known as the **diastolic pressure,** occurs when the heart muscle relaxes. Although the heart is relaxed, there is still pressure as the blood flows through the arteries.

Blood pressure is measured in millimeters of mercury (mm Hg) and is recorded as a fraction. The systolic pressure, which is higher, is recorded first, followed by the diastolic pressure, which is lower. For instance, if a person's systolic measurement is 110 mm Hg and his diastolic measurement is 72 mm Hg, then the blood pressure would be recorded as 110/72 mm Hg. The difference between the systolic and diastolic pressures is known as the **pulse pressure,** which in this case would be 38 mm Hg (110 − 72 = 38).

Blood pressure is considered a vital sign because it gives us important information about a person's health and risk for disease. Adequate blood pressure is necessary to keep blood flow constant to all of the tissues of the body. A blood pressure that is too low is a bad sign because it means the tissues of the body are not receiving enough oxygen and nutrients. On the other hand, a blood pressure that is too high forces the heart to do extra work, which, over time, damages the heart. High blood pressure also places stress on the kidneys, which can lead to kidney failure, and the blood vessels, which can lead to stroke. Blood pressure measurements allow health care workers to monitor existing problems and possibly even prevent future ones.

FACTORS AFFECTING BLOOD PRESSURE

The pressure that the blood puts on the arterial walls is controlled by three factors:

- **Cardiac output.** The cardiac output is the amount of blood that the heart is able to pump with each beat. If the heart is able to pump more blood into the vessel with each beat, then blood flow increases, leading to an increase in blood pressure. On the other hand, if the cardiac output is weak, then blood flow decreases, leading to a decrease in blood pressure.
- **Blood volume.** The amount of blood in the vessels at any given time influences the blood pressure. If the blood volume is low, for example, as a result of hemorrhage (see Chapter 12), then the blood pressure will decrease. Similarly, an increase in blood volume leads to an increase in blood pressure. In some people, a salty meal is enough to increase blood pressure, because the salt causes the body to store water, which increases the blood volume.
- **Resistance to blood flow.** Resistance is how hard it is for the blood to flow through the vessels. If the vessels are narrowed (for example, as a result of arteriosclerosis ["hardening of the arteries"]), then the resistance will be high and so will the blood pressure. Resistance is also increased when the blood is thick.

Blood pressure is also influenced by certain factors that we cannot do anything about, such as age, gender, and race:

- **Age.** Young people tend to have lower blood pressures than older people. Aging causes a decrease in the elasticity of the blood vessels (that is, the blood vessels' ability to stretch and bounce back as the blood pulses through). Decreased elasticity results in increased resistance and a higher blood pressure.
- **Gender.** Women tend to have lower blood pressures than men. However, women who take oral contraceptives ("birth control pills") may have a slightly increased blood pressure.
- **Race.** People of certain races (for example, African Americans) tend to have higher blood pressures than people of other races.

MEASURING BLOOD PRESSURE

Manually Operated Sphygmomanometers

Measuring and recording a person's blood pressure is a routine task for nursing assistants. There are many ways to measure a person's blood pressure. The most common method is by using a manually operated **sphygmomanometer** and a stethoscope. *Sphygmo-* is from the Greek word for "pulse," and *-manometer* means "a flat instrument used to measure pressure." A manual sphygmomanometer consists of:

- A cuff (a flat, cloth-covered inflatable pouch)
- A bulb, which is squeezed or pumped to fill the cuff with air
- A manometer (the device that measures the air pressure in the inflatable pouch)

Cuffs come in various sizes. The cuff must fit the person properly, or the blood pressure measurement will not be accurate. To find out what size cuff to use, measure around the person's upper arm, halfway between his or her elbow and shoulder. Cuff sizes are given in Table 16-2.

Two tubes are attached to the pouch within the cuff—one is attached to the bulb used to inflate the pouch, and the other is attached to the manometer. The manometer may be either aneroid or mercury (Fig. 16-9). An aneroid manometer is a small, round dial with a needle that indicates the pressure. A mercury manometer is a column of mercury that may be mounted on a wall or placed on a table. The manometer measures the pressure of the air in the cuff in millimeters of mercury (mm Hg). Long dashes mark increments of 10 mm Hg and the short dashes in between mark increments of 2 mm Hg.

The most common place to measure a person's blood pressure is on the brachial artery of the upper arm. However, the popliteal artery (which can be felt at the back of the person's knee) can be used as well. Measuring a blood

TABLE 16-2 ■ Blood Pressure Cuff Sizes	
Arm Measurement (cm)	Name of Cuff to Use
13 to 20	Child
24 to 32	Adult
32 to 42	Large Adult
42 to 50	Thigh

FIGURE 16-9

(*A*) A manual sphygmomanometer consists of a cuff, a bulb, and a manometer. The manometer may be either aneroid or mercury. Do you know which type of manometer is shown here? The tubes attach the inflatable pouch inside the cuff to the bulb and to the manometer. (*B*) An aneroid manometer. (*C*) A mercury manometer.

pressure is quite simple, once you have had some practice. The cuff is wrapped around the person's upper arm where the brachial artery is located. You can feel the brachial artery pulse in the antecubital space (the inner bend of the elbow) by straightening the person's arm and placing your fingers across the inside of the joint. After positioning the cuff, place the diaphragm of your stethoscope directly over where you felt the brachial artery in the antecubital space, and close the valve on the pumping bulb by turning it clockwise. Do not close the valve too tightly, or it will be difficult to release the air when you are ready. As you pump the bulb, air will enter the pouch in the cuff and you will see the needle (on an aneroid manometer) or the column of mercury (on a mercury manometer) move, indicating that the pressure of the air in the cuff is increasing.

Remember that you have two pressures that are measured within an artery, the systolic pressure (when the heart pumps) and the diastolic pressure (when the heart relaxes). When the pressure within the cuff becomes higher than the systolic pressure in the artery, it will essentially cut off the circulation and not allow any blood to flow through the brachial artery past the cuff. Continue pumping the bulb until the pressure in the cuff is 30 mm Hg higher than the systolic pressure. There are two ways to do this:

- Place the stethoscope over the brachial artery, and inflate the cuff slowly. After you have inflated the cuff a bit, you will start to

hear the pulse through your stethoscope. Continue inflating the cuff until you hear the pulse stop (this is the person's systolic pressure) and continue inflating the cuff 30 mm Hg more.
- Or, with your fingers on the person's radial pulse, you can inflate the cuff until you no longer can feel the pulse. The reading on the manometer will indicate the person's systolic pressure. Continue inflating the cuff 30 mm Hg more.

When the pressure in the cuff is 30 mm Hg higher than the systolic pressure, open the valve slightly (by turning it counter clockwise). Opening the valve slightly allows the slow release of air from the cuff, which lowers the pressure in the cuff. Under normal conditions, you may not be able to hear the brachial pulse, but under pressure, you will be able to hear the pulse through the stethoscope. As the pressure in the cuff falls (as indicated by the needle on the aneroid dial or the column of mercury) you listen for sounds, called **Korotkoff sounds** (Box 16-1), through the stethoscope. When the pressure in the cuff is equal to or slightly lower than the systolic pressure in the artery, blood will suddenly begin to flow through the brachial artery and you will start hearing the pulse. When you hear the first sound of the pulse, note the reading on the manometer. This is your systolic pressure. Now continue to listen to the pulse. When the pressure inside the cuff is less than the lowest arterial

BOX 16-1 Korotkoff Sounds

In some people, you will only be able to hear the beginning and ending sounds while auscultating the blood pressure, but in others, all of these sounds will be distinct.

Phase I: Faint but clear tapping sounds that gradually become louder. The first tapping sound is the systolic pressure.

Phase II: Muffled or swishing sounds that may actually disappear if a person has significant hypertension.

Phase III: Distinct, loud tapping sounds as the blood begins to flow more freely through the artery.

Phase IV: The sound may abruptly become muffled and soft. Keep listening.*

Phase V: The last sound heard before a period of continuous silence. This is the diastolic pressure.

---

*Occasionally, the tapping sounds of the pulse will be heard all the way down to zero. In this case, listening for the abrupt softening of phase IV will give you an approximate diastolic reading.

pressure, or diastolic pressure, the sound of the pulse will stop, because the artery is no longer under pressure. The last sound that you hear is the diastolic pressure, and is shown by the reading on the manometer.

Procedure 16-11 summarizes how to take a blood pressure. Guidelines for taking a blood pressure are given in Guidelines Box 16-1. Learning to take blood pressures takes time and practice. At first, you will need to concentrate on how to operate the equipment and control the rate at which the air leaves the cuff. Next, you will need to become familiar with the sounds that you will hear as the cuff deflates, and learn to recognize the beginning and ending sounds. Each person's blood pressure will sound slightly different. In some people, the blood pressure is easy to measure. In others, measuring the blood pressure will challenge even the most experienced nursing assistant. A good rule of thumb is if a person's brachial or radial pulse feels stronger in one arm over the other, you will have an easier time taking the blood pressure in the arm with the stronger pulse. Do not get discouraged if taking blood pressures is difficult at first. The more you practice, the more competent and confident you will

become. As with any skill you will learn, if you have difficulty taking a person's blood pressure or if you are unsure of a reading you get, always ask for a second opinion or help from another nursing assistant or a nurse. Your responsibility to the people you care for takes priority over your pride.

Automated Sphygmomanometers and Other Means of Measuring Blood Pressure

Your facility may use automated (electronic) sphygmomanometers instead of manual ones. Some automated models feature automatic inflation and deflation of the cuff, while others require the cuff to be manually inflated but will deflate it automatically. The blood pressure is displayed digitally.

A person's blood pressure can also be measured directly, by inserting a catheter into an artery, or possibly even the heart. Because this procedure is invasive (that is, something is inserted into a normally enclosed part of the person's body), it carries some risk for the person. This method of assessing blood pressure might be used when continuous blood pressure monitoring is required, such as during a surgical procedure or when a patient is critically ill.

NORMAL AND ABNORMAL FINDINGS

Normally, a person's blood pressure moves up and down within the range of normal during the course of a day. For example:

- Blood pressure readings are usually lowest in the morning, and can increase by as much as 10 mm Hg later in the day.
- Blood pressure is generally lower when a person is lying down, as compared to when he is sitting or standing.
- Blood pressure readings are usually slightly higher after a meal, especially a meal with a high salt content.
- Exercise will temporarily increase the systolic blood pressure.
- Stress, anxiety, fear, and pain will also temporarily raise a person's blood pressure.

Much medical research has been done related to the study of blood pressure and its effects on health. Studies have shown that for any individual, there is a wide range of blood pressure readings

GUIDELINES BOX 16-1
GUIDELINES FOR TAKING A PERSON'S BLOOD PRESSURE

What you do	Why you do it
Allow the person time to relax prior to taking the blood pressure.	Recent exercise and emotions (such as fear) can cause a blood pressure reading to be falsely elevated.
Make sure the manometer is properly calibrated (that is, it reads "0" when there is no air in the cuff).	A manometer that is not properly calibrated will not give an accurate pressure reading.
Use a cuff that is properly sized for the patient or resident.	A cuff that does not fit will not allow you to accurately measure the person's blood pressure. A cuff that is too small will result in a high reading, while a cuff that is too large will result in a low reading.
Make sure the cuff fits snugly around the person's arm before inflating it.	A cuff that is too loose can cause the skin to "pinch" under the cuff when the cuff is inflated, damaging the skin.
Do not place the cuff over a person's clothing.	Clothing will distort the Korotkoff sounds.
Do not take a blood pressure on an arm where an intravenous (IV) line is placed, or on an arm that is injured or in a cast.	Inflating the cuff can cause pain and swelling, and it may dislodge an IV line if one is present.
In a person who has had a mastectomy, do not take a blood pressure on the arm that is on the same side of the body as the breast that was removed.	Some people who have mastectomies also have the lymph nodes in the armpit removed, which disrupts fluid flow from the tissues in the hand and lower arm. This can lead to an inaccurate blood pressure reading.
Do not partially deflate the cuff and then reinflate it while taking a blood pressure measurement. If you make a mistake, release all of the air from the cuff and wait at least 30 seconds before trying again.	Not only is partially deflating and then reinflating the cuff uncomfortable for the patient or resident, it will result in an inaccurate reading.
If you are unable to hear the Korotkoff sounds, make sure the room is quiet and check your equipment: • Make sure the diaphragm of the stethoscope is active by gently tapping on it. • Make sure the diaphragm of the stethoscope is placed directly over the brachial pulse. • Make sure the earpieces of the stethoscope are seated properly in your ears.	Most difficulties with measuring blood pressure result from operator error. However, if you have checked your equipment and you still cannot hear the Korotkoff sounds, notify the nurse immediately. The person may have severe hypotension.

that can be considered "normal." When you are taking a person's blood pressure, it is important to allow that person time to relax or rest for a bit so that the blood pressure reading reflects the person's normal pressure, and not the changes that can occur from exertion or being emotionally upset. Also, as a nursing assistant, you must learn to recognize the range of blood pressure measurements that can be considered "normal" for each of your patients or residents, so that you will be able to recognize any changes. A person's blood pressure could rise or fall 20 to 30 mm Hg and still be within the range of what is considered normal for that person. However, a change in a person's blood pressure that is that large should be recognized and reported immediately to the nurse.

Accepted normal ranges for the systolic pressure are between 100 and 140 mm Hg, and for the diastolic pressure, between 60 and 90 mm Hg. If a person has a blood pressure that is consistently higher than 140 mm Hg (systolic) and/or 90 mm Hg (diastolic), then that person is said to have **hypertension** (high blood pressure). To diagnose a person with hypertension and start treatment for this condition, the person's blood pressure measurements must be taken and recorded over a period of time to show a pattern of constant elevation. Drugs that are taken for hypertension should be taken as ordered. If the person stops taking the drug or does not take it according to the prescribed schedule, the person's hypertension will usually return. Too often, a patient or resident will tell you that "I used to take medicine for my blood pressure, but the medicine brought my pressure back to normal, so I don't need to take it anymore." Measuring that person's blood pressure will usually tell a completely different story! Hypertension is often called the "silent killer" because a person with this condition does not feel ill, yet is at great risk for complications (and possibly even death) as a result of it.

A person who has a blood pressure that is consistently lower than 90 mm Hg (systolic) and/or 60 mm Hg (diastolic) is said to have **hypotension** (low blood pressure). Some people may have **orthostatic hypotension,** which is a sudden decrease in blood pressure that occurs when a person stands up from a sitting or lying position. When a person is sitting or lying down, the heart does not need to work as hard to pump blood throughout the body and the blood vessels are relaxed, so resistance is low. However, when the person stands up, the body needs to make up for the change in position. The heart pumps harder and the vessels constrict to bring the blood pressure back up to a normal level.

Until the body manages to make up for the sudden change in position, the person may feel lightheaded and faint. Some medications and aging can increase the time the body needs to adjust greatly. The lack of blood flow to the brain can cause the person to feel dizzy. This is why, when you are assisting a person to "dangle" (see Chapter 11), you must give the person a minute to adjust before proceeding. Always remind your patients or residents to first sit for a moment before standing up, to allow time for the body to adjust. Helping a person who experiences orthostatic hypotension to remember to take those extra few moments for the body to adjust can help prevent a fall.

For some patients or residents, you may be asked to take a sequence of blood pressures—usually first with the person lying down, then sitting, then standing. This is done to evaluate how well the person's body adapts to changes in position. Facility policy will state the order of the blood pressure measurements when a sequence of measurements is needed.

HEIGHT AND WEIGHT

Although height and weight are not technically vital signs, these measurements are taken periodically while a person is receiving care. The relationship of a person's weight to his height can provide insight into the person's overall health and nutritional status. In addition, a person's weight is often used to calculate medication dosages. In some cases, a change in a person's weight might indicate that the person's condition is getting worse, or that it is getting better. For all of these reasons, it is useful to obtain a "baseline" height and weight for each patient or resident, and to measure the person's weight periodically thereafter.

A person's height is measured only on admission. A person's weight is measured on admission, and on transfer or discharge. It may also be necessary to measure a person's weight at regular intervals throughout the person's stay. A person's weight is rechecked periodically for various reasons:

- Weight is an indicator of nutritional status.
- Weight is an indicator of heart and kidney function. If the heart or kidneys are not functioning well, the person will retain fluid, which will cause an increase in weight.
- Changes in weight can indicate disease. For example, one of the signs of some types of cancer is major, unexplained weight loss.
- Many medications are prescribed according to body weight. If a person gains or loses a great deal of weight, it may be necessary to adjust the person's medication dosages.

MEASURING HEIGHT AND WEIGHT

Height is measured in feet (') and inches (") or in centimeters (cm). Weight is measured in pounds (lbs) or kilograms (kg).

Measuring Height and Weight Using an Upright Scale

An upright scale is used to obtain height and weight measurements for a person who is able to stand on her own. An upright scale consists of a scale platform, a height scale, a height rod, and a balance bar (Fig. 16-10). The balance bar has two scale bars, and two weights. The heavier of the two weights slides along the lower scale bar, which is marked off in 50-pound increments. The lighter of the two weights slides along the upper scale bar, which is marked off in quarter-pound and pound increments. The tip of the balance bar is called the *balance pointer.* The balance pointer is centered between the two scale bars when the weight on the scales equals the person's weight. Procedure 16-12 describes how to use an upright scale to measure a person's height and weight.

Measuring Weight Using a Chair Scale

A chair scale (Fig. 16-11) is used to obtain a weight measurement for a person who cannot stand independently, but is able to get out of bed. One type of chair scale is for use with a wheelchair. The wheelchair is first weighed without the person in it to determine its weight. Next, the wheelchair, with the person in it, is rolled onto the scale. The weight of the empty wheelchair is subtracted from the weight of the wheelchair with the person in it to determine the person's weight. The other type of chair scale is simply a chair-like device that allows the person to sit while having his weight measured. Both types of chair scales display the weight digitally. Procedure 16-13 describes how to use a chair scale.

Measuring Height and Weight Using a Tape Measure and a Sling Scale

For a person who is totally bedridden, height and weight measurements may be taken while the person remains in bed, using a tape measure and a sling scale (Fig. 16-12). Procedure 16-14 describes how to obtain height and weight measurements

FIGURE 16-10

An upright scale is used to obtain height and weight measurements for people who are able to stand independently.

A   **B**

FIGURE 16-11

A chair scale is used to obtain weight measurements for a person who cannot stand up independently but is able to get out of bed. (*A*) A chair scale. (*B*) A chair scale for use with a wheelchair.

using a tape measure and a sling scale. Because sling scales from different manufacturers may vary greatly in their procedures for use, do not attempt to use a sling scale unless you have been trained in its use.

FIGURE 16-12

A sling scale is used to obtain weight measurements for a person who cannot get out of bed.

MEASURING VITAL SIGNS IN CHILDREN

The procedures for measuring vital signs are the same whether you are caring for children or adults. However, when you are measuring vital signs in a child, you will need to adjust your approach somewhat. Children can present their own challenges, depending on their age and ability to cooperate. For example, a toddler will prefer

TABLE 16-3 ■ Normal Pediatric Temperature Ranges		
Method Used to Obtain Temperature	Fahrenheit (°F)	Celsius (°C)
Oral	97–99	36–37
Rectal	98–100	37–38
Axillary	96–98	35–36
Aural	98–100	37–38

TABLE 16-4 ■ **Normal Pediatric Pulse, Respirations, and Blood Pressure Ranges**

Age of Child	Pulse Rate (beats/min)*	Respiration Rate (breaths/min)*	Blood Pressure (mm Hg)
Infant (0–1 year)	120–160	30–60	73/55
Toddler (1–3 years)	80–130	24–40	90/55
Preschooler (3–5 years)	80–120	22–34	94/60
School-age child (5–12 years)	75–110	15–25	100/75
Adolescent (12–20 years)	60–100	15–20	102/80

*The pulse and respiration rates are always measured for a full minute in children younger than 12 years.

to remain seated in his parent's lap while you are measuring his vital signs. He will be fascinated by your equipment and reach out to touch parts of it, such as the shiny stethoscope bell. Older children will expect a simple explanation of what you are going to do and how the procedure will feel. An adolescent will be very impressed that you are treating her as an adult if you tell her what the readings are as you take the vital signs.

Children who are younger than 5 years of age may not be able to cooperate fully for the measurement of an oral temperature, so an aural or axillary measurement will work best. Measure the child's pulse and respirations first, while the child is still cooperative, calm, and not suspicious of what you are doing. Make sure that you measure the pulse rate and respiratory rate for a full minute on children younger than 12 years. Blood pressure may be measured manually or with an electronic blood pressure device. The weight and age of the child determine cuff size. A cuff that is not the appropriate size will affect the accuracy of the reading.

The normal ranges for vital signs in children are given in Tables 16-3 and 16-4.

SUMMARY

▶ Vital signs provide essential information about a person's health.
  ■ The vital signs are body temperature, pulse, respirations, and blood pressure. A person's height and weight, although not technically vital signs, also provide insight into a person's overall health.
  ■ Measuring and recording vital signs is a routine part of a nursing assistant's daily duties.
    • Vital signs must be measured and recorded accurately because many people

rely on this information to make decisions about the person's care. In addition, a change in vital signs can be an important early sign that something is wrong.
  • Nursing assistants must be familiar with accepted normal ranges for all of the vital signs. In addition, nursing assistants must come to recognize what is "normal" for each of the patients or residents in their care.
  • Learning the skills associated with assessing vital signs takes practice. With practice, comes confidence.
▶ Body temperature is a measure of how hot the body is.
  ■ The body temperature can be measured using a number of devices in a number of places.
    • Types of thermometers include glass (mercury) thermometers, electronic thermometers, digital thermometers, tympanic thermometers, and temporal artery thermometers.
    • A person's temperature may be measured in the mouth, rectum, ear, armpit, or forehead.
  ■ An elevated temperature may be a sign of infection. Extreme changes in the environmental temperature can also affect a person's body temperature.
▶ The pulse reflects the rate, rhythm, and strength of the heartbeat, and therefore is a vital sign.
  ■ The pulse can be measured by feeling the radial artery (in the wrist) or by listening to the apical pulse (in the chest) with a stethoscope.
  ■ Tachycardia is an excessively rapid heartbeat. Bradycardia is an excessively slow heartbeat.
▶ The respiratory rate, rhythm, and depth are a reflection of how well the person is managing

gas exchange, or the intake of oxygen and the output of carbon dioxide.

- The respiratory rate is measured by counting the number of times the person inhales and exhales in 30 seconds (or 1 minute, if the respirations are irregular).
  - The chest rises with each inhalation and falls with each exhalation.
  - One respiration = one inhalation + one exhalation.
- Dyspnea is labored breathing. Tachypnea is a respiratory rate that is too fast, and bradypnea is a respiratory rate that is too slow.

▶ The blood pressure reflects the force the blood exerts against the arterial walls. Cardiac output, blood volume, and resistance affect the blood pressure.

- Blood pressure is most often measured in the brachial artery using a sphygmomanometer and a stethoscope.
- Korotkoff sounds are the sounds the blood makes as it rushes through the artery.
  - Phase I Korotkoff sounds signal the systolic pressure, or the pressure when the heart beats.
  - Phase V Korotkoff sounds signal the diastolic pressure, or the pressure when the heart relaxes.
  - Listening for and interpreting the Korotkoff sounds takes practice.
- Hypertension, or a consistently high blood pressure, can have serious long-term consequences if not treated.
- Orthostatic hypotension, or low blood pressure on changing positions, affects many people and is the reason people are encouraged to sit for a minute before standing up from a lying position.

▶ Height and weight are measured when a person enters a health care facility.

- Weight is measured periodically. Major weight loss or gain can be an early sign of disease. In addition, many medication dosages are calculated according to a person's body weight.
- A variety of devices, including upright scales, chair scales, and sling scales, can be used to measure a person's weight, depending on the person's situation.

Chapter 16 Procedures

Getting Ready Steps

a. **W**ash your hands and observe standard precautions as necessary.

b. **G**ather needed supplies.

c. **K**nock and introduce yourself.

d. **I**dentify the person and greet him or her by name.

e. **E**xplain the procedure.

f. **P**rovide privacy.

g. **S**ee to safety.

Finishing Up Steps

a. **C**onfirm **comfort** and good body alignment.

b. **L**eave the call light control within easy reach.

c. **S**ee to safety.

d. **O**pen the curtain and door.

e. **W**ash your hands.

f. **R**eport and record.

PROCEDURE 16-1

Measuring an Oral Temperature (Glass Thermometer)

Getting Ready **WGKIEPS**

1. Complete the "Getting Ready" steps **a** through **g**.

Supplies

- gloves
- paper towels
- tissues
- thermometer sheath (cover)
- glass thermometer

Procedure

2. Ask the person if he or she has eaten, consumed a beverage, chewed gum, or smoked within the last 15 minutes. If so, wait 15 to 30 minutes before proceeding (or follow facility policy).

3. If the thermometer has been soaking in a disinfectant solution, run cool water over the thermometer to rinse away the disinfectant. Dry the thermometer with a paper towel, and inspect it for cracks or chips.

4. Carefully shake down the thermometer so that the indicator material is below the 94° mark (if using a Fahrenheit thermometer) or the 34° mark (if using a Celsius thermometer). Cover the end of the thermometer stem with the thermometer sheath.

5. Ask the person to open his or her mouth. Slowly and carefully insert the thermometer, placing the bulb under the person's tongue, and to one side.

STEP 6 The person breathes through her nose while holding the thermometer in her mouth.

(continued)

PROCEDURE 16-1 (Continued)

Measuring an Oral Temperature (Glass Thermometer)

6. Ask the person to gently close his or her mouth around the thermometer, without biting down. If necessary, hold the thermometer in place. Ask the person to breathe through his or her nose.

7. Leave the thermometer in place for 3 to 5 minutes (or follow facility policy).

8. Ask the person to open his or her mouth. Remove the thermometer from the person's mouth.

9. Using a tissue, remove the thermometer sheath from the thermometer, being careful not to touch the bulb end of the thermometer. Dispose of the tissue and the thermometer sheath in a facility-approved waste container.

STEP 10 To read a glass thermometer, hold it horizontally by the stem at eye level.

11. To remove mucus or other debris, wipe the thermometer with a tissue, using a twisting motion and moving from the stem toward the bulb. To read the thermometer, hold it horizontally by the stem at eye level while facing a light source. Rotate the thermometer until you can see the level of the indicator material. Read the temperature.

11. Place the thermometer on a clean paper towel on the over-bed table.

12. Note the person's name, the time, the temperature, and the method on your notepad (or record the temperature and the method on the person's medical record, if it is kept at the bedside). Place an "O" (or the notation designated by your facility) next to the measurement to indicate that the measurement was taken orally. Report an abnormal temperature to the nurse immediately.

13. Shake down the thermometer, clean it according to facility policy, and return it to its disinfectant-filled case.

Finishing Up   CLSOWR

14. Complete the "Finishing Up" steps **a** through **f**.

PROCEDURE 16-2

Measuring an Oral Temperature (Electronic or Digital Thermometer)

Getting Ready   WCKIEpS

1. Complete the "Getting Ready" steps **a** through **g**.

Supplies

- probe sheath (cover)
- electronic or digital thermometer
- oral probe

Procedure

2. Ask the person if he or she has eaten, consumed a beverage, chewed gum, or smoked within the last 15 minutes. If so, wait 15 to 30 minutes before proceeding (or follow facility policy).

3. Cover the probe with the probe sheath. Turn the thermometer on and wait until the "ready" sign appears on the display screen.

4. Ask the person to open his or her mouth. Slowly and carefully insert the probe, placing the end of it under the person's tongue, and to one side.

5. Ask the person to gently close his or her mouth around the probe, without biting down.

(continued)

PROCEDURE 16-2 (Continued)

Measuring an Oral Temperature (Electronic or Digital Thermometer)

If necessary, hold the probe in place. Ask the person to breathe through his or her nose.

6. Leave the probe in place until the instrument blinks or beeps (usually just a few seconds).

7. Ask the person to open his or her mouth. Remove the probe from the person's mouth and read the temperature on the display screen.

8. Remove the probe sheath from the probe by pushing the button on the end of the probe. Direct the probe sheath into a facility-approved waste container.

9. Replace the probe. Turn the instrument off, if it does not automatically turn itself off. If you are using a digital thermometer, return it to its storage case. If you are using an electronic thermometer, place it in its charger.

(Always read the temperature before placing the thermometer in the charger because this action clears the display screen.)

10. Note the person's name, the time, the temperature, and the method on your notepad (or record the temperature and method on the person's medical record, if it is kept at the bedside). Place an "O" (or the notation designated by your facility) next to the measurement to indicate that the measurement was taken orally. Report an abnormal temperature to the nurse immediately.

Finishing Up

11. Complete the "Finishing Up" steps a through f.

PROCEDURE 16-3

Measuring a Rectal Temperature (Glass Thermometer)

Getting Ready

1. Complete the "Getting Ready" steps a through g.

Supplies

- gloves
- paper towels
- tissues
- thermometer sheath (cover)
- rectal thermometer
- lubricant jelly

Procedure

2. Make sure that the bed is positioned at a comfortable working height (to promote good body mechanics) and that the wheels are locked.

3. If the thermometer has been soaking in a disinfectant solution, run cool water over the thermometer to rinse away the disinfectant. Dry the thermometer with a paper towel, and inspect it for cracks or chips.

4. Carefully shake down the thermometer so that the indicator material is below the 94° mark (if using a Fahrenheit thermometer) or the 34° mark (if using a Celsius thermometer). Cover the end of the thermometer stem with the thermometer sheath.

5. Place the thermometer on a clean paper towel on the over-bed table. Open the

lubricant package and squeeze a small amount of lubricant onto the paper towel. Lubricate the bulb end of the thermometer to ease insertion.

6. If the side rails are in use, lower the side rail on the working side of the bed. The side rail on the opposite side of the bed should remain up. Lower the head of the bed so that the bed is flat (as tolerated).

7. Ask the person to lie on his or her side, facing away from you, in Sims' position. Help the person into this position, if necessary.

8. Fanfold the top linens to the foot of the bed. Adjust the person's hospital gown or pajama bottoms as necessary to expose the person's buttocks.

9. Put on the gloves.

10. With one hand, raise the person's upper buttock to expose the anus. Suggest that the person take a deep breath and slowly exhale as the thermometer is inserted. Using your other hand, gently and carefully insert the lubricated end of the thermometer into the person's rectum (not more than one inch for adults, or one-half inch for children). Never force the thermometer into the rectum. If you are unable to insert the thermometer, stop and call the nurse.

(continued)

PROCEDURE 16-3 (Continued)

Measuring a Rectal Temperature (Glass Thermometer)

11. Hold the thermometer in place for 3 to 5 minutes (or follow facility policy). Do not let go of the thermometer at any time!

STEP 10 Gently and carefully insert the lubricated end of the thermometer into the person's rectum.

12. Remove the thermometer from the person's rectum. Wipe the person's anal area with a tissue to remove the lubricant, and adjust the person's hospital gown or pajama bottoms as necessary to cover the buttocks.

13 Using a tissue, remove the thermometer sheath from the thermometer, being careful not to touch the bulb end of the thermometer. Dispose of the tissue and the thermometer sheath in a facility-approved waste container.

14. To remove feces or other debris, wipe the thermometer with a tissue, using a twisting motion and moving from the stem toward the bulb. To read the thermometer, hold it horizontally by the stem at eye level while facing a light source. Rotate the thermometer until you can see the level of the indicator material. Read the temperature.

15. Place the thermometer on a clean paper towel on the over-bed table.

16. Remove your gloves and dispose of them according to facility policy. Wash your hands.

17. Note the person's name, the time, the temperature, and the method on your notepad (or record the temperature and the method on the person's medical record, if it is kept at the bedside). Place an "R" (or the notation designated by your facility) next to the measurement to indicate that the measurement was taken rectally. Report an abnormal temperature to the nurse immediately.

18. Help the person back into a comfortable position, straighten the bottom linens, and draw the top linens over the person. Raise the head of the bed, as the person requests.

19. Make sure that the bed is lowered to its lowest position and that the wheels are locked. If the side rails are in use, return the side rails to the raised position.

20. Shake down the thermometer, clean it according to facility policy, and return it to its disinfectant-filled case.

Finishing Up CLSOWR

21. Complete the "Finishing Up" steps **a** through **f**.

PROCEDURE 16-4

Measuring a Rectal Temperature (Electronic or Digital Thermometer)

Getting Ready WCKIEpS

1. Complete the "Getting Ready" steps **a** through **g**.

Supplies

- gloves
- paper towels
- tissues
- probe sheath (cover)
- electronic or digital thermometer
- rectal probe
- lubricant jelly

Procedure

2. Make sure that the bed is positioned at a comfortable working height (to promote good body mechanics) and that the wheels are locked.

3. Cover the probe with the probe sheath. Open the lubricant package and squeeze a small amount of lubricant onto the paper towel. Lubricate the covered probe to ease insertion.

(continued)

PROCEDURE 16-4 (Continued)

Measuring a Rectal Temperature (Electronic or Digital Thermometer)

4. Turn the thermometer on and wait until the "ready" sign appears on the display screen.

5. If the side rails are in use, lower the side rail on the working side of the bed. The side rail on the opposite side of the bed should remain up. Lower the head of the bed so that the bed is flat (as tolerated).

6. Ask the person to lie on his or her side, facing away from you, in Sims' position. Help the person into this position, if necessary.

7. Fanfold the top linens to the foot of the bed. Adjust the person's hospital gown or pajama bottoms as necessary to expose the person's buttocks.

8. Put on the gloves.

9. With one hand, raise the person's upper buttock to expose the anus. Suggest that the person take a deep breath and slowly exhale as the thermometer is inserted. Using your other hand, gently and carefully insert the lubricated end of the probe into the person's rectum (not more than one inch for adults, or one-half inch for children). Never force the probe into the rectum. If you are unable to insert the probe, stop and call the nurse.

10. Hold the probe in place until the instrument blinks or beeps (usually just a few seconds).

11. Remove the probe from the person's rectum and read the temperature on the display screen. Wipe the person's anal area with a tissue to remove the lubricant, and adjust the person's hospital gown or pajama bottoms as necessary to cover the buttocks.

12. Remove the probe sheath from the probe by pushing the button on the side of the instrument. Direct the probe sheath into a facility-approved waste container.

13. Replace the probe. Turn the instrument off, if it does not automatically turn itself off. If you are using a digital thermometer, return it to its storage case. If you are using an electronic thermometer, place it in its charger. (Always read the temperature before placing the thermometer in the charger because this action clears the display screen.)

14. Remove your gloves and dispose of them according to facility policy. Wash your hands.

15. Note the person's name, the time, the temperature, and the method on your notepad (or record the temperature and method on the person's medical record, if it is kept at the bedside). Place an "R" (or the notation designated by your facility) next to the measurement to indicate that the measurement was taken rectally. Report an abnormal temperature to the nurse immediately.

16. Help the person back into a comfortable position, straighten the bottom linens, and draw the top linens over the person. Raise the head of the bed, as the person requests.

17. Make sure that the bed is lowered to its lowest position and that the wheels are locked. If the side rails are in use, return the side rail to the raised position on the working side of the bed.

Finishing Up CLSOWR

18. Complete the "Finishing Up" steps **a** through **f**.

PROCEDURE 16-5

Measuring an Axillary Temperature (Glass Thermometer)

Getting Ready WGKIEpS

1. Complete the "Getting Ready" steps **a** through **g**.

Supplies

- paper towels
- tissues
- thermometer sheath (cover)
- glass thermometer

Procedure

2. Ask the person if he or she has bathed or applied deodorant or antiperspirant within the last 15 minutes. If so, wait 15 to 30 minutes before proceeding (or follow facility policy).

(continued)

PROCEDURE 16-5 (Continued)

Measuring an Axillary Temperature (Glass Thermometer)

3. If the thermometer has been soaking in a disinfectant solution, run cool water over the thermometer to rinse away the disinfectant. Dry the thermometer with a paper towel, and inspect it for cracks or chips.

4. Carefully shake down the thermometer so that the indicator material is below the 94° mark (if using a Fahrenheit thermometer) or the 34° mark (if using a Celsius thermometer). Cover the end of the thermometer stem with the thermometer sheath.

5. Assist the person with removing his or her arm from the sleeve of his or her hospital gown or pajama top.

6. Pat the axilla (underarm area) gently with a paper towel.

7. Ask the person to lift his or her arm slightly. Position the bulb end of the thermometer in the center of the axilla, and ask the person to hold the thermometer in place by holding his or her arm close to the body (or by grasping the arm with the opposite hand).

STEP 7 The person holds the thermometer in place by grasping her arm with the opposite hand.

8. Leave the thermometer in place for 10 minutes (or follow facility policy).

9. Ask the person to lift his or her arm slightly. Remove the thermometer.

10. Using a tissue, remove the thermometer sheath from the thermometer, being careful not to touch the bulb end of the thermometer. Dispose of the tissue and the thermometer sheath in a facility-approved waste container.

11. To remove perspiration or other debris, wipe the thermometer with a tissue, using a twisting motion and moving from the stem toward the bulb. To read the thermometer, hold it horizontally by the stem at eye level while facing a light source. Rotate the thermometer until you can see the level of the indicator material. Read the temperature.

12. Place the thermometer on a clean paper towel on the over-bed table.

13. Note the person's name, the time, the temperature, and the method on your notepad (or record the temperature and the method on the person's medical record, if it is kept at the bedside). Place an "A" (or the notation designated by your facility) next to the measurement to indicate that the measurement was taken in the axilla. Report an abnormal temperature to the nurse immediately.

14. Help the person back into his or her hospital gown or pajama top.

15. Shake down the thermometer, clean it according to facility policy, and return it to its disinfectant-filled case.

Finishing Up

16. Complete the "Finishing Up" steps **a** through **f**.

PROCEDURE 16-6

Measuring an Axillary Temperature (Electronic or Digital Thermometer)

Getting Ready

1. Complete the "Getting Ready" steps **a** through **g**.

Supplies

- paper towels
- probe sheath (cover)
- electronic or digital thermometer
- oral probe

Procedure

2. Ask the person if he or she has bathed or applied deodorant or antiperspirant within the last 15 minutes. If so, wait 15 to 30 minutes before proceeding (or follow facility policy).

(continued)

PROCEDURE 16-6 (Continued)

Measuring an Axillary Temperature (Electronic or Digital Thermometer)

3. Cover the probe with the probe sheath. Turn the thermometer on and wait until the "ready" sign appears on the display screen.

4. Assist the person with removing his or her arm from the sleeve of his or her hospital gown or pajama top.

5. Pat the axilla (underarm area) gently with a paper towel.

6. Ask the person to lift his or her arm slightly. Position the covered probe in the center of the axilla, and ask the person to hold the probe in place by holding his or her arm close to the body (or by grasping the arm with the opposite hand).

7. Leave the probe in place until the instrument blinks or beeps (usually just a few seconds).

8. Ask the person to lift his or her arm slightly. Remove the probe and read the temperature on the display screen. Help the person back into his or her hospital gown or pajama top.

9. Remove the probe sheath from the probe by pushing the button on the end of the probe.

Direct the probe sheath into a facility-approved waste container.

10. Replace the probe. Turn the instrument off, if it does not automatically turn itself off. If you are using a digital thermometer, return it to its storage case. If you are using an electronic thermometer, place it in its charger. (Always read the temperature before placing the thermometer in the charger because this action clears the display screen.)

11. Note the person's name, the time, the temperature, and the method on your notepad (or record the temperature and method on the person's medical record, if it is kept at the bedside). Place an "A" (or the notation designated by your facility) next to the measurement to indicate that the measurement was taken in the axilla. Report an abnormal temperature to the nurse immediately.

Finishing Up CLSOWR
12. Complete the "Finishing Up" steps **a** through **f**.

PROCEDURE 16-7

Measuring an Aural Temperature (Tympanic Thermometer)

Getting Ready WGKIEpS

1. Complete the "Getting Ready" steps **a** through **g**.

Supplies

- tympanic probe sheath (cover)
- tympanic thermometer

Procedure

2. If the person wears a hearing aid, remove it carefully (see Procedure 29-1) and wait 2 minutes before taking the person's temperature.

3. Inspect the ear canal for excessive cerumen (ear wax). If you see excessive wax build-up in the ear canal, gently wipe the ear canal with a warm, moist washcloth.

4. Cover the cone-shaped end of the thermometer with the probe sheath. Turn the thermometer on and wait until the "ready" sign appears on the display screen.

5. Stand slightly to the front of, and facing, the person. To straighten the ear canal (which will ease insertion of the thermometer), grasp the top portion of the person's ear and gently pull:

   a. Up and back (in an adult)
   b. Straight back (in a child)

STEP 5a In an adult, grasp the top portion of the person's ear and gently pull up and back to insert the thermometer.

(continued)

PROCEDURE 16-7 (Continued)

Measuring an Aural Temperature (Tympanic Thermometer)

6. Insert the covered probe into the person's ear canal, pointing the probe down and toward the front of the ear canal (pretend that you are aiming for the person's nose). This will seal off the ear canal by seating the probe properly, leading to a more accurate temperature reading.

7. To take the temperature, press the button on the instrument. Keep the button depressed and the probe in place until the instrument blinks or beeps (usually 1 second).

8. Remove the probe and read the temperature on the display screen.

9. Remove the probe sheath from the probe by pushing the button on the side of the instrument. Direct the probe sheath into a facility-approved waste container.

10. Note the person's name, the time, the temperature, and the method on your notepad (or record the temperature and method on the person's medical record, if it is kept at the bedside). Place a "T" (or the notation designated by your facility) next to the measurement to indicate that the measurement was taken in the ear (i.e., using a tympanic thermometer). Report an abnormal temperature to the nurse immediately.

11. If your facility requires an aural temperature to be taken in both ears, repeat the procedure, using a clean probe cover for the other ear.

12. Turn the instrument off, if it does not automatically turn itself off. Place the thermometer in its charger. (Always read the temperature before placing the thermometer back in the charger because this action clears the display screen.)

Finishing Up   CLSOWR

13. Complete the "Finishing Up" steps **a** through **f**.

PROCEDURE 16-8

Taking a Radial Pulse

Getting Ready   WGKIEpS

1. Complete the "Getting Ready" steps **a** through **g**.

Supplies

- watch with second hand

Procedure

2. Rest the person's arm on the over-bed table or on the bed. Locate the radial pulse in the person's wrist using your middle two or three fingers. (TIP: The radial pulse will be on the person's "thumb" side.)

3. Note the strength and regularity of the pulse. Look at your watch and wait until the second hand gets to the "12" or "6." When the second hand reaches the "12" or the "6," begin counting the pulse.

   a. If the pulse rhythm is regular, count the number of pulses that occur in 30 seconds and multiply the result by 2 to arrive at the pulse rate.

   b. If the pulse rhythm is irregular, count the number of pulses that occur in 60 seconds. Counting each pulse that occurs over the course of 1 full minute is the only way to obtain a truly accurate pulse rate when the pulse is irregular.

STEP 2 Locate the radial pulse in the person's wrist using your middle two or three fingers.

(continued)

PROCEDURE 16-8 (Continued)

Taking a Radial Pulse

4. Note the person's name; the time; and the pulse rate, rhythm, and amplitude on your notepad (or record the pulse rate, rhythm, and amplitude on the person's medical record, if it is kept at the bedside). Report an abnormal pulse to the nurse immediately.

Finishing Up CLOSURE

5. Complete the "Finishing Up" steps **a** through **f**.

PROCEDURE 16-9

Taking an Apical Pulse

Getting Ready WGKIEPS

1. Complete the "Getting Ready" steps **a** through **g**.

Supplies

- alcohol wipes
- dual-sided stethoscope
- watch with second hand

Procedure

2. Help the person to a sitting position by raising the head of the bed.

3. Using alcohol wipes, clean the earpieces, the diaphragm, and the bell of the stethoscope. Place the earpieces in your ears.

4. Place the diaphragm (or the bell, if the person is a child or infant) of the stethoscope under the person's clothing, on the apical pulse site (located approximately 2 inches below the person's left nipple). The diaphragm or bell must be placed directly on the person's skin because clothing will distort the sound.

5. Using two fingers, hold the diaphragm or bell firmly against the person's chest. Look at your watch and wait until the second hand gets to the "12" or "6." When the second hand reaches the "12" or the "6," begin counting the heartbeat.

6. Count the number of heartbeats that occur in 60 seconds. Each time the heart beats, you will hear two sounds, best described as a "lubb" and a "dupp." Both sounds constitute one beat of the heart and should be counted as such.

STEP 5 Hold the diaphragm or bell firmly against the person's chest.

7. After 60 seconds, remove the diaphragm of the stethoscope from the person's chest. Adjust the person's clothing as necessary, and help the person back into a comfortable position. Lower the head of the bed, as the person requests.

8. Note the person's name; the time; the pulse rate, rhythm, and amplitude; and the method on your notepad (or record the pulse rate, rhythm, and amplitude and the method on the person's medical record, if it is kept at the bedside). Place an "a" (or the notation designated by your facility) next to the measurement to indicate that the measurement was taken apically. Report an abnormal pulse to the nurse immediately.

9. Using alcohol wipes, clean the earpieces, the diaphragm, and the bell of the stethoscope.

Finishing Up CLOSURE

10. Complete the "Finishing Up" steps **a** through **f**.

PROCEDURE 16-10
Counting Respirations

Getting Ready WCKIEPS

1. Complete the "Getting Ready" steps **a** through **g**.

Supplies

• watch with second hand

Procedure

2. Look at your watch and wait until the second hand gets to the "12" or "6." When the second hand reaches the "12" or the "6," look at the person's chest and begin counting each rise and fall of the chest as one breath.

   a. If the respiratory rhythm is regular, count the number of breaths that occur in 30 seconds and multiply the result by 2 to arrive at the respiratory rate.

   b. If the respiratory rhythm is irregular, count the number of breaths that occur in 60 seconds. Counting each respiration that occurs over the course of 1 full minute is the only way to obtain a truly accurate respiratory rate when the person's breathing is irregular.

3. Note the person's name, the time, and the respiratory rate on your notepad (or record the respiratory rate on the person's medical record, if it is kept at the bedside). Report abnormal respirations to the nurse immediately.

Finishing Up CLSOWR

4. Complete the "Finishing Up" steps **a** through **f**.

PROCEDURE 16-11
Measuring Blood Pressure

Getting Ready WCKIEPS

1. Complete the "Getting Ready" steps **a** through **g**.

Supplies

• alcohol wipes   • stethoscope
• sphygmomanometer

Procedure

2. Assist the person into a sitting or lying position. Position the person's arm so that the forearm is level with the heart, and the palm of the hand is facing upward. Assist the person with rolling up his or her sleeve so that the upper arm is exposed.

3. Using alcohol wipes, clean the earpieces, the diaphragm, and the bell of the stethoscope.

4. Stand no more than 3 feet away from the manometer. If it is not mounted on the wall, stand a mercury manometer upright on a flat surface, at eye level. Lay an aneroid manometer on a flat surface, directly in front of you, or leave it attached to the blood pressure cuff.

5. Squeeze the cuff to empty it of any remaining air. Turn the valve on the bulb clockwise to

close it; this will cause the cuff to inflate when you pump the bulb.

6. Locate the person's brachial artery in the antecubital space by placing your fingers at the inner aspect of the elbow.

STEP 6 Palpate the person's brachial artery in the antecubital space (inner aspect of the elbow).

7. Place the arrow mark on the cuff over the brachial artery. Wrap the cuff around the person's upper arm so that the bottom of the cuff is at least l inch above the person's elbow. The cuff must be even and snug.

(continued)

PROCEDURE 16-11 (Continued)

Measuring Blood Pressure

8. Place the stethoscope earpieces in your ears.

9. Hold the bulb in one hand and feel for the person's radial pulse (in his or her wrist) with the other hand. Inflate the cuff until you are no longer able to feel the radial pulse, and then inflate the cuff 30 mm Hg more.

STEP 9 Hold the bulb in one hand and feel for the person's radial pulse (in the wrist) with the other hand.

10. Position the diaphragm of the stethoscope over the brachial artery.

11. Turn the valve on the bulb slightly counter-clockwise to allow air to escape from the cuff slowly.

12. Note the reading on the manometer where the first Korotkoff sound is heard. This is the systolic reading.

13. Continue to deflate the cuff. Note the reading on the manometer where the last Korotkoff sound is heard. This is the diastolic reading.

14. Deflate the cuff completely and remove it from the person's arm. Remove the stethoscope from your ears.

STEP 12 With the diaphragm of the stethoscope over the person's brachial artery, allow the air to leave the cuff slowly while listening for the Korotkoff sounds and watching the manometer.

15. Note the person's name, the time, and the blood pressure on your notepad (or record the blood pressure on the person's medical record, if it is kept at the bedside). Report an abnormal blood pressure to the nurse immediately.

16. Return the sphygmomanometer to its case or wall holder.

17. Using alcohol wipes, clean the earpieces, the diaphragm, and the bell of the stethoscope.

Finishing Up CLSOWR

18. Complete the "Finishing Up" steps **a** through **f**.

PROCEDURE 16-12

Measuring Height and Weight Using an Upright Scale

Getting Ready WCKIEpS

1 Complete the "Getting Ready" steps **a** through **g**.

Supplies

- *upright scale*

Procedure

2. Ask the person to urinate. If necessary, assist the person to the bathroom or offer the bedpan or urinal (see Chapter 20, Procedures 20-1 and 20-2).

3. Move the weights all the way to the left of the balance bar.

4. Help the person onto the scale platform, so that she is facing the balance bar. Once the person is on the scale platform, do not allow her to hold on to you or to the scale.

5. Move the heavy weight on the bottom scale bar to the right to the weight closest to the

(continued)

PROCEDURE 16-12 (Continued)

Measuring Height and Weight Using an Upright Scale

person's prior weight. For example, if the person weighed 155 pounds the last time you weighed her, you would move the large weight to the "150" mark.

6. Move the light weight on the top scale bar to the right until the balance pointer is centered between the two scale bars.

7. Read the numbers on the top and the bottom scale bars where each weight has settled and add these two numbers together. This is the person's weight.

8. Have the person carefully turn around to face away from the scale bar. Slide the height scale up so that you can pull out the height rod, which extends from the top of the height scale. Be careful not to hit the person in the head with the height rod.

9. Slide the height rod down so that it lightly touches the top of the person's head. Read the number at the point where the height rod meets the height scale. This is the person's height.

10. Hold the height rod in your hand, and help the person step down from the scale.

11. Assist the person back to her room.

12. Note the person's name, the time, and the weight and height on your notepad (or record the weight and height on the person's medical record, if it is kept at the bedside). Report a change in the person's weight to the nurse.

STEP 9 Slide the height rod down so that it lightly touches the top of the person's head.

Finishing Up CLSOWR

13. Complete the "Finishing Up" steps **a** through **f**.

PROCEDURE 16-13

Measuring Weight Using a Chair Scale

Getting Ready WGKIEPS

1. Complete the "Getting Ready" steps **a** through **g**.

Supplies

• transfer belt   • wheelchair*

_____

*If you will be using a wheelchair scale to weigh the person, take the empty wheelchair to the wheelchair scale and weigh it before taking it to the person's room. Be sure to write down the weight of the unoccupied wheelchair.

Procedure

2. Ask the person to urinate. If necessary, assist the person to the bathroom or offer the bedpan or urinal (see Chapter 20, Procedures 20-1 and 20-2).

3. Assist or wheel the person to the scale, using a transfer belt, a wheelchair, or both.

4. Reset the scale to "0" by turning it on.

(continued)

PROCEDURE 16-13 (Continued)

Measuring Weight Using a Chair Scale

5. Help the person onto the scale.

   a. If a regular chair scale is being used, help the person to sit in the chair on the scale. Make sure the person is seated properly, with his buttocks against the back of the chair and his feet on the footrests.

   b. If a wheelchair scale is being used, roll the occupied wheelchair onto the platform and lock the wheels.

6. Read the weight on the display screen. If a wheelchair scale is being used, you must subtract the weight of the unoccupied wheelchair from this figure to determine the person's weight.

7. Help the person off of the scale.

   a. If a regular chair scale is being used, assist the person out of the chair and back into a wheelchair, if one was used for the transfer.

   b. If a wheelchair scale is being used, unlock the wheels and roll the wheelchair off the platform.

8. Assist the person back to his room.

9. Note the person's name, the time, and the weight on your notepad (or record the weight on the person's medical record, if it is kept at the bedside). Report a change in the person's weight to the nurse.

Finishing Up

10. Complete the "Finishing Up" steps a through f.

PROCEDURE 16-14

Measuring Height and Weight Using a Tape Measure and a Sling Scale

Getting Ready

1. Complete the "Getting Ready" steps a through g.

Supplies

- sling scale
- tape measure

Procedure

2. Ask the person to urinate. If necessary, assist the person to the bathroom or offer the bedpan or urinal (see Chapter 20, Procedures 20-1 and 20-2).

3. Position the sling scale next to the bed. Make sure that the bed is positioned at a comfortable working height (to promote good body mechanics) and that the wheels are locked. If the side rails are in use, lower the side rail on the working side of the bed. The side rail on the opposite side of the bed should remain up.

4. Fanfold the top linens to the foot of the bed.

5. Center the sling under the person. (To get the sling under the person, move the person as if you were making an occupied bed—see Procedure 15-2.)

6. Position the person in the supine position, or according to the manufacturer's instructions.

7. Move the release valve on the sling scale to the closed position.

8. Raise the sling scale so that it can be positioned over the person.

9. Spread the legs of the sling scale to provide a solid base of support. The legs must be locked in this position, or the scale could tip over, injuring you, the person you are trying to weigh, or both.

10. Move the scale into position over the person.

11. Fasten the sling to the straps or chains of the scale. Make sure the hooks face away from the person.

12. Cross the person's arms over her chest.

13. Slowly raise the sling until the person is clear of the bed.

14. Read the weight on the display screen. Note the person's name; the time; and the weight on your notepad (or record the weight on the person's medical record, if it is kept at the bedside). Report a change in the person's weight to the nurse.

(continued)

PROCEDURE 16-14 (Continued)

Measuring Height and Weight Using a Tape Measure and a Sling Scale

15. Gently lower the person to the bed and re-move the sling by gently rolling the person first to one side, then the other.

STEP 17 Using a pencil, mark the bottom sheet at the top of the person's head and at his heels.

16. Position the person in the supine position, with her arms by her sides and her legs straight.

17. Using a pencil, make a small mark on the bottom sheet at the top of the person's head. Make another small mark at her heels.

18. Using the tape measure, measure the distance between the pencil marks. This is the person's height.

19. Note the person's name; the time; and the height on your notepad (or record the height on the person's medical record, if it is kept at the bedside).

20. Make sure that the bed is lowered to its lowest position and that the wheels are locked. If the side rails are in use, return the side rails to the raised position.

Finishing Up

21. Complete the "Finishing Up" steps **a** through **f**.

What did you learn?

Multiple Choice

Select the single best answer for each of the following questions.

1. A stethoscope is used to determine the:
   a. Brachial pulse rate
   b. Carotid pulse rate
   c. Apical pulse rate
   d. Popliteal pulse rate

2. Which one of the following is the pressure exerted by the blood flowing through the arteries when the heart muscle relaxes?
   a. Diastolic pressure
   b. Pulse pressure
   c. Pulse deficit
   d. Systolic pressure

3. The most common site for counting the pulse is the:
   a. Brachial artery
   b. Radial artery
   c. Carotid artery
   d. Apex of the heart

4. When counting respirations, you should:
   a. Have the person exercise first to get a true reading
   b. Count five respirations and then check your watch
   c. Avoid telling the person what you are going to do
   d. Have the person count respirations while you take her pulse

5. You are using a glass Fahrenheit thermometer. When you shake it down, the mercury should be below the:
   a. 98.6°F mark
   b. Arrow

c. 100°F mark
   d. 94°F mark

6. Which of the following can cause an inaccurate oral temperature reading?
   a. The person exercised vigorously 15 minutes prior to having his temperature taken
   b. The nursing assistant failed to shake down the mercury thermometer
   c. The person drank a cup of hot coffee 15 minutes prior to having his temperature taken
   d. All of the above

7. One of your patients, Ms. Jones, has a temperature of 98.8°F, a pulse rate of 80 beats/min, and a respiratory rate of 30 breaths/min. Which finding should be reported to the nurse immediately?
   a. Ms. Jones' respiratory rate
   b. Ms. Jones' pulse rate
   c. Ms. Jones' temperature
   d. None of these findings needs to be reported to the nurse

8. Which one of the following could cause a decreased pulse rate?
   a. Pain
   b. Anger
   c. Certain medications
   d. Fever

9. What should you observe when taking a person's pulse?
   a. The rhythm and regularity of the pulse
   b. The number of beats per minute
   c. The strength of the pulse
   d. All of the above

10. If you notice a significant change in a person's vital signs, what should you do?
    a. Record the change with a special notation to indicate that the reading was different
    b. Mention the change to the nurse at the end of your shift
    c. Tell the patient or resident about the change
    d. Report the change to a nurse immediately
11. Which instrument is used to measure blood pressure?
    a. A temporal artery thermometer
    b. A sphygmomanometer
    c. An upright scale
    d. A watch with a second hand
12. Which one of the following conditions would prevent you from taking an oral temperature?
    a. The person has diarrhea
    b. The person has just had a mastectomy
    c. The person is unconscious
    d. The person is a 10-year-old child

Stop and think!

▶ You are assigned to take vital signs on all the residents in the north hall of your facility. Mrs. Tito, in room 102, has a cast on her left arm and an intravenous (IV) line in her right. How are you going to take Mrs. Tito's blood pressure?

▶ It is almost time for your shift to end, and you are having trouble getting a blood pressure reading on Mr. Hayes. You really need to leave work on time today, because your spouse is out of town and your daughter will be waiting for you to pick her up at school. Mr. Hayes is looking and acting the same way he always does so you have no reason to think that his blood pressure would be different today than it is any other day. Would it be acceptable to just copy yesterday's blood pressure measurement, since you really need to leave work on time? Why or why not? If not, what could you do to make sure that you still get out of work on time?

17

Cleanliness and Hygiene

What will you learn?

In this chapter, we will begin to explore the nursing assistant's role in helping people with **activities of daily living (ADLs),** or the routine tasks of daily life (such as bathing, eating, and grooming). Most people handle these tasks easily on their own, but people who are sick, injured, or otherwise disabled often need help with these basic activities. You will recall the discussion in Chapter 3 about how important good personal hygiene (cleanliness) is for both physical and emotional health. In this chapter, you will learn how to assist your patients or residents with keeping their skin and mouths clean, two activities that are key to maintaining personal hygiene. When you are finished with this chapter, you will be able to:

1. Describe the practices that make up personal hygiene.
2. Understand the importance of good hygiene in relation to a person's physical and emotional well-being.
3. Discuss how personal and cultural preferences influence a person's hygiene practices.
4. Describe practices that are considered to be a part of oral hygiene.
5. Explain situations that may require a person to need more frequent oral hygiene.
6. Discuss actions that promote the safe handling of a person's dentures.
7. Demonstrate proper technique for providing oral care for a person with natural teeth, for a person with dentures, and for an unconscious person.
8. Explain why perineal care is an essential aspect of daily hygiene.
9. Discuss sensitivity issues that a nursing assistant should be aware of when assisting with perineal care.
10. Demonstrate proper technique for providing perineal care for males and for females.

(continued)

Photo: A nursing assistant assists a resident in the tub room, following a shower.

11. Explain how bathing and skin care benefit a person's health.
12. List the methods of bathing a nursing assistant may be asked to assist with.
13. Describe observations that a nursing assistant should make while assisting a person with bathing and skin care.
14. Explain the benefits of massage.
15. Demonstrate proper technique for bathing a person (in bed or in a shower or bathtub), and giving a back massage.

Vocabulary

Use the CD in the back of your book to hear these terms pronounced, defined, and used in a sentence:

Activities of daily living (ADLs)	Evening (hour of sleep, hs) care	Pyorrhea	Circumcision
Early morning care	PRN (as-needed) care	Halitosis	Foreskin
Morning (A.M.) care	Diaphoretic	Edentulous	Deodorant
Afternoon care	Gingivitis	Perineal care (peri-care)	Antiperspirant
		Perineum	

THE BENEFITS OF PERSONAL HYGIENE

Personal cleanliness, also known as personal hygiene, helps to promote both physical and emotional health. The practices associated with personal hygiene—skin care (including bathing and moisturizing) and oral care (including brushing the teeth and flossing)—keep the skin and the mucous membranes of the mouth healthy. As you will remember from Chapter 7, the skin and mucous membranes of the body act as the first line of defense against infection. Caring for the skin and the mouth helps to prevent conditions such as rashes, dry skin, and cracked lips, which interrupt the body's first line of defense by creating a portal of entry for microbes. In addition, keeping the skin and mouth clean helps to reduce the number of microbes on these surfaces, which also helps to minimize the risk of infection.

In addition to promoting physical health, good personal hygiene promotes emotional health by helping a person to feel relaxed and well cared for. A person who feels relaxed and comfortable is able to rest better. Being clean and refreshed also helps a person meet his or her need for self-esteem (see Chapter 6) by preventing body and breath odors and making the person feel attractive to others.

SCHEDULING OF ROUTINE CARE

In many health care facilities and agencies, routine activities associated with personal hygiene are carried out at specific times throughout the day:

- **Early morning care** is provided after a person wakes up to prepare him or her for breakfast or early diagnostic testing or treatment. The person is assisted with using the toilet, washing of the face and hands, and mouth care. Dentures may need to be inserted prior to eating. Many people will want to have their hair brushed or combed. Residents of long-term care facilities may need help with dressing, in preparation for breakfast in the dining room.
- **Morning (A.M.) care** is when the morning personal hygiene routine is completed, to prepare the person for the day. During morning care, patients and residents are assisted with using the toilet, bathing, oral care, shaving, hair care, dressing, and putting on make-up. The degree of assistance each patient or resident will need in carrying out these activities will vary. In some facilities, the morning bath is followed by a back massage. General housekeeping

duties, such as tidying the person's room and changing the bed linens, are also performed during morning care. Facility policies differ regarding the frequency of bathing and linen changes.

- **Afternoon care** is care that is provided before and after lunch and dinner. Many people rest or receive visitors in the early afternoon. A general "freshening up" involves assistance with using the toilet, washing of the hands and face, and oral care.
- **Evening (hs, hour of sleep) care** is provided in preparation for sleep. During evening care, patients or residents are assisted with washing their hands and face, brushing their teeth, changing into pajamas, and using the toilet. Other bedtime preparations include straightening the bed linens and fluffing the pillows. Many residents in long-term care facilities may prefer to bathe in the evening instead of in the morning. "Extras," such as a bath, soft music and a back massage, or reading in bed for a while before turning out the light can help a person fall into a restful sleep. Allowing for these "extras" when providing evening care to your patients or residents shows a caring and compassionate attitude, because you are considering the person's preferences and honoring these wishes whenever possible.

The scheduling of routine personal care promotes efficiency and allows the nursing staff to plan these activities around other scheduled activities, such as meals, treatments, visiting hours, and social events. Sometimes, however, it is necessary to break from the schedule in order to accommodate a person's needs. **PRN (as-needed) care** is personal hygiene care that is provided whenever a patient or resident needs it, throughout the day or night. For example, a person in a coma needs frequent mouth care because he will tend to breathe through his mouth and he cannot take food or liquids orally, situations that put him at risk for a dry mouth. An incontinent person requires perineal care (peri-care), or cleansing of the genital and anal region, each time she loses control of her bowel or bladder. If her clothing or bedding is wet or soiled, these items will need to be changed as well. A person who is **diaphoretic** (that is, a person who has a medical condition that causes him to sweat a great deal) may need partial sponge baths, fresh linens, and a change of clothes frequently throughout the day. Any situation or condition that causes wetness or soiling of the skin, clothing, or bedding needs immediate attention.

RESPECTING THE INDIVIDUAL

In some situations, care is provided according to the facility's or agency's schedule, but adjustments are made in order to take into account the patient's or resident's personal preferences. For example, many long-term care facilities schedule baths as a routine part of the morning care, but some residents may prefer a bath later in the day or in the evening. Whenever possible, the resident's request should be granted. If you had always bathed in the evening, before bed, and then after entering a nursing home were told you had to bathe in the morning, how would you feel? Patients and residents may be required to change their normal routines to a certain extent to conform to the policies of the hospital or long-term care facility, but you can look for ways to accommodate each of your patient's or resident's personal preferences, while still following the rules of the facility. For example, asking a person whether he prefers to bathe in the morning or in the evening, allowing him to choose either bar soap or liquid soap, and permitting him to use the type of deodorant he is used to using will show that you care about the person as an individual. These actions will also help the person to maintain a sense of familiarity in an otherwise changed life. Certain cultural and religious beliefs may discourage bathing during certain times or may promote ritualistic bathing as part of a ceremony or spiritual service. Whenever possible, you should make an effort to accommodate these preferences as well.

Some patients or residents may refuse a personal care procedure, such as a bath, and they do have the right to refuse. For example, a resident may ask to skip his or her bath for many reasons: "I'm tired and I want to sleep," "I feel a cold coming on," "I don't feel up to it today." You could insist that the person bathe, creating tension and causing the person to feel unappreciated and disrespected. Or, you could offer to help the person "just freshen up a bit instead" and actually achieve the goal of bathing in a different manner. For example, you could assist the person with a partial bath at the sink instead of a complete bath in a tub or shower. With this approach, the person is clean but was allowed to refuse his or her bath (so to speak), and you have fulfilled your responsibility while also respecting the person's wishes.

For some patients and residents, such as those who have dementia or are confused, bath time can be very frightening. People who are confused or demented simply do not understand what you intend to do to them and they cannot remember what bathing is all about. Extra help from your coworkers and a calm, efficient attitude will help. Sometimes, singing to a confused person or playing soothing music will help to calm the person a bit. If a person refuses personal hygienic care consistently, report this to the nurse. If a person is unable to understand the consequences that can result from a lack of bathing or skin care, the decision may be made to bathe the person against his or her wishes out of respect for the person's health.

When assisting a patient or resident with personal hygiene, think about how you would feel if you were in that person's situation. You might feel embarrassed, because you have to rely on someone else to help you with one of life's most basic tasks. You might also feel exposed because another person (possibly of the opposite sex) is seeing and touching your body. It is very important that you acknowledge your patient's or resident's feelings and provide as much privacy and modesty as possible. A professional but compassionate attitude when performing intimate hygienic care is so important. For many reasons (such as cultural or religious beliefs, or a history of physical abuse), some people may object strongly to being touched by a member of the opposite sex, or even by a member of the same sex. Please respect your patient's or resident's wishes and work to find a suitable compromise, if at all possible.

At first, you may also feel embarrassed or uncomfortable when you need to help another person with personal hygiene. Having to bathe another adult or clean up someone else's bowel movement or urine may seem very unpleasant or awkward to you. But think of it this way—what if you were sick or injured to the point that you had wet yourself or had a bowel movement in the bed? Or you were simply too weak and sick to take a bath, and you were just lying in bed in a pool of your own sweat? Think of how wonderful it would feel to have someone clean you up, help you brush your teeth, change your clothes, and give you fresh bed linens. You would feel clean, refreshed, relaxed, and most importantly, cared for.

ASSISTING WITH MOUTH CARE

Keeping the mouth and teeth clean and healthy is an important part of personal hygiene. A clean, healthy mouth feels good and makes food taste better, and contributes to overall health. Poor oral hygiene can cause **gingivitis** (inflammation of the gums), which can lead to **pyorrhea** (gum disease). Gum disease is the main cause of tooth loss in people older than 35 years. Dental cavities and **halitosis** (bad breath that does not go away) are also caused by poor oral hygiene. Helping your patients and residents with oral care presents many opportunities for observation.

➡ *Tell the Nurse!*

While assisting a person with oral care, pay attention to the following:

➡ Dry, red, cracked, or bleeding lips

➡ Cold sores on the lips

➡ Red, irritated, swollen, or bleeding gums

➡ Cracked, chipped, or broken teeth; loose teeth; blackened teeth (possibly a sign of decay)

➡ Chipped, cracked, or poorly fitting dentures

➡ Red sores or canker sores inside the mouth; white spots inside the mouth; any areas of pus or infection

➡ Bad breath that does not improve after oral care

➡ Fruity-smelling breath (possibly a sign of diabetes mellitus)

➡ A red or swollen tongue or a white coating on the tongue

Oral care is usually provided on awakening, after meals, and before bed. People who are unable or not allowed to take food or fluids by mouth will need oral care as often as every 1 or 2 hours to keep their mouths fresh and moist. Most people can manage their own oral care, with assistance as needed. A person who is not allowed out of bed may still be able to brush and floss her own teeth, if you provide the necessary supplies. Occasionally a person will be too ill or weak to provide oral care for himself, and you will need to provide this care for him. Because the gums sometimes bleed as a result of routine oral care, it is important to practice standard precautions when assisting with brushing and flossing the teeth or cleaning dentures.

PROVIDING ORAL CARE FOR A PERSON WITH NATURAL TEETH

Natural teeth are best cleaned with a toothbrush and toothpaste, followed by flossing. Because bacteria in the mouth do the most damage to the teeth and gums after eating, the best time to brush is after meals. Brushing alone is not enough to remove food that lodges between the teeth, so flossing once a day is recommended as part of good oral hygiene. Many people like to use a mouthwash after brushing to complete their oral care routine. The use of mouthwash can further reduce harmful bacteria in the mouth.

Toothbrushes should have soft bristles and be small enough to reach all of the teeth. Electric toothbrushes are simple to use and effective, especially for people who have limited strength or use of their hands.

Procedure 17-1 describes how to assist a person with brushing and flossing the teeth.

PROVIDING ORAL CARE FOR A PERSON WITH DENTURES

Dentures and partial dentures take the place of a person's natural teeth, allowing the person to chew his or her food properly. Dentures that do not fit properly or that hurt the mouth when worn are not very useful for chewing. Proper care of the gums and dentures helps to keep the dentures fitting properly and comfortably.

Some people wear their dentures all of the time. Others may leave their dentures out at night or only wear them for meals. When a person has removed his dentures, the person is said to be **edentulous,** or without teeth. Personal preference for wearing dentures is to be respected, although it is important for a person who wears dentures to wear the dentures fairly consistently. If the dentures are not worn for a long period of time, the gum line can change, changing the way the dentures fit. If the dentures do not fit well, they will be uncomfortable and they will not work properly. Remember that people are more likely to wear their dentures if they are kept clean.

It is good practice to have a person rinse his or her dentures after every meal to remove any food that becomes trapped between the gums and dentures. Dentures must be handled carefully because they are expensive to replace. Dentures are cleaned over a water-filled sink lined with either a washcloth or paper towels. The towel acts as a cushion to help prevent breaking or chipping of the denture, should you accidentally drop it into the sink while cleaning it. A denture brush (or a toothbrush) and denture cleaner (or toothpaste) are used to clean all surfaces of the denture, and then the denture is rinsed with lukewarm water. Hot water should not be used because it can damage the dentures.

If the dentures are to be returned to the person's mouth, allow the person to rinse with water or mouthwash and use a soft toothbrush or a sponge-tipped swab to clean the person's gums and tongue and the insides of the cheeks before replacing the dentures. Wet dentures are easier to place in the person's mouth than dry ones. Dentures that are not being returned to the person's mouth should always be stored in a denture cup covered with lukewarm water, a 50/50 solution of mouthwash and lukewarm water, or a special denture solution, because the plastic that dentures are made from can dry out and warp if not kept wet. The denture cup should be identified with the person's name and room number. Procedure 17-2 describes how to provide oral care for a person who wears dentures.

PROVIDING ORAL CARE FOR AN UNCONSCIOUS PERSON

A person who is unconscious needs frequent mouth care to keep the mucous membranes of the mouth moist and healthy. An unconscious person breathes with her mouth open, which causes secretions to thicken and dry on the lips and in the mouth. These dried secretions, along with the intake of air through the mouth, can lead to cracking of the lips and tongue. Cracked, dry lips are very uncomfortable and they create a portal of entry for microbes. As always when caring for a person who is unconscious, remember to explain what you are doing, even though the person may not seem to be able to hear you.

Natural teeth are gently brushed with either a small amount of toothpaste or saline (salt water). If the person is edentulous, the gums, tongue, and inside of the cheeks are cleaned using a sponge-tipped swab moistened with saline or mouthwash. The mouth can be rinsed with a small amount of saline or water to clean out dried secretions. Care must be taken when performing oral care for an unconscious person to prevent aspiration of saline, water, toothpaste, mouthwash, or saliva. (Recall from Chapter 12 that aspiration is the inhalation of foreign material into the airway.) To prevent aspiration, turn the person on her side so that fluids run out of the mouth, not back toward the throat. You may need to place a padded tongue blade between the upper and lower back teeth to keep the mouth open during oral care (Fig. 17-1). Because an unconscious person may bite down involuntarily and without warning, never place your fingers in the person's mouth. Lubricant should be applied to keep the lips moist. Procedure 17-3 describes

FIGURE 17-1

It may be necessary to use a padded tongue blade to keep an unconscious person's mouth open while providing oral care. A padded tongue blade is made by folding a gauze square around two wooded tongue blades and taping the gauze in place.

how to provide oral care for a person who is unconscious.

ASSISTING WITH PERINEAL CARE

Perineal care (peri-care) is the cleaning of the **perineum** and associated structures (Fig. 17-2). In women, the perineum extends from the bottom of the vagina to the anus. In men, the perineum extends from the root of the penis to the anus. When nurses talk about "providing perineal care," they mean cleaning the perineum and anus, as well as the vulva (in women) and the penis (in men).

Making sure that the perineum, the vulva (in women), and the penis (in men) are clean is important for two main reasons:

- **Prevention of infection.** Because many microbes live in our digestive tracts and are passed from the body in the feces, there are always large numbers of microbes in and around the anus. The perineal area provides the perfect environment to support the growth of these microbes, because it is warm, dark, and moist. Because the perineum is close to the vulva (in women) and the penis (in men), these microbes can easily enter the vagina or urethra, causing infection. Therefore, inadequate hygiene in the perineal area puts the person at risk for infection.
- **Prevention of skin breakdown and odor.** The perineum, vulva, and penis are delicate, with many folds of skin. Feces, urine, and other body fluids, such as menstrual blood, can become trapped in these folds, leading to skin irritation and odor if they are not properly removed.

Perineal care is routinely performed at least once daily, as part of the bath. People with diarrhea or who are incontinent of urine or feces will need perineal care performed more frequently, as will women with vaginal bleeding (from surgery, childbirth, or menses) or vaginal discharge. Any person who can manage her own perineal care should be encouraged to do so to the best of her ability. A person who is unable to provide for her own self-care will need your help. When helping your patients and residents with perineal care, be aware of signs and symptoms that could indicate a health problem.

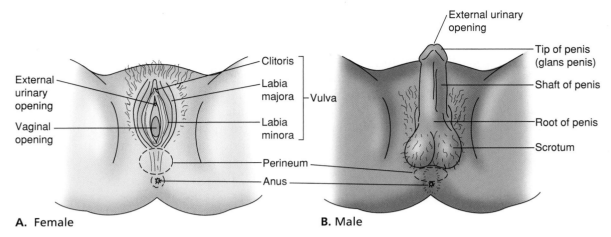

FIGURE 17-2

Perineal care refers to care of the perineum and associated structures. (*A*) The female perineum and associated structures. (*B*) The male perineum and associated structures.

![Tell the Nurse!]

▶ *Tell the Nurse!*

Tell the nurse immediately if you observe any of the following signs when providing perineal care for one of your patients or residents:

⟹ Any unusual redness, inflammation, or skin rashes in the perineal area

⟹ Any unusual discharge from the vagina or penis

⟹ Any bleeding from the vagina (especially in a postmenopausal woman) or the anus

⟹ Any abnormal odor

When you are providing perineal care for a person, you must have the person's consent for the procedure before beginning. For example, while helping a person with a bath, you may explain what you are about to do and ask the person's permission to go further. Make sure to explain the procedure completely, using professional yet understandable words (such as "crotch," "privates," "bottom," or "the area between your legs"). When there is a language barrier, stop and think. You may need an interpreter.

Perineal care can be embarrassing, both for the person receiving it and for the person providing it. Very few people are comfortable exposing their most private body parts to strangers, or seeing the private body parts of strangers. Draping the person's body with a bath blanket so that only the area to be cleaned is exposed helps to preserve the person's sense of modesty (Fig. 17-3). Another potential source of embarrassment for both

FIGURE 17-3

A bath blanket is used to preserve the person's modesty during perineal care. (*A*) The bath blanket is placed over the person's body so that one corner is pointing toward the person's head and the other is between the person's legs, covering the perineum. The other two corners are to the right and to the left, respectively. (*B*) The right corner is brought under and around the person's right leg, and then the same is done on the left.

the patient or resident and the nursing assistant is the fact that male patients or residents may become aroused during perineal care, simply from stimulation of the penis during washing. Acting in a professional, competent manner and using a gentle touch will help to ease embarrassment on the part of the patient or resident. Guidelines for providing perineal care are given in Guidelines Box 17-1.

PROVIDING PERINEAL CARE FOR FEMALE PATIENTS AND RESIDENTS

Procedure 17-4 describes how to assist a female patient or resident with perineal care.

PROVIDING PERINEAL CARE FOR MALE PATIENTS AND RESIDENTS

Male patients or residents may be circumcised or uncircumcised (Fig. 17-4). **Circumcision** is a procedure involving the removal of the **foreskin,** the fold of loose skin that covers the head of the penis. Male infants are often circumcised for religious or cultural reasons. When you are assisting an uncircumcised man with perineal care, it is important to pull the foreskin back so that the head of the penis can be cleaned thoroughly. After cleaning and rinsing the penis, always remember to pull the foreskin back up over the head of the penis. If the foreskin is not pulled back into place, it can create a band around the penis, causing pain and swelling. Procedure 17-5 describes how to assist a male patient or resident with perineal care.

ASSISTING WITH SKIN CARE

BATHING

Bathing serves many purposes. The act of bathing:
- Makes a person feel relaxed and refreshed
- Cleans the skin and eliminates body odors
- Exercises muscles that might otherwise not be used
- Stimulates blood flow to the skin (through touching and massaging of the skin), which helps to prevent skin breakdown

- Helps the patient or resident meet the needs of love and belonging and self-esteem
- Gives the nursing assistant an opportunity to observe for skin problems and to communicate and bond with the patient or resident

The frequency and method of bathing are determined by many factors, including:
- Personal choice
- The person's state of health
- The weather
- The person's level of activity
- The person's ability to care for himself
- The policies and procedures of the facility or agency

For example, people may bathe more often during the warmer months or when they are most active, and less often during the winter months or periods of physical inactivity. Hospital policy may state that patients receive daily baths, while the policy of a long-term care facility may call for residents to receive complete baths or showers two or three times weekly with partial baths on days in between.

Supplies for Bathing

Various supplies are used for bathing and skin care, many of which you are already familiar with:
- **Soap,** available in liquid or cake form, is used to clean the skin. The lather lifts away dirt, oil, microbes, and sweat. Because soap is drying to the skin, it is

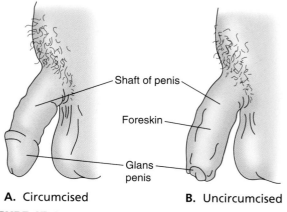

A. Circumcised   **B.** Uncircumcised

FIGURE 17-4

Male patients or residents may have a circumcised or uncircumcised penis. (*A*) A circumcised penis. (*B*) An uncircumcised penis.

What you do	Why you do it
Explain the procedure to the person, even if he or she is unconscious.	Many people find being touched in an intimate area by a stranger embarrassing, frightening, or even offensive. Explaining the procedure in a professional way helps to put the person at ease and reassures the person that he or she will be treated with respect.
Take care to protect the person's modesty.	Receiving perineal care can be very embarrassing. Properly draping the person may help to relieve some of the person's discomfort and feeling of being "exposed."
Always check the temperature of the water using a bath thermometer. The water temperature should be between 110°F (43.3°C) and 115°F (46.1°C).*	Water that is too cold is uncomfortable, and water that is too hot could scald the person. A bath thermometer provides *objective* information. Testing the water with your hand provides *subjective* information. (In other words, water that "feels all right" to your touch may, in reality, be much too hot or too cold. The only way to know that the water temperature is within the safe range is to measure it.)
Follow standard precautions when providing perineal care.	Providing perineal care places you at risk for exposure to urine, feces, and other body substances (for example, blood, vaginal secretions, semen).
Perineal care is the last part of a person's bathing routine. Washcloths, towels, and the water in the wash basin (if a bed bath is being given) are discarded and not used on any other body parts after the perineal care is completed.	The anus is a source of microbes and the perineum provides an environment that supports their growth. To prevent spread of these microbes to other parts of the body, where they may gain access and cause infection, the perineal area is washed last.
The vulva (in women) or the penis (in men) is cleaned before the perineum.	Because the anus opens onto the perineum, the perineum is often contaminated with microbes from the digestive tract. Therefore, this area is washed last to prevent microbes from the digestive tract from being introduced into the vagina or urethra, where they can cause infection.
Rinse the skin thoroughly to remove all soap.	The skin of the perineum and surrounding structures is very delicate. Soap is drying and can irritate the skin if not rinsed away. Squeezing clean, warm water from a washcloth held over the perineal area is a very effective method of rinsing when giving a bed bath.
Gently pat the skin dry. Do not rub vigorously. Dry the skin thoroughly.	The skin of the perineum and surrounding structures is very delicate. Vigorously rubbing the skin with a towel is uncomfortable for the person and can create friction, which in turn can cause skin breakdown. Moisture in areas where skin comes in contact with skin can also lead to skin breakdown.
Remove your gloves and wash your hands before touching clean clothing or linens.	Gloves worn while providing perineal care are considered contaminated.

*The water in the basin can be slightly hotter [110°F (43.3°C)] than the water in a tub or shower [105°F (40.5°C)] because it cools off quickly and the person will not be immersed in it.

important to rinse it away completely. For people with dry, fragile skin (such as elderly people), it may be better to use a soapless cleanser or just plain water.

- **Soapless cleansers.** Often, these products are supplied on premoistened disposable cloths. Many soapless cleansers do not need to be rinsed away. These products clean, moisturize, and protect the skin. Some of these products are for use specifically in the perineal area.
- **Bath oils** are added to the bath water to scent and moisten the skin. Because bath oils make the surface of the bathtub slippery, these products should be used with caution.
- **Lotions** and **creams,** which may be perfumed or unscented, are applied to skin that is still slightly damp to create a moisture barrier that helps to prevent drying and chapping. Lotions and creams are an especially important part of skin care for elderly people, because with aging, the skin secretes a reduced amount of natural oil, resulting in dryness and a loss of elasticity.
- **Body powder** can help absorb moisture and sweat and reduces friction between skin surfaces that touch. Powder should only be applied to skin that has been dried thoroughly. When using powder, sprinkle a small amount into the palm of your hand, and then gently pat it onto the person's skin. Avoid big clouds of powder—too much powder can irritate the skin, and if the person inhales it, then it can irritate the airways too. In addition, powder spilled on the floor can be very slippery.
- **Deodorants** and **antiperspirants** are often applied after bathing to help prevent body odor. **Deodorants** are products that cover or mask odor. **Antiperspirants** contain ingredients that stop or slow the secretion of sweat. Most antiperspirant products also contain a deodorant. Application of an antiperspirant or deodorant should be included as part of a person's hygiene routine if the person requests it.

Most people are particular about the skin care products they use. Some people are sensitive or allergic to ingredients commonly used in skin care products. If you notice that one of your patients or residents develops itching, redness, or a rash after using a skin care product, please report this observation to the nurse and stop use of that particular product until the source of the skin irritation has been determined. Always ask new patients or residents if they have particular preferences in skin care products, or if there are any products that cause problems for them.

In addition to skin care products, a variety of linens are used for bathing. Bath blankets are used to preserve a person's modesty during a bed bath or when providing perineal care. A washcloth is wrapped around the hand to form a "mitt" for cleansing the body (Fig. 17-5). A towel is used to dry the body, and can also be used to help preserve the person's modesty. A clean gown, pajamas, or change of clothes should be available for the patient or resident to put on after the bath.

Standard Bathing Techniques

A complete bath, or one that involves the entire body, is not always necessary. In some cases, a complete bath may not be allowed for medical reasons. For example, a person who has just had surgery may not be able to take a complete bath until her incision has healed. When a complete bath is not possible, a partial bath will provide many of the same health benefits and achieve the same goals of odor and infection control. During a partial bath, only the face, hands, axillae (armpits), back, buttocks, and perineal area are

FIGURE 17-5

Making a bath mitt from a washcloth.

washed. A partial bath can be done at the sink or, if the person cannot get out of bed, at the bedside. In long-term care facilities, a partial bath is often part of the morning care on days that the resident is not scheduled to have a complete bath. A partial bath can also be provided anytime a person needs to "freshen up."

The amount of assistance each resident or patient will need to bathe will vary according to the person's degree of disability. For people who can bathe themselves, you will only need to see that they have bathing supplies and clean clothes. Some people will only need your help to clean hard-to-reach areas, such as the back or feet. Others will need your help throughout the bath. You should encourage your patients or residents to do as much for themselves as possible during bathing and other personal care routines. Allowing a person to perform as much of her personal hygiene routine as possible on her own encourages feelings of independence and self-worth. It also provides a form of exercise, increasing the person's muscle tone, mobility, and circulation. General guidelines for assisting patients and residents with bathing are given in Guidelines Box 17-2.

Assisting your patients or residents with bathing provides an excellent opportunity for you to observe the patient's or resident's skin and body for any changes in condition that should be reported to the nurse. Because you will be caring for the person regularly, you will be more likely to notice changes that might go unnoticed by others.

▶ *Tell the Nurse!*

Tell the nurse immediately if you observe any of the following signs or symptoms while assisting a person with his or her bath:

⟾ New rashes, bruises, broken skin, bleeding, or unusual odors

⟾ Areas that are red, pale, or have a bluish cast (cyanosis)

⟾ Areas that are swollen or tender

⟾ Any complaints of burning or itching

⟾ New hair loss (anywhere on the body, not just on the head)

⟾ A flaking, itchy, or sore scalp or the presence of nits (head lice)

⟾ Redness or yellow discoloration of the sclera (that is, the whites of the eyes)

⟾ Yellowing or thickening of the fingernails or toenails

⟾ Changes in mental status and alertness (for example, disorientation, confusion)

Shower or Tub Baths

A shower or tub bath is the preferred method of bathing, because it allows for thorough cleaning and rinsing of the skin. Showers in many facilities have stalls that are large enough for a shower chair to fit inside, allowing a weak or unsteady person to sit down while taking a shower (Fig. 17-6). Some long-term facilities have whirlpool tubs that stimulate blood flow and relax muscles by the action of the water (Fig. 17-7). These tubs usually have chair-lift devices to allow for easy and safe transfer of residents into and out of the tub. The lift devices also allow people who are in a coma or who are severely physically disabled to receive the comfort and benefit of a whirlpool bath. Most tubs have a shower attachment so that hair can be washed during the bath. Many modern tub and shower units also have controls that pre-set the water temperature, ensuring that it is not too hot or too cold.

FIGURE 17-6

Shower stalls in health care facilities are usually wide enough to accommodate a shower chair. Use of a shower chair helps to reduce the risk of falling.

GUIDELINES BOX 17-2
GUIDELINES FOR BATHING

What you do	Why you do it
Follow the doctor's orders or the nursing care plan when determining what type of bath the person is to receive.	A person's medical condition may dictate the type of bath he or she can have. For example, a person with a spinal injury may not be permitted to have a whirlpool bath, whereas for a person with poor skin circulation, a whirlpool bath may be considered a type of therapy.
Before beginning the bath, explain to the person how the bathing procedure will be carried out (and how the person can assist in the process). In addition, explain the benefits of bathing (such as comfort, healthy skin).	Explaining the details of the bathing process may help to relieve the person's fears (for example, about potential exposure), and will help the person to see how he or she can participate in the process. Explaining the procedure is particularly important for people with memory problems, who may find the bathing experience very frightening because they cannot remember what bathing is or why it is important.
Collect all necessary equipment, linens, bath products, and clothing before beginning the bath. If the person will be taking a tub bath, check the tub room for cleanliness and prepare the tub before bringing the person into the room.	Being prepared and having all necessary supplies and equipment at hand will allow the bath to proceed efficiently. Efficiency is necessary to protect the person's modesty and to prevent chills.
Close all doors and windows in the room, and make sure the blinds are down or the curtains are drawn.	Closing doors and windows eliminate drafts in the room, which could cause the person to become chilled. In addition, closing doors and covering the windows protects the person's modesty and privacy.
Place a nonskid mat in the bathtub or on the shower floor. Encourage the person to use handrails. Provide a shower chair for people who are weak or unsteady.	These measures help to protect the person from falling.
Always keep the bathroom door unlocked.	Because you should never leave a person alone in the bathtub or shower, if you need help for any reason, you will have to call for someone to come to you. This person will need to be able to access the bathroom without your help.
Always check the temperature of the water using a bath thermometer. The water temperature should be between 105°F (40.5°C) and 115°F (46.1°C).	Water that is too cold is uncomfortable, and water that is too hot could scald the person. A bath thermometer provides *objective* information. Testing the water with your hand provides *subjective* information. (In other words, water that "feels all right" to your touch may, in reality, be much too hot or too cold. The only way to know that the water temperature is within the safe range is to measure it.)
When assisting a person to and from the tub room, always make sure that he or she is adequately covered.	The person's privacy and modesty must be protected at all times.
Always help the person into and out of the bathtub or shower.	A wet bathroom floor can be slippery, and can place the person at risk for falling.

GUIDELINES BOX 17-2
GUIDELINES FOR BATHING

What you do	*Why you do it*
Follow standard precautions when bathing a person.	Bathing a person places you at risk for coming into contact with non-intact skin or body fluids.
Wash from the cleanest to the dirtiest areas.	This approach prevents contamination of clean areas.
Touch the person's body gently yet deliberately, using long, firm strokes.	A gentle yet firm touch conveys to the person that this is a routine procedure being carried out by a professional, ensures that the skin is properly cleaned, and stimulates skin circulation.
Rinse the skin thoroughly to remove all soap.	Soap is drying and can irritate the skin if not rinsed away.
Gently pat the skin dry. Do not rub vigorously. Dry the skin thoroughly, especially in areas where skin touches skin (for example, underneath the breasts, between the legs).	The skin, especially that of elderly people, is fragile. Vigorously rubbing the skin with a towel is uncomfortable for the person and can create friction, which in turn can cause skin breakdown. Moisture in areas where skin comes in contact with skin can also lead to skin breakdown.

A

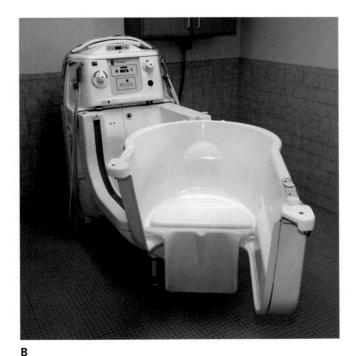

B

FIGURE 17-7

(*A*) Many long-term care facilities have whirlpool tubs, which help to stimulate circulation and massage the skin. (*B*) On this model, the front of the tub swings open to make it easier for the patient or resident to get into and out of the tub.

Procedure 17-6 describes how to assist with a tub bath or shower. After each use, the tub or shower stall (and the shower chair, if one was used) is disinfected. This is important to prevent the spread of infection. Facility policy will state who is responsible for cleaning and disinfecting the bathing equipment.

Bed Baths

Some patients and residents are simply too weak or ill to take a shower or tub bath. In this situation, bath supplies and a basin of warm water are brought to the bedside, and the person is assisted with bathing in bed (Fig. 17-8). A complete or partial bed bath is given, depending on the needs of the patient or resident (Procedures 17-7 and 17-8, respectively).

An alternative to the traditional bed bath is the use of a "bag bath." With this method, a plastic bag containing 8 to 10 washcloths soaked in a soapless cleanser is warmed in the microwave, and a different cloth is used to clean each main body part. "Bag baths" are very comfortable and refreshing for the patient or resident, and they are efficient and effective for the nursing staff (Fig. 17-9).

FIGURE 17-9
Many facilities use "bag baths" as a quick and efficient alternative to a traditional bed bath.

MASSAGE

Illness, disability that results in loss of mobility, and aging all contribute to a loss of blood flow (circulation) to the skin. A person who sits in a chair or wheelchair for long periods of time or who must remain in bed is at an increased risk for developing pressure ulcers (see Chapter 24) as a result of that lack of blood flow. Massaging the skin regularly helps to stimulate the circulation. It is also very relaxing for the patient or resident. A back massage is usually performed after a person's bath while rubbing lotion or cream into the skin, when repositioning a helpless person, or as a part of evening care to promote relaxation and sleep. Some studies have shown that slow, gentle massage can calm sick babies and confused or demented elderly people who become agitated easily.

An effective back massage takes approximately 4 to 6 minutes to complete and can be performed with the person in either the prone or the lateral position. The extra minutes spent massaging a patient's or resident's back are well worth the effort and are beneficial for both physical and emotional health. While performing a back massage, you have an excellent opportunity to observe the person's skin for potential problems.

FIGURE 17-8
When a shower or tub bath is not possible, a bed bath can be given. Some patients or residents, like the man shown here, will be able to bathe themselves with minimal assistance, whereas others will require a great deal of assistance.

▶ *Tell the Nurse!*

Skin breakdown can lead to pressure ulcers. Tell the nurse immediately if you observe any of the following early signs of skin breakdown:

➠ Reddened skin, especially over a bony area, that does not return to its normal color after a gentle massage

➠ Pale, white, or shiny skin over a bony area

➠ Areas of skin that are hot to the touch

➠ Areas of skin that are painful or tender

As with any personal care procedure, always check with a nurse or read the person's nursing care plan before beginning—a back massage should not be performed on a person with fractured ribs or a back injury, nor should it be performed on a person who has recently had back surgery. Procedure 17-9 describes how to give a back massage.

SUMMARY

▶ Cleanliness of the body is essential for a person's physical and emotional well-being.
  ■ Healthy skin and mucous membranes help protect the body from being invaded by infection-causing microbes.
  ■ Feeling clean also improves a person's self-esteem and increases comfort.
▶ Allowing people to participate in their own self-care helps to maintain independence, but assisting as necessary helps to ensure that hygiene is performed thoroughly. Assisting a person with personal hygiene activities provides many opportunities for observation.
▶ Activities associated with personal hygiene are usually carried out at scheduled times throughout the day.
  ■ When possible, adjustments are made to the schedule to accommodate personal preferences (for example, bathing in the evening versus the morning).
  ■ Assistance with personal hygiene is provided any time that a patient's or resident's condition warrants it. Wet or soiled skin, clothing, or bedding requires immediate attention.
▶ Mouth care involves caring for the teeth, gums, lips, and mucous membranes of the

mouth. A clean, healthy mouth makes food taste better, provides a line of defense against infection, and allows a person to chew his or her food properly.
  ■ Natural teeth should be brushed and flossed daily.
  ■ Dentures must be handled with care because they are expensive.
  ■ Standard precautions should be taken when providing oral care because contact with body fluids is possible. Droplet precautions should be taken if the patient or resident is known to have an infection caused by exposure to droplets released from the mouth or nose.
▶ Perineal care involves cleansing of the perineum, the anus, the vulva (in women), and the penis (in men).
  ■ Inadequate hygiene in the perineal area places a person at risk for infection and skin breakdown, and can lead to unpleasant odors.
  ■ Because receiving assistance with perineal care is embarrassing for most people, take extra care to preserve the person's modesty. Having a professional attitude when assisting a person with perineal care also demonstrates competence and helps to ease embarrassment on the part of the patient or resident.
  ■ Standard precautions should be taken when providing perineal care because contact with body fluids is likely.
  ■ Always wash toward the anus, away from the urethra. This helps to prevent the spread of microbes from the anus and perineum into the urethra or vagina, where they could cause infection.
▶ Skin care involves keeping the skin clean and moisturized. Skin care may also involve massage to enhance blood flow to the skin.
  ■ Bathing may be accomplished in a bathtub or shower, at the sink, or in bed.
  ■ During a partial bath, only the face, hands, axillae, back, buttocks, and perineum are washed.
  ■ A back massage is relaxing for the patient or resident and helps to prevent the development of pressure ulcers.

Chapter 17 Procedures

Getting Ready Steps

a. **W**ash your hands and observe standard precautions as necessary.

b. **G**ather needed supplies.

c. **K**nock and introduce yourself.

d. **I**dentify the person and greet him or her by name.

e. **E**xplain the procedure.

f. **P**rovide privacy.

g. **S**ee to safety.

Finishing Up Steps

a. **Confirm comfort** and good body alignment.

b. **L**eave the call light control within easy reach.

c. **S**ee to safety.

d. **O**pen the curtain and door.

e. **W**ash your hands.

f. **R**eport and record.

PROCEDURE 17-1
Brushing and Flossing the Teeth

Getting Ready WGKIEPS

1. Complete the "Getting Ready" steps **a** through **g**.

Supplies

- gloves
- paper towels
- straw (optional)
- paper cups
- emesis basin
- toothbrush
- toothpaste
- dental floss
- lip lubricant (optional)
- mouthwash (optional)
- towels

Procedure

2. Cover the over-bed table with paper towels. Place the oral care supplies on the over-bed table. Fill a paper cup with water. Put on the gloves.

3. Make sure that the bed is positioned at a comfortable working height (to promote good body mechanics) and that the wheels are locked.

4. If the side rails are in use, lower the side rail on the working side of the bed. The side rail on the opposite side of the bed should remain up.

5. Raise the head of the bed as tolerated. Place a towel under the person's chin.

6. Wet the toothbrush. Put a small amount of toothpaste on the toothbrush.

7. Brush the person's teeth as follows:

   a. Position the toothbrush at a 45° angle to the gums, against the outer surface of the top teeth. Starting at the back of the mouth, brush the outer surface of each tooth using a gentle circular motion. Repeat for the lower teeth. Allow the person to spit toothpaste into the emesis basin as necessary.

STEP 7a Clean the outer surfaces of the teeth.

   b. Position the toothbrush at a 45° angle to the gums, against the inner surface of the top teeth. Starting at the back of the mouth, brush the inner surface of each tooth using a gentle circular motion. Repeat for the lower teeth.

(continued)

PROCEDURE 17-1 (Continued)

Brushing and Flossing the Teeth

STEP 7b Clean the inner surfaces of the bottom teeth.

  c. Brush the chewing surfaces of the upper and lower teeth using a gentle circular motion.

STEP 13c Clean the chewing surfaces of the bottom teeth.

  d. Brush the tongue.

8. Offer the person the cup of water (and a straw, if desired) and ask her to rinse her mouth completely. Hold the emesis basin underneath the person's chin so that she can spit the water into the basin.

STEP 8 Hold the emesis basin underneath the person's chin so that she can spit.

9. Place the emesis basin on the over-bed table, and dry the person's mouth and chin thoroughly using a towel.

10. Cut a piece of dental floss measuring about 18 inches. Wrap the dental floss around the middle finger of each hand. Hold the dental floss between your thumb and index finger on each hand and stretch it tight.

STEP 10 Hold the dental floss between your thumb and index finger on each hand and stretch it tight.

11. Insert a segment of dental floss between two teeth, starting with the back upper teeth. Move the floss up and down gently, and then remove the dental floss from the person's mouth. Advance the floss a bit by releasing it from one middle finger and wrapping it around the other, and move on to the next two teeth. Use a new strand of dental floss as necessary. Offer the person the glass of water (and the straw, if desired) to rinse as necessary. Floss all of the person's teeth.

12. Offer the person the cup of water (and the straw, if desired) and ask her to rinse her mouth completely. Hold the emesis basin underneath the person's chin so that she can spit the water into the basin.

13. Place the emesis basin on the over-bed table, and dry the person's mouth and chin thoroughly using a towel.

14. Pour a small amount of mouthwash (approximately ¼ cup) into another paper cup and help the person to rinse, as the person requests.

15. Apply lip lubricant to the lips, as the person requests.

(continued)

PROCEDURE 17-1 (Continued)

Brushing and Flossing the Teeth

16. If the side rails are in use, return the side rails to the raised position. Lower the head of the bed as the person requests. Make sure that the bed is lowered to its lowest position and that the wheels are locked.

17. Gather the soiled linens and place them in the linen hamper or linen bag. Dispose of disposable items in a facility-approved waste container. Clean equipment and return it to the storage area.

18. Remove your gloves and dispose of them in a facility-approved waste container.

Finishing Up *CLSOWR*
19. Complete the "Finishing Up" steps **a** through **f**.

PROCEDURE 17-2

Providing Oral Care for a Person with Dentures

Getting Ready *WGKIEpS*

1. Complete the "Getting Ready" steps **a** through **g**.

Supplies

- gloves
- paper towels
- gauze squares (4″ × 4″)
- straw (optional)
- foam-tipped applicators (optional)
- emesis basin
- paper cups
- denture cup
- denture brush or toothbrush
- denture cleaner or toothpaste
- denture solution (optional)
- mouthwash (optional)
- lip lubricant (optional)
- towel
- washcloth

Procedure

2. Cover the over-bed table with paper towels. Place the oral care supplies on the over-bed table. Fill a paper cup with water. Put on the gloves.

3. Make sure that the bed is positioned at a comfortable working height (to promote good body mechanics) and that the wheels are locked. Raise the head of the bed as tolerated. Place a towel under the person's chin.

4. Ask the person to remove his dentures and place them in the emesis basin. If the person needs assistance with removing his dentures:

   a. Ask the person to open his mouth.

   b. Holding a gauze square between your thumb and index finger, grasp the upper denture, moving it up and down slightly to break the seal. Ease the denture down, forward, and out of the mouth. Place the denture in the emesis basin.

   c. Holding a gauze square between your thumb and index finger, grasp the lower denture. Turn the denture slightly, lifting it out of the mouth. Place the denture in the emesis basin.

5. Take the emesis basin, the washcloth, the denture cup, the denture brush or toothbrush, and the denture cleaner or toothpaste to the sink. Line the sink with the washcloth to provide extra cushioning. Fill the sink partially with lukewarm water. Do not place the dentures in the sink.

6. Wet the denture brush or the toothbrush. Put a small amount of toothpaste or denture cleaner on the denture brush or toothbrush. Working with one denture at a time, hold the denture in the palm of your hand, and brush it on all surfaces until it is clean. Rinse the denture thoroughly under lukewarm running water and place it in the denture cup. Repeat with the other denture.

STEP 6 Hold the denture in the palm of your hand, and brush it on all surfaces until it is clean.

(continued)

PROCEDURE 17-2 (Continued)

Providing Oral Care for a Person with Dentures

7. If the dentures are to be stored, fill the denture cup with lukewarm water, a mixture of one part mouthwash to one part lukewarm water, or a denture solution, so that the dentures are covered. Put the lid on the denture cup. Return the denture cup to the person's bedside table, making sure that it is within easy reach.

8. If the dentures are to be reinserted in the person's mouth, take the emesis basin, the denture cup, and the toothbrush to the over-bed table. If the side rails are in use, lower the side rail on the working side of the bed. The side rail on the opposite side of the bed should remain up.

   a. Offer the person the cup of water (and a straw, if desired) and ask him to rinse his mouth completely. Some people may wish to use mouthwash instead of water. Hold the emesis basin underneath the person's chin so that he can spit the water or mouthwash into the basin.

   b. Place the emesis basin on the over-bed table, and dry the person's mouth and chin thoroughly using a face towel.

   c. Gently clean the person's gums and tongue and the insides of the cheeks with the toothbrush or a foam-tipped applicator moistened with water or mouthwash. Use fresh applicators as needed.

   d. Ask the person to insert his dentures. If the person needs assistance with inserting his dentures:

   • Ask the person to open his mouth.
   • Gently lift the person's upper lip up. Grasp the upper denture between your thumb and index finger and insert it in the person's mouth. Press gently on the denture to be sure that it is seated properly.
   • Gently pull the person's lower lip down. Grasp the lower denture between your thumb and index finger and insert it in the person's mouth.

   e. Return the denture cup to the person's bedside table, making sure that it is within easy reach.

9. Dry the person's mouth and chin thoroughly using a towel. Apply lip lubricant to the lips, as the person requests.

10. Reposition the person comfortably, and lower the head of the bed if necessary. If the side rails are in use, return the side rails to the raised position. Make sure that the bed is lowered to its lowest position and that the wheels are locked.

11. Gather the soiled linens and place them in the linen hamper or linen bag. Dispose of disposable items in a facility-approved waste container. Clean equipment and return it to the storage area.

12. Remove your gloves and dispose of them in a facility-approved waste container.

Finishing Up CLSOWR

13. Complete the "Finishing Up" steps **a** through **f**.

PROCEDURE 17-3

Providing Oral Care for an Unconscious Person

Getting Ready WCKIEpS

1. Complete the "Getting Ready" steps **a** through **g**.

Supplies

- gloves
- paper towels
- sponge-tipped applicators
- padded tongue blade
- paper cups
- emesis basin
- toothbrush and toothpaste (if the person has natural teeth)
- lip lubricant
- saline (optional)
- mouthwash (optional)
- towels

Procedure

2. Cover the over-bed table with paper towels. Place the oral care supplies on the over-bed table. Fill the paper cup with water. Put on the gloves.

3. Make sure that the bed is positioned at a comfortable working height (to promote good body mechanics) and that the wheels are locked. If the side rails are in use, lower the side rail on the working side of the bed. The side rail on the opposite side of the bed should remain up.

(continued)

PROCEDURE 17-3 (Continued)

Providing Oral Care for an Unconscious Person

4. Raise the head of the bed as tolerated. Turn the person's head to the side facing you. If it is difficult to keep the person's head turned to the side, roll the person onto his or her side.

5. If the person's condition permits, gently lift the person's head and place a towel on the pillow. Place the emesis basin on the towel, level with the person's chin.

6. Open the person's mouth using the padded tongue blade. Be gentle; do not force the mouth open. Insert the tongue blade between the upper and lower teeth at the back of the mouth to hold the person's mouth open.

7. Clean the inside of the mouth:

STEP 7 Clean the inside of the person's mouth, using a padded tongue blade to keep the mouth open.

a. If the person has natural teeth, they should be gently brushed as described in Procedure 17-1.

b. If the person is edentulous, gently clean the person's gums and tongue and the insides of the cheeks with the toothbrush or a foam-tipped applicator moistened with water, saline, or mouthwash. Use fresh applicators as needed.

8. Dry the person's mouth and chin thoroughly using a towel. Apply lip lubricant to the lips. Reposition the person comfortably.

9. If the side rails are in use, return the side rails to the raised position. Lower the head of the bed. Make sure that the bed is lowered to its lowest position and that the wheels are locked.

10. Gather the soiled linens and place them in the linen hamper or linen bag. Dispose of disposable items in a facility-approved waste container. Clean equipment and return it to the storage area.

11. Remove your gloves and dispose of them in a facility-approved waste container.

Finishing Up CLSOWR

12. Complete the "Finishing Up" steps **a** through **f**.

PROCEDURE 17-4

Providing Female Perineal Care

Getting Ready WCKIEpS

1. Complete the "Getting Ready" steps **a** through **g**.

Supplies

- gloves
- paper towels
- bed protector
- bath thermometer
- wash basin
- bedpan
- soap
- bath blanket
- washcloths
- towels
- clean clothing
- clean linens
  (if necessary)

Procedure

2. Cover the over-bed table with paper towels. Place the wash basin, toiletries, clean clothing, and clean linens on the over-bed table. Put on the gloves.

3. Make sure that the bed is positioned at a comfortable working height (to promote good body mechanics) and that the wheels are locked.

4. Because bathing often stimulates the urge to urinate, offer the bedpan (see Chapter 20, Procedures 20-1 and 20-2). If the person uses the bedpan, empty and clean it before proceeding with the perineal care. Remove your gloves and dispose of them in a facility-approved waste container. Wash your hands and put on a clean pair of gloves.

5. Lower the head of the bed to a flat position (as tolerated).

(continued)

PROCEDURE 17-4 (Continued)

Providing Female Perineal Care

6. Fill the wash basin with warm water [110°F (43.3°C) to 115°F (46.1°C) on the bath thermometer]. Place the basin on the over-bed table.

7. If the side rails are in use, lower the side rail on the working side. The side rail on the opposite side of the bed should remain up.

8. Spread the bath blanket over the top linens (and the person). If the person is able, have her hold the bath blanket. If not, tuck the corners under the person's shoulders. Fanfold the top linens to the foot of the bed.

9. Assist the person with undressing (see Chapter 18, Procedures 18-3 and 18-4).

10. Ask the person to open her legs and bend her knees, if possible. If she is not able to bend her knees, help her spread her legs as much as possible.

11. Position the bath blanket over the person so that one corner can be wrapped under and around each leg (see Fig. 17-2).

12. Position the bed protector under the person's buttocks to keep the bed linens dry.

13. Lift the corner of the bath blanket that is between the person's legs upward, exposing only the perineal area.

14. Form a mitt around your hand with one of the washcloths (see Fig. 17-5). Wet the mitt with warm, clean water and apply soap.

15. Using the other hand, separate the labia. Clean the vulva by placing your washcloth-covered hand at the top of the vulva and stroking downward to the anus. First clean one side, then the other side, and finally the middle, using a different part of the washcloth each time, until the area is clean.

STEP 15 Clean the vulva by placing your washcloth-covered hand at the top of the vulva and stroking downward to the anus. First clean each side, then the middle.

16. Rinse the vulva and perineum thoroughly:

Method "A": Form a mitt around your hand with a clean, wet washcloth. Using the other hand, separate the labia. Rinse the vulva by placing your washcloth-covered hand at the top of the vulva and stroking downward to the anus. First rinse one side, then the other side, and finally the middle, using a different part of the washcloth each time, until the area is free of soap.

Method "B": Hold a clean washcloth saturated with clean, warm water over the vulva. Squeeze the water from the washcloth onto the vulva and allow it to run over the vulva and perineum. Repeat until the area is free of soap.

17. Dry the perineal area thoroughly using a towel.

18. Turn the person onto her side, so that she is facing away from you (see Chapter 11, Procedure 11-6). Help the person toward the working side of the bed, so that her buttocks are within easy reach. Adjust the bath blanket to keep the person covered.

19. Form a mitt around your hand with one of the washcloths (see Fig. 17-5). Wet the mitt with warm, clean water and apply soap.

20. Using the other hand, separate the buttocks. Place your washcloth-covered hand at the front of the body and stroke toward the back. First clean one side, then the other side, and finally the middle, using a different part of the washcloth each time, until the anal area is clean.

STEP 20 Clean the anal area by placing your washcloth-covered hand at the front of the body and stroking toward the back.

21. Rinse and dry the anal area thoroughly. Remove the bed protector from underneath the person.

(continued)

PROCEDURE 17-4 (Continued)

Providing Female Perineal Care

22. Remove your gloves and dispose of them in a facility-approved waste container. Put on a clean pair of gloves.

23. Assist the person into the supine position. Reposition the pillow under the person's head. Remove the bath blanket, and help the person into the clean clothing (see Chapter 18, Procedures 18-3 and 18-4).

24. If the bedding is wet or soiled, change the bed linens (see Chapter 15, Procedure 15-2).

25. If the side rails are in use, return the side rail to the raised position. Raise the head of the bed as the person requests. Make sure that the bed is lowered to its lowest position and that the wheels are locked.

26. Gather the soiled linens and place them in the linen hamper or linen bag. Dispose of disposable items in a facility-approved waste container. Clean equipment and return it to the storage area.

27. Remove your gloves and dispose of them in a facility-approved waste container.

Finishing Up   CLSOWR

28. Complete the "Finishing Up" steps **a** through **f**.

PROCEDURE 17-5

Providing Male Perineal Care

Getting Ready   WGKIEPS

1. Complete the "Getting Ready" steps **a** through **g**.

Supplies

- gloves
- paper towels
- bed protector
- bath thermometer
- wash basin
- bedpan or urinal
- soap
- bath blanket
- washcloths
- towels
- clean clothing
- clean linens (if necessary)

Procedure

2. Cover the over-bed table with paper towels. Place the wash basin, toiletries, clean clothing, and clean linens on the over-bed table. Put on the gloves.

3. Make sure that the bed is positioned at a comfortable working height (to promote good body mechanics) and that the wheels are locked.

4. Because bathing often stimulates the urge to urinate, offer the bedpan or urinal (see Chapter 20, Procedures 20-1 and 20-2). If the person uses the bedpan or urinal, empty and clean it before proceeding with the perineal care. Remove your gloves and dispose of them in a facility-approved waste container. Wash your hands and put on a clean pair of gloves.

5. Lower the head of the bed to a flat position (as tolerated).

6. Fill the wash basin with warm water [110°F (43.3°C) to 115°F (46.1°C) on the bath thermometer]. Place the basin on the over-bed table.

7. If the side rails are in use, lower the side rail on the working side. The side rail on the opposite side of the bed should remain up.

8. Spread the bath blanket over the top linens (and the person). If the person is able, have him hold the bath blanket. If not, tuck the corners under the person's shoulders. Fan-fold the top linens to the foot of the bed.

9. Assist the person with undressing (see Chapter 18, Procedures 18-3 and 18-4).

10. Ask the person to open his legs and bend his knees, if possible. If he is not able to bend his knees, help him spread his legs as much as possible.

11. Position the bath blanket over the person so that one corner can be wrapped under and around each leg (see Fig. 17-2).

12. Position the bed protector under the person's buttocks to keep the bed linens dry.

13. Lift the corner of the bath blanket that is between the person's legs upward, exposing only the perineal area.

14. Form a mitt around your hand with one of the washcloths (see Fig. 17-5). Wet the mitt with warm, clean water and apply soap.

15. Using the other hand, hold the penis slightly away from the body.

(continued)

PROCEDURE 17-5 (Continued)

Providing Male Perineal Care

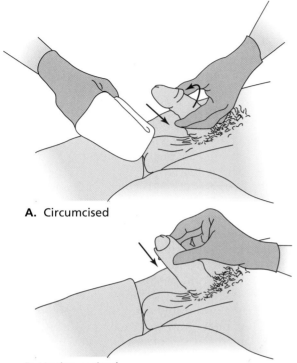

A. Circumcised

B. Uncircumcised

STEP 15 To wash the penis, pass the washcloth in a circular motion, moving from the tip of the penis to the base. (A) circumcised penis; (B) uncircumcised penis.

a. If the person is circumcised: Place your washcloth-covered hand at the tip of the penis and wash in a circular motion, downward to the base of the penis. Repeat, using a different part of the washcloth each time, until the area is clean. Rinse and dry the tip and the shaft of the penis thoroughly:

Method "A": Form a mitt around your hand with a clean, wet washcloth. Using the other hand, hold the penis slightly away from the body. Place your washcloth-covered hand at the tip of the penis and wipe in a circular motion, downward to the base of the penis. Repeat, using a different part of the washcloth each time, until the area is rinsed. Dry the penis thoroughly.

Method "B": Hold a clean washcloth saturated with clean, warm water over the area. Squeeze the water from the washcloth onto the area. Dry the penis thoroughly.

b. If the person is uncircumcised: Retract the foreskin by gently pushing the skin toward the base of the penis. Place your washcloth-covered hand at the tip of the penis and wash in a circular motion, downward to the base of the penis. Repeat, using a different

part of the washcloth each time, until the area is clean. Rinse and dry the tip and shaft of the penis thoroughly before gently pulling the foreskin back into its normal position.

16. Form a mitt around your hand with one of the washcloths (see Fig. 17-5). Wet the mitt with warm, clean water and apply soap. Wash the scrotum and perineum. Rinse and dry the scrotum and perineum thoroughly.

17. Turn the person onto his side, so that he is facing away from you (see Chapter 11, Procedure 11-6). Help the person toward the working side of the bed, so that his buttocks are within easy reach. Adjust the bath blanket to keep the person covered.

18. Form a mitt around your hand with one of the washcloths (see Fig. 17-5). Wet the mitt with warm, clean water and apply soap.

19. Using the other hand, separate the buttocks. Place your washcloth-covered hand at the front of the body and stroke toward the back. First clean one side, then the other side, and finally the middle, using a different part of the washcloth each time, until the anal area is clean.

20. Rinse and dry the anal area thoroughly. Remove the bed protector from underneath the person.

21. Remove your gloves and dispose of them in a facility-approved waste container. Put on a clean pair of gloves.

22. Assist the person into the supine position. Reposition the pillow under the person's head. Remove the bath blanket, and help the person into the clean clothing (see Chapter 18, Procedures 18-3 and 18-4).

23. If the bedding is wet or soiled, change the bed linens (see Chapter 15, Procedure 15-2).

24. If the side rails are in use, return the side rail to the raised position. Make sure that the bed is lowered to its lowest position and that the wheels are locked.

25. Gather the soiled linens and place them in the linen hamper or linen bag. Dispose of disposable items in a facility-approved waste container. Clean equipment and return it to the storage area.

26. Remove your gloves and dispose of them in a facility-approved waste container.

Finishing Up CLSOWR

27. Complete the "Finishing Up" steps **a** through **f**.

PROCEDURE 17-6
Assisting with a Tub Bath or Shower

OBRA ✓

Getting Ready   WORKTEPS

1. Prepare the tub room. Place a nonskid mat on the floor of the tub or shower. If the person will be taking a tub bath, fill the tub halfway with warm water (105°F [43.3°C] to 115°F [46.1°C] on the bath thermometer). Obtain a shower chair if necessary and place it in the shower. Place a towel on the chair in the tub room where the person will sit while drying off.

2. Complete the "Getting Ready" steps **a** through **g**.

Supplies

- gloves
- bath thermometer
- soap
- washcloth
- towels
- lotion (optional)
- powder (optional)
- deodorant or antiperspirant (optional)
- clean clothing

Procedure

3. Ask the person if he or she needs to use the bathroom before bathing.

4. Assist the person to the tub room.

5. If the person will be taking a tub bath, check the temperature of the water and make sure the nonskid mat is secure. If the person will be taking a shower, turn on the water and adjust the temperature until the water is comfortable.

6. Assist the person with undressing (see Chapter 18, Procedure 18-3, step 10, and Procedure 18-4). Assist the person into the bathtub or shower.

7. If the person is able to bathe himself, either partially or completely:

    a. Place bathing supplies within easy reach.

    b. Many facilities require you to remain in the room while the person bathes or showers. If facility policy permits you to leave the room, explain how to use the call light control and ask the person to signal when bathing is complete or when he has done as much as he can on his own and needs help completing the bath. Stay nearby and check on the person every 5 minutes. The person should not remain in the bathtub or shower for longer than 20 minutes. Return when the person signals. Remember to knock before entering.

8. If the person is unable to bathe himself, or requires assistance:

    a. Put on the gloves and form a mitt around your hand with one of the washcloths (see Fig. 17-5).

    b. If necessary, ask the person what parts of the body were not washed. Assist the person as needed with completing the bath. Wash the cleanest areas first and the dirtiest areas last:

- **Eyes.** Wet the mitt with warm, clean water. Ask the person to close his eyes. Place your washcloth-covered hand at the inner canthus (corner) of the eye and stroke gently outward, toward the outer canthus. Use a different part of the washcloth for each eye.
- **Face, neck, and ears.** Ask the person if you should use soap on the face. Rinse the washcloth and apply soap, if requested. Wash the face, neck, and ears, moving from the top of the head to the bottom (so that the nose and mouth are washed last). Rinse thoroughly.
- **Arms and axillae (armpits).** Rinse the washcloth and apply soap. Place your washcloth-covered hand at the shoulder and stroke downward, toward the hand, using long, firm strokes. Wash the hand. If necessary, assist the person with raising his arm so that you can wash the axilla. Repeat for the other arm and axilla.
- **Chest and abdomen.** Using long, firm strokes, wash the person's chest and abdomen.
- **Legs and feet.** Place your washcloth-covered hand at the top of the thigh and stroke downward, toward the foot, using long, firm strokes. Wash the foot. Repeat for the other leg.
- **Back and buttocks:** Wash the person's back and buttocks, moving from top to bottom and using long, firm strokes.
- **Perineal area:** Complete male or female perineal care as described in Procedures 17-4 and 17-5, respectively.

9. Make sure that soap is thoroughly rinsed from all parts of the body.

10. Remove your gloves and dispose of them in a facility-approved waste container. Put on a clean pair of gloves.

11. If the person is taking a tub bath, drain the water and carefully assist the person out of the tub and into the towel-covered chair. If the

(continued)

PROCEDURE 17-6 (Continued)

Assisting with a Tub Bath or Shower

person is taking a shower, turn the water off and assist the person into the towel-covered chair.

12. Wrap a towel around the person. Using another bath towel, help the person to dry off, patting the skin dry. Take care to ensure that areas where "skin meets skin" are dried thoroughly (for example, in between the toes, underneath the breasts).

STEP 12 Help the person to dry off, taking extra care to dry areas where "skin meets skin."

13. Help the person to apply lotion, powder, deodorant, antiperspirant, or other personal care products as the person requests.

14. Help the person into the clean clothing. If the person is wearing nightwear, help him into a robe. Help the person into his slippers.

15. Remove your gloves and dispose of them in a facility-approved waste container.

16. Assist the person back to his room.

Finishing Up CLSOWR

17. Complete the "Finishing Up" steps **a** through **f**.

18. Gather the soiled linens and place them in the linen hamper or linen bag. Dispose of disposable items in a facility-approved waste container. Clean equipment and return it to the storage area.

19. Clean the tub room and shower chair (if used), if housekeeping is not responsible for this task at your facility.

PROCEDURE 17-7

Giving a Complete Bed Bath

Getting Ready WGKIEPS

1. Complete the "Getting Ready" steps **a** through **g**.

Supplies

- gloves
- paper towels
- bed protectors
- oral hygiene supplies (see Procedures 17-1 through 17-3)
- bath thermometer
- wash basin
- bedpan or urinal
- soap
- lotion (optional)
- powder (optional)
- deodorant or antiperspirant (optional)
- washcloths
- towels
- bath blanket
- clean clothing
- clean linens (if necessary)

Procedure

2. Cover the over-bed table with paper towels. Place the wash basin, toiletries, clean clothing, and clean linens on the over-bed table. Put on the gloves.

3. Make sure that the bed is positioned at a comfortable working height (to promote good

body mechanics) and that the wheels are locked.

4. Because bathing often stimulates the urge to urinate, offer the bedpan or urinal (see Chapter 20, Procedures 20-1 and 20-2). If the person uses the bedpan or urinal, empty and clean it before proceeding with the bath. Remove your gloves and dispose of them in a facility-approved waste container. Wash your hands and put on a clean pair of gloves.

5. Assist the person with oral hygiene (see Procedures 17-1 through 17-3).

6. Remove the bedspread and blanket from the bed. If they are to be reused, fold them and place them on a clean surface, such as the chair.

7. Spread the bath blanket over the top linens (and the person). If the person is able, have her hold the bath blanket. If not, tuck the corners under the person's shoulders. Fanfold the top linens to the foot of the bed.

8. Assist the person with undressing (see Chapter 18, Procedures 18-3 and 18-4).

(continued)

PROCEDURE 17-7 (Continued)

Giving a Complete Bed Bath

9. Lower the head of the bed so that the bed is flat (as tolerated). Position the pillow under the person's head.

10. Fill the wash basin with warm water [110°F (43.3°C) to 115°F (46.1°C) on the bath thermometer]. Place the basin on the over-bed table.

11. If the side rails are in use, lower the side rail on the working side of the bed. The side rail on the opposite side of the bed should remain up.

12. Place a towel over the person's chest to keep the bath blanket dry.

13. To keep the bath water from becoming soapy too quickly, you can use two washcloths—one with soap for washing, and one without soap for rinsing. Form a mitt around your hand with one of the washcloths (see Fig. 17-2). Wet the mitt with warm, clean water. Ask the person to close his eyes. Place your washcloth-covered hand at the inner canthus (corner) of the eye and stroke gently outward, toward the outer canthus. Use a different part of the washcloth for each eye. Using a towel, dry the person's eyes.

STEP 13 Wash the person's eyes, moving from the inside corner toward the outer corner.

14. Ask the person if you should use soap on the face. Rinse the washcloth and apply soap, if requested. Wash the face, neck, and ears, moving from the top of the head to the bottom (so that the nose and mouth are washed last). Using the clean washcloth, rinse thoroughly, and pat the person's face, neck, and ears dry with a towel.

15. Place a bed protector under the person's far arm, to keep the linens dry. Form a mitt around your hand with the washcloth. Wet the mitt and apply soap. Place your

washcloth-covered hand at the shoulder and stroke downward, toward the hand, using long, firm strokes. Wash the hand. If necessary, assist the person with raising her arm so that you can wash the axilla. Rinse thoroughly, and pat the person's arm, hand, and axilla dry with a towel. Remove the bed protector from underneath the person's arm.

STEP 15 Wash the person's arm, moving from the shoulder to the wrist.

16. Repeat for the other arm.

17. Place a towel horizontally across the person's chest. (The person is now covered with both a bath blanket and a towel.) With the towel in place, fold the bath blanket down to the person's waist. Wet the mitt and apply soap. Reach under the towel and wash the person's chest, using long, firm strokes. Using the clean washcloth, rinse thoroughly, and pat the person's chest dry with a towel.

STEP 17 Reach under the towel and wash the person's chest.

18. With the towel still in place, fold the bath blanket down to the pubic area. Form a mitt around your hand with the washcloth. Wet the mitt and apply soap. Reach under the towel

(continued)

PROCEDURE 17-7 (Continued)

Giving a Complete Bed Bath

and wash the person's abdomen, using long, firm strokes. Rinse thoroughly, and pat the person's abdomen dry with a towel.

19. Replace the bath blanket by unfolding it back over the towel and the person's body. Slide the towel out from underneath the bath blanket.

20. Change the water in the wash basin if it is cool or soapy. (If the side rails are in use, raise the side rails before leaving the bedside.)

21. Fold the bath blanket so that the far leg is completely exposed. Place a bed protector under the person's far leg, to keep the linens dry. Wet the mitt and apply soap. Place your washcloth-covered hand at the top of the thigh and stroke downward, toward the foot, using long, firm strokes. Rinse thoroughly, and pat the person's leg dry with a bath towel.

22. Put the wash basin on the bed protector and place the person's foot in the basin. Wash the entire foot, including between the toes, with the soapy washcloth. Rinse thoroughly, and pat the person's foot dry with a towel. Be sure to dry between the toes. Remove the wash basin. Remove the bed protector from underneath the person's leg.

STEP 22 Put the wash basin on the bed protector and place the person's foot in the basin.

23. Repeat for the other leg and foot.

24. Change the water in the wash basin. (If the side rails are in use, raise the side rails before leaving the bedside.)

25. Turn the person onto his or her side, so that he or she is facing away from you (see Chapter 11, Procedure 11-6). Help the person toward the working side of the bed, so that his or her back is within easy reach. Adjust the bath blanket to keep the front of the person

covered (exposing only the back and buttocks). Place a bed protector on the bed alongside the person's back, to keep the linens dry.

26. Form a mitt around your hand with the washcloth. Wet the mitt and apply soap. Wash the person's back and buttocks, moving from top to bottom and using long, firm strokes. Rinse thoroughly, and pat the person's back and buttocks dry using a bath towel. At this point, a back massage may be given (see Procedure 17-9).

STEP 26 Wash the person's back and buttocks using long, firm strokes.

27. If the person is able to perform perineal care, assist the person into Fowler's position and adjust the over-bed table so that the bathing supplies are within easy reach. Place the call light control within easy reach and ask the person to signal when perineal care is complete. If the person is unable to perform perineal care, assist the person onto his or her back and complete male or female perineal care as described in Procedures 17-4 and 17-5, respectively.

28. Remove your gloves and dispose of them in a facility-approved waste container. Put on a clean pair of gloves.

29. Help the person to apply lotion, powder, deodorant, antiperspirant, or other personal care products as the person requests.

30. Help the person into the clean clothing.

31. If the bedding is wet or soiled, change the bed linens (see Chapter 15, Procedure 15-2).

32. Carry out range-of-motion exercises as ordered (see Chapter 25, Procedure 25-1).

(continued)

PROCEDURE 17-7 (Continued)

Giving a Complete Bed Bath

33. If the side rails are in use, return the side rails to the raised position. Raise or lower the head of the bed as the person requests. Make sure that the bed is lowered to its lowest position and that the wheels are locked.

34. Gather the soiled linens and place them in the linen hamper or linen bag. Dispose of disposable items in a facility-approved waste container. Clean equipment and return it to the storage area.

35. Remove your gloves and dispose of them in a facility-approved waste container.

Finishing Up   CLSOWR

36. Complete the "Finishing Up" steps **a** through **f**.

PROCEDURE 17-8

Giving a Partial Bed Bath

Getting Ready   WCKIEPS

1. Complete the "Getting Ready" steps **a** through **g**.

Supplies

- gloves
- paper towels
- bed protectors
- oral hygiene supplies (see Procedures 17-1 through 17-3)
- bath thermometer
- wash basin
- bedpan or urinal
- soap
- lotion (optional)
- powder (optional)
- washcloths
- towels
- bath blanket
- clean clothing
- clean linens (if necessary)

Procedure

2. Cover the over-bed table with paper towels. Place the wash basin, toiletries, clean clothing, and clean linens on the over-bed table. Put on the gloves.

3. Because bathing often stimulates the urge to urinate, offer the bedpan or urinal (see Chapter 20, Procedures 20-1 and 20-2). If the person uses the bedpan or urinal, empty and clean it before proceeding with the bath. Remove your gloves and dispose of them in a facility-approved waste container. Wash your hands and put on a clean pair of gloves.

4. Assist the person with oral hygiene (see Procedures 17-1 through 17-3). Remove your gloves and dispose of them in a facility-approved waste container. Wash your hands.

5. Fill the wash basin with warm water (110°F [43.3°C] to 115°F [46.1°C] on the bath thermometer). Place the basin on the over-bed table.

6. If the person will be bathing independently, make sure that the bed is lowered to its lowest position and that the wheels are locked. If you will be assisting the person with bathing, make sure that the bed is positioned at a comfortable working height (to promote good body mechanics) and that the wheels are locked. If the side rails are in use, lower the side rail on the working side. The side rails on the opposite side of the bed should remain up.

7. The bath may either be carried out with the person in Fowler's position, or the person can be assisted to sit on the edge of the bed (see Procedure 11-15). Help the person to undress as necessary.

8. If the person is able to bathe herself, either partially or completely:

   a. Place bathing supplies within easy reach.

   b. Many facilities require you to remain in the room while the person bathes. If facility policy permits you to leave the room, explain how to use the call light control and ask the person to signal when bathing is complete or when she has done as much as she can on her own and needs help completing the bath. Stay nearby and check on the person every 5 minutes. Return when the person signals. Remember to knock before entering.

9. If the person is unable to bathe herself, or requires assistance:

   a. Put on the gloves and form a mitt around your hand with one of the washcloths (see Fig. 17-5).

   b. If necessary, ask the person what parts of the body were not washed. Assist the person as needed with completing the bath. Wash the cleanest areas first and the dirtiest areas last:

(continued)

PROCEDURE 17-8 (Continued)

Giving a Partial Bed Bath

- **Face, neck, and ears.** Ask the person if you should use soap on the face. Rinse the washcloth and apply soap, if requested. Wash the face, neck, and ears, moving from the top of the head to the bottom (so that the nose and mouth are washed last). Rinse thoroughly, and pat the person's face, neck, and ears dry with a towel.
- **Hands.** Wash the hand. Rinse thoroughly, and pat the hand dry with a towel. Repeat for the other hand.
- **Axillae (armpits).** If necessary, assist the person with raising her arm so that you can wash the axilla. Rinse thoroughly, and pat the axilla dry with a towel. Repeat for the other axilla.
- **Back and buttocks.** Rinse the washcloth and apply soap. Wash the person's back and buttocks, moving from top to bottom and using long, firm strokes. Rinse thoroughly, and pat the back and buttocks dry with a towel.
- **Perineal area.** Complete male or female perineal care as described in Procedures 17-4 and 17-5, respectively.

10. Remove your gloves and dispose of them in a facility-approved waste container. Put on a clean pair of gloves.

11. Help the person to apply lotion, powder, deodorant, antiperspirant, or other personal care products as the person requests.
12. Help the person into the clean clothing.
13. If the bedding is wet or soiled, change the bed linens.
14. Carry out range-of-motion exercises as ordered (see Chapter 25, Procedure 25-1).
15. If the side rails are in use, return the side rails to the raised position. Raise or lower the head of the bed as the person requests. Make sure that the bed is lowered to its lowest position and that the wheels are locked.
16. Gather the soiled linens and place them in the linen hamper or linen bag. Dispose of disposable items in a facility-approved waste container. Clean equipment and return it to the storage area.
17. Remove your gloves and dispose of them in a facility-approved waste container.

Finishing Up
18. Complete the "Finishing Up" steps **a** through **f**.

PROCEDURE 17-9

Giving A Back Massage

Getting Ready

1. Complete the "Getting Ready" steps **a** through **g**.

Supplies
- gloves (if contact with broken skin is likely)
- wash basin
- lotion
- bath blanket
- towel

Procedure

2. Fill the wash basin with warm water. Place the bottle of lotion in the basin of warm water to warm it.
3. Make sure that the bed is positioned at a comfortable working height (to promote good body mechanics) and that the wheels are locked.
4. Lower the head of the bed so that the bed is flat (as tolerated). If the side rails are in use, lower the side rail on the working side of the bed. The side rail on the opposite side of the bed should remain up.
5. Help the person into the prone position, or turn the person onto his or her side, so that he or she is facing away from you (see Chapter 11, Procedure 11-6).
6. Reposition the pillow under the person's head, and adjust the bath blanket to keep the person covered, exposing only the back and buttocks.
7. Put on the gloves, if contact with broken skin is likely.
8. Pour some lotion into your cupped palm, and rub your hands together to distribute the lotion onto both palms.
9. Apply the lotion to the person's back with the palms of your hands. Massage the lotion into the person's skin, using long, gliding strokes (*effleurage*), moving up the center of the back

(continued)

PROCEDURE 17-9 (Continued)

Giving A Back Massage

from the buttocks to the shoulders, and then back down along the outside of the back. Do not directly rub any reddened areas. Repeat four times.

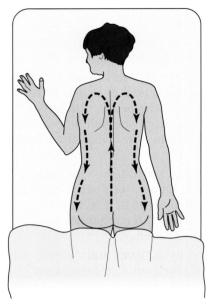

STEP 9 Move up the center of the back from the buttocks to the shoulders, and then back down along the outside of the back.

10. For the next set of strokes, move up the center of the back from the buttocks to the shoulders, and then back down along the outside of the back. On the downstroke, massage the person's shoulders and back using a small circular motion. Repeat four times.

STEP 10 For the next set of strokes, massage the person's shoulders and back using a small circular motion on the downstroke.

11. For the next set of strokes, move up the center of the back from the buttocks to the shoulders, and then back down along the outside of the back. On the downstroke, massage the person's shoulders, back, and buttocks using a small circular motion, paying special attention to the area at the base of the spine. Repeat four times.

STEP 11 For the final set of strokes, massage the person's shoulders, back, and buttocks using a small circular motion on the downstroke.

12. Finish with long, gliding strokes (*effleurage*), moving up the center of the back from the buttocks to the shoulders, and then back down along the outside of the back. Repeat four times.

13. Remove your gloves and dispose of them in a facility-approved waste container.

14. If the back massage is being given as part of a bath, assist the person onto his back and continue with the bath. If the back massage is being given before bed or at any other time, help the person back into his pajamas, nightgown, or hospital gown.

15. If the side rails are in use, return the side rails to the raised position. Make sure that the bed is lowered to its lowest position and that the wheels are locked.

16. Gather the soiled linens and place them in the linen hamper or linen bag. Dispose of disposable items in a facility-approved waste container. Clean equipment and return it to the storage area.

Finishing Up

17. Complete the "Finishing Up" steps **a** through **f**.

What did you learn?

Multiple Choice

Select the single best answer for each of the following questions.

1. As a safety measure, when you give mouth care to an unconscious person, you should position the person in which position?
   a. Semi-Fowler's position with head turned to side
   b. Supine position
   c. Fowler's position
   d. Prone position

2. Why do you line the sink with a washcloth when cleaning a person's dentures?
   a. To ensure that you always have a wet washcloth handy when you need one
   b. To protect the sink from scratches
   c. To guard against breaking the dentures
   d. To prevent contamination of the dentures

3. Which one of the following is within the range of appropriate temperatures for bath water?
   a. 98°F (36.6°C)
   b. 212°F (100°C)
   c. 120°F (48.9°C)
   d. 105°F (40.5°C)

4. When giving a complete bed bath, you should:
   a. Position yourself on one side of the bed and stay there
   b. Use the same water throughout the bath to minimize trips to the sink
   c. Avoid washing the person's perineal area because the person may be embarrassed
   d. Keep the person covered as much as possible

5. When assisting a man with perineal care, you should always:
   a. Hold the penis at a 90° angle to the body
   b. Wash from the base of the penis toward the tip
   c. Retract the foreskin if the man is uncircumcised
   d. Clean the scrotum first

6. When assisting a person with a shower, you should:
   a. Use a bath blanket to prevent falls
   b. Run the water until the temperature reaches 125°F (51.6°C)
   c. Wear waterproof personal protective equipment (PPE) to protect yourself from getting wet
   d. Use a shower chair if the person is weak or unsteady

7. Which one of the following actions must be taken to keep the skin healthy?
   a. Apply generous amounts of lotion after the bath
   b. Rinse the skin well and dry it thoroughly, especially in areas where "skin meets skin"
   c. Apply generous amounts of powder after the bath
   d. Rub the skin vigorously with the washcloth

8. How are natural teeth brushed?
   a. Using a circular motion
   b. For at least 10 minutes on each side
   c. Using an "up and down" motion
   d. All of the above

9. When assisting a woman with perineal care, you should always:
   a. Gently yet thoroughly dry the perineal area and vulva
   b. Clean the rectal area last
   c. Move the washcloth in a downward direction, from the urethra to the anus
   d. All of the above

10. What is the first thing you should do before assisting a person with a tub bath?
    a. Gather the necessary supplies
    b. Make sure the tub is clean
    c. Check the temperature of the water
    d. Check the nursing care plan to make sure the person is allowed to have a tub bath

11. Which of the following observations made while assisting with mouth care would you report to the nurse?
    a. Lips that are dry, cracked, swollen, or blistered
    b. Irritations, sores, or white patches in the mouth or on the tongue
    c. Bleeding, swelling, or redness of the gums
    d. All of the above

12. How long should a back massage last?
    a. 2 minutes
    b. 1 minute
    c. 4 to 6 minutes
    d. 15 minutes

Matching

Match each numbered item with its appropriate lettered description.

_____ **1.** Perineal care (peri-care)

_____ **2.** Activities of daily living (ADLs)

_____ **3.** Evening (hour of sleep, hs) care

_____ **4.** Gingivitis

_____ **5.** PRN (as-needed) care

_____ **6.** Antiperspirant

_____ **7.** Edentulous

a. Without teeth

b. Routine tasks of daily life, such as bathing, eating, and grooming

c. Care that is provided at any time of the day or night, when the person's condition warrants it

d. Inflammation of the gums, caused by poor oral hygiene

e. Stops or slows secretion of sweat

f. Care that is routinely provided at bedtime

g. Cleaning of the perineum, the anus, and the vulva or penis

? Stop and think!

▶ Mrs. Davis is a resident at your facility, which specializes in caring for people with Alzheimer's disease. As Mrs. Davis's disease has progressed, she has become progressively more lax about matters related to personal hygiene. She dislikes bathing, and if you do not remove her soiled clothes from her room she will continue to wear them every day. Today Mrs. Davis is scheduled to have a shower, and as you might have predicted, she tells you that she "will not take a shower today." What should you do?

▶ Mrs. Visknaya is from Russia and came to the United States to live near her daughter. She speaks very little English and understands even less. A male nursing assistant, Josh, has been assigned to care for Mrs. Visknaya today because Juanita, who usually cares for Mrs. Visknaya, is home sick with the flu. Josh comes to Mrs. Visknaya's room and announces with a big smile that it is "time for her bath." He explains the procedure to her, and she smiles back and nods her head. Unfortunately, she doesn't understand a word he is saying! When it comes time during the bath to assist Mrs. Visknaya with her perineal care, Josh lifts the corner of the bath blanket and attempts to separate Mrs. Visknaya's legs, and she starts to scream. What, if anything, did Josh do wrong? What could have been done to prevent this situation?

18

Grooming

What will you learn?

There are many types of personal care routines. In the previous chapter, you learned how to help people with the most basic aspects of personal care, those activities related to keeping the body clean and healthy. **Grooming,** or activities related to maintaining a neat and attractive appearance, goes beyond basic personal hygiene. The routine care of the hands and feet (including the nails), shampooing and styling of the hair, the application of make-up, and shaving are all grooming practices that, while not necessarily *essential* for health, certainly play a role in maintaining both physical and emotional health. Imagine that you are a patient or a resident, and you are unable to complete your regular grooming activities. Your hair is uncombed, you have not applied make-up (if you are a woman) or shaved (if you are a man), and you are not dressed for visitors, yet company arrives anyway. How would you feel? Would you be able to fully enjoy your guests, or would you be worried about your appearance? Helping your patients and residents with "putting their best face forward," the subject of this chapter, is part of providing holistic care. When you are finished with this chapter, you will be able to:

1. Discuss how grooming differs from hygiene.
2. Describe factors that influence a person's grooming habits.
3. Explain the effect that illness or disability may have on a person's grooming habits.
4. List changes that occur in a person's feet as a result of aging or illness.
5. Understand the importance of proper hand and foot care.
6. Demonstrate proper technique for assisting with hand and foot care.
7. Discuss the various dressing needs that a patient or resident may have.
8. Demonstrate different methods of helping a person to dress and undress.

(continued)

Photo: Grooming practices help people to feel more attractive and confident.

9. Discuss disorders a nursing assistant may observe when assisting with hair care.
10. Describe the different methods used to assist a person with shampooing his or her hair.
11. Describe methods used to style a person's hair.
12. Demonstrate proper technique for shampooing a bedridden person's hair and combing a person's hair.
13. Describe the tools and supplies used for shaving.
14. Demonstrate how to safely shave a man's face.
15. Explain how the use of make-up can affect a person's sense of well being.

Vocabulary

Use the CD in the back of your book to hear these terms pronounced, defined, and used in a sentence:

Grooming	Podiatrist	Seborrheic dermatitis	Pediculosis capitis
Hangnail	Dandruff	(cradle cap)	Nits
Tinea pedis	Tinea capitis	Alopecia	

A person's grooming practices may be very simple (for example, washing and combing the hair and applying a bit of moisturizing lotion to the skin). Or they may be very complex (for example, styling the hair with a blow dryer and curlers, applying full make-up, wearing perfume or cologne, and polishing the nails). Think for a moment about the routine grooming practices that you perform each day before you leave home to face the world. Have you ever overslept and had to go to school or work without your routine grooming accomplished? How did you feel? Did it affect your self-esteem?

People who are admitted to health care facilities or who are clients of health care agencies have personal grooming routines, just as you do. Like yours, their personal grooming practices are influenced by cultural and religious beliefs, upbringing, current fashion, level of income, and their feelings about their own sexuality. Many women feel more feminine if they are wearing lipstick and have polished nails, while others are quite happy with a freshly washed face and a ponytail. Men also have grooming routines that make them feel attractive and self-confident, such as shaving and applying cologne or aftershave, or caring for a beard or moustache. Illness or disability can affect a person's ability to complete his or her grooming practices, causing the person to feel unattractive and "not quite himself."

As a nursing assistant, you must provide holistic care for your patients and residents. This means looking after their physical needs, as well as their emotional needs. Helping a person to complete his or her routine grooming practices meets many of the person's emotional needs, as well as some physical ones. When you take the time and make the effort to style a person's hair attractively, polish her nails, or help apply make-up as part of morning care, you make that person feel extra special. Your actions help the person to meet the needs of love and belonging, because she feels cared for as the unique individual that she is. You also help the person to meet her need for self-esteem. Not only is she clean and comfortable, but she feels attractive too. As with any aspect of care, check with the nurse or check the person's nursing care plan to find out about any limitations or specifics related to grooming.

ASSISTING WITH HAND AND FOOT CARE

CARE OF THE HANDS

Soft, smooth skin and trimmed, filed fingernails feel wonderful and are important for overall health and comfort. Dryness and chapping of the skin on the hands causes discomfort and creates a portal of entry for microbes. Poorly cared for fingernails can become long and rough, placing the person at risk for accidentally scratching himself. For example, a person who is disoriented or semi-comatose can hurt himself if the fingernails are not kept short and smooth. For people who are alert and oriented, fingernail length and appearance is a personal choice, but the edges should be kept smooth.

A simple care routine is used to keep the skin of the hands healthy and the fingernails neat (Procedure 18-1). Even if a person can care for his or her own hands and fingernails, getting a manicure from someone else can really lift a person's spirits, especially if the person is not feeling his or her best (Fig. 18-1). In addition to making the person feel cared for, helping a patient or resident with hand and nail care gives you the chance to observe for signs of health. In a healthy person, the nailbeds are pink. There is no gap between the nail and the nailbed. When viewed from the side, the nails are convex (i.e., they curve slightly). The cuticles are smooth and unbroken.

Nail care is usually easiest to perform on nails that have been soaked for a short time in warm water. Therefore, during or immediately following a bath is an ideal time to perform nail care, because the water makes the nails soft and flexible. When nail care is to be provided at a time other than bath time, the nails can be softened by soaking the ends of the fingers for a short time in a small basin of warm water.

Fingernails are trimmed with clippers, not scissors, to a length no shorter than even with the

FIGURE 18-2

Nails are cut using nail clippers. Cut the nails straight across, being careful not to cut too close to the skin. Always make sure that it is within your scope of practice to trim a patient's or resident's fingernails or toenails. In many facilities, this task must be performed by a nurse.

ends of the fingers (Fig. 18-2). In some states and facilities, trimming a patient's or resident's fingernails is outside of the scope of practice for nursing assistants, so be sure to follow the policy at the facility where you work. After trimming, the nails are filed into an oval shape using an emery board. Pain or tenderness can result from **hangnails** (broken pieces of cuticle). Hangnails may need to be trimmed using cuticle scissors so that they do not rub or snag on clothing or linens. This can lead to tearing, bleeding, and inflammation.

An orange stick or the edge of a washcloth is used to gently push the cuticles back, and then the orange stick is used to clean underneath the tips of the nails. Some people like to use nail polish. If nail polish is not used, then the surfaces of the nails can be lightly buffed to give them shine. Applying hand cream helps to seal in moisture and prevent dryness of the skin and cuticles.

CARE OF THE FEET

Care of the feet is essential for good grooming as well as for good health. The feet tend to sweat, especially when slippers or shoes and socks are worn, leading to odors and a warm, moist environment that encourages the growth of microbes. For example, the disorder commonly known as "athlete's foot" **(tinea pedis)** is a fungal infection of the skin and nails. ("Pedis" is derived from the Latin word for foot, *pedalis*.) Toenails that are allowed to grow too long can make wearing footwear uncomfortable, and the nails may become ingrown (a condition where the nail curves down and back into the skin, causing injury and

FIGURE 18-1

Giving a person a manicure gives you the opportunity to spend "quality time" with a patient or resident.

pain). Finally, the feet are at risk for injury— how many times have you had your foot stepped on, stubbed your toes against a piece of furniture, or developed a blister as a result of shoes that did not fit properly?

Injuries such as cuts and blisters are painful for a person with normal blood flow to the feet and toes. For a person with poor blood flow (e.g., as a result of the normal aging process, a heart problem, or diabetes mellitus), a cut or a blister might develop into a life-threatening condition. Because blood flow to the wounded area is impaired, the area receives less oxygen and nutrients and fewer infection-fighting white blood cells. Healing is delayed, and the risk of infection is increased. To further complicate matters, impaired circulation usually goes hand-in-hand with impaired sensation. While you would certainly notice if a new pair of shoes made a blister on your heel, a person with reduced blood flow and sensation might not be aware of the blister, and a small blister could quickly become a dangerous infection. Helping a person with foot care allows you to observe the person's feet for small blisters, cracks in the skin, peeling of the skin between the toes or on the soles of the feet, ingrown toenails, and other problems. Red or tender areas should also be reported to the nurse immediately.

Like hand care, foot care is a grooming task that is easily added to the bathing routine. If foot care is to be done at a time other than bath time, the feet should first be bathed, rinsed, and dried thoroughly (especially between the toes). Prolonged soaking is not recommended. In most facilities, nursing assistants are not allowed to trim the toenails of patients or residents, because a small injury could carry the risk of a life-threatening infection. This task is usually performed by a nurse or a **podiatrist,** a doctor who specializes in the care of the feet. The attention of a podiatrist is especially necessary when the toenails are thick and difficult to trim (as a result of aging or poor blood flow; Fig. 18-3). If you are allowed to trim your patients' or residents' toenails, use clippers and cut the toenails straight across. Never try to trim or file corns or calluses.

After the toenails are trimmed, they are filed to remove rough edges. Applying foot powder or lotion to dry feet is refreshing and comforting. Cotton socks help to keep the feet warm and will absorb sweat. (Be careful when helping an elderly

FIGURE 18-3

Many elderly people have thick, yellowed toenails as a result of age or poor circulation. Because thickened toenails may be difficult to trim and an accidental injury can have serious consequences, many health care facilities require that a nurse or a podiatrist trim patients' or residents' toenails.

person to put on socks—roll the cuff of the sock down before putting it on the person's foot and take care not to accidentally scratch the person with your fingernails or jewelry when pulling the sock up over the heel). Encourage your patients or residents to wear appropriate footwear. Well-fitting, supportive shoes with nonskid soles help to protect the feet and make walking safer by helping to prevent falls and slipping. Procedure 18-2 describes how to assist a patient or resident with foot care.

▶ *Tell the Nurse!*

While providing hand and foot care, always be aware of potential signs and symptoms of illness or infection. Tell the nurse if you observe any of the following:

⮕ Nailbeds that are either very pale or blue, or bruised

⮕ Nails that are unusually yellow or white

⮕ Nails that are unusually thick

⮕ Nails that are broken or have been cut too short (especially if there is also bleeding or tenderness)

⮕ Nails that are ingrown

⮕ Cuticles that are torn, red, or swollen

⮕ Skin that is blistered, red, or tender (especially on the feet)

⮕ Any unusual rashes or odors

ASSISTING WITH DRESSING AND UNDRESSING

As a nursing assistant, you will be responsible for helping your patients or residents to change their clothes, possibly several times a day. Dressing is usually a routine part of morning and evening care. However, clothing should be changed any time that it becomes wet or soiled. The type of clothing worn by people receiving health care services differs according to the type of facility and the abilities of the person. If a resident of a long-term care facility is able to be out of bed during the day, he or she may wear street clothes during the day and a hospital gown, a nightgown, or pajamas at night. Procedure 18-3 describes how to assist a person with dressing in street clothes and nightwear. A patient in a hospital or acute care setting or a resident who has a specific physical disability or medical condition may wear a hospital gown or nightwear day and night. Procedure 18-4 describes how to change a hospital gown.

As with other personal care routines, the amount of help that each person needs for dressing will vary. Some people will need no assistance, except perhaps for some help tying their shoes or zipping a back zipper. Others may need a lot of assistance with every part of the process, from selecting clothes to putting them on. Allowing a person to choose the clothing he or she wishes to wear is a top priority when assisting with dressing (Fig. 18-4). When a person is unable to choose his or her own clothes, use good taste and common sense when choosing items for the person to wear. Dressing appropriately for the day's activities and with consideration for the season and environment will help residents and patients stay comfortable. If a person chooses an item of clothing that is not appropriate for the weather or the day's planned activities, you might tactfully steer him or her toward a more appropriate choice. Remember that some elderly or ill people may chill more easily than others and may need a sweater or jacket to remain warm, especially if there is air conditioning.

Comfort and ease of dressing help determine many wardrobe choices for the residents of long-term care facilities. Many residents are undergoing rehabilitation following an accident or a disabling illness, such as a stroke. The goal of rehabilitation is to return the person to the highest level of independent functioning as possible. In addition to selecting clothes that are easy to take on and off, a weak or disabled person may use one or more of the many assistive devices that are available to make dressing easier. For example, clothing that closes with a Velcro™ fastener instead of zippers or buttons allows a person with limited use of his or her fingers to manage dressing and toileting with little or no assistance (Fig. 18-5A). Long-handled shoehorns and graspers allow a person to put on his or her own socks and shoes (Fig. 18-5B). The use of these assistive devices can allow a person to maintain a large amount of personal independence in spite of disabilities.

Some patients or residents will, however, need your help with dressing and undressing. For example, consider the following situations:

- A person has an extremity (an arm or a leg) that is weak, paralyzed, in a cast, or splinted.
- A person has recently had surgery on an arm or a leg.
- A person has an intravenous (IV) line (Fig. 18-6).

These conditions may make helping the person to dress or undress a bit more challenging, but good planning on your part can simplify the situation. For example, if you place the garment's sleeve or leg onto the affected extremity first, dressing becomes much easier for both you and the person being dressed. (When it comes time to remove the garment, reverse the procedure—work with the strong arm or leg first and undress the affected extremity last.) If the person has an IV line, bring the IV bottle and tubing through the sleeve first

FIGURE 18-4

Whenever possible, a person should be permitted to choose which articles of clothing he or she will wear.

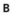

A   **B**

FIGURE 18-5

Assistive devices are available to help people with disabilities dress themselves independently. (*A*) Velcro fasteners on this shirt replace buttons or a zipper, which require more use of the fingers to manage. (*B*) A shoehorn makes it easier to put on shoes. (*Photos courtesy of Sammons Preston Rolyan, Bolingbroke, IL.*)

A   **B**

C

FIGURE 18-6

Helping a person who has an intravenous (IV) line in place get dressed is not as difficult as it may seem. (*A*) Put the IV bottle and tubing through the sleeve of the gown first, and place the IV bag on the hook. (*B*) Gently thread the sleeve down the tubing and gently bring the person's arm through the sleeve of the gown. (*C*) Bring the gown across the person's chest and guide the other arm through the other sleeve.

FIGURE 18-8

To foster independence and self-esteem, encourage your patients or residents to do as much as possible for themselves, while you stand by ready to offer assistance as needed.

FIGURE 18-7

Some facilities have on-site salons and barbershops for the convenience of residents. (*Catrina Genovese/Index Stock Imagery, Inc.*)

and then follow with the arm (see Fig. 18-6). Some hospitals and acute care units may have special hospital gowns with openings in the shoulder that make dressing and undressing with IV lines in place easier. You should not remove an IV line from an infusion pump or disconnect IV tubing when assisting a person to dress or undress. If you are unsure about how to manage an IV line or a bandage while helping a person to dress or undress, ask a nurse for assistance.

ASSISTING WITH HAIR CARE

Routine care is necessary to keep the hair clean and neat. For many people, the appearance of their hair affects how they feel about themselves. Think about how you have felt on the rare occasion when you have had a "bad hair day." Have you felt that you would rather walk around with a paper bag on your head than have other people see your hair dirty or poorly styled? Helping with hair care is an essential part of providing care for those who need you. Routine grooming of the hair consists of daily brushing, combing, and styling and is usually accomplished as part of early morning care, when a person arises. Additional

grooming may be necessary throughout the day, for example, after napping or before visiting times. Some health care facilities have on-site salons and barbershops where patients and residents can have their hair cut, washed, and professionally styled (Fig. 18-7).

The texture and length of the hair affect how a person cares for it. Hair that is straight and fine can be as hard to manage as hair that is curly and coarse. The hair of elderly people tends to be fragile. Personal preferences regarding hairstyle and the products used when grooming the hair vary and should be respected whenever possible. Asking a person about his or her usual hair care routine and preferred products will provide you with much useful information. Patients and residents should be encouraged to participate in caring for their own hair to their fullest ability. For example, a person with a paralyzed or injured arm can be encouraged to brush her hair on her "strong" side, and then you can complete the job on the other side (Fig. 18-8).

When assisting with grooming of the hair, it is important to observe the hair and scalp for any abnormalities. Common conditions of the hair and scalp that you may see in your patients or residents include the following:

- **Dandruff** is itching and flaking of the scalp. Daily brushing and using a medicated shampoo may be all that is needed to control dandruff.
- **Tinea capitis,** a fungal infection of the scalp, may also cause itching and flaking

of the scalp. ("Capitis" is derived from the Latin word for head, *caput*.)

- **Seborrheic dermatitis** (commonly referred to as **"cradle cap"** when it occurs in infants) causes severe scaling of the scalp. Thick, yellow, crusty patches are seen. The nurse may ask you to help shampoo the person daily with a medicated shampoo until the scaling is cleared up.
- **Alopecia,** or baldness, can be caused by many conditions. Alopecia is most commonly the result of an inherited trait in men and is rarely seen in women, although women may experience thinning of the hair with aging. Medications used to treat cancer (chemotherapy) and certain forms of radiation treatment can cause total baldness in both men and women. Stress, illness, and poor nutrition can also cause the hair to thin.
- **Pediculosis capitis,** or head lice, is particularly common in children. Lice, as you will recall from Chapter 7, are very small parasitic insects that feed on the blood of the host, or the person who is infected. The insects lay their eggs (called **nits**) on the hair shaft, near the root. The nits look like dandruff flakes or small pieces of lint, but cannot be brushed or shaken off the hair. Head lice are transmitted from person to person by direct contact with an infected person's hair. They may also be transmitted indirectly, through contact with clothing, bed linens, brushes and combs, and cloth-covered furniture (e.g., the back of a sofa or chair where an infected person has rested his or her head). Pediculosis is treated with medicated creams and shampoos. The person's clothing and bed linens must be washed in very hot water to prevent re-infection.

▶ *Tell the Nurse!*

When providing hair care, it is important to observe the condition of the person's hair and scalp. Make sure to report any of the following findings to the nurse immediately:

- ▶ Flaking, crusting, or scaling of the scalp
- ▶ Redness, itching, or tenderness of the scalp
- ▶ Unusual hair loss, especially if it is occurring in patches
- ▶ A foul smell
- ▶ Severely matted or tangled hair
- ▶ Nits ("flakes" that cannot be brushed or shaken off the hair)

SHAMPOOING THE HAIR

Hair should be washed as often as is necessary to keep it clean. The frequency of shampooing will vary according to personal preference and health status. People who are feverish or who have been sweating from an illness or from physical activity may welcome a non-scheduled shampoo to help them feel fresh and clean. Other people may only need their hair washed once or twice a week.

Many people in health care facilities can shampoo their own hair when they bathe. Others will need help. There are several ways to help a person shampoo his or her hair. Many bathtubs and showers have hand-held showerheads that make it easy to shampoo the hair during a person's bath. The hair can also be shampooed in a sink, either by having the person sit with his back to the sink and tilt his head backward, or by having the person face the sink and bend his head forward (Fig. 18-9). However, remember that for many elderly people, shampooing at the sink is either uncomfortable or impossible because it is more difficult for an older person to bend his or her neck to the degree required. When a person cannot get out of bed, a shampoo trough is used to wash the hair (Procedure 18-5).

As any trip down a drugstore or grocery store aisle will reveal, there are many different types of shampoos and conditioners to choose from. (Conditioners are used by many people to improve the hair's texture and reduce tangles.) Respecting personal preference in products is important. When a person is too ill to have regular shampoos, a "dry shampoo" product may be used instead. Before shampooing a patient's or resident's hair, always check with the nurse or the person's nursing care plan to find out necessary details, such as the frequency of shampoos, the method used, and the products preferred.

FIGURE 18-9

A person's hair can be shampooed at the sink, provided the person does not have neck or back problems.

STYLING THE HAIR

After the hair has been washed and towel-dried, the hair is dried and styled according to the person's wishes (Fig. 18-10). Most men and some women with shorter hair may prefer to allow their hair to air dry. Others may want to have their hair styled and dried with a blow dryer, or they may want their hair rolled on curlers and dried under a salon-style dryer. If you are using electric appliances to dry and style a person's hair, be sure to follow the safety precautions related to the use of electrical items as described in Chapter 9—for example, check for frayed cords and never use an electrical appliance near water. Be very careful not to burn the person's scalp with the dryer or curling iron. It is best to use a low heat setting.

The time and attention you spend helping your patients or residents style their hair will help to make those in your care feel and look attractive, which will certainly have a positive effect on their well-being. Stop and think for a moment how you felt the last time you had the opportunity to get your hair professionally done, or a friend offered to wash and style your hair. That is how well-cared for and pampered your patients or residents will feel when you provide these services for them!

PREVENTING TANGLES

Regular brushing and combing of the hair helps to keep hair soft and tangle-free. The scalp produces oil that keeps the hair shiny and soft. Brushing distributes this oil throughout the hair. Hair that is long, curly, or kinky may need to be braided after it is brushed to help prevent tangling (Fig. 18-11). Many African-American people have curly or kinky hair and a very dry scalp. African-American hair may require braiding and the application of a moisturizing product to keep the hair soft and pliable. The use of barrettes,

FIGURE 18-10

After shampooing, some people may like to have their hair dried and styled.

FIGURE 18-11

Braiding helps to prevent tangles in hair that is long, curly, or kinky.

headbands, and clips can be both functional (by keeping hair out of the face) and decorative.

Sometimes the hair becomes tangled, especially if the person has been restricted to bed for a period of time. To remove tangles from the hair, use a wide-tooth comb and start at the ends of the hair, one section at a time, gently working up toward the scalp (Procedure 18-6). Hair that is very tangled or matted may need to be cut, but the nurse must first obtain permission from the person or his or her legal guardian to cut the hair.

ASSISTING WITH SHAVING

ASSISTING MEN

Shaving is a routine grooming practice among most men. Shaving a man's face should be a part of either morning or evening care, depending on the person's preference (some men prefer to shave before going to bed). Prior to shaving, the face should be cleaned and the beard softened, making bath time an ideal time to complete the shave. The frequency of shaving depends on how fast the beard grows and personal preference.

The type of shaving tool used also varies (Fig. 18-12). Many men prefer to use a safety razor, which may be disposable or have a changeable blade unit. Blades that become dull pull at the beard and do not cut the hair smoothly and should be changed. Disposable razors are used once and then discarded. Used blades and disposable razors should always be disposed of in a sharps container, not in a wastebasket. When

A   **B**

FIGURE 18-12

Shaving supplies. (*A*) A safety razor is used with shaving cream or gel or shaving soap. (*B*) An electric razor is used with a pre-shave lotion. An electric razor carries less risk of cuts or nicks, and therefore is preferred for a person who is taking medications that affect the blood's ability to clot.

using a safety razor, the beard is softened with warm water and a shaving cream or gel is applied to retain the moisture and reduce the friction of the blade against the skin. Some men may prefer to use shaving soap instead of a shaving cream or gel. In this case, a shaving brush is used to lather the soap and apply it to the beard. Procedure 18-7 describes how to shave a man's face using a blade razor and shaving cream, gel, or soap.

Other men like to use electric razors. People who are taking drugs that decrease the blood's ability to form a clot should always use an electric razor, because electric razors are less likely to cut or nick the skin. If an electric razor is being used, a pre-shave lotion is applied to soften the whiskers and allow the razor to glide smoothly across the face. The usual safety precautions that are taken with all electrical appliances should be taken when using an electric razor. The electric razor is cleaned after each use.

If a person is able, he should be encouraged to do his own shaving. You should provide whatever assistance is necessary, which may range from placing a chair and a mirror near the sink or bringing supplies and water to the bedside, to completing the shave in full. When shaving a person, always remember to wear gloves because a cut or a nick will put you at risk for exposure to bloodborne pathogens. Always ask the nurse or check the nursing care plan to determine if there are any limitations or special instructions for a person's shave.

A man may prefer to have a beard or mustache instead of being clean-shaven. Beards and mustaches need routine grooming care also. They must be kept clean and free of food and drink and will need to be combed or brushed and trimmed regularly. Never shave off a person's beard or mustache unless the person requests that you do so. Be careful when shaving near the mustache or beard to avoid accidentally shaving part of the facial hair off.

ASSISTING WOMEN

Shaving the legs, underarms, or both makes many women feel feminine and attractive. In addition, some women experience the growth of coarse facial hair as they age and may request your help with removing this unwanted hair. If a woman is unable to shave her legs, armpits, or face and wants to do so, you should help her as necessary.

Many of the same principles used when assisting men to shave apply to women as well. The hair should be softened with warm water first, making bath time the ideal time to shave. A safety razor or an electric razor may be used. If a safety razor is used, shaving cream or gel should be applied first. Like men, many women will have clear preferences regarding the type of razor and shaving products that are used, and respecting the person's preferences is important. A woman's face is shaved in the same manner as a man's. When shaving the armpits, it is best to move in the direction of hair growth. When shaving the legs, start at the ankle and move upward, against the direction of hair growth. Many women shave their legs only below the knee, while others may shave the thigh as well.

ASSISTING WITH THE APPLICATION OF MAKE-UP

Since ancient Egyptian times, people have been applying make-up with the goal of looking more beautiful, feeling younger, preventing wrinkles, and attracting the opposite sex. In the United States today, the cosmetics industry has sales of approximately 8 *billion* dollars each year. Clearly, the ability of make-up to make us feel more confident, attractive, and healthy has powerful appeal.

A person's culture, religion, age, and feelings about his or her own sexuality all contribute to that person's feelings about, and use of, make-up. Many times, the types of make-up a person likes and the way she applies them are influenced greatly by the time in that person's life when she felt most attractive. For example, many of your elderly ladies will insist on wearing dark lipstick and heavy face powder because that was the style that was popular during their younger years. Other women may insist that a certain type of mascara or a certain shade of eye shadow is an essential grooming item.

Helping a person to continue with her normal personal grooming routine has an enormous impact on the person's continued well-being. For some people, wearing make-up increases their self-esteem and feelings of self worth. When you help a person who likes to wear make-up to complete this part of her grooming routine, the person will feel that you take special care of her and that you value her as the unique human being that she is. This idea is at the heart of holistic care.

SUMMARY

▶ Caring for the hands and feet (especially the fingernails and toenails), selecting an outfit to wear, shampooing and styling the hair, shaving, and applying make-up are grooming practices that people may engage in to make themselves feel more attractive and confident.

- Grooming practices differ from hygiene practices in that grooming practices are performed mainly for the sake of appearance. Therefore, good grooming is more essential for emotional health than for physical health. However, grooming practices do benefit physical health as well.

- Personal grooming practices are highly variable and are influenced by many factors, including culture, religion, upbringing, level of income, current fashion, and a person's feelings about his or her own sexuality. Respecting your patient's or resident's personal preferences is an important part of providing holistic care. Remembering this is very important when assisting with grooming.

▶ Care of the hands and feet focuses on keeping the skin and nails clean and healthy.

- Assisting with hand and foot care gives the nursing assistant the chance to observe for potential health problems, including poor blood flow and fungal infections.

- Poor blood flow to the feet is associated with many health problems, including decreased sensation and an increased risk for a life-threatening infection. Circulatory problems may be caused by heart disease, diabetes mellitus, or the normal aging process.

- Trimming a person's toenails is usually beyond the nursing assistant's scope of practice. Instead, this task is performed by a nurse or a podiatrist.

▶ Dressing daily is necessary for warmth and modesty, and it gives people a sense of purpose.

- For many people, dressing is a way of expressing themselves. Therefore, a person's preferences regarding outfit selection should be followed whenever possible. Sometimes, due to disability or illness, a person will be required to wear a hospital gown or nightwear during the day.

- Wet or soiled garments must be exchanged for dry, clean ones as often as necessary.

- Assistive devices, such as Velcro™ fasteners, shoehorns, and graspers, increase a disabled person's independence. With increased independence comes increased self-esteem.

- Certain conditions (e.g., a weak, paralyzed, or injured arm or leg or an IV line) can make dressing more challenging but by no means impossible.

▶ Most people feel best when their hair is clean, free of tangles, and styled in a familiar style.

- Assisting with hair care gives the nursing assistant an excellent chance to observe for conditions of the scalp and hair, including dandruff, tinea capitis, seborrheic dermatitis (cradle cap), alopecia, and pediculosis capitis (head lice).

- Hair may be shampooed as part of a tub or shower bath, at the sink, or in bed, using a shampoo trough.

- Styling tools include blow dryers, curling irons, hot curlers, and salon-style hairdryers. Caution must be used when operating these electrical appliances.

- Regular brushing and combing keeps the hair shiny and tangle-free.

▶ Most men shave their faces daily, either completely or partially. Many women shave their legs, their underarms, or both.

▶ Many women, and some men, consider the application of make-up to be an essential grooming activity.

Chapter 18 Procedures

Getting Ready Steps

a. **W**ash your hands and observe standard precautions as necessary.

b. **G**ather needed supplies.

c. **K**nock and introduce yourself.

d. **I**dentify the person, and greet him or her by name.

e. **E**xplain the procedure.

f. **P**rovide privacy.

g. **S**ee to safety.

Finishing Up Steps

a. **C**onfirm comfort and good body alignment.

b. **L**eave the call light control within easy reach.

c. **S**ee to safety.

d. **O**pen the curtain and door.

e. **W**ash your hands.

f. **R**eport and record.

PROCEDURE 18-1
Assisting with Hand Care

Getting Ready WGKIEPS

1. Complete the "Getting Ready" steps **a** through **g**.

Supplies

- gloves (if contact with broken skin is likely)
- paper towels
- orange stick
- nail clippers
- emery board (nail file)
- bath thermometer
- emesis basin
- soap
- lotion
- nail polish remover (optional)
- nail polish (optional)
- cotton balls (optional)
- washcloth
- towel

Procedure

2. Make sure that the bed is lowered to its lowest position and that the wheels are locked.

3. Cover the over-bed table with paper towels. Pour some liquid soap into the emesis basin, and fill the basin with warm water (100°F [37.7°C] to 115°F [46.1°C] on the bath thermometer). Place the emesis basin on the over-bed table, along with the nail care supplies and clean linens. Put on the gloves if contact with broken skin is likely.

4. If the side rails are in use, lower the side rail on the working side of the bed. The side rail on the opposite side of the bed should remain up.

5. Help the person to transfer from the bed to a bedside chair (see Procedure 11-9), assist the person to sit on the edge of the bed (see Procedure 11-15), or raise the head of the bed as tolerated.

6. If the person is wearing nail polish and wants it removed, remove the nail polish by putting a small amount of nail polish remover on a cotton ball and gently rubbing each nail.

7. Help the person to position the tips of his or her fingers in the basin to soak. Let the person soak his or her fingers for about 5 minutes.

STEP 7 Soak the nails to soften them.

(continued)

PROCEDURE 18-1 (Continued)

Assisting with Hand Care

8. Working with one hand at a time, lift the person's hand out of the basin and wash the entire hand, including between the fingers, with the soapy washcloth. Use the orange stick to gently clean underneath the person's fingernails. Rinse thoroughly, and pat the person's hand dry with a face towel. Be sure to dry between the fingers. Repeat with the other hand.

STEP 8 Clean under the person's nails using the orange stick.

9. Remove the emesis basin and dry the person's hands thoroughly. If facility policy allows it, gently push the cuticles back with the orange stick.

10. If facility policy allows it, use the nail clippers to cut the person's fingernails (see Fig. 18-2). If the person's nails need to be trimmed but this task is outside of your scope of practice, report this need to the nurse.

11. Use the emery board to file the fingernails into an oval shape and smooth the rough edges.

12. Apply lotion to the person's hands and gently massage it into the skin.

13. Apply nail polish as the person requests.

14. If necessary, help the person return to bed. If the side rails are in use, return the side rails to the raised position. Lower the head of the bed as the person requests.

15. Gather the soiled linens and place them in the linen hamper or linen bag. Dispose of disposable items in a facility-approved waste container. Clean equipment and return it to the storage area.

16. Remove your gloves and dispose of them in a facility-approved waste container.

Finishing Up

17. Complete the "Finishing Up" steps **a** through **f**.

PROCEDURE 18-2

Assisting with Foot Care

Getting Ready

1. Complete the "Getting Ready" steps **a** through **g**.

Supplies

- gloves (if contact with broken skin is likely)
- paper towels
- bed protector
- orange stick
- nailbrush
- nail clippers
- emery board (nail file)
- wash basin
- bath thermometer
- soap
- lotion
- nail polish remover (optional)
- nail polish (optional)
- cotton balls (optional)
- washcloth
- towels

Procedure

2. Make sure that the bed is lowered to its lowest position and that the wheels are locked.

3. Cover the over-bed table with paper towels. Pour some liquid soap into the wash basin, and fill the basin with warm water (100°F [37.7°C] to 115°F [46.1°C] on the bath thermometer). Place the wash basin on the over-bed table, along with the nail care supplies and clean linens. Put on the gloves if contact with broken skin is likely.

4. If the side rails are in use, lower the side rail on the working side of the bed. The side rail on the opposite side of the bed should remain up.

5. If the person is able to get out of bed, help the person to transfer from the bed to a bedside chair (see Procedure 11-9). If the person is not able to get out of bed, raise the head of the bed as tolerated. Fanfold the top linens to the foot of the bed.

(continued)

PROCEDURE 18-2 (Continued)

Assisting with Foot Care

6. If the person is wearing nail polish and wants it removed, remove the nail polish by putting a small amount of nail polish remover on a cotton ball and gently rubbing each nail.

7. Place a bed protector on the floor in front of the chair (if the person is out of bed) or on the bottom sheet (if the person is in bed). Place the wash basin on the bed protector.

8. Help the person to position his or her feet in the basin to soak. Let the person soak his or her feet for about 5 minutes.

9. Working with one foot at a time, lift the person's foot out of the basin and wash the entire foot, including between the toes, with the soapy washcloth. Apply soap to the nailbrush and gently scrub any rough areas. Use the orange stick to gently clean underneath the person's toenails. Rinse thoroughly, and pat the person's foot dry with a towel. Be sure to dry between the toes. Repeat with the other foot.

10. If facility policy allows it, use the nail clippers to cut the person's toenails (see Fig. 18-2). If the person's nails need to be trimmed but this task is outside of your scope of practice, report this need to the nurse.

11. Use the emery board to smooth the rough edges of the toenails.

12. Apply lotion to the person's feet and gently massage it into the skin.

13. Apply nail polish as the person requests.

14. If necessary, help the person return to bed. If the side rails are in use, return the side rails to the raised position. Lower the head of the bed as the person requests.

15. Gather the soiled linens and place them in the linen hamper or linen bag. Dispose of disposable items in a facility-approved waste container. Clean equipment and return it to the storage area.

Finishing Up CLSOWR

16. Complete the "Finishing Up" steps a through f.

PROCEDURE 18-3

Assisting a Person with Dressing

Getting Ready WGKIEPS

1. Complete the "Getting Ready" steps a through g.

Supplies

- gloves (if contact with broken skin is likely)
- bath blanket
- clean clothing

Procedure

2. Make sure that the bed is positioned at a comfortable working height (to promote good body mechanics) and that the wheels are locked.

3. Lower the head of the bed so that the bed is flat (as tolerated). If the side rails are in use, lower the side rail on the working side of the bed. The side rail on the opposite side of the bed should remain up.

4. Put on the gloves if contact with broken skin is likely.

5. Spread the bath blanket over the top linens (and the person). If the person is able, have him or her hold the bath blanket. If not, tuck the corners under the person's shoulders. Fanfold the top linens to the foot of the bed.

6. Assist the person with undressing:

   a. **Hospital gown.** See Procedure 18-4, steps 5 through 9.

   b. **Garments that fasten in the back.** Undo any fasteners, such as buttons, zippers, snaps, or ties. Gently lift the person's head and shoulders and gather the garment around the person's neck. Working with the person's strongest side first, gently remove the arm from the garment by sliding the garment down the arm. Repeat with the other arm. (If it is not possible to lift the person's head and shoulders, roll the person onto his or her side, facing away from you. Working with the person's strongest side first, gently remove the arm from the garment. Roll the person onto his or her other side, facing you, and remove the other arm from the garment.) Remove the garment completely by lifting it over the person's head.

(continued)

PROCEDURE 18-3 (Continued)

Assisting a Person with Dressing

c. **Garments that fasten in the front.** Undo any fasteners, such as buttons, zippers, snaps, or ties. To remove the top, gently lift the person's head and shoulders. Working with the person's strongest side first, gently remove the arm from the garment by sliding the garment over the shoulder and down the arm. Gather the garment behind the person and remove the garment completely by sliding the other sleeve over the weak shoulder and arm. To remove the bottoms, undo any fasteners, such as buttons, zippers or snaps. Ask the person to lift his or her buttocks off the bed and gently slide the pants down to the ankles and over the feet. (If the person cannot raise his buttocks off the bed, help the person to roll first to his strong side, allowing you to pull the bottoms down on the weak side. Then roll the person to his weak side and finish pulling the bottoms down.)

7. Assist the person with putting on his or her undergarments:

a. **Underpants.** Facing the foot of the bed, gather the underpants together at the leg opening and at the waistband. Working with one foot at a time, slip first one foot and then the other through the waistband and into the leg openings. Slide the underpants up the person's legs as far as they will go, and then ask the person to lift his or her buttocks off the bed. Gently slide the underpants up over the buttocks. (If the person cannot raise his buttocks off the bed, help the person to roll first to his strong side, allowing you to pull the underpants up on the weak side. Then roll the person to his weak side and finish pulling the underpants up.) Adjust the underpants so that they fit comfortably.

b. **Bra.** Working with the person's weak side first, slip the arms through the straps and position the straps on the shoulders so that the front of the bra is covering the person's chest. Adjust the cups of the bra over the person's breasts. Raise the person's head and shoulders and help the person to lean forward so that you can fasten the bra in the back.

c. **Undershirt.** Facing the head of the bed, gather the top and the bottom of the undershirt together at the neck opening. Place the undershirt over the person's

head. Working with the person's weak side first, slip the arms through the arm openings. Raise the person's head and shoulders and help the person to lean forward so that you can pull the undershirt down, smoothing out any wrinkles.

8. Assist the person with putting on his or her outerwear:

a. **Pants.** Assist the person with putting on his or her pants by following the same procedure as that used for putting on underpants (see step 7a). Fasten any buttons, zippers, snaps, or ties.

b. **Shirts and sweaters that fasten in the front.** Facing the head of the bed, place your hand and arm through the wristband of the garment. Working with the person's weak side first, grasp the person's hand and slip the garment off of your hand and arm, gently guiding the person's arm into the sleeve. Pull the sleeve up, adjusting it at the shoulder. Raise the person's head and shoulders and help the person to lean forward so that you can bring the other side of the garment around the back of the person's body. Guide the person's strong arm into the sleeve of the garment. Fasten any buttons, zippers, snaps, or ties.

c. **Sweatshirts and pullover sweaters.** Assist the person with putting on a sweatshirt or pullover sweater by following the same procedure as that used for putting on an undershirt (see step 7c). Fasten any buttons, zippers, snaps, or ties.

d. **Blouses that fasten in the back.** Facing the head of the bed, place your hand and arm through the wristband of the garment. Working with the person's weak side first, grasp the person's hand and slip the garment off of your hand and arm, gently guiding the person's arm into the sleeve. Pull the sleeve up, adjusting it at the shoulder. Repeat for the other side. Raise the person's head and shoulders and help the person to lean forward so that you can bring the sides of the garment around to the back. Fasten any buttons, zippers, snaps, or ties.

9. Assist the person with putting on footwear:

a. **Socks or knee-high stockings.** Gather the sock or stocking, bringing the toe area and the opening together. With the toe area fac-

(continued)

PROCEDURE 18-3 (Continued)

Assisting a Person with Dressing

ing up, slip the sock or stocking over the person's foot. Smooth the heel of the sock or stocking over the person's heel, and pull the sock or stocking up into position. Adjust the sock or stocking so that it fits comfortably. Repeat for the other foot.

b. **Shoes or slippers.** If the shoe has laces, loosen them completely to make it easier to slip the shoe onto the foot. Guide the person's foot into the shoe or slipper. A shoehorn may be used to help ease the person's heel into the shoe. Make sure that the foot is seated properly in the shoe. Socks or stockings should not be bunched

at the toe. If necessary, tie the shoe or fasten the Velcro™ fasteners securely.

10. If the person will be remaining in bed and the side rails are in use, return the side rails to the raised position. Raise the head of the bed as the person requests.

11. Gather the soiled garments and place them in the linen hamper or linen bag.

12. Remove your gloves and dispose of them in a facility-approved waste container.

Finishing Up C L S O W R

13. Complete the "Finishing Up" steps **a** through **f**.

PROCEDURE 18-4

Changing a Hospital Gown

Getting Ready W C K I E P S

1. Complete the "Getting Ready" steps **a** through **g**.

Supplies

- gloves (if contact with broken skin is likely)
- clean hospital gown

Procedure

2. Make sure that the bed is positioned at a comfortable working height (to promote good body mechanics) and that the wheels are locked.

3. Put on the gloves if contact with broken skin is likely.

4. Lower the head of the bed so that the bed is flat (as tolerated). If the side rails are in use, lower them on the working side of the bed. The side rails on the opposite side of the bed should remain up.

5. Have the person turn onto his or her side, facing away from you, so that you can untie the gown at the neck and waist. Assist the person back into the supine position. If the person cannot turn onto his or her side, reach under the person and untie the gown.

6. Loosen the gown from around the person's body.

7. Unfold the clean gown and lay it over the person's chest.

8. Working with the person's strongest side first, remove one sleeve at a time, leaving the old gown draped over the person's body.

9. Working with the person's weakest side first, slide the arm through the sleeve of the clean gown. Repeat for the other arm.

STEP 9 Slide the person's arm through the sleeve of the clean gown.

10. Remove the soiled gown from underneath the clean gown and place it in the linen hamper or linen bag.

11. Have the person turn onto his or her side, facing away from you, so that you can tie the

(continued)

PROCEDURE 18-4 (Continued)

Changing a Hospital Gown

gown at the neck and waist (or reach under the person and tie the gown). Adjust the gown so that it fits comfortably.

12. If the side rails are in use, return the side rails to the raised position. Raise the head of the bed as the person requests.

13. Remove your gloves and dispose of them in a facility-approved waste container.

Finishing Up CLSOWR

14. Complete the "Finishing Up" steps **a** through **f**.

PROCEDURE 18-5

Shampooing a Person's Hair in Bed

Getting Ready WGKIEpS

1. Complete the "Getting Ready" steps **a** through **g**.

Supplies

- gloves (if contact with broken skin is likely)
- paper towels
- bed protector
- wash basin
- water pitcher
- bath thermometer
- shampoo trough
- comb
- brush
- blow dryer (optional)
- shampoo
- conditioner (optional)
- washcloth
- towels

Procedure

2. Make sure that the bed is positioned at a comfortable working height (to promote good body mechanics) and that the wheels are locked.

3. Fill the water pitcher with warm water (100°F [37.7°C] to 115°F [46.1°C] on the bath thermometer).

4. Cover the over-bed table with paper towels. Place the hair care supplies and clean linens on the over-bed table. Put on the gloves if contact with broken skin is likely.

5. Raise the head of the bed as tolerated. Comb the person's hair to remove snarls and tangles (see Procedure 18-6).

6. Lower the head of the bed so that the bed is flat (as tolerated). If the side rails are in use, lower the side rail on the working side of the bed. The side rail on the opposite side of the bed should remain up.

7. Gently lift the person's head and shoulders and reposition the pillow under the person's shoulders. Cover the head of the bed and the

pillow with the bed protector, and place the shampoo trough on the bed protector. Help the person to rest his or her head on the shampoo trough. Place a towel across the person's shoulders and chest.

8. Place the wash basin on the floor beside the bed to catch the water as it drains from the shampoo trough.

9. Ask the person to hold the washcloth over his or her eyes.

10. Holding the water pitcher in one hand, slowly pour water over the person's hair until the hair is completely wet. Use your other hand to help direct the flow of water away from the person's eyes and ears.

STEP 10 Wet the person's hair, being careful to keep the water out of her eyes.

11. Apply a small amount of shampoo to the wet hair. Lather the hair and massage the scalp to help stimulate the circulation.

12. Using the water pitcher, rinse the hair thoroughly.

(continued)

PROCEDURE 18-5 (Continued)

Shampooing a Person's Hair in Bed

13. Apply conditioner, as the person requests. Rinse the hair thoroughly.

STEP 11 Apply a small amount of shampoo and work it into a lather.

14. Gently lift the person's head and shoulders and remove the shampoo trough and bed protector. Wrap the person's hair in a towel.

15. Raise the head of the bed as tolerated. Gently pat the person's face, neck, and ears dry, and finish towel drying the hair.

16. Replace any wet or soiled linens. (If the side rails are in use, raise the side rails before leaving the bedside to get the necessary replacement linens.)

17. Comb the person's hair to remove snarls and tangles (see Procedure 18-6).

18. Dry and style the hair with the brush and blow dryer, as the person requests. Use the cool setting and take care not to burn the person's scalp or face.

19. Reposition the pillow under the person's head and straighten the bed linens. If the side rails are in use, return the side rails to the raised position. Lower the head of the bed as the person requests.

20. Gather the soiled linens and place them in the linen hamper or linen bag. Dispose of disposable items in a facility-approved waste container. Clean equipment and return it to the storage area.

21. Remove your gloves and dispose of them in a facility-approved waste container.

Finishing Up

22. Complete the "Finishing Up" steps **a** through **f**.

PROCEDURE 18-6

Combing a Person's Hair

Getting Ready

1. Complete the "Getting Ready" steps **a** through **g**.

Supplies

- paper towels
- wide-toothed comb or pick
- brush
- mirror
- hair accessories (optional)
- detangler or leave-in conditioner (optional)
- towels

Procedure

2. Make sure that the bed is positioned at a comfortable working height (to promote good body mechanics) and that the wheels are locked.

3. Cover the over-bed table with paper towels. Place the hair care supplies and clean linens on the over-bed table.

4. Raise the head of the bed as tolerated. Gently lift the person's head and shoulders and cover the pillow with a towel. Drape another towel across the person's back and shoulders.

5. If the side rails are in use, lower the side rail on the working side of the bed. The side rail on the opposite side of the bed should remain up.

6. If the hair is tangled, work on the tangles first. Put a small amount of detangler or leave-in conditioner on the tangled hair. Begin at the ends of the hair and work

(continued)

PROCEDURE 18-6 (Continued)

Combing a Person's Hair

toward the scalp. Hold the lock of hair just above the tangle (closest to the scalp) and use the wide-tooth comb to gently work through the tangle.

7. Using the brush and working with one 2-inch section at a time, gently brush the hair,

STEP 7 Hold the lock of hair just above the tangle.

moving from the roots of the hair toward the ends.

8. Secure the hair using barrettes, clips, or pins or braid the hair, as the person requests. Offer the person the mirror to check his or her appearance when you are finished.

9. Reposition the pillow under the person's head and straighten the bed linens. If the side rails are in use, return the side rails to the raised position. Lower the head of the bed as the person requests.

10. Gather the soiled linens and place them in the linen hamper or linen bag. Dispose of disposable items in a facility-approved waste container. Clean equipment and return it to the storage area.

Finishing Up CLSOWR

11. Complete the "Finishing Up" steps **a** through **f**.

PROCEDURE 18-7

Shaving a Person's Face

Getting Ready WCKIEPS

1. Complete the "Getting Ready" steps **a** through **g**.

Supplies

- gloves
- paper towels
- safety razor
- shaving cream/gel/ soap
- shaving brush (if using shaving soap)
- aftershave lotion (optional)
- wash basin
- bath thermometer
- mirror
- washcloth
- towels

Procedure

2. Make sure that the bed is lowered to its lowest position and that the wheels are locked.

3. Fill the wash basin with warm water (100°F [37.7°C] to 115°F [46.1°C] on the bath thermometer).

4. Cover the over-bed table with paper towels. Place the wash basin, shaving supplies, and clean linens on the over-bed table. Put on the gloves.

5. If the side rails are in use, lower the side rail on the working side of the bed. The side rail on the opposite side of the bed should remain up.

6. Help the person to transfer from the bed to a bedside chair (see Procedure 11-9), assist the person to sit on the edge of the bed (see Procedure 11-15), or raise the head of the bed as tolerated.

7. Place a towel across the person's shoulders and chest.

8. Wet the washcloth with warm, clean water. Soften the beard by holding the washcloth against the person's face for 2 to 3 minutes.

9. Apply shaving cream, gel, or soap to the beard.

10. Shave the person's cheeks:

   a. Stand facing the person.

   b. Gently pull the skin tight and shave downward, in the direction of hair growth (i.e., toward the chin). Use short, even strokes, rinsing the razor frequently in the wash

(continued)

PROCEDURE 18-7 (Continued)

Shaving a Person's Face

basin. Repeat until all of the lather on the cheek has been removed.

c. Repeat for the other cheek.

STEP 10 Shave downward, in the direction of hair growth.

11. Shave the person's chin:

a. Ask the person to "tighten the chin" by drawing the lower lip over the teeth.

b. Shave the chin using short, even, downward strokes. Repeat until all of the lather on the chin has been removed, rinsing the razor frequently in the wash basin.

12. Shave the person's neck:

a. Ask the person to tip his head back.

b. Gently pull the skin tight and shave upward, in the direction of hair growth (i.e., toward the chin). Use short, even strokes, rinsing the razor frequently in the wash basin. Repeat until all of the lather on the neck has been removed.

13. Shave the area between the person's nose and upper lip:

a. Ask the person to "tighten his upper lip" by drawing the upper lip over the teeth.

b. Shave the area between the nose and the upper lip using short, even downward strokes. Repeat until all of the lather has been removed, rinsing the razor frequently in the wash basin.

14. Change the water in the wash basin. (If the side rails are in use, raise the side rails before leaving the bedside.) Form a mitt around your hand with the washcloth and wet the mitt with warm, clean water. Wash the person's face and neck. Rinse thoroughly, and pat the person's face, neck, and ears dry with the face towel.

15. Apply aftershave lotion, as the person requests.

16. If you have accidentally nicked the skin and the person is bleeding, apply direct pressure with a tissue until the bleeding stops. Report the incident to the nurse.

17. If necessary, help the person return to bed. If the side rails are in use, return the side rails to the raised position.

18. Gather the soiled linens and place them in the linen hamper or linen bag. Dispose of disposable items in a facility-approved waste container. Clean equipment and return it to the storage area.

19. Remove your gloves and dispose of them in a facility-approved waste container.

Finishing Up

20. Complete the "Finishing Up" steps **a** through **f**.

What did you learn?

Multiple Choice

Select the single best answer for each of the following questions.

1. You are a nursing assistant in a long-term care facility. Which one of the following procedures may be beyond your scope of practice?
   a. Assisting a resident with bathing
   b. Polishing a female resident's fingernails
   c. Trimming the toenails of a resident with diabetes
   d. Assisting a resident with oral hygiene

2. When helping a person to dress, which item of clothing would you put on first?
   a. Underpants
   b. Socks
   c. Slacks
   d. Sweater

3. Mrs. Dinksley, one of your residents, had a stroke that caused her left side to become weak. You are helping Mrs. Dinksley put on a cardigan sweater. Which arm should you put in the sleeve first?
   a. The left arm
   b. The right arm
   c. Either arm; it makes no difference
   d. Neither arm; Mrs. Dinksley should not be wearing a cardigan sweater

4. Mr. Bush has just been admitted to the long-term care facility where you work. You are telling him about the facility's policies. One of these policies is that residents are bathed on Monday, Wednesday, and Friday mornings. Mr. Bush looks worried, and says that he always bathes and shaves before he goes to bed, and he likes to do this every night. How do you react to this?
   a. You tell Mr. Bush that you're sorry, but he has to follow facility policy.
   b. You tell Mr. Bush "OK" but then schedule him for a bath every Monday, Wednesday, and Friday morning, just like everyone else.
   c. You respect Mr. Bush's choice and schedule him for a bath and a shave as part of evening care, every evening.
   d. You report Mr. Bush to the nurse because he is being difficult.

5. Brushing the hair is important to:
   a. Make it grow faster
   b. Make it soft and shiny and prevent tangles
   c. Keep it clean
   d. Keep it free from lice

6. When shaving a man's face with a safety razor and shaving cream, you should:
   a. Soften the beard with warm water before applying the shaving cream
   b. Apply aftershave lotion after the shave is complete, if the man requests it
   c. Give the man a mirror so that he can check his appearance when you are finished
   d. All of the above

7. When shaving a man's face, you should:
   a. Apply shaving cream sparingly
   b. Use upward strokes when shaving the cheeks
   c. Apply an antiseptic to any cuts or nicks
   d. Use downward strokes to shave the chin

8. Which one of the following statements about nail care is true?
   a. Scissors are used to trim the nails.
   b. Elderly people do not need nail care because their nails do not grow as fast.
   c. Providing nail care allows you to examine the hands and feet for signs of health and disease.
   d. Nail care is an activity that can be skipped if there is not enough time.

9. Which one of the following benefits does a patient or resident enjoy when you shampoo his or her hair?
   a. Improved circulation (blood flow) to the scalp
   b. A clean, neat appearance
   c. Increased feelings of well-being
   d. All of the above

10. Which one of the following statements about helping a resident to dress is true?
    a. Residents like staff members to decide what they are going to wear.
    b. Residents are used to being dressed in front of others.
    c. Residents care about how they look.
    d. Residents who are disabled do not need to dress in street clothes.

11. One of your residents, Mrs. Ament, has diabetes. Why is providing foot care an important part of caring for Mrs. Ament?
    a. The circulation to her feet is likely to be poor, which puts her at risk for infection and other complications.
    b. Diabetes makes the toenails grow faster.
    c. People with diabetes usually do not take good care of their feet.
    d. All of the above.

12. You must remove a soiled gown from a patient who has an intravenous (IV) line. What is the best way to do this?
    a. Remove the gown from the arm with the IV first.
    b. Ask the nurse to disconnect the bag and tubing before beginning.
    c. Disconnect the bag and tubing before beginning.
    d. Remove the opposite arm from the gown first.

Matching

Match each numbered item with its appropriate lettered description.

_____ **1.** Pediculosis
_____ **2.** Alopecia
_____ **3.** Podiatrist
_____ **4.** Tinea pedis
_____ **5.** Tinea capitis

a. A fungal infection of the scalp
b. Loss of hair
c. A fungal infection of the feet
d. Head lice
e. A doctor who specializes in care of the feet

? *Stop and think!*

▶ You have been assigned to take care of Mr. Wiseman, an Orthodox Jewish rabbi who is recovering from a stroke. As you are assisting Mr. Wiseman with his morning care, you note that his long beard is matted and he has food crusted in it. You try combing and brushing the beard, but you are not making much progress. Then you notice white spots on the hairs of the beard. Having recently graduated from your nursing assistant training program, you suspect that these spots are nits, or lice eggs. You look out into the hall for a nurse. Seeing no one, you decide to trim Mr. Wiseman's beard yourself, because you know that lice are transmitted easily from person to person. Not being a barber (or having had much experience with shaving another person's face!), you get carried away and end up shaving off Mr. Wiseman's entire beard. As you are finishing up, the medication nurse arrives in the room and realizes with horror what has happened. She says to you, "Oh, no! Didn't you realize that Mr. Wiseman's beard is part of his religion? What are we going to tell his wife?" What did you do wrong? What could you have done to prevent this mistake?

19

Basic Nutrition

What will you learn?

Few things are more satisfying than a good meal—you know, one that is made up of your favorite foods, all cooked to perfection, just like Mom's home cooking. Eating meets many needs for people, both emotionally and physically. In this chapter, you will learn about what we need to eat to keep our bodies healthy. You will also learn how to help your patients and residents to meet their own nutritional needs. When you are finished with this chapter, you will be able to:

1. Define the term *nutrition* and explain why our bodies need adequate nutrition.
2. List the general types of nutrients and describe how the body uses them.
3. Discuss how the Food Guide Pyramid can be used to help plan and provide better nutrition for a person.
4. Explain factors that influence a person's food preferences.
5. List and describe common special diets.
6. Discuss the importance of making meals attractive and the dining experience pleasant.
7. Explain the steps that are taken to help prepare a person for meal time.
8. Describe ways that a nursing assistant may need to help a person during meal time.
9. Demonstrate proper technique for feeding a person who cannot feed herself.
10. Describe how the amount of solid food eaten is recorded.
11. Discuss other ways of providing nutrition for people who are unable to take food by mouth.
12. Explain the fluid needs of the body and factors that affect the body's fluid balance.
13. Demonstrate methods used to measure and record fluid intake and output.

Photo: Meal time is as much about socializing as it is about eating.
(ThinkStock LLC.)

Vocabulary

Use the CD in the back of your book to hear these terms pronounced, defined, and used in a sentence:

Nutrients	Food Guide Pyramid	Nasointestinal tube	Fluid balance
Nutrition	Nutritional Labeling	Gastrostomy tube	Dehydration
Ingestion	and Education Act	Jejunostomy tube	Edema
Digestion	Appetite	Percutaneous	NPO status
Absorption	Anorexia	endoscopic	Intake and output
Calories	Dietitian	gastrostomy (PEG)	(I&O) flow sheet
Glucose	Nutritional supplement	tube	Graduate
Amino acids	Intravenous (IV) therapy	Total parenteral	
Fat-soluble	Enteral nutrition	nutrition (TPN,	
Water-soluble	Nasogastric tube	hyperalimentation)	

FOOD AND HOW OUR BODIES USE IT

All living things eat. The food that we take into our bodies is broken down into essential elements, called **nutrients**. The body uses these nutrients to grow, to repair itself, and to carry out processes essential for living. **Nutrition,** or the process of taking in and using food, involves the following steps:

- **Ingestion,** or the intake of food
- **Digestion,** or the breaking down of food into simple elements (nutrients)
- **Absorption,** or the transfer of these nutrients from the digestive tract into the bloodstream
- **Metabolism,** or the process that occurs in cells to convert the nutrients into energy

To function, the body needs a continuous supply of energy, which it gets from the metabolism of food. You know that your body uses energy when you run to catch a bus, reposition a patient or resident, or climb a flight of stairs. But did you also know that your body uses energy even when you are sitting perfectly still? Every time you blink, or your heart beats, or your lungs expand to take in air, you are using energy. The energy to power our bodies comes from food, especially food that is high in carbohydrates, protein, or fat. Energy is measured in units called kilocalories, more commonly known as **calories.**

In addition to providing us with energy, food provides us with other substances our bodies need to function properly. Other substances found in food that benefit us include vitamins and minerals, fiber, and water:

- **Vitamins** and **minerals** are small molecules that help to regulate body processes and form structures within the body. For example, vitamin K helps the blood to clot, and calcium, a mineral, helps to build strong bones. Table 19-1 lists some of the common vitamins and minerals and describes how they benefit the body.
- **Fiber** is found in fruits, vegetables, and whole grain cereals and breads. Fiber may be soluble, which means that it can be broken down, or digested. Or it may be insoluble, which means that it cannot be digested. Insoluble fiber helps to prevent problems with bowel movements by adding bulk to the feces.
- **Water,** which will be discussed in more detail later in this chapter, plays many important roles in helping the body to function well.

TYPES OF NUTRIENTS

There are six general types of nutrients. Three of these nutrient types (carbohydrates, proteins, and fat) supply energy. The remaining three (minerals, vitamins, and water) regulate body processes.

Carbohydrates

Foods containing carbohydrates form the basis of many diets throughout the world because these foods tend to be plentiful and inexpensive. Carbohydrates are found in bread, cereal, fruit,

TABLE 19-1 ■ Vitamins and Minerals

Nutrient	Sources	Function
VITAMINS		
Vitamin A	Liver, carrots, egg yolks, fortified milk	Helps us to see in dim light Keeps skin and mucous membranes healthy
Vitamin B_1 (thiamin)	Pork, liver, whole and enriched grains, legumes	Helps produce energy from glucose Assists with nerve function
Vitamin B_2 (riboflavin)	Milk, organ meats (e.g., brain, kidneys, liver), enriched grains, green vegetables	Assists with the metabolism of carbohydrates, protein, and fat
Vitamin B_3 (niacin)	Kidneys, grains, lean meats, nuts	Assists with the metabolism of carbohydrates, protein, and fat
Vitamin B_{12}	Meat (including organ meats), eggs, milk, cheese	Assists with the formation of hemoglobin (the molecule that carries oxygen throughout the body) and red blood cells
Folic acid	Green leafy vegetables, meats, and whole grains	Assists with protein metabolism and the formation of red blood cells
Vitamin C (ascorbic acid)	Citrus fruits, broccoli, green peppers, strawberries, green leafy vegetables	Assists with tissue healing, building red blood cells, and iron absorption
Vitamin D	Sunlight, fortified milk, fish liver oils	Assists with the absorption of calcium and phosphorus to strengthen bones
Vitamin E	Vegetable oils, wheat germ, whole grains	Assists with the formation of red blood cells Assists with the reproductive system
Vitamin K	Vegetable oils, wheat germ, whole grains, liver, green leafy vegetables, eggs	Assists with metabolism of the proteins necessary for normal blood clotting
MINERALS		
Calcium	Milk, cheese, canned fish with bones, green leafy vegetables	Keeps the teeth and bones strong Assists with blood clotting Assists with nerve function and contraction of the heart and skeletal muscles
Phosphorus	Milk, soft drinks, meat, nuts, peas, and beans	Keeps the teeth and bones strong Assists with the metabolism of carbohydrates, protein, and fat
Iron	Liver, lean meats, enriched and whole-grain breads, and cheese	Used to produce hemoglobin (the molecule that carries oxygen throughout the body)
Iodine	Table salt and seafood	Used by the thyroid gland to produce hormones for cell metabolism
Sodium	Table salt	Assists with fluid balance, nerve function, and contraction of the heart and skeletal muscles
Potassium	Whole grains, fruits, green leafy vegetables	Assists with fluid balance, nerve function, and contraction of the heart and skeletal muscles

vegetables, and table sugar. Carbohydrates are the source of the body's most basic type of fuel, **glucose**. Glucose, sometimes called "blood sugar," is carried in the blood and rapidly absorbed by every cell in the body. The cells use the glucose to "run," much like your car uses gas. Glucose is a simple carbohydrate, or sugar, which means that it passes quickly from the digestive tract into the bloodstream. Other carbohydrates, known as complex carbohydrates, or starches, must be broken down into simple sugars before the body can use them. Extra carbohydrates that are not used immediately as fuel are either stored in the liver or converted to fat and stored elsewhere in the body. Each gram of carbohydrate provides the body with 4 calories, or energy units.

Protein

Protein is found in foods such as milk and cheese, meat, poultry, fish, eggs, nuts, and dried peas and beans. Proteins contain **amino acids,** small molecules that are the "building blocks" of all of the body's cells. Therefore, foods containing protein help the body to rebuild tissue that breaks down from normal use and to grow new tissue after illness or injury. In addition to providing amino acids, protein is a source of fuel. Like carbohydrate, protein provides the body with 4 calories per gram.

Fats (Lipids)

Fats are found in butter, cooking oils, whole milk, cheese, meat, egg yolks, nuts, shortening, and lard. Fats make food taste better and satisfy the appetite longer because they take longer to digest than most other food sources. Although a "low-fat" diet is recommended for most people to maintain health, not all fats are bad. In fact, the body requires a certain amount of dietary fat to function properly. For example, some vitamins will dissolve only in fat, not water (that is, they are **fat-soluble**). This means that fat must be present in order for the body to use the vitamins. Fat also protects our organs and helps us to stay warm. Finally, fats are the most concentrated source of energy, providing 9 calories per gram.

Vitamins

Vitamins, as described earlier and in Table 19-1, play a key role in many body processes. Vitamins are classified as water-soluble or fat-soluble. **Water-soluble** vitamins dissolve in water. Water-soluble vitamins (vitamin C and the B-complex vitamins) are absorbed directly from the digestive tract into the bloodstream. The body cannot store water-soluble vitamins. Instead, any extra amounts of these vitamins are passed from the body in the urine. This means that water-soluble vitamins must be replenished daily for use by the body.

Fat-soluble vitamins (vitamins A, D, E, and K) are absorbed and stored in the body's fat, where they can be used as needed. Unlike water-soluble vitamins, fat-soluble vitamins are not easily passed from the body. For this reason, consuming too much of a fat-soluble vitamin can be as harmful as not consuming enough, because the vitamin builds up in the body. In some cases, this build-up may actually be harmful.

Minerals

Minerals help provide structure within the body. For example, fluorine strengthens the teeth and calcium strengthens the bones. Minerals also regulate body processes. For example, red blood cells need iron in order to do their job of carrying oxygen to all of the cells in the body. Key minerals that the body needs to function properly are summarized in Table 19-1.

Water

Water is provided in the diet in the form of beverages, such as juice, soda, milk, coffee, tea, and, of course, water! Water is also found in many foods, such as fruits and vegetables. Water provides no calories or nutritional value, but may be more essential to life than food. You can live for quite a long time without food, but only for 3 to 7 days without water. Every cell in your body contains water, which is why water accounts for approximately 50% to 60% of your body weight! Water does the following things for our bodies:

- The nutrients found in food must be dissolved in fluid and circulated throughout the body. Water forms the basis for this fluid.
- Water transports waste products out of the body, by way of the urine and feces.
- Water keeps us cool when it evaporates from our skin in the form of sweat.

- Water keeps the mucous membranes moist.
- Water forms the basis of the fluid that helps our joints to move smoothly.

A BALANCED DIET

Some foods contain many nutrients that our bodies need to remain healthy, whereas other foods have little or no nutritional value. Although some nutrients play very specific roles within the body, most nutrients work best when combined with a variety of other nutrients. For the best health, you must follow a diet that provides your body with a balanced amount of the essential nutrients. Two tools are available to help you achieve this goal—the Food Guide Pyramid and the nutrition labels on food.

Food Guide Pyramid

The United States Department of Agriculture's **Food Guide Pyramid** (Fig. 19-1) is a guide for making daily food choices. This Food Guide Pyramid applies for all healthy people older than 2 years. The foods that we should eat the most of are at the bottom of the pyramid, forming its solid base. The foods that we should eat the least of are found near the top of the pyramid, forming its tip. Let's take a look at the levels of the pyramid:

- **Bread, cereal, rice, and pasta group.** According to the pyramid, the base of a sound diet is 6 to 11 servings of grains, such as bread, cereal, rice, and pasta. These foods supply our bodies with carbohydrates, which are easily converted to energy. Each of the following counts as one serving: 1 slice of bread; one half of an English muffin; ½ cup of cooked rice, pasta, or cereal; or 1 ounce of ready-to-eat cereal. Although 6 to 11 servings a day may seem like a lot, note that these servings are small (Fig. 19-2).
- **Fruit and vegetable groups.** The next level of the pyramid is made up of the fruit and vegetable groups. Fruits and vegetables supply carbohydrates, vitamins, and minerals, as well as fiber to aid in elimination. The government recommends that we eat 3 to 5 servings of vegetables and 2 to 4 servings of fruit each day. A serving of vegetables consists of ½ cup of chopped raw or cooked vegetables, or 1 cup of leafy raw vegetables. A serving of fruit consists of 1 medium-sized piece of fruit, ¾ cup of fruit juice, ½ cup of canned fruit, or ¼ cup of dried fruit.
- **Milk and meat groups.** The third level of the pyramid contains the "animal-based"

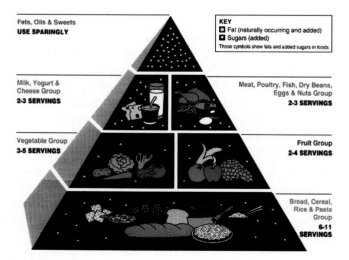

FIGURE 19-1

The Food Guide Pyramid. This guide shows the recommended number of servings from each food group that should be consumed each day in order to ensure the best nutrition. This pyramid was designed for healthy people older than 2 years. (*Courtesy of the United States Department of Agriculture and the United States Department of Health and Human Services.*)

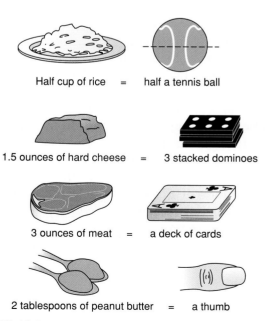

Half cup of rice   =   half a tennis ball

1.5 ounces of hard cheese   =   3 stacked dominoes

3 ounces of meat   =   a deck of cards

2 tablespoons of peanut butter   =   a thumb

FIGURE 19-2

What is a "serving"?

food groups, the dairy group (milk, yogurt, cheese) and the meat group (red meat, poultry, fish, beans, eggs, and nuts). Foods from these groups supply the body with protein and minerals, such as calcium, iron, and zinc. According to these guidelines, a healthy person needs 2 to 3 daily servings from both the dairy group and the meat group. A serving from the dairy group consists of 1 cup of milk or yogurt, 1½ ounces of natural cheese, or 2 ounces of processed cheese. A serving from the meat group consists of 2½ to 3 ounces of cooked lean meat, poultry, or fish; ½ cup of cooked beans; 1 egg; or 2 tablespoons of peanut butter (see Fig. 19-2). Although protein is an essential nutrient, most people in North America consume twice the recommended daily amount of protein.

- **Fats, oils, and sweets group.** The very top of the pyramid is represented by a food group that should be used sparingly—fats, oils, and sweets. These foods provide little nutrition, but have many calories. Examples of foods in this group include salad dressings and oils, cream, butter, margarine, sugar, soft drinks, candy, cakes, and cookies. No one wants to eat a salad without dressing, or to skip dessert all of the time. However, foods from this category should be eaten in moderate amounts.

This Food Guide Pyramid is just that, a guide. Nutritional requirements vary at different times throughout a person's life. For example, infants and very small children have an increased need for calories and iron because they are growing rapidly. Similarly, teenagers going through "growth spurts" have increased caloric and nutritional needs. Pregnant and breast-feeding women need more protein and calcium. People who are recovering from physical trauma, such as that caused by burns or surgery, have different nutritional requirements from healthy people. Likewise, some illnesses change the nutritional requirements of the body, including chronic conditions such as diabetes, kidney disease, or alcoholism.

Modifications of the United States Department of Agriculture's Food Guide Pyramid have been developed that take into account special groups of people, such as people from other cultures who may prefer other types of food, and

people older than 70 years. The physical changes that occur with normal aging affect a person's nutritional requirements. For example, older people do not need as many calories as younger people, because they are usually less physically active. They also may not feel thirsty as often, although the need for water and other fluids increases with age. As a result of much research into the nutritional needs of elderly people, Tufts University created the Food Guide Pyramid for Older Adults (Fig. 19-3). On this version of the pyramid, also known as the "70+ Food Guide Pyramid," the number of servings has been reduced in some food groups to meet the decreased caloric need, while water now forms the base of the pyramid to show the importance of drinking fluids. The total pyramid focuses on foods in each group that are high in nutrients but lower in fat and calories. A flag has been added to the top of

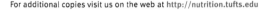

For additional copies visit us on the web at http://nutrition.tufts.edu

FIGURE 19-3

The Tufts Food Guide Pyramid for Older Adults. This pyramid takes into account the special nutritional needs of people 70 years of age and older. (*Courtesy of Tufts University.*)

the pyramid to represent the possible need for vitamin and mineral supplements. Like the standard Food Guide Pyramid, the 70+ Food Guide Pyramid contains recommendations for *healthy* people. Factors such as illness can change a person's nutritional requirements.

Food Labels

There is a second tool available to help you plan a balanced diet—the nutrition labels that appear on most foods offered for sale at the grocery store. Education about proper nutrition and diet planning is one of the most effective ways of promoting health and helping to prevent some illnesses. In recognition of this fact, the United States Congress passed the **Nutritional Labeling and Education Act** in 1990, which requires that the labels of all packaged foods include information about the food's nutritional value, approximate serving size, and any related health claims (Fig. 19-4). By reading the nutrition label, you can see how the food can help you to achieve your nutrition goals for the day.

RESPECTING THE INDIVIDUAL

The Food Pyramid and food labels help us to make wise food choices. However, factors other than the nutritional content of a food often affect the choices we make about what we eat and when we eat it. Some people prefer a hot, hearty breakfast to start the day whereas others may want only a bowl of cereal or coffee and toast. Some people like a light meal at lunchtime whereas others eat their main meal at mid-day. Dinner may consist of a light snack for some whereas others routinely have a seven-course meal. Listed below are some of the factors that affect a person's food choices and eating habits. Think about your own eating habits and food likes and dislikes. Are any of your personal preferences related to the factors listed here?

- **Religion.** Dietary restrictions are a part of many religions. Some of these restrictions are specific to certain days (for example, the Roman Catholic custom of avoiding meat on Fridays during Lent, or the Jewish tradition of avoiding flour-based foods during Passover). Other dietary restrictions are in effect all of the time (for example, some Jewish people keep a kosher kitchen).

FIGURE 19-4

The law requires all packaged foods to have a nutrition label like this one. (*Courtesy of Sunsweet Growers, Inc.*)

- **Culture and geography.** People often like certain foods because they are associated with their culture, or the area where they grew up. For example, a person who was raised in the southern United States may have grown up eating "grits" (corn mush) for breakfast instead of oatmeal. Now imagine that this person has moved to a long-term care facility in the Northeast to be closer to a son or daughter, where the typical "northern" dish of oatmeal is served for breakfast. Although the person might like oatmeal just fine, she might prefer grits because they are familiar and they remind her of "home." Cultural preferences are a combination of heritage, religion, geography, and all of the characteristics that make a person unique. Some people are willing to try new foods, while others prefer to stay with what they know. This desire for familiar foods is one reason why chain restaurants are so popular in the United States.

- **Economics.** There is no doubt about it—food is expensive! The grocery bill takes a major chunk out of any family's budget. People who are on a fixed income, especially disabled or elderly people, may find it difficult to afford foods that supply good nutrition. Often, fresh fruits and vegetables and lean cuts of meat are among the most expensive items in the grocery cart. Milk and cheese, which are also packed with nutrition, may also be out of many people's price range. Instead, people in the lower economic levels often rely on cheaper foods that are high in calories and carbohydrates, but low in many nutrients. Fortunately, a small food budget does not necessarily make it impossible to eat healthy foods. With information and planning, it is possible to afford nutritionally sound food, even on a fixed income.

- **Individual taste.** Do you like lima beans? Some people find certain foods delicious whereas others could barely swallow a bite. Some people may not like a certain food because of its texture, or the degree of spiciness. Others will avoid a food because of the way it looks or smells. Many people are unable to eat certain foods, no matter how much they love them, because of food allergies. As you certainly know from your own experience, individual tastes vary greatly, even among people who belong to the same culture (or the same family)!

- **Appetite.** Appetite is simply the desire for food. Appetite is both physically driven (by the feeling of hunger) and emotionally driven. Have you ever had your television show interrupted by a commercial for some type of food, where the food looked so good you actually started to feel hungry? You may not have actually been physically hungry, but the sight of the food and the thought of how it would taste stimulated your appetite. The opposite can be true as well. For example, a person who is ill or under emotional stress may be physically hungry, but have no appetite for any food. This loss of appetite is called **anorexia.** Although illness may cause anorexia, a person who is ill usually needs *more* calories and nutrients than he or she normally would in order to heal and become healthy again. Part of providing holistic care is encouraging your patients or residents to eat adequate amounts of food, even when they have no appetite.

Meals prepared for people in health care facilities are specific to each person's individual needs. Some patients and residents are on special diets because of surgery, illness, or chronic health conditions. Personal preferences are taken into account when planning meals. No matter how tasty that ham steak may look, a person who does not like ham will not eat it. In order to find out as much as possible about the patient's or resident's eating habits and food likes and dislikes, a nurse completes a dietary assessment as part of the admissions process. During the assessment, the nurse asks the person (or his family members, if the person cannot answer for himself) about eating habits, favorite foods, and foods that should be avoided. This information is shared with the **dietitian,** a person who has a degree in nutrition. The dietitian uses the information from the dietary assessment, as well as her knowledge of nutrition, to plan a diet for the person that he will enjoy eating and that will keep him healthy.

As a nursing assistant, you will play a key role in the ongoing evaluation of your patients' or residents' dietary status. Of all the nursing team members, you will have the most contact with your patients or residents during meal times. You will see which foods are eaten readily and which are left on the tray. When you notice that a food has not been eaten, you might talk to the person about it. For example:

Nursing assistant: Hi, Mr. Wheeling! How was your lunch? (*Noticing that the dessert has not been eaten*) Oh! I see you didn't eat your dessert. Are you full, or do you just not like vanilla tapioca?

Mr. Wheeling: Well, actually, I am pretty full, so I decided to skip the tapioca today. It's not my favorite anyway. (*Wrinkling nose*) I don't like the lumps.

FIGURE 19-5

Respecting a person's preferences when it comes to food lets the person know that you care about him or her as an individual.

Nursing assistant: Well, I'm glad you told me! We ought to be able to avoid 'lumpy' desserts in the future...maybe vanilla pudding or ice cream would be better instead?

Mr. Wheeling *(smiling):* Thanks, Nancy. That would be great. I do look forward to dessert!

Talking with the person about why a food was not eaten serves two purposes. First, it allows you to give the nurse information that she and the dietitian can use to plan future meals for the person. Second, when you notice that a food has gone untouched and take the time to ask the person about it, you let the person know that you care about him as an individual (Fig. 19-5).

As you might expect, long-term care facilities that receive government funding must follow Omnibus Budget Reconciliation Act (OBRA) regulations pertaining to meals. OBRA requires that meals meet the individual nutritional needs of each resident. Foods must be served at the proper temperature. They must be appealing to look at, and seasoned to the individual resident's preference. Special diets, such as those followed for health or religious reasons, are provided for those residents who need them. Dining in the company of other residents is also recommended.

SPECIAL DIETS

The type of diet that is ordered for a person in a health care setting is determined by many factors. People with illnesses such as diabetes, heart disease, or kidney disease require special diets. People who are recovering from surgery or trauma may require liquid or high-calorie diets for a period of time. Just the normal changes in the digestive system that accompany aging may require foods that are easier to chew, easier to digest, and have added fiber to help prevent constipation. Specific diets are ordered by a doctor and prepared by a dietitian.

Brief descriptions of some of the special diets that you may see ordered in a health care facility are provided here. It is important for you to familiarize yourself with your facility's specific diets and the foods that they include. That way, if a mistake is made in the kitchen and the wrong meal is sent up for one of your patients or residents, you will be able to recognize that an error has been made. Diets that are commonly seen in health care facilities include the following:

- **Regular ("house") diet.** This is simply a well-balanced diet. There are no restrictions on specific foods or condiments (for example, salt, pepper, ketchup, salad dressing). A person on a regular diet is usually allowed to eat foods prepared and brought by friends and family members. There are many variations to the regular diet. For example, a high-calorie or low-calorie version may be ordered to promote weight gain or weight loss. A low-residue or high-fiber version may be ordered to either decrease or increase dietary fiber for people with certain digestive problems. A bland diet contains foods that are easy to digest and will not irritate the digestive tract.

- **Clear liquid diet.** Clear liquids are substances that can be poured at room or body temperature and that you can see through. Foods that are considered clear liquids include water, gelatin, fat-free broth or bouillon, popsicles, clear juices (for example, apple, cranberry, grape), clear carbonated sodas, and coffee and tea (without cream). A person who is nauseous or vomiting, or who has just had surgery or is recovering from an acute illness or trauma, may be ordered to have a clear liquid diet initially. Clear liquids do not contain enough nutrients to maintain health for very long, so a person is usually progressed into a more nutritious diet as soon as the body can tolerate it.

- **Full liquid diet.** A full liquid diet is the clear liquid diet, plus any food that can be poured at room or body temperature. For example, milk, plain frozen desserts (such as popsicles, ice cream, or frozen yogurt), pasteurized eggs (egg custard or eggnog), cereal gruels, and strained soups and juices are all considered full liquids. Full liquids contain more nutrition than clear liquids, but a high-calorie, high-protein liquid dietary supplement may be added if the person must be on a full-liquid diet for more than 3 days.

- **Soft diet.** Soft diets are usually regular diets that have been changed slightly to remove foods that are hard to chew or digest. The soft diet is used for people who have difficulty chewing or swallowing their food. The soft diet is not highly seasoned and does not contain foods that are fried or high in fiber. Soft diets contain adequate nutrition. Therefore, a person can remain on a soft diet for as long as is necessary.

- **Diabetic diet (consistent-carbohydrate diabetes meal plan).** This diet regulates the amount of fat, carbohydrate, and protein that a person with diabetes mellitus consumes. The person's specific energy and nutritional requirements determine the amounts of fat, carbohydrate, and protein that are permitted. The diet is different for each person. A person with diabetes who is receiving insulin injections must eat enough to prevent her blood sugar levels from dropping. When caring for patients or residents who have diabetes, you must make special note of the amount of food the person eats at each meal.

- **Sodium-restricted diet.** Sodium restriction is helpful for the treatment of certain types of heart disease, hypertension (high blood pressure), and kidney disease. A person on a sodium-restricted diet may be allowed to have a small amount of salt, or none at all. For example, some people may be able to eat foods that have some salt in them, but they will not be allowed to add extra salt at the table or eat very salty foods, such as pickles. Other people may have severe restrictions placed on their salt intake. For these people, food will be prepared without any salt at all, and of course, the person will not be able to add salt to the food at the table. Some people on sodium-restricted diets may use salt substitutes. If you have a patient or resident who has been placed on a sodium-restricted diet, make sure you know whether he is allowed to use a little bit of salt or a salt substitute, or none at all.

- **Low-cholesterol diet.** Following a diet that is low in saturated fats and cholesterol is good advice for everybody, but it is especially good advice for a person with heart disease. Foods are chosen that are lower in animal fat and prepared in ways that do not add additional fats. The addition of butter, shortening, and margarine to foods is avoided, and foods such as fruits and vegetables, whole grains, and skim milk are encouraged.

Some of your patients or residents will have **nutritional supplements** that are either offered with the meal or as an in-between meal snack. These nutritional supplements, which can be used to supply extra calories or protein, often take the form of a flavored shake or drink. These drinks are convenient and easy to serve. People with diabetes mellitus may require snacks in between meals to keep their blood sugar levels stable. The dietitian will plan for the nutritional supplements. It is usually the nursing assistant's responsibility to serve these nutritional supplements at specific times throughout the day and record that the supplements have been consumed. If your patient or resident refuses to eat an ordered supplement, report this to a nurse.

As you can see, the people you are caring for could be placed on any number of special diets for a variety of reasons. Take the time to learn about a person's medical condition, and the reason a particular diet was ordered for that person. For example, you could ask the nurse if she knows of any articles you could read about the person's condition. This additional information will give you the insight you need to make good observations about a person's dietary habits. Your patients or residents will benefit, and so will you, because you will become a more effective member of the health care team.

MEAL TIME

A tasty meal, good company, and a relaxed dining atmosphere satisfy physical needs (hunger) as well as emotional ones (the need for love and

FIGURE 19-6

In most cultures, food plays a central role at social events.

belonging). In most cultures, eating is a social event. We eat at parties and celebrations, we eat on dates, we eat certain foods on certain holidays, and we look forward to catching up with family members and friends over the dinner table (Fig. 19-6). Now imagine that you have just moved into a long-term care facility or been admitted to the hospital. Who will you share your meals with? Would you miss one special dish that your family always has for Sunday dinner? You might find yourself feeling a little lonely and homesick.

Meal times can be emotionally difficult for people who are receiving health care. For example, many clients of home health care agencies live alone. People who live alone often eat with the television for company. These people may feel lonely and not have much of an appetite. Or, they may eat too much because they are lonely. People who become patients in hospitals or residents in long-term care facilities may feel that all personal choice is lost when it comes to meals. Injury, illness, or surgery may demand specific dietary restrictions. Meals are served at specific times. Often, the menus offer limited choices. Pain, anxiety, illness, and medication side effects can cause a person to have little or no appetite. Sometimes, people have physical disabilities that make it difficult for them to feed themselves, and they feel embarrassed because they need help. Meal times and the act of eating may take on a whole different meaning for a person who needs health care.

By providing companionship and assistance as needed, you can help to make sure that meal time remains a pleasant part of your patient's, resident's, or client's daily routine. You must make an effort to make the dining experience as pleasant as possible. Food should be presented in a way that will stimulate the appetite. Offering small portions of favorite foods frequently throughout the day can help increase a person's desire to eat. A clean, fresh mouth makes food taste better. A comfortable position, whether the person is using an over-bed table in bed or is seated at a regular table in the dining room, keeps the person focused on the food. If the person uses glasses or a hearing aid, make sure that these aids are in place. Provide pleasant conversation. All of these measures help to set a relaxed overall atmosphere and stimulate the appetite.

PREPARING FOR MEAL TIME

You will need to help your patients and residents get ready for each meal. Be sure to give your patients or residents ample time to prepare for meals. Allowing time to prepare is especially important before breakfast, because early morning care must be completed before the meal. In a long-term care facility, the residents are assisted to the dining room to eat. In a hospital, the patients usually take their meals in their rooms. The assistance you provide will vary, depending on the person you are helping. Some people only need to be reminded that it is "almost time for lunch" and they will prepare themselves to eat. Others will need your help to get ready for the meal. The following actions are taken to help prepare a person for meal time:

- Assist the person with toileting. Help him to the bathroom, or offer the bedpan or urinal.
- Assist the person with basic hygiene. Help him to wash his hands and face, and brush his teeth. If the person wears dentures, glasses, or a hearing aid, make sure these items are clean and in place.
- Position the person for eating. Residents in long-term care facilities are walked to the dining room, or taken in a wheelchair. In many facilities, the resident is helped from the wheelchair into a standard dining

chair for the meal. If the person will be eating his meal in bed, smooth the bed linens and position the bed in a high Fowler's position if permitted. Clear the over-bed table of clutter and wipe down the surface if necessary.

- Provide a pleasant environment. Remove any offensive or odorous items, such as bedpans or emesis basins, from the room. Adjust the lighting for comfort and turn on the radio or television if the person asks you to. Many people like to listen to music or watch a favorite program while they eat.

ASSISTING WITH MEALS

Once these preparations are completed, it is time to eat! Meals should be served as soon as they are sent up from the kitchen. This helps to ensure that hot foods are hot and cold foods are cold. Check that the name on the meal tray matches the name of the resident or patient who will be receiving it (Fig. 19-7). Also make sure that the diet noted on the tray matches the diet noted on the person's medical chart or nursing care plan. If the meal is not as ordered, ask a nurse to confirm that a mistake has in fact been made, and then return the meal to the kitchen. The kitchen will replace the meal with the correct one.

In many facilities, especially long-term care facilities, a cloth or paper clothing protector is used. This protector is placed over the person's chest to prevent the clothing from being soiled with food during the meal. Wearing a clothing protector is a matter of personal choice, so always ask the resident if it is all right for you to put the clothing protector on her before the meal. Please do not refer to the clothing protector as a "bib." An adult, especially one who is already feeling self-conscious because she needs help eating, will not appreciate being likened to a helpless baby! Think for a moment—when you are hungry, you sit down and eat. You cut your juicy steak, butter your hot rolls, and never give the act of eating a second thought. How would it feel to have to rely on another person to feed you, or cut up your food? Would you feel like a small child again, or a burden, or just useless? Be sensitive to your patients' or residents' feelings as you assist them with meals. Realize how very much they would like to be able to perform routine activities like eating without a second thought, just like you do.

Help the person to eat as necessary. Encourage your patients or residents to do as much for themselves as possible to help promote their independence. The nursing care plan will have basic information about the type of assistance the person needs, or you can ask the nurse. First, remove the cover from the tray and tell the person what foods are on the tray. No one likes "mystery meat" for dinner! Depending on the situation, you may also need to help the person with opening milk cartons or removing silverware from its wrapper, buttering bread, or cutting up meat (Fig. 19-8). If the

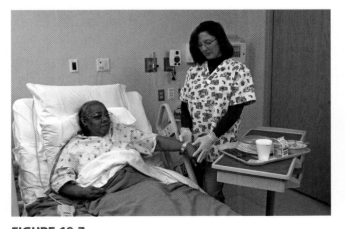

FIGURE 19-7

Always make sure that the right meal tray is being delivered to the right person.

FIGURE 19-8

Some people will be able to eat on their own if you give them a little bit of assistance.

person needs help seasoning the food, make sure that you add salt, pepper, and condiments according to the patient's or resident's tastes, not your own. If the person has poor eyesight, you will need to tell her where items are on the tray. Describe the food and help the person to find it on the plate by referencing a clock face (Fig. 19-9). For example, you might say, "Okay, Mr. Diaz—your pork chop is at 12 o'clock. The potatoes are at 3 o'clock, the green beans are at 6 o'clock, and the corn is at 9 o'clock. Your milk is on the upper right corner of the tray and your roll is on a bread plate to the left of your dinner plate."

Many of the people in your care will have some sort of physical disability that affects their ability to feed themselves. Special forks, knives, spoons, plates, and cups can help people with physical disabilities regain their independence. For example, many people who have had a stroke may have limited use of their hands and arms. They may be able to make big, sweeping movements, but small, delicate movements, such as those needed to hold and use regular silverware, are difficult. Specially made eating utensils, like those shown in Figure 19-10, allow the person to overcome these difficulties and feed himself. A person who has lost the use of one hand will have to learn to eat using only the other hand. In this situation, a plate with a raised rim is very helpful. The rim is used to help guide food, much as you would use a knife to steer peas onto your fork. Special holders that fit around drinking glasses make it easier to hold the glass. All of these assistive devices help

FIGURE 19-9
You can help a person with poor eyesight locate food on the plate by describing its location in terms of a clock face.

a disabled person regain independence, which is important for self-esteem.

FEEDING DEPENDENT PATIENTS AND RESIDENTS

Some people may not be able to feed themselves at all (Fig. 19-11). Even though these patients and residents will depend on you to do most of the work, it is very important that you involve them as much as possible in the process of eating. For example, you might ask the patient or resident to help you by holding her own napkin. Remember that meal time is a very social time in a person's day. It is important to talk to the person you are feeding, even if the person does not answer you. Hearing your voice and knowing that you care about him or her will increase the person's appetite and aid digestion.

The types of food served will differ according to the person's chewing and swallowing abilities. Some people may be able to eat solid food whereas others will require semi-solid or liquid food. When feeding another person, always use a spoon, not a fork, because the blunt edge of the spoon is safer than the sharp tines of the fork. Fill the spoon only about one-third full for each bite, and offer the bites slowly to prevent choking. Never rush the person through eating. Be sure to tell the person what foods you are offering her. If the person is alert and able to respond, ask her in what order she would like to try the food on the plate. Make sure you have seasoned the food according to the person's preference. If she is unable to tell you her preference, season the food mildly. Give the person enough time to chew and swallow each bite. You may need to gently remind the person to chew and swallow, especially if the person has dementia.

Offer liquids frequently, between bites. Some people find drinking through a straw to be easiest. Some people may have difficulty swallowing as the result of a stroke, injury, or dementia. These people can choke easily on liquids, so always offer liquids slowly. Sometimes the doctor orders the use of an additive that will thicken the liquid, making it easier to swallow. The nurse or therapist will show you how to use these additives to thicken liquids if this is necessary for one of your patients or residents.

A. Plate guard

B. Knife with a rounded blade

C. Cup holder

FIGURE 19-10

Assistive eating utensils help people with physical disabilities feed themselves. (*A*) Plate guards help to keep food on the plate and provide an "extra hand" for pushing food onto the fork. (*B*) A knife with a rounded blade can be rocked back and forth to cut food. This knife prevents the food from sliding on the plate. (*C*) A cup holder fits around a drinking glass, giving the person a firmer grip. (*Photos courtesy of Sammons Preston Rolyan, Bolingbrook, IL.*)

FIGURE 19-11

Some people may not be able to feed themselves.

Procedure 19-1 gives the steps for feeding a patient or resident who needs complete assistance with eating.

MEASURING AND RECORDING FOOD INTAKE

Most long-term care facilities and some hospitals will require you to record the amount of food that the person eats. In some facilities, you will just have to note the portion of the total meal that was consumed (for example, Mrs. Wells ate 60% of her breakfast, 80% of her lunch, and 30% of her dinner). Many facilities will want you to tell the nurse if one of your patients or residents eats less than 70% of his or her meal.

In other facilities, you will have to note what percentage of *each* food was eaten (for example, At dinner, Mr. Sommers ate 100% of his mashed potatoes, 50% of his salad, and 75% of his chicken breast). The nurse or dietitian will then convert the percentages that you provide into "total calories consumed," and this number is recorded on the person's chart.

OTHER WAYS OF PROVIDING FLUIDS AND NUTRITION

Drinking water and chewing, swallowing, and digesting food are the best ways to obtain fluids and nutrients. However, sometimes drinking and eating "the regular way" are simply not possible. For people who have problems chewing, swallowing, or digesting their food, fluids and nutrients must be provided another way. Three alternate methods of providing fluids and nutrition include intravenous (IV) therapy, enteral nutrition, and total parenteral nutrition (TPN, hyperalimentation).

INTRAVENOUS (IV) THERAPY

In **intravenous (IV) therapy,** fluids are given through a small catheter (tube) that is inserted into a vein (*intra* = in; *venous* = vein). The IV tubing (sometimes called an "IV line") is connected to a bag that contains the IV fluid (Fig. 19-12). The fluid slowly drips through the tubing and into the vein. Usually the IV line, which is thin, is inserted into one of the small veins in the arm or the back of the hand.

IV therapy is not a source of complete nutrition, but it is useful when a person needs fluids. In addition to water, the IV fluid usually contains glucose, vitamins, and minerals. Drugs, such as pain medications or antibiotics, may also be added to the IV fluid. Sometimes, blood is given through an IV line.

You will not be responsible for managing IV therapy, but you may care for many people who have an IV line in place.

 Tell the Nurse!

When caring for a person with an IV line, report any of the following observations to the nurse immediately:

- The tubing has become disconnected
- The fluid bag is empty
- The IV fluid is not dripping into the drip chamber
- Blood has backed up into the IV tubing
- The person complains of pain at the IV site
- There is swelling or redness at the IV site

ENTERAL NUTRITION

The word "enteral" comes from the Greek word for "intestines," *enteron.* **Enteral nutrition** involves placing food directly into the stomach or intestines, which eliminates the need for the person to chew or swallow. For example, a person who is in a coma is not able to chew and swallow. Certain injuries to the head and neck may prevent a person from chewing and swallowing, as might certain cancers. As suggested earlier, sometimes people in the advanced

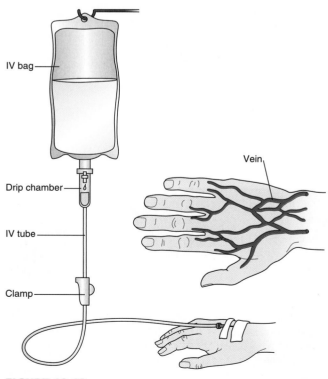

FIGURE 19-12

Intravenous (IV) therapy is used to give fluids. The IV fluid drips from the bag, into the tubing, and into the person's vein. The nurse uses the clamp to control the rate of flow.

stages of dementia "forget" how to swallow. All of these people may require enteral nutrition.

Enteral nutrition is sometimes called "tube feeding" because food, in the form of a formula-like fluid, is delivered through a tube that has been passed into the digestive tract. There are many ways to access the digestive tract with the feeding tube (Fig. 19-13):

- A **nasogastric tube** is inserted through the nose (*naso-*), down the throat, and into the stomach (*gastric*).
- A **nasointestinal tube** is inserted through the nose (*naso-*), down the throat, and into the small intestine (*intestinal*).

- A **gastrostomy tube** is inserted into the stomach (*gastro-*) through a surgical incision (*stoma*). The incision is made in the abdomen.
- A **jejunostomy tube** is inserted into the jejunum (part of the small intestine) through a surgical incision (*stoma*). The incision is made in the abdomen.
- A **percutaneous endoscopic gastrostomy (PEG) tube** is a special type of gastrostomy tube that is inserted into the stomach with the aid of an *endoscope*, a lighted, flexible tool that allows the doctor to see inside the body. The endoscope is passed through the mouth, down the throat, and into the stomach to help the doctor determine where to make the incision for the PEG tube (Fig. 19-14). Placement of a PEG tube is faster, cheaper, and less risky for the patient than placement of a regular gastrostomy tube because open abdominal surgery is not needed.

When a person needs enteral nutrition for only a short time, a nasogastric or nasointestinal tube is usually used. These tubes do not require a surgical incision for placement. However, they can cause irritation of the nose and the back of the throat and may be difficult for the person to tolerate. The tube can be easily displaced, especially if the person vomits, coughs, or pulls on the tube. Because it is possible for the tube to become displaced during feeding, nurses are responsible for feeding people with nasogastric or nasointestinal tubes.

When a person needs enteral nutrition for more than a few days, a gastrostomy, jejunostomy, or PEG tube is used. These tubes are inserted through an incision in the abdomen, so irritation of the nose and throat is not a problem. Gastrostomy, jejunostomy, and PEG tubes are not as easily dislodged from their position as nasogastric or nasointestinal tubes are. However, they can come loose when a person moves, or during repositioning. People who are disoriented or confused may also pull them out by accident.

Enteral feedings may be given at scheduled times, or continuously by an infusion pump (Fig. 19-15). A person who is receiving nourishment through an enteral tube is at high risk for aspiration (inhalation of foreign material into the

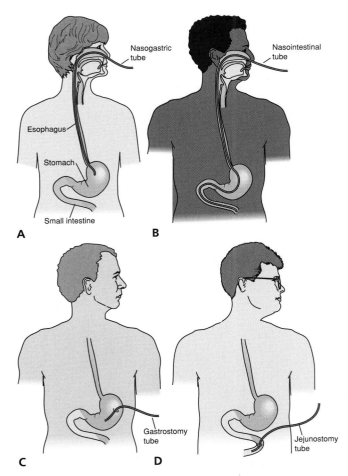

FIGURE 19-13

Enteral feeding tubes are inserted directly into the stomach or intestines. (*A*) A nasogastric tube is passed through the nose, down the throat, and into the stomach. (*B*) A nasointestinal tube is passed through the nose, down the throat, and into the small intestine. (*C*) A gastrostomy tube is inserted into the stomach through a surgical incision. (*D*) A jejunostomy tube is inserted into the small intestine through a surgical incision.

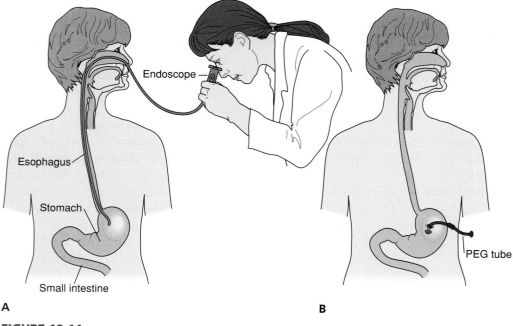

Esophagus

Stomach

Small intestine

A

Endoscope

B

PEG tube

FIGURE 19-14

A percutaneous endoscopic gastrostomy (PEG) tube is a type of gastrostomy tube that is placed using an endoscope. (*A*) The endoscope is passed through the nose, down the throat, and into the stomach. A small incision is made for inserting the PEG tube, and then the endoscope is withdrawn. (*B*) The PEG tube in place.

lungs). Aspiration can occur if the person regurgitates (vomits) the feeding formula and it goes down the windpipe and into the lungs. To help avoid regurgitation and aspiration, the head of the bed is raised during the feeding and for a period of time afterwards.

Tell the Nurse!

Notify the nurse if you suspect that a person who is receiving enteral nutrition has regurgitated or aspirated the feeding or if you think that the feeding tube has become displaced. (Remember that only nurses can reconnect tubing that has been displaced.) Signs and symptoms of problems with enteral feeding devices include:

⟹ Nausea, bloating, or pain during the feeding

⟹ Coughing, gagging, or vomiting during the feeding

⟹ Abdominal distention (a swollen abdomen)

⟹ Diarrhea

⟹ Drainage from around the tube insertion site

⟹ Disconnected tubing

FIGURE 19-15

This patient is receiving enteral nutrition through a continuous infusion pump.

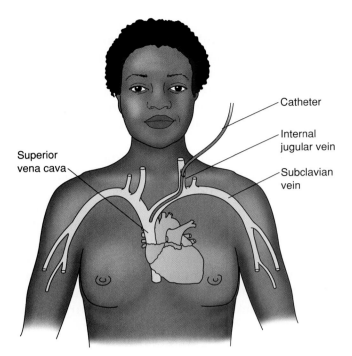

Superior vena cava

Catheter

Internal jugular vein

Subclavian vein

FIGURE 19-16

Total parenteral nutrition (TPN) delivers nutrients directly to the bloodstream. A large catheter (or "central line") is inserted into a large vein near the heart.

TOTAL PARENTERAL NUTRITION (TPN, HYPERALIMENTATION)

People who are very ill, injured, or recovering from surgery, especially gastrointestinal surgery, may not be able to tolerate food in the digestive tract. For these people, nourishment is delivered directly into the bloodstream through a large catheter (tube) inserted into a large vein near the heart (Fig. 19-16). This method of nutrient delivery is called **total parenteral nutrition (TPN)** or **hyperalimentation.** *Parenteral* means "by some way other than through the digestive tract." And *hyperalimentation* means "above (*hyper*) the alimentary (or digestive) tract." So you can see that both terms refer to a method of feeding that does not involve the digestive tract.

As you will recall from the beginning of the chapter, the digestive tract breaks food down into nutrients, and then these nutrients are absorbed into the bloodstream. If a person is receiving TPN, then the nutrients must be delivered to the bloodstream in their smallest form, because digestion does not occur. Water, glucose, vitamins, and minerals are small molecules. But proteins and fats are bigger. This is why a large catheter is used for TPN, instead of

an IV line. The large catheter used for TPN is wider and allows the bigger fat and protein molecules to pass through. An IV line is smaller and only allows smaller molecules, such as water, glucose, vitamins, minerals, and medications to pass. The ability to administer fats and proteins, as well as the other four classes of nutrients, is where the "total" comes from in the term *total parenteral nutrition.*

As a nursing assistant, you will not be responsible for giving TPN feedings, but you may care for people receiving them.

FLUIDS AND HYDRATION

FLUID BALANCE

As you learned earlier, water is just as necessary to life as food, if not more so. A healthy adult needs to drink between 1.5 to 3 quarts (48 to 96 ounces) of fluid each day just to keep up with the fluid that normally leaves the body in urine, feces, sweat, and the air we exhale. Most of these fluid needs are met by drinking water, juice, milk, and other beverages. However, certain foods, such as cucumbers, watermelon, grapes, and soup, have high water contents as well and provide for some of the fluid needed by the body.

When the amount of fluid taken into the body equals the amount of fluid that leaves the body, a state of **fluid balance** occurs. Fluid balance is important for health. **Dehydration** occurs when there is too little fluid in the tissues of the body. Causes of dehydration include diarrhea, vomiting, hemorrhage, severe burns, diaphoresis (excessive sweating), and simply not drinking enough fluids. In all of these situations, the amount of fluid that leaves the body is greater than the amount of fluid taken in. Older people are often at risk for dehydration because they do not feel thirsty as often as younger people do. (Recall that water forms the base of the 70+ Food Pyramid to remind older people to drink water even if they are not thirsty). People in comas and people with dementia are also at risk for dehydration because they may not be able to ask for a drink.

The opposite of dehydration, **edema,** occurs when there is too much fluid in the tissues of the body. Kidney disease and certain types of heart disease can make it hard for the body to get rid of extra water, resulting in edema. In these situations, the amount of fluid that leaves the body is less than the amount of fluid taken in. For a person with edema, the doctor may restrict the person's fluid intake or order certain medications to help the body rid itself of the excess fluid.

OFFERING FLUIDS

Nursing assistants are responsible for providing fresh drinking water and other fluids to patients and residents. Many of your patients or residents will be allowed to have as much water as they like, and should be encouraged to drink (Fig. 19-17). If a person is allowed to have ice water, make sure that the water pitcher is filled with fresh, cold water. Replace the water when the ice melts or when the pitcher is almost empty. People are more likely to drink fluids that taste good and are served at the appropriate temperature. Remember to also offer a drink regularly to people who are elderly, bed-bound, confused, or taking pain medications. These people might not remember to drink fluids often enough, or they may feel that they are being a burden to you by asking for a drink.

Sometimes, the doctor may either increase or restrict a person's fluid intake. An order to encourage fluids (sometimes called "force fluids") means that the person should increase his or her fluid intake. The nurse will give you information about the amount and type of fluids that should be offered. Most people do not enjoy having to drink a large amount of liquid all at once. Often, offering small amounts of a drink that the person likes frequently throughout the day is a better approach. Make sure that the fluids you offer are cold or hot, and fresh. Not many people like room-temperature water, flat soda, or lukewarm tea.

Offering small amounts of fluids at regular times throughout the day is also a good approach when the doctor has restricted a person's fluid intake. This approach helps to make sure that the person is never too thirsty, by spreading out his or her fluid intake over the course of the day. Frequent oral hygiene also helps to keep the person comfortable and prevent "dry mouth." Recording the amount of fluid taken in is an important part of your duties when you are either encouraging or restricting fluids for a person.

Some patients or residents will not be allowed to have any fluids at all in preparation for surgery or a diagnostic procedure. A person who is not allowed to have any fluids at all is said to be on **"NPO status."** *NPO* stands for *nils per os*, or "nothing by mouth" in Latin. NPO means exactly what it stands for—no fluids (not even water or ice chips), no food, no hard candy, no gum. If one of your patients or residents has been placed on NPO status, empty his water pitcher and store it out of sight. You might also want to gently remind visitors that the person is not allowed to have anything to eat or drink, and suggest that they enjoy their own snacks and beverages in another room. Being on NPO status can be extremely uncomfortable. Think of all of those cartoons where a man lost in a hot desert keeps imagining that he sees a big frosty glass of water "just ahead." Being thirsty and not being able to drink is difficult. Frequent oral care helps to relieve some of the discomfort until the person is allowed to have fluids again.

MEASURING AND RECORDING INTAKE AND OUTPUT

As described earlier, certain medical conditions can make monitoring a person's fluid balance very important. For those people, an order to "maintain intake and output measurements" will be followed. All of the fluids that enter and leave

FIGURE 19-17

Water is essential to life.

the body are measured and recorded on an **intake and output (I&O) flow sheet.** In health care facilities, fluids are measured and recorded in milliliters (mL) or cubic centimeters (cc). One mL is the same as one cc. One fluid ounce is equal to 30 mL or 30 cc.

Each time the person takes in fluids, or fluids leave the body, the amount is recorded. The amounts are totaled at the end of the shift and again at the end of the 24-hour reporting period. The amount of intake can then be compared with the amount of output to monitor the person's fluid balance.

Measuring Fluid Intake

Fluid intake includes all of the fluids that a person drinks, including those foods that are liquid at room or body temperature (such as gelatin, ice cream, pudding, and popsicles). Other fluids that are considered as part of a person's total intake include enteral or TPN feedings and IV fluids, but the nurse will be responsible for recording these amounts. The health care facility where you work will have a listing of the amount of fluid in common servings, and you will need to become familiar with the amount of fluid contained by the cups, glasses, and bowls used in your facility. Remember that 30 mL (30 cc) is equal to 1 fluid ounce, so an 8-ounce carton of milk would equal 240 mL (8 × 30 = 240). But what if the person did not drink the entire carton of milk? In this case, you can estimate how much fluid was taken in. For example, if the person drank half of the carton of milk, then half of 8 ounces is 4, so 4 × 30 would be 120 mL. (Another way to arrive at this figure is to calculate what the total carton is worth in milliliters, and then divide by the amount consumed: 240/2 = 120 mL.)

Sometimes it is necessary to calculate intake exactly. In this situation, you would calculate how many fluids were offered to the person before he or she started to eat. For example, let's say a person's meal tray contained 150 mL of orange juice, 240 mL of milk, and 90 mL of water at the beginning of the meal. This would mean that 480 mL of fluid were offered (150 + 240 + 90 = 480). After the person has finished with the meal, you would take all of the fluids left in the glasses and pour them into a **graduate** (a measuring device) to measure the amount left (Fig. 19-18). Let's say

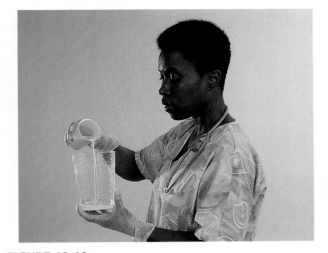

FIGURE 19-18

A graduate is a measuring device that is used to measure fluids. The graduate is marked with lines that indicate milliliters (mL) on the left and ounces (oz) on the right. (*Copyright B. Proud.*)

that 40 mL of fluid are left. You would subtract the amount left (40 mL) from the total amount offered (480 mL) and record the total consumed as 440 mL.

Measuring Fluid Output

Fluids that are considered output are urine, vomit, blood, wound drainage, and diarrhea. Output is measured and recorded the same way that intake is. A person who is on I&O status will need to be reminded to urinate into a measuring device. The urine cannot be discarded until you have had a chance to measure and record the amount. Urine collection devices are available that can be used on a regular toilet, or with a bedside commode (Fig. 19-19). Urinals have measurements marked on the side so that you can easily see the amount that they contain. Urine from a bedpan or a urinary catheter drainage bag is poured into a graduate for measurement. (Urinary catheters are discussed in detail in Chapter 20.)

If a person vomits, the amount can be measured using the markings on the emesis basin. If the person vomited somewhere other than in the emesis basin (for example, on the floor or bed linens), then the nurse will estimate the amount of vomit. Blood and wound drainage is either

FIGURE 19-19

A collection device (sometimes called a "commode hat") is placed over the toilet seat before the person urinates, to contain and measure the amount of urine. (*Photograph courtesy of Medline Industries, Inc.*)

estimated by the nurse or measured in a graduate if it is collected into a drainage device. Diarrhea is estimated for amount also.

Always remember to wear gloves when measuring output.

SUMMARY

▶ Food and fluids are necessary for life.
  ■ Food provides us with energy and nutrients that our bodies need to work properly.
  ■ The six types of nutrients are carbohydrates, proteins, fats, vitamins, minerals, and water.
    • Carbohydrates, proteins, and fat provide energy.
    • Vitamins, minerals, and water regulate body processes.
  ■ Water is more essential to life than food.
▶ In order to be healthy, we need to eat a variety of nutritious foods every day.
  ■ Not all foods are equally nutritious.
  ■ Nutrients work best in combination with other nutrients.
  ■ The Food Guide Pyramid and nutrition labels on packaged foods can be used to plan a healthy diet.
  ■ People in health care settings often have special needs as far as nutrition is concerned.

▶ Factors that influence a person's eating habits include religion, culture, geography, economics, food likes and dislikes, and appetite. The dietary assessment and the nursing assistant's observations about a person's food preferences assist with meal planning.
▶ Eating helps us to meet both physical and emotional needs.
  ■ Helping a person to prepare for meal time and serving meals promptly contributes to comfort and a relaxed atmosphere.
  ■ Respecting the individual's preferences is important when it comes to food.
  ■ Talking with the person as you assist with the meal is important, even if the person cannot answer you.
  ■ When our emotional needs are met, it is easier for us to meet our physical needs. Ensuring that meal time is pleasant can help improve a person's appetite.
▶ Nursing assistants assist people with meals as necessary.
  ■ Patients and residents are encouraged to do as much as they can for themselves.
  ■ Assistive devices are available to help people with physical impairments to eat on their own.
  ■ Some people will need to be fed.
▶ When a person cannot take food or fluids by mouth, nutrition and fluids are provided in other ways.
  ■ Intravenous (IV) therapy provides fluids, glucose, vitamins, and minerals through a small catheter inserted into one of the small veins of the arm or hand. IV therapy does not provide complete nutrition.
  ■ Enteral nutrition is provided by a tube that is placed directly into the stomach or intestines.
    • Nasogastric tubes, nasointestinal tubes, gastrostomy tubes, jejunostomy tubes, and percutaneous endoscopic gastrostomy (PEG) tubes are used for enteral feeding.
    • Formula-like food is usually delivered through an infusion device, either continuously or at specified times.
  ■ Total parenteral nutrition (TPN, hyperalimentation) involves the delivery of all six classes of nutrients through a catheter inserted into a large vein near the heart.
▶ Maintaining proper fluid balance is important for health.

- The amount of fluids taken into the body should equal the amount of fluids that leave the body.
  - If the amount of fluid leaving the body is greater than the amount taken in, dehydration can occur.
  - If the amount of fluid leaving the body is less than the amount taken in, edema can occur.

- A doctor may order a person's fluid intake to be increased or restricted. People who have no fluid restrictions should be encouraged to drink frequently.
- A person's fluid balance is monitored by measuring and recording fluid intake and output. One fluid ounce = 30 milliliters (mL) = 30 cubic centimeters (cc).

Chapter 19 Procedure

Getting Ready Steps

a. **W**ash your hands and observe standard precautions as necessary.

b. **G**ather needed supplies.

c. **K**nock and introduce yourself.

d. **I**dentify the person, and greet him or her by name.

e. **E**xplain the procedure.

f. **P**rovide privacy.

g. **S**ee to safety.

Finishing Up Steps

a. **C**onfirm comfort and good body alignment.

b. **L**eave the call light control within easy reach.

c. **S**ee to safety.

d. **O**pen the curtain and door.

e. **W**ash your hands.

f. **R**eport and record.

PROCEDURE 19-1

Feeding a Dependent Person

Getting Ready **WGKIEPS**

1. Complete the "Getting Ready" steps **a** through **g**.

Supplies

- gloves
- paper towels
- clothing protector
- oral hygiene supplies (see Procedures 17-1 through 17-3)
- wash basin
- bedpan or urinal
- towel
- washcloth

Procedure

2. Cover the over-bed table with paper towels. Place the oral hygiene supplies on the over-bed table. Fill the wash basin with warm water (110°F [37.7°C] to 115°F [46.1°C] on the bath thermometer). Place the basin on the over-bed table. Put on the gloves.

3. If the side rails are in use, lower the side rail on the working side of the bed. The side rail on the opposite side of the bed should remain up. Raise the head of the bed. Make sure that the bed is positioned at a comfortable working height (to promote good body mechanics) and that the wheels are locked.

4. Assist the person with oral hygiene (see Procedures 17-1 through 17-3).

5. Offer the bedpan or urinal (see Chapter 20, Procedures 20-1 and 20-2). If the person uses the bedpan or urinal, empty and clean it before proceeding with the meal. Remove your gloves and dispose of them in a facility-approved waste container. Wash your hands.

6. Wash the person's hands and face (see Procedure 17-8).

7. Clear the over-bed table and position it over the bed, at the proper height for the person.

8. Get the meal tray from the dietary cart. (If the side rails are in use, raise the side rails before leaving the bedside.) Check the meal tray to make sure that it has the person's name on it and that it contains the correct diet for the person. Place the meal tray on the over-bed table.

9. Ask the person if he or she would like to use a clothing protector. Put the clothing protector on the person, if desired.

10. Uncover the meal tray, and prepare the food for eating (for example, cut the meat, butter the bread, open any containers). Tell the person what is on the tray.

(continued)

PROCEDURE 19-1 (Continued)

Feeding a Dependent Person

11. Take a seat.

12. Allow the person to choose what he or she would like to taste first. Using a spoon, offer a small bite to the person (fill the spoon no more than one-third full). Allow the person enough time to swallow the food.

13. Offer the person something to drink every few bites. Use the napkin to wipe the person's mouth and chin as often as necessary. Allow the person to assist with the eating process to the best of his or her ability.

14. Continue in this manner until the person is finished. Encourage the person to finish the food on the tray, but do not force the person to eat.

15. Remove the tray and the clothing protector when the person has finished eating.

16. Put on a clean pair of gloves. Assist the person with oral hygiene (see Procedures 17-1 through 17-3).

17. If the side rails are in use, return the side rails to the raised position. Lower the head of the bed as the person requests. Make sure that the bed is lowered to its lowest position and that the wheels are locked.

18. Gather the soiled linens and place them in the linen hamper or linen bag. Dispose of disposable items in a facility-approved waste container. Clean equipment and return it to the storage area.

19. Remove your gloves and dispose of them in a facility-approved waste container.

20. Record the percentage of food eaten and the amount of fluid intake in the person's medical record, per your facility's policy. Report an abnormal appetite to the nurse (for example, less than 70% of the total meal consumed).

Finishing Up

21. Complete the "Finishing Up" steps **a** through **f**.

What did you learn?

Multiple Choice

Select the single best answer for each of the following questions.

1. When assisting a person with eating, one of the first things you should do is
   a. Provide the person with privacy
   b. Butter the person's muffin
   c. Wash your hands and the person's hands
   d. Cut the food into large pieces

2. Mrs. Wellington is blind. Which one of the following should she have during meal time?
   a. A soft diet
   b. Help identifying the location of the food on the plate
   c. A large spoon
   d. A cup holder

3. Mr. Jones is 98 years old and has no food restrictions on his diet. However, he is missing several teeth. Which one of the following menus would be the best choice for Mr. Jones?
   a. Spare ribs, macaroni and cheese, coleslaw, and fruit cocktail
   b. Hamburger, french fries, corn on the cob, and ice cream
   c. Baked fish, mashed potatoes, spinach soufflé, and tapioca
   d. Fried chicken, baked potato, green beans, and chocolate chip cookies

4. Which one of the following lists only items that would be included in fluid intake?
   a. Orange juice, soft boiled egg, toast
   b. Milk, soup, gelatin
   c. Water, mashed potatoes, egg custard
   d. Milk, ham sandwich, ice cream bar

5. Miss Lee drank one third of an 8-ounce glass of iced tea. How many milliliters of fluid did Miss Lee drink?
   a. 60 mL
   b. 80 mL
   c. 100 mL
   d. 240 mL

6. Which one of the following lists foods that are good sources of protein?
   a. Steak, chicken, fish
   b. Spinach, carrots, beets

   c. Bread, cereal, rice
   d. Apples, oranges, bananas

7. Which one of the following nutrients accounts for 50% to 60% of our total body weight?
   a. Vitamin A
   b. Glucose
   c. Water
   d. Calcium

8. At the beginning of your shift, you give Mr. Gibson a water pitcher containing 270 mL of water. At the end of your shift, you note that 35 mL of water are left in the pitcher. How much water did Mr. Gibson drink?
   a. 35 mL
   b. 175 mL
   c. 235 mL
   d. 140 mL

9. Which of the following lists foods that are good sources of carbohydrates?
   a. Liver, fish, chicken
   b. Cereal, fruit, bread
   c. Milk, beans, cheese
   d. Water, soda, butter

10. Which one of the following can be harmful if too much is consumed?
    a. Folic acid
    b. Water-soluble vitamins (for example, vitamins C and B_{12})
    c. Fat-soluble vitamins (for example, vitamins A, D, E , and K)
    d. None of the above

11. Which health care professional is specially trained to plan for the patient's or resident's nutritional needs and teach about good nutrition?
    a. The nurse
    b. The dietitian
    c. The nursing assistant
    d. The doctor

12. Which one of the following can affect a person's food likes and dislikes?
    a. The person's religious beliefs
    b. The person's culture
    c. Where the person lives
    d. All of the above

Matching

Match the amount of fluid in milliliters (mL) with the same amount in ounces (oz).

_____ **1.** 240 mL

_____ **2.** 180 mL

_____ **3.** 300 mL

_____ **4.** 30 mL

_____ **5.** 120 mL

_____ **6.** 150 mL

a. 10 oz
b. 5 oz
c. 8 oz
d. 4 oz
e. 1 oz
f. 6 oz

Stop and think!

▶ You are a home health care nurse. You first started caring for the Giovannis, a couple in their 70s, a few years ago, when Mrs. Giovanni's Alzheimer's disease started to worsen. Mr. Giovanni had health problems of his own that did not allow for him to care for his wife alone, so he called the home health care agency where you work. You have been going to the Giovannis' home regularly ever since. Two weeks ago, Mrs. Giovanni died suddenly from complications of pneumonia. You have been to see Mr. Giovanni four times since then and you have noticed that at dinner time, he just pushes his food around on the plate. What could be causing Mr. Giovanni's loss of appetite? What could you do to help him get it back?

▶ You work in an assisted living facility, and one of your residents, Mr. Wayne, has severe arthritis in his hands. The arthritis makes it hard for Mr. Wayne to use his silverware, but he refuses to let you help him eat. He says that he'll let you feed him "if and when they cut off both of my hands!" Lately, the arthritis has gotten much worse and Mr. Wayne is having more and more difficulty eating. Most of the food winds up beside the plate, instead of in his mouth, and what little food makes it to his mouth is ice-cold by the time it gets there. You know that Mr. Wayne has to eat to maintain his health. What can you do to assist Mr. Wayne in feeding himself? What member of the staff could you ask to assist you?

20

Assisting With Urinary and Bowel Elimination

What will you learn?

In Chapter 19, you learned about how we take in food and convert it to energy in a process called *metabolism.* During this conversion process, waste materials (or by-products) are created. These waste products must be removed from our bodies, or we will become sick. Wastes are eliminated from the body in various forms. The urinary system rids the body of waste products that have been filtered from the bloodstream, along with excess fluid, in the form of urine. The digestive system rids the body of the solid waste that is left over from the foods that we eat, in the form of feces, or bowel movements. Although there are other ways the body rids itself of waste, urinary and bowel elimination is the subject of this chapter.

Your patients or residents may have physical or mental difficulties that affect their ability to manage urinary or bowel elimination, or both. As a nursing assistant, you will need to assist your patients or residents with elimination as necessary. When you are finished with this chapter, you will be able to:

1. Describe two methods the body uses to eliminate waste products.
2. Discuss attitudes that people may have regarding the processes of urinary or bowel elimination.
3. Discuss actions the nursing assistant can take to promote normal urinary and bowel elimination, and explain why normal urinary and bowel elimination is essential to health.
4. Define terminology associated with urinary elimination and list normal characteristics of urine.
5. Demonstrate methods used to measure and record urinary output.
6. Describe the use of urinary catheters and demonstrate how to provide routine catheter care.
7. Discuss problems associated with urinary elimination and methods the nursing assistant uses to assist people having those problems.
8. Understand the underlying principles of bladder training.
9. Discuss the process of bowel elimination and characteristics of normal stool.
10. Define terms related to abnormal bowel function.
11. List the types of enemas and discuss their indications for use.
13. Demonstrate proper technique for assisting with urinary and bowel elimination, obtaining urine and stool samples, providing catheter care, and administering enemas.

Photo: Nursing assistants help their patients or residents to meet their elimination needs by providing assistance as necessary.

Vocabulary

Use the CD in the back of your book to hear these terms pronounced, defined, and used in a sentence:

Bedside commode	Occult	Suprapubic catheter	Constipation
Bedpan	Frequency	Catheter care	Laxative
Fracture pan	Urgency	Urinary incontinence	Stool softener
Urinal	Nocturia	Urinary retention	Fiber supplement
Urinalysis	Dysuria	Condom catheter	Fecal impaction
Midstream ("clean	Oliguria	Chyme	Digital examination
catch") urine	Polyuria	Peristalsis	Flatulence
specimen	Diuresis	Feces	Fecal (bowel)
Urination	Anuria	Defecate	incontinence
Voiding	Catheter	Stool	Enema
Micturition	Straight catheter	Flatus	
Hematuria	Indwelling catheter	Diarrhea	

ASSISTING WITH ELIMINATION

ELIMINATION EQUIPMENT

Many of your patients or residents will need no more assistance with elimination than a steady arm to lean on during the trip to the bathroom. The bathrooms in many health care facilities have special features that make them easier for people with physical disabilities to use (Fig. 20-1A). For example, hand rails attached to the walls alongside the toilet or onto the toilet itself make it easier for the person to sit down and get back up. Some toilets have higher seats, so the person does not have to bend her knees as much to sit down and get back up. Modifications like these allow many patients or residents to use the toilet in the bathroom with very little assistance from you. However, some of your patients or residents may not be able to get out of bed at all, or they may be too weak or ill to walk to the bathroom. These people will need more help with elimination, and special equipment.

A

B

FIGURE 20-1

(*A*) Many toilets in health care facilities have special modifications that make them easier to use. (*B*) A bedside commode can be used if a person can get out of bed but is not capable of walking the distance to the bathroom.

Bedside Commodes

For a person who is able to get out of bed, but who is not able to walk to the bathroom, a bedside commode can make toileting easier (see Fig. 20-1B). The **bedside commode** consists of a chair frame with a toilet seat and a removable collection bucket. If the person is weak or unsteady, you will need to help her get out of bed and over to the bedside commode.

Bedpans

A **bedpan** is used for elimination when a person is unable to get out of bed at all (Fig. 20-2A). A woman who cannot get out of bed uses a bedpan to urinate, and for bowel movements. A man who cannot get out of bed uses a bedpan for bowel movements, and a urinal to urinate (see next section).

Bedpans, while sometimes necessary, must be used with extreme care. It is very easy to bruise or tear the fragile skin of an elderly or disabled person. In addition to causing immediate pain to the person, an injury like this can also lead to the formation of a pressure ulcer later on. Arthritis can make using a bedpan very painful, as can fractures of the back or legs. If a person has an injury or disability that makes it too uncomfortable or dangerous to use a regular bedpan, a special bedpan called a fracture pan is used. The **fracture pan,** which is wedge-shaped, is placed underneath the person's buttocks with the thin edge toward the person's back (Fig. 20-2B).

Using a bedpan is very uncomfortable, and the discomfort alone can cause the person to have difficulty using it. Many facilities use disposable bedpans that are made from molded plastic. However, some facilities still use bedpans made from stainless steel. If the facility where you work uses metal bedpans, be sure to warm the bedpan before offering it to the patient or resident. You can do this by wrapping the bedpan in a warm towel, or running warm water over the seat area and then drying it before use. If the person's condition allows, raise the head of the bed to promote a more natural elimination position. Provide as much privacy as safely possible. Pro-

A. Regular bedpan

B. Fracture pan

FIGURE 20-2

Bedpans are used for women who cannot get out of bed to urinate. A bedridden man also uses a bedpan for bowel movements. (*A*) A standard bedpan. Position a standard bedpan like a regular toilet seat—the buttocks are placed on the wide, rounded shelf, with the open end pointed toward the foot of the bed. (*B*) A fracture pan. Position a fracture pan with the thin edge toward the head of the bed.

cedure 20-1 describes how to help a person to use a bedpan.

Urinals

A man uses a **urinal** to urinate when he cannot get out of bed. The urinal is designed to fit between the man's legs. To urinate, the man puts his penis in the opening of the urinal (Fig. 20-3). If the man is very weak or disabled, you may need to place his penis inside the opening of the urinal for him. Procedure 20-2 describes how to help a man to use a urinal.

PROMOTING NORMAL ELIMINATION

Everyone urinates and has bowel movements. However, most people consider elimination a very private activity and would prefer not to discuss it with others. In a health care facility, people may be forced to think about and discuss elimination much more than they would normally care to! Think about how it would affect you to be a patient or a resident in a health care facility. Nurses and nursing assistants ask you about your bathroom patterns. They want to know if you have had a bowel movement today, how big it was, and what it looked like. They want you to urinate into a cup and then carry the sample to the nurses' station in full view of everyone. You may have to share a bathroom, or worse yet, use a bedpan while being separated from other people in the room by only a curtain! Elimination, especially when it must take place in a fairly public way, is very embarrassing for many people.

A person who is a patient or a resident in a health care facility may have difficulty with elimination, especially if elimination must occur under conditions that are not as private as the person would like. Regardless of the amount of assistance that your patients or residents need, privacy and consideration for individual preferences are essential. Provide privacy to the extent possible with regard to the safety of the person. Close the bathroom door, or close the privacy curtains and the door to the room, if the person cannot use the regular toilet. Always make sure the call light is in reach so that the person can call you when he is ready for assistance. Some people are too weak or unsteady to be left alone while they urinate or have a bowel movement. In fact, some people will actually need for you to help hold them in the correct position during elimination. Being professional, kind, and straightforward about the "business at hand" will help to ease your patient's or resident's embarrassment.

Similarly, it is important to help your residents or patients keep their sense of dignity. For many people, needing assistance with this most private of bodily functions is humiliating. Feelings of embarrassment and shame are made worse when patients or residents accidentally soil themselves, their bed linens, or their clothing with urine or feces. This is a fairly common occurrence in health care facilities. The effects of medications, being in a strange place, reluctance to ask for help, and physical or mental disabilities can all lead to accidents. Again, kindness, empathy, and a professional attitude can go a long way toward easing the patient's or resident's embarrassment.

Being in a health care facility can change a person's normal elimination patterns, which can cause health problems. The most effective method of treating urinary and bowel problems is to prevent them from happening in the first place. As a nursing assistant, you can help promote

FIGURE 20-3

Men who cannot get out of bed to urinate can use a urinal.

normal urinary and bowel function for your patients or residents. The following tips are simple, but effective.

- Encourage plenty of fluids, unless a person has a medical condition that requires fluid restriction. Drinking plenty of fluids helps the kidneys to work properly, and regular urination flushes harmful bacteria from the bladder, helping to prevent urinary tract infections. In addition, drinking enough fluids helps to keep the feces soft, making bowel movements easier.

- Answer call lights promptly and take people to the bathroom or provide them with a bedpan or urinal as soon as they ask you to. Many residents and patients do not want to "bother" the nursing staff and will wait until the last minute to signal for assistance with the bedpan or for help getting to the bathroom. If the person must wait too long for help to arrive, he or she may have an accident.

- Encourage your patients or residents to call when they first feel the urge to void. This can help to prevent accidents. In addition, "holding" urine or feces is not only uncomfortable, it can lead to problems such as constipation.

- Offer people the chance to eliminate frequently, especially if they are bed-bound or require assistance. Some people may find it easier to accept an offer of assistance than to ask for help.

- Provide for privacy and comfort. A person is able to urinate or have a bowel movement much more easily if she is warm enough, in a comfortable position, and ensured of as much privacy as possible. Most women urinate and have bowel movements in a sitting or squatting position. Help a woman to sit upright by elevating the head of the bed (if she is using a bedpan), or have her lean forward a bit while seated on the toilet or bedside commode. Most men stand up to urinate and sit down to have a bowel movement. Some men have no difficulty using a urinal while lying down, but others will need to sit up or even to stand. In this case, you may need to help the man to sit or stand up.

If a person is having difficulty urinating, there are some things you can do to help. For example, try turning on the faucet and allowing water to run into the sink. The sound of running water, which accompanied many of our early toilet training lessons, can help a person relax enough to start the urine stream. The sound of the running water also helps to cover up the sounds of urination, which may put some people more at ease. Putting the person's fingers in a basin of warm water can also help stimulate urination.

If a person is having difficulty moving his bowels, make sure that the person does not feel rushed. Many people like to read while having a bowel movement. Some people find that drinking warm fluids (such as coffee, tea, or warm water with lemon) helps stimulate the bowels to empty. Finally, regular exercise and foods that contain insoluble fiber help to promote regular bowel movements.

General guidelines for assisting a person with elimination are given in Guidelines Box 20-1.

OBTAINING URINE AND STOOL SPECIMENS

Because the contents of a person's urine or feces can provide a doctor with clues about the person's overall health status, you may be asked to obtain a urine or stool specimen (sample) for laboratory study. When assisting with specimen collection, it is very important to make sure that the specimen cup is properly labeled with the person's name and room number. Otherwise, a person may be diagnosed with, and receive treatment for, a condition he or she does not have! It is also important to make sure that the specimen is handled correctly after you obtain it. For example, in certain situations, the specimen may need to be delivered to the laboratory while it is still warm, or placed in a special plastic transport bag. If a specimen is not being delivered to the laboratory right away, then it needs to be stored properly until the scheduled pick-up time. Before collecting *any* specimen—of urine, feces, or any other body fluid—always ask yourself the following questions:

- Do I have the right person?
- Do I have the right laboratory requisition slip? (The laboratory requisition slip states the person's name, the date, and the type

GUIDELINES BOX 20-1
GUIDELINES FOR ASSISTING WITH ELIMINATION

What you do	Why you do it
Always honor a person's request for assistance with elimination as quickly as possible.	Answering call lights quickly builds trust and prevents accidents. If a person who is bed-bound must wait too long for assistance, he could have an accident in the bed. A weak or unsteady person may try to make it to the bathroom on her own, rather than waiting for help to arrive. This puts the person at risk for a fall. Finally, it is very uncomfortable to "hold" urine or feces for a long time, and doing so can change the normal elimination patterns, causing health problems.
Always provide the person with as much privacy as safety considerations will allow.	Regular elimination is essential to health, so it is important to make this process as normal as possible for your patients or residents. Many people have difficulty urinating or having a bowel movement if they think that someone else can hear them, or if someone else is in the bathroom with them.
If you leave the person alone, always make sure that the call light control is within easy reach of the person.	The person will need the call light control to let you know when she is finished, or if she needs help.
Make sure the toilet paper is within easy reach of the person. If the person is unable to wipe himself, assist with this task.	Wiping promotes comfort and helps to prevent irritation, odors, and infection.
Be sure to provide good perineal care as necessary, especially after bowel movements (see Chapter 17).	Good perineal care promotes comfort and helps to prevent irritation, odors, and infection.
Provide the person with the chance to wash his hands after elimination. This can be accomplished by stopping by the sink if the person is in the bathroom, or by providing a warm, wet washcloth after assisting the person from the bedside commode or removing the bedpan or urinal.	Most people prefer to wash their hands after using the toilet. Allowing people to follow their normal routines whenever possible is important, especially when other aspects of the routine need to be altered. In addition, handwashing is important for hygiene.
Always wear gloves when assisting a person with elimination, or when handling a bedpan, bedside commode bucket, or urinal that contains waste.	Urine and feces are considered "body fluids" and may contain pathogens.
Before disposing of waste, observe the feces or urine for amount and any unusual characteristics. Report and record your observations.	Abnormalities in the urine or feces could indicate a health problem.
Never place a bedpan or urinal on an over-bed table or bedside table, even if the bedpan or urinal is clean. Dirty bedpans and urinals are taken to the bathroom immediately after use and cleaned and disinfected according to facility policy. Clean bedpans are either stored in a cabinet underneath the bedside table or returned to the equipment room. Clean urinals may be hung over the side rail, stored in a cabinet, or returned to the equipment room.	The over-bed table and bedside table are considered "clean" areas. Even if the bedpan or urinal is clean, most people do not want items associated with elimination placed on surfaces where they eat or have personal items displayed.

(continued)

GUIDELINES BOX 20-1 (Continued)
GUIDELINES FOR ASSISTING WITH ELIMINATION

What you do	Why you do it
If there are odors in the room as a result of elimination, use an air freshener.	Most people will appreciate the use of an air freshener to make the air in the room smell fresher. Just be professional in any remarks you may make about the odor.
Disinfect equipment used for elimination carefully, according to facility policy.	Bedpans, urinals, and bedside commode buckets can act as fomites (that is, non-living objects that can transmit pathogens and cause infection) if they are not properly disinfected.

of test to be done. It is filled out by the nurse and sent with the specimen to the laboratory.)

- What method is to be used to collect the specimen?
- Do I have the right type of specimen cup?
- Is the specimen cup properly labeled?
- What is the correct date and time?
- What storage and delivery method must I use?

Finally, always remember to wear gloves when assisting with specimen collection and when handling the specimen cups.

Obtaining a Urine Specimen

Urinalysis, or examination of the urine under a microscope and by chemical means, is a commonly used diagnostic tool in the health care setting. Substances found in urine during urinalysis can help doctors diagnose kidney disease, certain metabolic diseases, and infections. The collection and analysis of urine over the course of 24 hours allows for evaluation of kidney function. In order to perform urinalysis, a urine specimen must be obtained.

Depending on the situation, the method of collecting a urine sample may vary. For routine urinalysis, no special collection procedures are necessary. The person is asked to urinate directly into the specimen cup, if possible. If this is difficult for the person, he or she can urinate into a specimen collection device ("commode hat;" see Chapter 19, Fig. 19-19), or into a bedpan or urinal. The person must not have a bowel movement at the same time the urine is

being collected, or place toilet paper in the collection device, because these actions will change the urinalysis results. The urine is then poured from the collection device, bedpan, or urinal into the specimen cup. The procedure for obtaining a routine urine sample is described in Procedure 20-3.

In some situations, it may be necessary to obtain a **midstream ("clean catch") urine specimen** using a sterile specimen cup. This method of collecting urine prevents contamination of the urine by the bacteria that normally live in and around the urethra. A midstream ("clean catch") urine specimen is usually ordered when the doctor suspects a urinary tract infection. This way, if any bacteria are found in the urine sample, the doctor knows that they are the ones most likely responsible for the infection. When a midstream ("clean catch") urine specimen is requested, the person is asked to clean the area around the urethral opening with a special cleansing wipe. The urine flow is started, then stopped, then started again. The urine sample is collected from the restarted flow. Procedure 20-4 describes how to assist a person with obtaining a midstream ("clean catch") urine specimen.

Your facility or agency may train you to do a type of routine urine testing that involves dipping chemically treated paper strips into a urine sample. Chemicals on the paper react with certain substances that may be found in the urine, causing the chemical blocks on the paper to change color if these substances are present in the urine. The paper is then compared with a color chart that comes with the strips (Fig. 20-4), and the results are recorded in the person's chart and reported to the nurse.

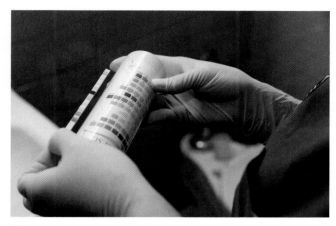

FIGURE 20-4

Chemically treated reagent strips are used to test urine for some substances. Your facility may train you to do this type of urinalysis.

Obtaining a Stool Sample

Stool can be analyzed for the presence of blood, pathogens (such as parasites or bacteria), fat, and other things that are not normally found in feces. Because people do not have bowel movements as often as they urinate, if a stool sample is needed, the person should be notified well in advance so that the specimen can be collected when it becomes available. Ask the nurse if there are any particular collection methods that should be used. Stool can be collected in a bedpan, bedside commode, or in a collection device placed into a regular toilet. The person must not urinate at the same time the stool sample is being collected, or place toilet paper in the collection device, because these actions will change the test results. The procedure for collecting a stool sample is given in Procedure 20-5.

URINARY ELIMINATION

The urinary system, which is discussed in more detail in Chapter 32, is made up of the kidneys, urinary bladder, ureters, and urethra (Fig. 20-5). Blood passes through the kidneys, which remove waste products and excess fluid, forming urine. It takes the kidneys approximately one half hour to process the body's total blood volume. As it forms, the urine flows from the kidneys through the ureters and is stored in the

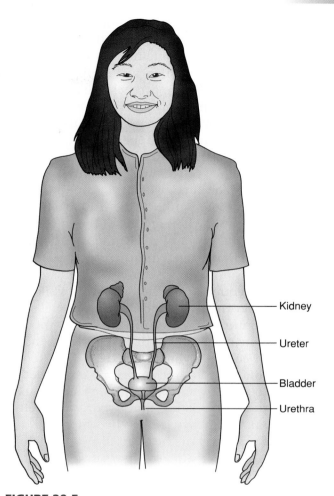

FIGURE 20-5

The urinary system.

urinary bladder. As the bladder fills, we begin to feel the urge to urinate. Urine leaves the body through the urethra.

The process of passing urine from the body is known by several terms, including **urination, voiding,** and **micturition.** Many of your patients or residents will have their own terms for urinating, such as "peeing" or "passing water." When talking about urination with a patient or resident, you should use words that the person is familiar with. This is especially important when talking with children.

In healthy people, urine is clear, without cloudiness or particles. Sometimes urine that has been in a container for a while will become cloudy as it cools. Healthy urine is pale yellow, straw-colored, or dark gold (amber) in color, with a slight odor. A slight red tinge to the urine may indicate **hematuria,** or the presence of blood in the urine. This is an abnormal finding. Sometimes hematuria is **occult** (that is, hidden) and must be detected using urinalysis. Some foods and drugs can also affect the color and odor of urine. When you are helping a patient or resident with urination, observe the urine and report any abnormalities to the nurse. Urine with an unusual odor or appearance could be a sign of illness or infection.

The frequency of voiding, and the amount of urine voided each time, will differ from person to person. Many factors influence a person's urinary pattern, including the amount of fluids the person drinks, the types of medications the person takes, the person's age, and the person's lifelong elimination habits. For example, some people void quite frequently, at the first urge, while others may hold their urine for as long as possible, even if a bathroom is readily available. You will soon become aware of the urinary pattern that is normal for each person in your care. This knowledge will allow you to recognize any changes that may occur. For example, **frequency** is the term used to describe voiding that occurs more often than usual. Frequency is often accompanied by a feeling of **urgency,** or the need to urinate immediately. A person with a urinary tract infection may experience frequency and urgency. **Nocturia** is the need to get up more than once or twice during the night to urinate, to the point where sleep is disrupted. Nocturia can be a sign of pain or depression; a prostate or bladder disorder; or heart failure.

Urination should not cause discomfort. **Dysuria** is difficulty voiding that may or may not be associated with pain. Some people describe the discomfort they feel during urination as a "burning" or "cramping" sensation. Dysuria is often associated with bladder infections, prostate problems, and some sexually transmitted diseases (STDs).

▶ Tell the Nurse!

Changes in the quality of a person's urine or pattern of urination can be a sign that something is wrong. Be sure to report the following observations to the nurse immediately:

⯈ The urine is cloudy or contains particles, is an abnormal color, or has an abnormal odor

⯈ The person complains that the urine is difficult or painful to pass (that is, the person has dysuria)

⯈ The person is experiencing frequency, urgency, or both

⯈ The person needs to get up more frequently than usual to use the bathroom during the night

MEASURING URINE OUTPUT

As you learned in Chapter 19, urine output is a key indicator of fluid balance. In a person who is maintaining a good fluid balance, urine output is neither too high nor too low.

- **Oliguria** is the state of voiding a very small amount of urine over a given period of time (for example, voiding only 100 to 400 mL of urine over 24 hours). *Olig-* means "few" and *-uria* means "urine." A person who is dehydrated might become oliguric (that is, have a urine output that is well below normal).
- **Polyuria** (*poly-* means "many") is excessive urine output. Polyuria, also known as **diuresis,** can be a sign of a health problem. For example, polyuria can be a symptom of poorly controlled diabetes. Or, polyuria may be the desired effect of a medication. For example, a person who is retaining excessive amounts of fluid (for example, as the result of a heart disorder) may be put on a medication called a diuretic to help rid the body of the extra fluid. The polyuria that results is a sign that the medication is having the desired effect.

Evaluating a person's urine output is also a good way to determine how well a person's kidneys are working. **Anuria** (*an-* means "none") is defined as the state of voiding less than 100 mL of urine over the course of 24 hours. Anuria usually indicates that a person is in kidney failure.

Not all of the people you care for will need to have their urine output measured and recorded, but people who have illnesses or take medications that may alter their body's ability to maintain a healthy fluid balance will need to have their urine output measured regularly. Some people who are critically ill will have their urine output measured and recorded every hour, but most people in the health care setting have routine orders for their urine output to be measured and recorded each shift.

If a person uses a regular toilet, you will need to remind the person to void into a specimen collection device ("commode hat") and to call you after he or she has finished voiding so that you can measure and record the amount of urine. Specimen collection devices, urinals, and the drainage bags used with urinary catheters often have markings that make measuring urine output easy. If they do not, then the urine output can be measured by pouring it into a graduate (Fig. 20-6). A graduate is also used to measure urine output if a person voids into a bedpan or bedside commode bucket.

If the urine output of one of your residents or patients is being monitored, you will need to keep a record of the amount of urine passed at each voiding. Some intake and output (I&O) flow sheets will have spaces to record the amount of each individual voiding, while others may only have a space to record the end-of-shift amount. To obtain the end-of-shift amount, simply add the individual amounts together and record the total in the appropriate space.

URINARY CATHETERIZATION

Sometimes a person is unable to urinate using a toilet, bedpan, urinal, or bedside commode, due to disability or illness. In these situations, a urinary catheter is used. A **catheter** is a tube that is inserted into the body for the purpose of administering or removing fluids. A urinary catheter is inserted into the bladder through the urethra (or through an incision made in the abdominal wall) to allow the urine in the bladder to drain out. A urinary catheter is used in many different situations:

- A urinary catheter may be inserted to drain the bladder before or during a surgical procedure, during recovery from a serious illness or injury, or to collect urine for testing.
- A urinary catheter may be used for a person who is incontinent of urine, if the person has wounds or pressure ulcers that would be made worse by contact with urine.
- A urinary catheter is necessary when a person is unable to urinate because of an obstruction in the urethra.

Usually, inserting a urinary catheter is beyond the scope of practice for a nursing assistant, although in some facilities, nursing assistants are provided with additional training that allows them to catheterize residents or patients. Inserting a catheter is a procedure that requires sterile technique because it involves putting a foreign object (that is, the catheter) into a person's body. If sterile technique is not used, the catheter can introduce infection-causing bacteria into the bladder. Regardless of whether or not you are trained to actually insert urinary catheters, caring for people who have urinary catheters in place will almost certainly be a part of your daily duties.

Types of Urinary Catheters

You will see many different types of urinary catheters in use.

- A **straight catheter,** also known as a Robinson, Rob-Nel, or Red Rubber catheter, is used when the catheter is to be inserted and removed immediately. The catheter is introduced into the bladder, the urine is allowed to drain out, and the catheter is removed (Fig. 20-7A). This type of catheterization is commonly used to obtain a sterile urine specimen from a woman, before or after surgery, after a vaginal delivery, or when a person needs to empty his bladder but cannot as a result of pain or swelling that is temporary.

FIGURE 20-6

To measure urine output, the urine is poured into a measuring device called a graduate. The graduate is held at eye level to properly determine the amount of fluid it contains.

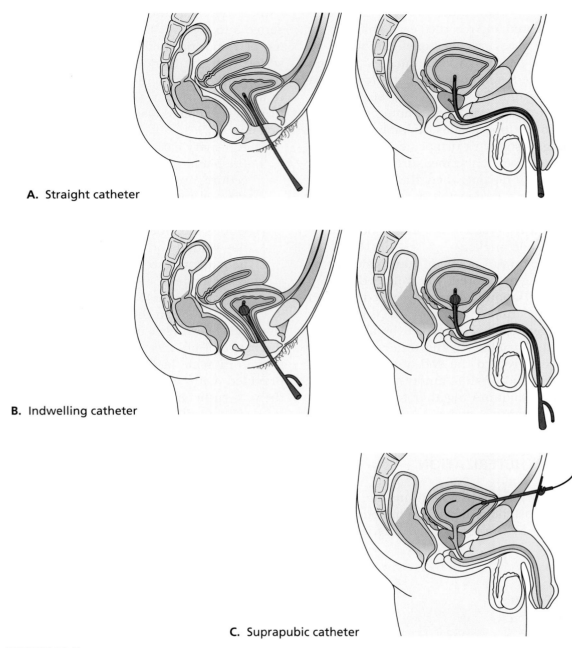

A. Straight catheter

B. Indwelling catheter

C. Suprapubic catheter

FIGURE 20-7

Types of catheters. (*A*) A straight catheter is inserted into the bladder, the urine is drained, and then the catheter is removed. (*B*) An indwelling catheter, also known as a Foley catheter or a retention catheter, remains in the body and urine drains continuously into a drainage bag. (*C*) A suprapubic catheter is inserted into the bladder through a surgical incision made above the pubic bone (*supra-* means "above"). A suprapubic catheter is a bit less likely to promote urinary infections because its location keeps the opening away from the contaminated perineal area.

- An **indwelling catheter,** also known as a retention or Foley catheter, is left inside the bladder to provide continuous urine drainage. An indwelling catheter has a soft balloon that is inflated inside the bladder to keep the catheter from sliding out of the urethra (see Fig. 20-7*B*). Urine collects in a drainage bag, which is attached to the indwelling catheter by a length of tubing.

- A **suprapubic catheter** is a type of indwelling catheter. The suprapubic catheter is inserted into the bladder through a surgical incision made in the abdominal wall, right above the pubic bone (see Fig. 20-7C). This type of catheter is most often used for people with blocked urethras, and for men. Men typically are not able to use an indwelling urinary catheter that is inserted through the urethra for long periods of time due to the anatomy of the male urethra. Whereas a woman's urethra is straight and only about 2 inches long, a man's urethra is curved in an "S" shape and is about 6 inches long (see Fig. 20-7B). In men, the pressure of the indwelling catheter can cause erosion of the mucous membrane that lines the urethra in the curved areas.

Caring for a Person With an Indwelling Urinary Catheter

Indwelling urinary catheters are connected by a length of tubing to a urine drainage bag. Urine drains continuously from the bladder, through the catheter, into the tubing, and into the drainage bag (Fig. 20-8). There are several different types of urine drainage bags that you will encounter in the health care setting. Some urine drainage bags have a long length of tubing that allows them to be carried or secured to a bed frame or the back of a wheelchair. Other urine drainage bags, called "leg bags," are connected to the catheter by a short length of tubing and secured to the person's thigh with rubberized straps. Leg bags are useful because they can be concealed underneath a person's clothing and they allow the person to move around freely.

When a regular urine drainage bag with a long length of tubing is being used, the tubing is secured loosely to the person's body near the insertion site using a catheter strap or adhesive tape. Securing the tubing to the person's body prevents the catheter from being accidentally pulled out during repositioning. In women, the tubing is attached to the thigh. In men, the tubing is attached to the thigh or lower abdomen (Fig. 20-9). A little bit of slack is left in the tubing to prevent the catheter from pulling against the bladder outlet and the urethral opening. The remaining length of

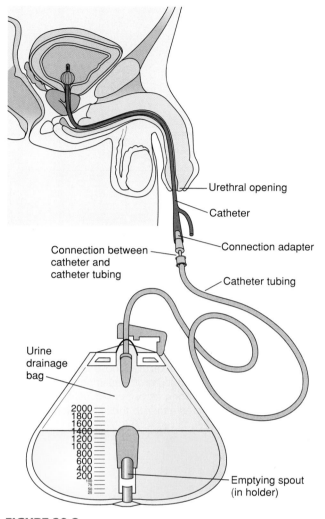

FIGURE 20-8

The indwelling urinary catheter drainage system consists of a catheter that is connected to a urine drainage bag by way of a length of tubing. The urine drainage bag has a connection adapter, where the tubing attaches, and an emptying spout, which is unclamped to allow the urine to drain from the bag. When not in use, the emptying spout is stored in a holder that is part of the bag.

tubing is then gently coiled and secured to the bed linens using a plastic clip or safety pin (Fig. 20-10). Coiling the tubing prevents the tubing from becoming bent or kinked, which would stop the free flow of urine into the drainage bag. Coiling the tubing and securing it to the bed linens also keeps the weight of the tubing from pulling against the person's body. The drainage bag is then secured to the bed frame or the back of the person's wheelchair, at a level lower than the person's bladder (Fig. 20-11). If the drainage bag and tubing are higher than the person's bladder, then gravity

A. Women   **B.** Men

FIGURE 20-9

The catheter tubing is secured loosely to the person's body to prevent tension on the tubing and catheter, which could cause discomfort. Securing the tubing also prevents the catheter from accidentally being pulled out of the body during repositioning. (*A*) In women, the tubing is secured to the inner thigh. (*B*) In men, the tubing is connected either to the inner thigh or the lower abdomen.

could cause old, contaminated urine to run back down the tubing and into the person's bladder, causing an infection.

All urine drainage bags have a connection adapter (where the catheter tubing attaches)

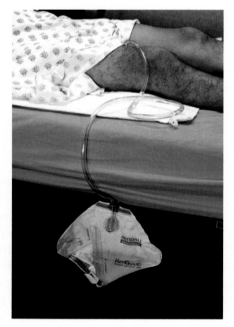

FIGURE 20-10

The catheter tubing is gently coiled (to prevent it from kinking) and secured to the bed linens with a plastic clip or safety pin.

FIGURE 20-11

When a person with an indwelling urinary catheter system is in a wheelchair, the urine drainage bag is attached to the back of the person's wheelchair, away from the wheels and at a level that is lower than the person's bladder. When the person is in bed, the urine drainage bag is attached to the bed frame (see Fig. 20-10).

and an emptying spout that is opened to allow urine to drain from the bag. Because the inside of the catheter and tubing are sterile, it is safer for the person if the bag is not disconnected from the tubing once the catheter is in place. Disconnecting the bag from the tubing can allow harmful bacteria to enter the catheter. Occasionally, the tubing has to be disconnected from the bag (for example, to change the bag if it is leaking, to replace a regular drainage bag with a leg bag, or to perform certain procedures). If you must disconnect the tubing from the bag, be sure to prevent the end of the tubing from touching anything, and wipe the exposed tubing with an antibacterial wipe before reconnecting the drainage bag. General guidelines for caring for a person with an indwelling catheter are given in Guidelines Box 20-2.

GUIDELINES BOX 20-2
GUIDELINES FOR CARING FOR PEOPLE WITH INDWELLING CATHETERS

What you do	Why you do it
Loosely secure the catheter tubing to the person near the insertion site, using a catheter strap or adhesive tape.	Securing the catheter tubing helps to prevent the catheter from being pulled out during repositioning. Allowing a little bit of slack helps to prevent the catheter from pulling against the bladder outlet and the urethral opening.
The remaining length of tubing is gently coiled and secured to the bed linens using a plastic clip or safety pin.	Coiling the tubing helps to prevent kinking, which could stop the free flow of urine into the drainage bag. It also keeps the weight of the tubing from pulling against the area where the tubing is secured to the person's body.
When repositioning a person who has an indwelling catheter, always make sure to unclip the coiled tubing from the linens before beginning the procedure. When you are finished with the procedure, secure the coiled tubing to the linens again.	The person needs to be able to move freely during procedures such as repositioning. If you try to move a person in the direction opposite from the length of tubing, and the length of tubing is still attached to the bed linens, then the resulting opposing forces could cause the catheter to be pulled out of the person's body.
Make sure that the person is not lying on the coiled tubing.	This would be uncomfortable for the person. In addition, the weight of the person's body on the tubing could stop the free flow of urine into the drainage bag.
Always make sure the urine drainage bag is placed at a level lower than that of the person's bladder.	Raising the urine drainage bag up higher than the bladder can cause old, contaminated urine to run back into the bladder, which can lead to infection.
Never attach a urine drainage bag to a side rail. Instead, attach the drainage bag to the bed frame.	Raising the side rail would raise the drainage bag to a level that is higher than the person's bladder. The bed frame does not move; therefore, the level of the drainage bag cannot change.
Keep the drainage bag off the floor. When emptying the drainage bag, be sure that the open emptying spout does not touch anything.	Bacteria can enter the closed drainage system in this manner. The presence of bacteria in the system can lead to nosocomial urinary tract infections in people with indwelling catheters.
Always wear gloves when emptying the urine drainage bag.	Urine is a body fluid and may contain pathogens.

Providing Catheter Care

Although you may not be permitted to catheterize your patients or residents, you will most likely be responsible for providing catheter care. **Catheter care** involves thorough cleaning of the perineal area (especially around the urethra) and the catheter tubing that extends outside of the body, to prevent infection. Providing good catheter care is important because the presence of the catheter in the urethra provides a pathway for bacteria to travel up from the perineum into the bladder, where they can cause infection. In addition, having a catheter in place eliminates the "flushing" action of normal urination, which helps to remove bacteria from the urinary tract naturally. Because bacteria can be introduced into the body both when a urinary catheter is inserted and after it is in place, urinary tract infections in catheterized people are one of the most common nosocomial infections. (Remember that *nosocomial* refers to an infection that is acquired in the health care setting.)

In an effort to reduce the risk of nosocomial infection in people who are catheterized, many facilities require catheter care to be provided routinely (for example, once or twice daily), and again whenever the perineal area becomes soiled (such as when a person is incontinent of feces). Soap and water or a special antibacterial solution may be used when providing catheter care. The procedure for providing catheter care is given in Procedure 20-6.

Emptying Urine Drainage Bags

Urine drainage bags are routinely emptied and the urine measured at the end of each shift unless ordered otherwise. Urine drainage bags should also be emptied if they become too full. Leg bags need to be emptied frequently because they are smaller and hold less urine. The procedure for emptying a urine drainage bag is given in Procedure 20-7.

⏩ Tell the Nurse!

When caring for a catheterized person, make sure you report any of the following observations to the nurse immediately:

⏩ Changes in the color, clarity, or odor of the urine

⏩ Failure of urine to flow freely through the tubing (make sure that the tubing is not kinked or bent)

⏩ The person complains of pain or discomfort as a result of the catheter

⏩ Redness, swelling, or discharge from the catheter insertion site

⏩ Leaking of urine around the catheter insertion site

Preparing for Removal of an Indwelling Catheter

Use of an indwelling catheter can lead to temporary urinary incontinence when the catheter is removed, because the catheter allows the bladder to become "lazy." While the catheter was in place, urine drained out of the body continuously. The bladder did not have to fill up and then empty itself. This lack of activity can decrease the muscle tone of the bladder, leading to incontinence. To prepare the bladder for removal of the catheter and prevent temporary incontinence from developing, it is common to clamp the tubing of the catheter for a period of time to allow the urine to fill the bladder. The tubing is then unclamped and the urine is allowed to drain from the bladder. This procedure is repeated over a period of time, with the time intervals between clamping and emptying becoming increasingly longer. Then the catheter is removed and the person is allowed to void normally. The nurse will let you know if you are to help prepare a person for removal of an indwelling catheter.

URINARY INCONTINENCE

Urinary incontinence is the inability to hold one's urine, or the involuntary loss of urine from the bladder. Urinary incontinence may be temporary or permanent. Temporary urinary incontinence can occur as a result of a bladder infection, or after an indwelling catheter that has been in place for a long time is removed. Permanent urinary incontinence can be caused by many things, including:

• Decreased muscle tone in the bladder or the muscles that support the bladder, such as occurs after childbirth or from obesity

- Injuries or illnesses that affect the spinal cord, the brain, or the nerves that control bladder function
- Dementia

Urinary incontinence can be emotionally devastating for both the incontinent person and the person's caregivers. For the person who is incontinent, having wet clothes or smelling like urine can be very embarrassing. In addition, being incontinent of urine places a person at risk for developing skin problems (such as rashes and pressure ulcers) and for falling (as the person rushes to the bathroom to avoid having an accident). For the caregiver, caring for a person who is incontinent of urine can be frustrating and emotionally draining. It is not uncommon to change a person's clothes or bedding, only to have the person wet herself all over again. Because caring for an incontinent person can be so emotionally trying and time consuming, incontinence is the factor that most often leads family members to have a relative admitted to a long-term care facility.

Types of Urinary Incontinence

There are many types of urinary incontinence.

- **Stress incontinence** is probably the most common type of urinary incontinence. In stress incontinence, urine leaks from the bladder when the person coughs, sneezes, or exerts herself. Stress incontinence can also occur if a person delays voiding and the bladder becomes too full. Childbirth, obesity, and loss of muscle tone as a result of aging are all factors that can contribute to stress incontinence. Stress incontinence can also occur in men after prostate surgery. Stress incontinence can often be corrected with exercises or surgery.
- **Urge incontinence** is the involuntary release of urine right after feeling a strong urge to void. This type of incontinence is common in people with urinary tract infections because irritation of the bladder causes the bladder muscle to spasm, expelling the contents of the bladder with little warning. Other conditions that decrease the ability of the bladder to hold urine, such as an enlarged prostate gland

or increased intake of caffeinated beverages or alcohol, can also cause urge incontinence.

- **Functional incontinence** occurs in the absence of physical or nervous system problems affecting the urinary tract. The person just cannot make it to the bathroom in enough time, or wait until a bedpan or urinal is provided. It is thought that being in a strange environment (as a hospital or long-term care facility would be to someone who has just been admitted) contributes to functional incontinence. Confusion, disorientation, and loss of mobility are also contributing factors.
- **Overflow incontinence** occurs when the bladder is too full of urine. Overflow incontinence is associated with **urinary retention,** which is the inability of the bladder to empty either completely during urination, or at all. Urinary retention can result from blockage of the bladder outlet (such as occurs with an enlarged prostate gland or from swelling of the urethra during labor or childbirth), or from pain following a surgical procedure. Some injuries that involve the spinal cord can also keep the bladder from emptying fully, leading to urinary retention. Because the bladder does not empty completely when the person voids, it refills with urine quickly, and the urine simply overflows. A person with overflow incontinence may "dribble" urine in between visits to the bathroom. If a person cannot empty his bladder completely, it may be necessary to insert a catheter (either temporarily or permanently) to allow urine to drain from the bladder and prevent urinary retention and overflow incontinence from occurring.
- **Reflex incontinence** occurs when there is damage to the nerves that enable the person to control urination. The bladder fills, but the person does not feel the urge to urinate. When the bladder is completely full, it empties reflexively (that is, automatically). Some people with certain disorders of the nervous system, such as paralysis from a spinal cord injury, will catheterize

themselves with a straight catheter on a regular basis to prevent reflex urinary incontinence.

Managing Urinary Incontinence

Many products are available to help manage urinary incontinence, including incontinence pads, incontinence briefs, and condom catheters. In addition, techniques such as bladder training may be used to help a person overcome certain types of incontinence. For some people, temporary or permanent catheterization may be necessary to manage the incontinence.

Incontinence Pads and Briefs

Products made for urinary incontinence are available to help prevent soiling of clothes and furniture (Fig. 20-12). Incontinence pads and briefs are specially made to absorb urine and hold it away from the person's skin. Keeping the skin dry helps to reduce the skin problems that can occur from prolonged contact with urine. Incontinence pads are placed inside the person's underpants to prevent wetting of the clothes and to draw the moisture away from the person's body. Incontinence briefs are worn instead of underpants. Incontinence pads and briefs are very useful for active people.

For a person who is confined to bed, special bed protectors are used to help to keep the bed linens and mattress dry and to wick urine away from the person's skin. Many facilities have policies that specify that incontinence briefs are to be used only when the person is out of bed, and that bed protec-

tors are to be used when the person is sleeping. Incontinence briefs tend to fit closely, which makes it difficult for air to reach the skin. Switching between briefs and bed protectors helps to prevent skin breakdown by allowing the skin to be exposed to the air at night. As a nursing assistant, you must make sure that these incontinence products are changed frequently and that urine is cleaned from the skin whenever the change occurs. (See Chapter 17 for a discussion of providing perineal care, which is especially important in people who are incontinent of urine, feces, or both.)

Condom Catheters

A **condom catheter** can be used to manage incontinence in men. A condom catheter is not a true catheter because it is not placed inside the body. It consists of a soft plastic or rubber sheath, tubing, and a collection bag for the urine (Fig. 20-13). The sheath is placed over the penis and the collection bag is attached to the leg. The

Tape to hold catheter in place

FIGURE 20-13

A condom catheter can be used to manage urinary incontinence in men. If tape is used to secure the condom catheter to the penis, it should be applied in a spiral fashion, not a circular fashion.

A   **B**

FIGURE 20-12

Incontinence pads and briefs are worn under clothing to absorb moisture and keep it away from the body. (*A*) DEPEND Guards for men. (*B*) DEPEND Extra Absorbency Underwear. (*Photographs courtesy of Kimberly-Clark Worldwide, Inc., Neenah, WI.*)

urine flows through the tubing into the collection bag, allowing the man to urinate at will.

The condom must fit the penis. It should be fastened securely enough to prevent leaking, but not so snugly as to restrict circulation. Many condom catheters have adhesive material on the inside of the condom that allows for a good seal. Others must be secured with tape, the most effective type being elastic. The tape strip is applied in a spiral fashion to allow for changes in the size of the penis (see Fig. 20-13). Applying the tape in an overlapping, circular fashion would compromise blood flow if the man had an erection, possibly causing permanent damage to the penis.

Use of a condom catheter requires good skin care. The penis must be cleaned, and the condom apparatus changed, daily.

Bladder Training

Bladder training is commonly used to help people relearn how to control their urinary elimination patterns. For example, a person may be encouraged to use the bedpan, urinal, or commode at scheduled times. Scheduling of elimination helps promote regular emptying of the bladder. The primary goal is for the person to be able to control involuntary urination. If this is not possible, then the person may still at least be able to get to the bathroom in time to avoid accidents, because she will know when voiding is due to occur. The person's care plan will note any special bladder training techniques that are being used and the nurse will instruct you on any specific duties you will be assigned as part of that training.

BOWEL ELIMINATION

The digestive tract, which is discussed in more detail in Chapter 32, consists of the mouth, esophagus, stomach, small intestine, large intestine, rectum, and anus (Fig. 20-14). The rectum is actually part of the large intestine, and together, the large and small intestines are sometimes referred to as "bowels." Essentially, the digestive tract is a long, hollow tube. The food and fluids that we take in are broken down into smaller pieces and mixed together in the stomach, forming a partially digested food and fluid mixture known as **chyme.** From the stomach, the

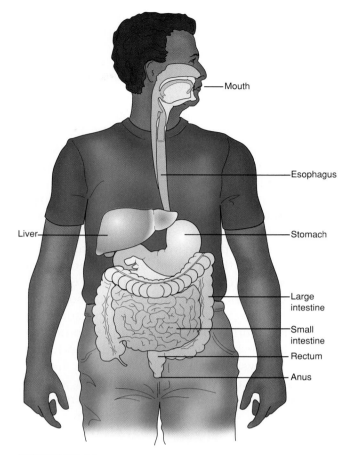

FIGURE 20-14

The digestive tract consists of the mouth, esophagus, stomach, small intestine, large intestine, rectum, and anus.

chyme passes slowly into the small intestine, where more digestion occurs and nutrients and fluid are absorbed, and then into the large intestine. Wave-like muscular movements, called **peristalsis,** move the chyme through the intestines. Finally, the chyme reaches the last part of the large intestine, called the rectum. At this point, all of the nutrients have been removed, and what remains is a semi-solid waste material, called **feces.** The presence of feces in the rectum stimulates the urge to **defecate** (that is, have a bowel movement), and the feces leave the body through the anus, the very end of the digestive tract. Sometimes fecal material is referred to as **"stool"** after it leaves the body.

Flatus (or gas) is a natural byproduct of digestion, just as feces are. Eating certain foods, such as beans, broccoli, cabbage, cauliflower, and onions, can lead to the formation of flatus. The passing of flatus may be quite noisy and depending on what was eaten, the flatus may have a foul odor. For some people, passing flatus is very embarrassing.

In healthy people, feces are soft, brown, moist, and formed, with a distinct odor. Certain foods and medications can affect the color and odor of feces. When you are helping a patient or resident with defecation, observe the feces and report any abnormalities to the nurse. Feces with an unusual odor or appearance could be a sign of illness or infection.

The frequency of a person's bowel movements, and the amount of feces passed each time, will differ from person to person. Many factors influence a person's bowel elimination pattern, including the amount of fluid the person drinks and the type of food he or she eats, the types of drugs the person takes, the person's age, the person's level of activity, and the person's lifelong elimination habits. For example, some people are in the habit of retiring to the bathroom with the newspaper after breakfast to have a bowel movement. Other people are not so predictable. For some people, one or two bowel movements a day is normal. For others, one bowel movement every 2 or 3 days is normal. You will soon become aware of the bowel elimination pattern that is normal for each person in your care. This knowledge will allow you to recognize any changes that may occur.

PROBLEMS WITH BOWEL ELIMINATION

Problems with bowel elimination that are often seen in the health care setting include diarrhea, constipation, fecal impaction, flatulence, and fecal incontinence.

Diarrhea

Diarrhea is the passage of liquid, unformed stool. Diarrhea may occur frequently and can be accompanied by abdominal cramping. If diarrhea is frequent or excessive, the loss of fluid from the body can quickly cause dehydration, especially in young or elderly people. When caring for a person with diarrhea:

- Practice good infection control techniques. A common cause of diarrhea is a bacterial or viral infection. Because the pathogen that caused the diarrhea will be present in the feces, it is important to use good infection control techniques when caring for a person with diarrhea.
- Answer the call light quickly to provide access to the toilet, commode, or bedpan. A normally continent person can have temporary fecal incontinence from diarrhea, which can be very humiliating. Being quick to respond, compassionate, and supportive can help the person to feel better.
- Provide gentle, thorough skin care after each bowel movement to prevent skin breakdown.
- Make sure to record and report the frequency and amount of each incident of diarrhea.

Constipation

The opposite of diarrhea is constipation. **Constipation** occurs when the feces remain in the intestines for too long. The delay allows too much fluid to be reabsorbed by the intestines, resulting in hard, dry feces that are difficult to pass. Constipation is a fairly common occurrence among people who are patients and residents in health care facilities. Risk factors for developing constipation include:

- Taking medications that slow peristalsis (for example, pain medications)
- Not taking in enough dietary fiber or fluids
- Not getting enough exercise
- Delaying having a bowel movement after the urge occurs
- Lack of privacy

As you learned earlier in this chapter, there are many things a nursing assistant can do to help a patient or resident maintain normal bowel function and prevent constipation. For example, eating fiber-rich foods, drinking plenty of fluids, and exercising regularly are all habits that help to keep the bowels functioning regularly. However, if a person is constipated and all other methods of promoting normal bowel function have failed, a laxative, stool softener, or fiber supplement may need to be used.

- A **laxative** is a medication that chemically stimulates peristalsis so that material inside the intestines moves through at a faster pace. The resulting bowel movement is soft (or possibly liquid) and occurs within a few hours of taking the laxative, or overnight. Laxatives are acceptable for occasional use, but should not be used regularly. The problem with regular laxative use is that laxatives cause the chyme to pass through the intestines too quickly for nutrients and fluids to be absorbed. This can result in poor nutrition and dehydration. The intestines also become used to being chemically stimulated to move and can become dependent on the laxative.

- **Stool softeners** help to keep fluid in the feces and are used to help prevent constipation for some people. Unlike laxatives, stool softeners do not chemically stimulate the intestines to cause a bowel movement.
- **Fiber supplements,** in the form of tablets or drink additives, can add bulk to the feces, causing it to hold fluid and preventing constipation.

FIGURE 20-15

Digital examination. A finger is inserted into the person's rectum to check for a fecal impaction.

Fecal Impaction

A **fecal impaction** occurs when constipation is not relieved. The feces build up in the rectum and become harder and harder as more and more fluid is absorbed. Eventually, it becomes almost impossible to pass the feces normally. The impaction blocks the passage of normal stool, but liquid stool may go around the impacted mass. A person with an impaction is usually very uncomfortable, and may complain of abdominal or rectal pain or of liquid feces "seeping" out of the anus. The person's abdomen may be swollen.

If a person is thought to have a fecal impaction, a **digital examination** is done (Fig. 20-15). During the digital examination, a finger is inserted into the person's rectum to feel for the impacted mass (*digital* means "finger"). The impaction is then removed by using the finger to break the impacted feces apart and scoop it out of the rectum piece by piece. The doctor may also order the use of an oil retention enema or drugs to help remove the impaction. Digital removal of a fecal impaction is very uncomfortable and embarrassing for most patients and residents. Many facilities require that a nurse remove an impaction, but your assistance will be necessary. If you are allowed to remove an impaction, make sure you have been adequately trained for the procedure and that it is part of your job description.

Flatulence

Flatulence is the presence of excessive amounts of flatus (gas) in the intestines, causing abdominal distension (swelling) and discomfort. Sometimes people have difficulty passing flatus because of a lack of activity or a recent surgical procedure. Getting out of bed and walking might be all that is needed to help the person to expel the gas. If walking is not allowed, positioning the person on her left side may help. If the flatulence cannot be relieved with these methods, a nurse may insert a rectal tube to help the gas escape (Fig. 20-16).

Fecal Incontinence

Fecal (bowel) incontinence is the inability to hold one's feces, or the involuntary loss of feces from the bowel. Like urinary incontinence, fecal incontinence can be temporary or permanent. Temporary fecal incontinence can accompany a severe case of diarrhea, simply because the person might not be able to get to the bathroom quickly enough. Some people experience temporary fecal incontinence if the call light is not answered soon enough. Diseases or injuries that affect the nervous system can also result in temporary or permanent fecal incontinence. A person who is unconscious will be incontinent of feces. A person who has dementia will develop fecal incontinence as the disease progresses.

FIGURE 20-16

A rectal tube may be placed to relieve flatulence (excess gas in the intestines) if the gas cannot be passed naturally. The small bag connected to the end of the rectal tube is used to collect any liquid stool that may escape with the flatus.

Bowel training is very similar to bladder training and works to promote regular, controlled bowel movements. Offering the commode or bedpan at regular scheduled intervals is a common method of bowel training. Bowel training is often started by keeping track of when an incontinent person usually has a bowel movement, then making sure to provide the appropriate toilet facilities during that time period.

⟩ **Tell the Nurse!**

Changes in the quality of a person's feces or pattern of defecation can be a sign that something is wrong. Be sure to report the following observations to the nurse immediately:

⟩ The person has diarrhea or is constipated

⟩ There is blood or mucus in the stool

⟩ The stool is black or dark green

⟩ The stool is foul-smelling

⟩ The person complains that the feces are painful or difficult to pass

⟩ There is bleeding from the anus during or after a bowel movement

⟩ The person has a swollen abdomen or complains of abdominal pain

⟩ The person complains of liquid feces "seeping" from the anus

⟩ The person has excessive flatus (gas)

ENEMAS

An **enema** is the introduction of fluid into the large intestine by way of the anus for the purpose of removing stool from the rectum. There are several reasons a person would be given an enema. Enemas are used to relieve constipation and fecal impactions and to empty the intestine of fecal material before surgery or certain diagnostic tests. Sometimes enemas are used as part of a bowel training program.

Types of Enemas

Several types of enemas are used in the health care setting (Fig. 20-17). Some are prepared by the nurse or nursing assistant, and others come prepackaged. The solution that is placed into the anus varies according to the reason the enema was ordered.

- **Cleansing enemas.** Cleansing enemas are primarily used to remove feces from the lower large intestine. **Tap water enemas** and **saline (salt water) enemas** help soften the stool and stimulate peristalsis. Enemas containing these solutions should not be given repeatedly because the intestine can absorb the solution, causing a fluid imbalance in the body. **Soapsuds enemas** consist of water and a small amount of a very gentle soap called *castile soap*. The soap solution irritates the lining of the bowel, stimulating peristalsis. These, too, must be used with caution because too much soap can cause damage to the lining of the intestines.
- **Oil retention enemas.** An oil retention enema contains mineral, olive, or cottonseed oil. The oil lubricates the inside of the intestine and any stool that is present, making the stool easier to pass or remove. Oil retention enemas are useful for helping to remove fecal impactions.
- **Commercial enemas.** Commercially prepared and packaged enemas usually

A

B

FIGURE 20-17

There are many different types of enema solutions. (*A*) Commercially prepared enema solutions. (*B*) A soap-suds enema is prepared using castile soap and water (not shown) and administered using an enema bag.

contain 120 mL of a solution that irritates the intestinal mucosa to promote peristalsis. Some commercial enemas contain a solution that is absorbed into the stool to make it softer and easier to pass.

Administering Enemas

Enemas are ordered by a doctor and usually given by a nurse. Some facilities allow nursing assistants to administer enemas after adequate training. Make sure you are familiar with your facility's policies on the administration of enemas. If you are permitted to give enemas, be sure to follow proper procedure and the doctor's orders closely. Make sure the solution is correct for the person, that you have the correct amount of solution, and that the solution is at the proper temperature. Enema solutions that are too cool can cause abdominal cramping and pain, whereas solutions that are too hot can cause serious injury and possibly even death. When you are assisting with the administration of an enema, make sure that a bed protector and bedpan are in place, or that the path to the bathroom is clear. When it comes time for the person to expel the enema, she will need immediate access to toilet facilities.

An enema is given with the person on her left side in Sims' position. When a person is lying on her left side in Sims' position, the intestine is positioned to take the best advantage of gravity. The solution will flow downward to clean a longer segment of bowel (Fig. 20-18). Having the person lie on her right side in Sims' position is not as effective because the enema solution flows only as far as the rectum and does not clean as much of the bowel. After the enema has been administered, the person is asked to hold the solution in the bowel for the specified amount of time, and then to expel the solution. The doctor may order a cleansing enema to be administered "until clear," which means that enemas are to be given until the enema return from the person does not contain any fecal material. If you are responsible for giving a cleansing enema, make sure to ask the nurse how many enemas are allowed to be given during a particular session.

Receiving an enema can be uncomfortable and embarrassing. To make the procedure easier for the person, keep the person covered as much as possible and ensure that she has as much privacy as possible. Having the person take a few slow, deep breaths as the enema tubing is inserted into

FIGURE 20-18

The left Sims' position is used when a person is to receive an enema. This position exposes the greatest amount of the bowel to the enema solution.

the rectum may help to relax the person and make insertion easier. The procedure for administering an enema is given in Procedure 20-8.

RECTAL SUPPOSITORIES

A **rectal suppository** is a small, wax-like cone or oval that is inserted into the anus. The wax-like substance dissolves at body temperature, stimulating peristalsis or lubricating and softening the stool. Glycerin rectal suppositories are often used to help with bowel elimination before resorting to an enema. Some rectal suppositories also contain medication. These should only be inserted by a nurse.

SUMMARY

▶ The elimination of waste products from the body is one of the most basic physical needs.
   ■ Although elimination is a natural function, many people are not comfortable discussing it or doing it in front of others. A person's culture and upbringing influence how comfortable he is with the body processes involved in elimination.
   ■ Normal urinary and bowel elimination can be promoted by encouraging fluids, answering the call light promptly, and providing for the person's privacy and comfort.
   ■ Incontinence is the inability to hold one's urine, feces, or both until a suitable receptacle (for example, a toilet, bedside commode, or bedpan) is made available. Incontinence has many causes and may be temporary or permanent.
      ● Incontinence is difficult emotionally for both the person who is incontinent and that person's caregiver.
      ● Being incontinent of urine or feces places a person at risk for skin breakdown. Providing good perineal care is essential when caring for a person who is incontinent of urine, feces, or both.
▶ The urinary system rids the body of waste products that have been filtered from the bloodstream.
   ■ Normal urine is clear, pale yellow to dark gold in color, with a characteristic odor. Urinary patterns vary among individuals. Any abnormal observations should be reported to the nurse.
   ■ A person who is having trouble urinating for physical or emotional reasons may need to have a urinary catheter placed to remove the urine from the bladder.
      ● Urinary catheters may be left in place for an extended period of time, or inserted and then removed as soon as the bladder has been drained.
      ● Providing good catheter care is essential to prevent nosocomial infection. The use of urinary catheters is the leading cause of nosocomial infection.
▶ The digestive system rids the body of waste products that are left over from digestion.
   ■ Normal stool is soft, brown, moist, formed, and has a distinct odor. Bowel elimination patterns vary among individuals. Any abnormal observations should be reported to the nurse.
      ● Constipation occurs when feces remain in the intestine too long and excess fluid is

absorbed, leaving the stool hard and difficult to pass. Fecal impaction can result if constipation is not relieved.

- Diarrhea is the passage of liquid, unformed stool. Diarrhea can lead to dehydration.

■ An enema is the introduction of solution into the large intestine. An enema is sometimes ordered by a doctor to treat or prevent bowel elimination problems.

- The type of enema solution used is determined by the reason the enema has been ordered.

- Enemas are usually given by a nurse. However, in some facilities, enema administration is within the scope of practice of the nursing assistant. Enemas must be administered correctly, with special attention paid to the position of the person.

Chapter 20 Procedures

Getting Ready Steps

a. **W**ash your hands and observe standard precautions as necessary.

b. **G**ather needed supplies.

c. **K**nock and introduce yourself.

d. **I**dentify the person, and greet him or her by name.

e. **E**xplain the procedure.

f. **P**rovide privacy.

g. **S**ee to safety.

Finishing Up Steps

a. **C**onfirm comfort and good body alignment.

b. **L**eave the call light control within easy reach.

c. **S**ee to safety.

d. **O**pen the curtain and door.

e. **W**ash your hands.

f. **R**eport and record.

PROCEDURE 20-1

Assisting a Person with Using a Bedpan

Getting Ready

1. Complete the "Getting Ready" steps **a** through **g**.

Supplies

- gloves
- bed protector
- toilet paper
- bedpan
- bedpan cover (or
- paper towels)
- perineal care supplies
- washcloth
- towel

Procedure

2. Make sure that the bed is positioned at a comfortable working height (to promote good body mechanics) and that the wheels are locked. If the side rails are in use, lower the side rail on the working side of the bed. The side rail on the opposite side of the bed should remain up. If necessary, lower the head of the bed so that the bed is flat (as tolerated).

3. Fanfold the top linens to the foot of the bed. Place the bed protector on the bed. Adjust the person's hospital gown or pajama bottoms as necessary to expose the person's buttocks.

4. Place the bedpan underneath the person's buttocks. This can be accomplished by either

STEP 4 Place the bedpan against the person's buttocks and help the person to roll back onto it.

helping the person to lie on her side, facing away from you, or by asking the person to bend her knees, lift her buttocks, and press her heels into the mattress. Slide the bedpan underneath the person (if the person is holding her buttocks away from the bed by bending her knees), or place the bedpan against the person's buttocks and help the person to roll back onto it.

a. A standard bedpan is positioned like a regular toilet seat.

(continued)

PROCEDURE 20-1 (Continued)

Assisting a Person with Using a Bedpan

b. A fracture pan is positioned with the narrow end pointed toward the head of the bed.

5. Raise the head of the bed as tolerated. Draw the top linens over the person for modesty and warmth.

6. Make sure that the toilet paper and the call light control are within reach.

7. If the side rails are in use, return the side rails to the raised position. If safety permits, leave the room and ask the person to call you when she is finished. Remember to close the door on your way out.

8. Return when the person signals. Remember to knock before entering.

9. If the side rails are in use, lower the side rail on the working side of the bed. Lower the head of the bed so that the bed is flat (as tolerated).

10. Put on the gloves.

11. Fanfold the top linens to the foot of the bed.

12. Ask the person to bend her knees, lift her buttocks, and press her heels into the mattress so that you can remove the bedpan and bed protector. (Or help the person to roll onto her side, facing away from you, while you hold the bedpan securely in place against the mattress to prevent the contents from spilling. Remove the bedpan and bed protector, and then help the person to roll back.) If necessary, help the person to use the toilet paper.

13. Cover the bedpan with the bedpan cover or paper towels. Take the bedpan to the bathroom. (If the side rails are in use, raise them before leaving the bedside.)

14. Remove your gloves and dispose of them in a facility-approved waste container. Wash your hands.

15. Return to the bedside. Give the person a wet washcloth and help the person to wash her hands. Make sure the person's perineum is clean and dry. If necessary, provide perineal care.

16. Adjust the person's hospital gown or pajama bottoms as necessary to cover the buttocks. Help the person back into a comfortable position, straighten the bottom linens, and draw the top linens over the person. Raise the head of the bed, as the person requests. Make sure that the bed is lowered to its lowest position and that the wheels are locked.

17. Return to the bathroom. Put on a clean pair of gloves. If the person is on intake and output (I&O) status, measure the urine. Note the color, amount, and quality of the urine or feces before emptying the contents of the bedpan into the toilet. (If anything unusual is observed, do not empty the bedpan until a nurse has had a chance to look at its contents.)

18. Gather the soiled linens and place them in the linen hamper or linen bag. Dispose of disposable items in a facility-approved waste container. Clean equipment and return it to the storage area.

19. Remove your gloves and dispose of them in a facility-approved waste container.

Finishing Up CLSOWR

20. Complete the "Finishing Up" steps **a** through **f**.

PROCEDURE 20-2

Assisting a Man with Using a Urinal

Getting Ready WCKIEDS

1. Complete the "Getting Ready" steps **a** through **g**.

Supplies

- gloves
- toilet paper
- urinal
- washcloth
- towel

Procedure

2. Ask the man what position he prefers—lying, sitting, or standing. If necessary, raise the head of the bed as tolerated. If the man would prefer to stand, help him to sit on the edge of the bed, and then to stand up (see Chapter 11, Procedure 11-15).

3. Hand the man the urinal. If necessary, assist him in positioning it correctly.

4. Make sure that the toilet paper and the call light control are within reach.

5. If safety permits, leave the room and ask the man to call you when he is finished. Remember to close the door on your way out.

(continued)

PROCEDURE 20-2 (Continued)

Assisting a Man with Using a Urinal

6. Return when the man signals. Remember to knock before entering.

7. Put on the gloves. Have the man hand you the urinal, or remove it if he is unable to hand it to you. Put the lid on the urinal and hang it on the side rail while you assist the man with handwashing and perineal care as needed. Lower the head of the bed as the man requests.

8. Take the urinal to the bathroom. If the man is on intake and output (I&O) status, measure the urine. Note the color, amount, and quality of the urine before emptying the contents of the urinal into the toilet. (If anything unusual is observed, do not empty the urinal until a nurse has had a chance to look at its contents.)

9. Gather the soiled linens and place them in the linen hamper or linen bag. Dispose of disposable items in a facility-approved waste container. Clean equipment and return it to the storage area.

10. Remove your gloves and dispose of them in a facility-approved waste container.

Finishing Up CLSOWR

11. Complete the "Finishing Up" steps **a** through **f**.

PROCEDURE 20-3

Collecting a Routine Urine Specimen

Getting Ready WGKIEpS

1. Complete the "Getting Ready" steps **a** through **g**.

Supplies

- gloves
- paper towel
- toilet paper
- specimen cup and label
- plastic transport bag (if required at your facility)
- plastic bag or waste container
- specimen collection device ("commode hat"), bedpan, or urinal

Procedure

2. Complete the label with the person's name, room number, and other identifying information. Put the completed label on the specimen cup. Take the specimen cup to the bathroom. Place a paper towel on the counter. Open the specimen cup and place the lid on the paper towel, with the inside of the lid facing up.

3. If the person will be using a regular toilet or bedside commode, fit the specimen collection device underneath the toilet or commode seat. Otherwise, provide the person with a bedpan or urinal, as applicable.

4. Assist the person with urination as necessary (see Procedures 20-1 and 20-2). Before leaving the room, remind the person not to have a bowel movement or place toilet paper into the specimen collection device, bedpan, or urinal. Provide a plastic bag or waste container for the used toilet paper.

5. Return when the person signals. Remember to knock before entering.

6. Put on the gloves.

7. If the person used a regular toilet or bedside commode, assist the person with handwashing and perineal care as necessary, and then help the person to return to bed. If the person used a bedpan or urinal, cover and remove the bedpan or urinal and assist the person with handwashing and perineal care as necessary.

8. Take the covered bedpan, urinal, or specimen collection device (if the person used a bedside commode) to the bathroom. (If the side rails are in use, raise the side rails before leaving the bedside.)

9. If the person is on intake and output (I&O) status, measure the urine. Note the color, amount, and quality of the urine.

10. Raise the toilet seat. While holding the specimen cup over the toilet, carefully fill it about three-quarters full with urine from the

(continued)

PROCEDURE 20-3 (Continued)

Collecting a Routine Urine Specimen

specimen collection device, bedpan, or urinal. Discard the rest of the urine into the toilet.

STEP 10 Hold the specimen cup over the toilet and fill it about three-quarters full with urine.

11. Put the lid on the specimen cup. Make sure that the lid is tight. Put the specimen cup on the paper towel on the counter.

12. Remove one glove and dispose of it in a facility-approved waste container. Holding the plastic transport bag in your ungloved hand, place the specimen cup into the transport bag with your gloved hand. Avoid touching the outside of the transport bag with your glove.

STEP 12 Place the specimen cup into the transport bag with your gloved hand.

13. Remove the other glove and dispose of it in a facility-approved waste container.

14. Gather the soiled linens and place them in the linen hamper or linen bag. Dispose of disposable items in a facility-approved waste container. Clean equipment and return it to the storage area.

15. Take the specimen cup to the designated location.

Finishing Up   CLSOWR

16. Complete the "Finishing Up" steps **a** through **f**.

PROCEDURE 20-4

Collecting a Midstream ("Clean Catch") Urine Specimen

Getting Ready   WGKIEps

1. Complete the "Getting Ready" steps **a** through **g**.

Supplies

- gloves
- paper towel
- toilet paper
- specimen cup and label
- "clean catch" kit
- plastic transport bag (if required at your facility)
- bedpan or urinal (if necessary)

Procedure

2. Complete the label with the person's name, room number, and other identifying information. Put the completed label on the specimen cup.

3. If the person will be using a regular toilet or bedside commode, help the person to the bathroom or bedside commode. Otherwise, provide the person with a bedpan or urinal, as applicable.

4. Put on the gloves.

5. Place a paper towel on the counter (if the person is in the bathroom) or on the over-bed table (if the person is using a bedside commode, bedpan, or urinal). Open the specimen cup and place the lid on the paper towel, with the inside of the lid facing up.

(continued)

PROCEDURE 20-4 (Continued)

Collecting a Midstream ("Clean Catch") Urine Specimen

6. Open the "clean catch" kit. Have the person clean his or her perineum using the wipes in the kit. Assist as necessary:

   a. **If the person is a woman:** Use one hand to separate the labia. Hold the wipe in the other hand. Place your wipe-covered hand at the top of the vulva and stroke downward to the anus.

   b. **If the person is a circumcised man:** Use one hand to hold the penis slightly away from the body. Hold the wipe in the other hand. Place your wipe-covered hand at the tip of the penis and wash in a circular motion, downward to the base of the penis.

   c. **If the person is an uncircumcised man:** Retract the foreskin by gently pushing the skin toward the base of the penis. Place your wipe-covered hand at the tip of the penis and wash in a circular motion, downward to the base of the penis.

7. Assist the person with urination as necessary (see Procedures 20-1 and 20-2). Before leaving the room:

   a. Make sure that the toilet paper, call light control, and specimen cup are within reach.

   b. Remind the person that he or she must start the stream of urine, then stop it, then restart it. The urine sample is to be

collected from the restarted flow. If the person is a woman, she must hold the labia open until the specimen is collected. If the person is an uncircumcised man, he must keep the foreskin pulled back until the specimen is collected.

8. Remove your gloves and dispose of them in a facility-approved waste container.

9. Return when the person signals. Remember to knock before entering.

10. Put on a clean pair of gloves.

11. If the person used a regular toilet or bedside commode, assist the person with handwashing and perineal care as necessary, and then help the person to return to bed. If the person used a bedpan or urinal, remove the bedpan or urinal and assist the person with handwashing and perineal care as necessary.

12. Put the lid on the specimen cup, being careful not to touch the inside of the lid or container. Make sure that the lid is tight. Put the specimen cup on the paper towel on the counter or over-bed table.

13. Remove one glove and dispose of it in a facility-approved waste container. Holding the plastic transport bag in your ungloved hand, place the specimen cup into the transport bag with your gloved hand. Avoid touching the outside of the transport bag with your glove.

14. Remove the other glove and dispose of it in a facility-approved waste container.

15. Gather the soiled linens and place them in the linen hamper or linen bag. Dispose of disposable items in a facility-approved waste container. Clean equipment and return it to the storage area.

16. Take the specimen cup to the designated location.

STEP 7b Women must hold the labia open while voiding to prevent contamination of the urine sample. Uncircumcised men must keep the foreskin pulled back.

Finishing Up CL3OWR

17. Complete the "Finishing Up" steps **a** through **f**.

PROCEDURE 20-5
Collecting a Stool Specimen

Getting Ready

1. Complete the "Getting Ready" steps **a** through **g**.

Supplies

- gloves
- paper towel
- tongue depressor
- toilet paper
- specimen cup and label
- plastic transport bag

- (if required at your facility)
- plastic bag or waste container
- specimen collection device ("commode hat") or bedpan

Procedure

2. Complete the label with the person's name, room number, and other identifying information. Put the completed label on the specimen cup. Take the specimen cup to the bathroom. Place a paper towel on the counter. Open the specimen cup and place the lid on the paper towel, with the inside of the lid facing up.

3. If the person will be using a regular toilet or bedside commode, fit the specimen collection device underneath the toilet or commode seat. Otherwise, provide the person with a bedpan.

4. Assist the person with defecation as necessary (see Procedure 20-1). Before leaving the room, remind the person not to urinate or place toilet paper into the specimen collection device or bedpan. Provide a plastic bag or waste container for the used toilet paper.

5. Return when the person signals. Remember to knock before entering.

6. Put on the gloves.

7. If the person used a regular toilet or bedside commode, assist the person with handwashing and then help the person to return to bed. Provide perineal care as necessary. If the person used a bedpan, cover and remove the bedpan and assist the person with handwashing and perineal care as necessary.

8. Take the covered bedpan or specimen collection device (if the person used a bedside commode) to the bathroom. (If the side rails are in use, raise the side rails before leaving the bedside.)

9. Note the color, amount, and quality of the feces. Using the tongue depressor, take two tablespoons of feces from the bedpan or specimen collection device and put them into the specimen cup. Dispose of the tongue depressor in a facility-approved waste container. Empty the remaining contents of the bedpan or specimen collection device into the toilet.

10. Put the lid on the specimen cup. Make sure that the lid is tight. Put the specimen cup on the paper towel on the counter.

11. Remove one glove and dispose of it in a facility-approved waste container. Holding the plastic transport bag in your ungloved hand, place the specimen cup into the transport bag with your gloved hand. Avoid touching the outside of the transport bag with your glove.

12. Remove the other glove and dispose of it in a facility-approved waste container.

13. Gather the soiled linens and place them in the linen hamper or linen bag. Dispose of disposable items in a facility-approved waste container. Clean equipment and return it to the storage area.

14. Take the specimen cup to the designated location.

Finishing Up

15. Complete the "Finishing Up" steps **a** through **f**.

PROCEDURE 20-6
Providing Catheter Care

Getting Ready   WCKIEpS

1. Complete the "Getting Ready" steps **a** through **g**.

Supplies

- gloves
- paper towels
- bed protector
- bath thermometer
- wash basin
- soap or antiseptic solution
- bath blanket
- washcloths
- towels
- clean clothing

Procedure

2. Cover the over-bed table with paper towels.

3. Lower the head of the bed so that the bed is flat (as tolerated). Make sure that the bed is positioned at a comfortable working height (to promote good body mechanics) and that the wheels are locked.

4. Fill the wash basin with warm water (110°F [43.3°C] to 115°F [46.1°C] on the bath thermometer). Place the wash basin, soap, towels, and washcloths on the over-bed table. Put on the gloves.

5. If the side rails are in use, lower the side rail on the working side of the bed. The side rail on the opposite side of the bed should remain up.

6. Spread the bath blanket over the top linens (and the person). If the person is able, have him or her hold the bath blanket. If not, tuck the corners under the person's shoulders. Fanfold the top linens to the foot of the bed.

7. Adjust the person's hospital gown or pajama bottoms as necessary to expose the person's perineum.

8. Ask the person to open his legs and bend his knees, if possible. If the person is not able to bend his knees, help the person to spread his legs as much as possible.

9. Position the bath blanket over the person so that one corner can be wrapped under and around each leg.

10. Position a bed protector under the person's buttocks to keep the bed linens dry.

11. Lift the corner of the bath blanket that is between the person's legs upward, exposing only the perineal area.

12. Form a mitt around your hand with one of the washcloths. Wet the mitt with warm, clean water and apply soap or antiseptic solution.

  a. **If the person is a woman:** Using the other hand, separate the labia. Place your washcloth-covered hand at the top of the vulva and stroke downward to the anus. Repeat, using a different part of the washcloth each time, until the area is clean. Rinse and dry the vulva and perineum thoroughly.

  b. **If the person is a circumcised man:** Place your washcloth-covered hand at the tip of the penis and wash in a circular motion, downward to the base of the penis. Repeat, using a different part of the washcloth each time, until the area is clean. Rinse and dry the tip and the shaft of the penis thoroughly.

  c. **If the person is an uncircumcised man:** Retract the foreskin by gently pushing the skin toward the base of the penis. Place your washcloth-covered hand at the tip of the penis and wash in a circular motion, downward to the base of the penis. Repeat, using a different part of the washcloth each time, until the area is clean. Rinse and dry the tip and the shaft of the penis thoroughly before gently pulling the foreskin back into its normal position.

STEP 13 Clean the catheter tubing, starting at the body and moving outward.

(continued)

PROCEDURE 20-6 (Continued)

Providing Catheter Care

13. Using a clean part of the washcloth, clean the catheter tubing, starting at the body and moving outward from the body about four inches.* Hold the catheter near the opening of the urethra. This will help to prevent tugging on the catheter as you clean it.

14. Dry the perineal area thoroughly using a towel.

15. Check that the catheter tubing is free from kinks. Make sure that it is securely taped to the person's leg.

16. Remove your gloves and dispose of them in a facility-approved waste container.

---

*In some facilities, disposable antiseptic wipes may be used instead of a washcloth to clean the catheter tubing.

17. Assist the person into the supine position. Remove the bath blanket, and help the person into the clean clothing (see Chapter 18, Procedures 18-3 and 18-4).

18. If the side rails are in use, return the side rails to the raised position. Raise the head of the bed as the person requests. Make sure that the bed is lowered to its lowest position and that the wheels are locked.

19. Gather the soiled linens and place them in the linen hamper or linen bag. Dispose of disposable items in a facility-approved waste container. Clean equipment and return it to the storage area.

Finishing Up CLSOWR

20. Complete the "Finishing Up" steps **a** through **f**.

PROCEDURE 20-7

Emptying a Urine Drainage Bag

Getting Ready WGKIEpS

1. Complete the "Getting Ready" steps **a** through **g**.

Supplies

- gloves
- paper towels
- alcohol wipes (optional)
- graduate

Procedure

2. Put on the gloves.

3. Place a paper towel on the floor, underneath the urine drainage bag. Unhook the drainage bag emptying spout from its holder on the urine drainage bag. Position the graduate on the paper towel, underneath the emptying spout.

4. Unclamp the emptying spout on the urine drainage bag and allow all of the urine to drain into the graduate. Avoid touching the tip of the emptying spout with your hands or the side of the graduate.

5. After the urine has drained into the graduate, wipe the emptying spout with an alcohol wipe (or follow facility policy). Reclamp the emptying spout and return it to its holder.

6. If the person is on intake and output (I&O) status, measure the urine. Note the color,

amount, and quality of the urine before emptying the contents of the graduate into the toilet. (If anything unusual is observed, do not empty the graduate until a nurse has had a chance to look at its contents.)

STEP 4 Unclamp the emptying spout on the urine drainage bag and allow the urine to drain into the graduate.

7. Dispose of disposable items in a facility-approved waste container. Clean equipment and return it to the storage area.

8. Remove your gloves and dispose of them in a facility-approved waste container.

Finishing Up CLSOWR

9. Complete the "Finishing Up" steps **a** through **f**.

PROCEDURE 20-8

Administering a Soapsuds Enema

Getting Ready   WGKIEDS

1. Complete the "Getting Ready" steps **a** through **g**.

Supplies

- gloves
- paper towel
- toilet paper
- bed protector
- lubricant jelly
- 5-mL packet of castile soap
- bedpan
- bedpan cover
- enema bag with tubing and clamp
- IV pole
- bath thermometer
- bath blanket
- perineal care supplies

Procedure

2. Make sure that the bed is positioned at a comfortable working height (to promote good body mechanics) and that the wheels are locked.

3. Prepare the enema solution in the bathroom or utility room. Clamp the tubing, and then fill the enema bag with warm water (105°F [40.5°C] on the bath thermometer) in the specified amount (usually from 500 to 1500 mL). Add the castile soap packet and mix by gently rotating the enema bag. Do not shake the solution vigorously.

4. Release the clamp on the tubing and allow a little water to run through tubing into the sink or bedpan. This will remove all of the air from the tubing. Reclamp the tubing.

5. Hang the enema bag on the IV pole and bring it to the person's bedside. Adjust the height of the IV pole so that the enema bag is hanging no more than 18 inches above the person's anus.

6. Put on the gloves.

7. If the side rails are in use, lower the side rail on the working side of the bed. The side rail on the opposite side of the bed should remain up. Lower the head of the bed so that the bed is flat (as tolerated).

8. Spread the bath blanket over the top linens (and the person). If the person is able, have her hold the bath blanket. If not, tuck the corners under the person's shoulders. Fanfold the top linens to the foot of the bed.

9. Ask the person to lie on her left side, facing away from you, in Sims' position. Help the person into this position, if necessary.

STEP 9 Position the person in the left Sims' position. The enema bag should hang no more than 18 inches above the person's anus.

10. Adjust the bath blanket and the person's hospital gown or pajama bottoms as necessary to expose the person's buttocks. Position the bed protector under the person's buttocks to keep the bed linens dry.

11. Open the lubricant package and squeeze a small amount of lubricant onto a paper towel. Lubricate the tip of the enema tubing to ease insertion.

12. Suggest that the person take a deep breath and slowly exhale as the enema tubing is inserted. With one hand, raise the person's upper buttock to expose the anus. Using your other hand, gently and carefully insert the lubricated tip of the tubing into the person's rectum (not more than 3 to 4 inches for adults). Never force the tubing into the rectum. If you are unable to insert the tubing, stop and call the nurse.

13. Unclamp the tubing and allow the solution to begin running. Hold the enema tubing firmly with one hand so that it does not slip out of the rectum. If the person complains of pain or cramping, slow down the rate of flow by tightening the clamp a bit. If the pain or cramping does not stop after slowing the rate of flow, stop the procedure and call the nurse.

14. When the fluid level reaches the bottom of the bag, clamp the tubing to avoid injecting air into the person's rectum. Ask the person to retain the solution for the designated amount of time.

(continued)

PROCEDURE 20-8 (Continued)

Administering a Soapsuds Enema

15. Remove the tubing from the person's rectum and place it inside the enema bag. Gently place several thicknesses of toilet paper against the person's anus to absorb any fluid.

16. Assist the person with expelling the enema as necessary, using the bedpan, bedside commode, or toilet. If the person is using a regular toilet, ask him or her not to flush the toilet after expelling the enema.

17. If the person used a regular toilet or bedside commode, assist the person with handwashing and then help the person to return to bed. Provide perineal care as necessary. If the person used a bedpan, cover and remove the bedpan and assist the person with handwashing and perineal care as necessary.

18. Raise the head of the bed as the person requests. Make sure that the bed is lowered to its lowest position and that the wheels are locked. (If the side rails are in use, raise the side rails before leaving the bedside.)

19. Take the covered bedpan or commode bucket (if the person used a bedside commode) to the bathroom.

20. Note the color, amount, and quality of feces before emptying the contents of the bedpan or commode bucket into the toilet. (If anything unusual is observed, do not empty the bedpan or commode bucket until a nurse has had a chance to look at its contents.)

21. Gather the soiled linens and place them in the linen hamper. Dispose of disposable items in a facility-approved waste container. Clean equipment and return it to the storage area.

22. Remove your gloves and dispose of them in a facility-approved waste container.

Finishing Up   CLSOWR

23. Complete the "Finishing Up" steps **a** through **f**.

What did you learn?

Multiple Choice

Select the single best answer for each of the following questions.

1. The perineum (perineal area) is cleaned before collecting a
   a. 24-hour urine specimen
   b. Clean-catch urine specimen
   c. Random urine specimen
   d. Stool specimen

2. The most comfortable position for using a bedpan is
   a. Fowler's position
   b. Sims' position
   c. Prone position
   d. Supine position

3. How far is an enema tube inserted into the rectum in an adult?
   a. 3 to 4 inches
   b. 5 to 6 inches
   c. 7 to 8 inches
   d. 12 to16 inches

4. One of your residents needs to have an enema administered. How should you position the resident in preparation for the enema?
   a. Left Sims' position
   b. Fowler's position
   c. Supine position
   d. Right Sims' position

5. In a person with an indwelling urinary catheter, why must the urine drainage bag be kept lower than the person's bladder?
   a. Keeping the drainage bag below bladder level will prevent a bedridden person from seeing the bag, which he or she might find embarrassing
   b. Keeping the drainage bag below bladder level will keep the person comfortable in bed
   c. Keeping the drainage bag below bladder level will prevent urine from returning to the bladder, where it could cause infection

   d. Keeping the drainage bag below bladder level will prevent the urine from leaking out

6. Which one of the following describes normal urine?
   a. Cloudy with a strong odor
   b. Well-formed
   c. Red-tinged
   d. Clear, light yellow, or golden with a slight odor

7. A healthy person's feces will be:
   a. Black and tarry
   b. Soft, brown, formed, and moist with a distinct odor
   c. Hard and pellet-like
   d. Long and stringy

8. To help your residents or patients to maintain healthy bowel function, it is important to
   a. Answer call lights promptly
   b. Encourage them to eat a well-balanced diet and drink plenty of fluids
   c. Assist them with exercise
   d. All of the above

9. When caring for a person who is incontinent of urine or feces, it is important to:
   a. Provide good perineal care
   b. Let the person know that his or her behavior is inappropriate, so it will stop
   c. Take the person to the bathroom once daily
   d. Restrict fluids to reduce the chance of an accident

10. When caring for a person with an indwelling catheter, always remember to:
    a. Leave the drainage bag above the level of the bladder, while the person is in bed
    b. Tape any leaks at the connection site
    c. Wear gloves when providing daily catheter care
    d. Tape the drainage tube under the leg

Matching

Match each numbered item with its appropriate lettered description.

_____ **1.** Hematuria

_____ **2.** Peristalsis

_____ **3.** Micturition

_____ **4.** Defecation

_____ **5.** Nocturia

_____ **6.** Dysuria

_____ **7.** Urinalysis

_____ **8.** Anuria

_____ **9.** Oliguria

_____ **10.** Polyuria

a. Excessive urine production

b. Excessive urination at night

c. Difficulty urinating

d. No urine production

e. Urination

f. Passing of feces

g. Routine urine test

h. Inadequate urine production

i. Blood in the urine

j. Wave-like muscular movement of the intestines

? Stop and think!

▶ You are a nursing assistant in a hospital. One of your patients, Mrs. Walker, must use a bedpan because she is confined to bed, but she is having a hard time relaxing enough to urinate "in bed." What sorts of things could you do to help make using a bedpan easier for Mrs. Walker?

▶ You are caring for Miss Smiley, who has an indwelling catheter. When you are making your end-of-shift rounds, you note that Miss Smiley's urinary drainage bag has very little urine in it. You know that the drainage bag was emptied right before you started your shift, and the output was not significant at that time. That was almost 12 hours ago. What concerns do you have regarding Miss Smiley's urine output? What would you do?

Nursing Assistants Make a Difference!

"My name is Philip and I came to live here at the Emerald Isle Nursing Facility after I had a stroke, about 6 months ago. The stroke darn near killed me, but I pulled through like the tough old bird that I am. Now my right side is paralyzed, but I have had lots of rehabilitation to help me regain some of the skills I lost and learn how to move myself in and out of my wheelchair. *You've come a long way*, Wanda would say. Wanda was my wife of 53 years. She passed away 2 years ago and I really miss her. When Wanda and I married, she asked me to grow a moustache so I would look old enough to be her husband and not her younger brother. I humored her and I've kept this hair on my lip for all those years...it reminds me of her when I look in the mirror.

When I came to live here, I was pretty worried that I would have to shave off my moustache, because I am very right-handed. With my bum arm, I couldn't trim and maintain my moustache any longer, and I wondered if the staff here would have the time or desire to help an old man keep a memory growing on his lip. Betty, one of the nursing assistants, took one look at me right after I was admitted and asked me what kind of animal I had growing out of my nose! Even though I laughed (because my moustache *had* become pretty bushy in the hospital), I felt a lump in my throat because I figured that she was getting ready to shave it off. Instead, Betty shaved my face and trimmed my mustache up just right. Then she told me how handsome the mustache made my face look and it brought tears to my eyes. I told her about my dear wife and how important my moustache was to me. She sat there and held my hand and told me that she would help me keep my whiskers. At that moment, Betty became my favorite nursing assistant! Since then, Betty has started bringing new nursing assistants and students by to show them how to care for a moustache, and its owner. Betty makes me feel special, and for that reason, she is special to me."

You can listen to more stories about how nursing assistants make a difference on the CD in the back of your book.

Death and Dying

Do not go gentle into that good night,
Old age should burn and rave at close of
*   day*
Rage, rage against the dying of the light.

—From Do Not Go Gentle into That Good Night
by Dylan Thomas

In this poem by the Welsh poet Dylan Thomas (1914–1953), the speaker begs his father to fight, rather than accept, death. Although everyone who lives must die, accepting the certainty of our own death, or the death of someone we care about, is rarely easy. In Unit 4, we will look at the final stages of life and the role the nursing assistant plays in providing compassionate care to those who are dying, and their families.

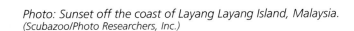

Photo: Sunset off the coast of Layang Layang Island, Malaysia.
(Scubazoo/Photo Researchers, Inc.)

443

21

Caring for People Who Are Terminally Ill

What will you learn?

This chapter focuses on caring for people with a terminal illness (an illness that will end in death). You will learn about the stages of grief a dying person experiences, and the role hospice workers play in caring for a dying person. You will also learn about care considerations for the terminally ill person's family, and the effects of caring for a terminally ill person on the caregiver. When you are finished with this chapter, you will be able to:

1. Define the term *terminal illness* and give examples of specific illnesses that are considered terminal.
2. List the stages of grief and discuss their effects on the terminally ill person.
3. Describe the effects of a terminal illness on the person's family.
4. Define the term *advance directives* and list examples of ways a terminally ill person specifies end-of-life care wishes.
5. Discuss the role of hospice in the care of the terminally ill person.
6. Describe care concerns when providing for the needs of the person with a terminal illness.
7. Explain how caring for terminally ill people can affect the nursing assistant.

Photo: A hospice nurse cares for one of her terminally ill patients.
(Photograph courtesy of Wuesthoff Brevard Hospice & Palliative Care/Brenda Spakes.)

Vocabulary

Use the CD in the back of your book to hear these terms pronounced, defined, and used in a sentence:

Grief	Hope	Patient Self-	No code or do not
Denial	Will	Determination Act of	resuscitate (DNR)
Anger	Advance directive	1990	order
Bargaining	Living will	Supportive care	Palliative care
Depression	Durable power of attor-	Life-sustaining	
Acceptance	ney for health care	treatment	

People die from many different causes and at many different ages. Some people die suddenly of accidents or acute illnesses; others die simply as a result of the natural aging process. Still others die from a terminal illness, an illness or condition for which there is no cure. There are many types of terminal illnesses. Acquired immunodeficiency syndrome (AIDS), as well as certain cancers, heart conditions, chronic respiratory disorders, kidney disorders, and liver disorders are all examples of conditions that can become terminal.

In years past, the person with a terminal illness was cared for in the home, surrounded by family and friends and treated by a family doctor or private-duty nurse. The caregivers focused on making the ill person comfortable and filling his or her last days with love and compassion. As medical technology became more advanced, the emphasis for health care workers slowly shifted from "care" to "cure" (Fig. 21-1). Although the treatments that are available to us through modern medicine are certainly wonderful, we must be careful not to forget the "old-fashioned" aspect of caring for the terminally ill, which focused on allowing the person to live (and to die) with dignity. A primary focus of this book, and of the health care industry today, is holistic care—caring for the whole person by attending to the person's physical, as well as emotional and spiritual, needs. Applying the concept of holistic care is very important when you are caring for people at the end of life's journey.

Some of you will have experienced life events, such as the death of someone close to you, that inspired you to enter the health care industry. However, many of you are entering the nursing assisting profession with little or no exposure to death and the process of grieving. Caring for a terminally ill person can be very rewarding, but it can also be emotionally draining. To become emotionally secure enough to be supportive of a terminally ill person and her family members, you will need to explore your own feelings and emotions regarding death and dying. However, you must also remember that everyone has her own beliefs and ideas about death, and that these beliefs and ideas are just as important and meaningful to that person as yours are to you. (See Chapter 22, "Caring for People Who Are Dying," for a more detailed discussion of beliefs and practices related to death and dying across various religions and cultures.)

When you are caring for people who are dying, you should be aware of the power of listening and touch. In many cases, it is not necessary to say anything at all—your presence will be noticed and will be reassuring for the dying person. Listen to whatever the person needs to say, without imposing your own opinions or beliefs. Remember that this is your patient's or resident's grief, and he or she must work through it on his own terms.

STAGES OF GRIEF

Anyone experiencing any type of loss, be it the loss of health, loss of a marriage, loss of a loved one, or the impending loss of his own life will experience grief. **Grief** is defined as mental anguish, specifically associated with loss. Dr. Elisabeth Kübler-Ross (1926–), a Swiss-born doctor who came to the United States in the 1950s, is the author of a famous book called *On Death and Dying.* Dr. Kübler-Ross, a psychiatrist, chose to work

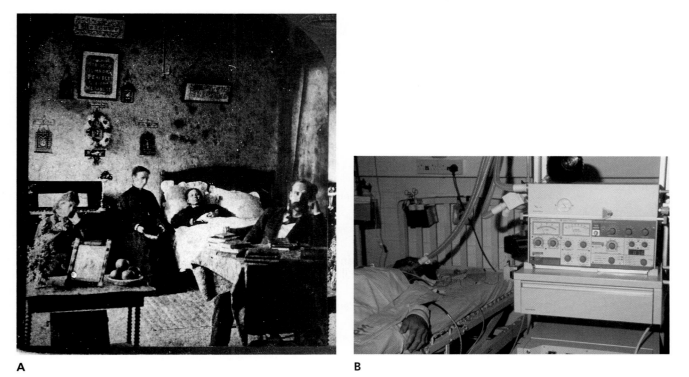

A   **B**

FIGURE 21-1

Providing care to the dying (A) the "old-fashioned" way and (B) the "modern" way. (A © Stanley B. Burns, M.O./The Burns Archive; B © Sue Ford/Photo Researchers, Inc.)

with terminally ill people. During her conversations with her patients, they expressed to her their feelings about what they were going through. These conversations formed the basis for many of the ideas in *On Death and Dying.* One key idea of Dr. Kübler-Ross, outlined in *On Death and Dying,* is the idea that dying people experience distinct stages of grief. Interestingly, these same stages are also seen to some degree in people who are diagnosed with chronic illnesses, especially those illnesses that will greatly affect the person's way of living. For example, a person who has recently been told he has diabetes, heart disease, or hypertension may go through the same stages of grief that a person who has been told he is dying goes through. The stages of grief that Dr. Kübler-Ross identified are denial, anger, bargaining, depression, acceptance, and hope.

Denial, the first stage of grief, occurs when a person is told that he has a terminal illness. The person refuses to accept the diagnosis or feels that a mistake has been made. He may ask for a second opinion, or act as if nothing is wrong and avoid returning to the doctor for a period of time. Denial helps to protect a person emotionally from

overwhelming grief. This stage of grief can last only a few minutes, or it may last until the person actually dies. As a nursing assistant, it is not your place to convince the person that his illness exists, or to argue with the person about treatment or care issues. Instead, recognize that denial is a normal part of the grieving process, respond to the person in an honest yet neutral way, and communicate your observations to the nurse (Table 21-1). Be sure to tell the nurse if the person refuses medication or other medical treatment.

Anger occurs when the person realizes that he is actually going to die. People may feel angry for different reasons, and each person handles anger differently. Some people may be angry with themselves for not seeking help sooner, or for making a lifestyle choice that contributed to the illness, such as smoking. People express anger differently. Some people become moody and withdrawn, or uncooperative and hostile. Others may yell, or throw objects. If the person is religious, he may lose faith. Some people take their anger out on family members. Others may direct their anger toward health care professionals, feeling that the

TABLE 21-1 ■ Stages of Grief

Stage	Sample Dialogue	Appropriate Response from Nursing Assistant
Denial	**Patient:** "They don't know what they're talking about. I can't possibly have an incurable brain tumor." **Nursing assistant:** "I'm sorry; it must have been very hard for you to learn the results of the MRI."	Acknowledges what the person is saying by responding in an honest, yet neutral way
Anger	**Patient:** "If you medical people weren't so incompetent, I wouldn't be so sick!" **Nursing assistant:** "Mr. Smith, you seem so angry."	Acknowledges the person's anger and allows him to talk about it; by practicing empathy, avoids feeling defensive or taking the person's anger personally
Bargaining	**Patient:** "If I could just hang on until my sister arrives..." **Nursing assistant:** "We'll do all we can to help you do that. But until then, I'll be with you."	Offers support that she can realistically provide, and reassures the person that he will be cared for
Depression	**Patient:** "I don't want to die....I'm so sad." **Nursing assistant** (sitting quietly and holding the patient's hand): "I'm here for you."	Offers comfort in the form of touch and silence; does not attempt to "cheer the person up"; if the person is refusing food or not sleeping, could offer to obtain whatever foods appeal to the person's appetite or to talk to the nurse about arranging for medication to aid sleep
Acceptance	**Patient:** "It won't be long until I'm going on to my reward." **Nursing assistant:** "You're going on to your reward?"	Uses communication techniques that encourage the person to talk, such as rephrasing the person's statement as an open-ended question
Hope	**Patient:** "I really think this treatment is helping." **Nursing assistant:** "You must be feeling stronger!"	Acknowledges and nurtures the person's hope without being unrealistic

people they have placed so much trust in have somehow failed them. You must not take the anger personally—doing so can hurt your emotional well-being, as well as your ability to care for the person.

Bargaining is typically done on a very private basis by the terminally ill person. The person wants to "make a deal" with someone he feels has control over his fate, such as God or a health care provider. The person may want to live long enough to accomplish a goal, or to witness a specific event, such as the birth of a child, a wedding, or an anniversary celebration. The will to live can be a very powerful force, and may, in fact, extend the person's life by a few months. As a nursing assistant, it is important for you to allow the terminally ill person to experience the feeling of hope that accompanies this stage of grieving.

Depression is the stage in which the person fully realizes that death will be the end result of the

illness. The person will be sad and may have regrets about things he was not able to accomplish during his lifetime. Some people are quite withdrawn and may say little, while others may want to openly mourn for their loss. Recognize that depression is a normal part of the grieving process, and be supportive. Let the person know that it is all right for him to be feeling the way he is feeling. Tell the nurse if a grieving person's depression causes the person to cry constantly, refuse food, or fail to sleep. Some people will require medical intervention to treat their depression.

Acceptance occurs when a terminally ill person comes to terms with the reality of his own death, and is finally at peace with this knowledge. Typically, people who have reached the acceptance stage will demonstrate their acceptance by completing unfinished business and saying their goodbyes. Many will plan their funeral service or write a poem or letter to be read after they are gone. Often, they will want to talk about their death, in an effort to help family members accept it also. The acceptance stage does not necessarily occur when death is near; some people gain acceptance months or even years prior to their eventual death from the illness.

Terminally ill people may not pass through all the stages of grief, and they may not pass through them in order. Many people work through the first five stages of grief, only to "relapse" and experience some of the earlier stages again. Throughout the grieving process, the one thing that usually persists is **hope**. Even the most realistic and accepting patients hold onto the hope that a new drug will be developed, or that a new research project will yield a cure. Hope is what helps a terminally ill person face another day or another painful treatment. It is what drives the person to keep up with normal activities, such as eating and praying, when she might otherwise feel like giving up entirely. As a nursing assistant, you must be responsive to, and nurture, a patient's hope, without being unrealistic.

One factor that influences how a person handles the grieving process is where the person is in his or her life in terms of responsibilities, commitments, accomplishments, hopes, and dreams. For example, a mother with young children will have different concerns than a grandmother whose children are grown and independent. A terminally ill person who is able to view her life with a feeling of satisfaction may act very differently from a person who has regrets about choices made, opportunities lost, or goals unmet. A child will handle a terminal illness very differently from an adult (often, children reach the acceptance stage faster than adults). It is important for you to recognize the stages of grief and understand that, although these stages have been identified, each person will experience them, and react to them, differently. Being able to recognize the stages of grief will enable you to provide better care to your patients or residents, because you will have a better understanding of what they are going through. This understanding will help you to be more effective in determining what your patients or residents need from you.

The family and loved ones of a terminally ill person will also go through the stages of grief as they prepare for their loss. Remembering this will help you to understand behavior that may not seem fair or appropriate. For example, a family member of a terminally ill person may direct her anger at you, but the family member is not necessarily angry with you—she is angry that

she is losing someone she loves. Like the dying person, the family members will each pass through the stages of grief individually and at their own order and pace. Sometimes there is emotional upset within a family when the members of the family (including the patient) are at different stages of the grieving process. Reporting your observations of this turmoil to the nurse will be helpful. Arranging for the assistance of clergy or other professionals experienced in grief counseling may be of great comfort to the patient and the family (Fig. 21-2).

▶ *Tell the Nurse!*

When caring for a terminally ill person, pay attention to the person's emotional well-being, as well as his or her physical well-being. Report any of the following observations to the nurse immediately:

⟶ The person refuses medications, or other medical treatment

⟶ The person cries constantly, refuses food, or cannot sleep

⟶ There is tension and disagreement within the family

⟶ The person or a family member requests the assistance of clergy or a grief counselor

⟶ The person expresses interest in having a will made

WILLS

A **will** is a legal statement that expresses a person's wishes for the management of his or her affairs after death (Fig. 21-3). For a will to be valid, the person must be deemed competent, or "of sound mind," at the time the will is made. If a patient or resident expresses a desire to make a will, you should relay this information to the nurse so that arrangements can be made for the person to talk with a lawyer. As a nursing assistant, you may be asked to sign a will as a witness. When you sign as a witness, your signature means that you saw the person sign the document and that, to the best of your knowledge, the document accurately expresses that person's wishes. You

FIGURE 21-2

Grief counseling may be a comfort to the patient and the family. (*Mark Gibson.*)

should never sign a will as a witness if you have been named as a benefactor of the will. A benefactor is a person who will receive money or other items belonging to the person who has died when the will is read.

DYING WITH DIGNITY

ADVANCE DIRECTIVES

All people have the right to die in a way that is as peaceful and dignified as possible. For many people, this means choosing to avoid "heroic measures" that will prolong life, if by taking these heroic measures, their quality of life will be compromised. Many people make their wishes known through advance directives. An **advance directive** is a document that allows a person to make his wishes regarding health care known to family members and health care workers, in case the

time comes when he is no longer able to make those wishes known himself. Examples of advance directives include living wills and durable powers of attorney for health care. A **living will** requests that death not be artificially postponed. A **durable power of attorney for health care** transfers the responsibility for handling a person's affairs and making medical decisions to a family member, friend, or other trusted individual, in the event that the person is no longer able to make these decisions on his or her own behalf. Many people, not just the terminally ill, arrange for living wills, durable powers of attorney, or both as a way of ensuring that their wishes regarding their own health care are known and honored.

The **Patient Self-Determination Act of 1990** was passed to ensure that the wishes patients and their family members have regarding measures to be taken on their own behalf (or on the behalf of their loved one) are followed. This act requires health care facilities and providers to educate

LF235-04
R235-04

LAST WILL AND TESTAMENT

BE IT KNOWN that I, _____, a resident of _____, County of _____, in the State of _____, being of sound mind, do make and declare this to be my Last Will and Testament expressly revoking all my prior Wills and Codicils at any time made.

I.   **PERSONAL REPRESENTATIVE:**

I appoint _____ of _____, as Personal Representative of this my Last Will and Testament and provide that if this Personal Representative is unable or unwilling to serve then I appoint _____ of _____, as alternate Personal Representative. My Personal Representative shall be authorized to carry out all provisions of this Will and pay my just debts, obligations and funeral expenses. I further provide my Personal Representative shall not be required to post surety bond in this or any other jurisdiction, and direct that no expert appraisal be made of my estate unless required by law.

II.   **GUARDIAN:**

In the event I shall die as the sole parent of minor children, then I appoint _____ as Guardian of said minor children. If this named Guardian is unable or unwilling to serve, then I appoint _____ as alternate Guardian.

III.   **BEQUESTS:**

I direct that after payment of all my just debts, my property be bequeathed in the manner following:

_____ Testator's Initials

Page ____ of ____ pages

Execute and attest before a notary.
Caution: Louisiana residents should consult an attorney before preparing a will.

IN WITNESS WHEREOF, I have hereunto set my hand this ____ day of ____ (year), to this my Last Will and Testament.

_____
Testator Signature

IV.   **WITNESSED:**

The testator has signed this will at the end and on each other separate page, and has declared or signified in our presence that it is his/her last will and testament, and in the presence of the testator and each other we have hereunto subscribed our names this ____ day of ____, 20 ___.

_____   _____
Witness Signature   Address

_____   _____
Witness Signature   Address

_____   _____
Witness Signature   Address

ACKNOWLEDGMENT

State of _____ }
County of _____

We, _____, _____,
_____, and _____,
the testator and the witnesses, respectively, whose names are signed to the attached and foregoing instrument, were sworn and declared to the undersigned that the testator signed the instrument as his/her Last Will and that each of the witnesses, in the presence of the testator and each other, signed the will as a witness.

Testator: _____   Witness _____

Witness _____

Witness _____

On _____ before me, _____, appeared _____ personally known to me (or proved to me on the basis of satisfactory evidence) to be the person(s) whose name(s) is/are subscribed to the within instrument and acknowledged to me that he/she/they executed the same in his/her/their authorized capacity(ies), and that by his/her/their signature(s) on the instrument the person(s), or the entity upon behalf of which the person(s) acted, executed the instrument.
WITNESS my hand and official seal.

Signature _____
Signature of Notary

Affiant ____Known ____Produced ID
Type of ID _____
(Seal)

Page ____ of ____ pages

FIGURE 21-3

Writing a will is as simple as obtaining a form from an office supply store, completing it, and having it notarized.

patients about advance directives, and to offer them the opportunity to establish either a living will or a durable power of attorney, or both. It is particularly important for terminally ill people, who not only have knowledge of their own imminent death, but in many cases have conditions that will cause their suffering to increase as time goes on, to have the opportunity to make their wishes regarding supportive care and life-sustaining treatment known.

Supportive care is offering treatments that will not prolong life, but will make a person more comfortable, such as oxygen therapy, nutritional supplementation, pain medication, range-of-motion exercises, grooming and hygiene, and positioning assistance. (Supportive care is discussed in detail in Chapter 22.) Examples of **life-sustaining treatments,** which tend to be more aggressive, include respiratory ventilation, cardiopulmonary resuscitation (CPR), and the placement of a feeding tube or intravenous (IV) line for the provision of nutrition. A terminally ill person who has made the decision to receive only supportive care at the end of her life will have a **no-code** or **do not resuscitate (DNR) order** written on her chart. This means that the usual efforts to save the person's life will not be made. The entire health care team should be aware of this order so that the person will be allowed to pass on with the compassion and dignity she has requested.

HOSPICE CARE

Hospice agencies and facilities are organizations that have the mission of offering the terminally ill person the best quality of life possible, and ensuring his or her comfort and dignity as death approaches. Hospice care is provided by a multidisciplinary team (made up of nurses, nursing assistants, clergy, social workers, doctors, mental health providers, and other professionals). The team seeks to meet the terminally ill person's, and his or her family members', physical, emotional, and spiritual needs. After the person's death, hospice provides grief counseling and other types of assistance for the family. Hospice care is available to patients and families 24 hours a day, 7 days a week, and can be provided to a terminally ill person in his or her home, a long-term care facility, or the hospital. In addition, there are a few special facilities that specialize in providing hospice care. People become eligible for hospice care when their doctors tell them they have approximately 6 months left to live.

The first hospice program, St. Christopher's Hospice in London, was opened in 1974 to provide supportive care and palliative care to terminally ill people. **Palliative care** focuses on relieving uncomfortable symptoms, not on curing the problem that is causing the symptoms (Fig. 21-4). Examples of palliative treatments include the administration of medications to control pain, the use of chemotherapy or radiation to shrink a tumor (thereby making a person more comfortable), and the use of oxygen therapy to help keep a person with breathing problems comfortable. Surgical procedures can also be of a palliative nature. For example, surgery to remove a tumor that is blocking the intestines may be done primarily to increase the person's comfort, not to cure the cancer. Although hospice care focuses on pain and symptom control and not curative measures, it in no way asks that a terminally ill person give up hope for recovery or a cure from his or her illness.

In addition to providing palliative and supportive care, hospice organizations can assist with having special equipment (such as a hospital bed or bedside commode) brought into a person's home. This special equipment often makes it easier for family members and other caregivers to meet the person's physical needs. The primary focus of the hospice team's efforts is to honor the wishes of the terminally ill person and the family. If a person wishes to die at home or at the hospital, the hospice organization will make every effort to honor these wishes. A terminally ill person can take much comfort in knowing that his or her wishes for a dignified and peaceful death will be honored and that hospice is there to offer support and comfort to the family.

EFFECTS OF CARING FOR THE TERMINALLY ILL ON THE CAREGIVER

Caring for a terminally ill person will affect you. As we work with patients and residents, we become part of their lives and they become part of ours. When one of our patients or residents is diagnosed with a terminal illness, we go through a grief process very similar to that experienced by the person and the family. Additionally, because members of the health care profession feel a great need to be able to help others, we often feel inadequate when we must watch others suffer and grieve, and there is little we can do to relieve their pain. We may even question our professional calling. Regardless of how long you work in the medical profession, terminal illness and death will impact you emotionally.

Taking time for yourself is very important. Doing this will help you to keep your feelings and emotions in perspective and it will allow you to continue to give of yourself to others. Talking to your supervisor, a clergy member, or a mental health counselor about questions and fears you have about death can help you to clarify your feelings about death and dying (Fig. 21-5). In addition, you might find seeking advice from an "expert" helpful when you are trying to work

FIGURE 21-4

Hospice organizations can provide palliative care. Here, a nurse applies a skin patch used for pain control to the chest of a patient with cancer. (© *Samuel Ashfield/Photo Researchers, Inc.*)

FIGURE 21-5

Clarifying your beliefs and confronting your fears about death and dying can help you to care for your patients and residents more effectively.

through feelings concerning a specific situation with a patient or resident.

SUMMARY

▶ As health care providers, we must strive to meet not only the physical needs, but also the spiritual and emotional needs, of the terminally ill people who trust us to care for them.

▶ Caring for people with a terminal illness requires an understanding of the ways in which people grieve.

  ■ Dr. Elisabeth Kübler-Ross, a noted authority on death and dying, has identified six stages of grief that a person who is dying from a terminal illness experiences: denial, anger, bargaining, depression, acceptance, and hope.

  ■ Having an understanding of these stages and what the person is feeling during each one enables us to be more compassionate and understanding toward both the person and the family.

▶ Advance directives and hospice care seek to preserve the terminally ill patient's right to die in as peaceful and dignified a manner as possible.

▶ Caring for a terminally ill person and his or her family members can be very rewarding. It can also be very difficult, emotionally.

  ■ Exploring your own feelings about death (with the help of a professional, if necessary) can help to prepare you for the loss of a patient or resident.

  ■ When caring for a terminally ill person, recognize that you will also go through the grieving process as part of caring for the person, and make allowance for this.

What did you learn?

Multiple Choice

Select the single best answer for each of the following questions.

1. Denial is:
   a. The stage of the grieving process in which the person becomes very depressed
   b. A form of bargaining with God for more time
   c. The final step of the grieving process
   d. The time during the grieving process when the person believes the diagnosis is incorrect

2. An agency that cares only for people who are dying is a:
   a. Skilled facility
   b. Sub-acute-care unit
   c. Long-term care facility
   d. Hospice organization

3. The stage of grief when a person begins to say goodbye and make arrangements for his or her death would be the:
   a. Bargaining stage
   b. Anger stage
   c. Denial stage
   d. Acceptance stage

4. Hospice care is designed to:
   a. Keep the person comfortable
   b. Prolong the person's life
   c. Treat the person aggressively
   d. All of the above

5. A patient with terminal cancer says he plans to live long enough to walk his daughter, who is getting married, down the aisle. This is an example of:
   a. Acceptance
   b. Depression
   c. Bargaining
   d. Denial

6. A legal document that expresses a person's wishes for the management of his or her affairs after death is a/an:
   a. Advance directive
   b. Living will
   c. Durable power of attorney
   d. Will

True or False?

Indicate whether each statement is "true" (T) or "false" (F).

1. Terminal illness is an illness or injury from which the person is not likely to recover.
   T or F ?

2. Family members move through the same emotional stages of dying as the patient or resident.
   T or F ?

3. During the grieving process, the patient or resident may become angry with the nursing assistant.
   T or F ?

> **?** **Stop and think!**
>
> ▶ Mrs. Brown has a history of depression, and years ago, she attempted suicide. Mrs. Brown's husband has been told that his wife has terminal cancer. He does not want her to know her diagnosis, because he thinks she will become depressed and attempt suicide again. When you are giving Mrs. Brown a bed bath, she asks you if she is dying. How would you respond?

22

Caring for People Who Are Dying

What will you learn?

Each person is born to one possession which outvalues all the others—his last breath.
—*Mark Twain*

Most of us give little, if any, thought to what our "last breath" will be like. Sure, we read death notices in the newspaper and hear stories on the evening news about murders and fatal accidents, but do we ever really think about what the person who died experienced during her last moments alive? Was the person in pain, was she lonely, did someone hold her hand, was someone there to hear the person's last words? In the quote above, the American writer Mark Twain (1835–1910) suggests that the very end of life is an important life experience, just like all of the experiences leading up to that moment. As a nursing assistant, you will certainly find yourself in the position of caring for a patient or resident who is dying. In this chapter, you will learn how you can help the dying person, and his or her family, in the time leading up to the person's "last breath," so that when the time comes, it is as peaceful as possible. You will also learn how to care for a person's body after death occurs. When you are finished with this chapter, you will be able to:

1. Discuss how a nursing assistant's own feelings about death can affect the care given to a dying patient or resident.
2. Describe the physical signs that frequently signal impending death.
3. Describe ways in which the nursing assistant can provide comfort for the dying person.

(continued)

Photo: Sometimes, a simple gesture like holding someone's hand is the best thing you can do.

4. Discuss how cultural and religious influences can affect how the dying person views death.
5. Describe the different ways in which family members may show grief.
6. Describe ways that a nursing assistant can help the family of a dying person.
7. Discuss the various responsibilities that a nursing assistant may have following the death of a patient or resident.

Vocabulary

Use the CD in the back of your book to hear these terms pronounced, defined, and used in a sentence:

Cyanotic
Cheyne-Stokes
  respiration
Afterlife
Reincarnation

Postmortem care
Rigor mortis
Autopsy
Shroud

As you learned in Chapter 12, biological death occurs when all vital body functions stop. Usually, we consider a person "dead" when the heart stops beating and cannot be started again. However, a doctor can also declare a person dead when there has been a permanent loss of brain function. In order to be declared "brain dead," a person must show no brain activity for a period of time specified by the law (usually 24 hours or more). Brain activity is monitored using sophisticated equipment, and several examinations are performed before the person is declared dead.

Many people die suddenly. However, often there is some warning of approaching death. As death draws near, a person may show certain characteristic physical signs, caused as the body begins to "shut down." These signs may appear over the course of a few hours or a few days, or within the space of a few minutes. Some people may not show these signs. However, recognizing these physical signs and understanding why they occur will help you to know what type of care to offer the dying person. Family members may also notice these signs, and become concerned. In this case, you will need to reassure them that these signs are normal signs of dying. (Any specific questions regarding the person's condition should be directed to the

nurse.) Physical signs of impending death include the following:

- As circulation fails, the blood pressure drops and the pulse becomes rapid and weak. The skin feels cool and clammy, even though the body temperature is rising. The person may perspire heavily and the skin may appear mottled (blotchy), very pale, **cyanotic** (blue-tinged), or grayish. Although you may be tempted to cover the person warmly, he or she will need only light bed coverings.
- The respiratory pattern changes. The person may take very irregular, shallow breaths, in an alternating fast–slow pattern. This pattern of breathing is called **Cheyne-Stokes respiration.** As the person weakens, fluid or mucus may collect in the air passages, causing the noisy, rattling breathing that is often known as the "death rattle."
- The digestive system slows down. The person may experience nausea, vomiting, abdominal swelling, fecal impaction, or bowel incontinence. The person may not want food or water. Offering ice chips and providing frequent oral hygiene helps to keep the mouth moist.
- Urine output decreases as the kidneys respond to the lack of blood flow. In addition, the person may become incontinent of urine.
- Nervous system changes result in decreased muscle tone and sensation. The muscles relax and the person may be too weak to reposition himself. Some people lose the ability to speak. The person may lose sensation in his arms or legs, and pain may diminish. Vision may become blurred. (You may notice that the person will turn toward a light in an effort to see better.) Hearing, however, usually remains normal until the moment of death.

- Consciousness may be altered. Some dying people lose consciousness and become comatose as death approaches. As consciousness diminishes, pain usually does too. Some people remain conscious and oriented until the moment of death. It is not uncommon for a person who has drifted into and out of a semi-comatose state to become perfectly alert and oriented right before he or she dies.

When you are caring for a person who is dying, take note of any physical changes that you observe. Report these changes to the nurse and record them in the person's medical chart, per facility policy.

CARING FOR A DYING PERSON

A holistic approach to care is taken with a dying person, just as with any other person (Fig. 22-1). Dying people, like everyone else, have physical and emotional needs. These needs may change dramatically as the time of death approaches, and will vary greatly depending on the person. Every person has the right to die peacefully and with dignity (Box 22-1). As a nursing assistant, it is your job to do everything you can to ensure that this right is honored.

Many nursing assistants (especially new nursing assistants) compromise the care they give to a dying patient or resident, without being fully aware that they are doing so. For example, a nursing assistant might not check in on the dying person as often as he checks in on his other patients or residents. He might provide only the necessary care and then leave the person's room quickly, because he is afraid that if he stays, the person will want to talk about death. Or he may be overly cheerful around the person. These avoidance behaviors usually occur because the nursing assistant has not yet explored his own feelings about death. Many people who are new to the health care profession express concerns such

FIGURE 22-1

The nursing assistant provides for the dying person's physical and emotional comfort. Examples of physical comfort measures include providing frequent oral hygiene and back massages. Examples of emotional comfort measures include caring for the family, helping the person to meet spiritual needs (for example, by reading aloud from a book that has special meaning for the person), and simply spending quiet time with the person.

BOX 22-1 The Dying Person's Bill of Rights

I have the right to be treated as a living human being until I die.

I have the right to maintain a sense of hopefulness, however changing its focus may be.

I have the right to be cared for by those who can maintain a sense of hopefulness, however changing this might be.

I have the right to express my feelings and emotions about my approaching death in my own way.

I have the right to participate in decisions concerning my care.

I have the right to expect continuing medical and nursing attention even though "cure" goals must be changed to "comfort" goals.

I have the right not to die alone.

I have the right to be free from pain.

I have the right to have my questions answered honestly.

I have the right not to be deceived.

I have the right to have help from and for my family in accepting my death.

I have the right to die in peace and dignity.

I have a right to retain my individuality and not be judged for my decisions, which may be contrary to beliefs of others.

I have the right to discuss and enlarge my religious and/or spiritual experiences, whatever these may mean to others.

I have the right to expect that the sanctity of the human body will be respected after death.

I have the right to be cared for by caring, sensitive, knowledgeable people who will attempt to understand my needs and will be able to gain some satisfaction in helping me face my death.

(Created at the workshop *The Terminally Ill Patient and the Helping Person*, in Lansing, Michigan, sponsored by the Southwestern Michigan Inservice Education Council and conducted by Amelia J. Barbus, Associate Professor of Nursing, Wayne State University, Detroit.)

as, "I'm afraid I'll cry if my resident dies," "I don't want to get too attached," or "I've never touched a dead person before and I'm scared." All of these are normal fears that new nursing assistants have. As noted in Chapter 21, talking to your supervisor, a clergy member, or a mental health counselor can help you to come to terms with your own feelings and beliefs about death. This knowledge of your own feelings will serve you well as you care for others who are dying.

Facing the death of a patient or resident never gets any easier. You will become very attached to your patients or residents. Although the relationship you have with your patient or resident can make providing end-of-life care very emotionally difficult for you, it is this relationship that will allow you to provide the holistic care that the dying person needs so much.

MEETING THE DYING PERSON'S PHYSICAL NEEDS

A dying person becomes more and more dependent on others for basic physical care as the time of death approaches. As the focus of care becomes comfort, the nursing assistant has an excellent chance to help the person feel that he is not alone in this last stage of life. Basic aspects of physical care for the dying person include the following:

- **Care of the skin.** More frequent skin care and linen changes are needed because of the urinary or bowel incontinence and the moist skin that often occur as the person nears death. The person will need to be checked regularly for incontinence of both urine and feces. His skin will need to be cleaned gently, and soiled clothing and linens must be changed. Bed protectors or indwelling urinary catheters may be needed to assist with incontinence problems.

- **Care of the mucous membranes.** Frequent mouth care helps keep the mouth moist and more comfortable, especially if the person is comatose or not taking food or drink. Sometimes as death nears, the person does not blink as often, and a mucus crust may form around the eyelids. Gentle cleaning with a warm, wet washcloth helps to remove the dried mucus. The nurse may apply an ointment to keep the eyes moist. If the person is comatose, moist eye pads may be used for protection. Medical equipment, such as oxygen cannulas and nasogastric tubes, may cause irritation and crusting of mucus around the nostrils. Gently removing the mucus crust with a warm, wet washcloth and applying a lubricant can help to keep the person comfortable.

- **Positioning.** As the person's condition worsens, she may not be able to reposition herself without assistance. Frequent, regular position changes help to prevent pressure ulcers and promote comfort. The use of pillows or other positioning devices helps to maintain the body in proper alignment. If the person is in pain, you will need to be extra gentle and slow with position changes. Always notify the nurse of your observations of pain so that necessary medications can be administered. A person who is having difficulty breathing will probably be more comfortable positioned with her head elevated.

- **Other comfort measures.** Receiving a back massage, listening to soft music, or being read to are all activities that can help a person to rest and feel better. Enemas may be necessary to assist with bowel elimination. Secretions may collect in the person's airways, making breathing difficult. If you notice that a person is having difficulty breathing, report this to the nurse. The nurse will be able to provide suctioning and oxygen therapy, measures that can make breathing easier and more comfortable for the person. Keep the room well lit and ventilated. Remove soiled linens, bedpans, or emesis basins and use air freshener to help eliminate unpleasant odors.

As death nears, there may be changes in the dying person's ability to communicate with others. Therefore, when caring for a dying person, you must be very observant of the person's physical needs. As the person's ability to communicate pain, thirst, or other physical needs decreases, he will rely more and more on the nursing team to notice those needs and take care of them. In addition, you must take measures to make communication easier:

- Remember that as death approaches, the person's vision may become blurry. Keep the room well lit to help the person to see better. Also, make sure you introduce yourself when entering the room and encourage family members to do the same. Imagine how you would feel if you could no longer see well, and you could not tell who was entering and leaving your room!

- Speaking may become difficult for the person. In this case, asking simple "yes or no" questions will make communication more effective.

- Hearing usually remains quite sharp up until the time of death, even if the person is comatose. Always talk to the person as if he is able to hear you, even if he cannot respond. Explain procedures to the person and offer reassurance that you are there and will return soon when you leave the room. Gently remind family members that the person may still be able to hear their conversations, and encourage them to talk to the person. Hearing the voices of family members can be comforting for the dying person. However, family members should be advised that potentially upsetting topics should be discussed elsewhere, out of earshot of the dying person.

A person's family members may wish to assist in providing physical care. If a family member says that she would like to be involved in caring for the dying person, encourage this by suggesting ways that the family member can help. For example, you might ask the family member if she would be willing to help you out by giving the person ice chips, and then show the family member how to do this (Fig. 22-2). Family members often feel

FIGURE 22-2

Sometimes, family members want to assist in meeting a dying person's physical needs. Here, a nursing assistant is showing a family member how to ease the person's thirst by giving ice chips.

FIGURE 22-3

Many people have fears related to death, such as a fear of dying alone or of dying in pain. As a nursing assistant, you can help to relieve some of these fears.

FIGURE 22-4

A nursing assistant helps to meet a dying person's emotional needs by being a good listener. Although you may think that the dying person is the one who benefits the most from these times spent together, quite frequently you will find that you benefit too. These moments spent listening can help you to understand yourself better, as well as your patients or residents.

useless or helpless when it becomes clear that there is nothing left to do except wait for death to arrive. Participating in the care of a dying loved one can help a family member to feel better about the situation.

MEETING THE DYING PERSON'S EMOTIONAL NEEDS

Emotionally, people prepare for death very individually. People may have many fears regarding death, such as a fear of the unknown or a fear of losing dignity and self-control. Some may fear that death will be painful, or worry about the effects of their death on the people left behind. Some people have concerns about unfinished business. Another concern that many dying people have is a fear of facing death alone (Fig. 22-3). Some people are able to speak of their fears, while others remain silent, afraid to even speak of what frightens them the most.

A nursing assistant can help meet a dying person's emotional needs by being a good listener (Fig. 22-4). A dying person may want to talk about her fears related to dying, or what she expects the afterlife to be like. Or, the person might just want to remember significant events in her life, and share those memories with you now. If you sense that a person wants to talk, use the communication techniques you learned in Chapter 5 to encourage her and let her know that you are there to listen. Even though you may be uncomfortable at

first when a patient or resident brings up the subject of death, do not change the subject, make yourself "busy," or simply pat the person on the hand and say, "Oh, don't worry, honey; you've got lots of time left." Many dying people are very well aware of their situation and they may tell you that their time here is very short. Do not avoid spending time with a dying person because you are afraid that the person will bring up a subject and you will not know what to say in response. You do not need to say anything—you just need to listen to what the person wants to tell you.

Other dying people do not want to talk and can become annoyed at your attempts to make small talk. Use your observation skills to note when a person would prefer not to talk. Although the person may not want to have a conversation, she will still want to know that you are nearby and watching out for her. Check on the person frequently and regularly and remind her that you are close by if she needs anything. Many dying people genuinely appreciate it when someone takes the time to sit near them quietly. Touch can convey so much more than words can in a situation like this. Gently hold the person's hand or touch her shoulder when you are speaking to her. Gently smooth the person's hair after you have finished straightening the bed linens or repositioning the pillow, or comfort the person with a back massage. All of these actions let a person know that she is cared for and not alone.

As you learned in Chapter 6, a person's culture and religion often influence how the person responds to illness and other life experiences, including death. Cultural and religious beliefs influence how a person feels about death and prepares for it. For example, some people may not feel comfortable talking about dying, because in their culture, death is considered a very private matter. On the other hand, some people may seem very accepting of death, because their culture or religion has taught them that death is not to be feared.

Many dying people find peace and comfort in their religious faith. They may wish to visit with clergy members, surround themselves with religious items, or spend time alone in prayer, meditation, and reading of religious scriptures. Some people may ask you to read to them. Although you may not share the person's religious beliefs, you should honor this request. For the dying person, hearing familiar words that reflect his or her deepest beliefs can bring great comfort. You must respect the beliefs of other people, even if you do not share these beliefs. Remember that your patient's or resident's faith is just as precious to her as yours is to you.

A dying person may request that you call a clergy member to administer religious blessings or "last rites." If such a request is made, report it immediately to the nurse so that the necessary arrangements can be made. When the clergy member arrives, make sure that there is a place for him or her to sit, and ensure privacy. As part of preparing for death, people often want to confess to a clergy member, and they will want privacy to do this.

Religion is but one aspect of spirituality and many people are very spiritual without belonging to any particular religious group. Most people who are "spiritual" believe that a higher being or spirit offers hope and peace, although this higher being may not necessarily be one that is recognized by the world's various religions. Spirituality gives a person inner strength to face life's challenges. It gives meaning to a person's life. Many people exhibit their inner spirituality by listening to music, reading poetry, or just watching a sunset.

When cultural and religious or spiritual beliefs provide an explanation for what happens to a person after death, they can be a source of comfort for the dying person (as well as for the person's family members). For example, many people believe in an **afterlife,** a state of being where the dead meet again with loved ones who have passed on before them. Other people believe in **reincarnation,** the idea that a person's spirit or soul will live again on Earth in the form of an animal or human being yet to be born.

CARE OF THE FAMILY

Knowing that a loved one will die soon can be very difficult for family members. Family members must cope with their own grief, and possibly that of other family members as well. Remember that the stress and grief experienced by family members can cause them to act in ways that may seem strange to you. For example, some people may treat you rudely, or snap at you in anger. Be polite and do not take offensive actions or words personally. Usually, these offensive behaviors are just a result of the person's grief. If a family member seems to be getting overly agitated or angry, or if arguing or aggression between family members occurs, notify the nurse immediately.

As a nursing assistant, you may feel overwhelmed at the thought of caring for the family as well as for the patient or resident. However, there are many simple things you can do to comfort the family (Fig. 22-5).

- **Ensure good communication between the family members and the health care**

FIGURE 22-5

Family members will often seek reassurance and comfort from the nursing staff. As a nursing assistant, there are many simple kindnesses you can extend to the family that will help make this ordeal easier for them. Here, a nursing assistant has brought in an extra chair for a family member who has just arrived at the bedside.

team. Often, family members will have worries or fears related to the person's care or condition, and they may want to discuss these with you or another member of the health care team. If a family member asks you a question that you do not know the answer to or are not qualified to answer, make sure to relay this request for information to the nurse so that the family member's concerns can be addressed.

- **Allow family members to stay with the dying person, and to participate in the person's care if they want to.** When a person is dying, many families wish to remain close by. Visiting hours are usually relaxed, allowing family members to stay with the dying person for as long as they like. Encourage family members to talk to the dying person and to help with the person's care. However, do not push family members to do this if they seem hesitant. Although you have responsibilities to the family, your first responsibility is to your patient or resident. When providing physical care to the dying person, please ask the family members to step outside for a moment (unless they have chosen to help you) and close the curtains to help maintain the person's dignity. Also, too many visitors for too long a period of time can be tiring for some patients or residents. If you suspect that the number of visitors or the length of time that they are staying is causing your patient or resident to become overly tired, please report your observations to the nurse.

- **Ensure that the family members' basic needs are met.** Make sure that there are enough chairs in the room, so that everyone can sit down. Encourage family members to rest and take meals as necessary. Show them how to find the restrooms, public telephones, vending machines, and cafeteria. If a family member is showing signs of weariness, offer to stay at the dying person's side while the family member takes a short walk outside or down the hall to grab a cup of coffee.

- **Be readily available to provide needed care to the patient or resident without being intrusive of the family's privacy.** Often, the most comforting thing to family members is knowing that their loved one is receiving competent, compassionate care.

POSTMORTEM CARE

If you are present when one of your patients or residents dies, you must notify the nurse that the person has died, and note the time. You may need to document the absence of vital signs. A doctor must be called to legally pronounce the person dead. The time of death is recorded on the person's death certificate. After the doctor has pronounced the person dead, you may be required to assist the nurse in giving postmortem care, depending on the policy at the facility or agency where you work.

Postmortem care is the care of a person's body after the person's death. Cultural and religious beliefs often dictate how the body is to be cared for after death (and by whom). In some cultures, family members help to clean and prepare the body for whatever lies ahead, in accordance with cultural and religious traditions.

Postmortem care is necessary to keep the body in proper alignment and to prevent skin damage and discoloration. The skin is cleaned of any mucus, urine, feces, or other fluids. Standard precautions are followed when performing postmortem care, because bodily fluids are still potentially infectious, even after death. The body is placed in proper alignment before rigor mortis occurs. **Rigor mortis** is the stiffening of the muscles that usually develops within 2 to 4 hours of death. Once rigor mortis occurs, it is difficult to reposition the body. It is not uncommon for air that has been trapped in the lungs or the digestive tract to be released from the body when the body is repositioned as part of postmortem care. It may sound like the person has sighed or moaned. This natural occurrence may frighten you, unless you are aware of its cause.

In some cases, an autopsy may be required to confirm or identify the cause of the person's death. An **autopsy** is an examination of the person's organs and tissues after the person has died. In most cases, the doctor is responsible for obtaining a family member's permission to perform an autopsy. If an autopsy is to be performed, medical devices such as tubes, drains, catheters, and intravenous (IV) lines are not

FIGURE 22-6

The body is placed in the supine position for viewing by the family. A pillow is placed under the person's head and shoulders.

FIGURE 22-7

A shroud may be placed on the body after the family has left and before the body is taken to the morgue or funeral home. (*A*) The shroud is unfolded on the bed, and the body is placed on the shroud. (*B*) The top of the shroud is brought over the person's head. (*C*) The bottom of the shroud is brought over the person's feet. (*D*) The sides of the shroud are folded over the person's body and pinned, taped, or tied together. An identification tag is secured to the outside of the shroud.

removed as part of postmortem care. If an autopsy is not necessary, the nurse will usually remove these medical devices as part of the postmortem care procedure.

Many facilities only prepare the person's body for the family to view before sending it to the morgue or funeral home, where the funeral director completes the postmortem care procedure. In this case, the bed linens are straightened (or changed, if they are soiled). The body is cleaned, dressed in a clean gown or pajamas, and positioned in a natural position on the bed (Fig. 22-6). Draw the top sheet up to the person's shoulders and cuff it neatly. (Do not cover the person's face with the sheet. This can be very disturbing for family members.) Make sure that the room is neat, and adjust the lights so that they are not too bright. As always, provide for privacy. You will need to help collect the person's personal belongings to be sent with the family. Dentures are either placed in the person's mouth, or labeled and sent with the body to the funeral home.

After the family has viewed the body and left, the body may be wrapped in a **shroud** ("body bag") for transport to the morgue or funeral home (Fig. 22-7). A shroud is contained in the preassembled postmortem kits used by many facilities (Fig. 22-8). The postmortem kit also usually contains safety pins or tape for securing the shroud, ties for holding the person's hands together, identification tags, a chin strap for securing the person's jaw, a plastic bag or envelope for the person's belongings, and 12″ × 12″ gauze pads to absorb drainage. The procedure for postmortem care is given in Procedure 22-1. You

show your respect for the person and the person's family by working quietly and preserving the person's privacy, even after death.

Providing postmortem care can be emotionally difficult. Health care workers often become very attached to their patients or residents and grieve when they die. It is not uncommon to feel frustrated at death when the focus of health care seems to be mostly on curing disease. It is

Tags

Plastic bag (for personal belongings)

Gauze pads

Safety pins

Ties

Shroud

Chin strap

FIGURE 22-8

The contents of the postmortem kit vary, but most contain a shroud, something for securing the shroud, ties, gauze pads, a chin strap, identification tags, and a plastic bag or envelope for the person's belongings.

perfectly acceptable to feel sad and cry at the passing of a patient or resident. You might be surprised to know that even the most experienced health care workers often seek a "shoulder to cry on." Talking about your feelings with a coworker, supervisor, clergy member, or counselor can help you work through your own grief. Allow yourself to be a human being and to feel emotions. It might also help to think of providing postmortem care as a way of paying your last respects to the dead person. In this way, the ritual of providing this care becomes a way of coping with your grief.

SUMMARY

▶ Providing holistic care is as important at the end of life as it is at any other time. Nursing assistants must take steps to prevent their own discomfort with the subject of death from compromising their ability to care for dying people.

- A dying person becomes very dependent on others for basic physical care. Recognizing the physical signs of impending death helps the nursing assistant to provide the necessary care.

- A dying person will need assistance to meet emotional and spiritual needs as well.
  - Emotionally, people prepare for death in their own individual ways. Cultural and religious beliefs and traditions greatly influence a person's response to illness and death.
  - Often, the best thing a nursing assistant can do is listen if the person wants to talk, or spend quiet time with the person if he or she does not want to talk.

▶ Family members of a dying person require support as well.

- Being respectful, thoughtful, and kind can do much to make family members feel better.

- Some family members react poorly to grief and stress and may take out their frustrations on nursing assistants or other members of the health care team.

▶ Postmortem care is done to prepare the body for the morgue or funeral home. In some facilities, the body is prepared for immediate viewing by the family, and then postmortem care is done at the morgue or funeral home.

Chapter 22 Procedure

Getting Ready Steps

a. **W**ash your hands and observe standard precautions as necessary.

b. **G**ather needed supplies.

c. **K**nock and introduce yourself.

d. **I**dentify the person, and greet him or her by name.

e. **E**xplain the procedure.

f. **P**rovide privacy.

g. **S**ee to safety.

Finishing Up Steps

a. **C**reate comfort and good body alignment.

b. **L**eave the call light control within easy reach.

c. **S**ee to safety.

d. **O**pen the curtain and door.

e. **W**ash your hands.

f. **R**eport and record.

PROCEDURE 22-1
Providing Postmortem Care

Getting Ready   WGKIEPS

1. Complete the "Getting Ready" steps **a** through **g**.

Supplies

- gloves
- paper towels
- cotton balls
- bed protector
- postmortem kit
- wash basin
- soap
- comb
- bath blanket
- washcloth
- towel
- clean gown
- clean linens (if necessary)

Procedure

2. Cover the over-bed table with paper towels. Place your supplies on the over-bed table.

3. Make sure that the bed is positioned at a comfortable working height (to promote good body mechanics) and that the wheels are locked. Lower the head of the bed so that the bed is flat. Fanfold the top linens to the foot of the bed.

4. Put on the gloves.

5. If instructed to by the nurse, remove or turn off any medical equipment.

6. Place the body in the supine position. Position the pillow under the person's head and shoulders. Undress the body, and cover it with the bath blanket.

7. Close the eyes. Put a moistened cotton ball on each eyelid if the eyes do not stay closed. If the person has an artificial eye, this should be in place, unless you are instructed otherwise.

8. Replace the person's dentures, unless you are instructed otherwise. Close the mouth and, if necessary, gently support the jaw with the chin strap, a light bandage, or a rolled hand towel.

9. Remove any jewelry and place it in a plastic bag or envelope for the family. List each piece of jewelry as you remove it. Do not remove engagement or wedding rings, unless it is your facility's policy to do so.

10. Fill the wash basin with warm water. Place the basin on the over-bed table. Wash the body and comb the hair.

11. If the family is to view the body, dress the body in a clean gown. If the bedding is wet or soiled, change the bed linens. Draw the top linens over the person, forming a cuff at the

(continued)

PROCEDURE 22-1 (Continued)

Providing Postmortem Care

shoulders. (Do not cover the person's face.) Straighten the room, lower the lights, and provide for the family's privacy.

12. After the family leaves, collect all of the person's belongings, noting each item on your list.

13. Fill out three identification tags:

   a. Attach one to the right great toe or the right ankle.

   b. Attach one to the person's belongings.

   c. Save the last to be attached to the outside of the shroud (if used).

14. If a shroud is to be used, apply it now (see Fig. 22-7) and attach the third identification tag to the outside of the shroud.

15. Gather the soiled linens and place them in the linen hamper. Dispose of disposable items in a facility-approved waste container. Clean equipment and return it to the storage area.

16. Remove your gloves and dispose of them in a facility-approved waste container.

17. Transfer the body from the bed to a stretcher for transport to the morgue, if appropriate. If the family has made funeral arrangements, leave the body in the room with the door or curtain closed.

18. Report the time the body was transported and the location of the person's belongings to the nurse.

Finishing Up C L S O W R

19. Complete the "Finishing Up" steps **a** through **f**.

What did you learn?

Multiple Choice

Select the single best answer for each of the following questions.

1. When caring for a person who is dying, you should:
   a. Keep family members away from the dying person
   b. Keep the room dark
   c. Provide for the person's physical and emotional needs
   d. Change the subject if the person starts to talk about death or dying

2. A common sign of approaching death is:
   a. Severe pain that gets worse
   b. Normal or increased vital signs
   c. Cool, moist skin
   d. Increased appetite

3. Postmortem care is done:
   a. Right before the person dies
   b. After the doctor pronounces the person dead
   c. After rigor mortis sets in
   d. If there is time

4. As death approaches, the last sense to be lost is:
   a. Sight
   b. Hearing
   c. Smell
   d. Taste

5. Which one of the following is a true statement about providing postmortem care?
   a. Standard precautions are used because the body may be infectious
   b. Dentures are removed from the mouth and given to the family to take home
   c. There is no need for privacy because the person is dead
   d. All of the above

6. In caring for the dying person, the nursing assistant also needs to care for the family. Which of the following can the nursing assistant do to support the family?
   a. Allow family members to stay with the dying person
   b. Be respectful of the family
   c. Provide the family with privacy
   d. All of the above

7. You are helping to care for Mrs. Winger, who has a terminal illness. One day when you are in Mrs. Winger's room, she tells you that during difficult times she has always found comfort in reading poems by her favorite poets. What is this an example of?
   a. Culture
   b. Spirituality
   c. Religion
   d. Reincarnation

8. Which of the following meets a dying person's physical needs?
   a. Providing frequent skin care
   b. Listening if the person wants to talk
   c. Preventing rigor mortis
   d. All of the above

Matching

Match each numbered item with its appropriate lettered description.

_____ 1. Reincarnation

_____ 2. Cheyne-Stokes respiration

_____ 3. Rigor mortis

_____ 4. Postmortem care

_____ 5. Autopsy

a. Examination of a person's tissues and organs after death
b. Stiffening of the muscles that occurs 2 to 4 hours after death
c. Care of a body after death
d. The belief that the soul of a dead person returns to Earth in the form of another human being or animal yet to be born
e. Pattern of rapid–slow respirations

Stop and think!

▶ Wendy has been caring for Mr. Cole, who is dying, for the last 6 weeks. Mr. Cole's demanding daughter, Maria, has not made these last 6 weeks easy for Wendy. Maria feels that Wendy is not doing enough for her father, and she has taken every opportunity to point that out to Wendy. However, Wendy has in fact provided Mr. Cole with excellent care—during her shift, she has always taken care to make sure that all of Mr. Cole's physical needs are met, and she has spent a lot of time just sitting with Mr. Cole and holding his hand. One day, during Wendy's shift, Mr. Cole's vital signs start to decline. Wendy knows that this probably means that Mr. Cole will die soon. Maria is also present, and she also notices the change in her father's condition. She says impatiently to Wendy, "Why are you just standing there? Go get a doctor! I won't have my father die like this!" What should Wendy do? Mr. Cole has told her on several occasions that he is tired of suffering and ready to die, and she knows that there is a "do not resuscitate" (DNR) order in his chart.

Nursing Assistants Make a Difference!

"My mother recently passed away at Clayton County Nursing Home. Although Mom had been in poor health for some time, her death was hard on me. I must say, though, that the staff at Clayton County made this difficult time more bearable through their kindness and competence.

Last Monday night around midnight, the phone rang and it was Elaine, one of the night nurses on duty. Elaine said that we needed to gather the family and come out, that Mom was dying. Soon, we had quite a crowd in Mom's room. I guess the staff was expecting us, because they had moved Mom's roommate to another room and brought in chairs so we would all have someplace to sit. One of the nursing assistants, Patty, was so great. She actually brought us a tray with a pot full of hot coffee, coffee cups, sugar, and creamer on it! We sat with Mom throughout the night and morning hours as she slowly weakened. Patty checked in with us often and would help turn Mom and change her when she soiled the bed. Sometimes she brought the nurse in to suction Mom when she started having trouble breathing. Although Mom could not talk to us, she regained consciousness about an hour before she died and looked us each in the eyes as we said our tearful good-byes.

When Mom took her last breath, we all sort of knew what had happened. My sister went out into the hall to look for help. Luckily, Patty was nearby, and she quickly returned to the room to check Mom's vital signs. Then the doctor came in, and pronounced Mom dead. I asked if I could help Patty wash Mom's body and get her into a clean gown, and Patty said that would be fine. Together, Patty and I prepared Mom for the funeral home. My family and I were allowed to stay in the room for a while after Mom died, just to reflect on things and finish making plans for the funeral.

Patty was really a godsend to me and my family during this difficult time. The excellent way Patty handled Mom's death spoke volumes about the care she gave to Mom while she was alive."

You can listen to more stories about how nursing assistants make a difference on the CD in the back of your book.

Structure and Function of the Human Body

The human body has amazing capabilities. Our bodies allow us to fully experience the world around us, to move, to think, to create. Perhaps even more amazing than what our bodies allow us to do is what our bodies do for us automatically. For example, think about how many times a day your heart beats or your lungs inhale and exhale. What would it be like if you had to remember to do this on your own? Or think about the last time you had a cold or the flu, and your body fought off the infection. The human body is truly remarkable in its ability to maintain health and to heal from disease.

In this unit, we will explore how each organ system functions normally, as well as how disease or injury affects the function of the organ system. We will also explore the measures that are taken to help the body return to its best level of functioning after injury or illness. Knowing how the body works when it is healthy helps us to understand how to help the body heal and function more effectively during illness.

Photo: The human body has amazing capabilities.
(David Scott/Index Stock Imagery, Inc.)

471

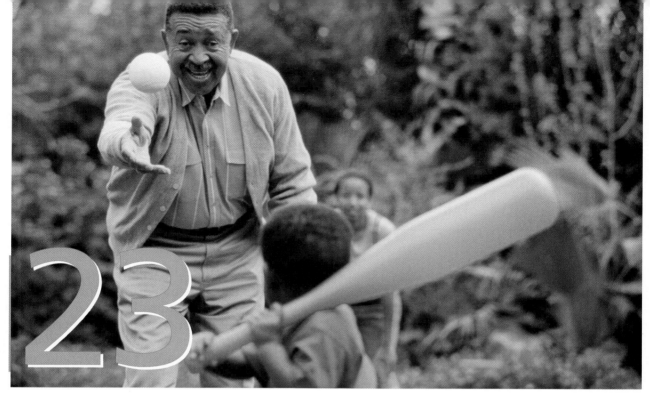

23

Basic Body Structure and Function

What will you learn?

The human body is a wonder of design. In a healthy person, all of the body's parts work together effortlessly, like those of a highly efficient machine. To understand how a machine works, a mechanic studies the machine's parts and how they work together. The same is true of people who want to know how the human body works. **Anatomy** is the study of what body parts look like, where they are located, how big they are, and how they connect to other body parts. **Physiology** is the study of how the body parts work. In this chapter, we will take a look at the body as a whole, functioning unit. You will learn about how changes in a person's normal anatomy or physiology can lead to disease or disabilities, and about the body's remarkable ability to correct small problems before they become large ones. In addition, you will learn about the important role the health care team plays in helping people to achieve their best possible level of functioning. When you are finished with this chapter, you will be able to:

1. Define the terms *anatomy* and *physiology.*
2. List and describe the basic organizational levels of the body.
3. Define the term *homeostasis* and give examples of how the body maintains the balance necessary for life.
4. Discuss how the body's inability to maintain homeostasis affects a person's health.
5. Describe the categories of disease and list some factors that may put a person at risk for developing a certain disease.
6. Explain the goal of rehabilitation.
7. Describe how the concept of holistic care applies to rehabilitation.
8. Understand the nursing assistant's responsibilities related to providing restorative care.

Photo: When we are healthy, our bodies allow us to do the things we like to do.

Vocabulary

Use the CD in the back of your book to hear these terms pronounced, defined, and used in a sentence:

Anatomy	Cytoplasm	Organ system	Restorative care
Physiology	Nucleus	Homeostasis	Supportive device
Organism	Cell membrane	Disease	Assistive device
Cell	Tissue	Disability	Prosthetic device
Organelles	Organ	Rehabilitation	

HOW IS THE BODY ORGANIZED?

All living things, from a jellyfish that washes up on the beach to the largest elephant roaming the plains of Africa, share the same general organization. The basic unit of life is the cell. Cells group together to form tissues. Tissues group together to form organs, and organs group together to form organ systems. These levels of organization are shared by every living thing, or **organism,** whether it is an animal or a plant (Fig. 23-1). The reason not all living things look alike or function alike is because at each level, there are variations specific to the type of organism. Let's take a closer look now at the levels of organization that make up each organism—cells, tissues, organs, and organ systems.

CELLS

A **cell** is the basic unit of life. As you will remember from Chapter 7, a cell is so small that it can only be seen with a microscope. A single cell, as small as it is, has all of the characteristics of life. It is capable of organization, which means that it can join with other similar cells to perform a common function. It is capable of metabolism, which means that it takes in "raw materials" and converts them into the energy it needs to stay alive. It is capable of growth, which means that it changes in size over time. And finally, it is capable of reproduction, which means that it can make a copy of itself. Organization, metabolism, growth, and reproduction are basic qualities that make a living thing different from a non-living thing.

The human body is made up of millions of cells, of all different shapes, sizes, and functions (Fig. 23-2). Some cells cover the body and line the body openings that are exposed to the outside world, offering us protection (epithelial cells). Some cells produce movement (muscle cells) or transmit signals from the nervous system (nerve cells), whereas others secrete chemicals to help us digest the food we eat (pancreas cells). Some cells transport oxygen throughout the body (red blood cells), whereas others actually eat pathogens that could make us sick (white blood

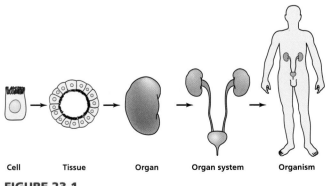

Cell   Tissue   Organ   Organ system   Organism

FIGURE 23-1

All living things (organisms) share the same basic levels of organization. Cells form tissues, tissues form organs, and organs form organ systems.

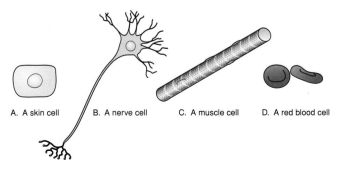

A. A skin cell   B. A nerve cell   C. A muscle cell   D. A red blood cell

FIGURE 23-2

Cells come in different shapes and sizes, and perform many different functions. (*A*) A skin cell. (*B*) A nerve cell. (*C*) A muscle cell. (*D*) A red blood cell.

cells). Each type of cell in the body has a specific duty. Our overall health depends on the ability of the cells of the body to do their jobs.

To function properly, cells require oxygen, water, nutrition, and the ability to eliminate waste products. Structures inside of the cell, called **organelles,** help the cell to make the energy it needs to stay alive and to rid itself of waste products (Fig. 23-3). The organelles float in a jelly-like substance called **cytoplasm.** In addition to organelles and cytoplasm, the cell contains a nucleus. The **nucleus** of the cell is like the cell's "brain." It contains all of the information the cell needs to do its job, grow, and reproduce. A **cell membrane** surrounds the cytoplasm and gives the cell its shape.

TISSUES

When cells that are similar in structure and specialized to perform a specific function join together, they form **tissue** (Fig. 23-4). There are four main types of tissue in the human body:

- **Epithelial tissue** covers the outside of the body, lines its internal structures, and forms glands. The purpose of epithelial tissue is protection. Epithelial tissue forms the outer part of the skin. It forms the mucous membranes that line our digestive, respiratory, urinary, and reproductive systems. It also covers organs such as the lungs and heart, and lines the inside of the blood vessels, abdominal cavity, and chest cavity.

FIGURE 23-3

An artist's representation of the inside of an animal cell. A cell contains organelles and a nucleus, which float in a jelly-like substance called cytoplasm. A cell membrane surrounds the cytoplasm and gives the cell its shape. (*Photo Researchers, Inc.*)

FIGURE 23-4

Cells join together to form tissues. (© *Scott Camazine/Photo Researchers, Inc.*)

- **Connective tissue** does what its name suggests—it connects other tissues together. Connective tissue supports and forms the framework for all of the parts of the body. Examples of connective tissue include bone, cartilage, ligaments, tendons, and fatty tissues. Blood is also considered a form of connective tissue.
- **Muscle tissue** produces movement. There are three types of muscle tissue found in the body (Table 23-1). Skeletal muscle allows you to move your arms, legs, and other parts of the body. Because you can decide when and how to move the parts of your body that contain skeletal muscle, skeletal muscle is said to be "voluntary," or under the control of the individual. The second type of muscle tissue, smooth muscle, lines the walls of organs such as the intestines, the stomach, and the blood vessels. The movement provided by smooth muscle is involuntary, or out of your control. For example, it is the smooth muscle in the walls of the intestines that produces peristalsis (the wave-like movements that pass digested food through the intestines). You do not need to think about moving food through your intestines. Instead, this action occurs automatically. The third type of muscle tissue, cardiac muscle, forms the heart. Contraction and relaxation of the cardiac muscle pumps blood through-

out the body. Like smooth muscle, cardiac muscle is involuntary.
- **Nervous tissue** conducts information. The brain, spinal cord, and nerves are made of nervous tissue. Nervous tissue allows one part of the body to "talk" to another part. For example, nerves carry information to the brain to be processed and interpreted. In addition, the brain sends commands to other parts of the body through the nerves.

ORGANS

A group of tissues functioning together for a similar purpose form an **organ.** For example, the heart is composed of all four tissue types, and its main function is to pump blood throughout the body. Other examples of organs include the stomach, liver, kidneys, and lungs. An organ may have one specific function, or it may have several.

ORGAN SYSTEMS

An **organ system** is a group of organs that work together to perform a specific function for the body. In order for the organ system to work properly, each organ within the system must function well. Human beings have ten main organ systems (Fig. 23-5):

- The **integumentary system** includes the skin and its glands, the hair, and the nails. The function of the integumentary system is to protect the body.
- The **skeletal system** includes the bones. The function of the skeletal system is to provide a frame for the body and to give the body shape.
- The **muscular system** includes the muscles. The muscular system works along with the skeletal system to enable the body to move. Sometimes the muscular system and the skeletal system together are called the musculoskeletal system.
- The **respiratory system** includes the lungs and the airways. The respiratory system allows for the exchange of gases with the environment. In other words, it allows us to take in oxygen and get rid of carbon dioxide, a waste product of cellular metabolism.

TABLE 23-1 ■ Types of Muscle Tissue

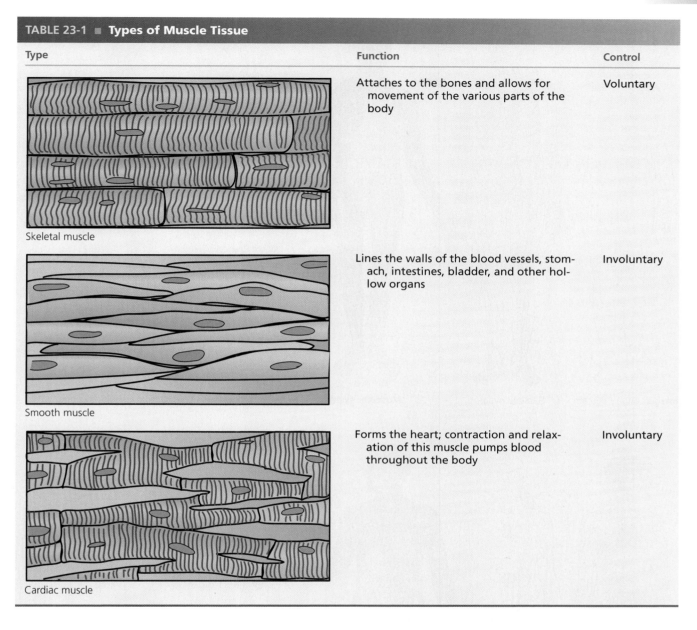

Type	Function	Control
Skeletal muscle	Attaches to the bones and allows for movement of the various parts of the body	Voluntary
Smooth muscle	Lines the walls of the blood vessels, stomach, intestines, bladder, and other hollow organs	Involuntary
Cardiac muscle	Forms the heart; contraction and relaxation of this muscle pumps blood throughout the body	Involuntary

- The **cardiovascular system** is made up of the blood, the heart, and the blood vessels. The cardiovascular system transports nutrients and oxygen to the cells of the body, and carries waste products away.
- The **nervous system** includes the brain, spinal cord, and nerves. The nervous system controls the functioning of the other organ systems. It also allows us to interact with our environment through the **special senses** (sight, hearing, smell, taste, and touch).
- The **endocrine system** consists of glands throughout the body. These glands secrete chemical substances called hormones, which control the function of certain organs.
- The **digestive system** consists of the teeth, salivary glands, tongue, esophagus, stomach, small intestine, large intestine, liver, pancreas, and gallbladder. As you learned in Chapter 19, the digestive system allows us to take in food and water, digest the food into nutrients, and absorb the nutrients into the bloodstream. The digestive system also removes solid waste from the body in the form of feces.
- The **urinary system** consists of the kidneys, the bladder, the ureters, and the urethra. As you learned in Chapter 20, the

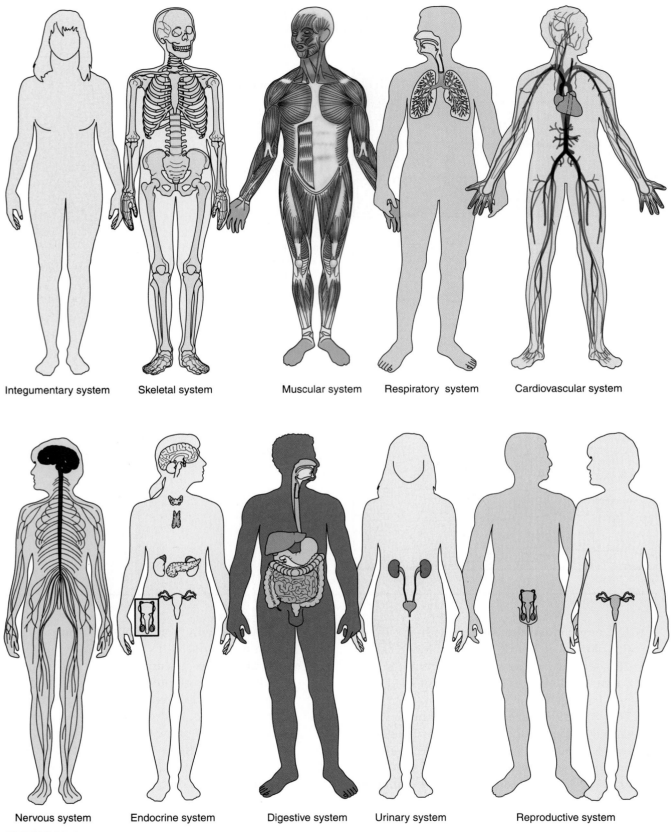

Integumentary system   Skeletal system   Muscular system   Respiratory system   Cardiovascular system

Nervous system   Endocrine system   Digestive system   Urinary system   Reproductive system

FIGURE 23-5

There are ten organ systems in the human body.

urinary system removes liquid waste from the body in the form of urine.

- The **reproductive system** allows the human body to produce new life. Without a means of reproduction, human life would cease to exist.

As you can see, organ systems do not work alone. They work together to maintain the life of the organism.

HEALTH AND DISEASE

All of the organ systems work together to maintain **homeostasis,** or balance. Homeostasis is a basic concept in physiology. The word comes from the Greek words *homoios,* which means "same," and *stasis,* which means "standing." So homeostasis means "staying the same." For an organism to stay alive, certain conditions within the body must remain the same, within a range of normal limits. You were introduced to this idea in Chapter 16, when we discussed vital signs. For example, the body temperature must remain within a certain range. The blood pressure must remain within a certain range. The fluids that keep our cells moist and healthy must not be too acidic or too basic. Our blood must contain the right amount of oxygen, nutrients, and other substances needed for metabolism at all times.

All of the organ systems are constantly working together to maintain a state of balance. When the external or internal environment changes, the organ systems must make adjustments to compensate for the change. For example, imagine that you are playing basketball at the park with your friends on a very hot day. You begin to sweat. This is your body working to cool you down. As you continue to play and sweat, you begin to get thirsty. This is your body telling you that it needs more water. As you run back and forth on the court, you breathe harder and your heart rate increases, as your respiratory and circulatory systems work to send extra oxygen to your tissues. Your tissues need the extra oxygen because they use it to help produce the energy that allows you to keep playing.

Most of the time, you are not even aware of the adjustments your body is making to keep everything within the normal range. Even when you are sitting perfectly still, little adjustments are being made to keep the internal environment stable. Perhaps you are wondering how your body "knows" that an adjustment is needed. The answer is, through a feedback mechanism. Although all of the organ systems play a role in maintaining homeostasis, most of these feedback mechanisms are controlled by the nervous and endocrine systems.

The body's ability to maintain balance is an indicator of good health. There are times when the body's ability to maintain homeostasis is altered. This imbalance is usually the result of a disease. A **disease** occurs when the structure or function of an organ or an organ system is abnormal. Diseases can be acute (temporary) or chronic (long-term). They can be mild or severe. Sometimes, the same disease may be severe in one person but mild in another. There are several common categories of disease. A disease may belong to more than one of these categories. Common categories of disease include:

- **Infectious diseases.** Infections are believed to play a role in approximately half of all illnesses.
- **Degenerative diseases.** To degenerate means to "break down." Degenerative diseases occur when the tissues of the body wear out or break down. Arthritis, muscular dystrophy, osteoporosis, and Alzheimer's disease are examples of degenerative diseases. These diseases can be inherited, or they can be caused by infection, injury, or aging. Sometimes there is no known cause.
- **Nutritional disorders.** These disorders occur when a person's diet lacks certain nutrients. Consuming too much of any one nutrient (for example, vitamins) or too many calories can also cause nutritional disorders. For example, obesity is a nutritional disorder.
- **Metabolic (endocrine) disorders.** Metabolic disorders, such as diabetes, occur when the body is unable to metabolize or absorb certain nutrients. Metabolic disorders often occur when the body secretes either too much of one type of hormone, or not enough. Because the hormone is responsible for controlling the function of a particular organ, the organ does not function properly and an imbalance in homeostasis occurs.

- **Immune disorders.** These disorders change the way the immune system behaves. Sometimes, as in acquired immunodeficiency syndrome (AIDS), the disease reduces the immune system's ability to fight off infection. Other times, the disease causes the immune system to start attacking the body's own tissues.
- **Neoplastic diseases.** The word neoplasm means "new growth." Many people use the word "cancer" or "tumor" when they are talking about neoplastic disease. Neoplasms cause problems by invading otherwise healthy tissues. The presence of the new growth prevents the tissues from functioning properly.
- **Psychiatric disorders.** Mental disorders that affect a person's ability to function normally, such as depression, are also considered diseases.

Why do some people get certain diseases and others do not? Why does a certain disease affect one person very mildly but totally destroy the health of another person? As a nursing assistant, one of your many responsibilities will be to help improve or maintain the health of your patients or residents. To do that, you need to know about the factors that can put a person at risk for disease, or negatively affect his or her ability to recover from disease. Some of these factors include the following:

- **Age.** Some disorders are more likely to occur in certain age groups. For example, chickenpox, a viral infection, is more common in children. Age can also influence how a person reacts to disease. For example, when an adult gets the chickenpox, the infection is usually much more severe. In general, older people are more at risk for certain diseases because the process of aging causes a lot of wear and tear on the body's tissues and organs.
- **Gender.** A person's gender can put the person at risk for certain diseases. For instance, breast cancer is much more common in women than in men. Women are also more likely than men to develop diabetes. However, men are more likely to have heart disease.
- **Heredity.** The genes that we inherit from our parents may put us at risk for developing certain diseases. For example, scientists now know that some types of cancer, diabetes, and heart disease are inherited.
- **Lifestyle.** A person's living conditions and health habits play a major role in the person's overall health status. For example, a person who is homeless is more likely to get sick than a person who has shelter from the weather. A person who gets too little rest and has poor nutritional habits is more likely to become ill than a person who gets enough sleep and eats well. A person who smokes is more likely to develop cancer, lung disease, or heart disease than a person who does not. A person who likes a deep, dark tan in the summer is more at risk for developing skin cancer than a person who uses sunscreen. These are just examples of the many ways in which lifestyle influences health.
- **Occupation.** Many jobs put a person at risk for certain diseases. For example, constant exposure to coal dust puts coal miners at risk for developing "black lung disease." Health care workers who do not take care to protect themselves are at risk for certain infections, such as human immunodeficiency virus (HIV) or hepatitis.
- **Chronic disease.** A person who has a chronic disease, such as diabetes or high blood pressure, is at increased risk for developing another disease. For example, a person who does not manage his diabetes well is likely to develop heart disease, blindness, or kidney failure. In addition, a person who has a chronic disease is often more likely to experience more severe problems from something that would not really affect a healthy person. For example, an ingrown toenail will cause discomfort and inconvenience in a healthy person. However, in a person with diabetes, the ingrown toenail could cause a severe infection, because diabetes changes the internal environment of the body, making it more at risk for infection.
- **Emotional health.** A person's emotional health can directly affect her physical health. Emotional stress can create physical problems such as headaches, digestive disorders, and muscle strain. In addition, stress makes the body more at risk for

infection. If you remember from Chapter 6, just becoming a patient or resident of a health care facility can significantly increase a person's level of emotional stress and make coping with physical illness or disability more difficult.

Awareness of the factors that can put your patients or residents at risk for disease will help you to better meet their individual needs. When you meet your patient's or resident's specific needs, or observe and report signs that indicate that the person's body is struggling to return to a balanced state, you are making a very important contribution to the person's health.

REHABILITATION AND RESTORATIVE CARE

Clearly, not all diseases and injuries result in death. But many of them leave the person with a **disability,** or impaired function. The disability can be physical, emotional, or both. Like diseases, some disabilities are acute while others are chronic. Some may be permanent (Fig. 23-6). A person with a disability may need minimal help with activities of daily living (ADLs) or total physical care, depending on how severe the disability is. One of the goals of health care workers is to help patients and residents learn to manage their disabilities and regain as much independence as possible.

Rehabilitation is the process of helping a person with a disability to return to his highest level of physical, emotional, or economic function. Rehabilitation is achieved through **restorative care,** or the measures that health care workers take to help a person regain health, strength, and function. Restorative care involves treatment, education, and the prevention of further disability. Like any other type of health care, restorative care is achieved through a team effort. Members of the team include the patient or resident and her family members, the nurse, the nursing assistant, a doctor, and any number of other specialists, depending on the type of rehabilitation and the goals of the effort.

The rehabilitative effort focuses on the individual needs and capabilities of the patient or resident. For example, following rehabilitation, some people will be able to leave the health care

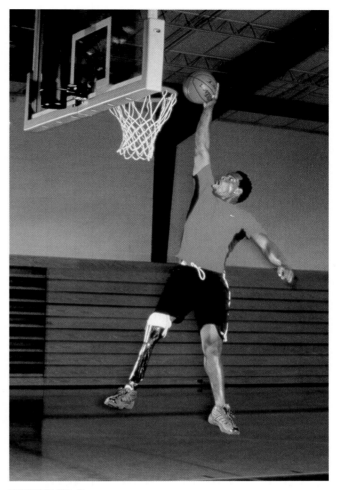

FIGURE 23-6

This young man has lost a leg, resulting in a permanent disability. However, he has adapted to the loss of the leg and is able to do everything that a person with two legs is able to do. (© *Richard T. Nowitz/Photo Researchers, Inc.*)

facility and return to independent, productive lives. Others will always be dependent to some degree on others for help with their ADLs, but following rehabilitation, they will be less dependent than they were before. Some people will require many months, or even years, of rehabilitation to return to their best level of functioning.

Rehabilitation services are offered by many types of facilities. Hospitals may offer a variety of rehabilitative services, from physical therapy to mental counseling. The Omnibus Budget Reconciliation Act (OBRA) requires long-term care facilities to provide rehabilitative services that meet the specific needs of the residents who live in the facility. Some facilities provide only rehabilitative services for people with specific types of disabilities. For example, a facility may have the mission of helping people to cope with disabilities caused by head or spinal cord injuries, burns, or birth defects.

TAKING A HOLISTIC APPROACH

Rehabilitation must focus on the whole person—his needs, well-being, and abilities—not just on his disabilities. As you learned in Chapter 6, each of your patients and residents has unique emotional, social, and spiritual needs in addition to her physical needs. An illness or injury that results in a disability can affect a person's ability to care for herself physically, as well as her ability to function emotionally. Think for a moment how a disability might affect you. How would it feel to have to rely on someone else for transportation? To lose your job? To be embarrassed by your appearance? People who become disabled in some way often feel inadequate, helpless, or resentful of other "normal" people, especially at first. A person who is depressed or feels that he is a burden to others may have very little energy left to focus on physical therapy.

During rehabilitation, providing emotional and spiritual care is just as important as providing physical care. A person who has become disabled may feel frustrated, depressed, or guilty about her inability to do the things she used to be able to do. The person may become angry with caregivers, family, or herself because of these feelings. A holistic approach—consideration of the person's emotional needs, as well as his or her physical ones—is essential for the rehabilitative effort to be effective.

THE ROLE OF THE NURSING ASSISTANT

The nursing assistant plays a key role in the successful rehabilitation of a patient or resident. Although other health care professionals evaluate the person's rehabilitation needs and then plan the restorative care, the nursing assistant plays a key role in helping to carry out the plan. Because of the unique relationship that develops between a nursing assistant and the people he cares for, the nursing assistant becomes the "eyes and ears" of the rehabilitation team.

You will be able to observe the patient or resident for any physical changes, positive or negative, that are related to the rehabilitation. You will be the one who notices that a new splint or sup-

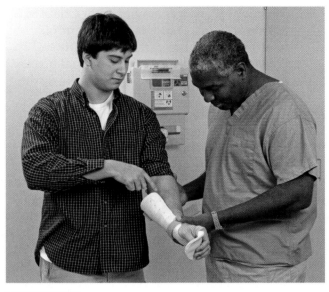

FIGURE 23-7

The nursing assistant is the "eyes and ears" of the rehabilitation team.

portive device has caused chafing or redness of the skin (Fig. 23-7). You will document the results of a bowel or bladder training plan, and it will be your responsibility to make sure that the person is taken to the bathroom on schedule. You will be the person responsible for adding the thickening powder to a person's liquids to help him swallow without choking. You will reassure, encourage, listen to, and praise the people you care for as they struggle with the challenges that rehabilitation brings.

Ask questions about new rehabilitation measures that have been planned for a resident or patient. Have the nurse or therapist explain how to use new equipment and show you how to help your patient or resident to use it (Fig. 23-8). Make sure you document and report your observations. If a new rehabilitation measure does not seem to be working for the person, perhaps a change is necessary. Your input can help initiate that change.

It is also important for you to monitor the person's emotional status. Rehabilitation, which in some cases can take a very long time, can be extremely frustrating for the person who is trying to overcome a disability. If you sense that one of your patients or residents is becoming depressed, angry, or frustrated, report this to the nurse. The nurse and the other members of the rehabilitation team will be able to help the person work

FIGURE 23-8

Ask the nurse or physical therapist to show you how to use assistive devices. This will allow you to help your patient or resident use the assistive device more effectively. Here, a physical therapist is showing a nursing assistant how to assist a resident with using a wrist supporter with a spoon attached.

through these feelings, so that he can again focus on recovery. You, too, may find yourself feeling frustrated with a patient or resident who is struggling with rehabilitation. If this occurs, please talk to the nurse. You may need a break or a short reassignment from that person.

TYPES OF REHABILITATION

There are many types of rehabilitation. The type of rehabilitation depends on the person's specific disability and the individual needs of that person. In many cases, a person may need a combination of different types of rehabilitation. For example, imagine a patient named Mr. Hayes. Mr. Hayes was involved in a car accident that killed his wife and resulted in the loss of his own leg. Mr. Hayes now needs to learn to walk with a false (prosthetic) leg. He also needs to overcome the emotional crisis associated with the loss of his wife. Depending on what sort of job Mr. Hayes had before the accident, he may also need to learn new job skills so that he can work again. In this example, learning to walk with the false leg would be achieved through physical rehabilitation. Overcoming the grief and guilt caused by his wife's death would

require emotional rehabilitation. Learning the skills needed to return to work would be achieved through vocational rehabilitation.

Physical Rehabilitation

Helping people to overcome physical disabilities is a common function of most health care facilities. Physical therapy helps to restore strength and function to limbs that have been affected by illness and injury. Exercise, combined with supportive devices, assistive devices, prosthetic devices, or all three can help a person regain function.

- **Supportive devices,** such as splints and braces, help to stabilize a weak joint or limb.
- **Assistive devices** make certain tasks, such as transferring, walking, eating, or dressing, easier (Fig. 23-9). You have already learned about many assistive devices in previous chapters.
- **Prosthetic devices** are artificial replacements for legs, feet, arms, or other body parts.

Although a person's disability may prevent him from ever doing some things again, there will be many things that he will be able to do independently following physical rehabilitation. The ability to function independently is very important for a person's self-esteem.

FIGURE 23-9

Physical rehabilitation focuses on helping a person regain the physical ability to do certain tasks. Learning how to use assistive devices is part of physical rehabilitation. Assistive devices help a person to become more independent. For example, this woman is using a transfer board to transfer herself from her wheelchair to her bed. (*Copyright B. Proud.*)

Another major focus of physical rehabilitation is to prevent complications that can result from the loss of function. When a person does not use a part of the body for a long time, he loses muscle mass in that part. As the muscle mass is lost, so is the person's strength. For example, have you ever had a cast put on an arm or a leg for a long period of time? When the cast finally came off, your arm or leg probably looked skinny and felt weak. That was because during the time your arm or leg was in the cast, you were not able to move it, and your muscle mass decreased. When a person cannot use an arm or a leg, exercising the arm or leg helps to keep it working properly. Imagine that Mr. Gibbons has been in a coma for several months. Finally, after weeks of unconsciousness, Mr. Gibbons comes out of the coma. Fortunately, the people caring for Mr. Gibbons while he was in the coma took care to exercise his arms and legs for him. If they had not done this, complications associated with immobility, such as contractures and muscle atrophy, could have caused permanent disability. By preventing these complications from occurring, the health care team ensured that Mr. Gibbons would be able to be rehabilitated successfully.

Rehabilitative measures are also used to help people learn about and recover from chronic and acute illnesses. A person with diabetes will learn how to control her condition through a combination of exercise and diet. Cardiac rehabilitation involves the use of closely monitored exercise and dietary changes to help a person recover from a heart attack.

Emotional Rehabilitation

The stresses that accompany disability can interfere with a person's ability to cope emotionally. Feelings of despair and a loss of self-esteem often accompany conditions that cause a disability. The loss of ability, the loss of a "normal" appearance, the loss of income, and the loss of independence will affect each person differently. You will see some people rally in the face of disability and actually find a new focus for their life, while others withdraw emotionally and use the disability as a reason to not try to improve. Some people who have experienced a devastating illness or injury may even talk of suicide. If you think that one of your patients or residents is experiencing emotional distress, report your concerns to the nurse. The nurse will arrange for

FIGURE 23-10

Emotional rehabilitation helps the person learn to cope with the losses caused by the disability. Many people with disabilities benefit from talking to a professional therapist or a clergy member. (© CC Studio/Photo Researchers, Inc.)

emotional counseling to help the person overcome his grief and learn to accept and work with his disability (Fig. 23-10).

When you are caring for a person with a disability, there is a lot you can do to help meet the person's emotional needs. Focus on the person's abilities. Encourage and reassure the person, but be careful not to compare the person with someone else. For example, do not say, "Well, if Mr. Smith can learn to walk again, surely you can too!" Instead, say "Mr. Williams, I am so impressed by your progress! You've gone so much further this week than you did last week!" Be realistic in your encouragement. Do not say things like, "Oh, keep on working and you'll be back to normal in no time" if it is unlikely that the person will ever be able to return to the level of function she had before the injury or illness. However, allow the person to hope for cures, new treatments, and advances in medical technology that can improve her quality of life.

Vocational Rehabilitation

A *vocation* is a job. The goal of vocational rehabilitation is to return a person to gainful employment. Gainful employment is a job or career that

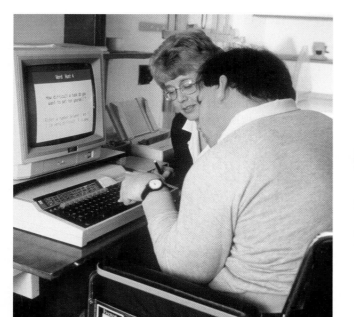

FIGURE 23-11

Vocational rehabilitation helps a person learn or re-learn the skills he will need to return to work. (© *Simon Fraser/Disability Research, Hunters Moor Hospital/ Photo Researchers, Inc.*)

will provide enough income for the person to live, without being dependent on financial assistance to survive. Vocational rehabilitation is used when a person's disability causes her to lose the skills she needs to do the job she had prior to becoming disabled. In some cases, the person may just need vocational rehabilitation to relearn the skills she had before. In other cases, the person will need to learn a completely new set of skills that will enable her to get another type of job (Fig. 23-11). Assistance may also be available to help the person locate a new job, new living arrangements, or a new mode of transportation that will allow her to become independent again.

▷ *Tell the Nurse!*

When you are caring for a person receiving rehabilitative therapy, you should report the following observations to the nurse immediately:

▷ A supportive device is broken or not working properly

▷ The person has a change in vital signs during or after the rehabilitation activity

▷ The person has pain, swelling, redness, or signs of inflammation around braces, prosthetics, or supportive devices

▷ The person is showing signs of depression or excessive frustration, such as crying, withdrawal, anger, or talk of suicide

▷ The person is having excessive difficulty with a new rehabilitation technique or treatment

SUMMARY

▶ Understanding how the healthy body works helps us to understand and treat disease.

▶ All living things share the same levels of organization.

■ A cell is the basic unit of life.

■ A group of cells that is similar in structure and specialized for a specific function forms tissue.

■ A group of tissues functioning together for a similar purpose forms an organ.

■ A group of organs that function together for the same general purpose forms an organ system.

■ A group of organ systems working together for the purpose of maintaining life forms an organism.

▶ All of the organ systems work together to maintain a state of homeostasis, or balance.

■ When the body's ability to maintain homeostasis is altered, disease or illness can result.

• There are several common categories of disease. These categories often overlap.

• Certain factors put some people more at risk for disease than others.

■ A nursing assistant who is aware of the factors that put a person at risk for disease is able to provide better care for her patients or residents, because she has a better understanding of each individual's needs.

▶ A primary focus of the health care industry is to help a person recover from an illness or injury and regain independence. Rehabilitation is the process that helps a person with a disability return to the highest level of physical, emotional, and economic function possible.

■ Rehabilitation must focus on the whole person—his needs, well-being, and abilities—not just on the person's disabilities.

■ Rehabilitation involves a team of people working together to address the needs of the patient or resident. Because of the unique relationship that develops between a nursing assistant and the people he cares for, the nursing assistant becomes the "eyes and ears" of the rehabilitation team.

■ Many types of rehabilitation are used to help a disabled person regain function.

- Physical rehabilitation focuses on regaining physical function through the use of exercise, supportive devices, assistive devices, and prosthetic devices.

- Emotional rehabilitation focuses on helping the person come to terms with the disability and cope with loss.

- Vocational rehabilitation focuses on providing the person with the skills he or she needs in order to get a job and achieve financial independence.

What did you learn?

Multiple Choice

Select the single best answer for each of the following questions.

1. The process that helps a person with a disability to return to her highest level of physical, emotional, or economic function is called:
   a. Homeostasis
   b. Metabolism
   c. Prosthetics
   d. Rehabilitation
2. Which of the following is a factor that might put a person at risk for disease?
   a. Age
   b. Heredity
   c. Gender
   d. All of the above
3. What is the purpose of epithelial tissue?
   a. To provide a frame for, and give shape to, the body
   b. To connect other types of tissue together
   c. To cover the body and line its cavities
   d. To conduct nerve impulses
4. Which one of the following would you be responsible for when providing a patient or resident with rehabilitative care?
   a. Adding a thickener to the person's drink to make the liquid easier to swallow
   b. Documenting the results of bladder training
   c. Observing the person for changes in ability, positive or negative
   d. All of the above

Matching

Match each numbered item with its appropriate lettered description.

_____ 1. Anatomy

_____ 2. Organ

_____ 3. Vocational rehabilitation

_____ 4. Cell

_____ 5. Emotional rehabilitation

_____ 6. Physical rehabilitation

_____ 7. Tissue

_____ 8. Physiology

_____ 9. Homeostasis

_____ 10. Organ system

_____ 11. Organism

a. Used when a person's disability causes her to lose the skills she needs to do the job she had prior to becoming disabled
b. Study of how the body parts work
c. Used to restore strength and function to limbs that have been affected by illness and injury
d. Basic unit of life
e. Used to help a person manage the feelings caused by a disability
f. Study of what body parts look like, where they are located, how big they are, and how they connect to other body parts
g. A group of organs that work together to perform a specific function for the body
h. A state of balance
i. A living thing, formed by a group of organ systems working together for the purpose of maintaining life
j. A group of tissues functioning together for a similar purpose
k. Formed when cells that are similar in structure and specialized to perform a specific function join together

? Stop and think!

▶ Jacob is working in the rehabilitation unit of his nursing facility. He has been assigned to care for Mr. Huff, who has recently had his right leg amputated (removed) above the knee. Jacob is to assist Mr. Huff in his transfers until he is able to do them himself. Mr. Huff is to do all of his own activities of daily living (ADLs), such as bathing, feeding, and dressing himself, with minimal help from Jacob. This morning when Jacob enters the room, he finds Mr. Huff on the floor between the bed and the wheelchair. Mr. Huff is struggling to climb into his wheelchair. When Jacob approaches him to help, Mr. Huff says angrily, "Leave me alone; I can do this. I'm OK, just leave me alone." Aside from helping Mr. Huff into his wheelchair, what could Jacob do to help Mr. Huff? What do you think about Mr. Huff's attempt to move from the bed to the wheelchair by himself?

▶ Amanda is assigned to care for Mrs. Webb, who recently had a stroke. When the stroke occurred, Mrs. Webb had been preparing dinner at the stove. As a result, when she fell, she also suffered severe burns on her arms. Now Mrs. Webb is receiving rehabilitation therapy for her left-sided weakness, in addition to recovering from the skin grafts used to treat the burns on her arms. Mrs. Webb is a widow and her children live out of state. She cries frequently because she says there is "no one to help her and she will probably end up staying in the nursing home for the rest of her life." Every time Amanda tries to get Mrs. Webb to participate in bathing and feeding herself, Mrs. Webb shakes her head and says she "just doesn't feel up to the effort today." Mrs. Webb's grafts are healing well and she is doing great in therapy. Is there anything Amanda can do to help Mrs. Webb not feel so helpless? What can she say to her to encourage her to do more for herself and be less dependent?

24

The Integumentary System

What will you learn?

What is the largest organ in your body? Your skin! Just think—your body is covered in about 22 square feet of skin, and your skin alone weighs between 8 and 10 pounds. You already know that a major function of this very large organ is to cover and protect your body. But did you also know that the skin give us clues about what is going on inside of a person's body? In this chapter, you will learn about the skin and the other organs that make up the integumentary system. You will learn about the importance of observing this organ system for changes that may indicate illness, and about actions you can take to help keep the skin (and its wearer!) healthy. When you are finished with this chapter, you will be able to:

1. List the layers of the skin.
2. Describe the accessory structures of the skin.
3. Discuss the major functions of the integumentary system.
4. Describe how normal aging processes affect the integumentary system.
5. Explain how pressure ulcers are formed and what conditions may increase a patient's or resident's risk of developing a pressure ulcer.
6. Describe how the nursing assistant helps to prevent residents and patients from developing pressure ulcers.
7. Describe the different types of wounds that a patient or resident might have.
8. Discuss the nursing assistant's duties regarding wound care.
9. Define terms used to describe skin lesions.

Photo: Your integumentary system includes your skin, hair, and nails.

Vocabulary

Use the CD in the back of your book to hear these terms pronounced, defined, and used in a sentence:

Jaundice	Subcutaneous tissue	Unintentional wound	Vesicle
Pallor	Sebum	Lesion	Pustule
Flushing	Collagen	Rash	Excoriation
Cyanosis	Bony prominences	Dermatitis	Fissure
Epidermis	Necrosis	Eczema	Ulcer
Keratin	Pressure points	Erythema	
Melanin	Wound	Macule	
Dermis	Intentional wound	Papule	

The integumentary system gets its name from the Latin word *integumentum,* which means "a covering." The integumentary system is made up of the skin, which covers the body, and the structures that develop from it, called *accessory structures* or *appendages.* The accessory structures of the skin are the nails, the hair, the sebaceous glands (which secrete oils to keep the skin moist), and the sweat glands.

Of all the body's organ systems, the integumentary system is the most easily observed. Healthy skin is glowing and vibrant, and may range in color from very light to very dark. A change in a person's normal skin color can indicate a serious health problem and should be reported to the nurse immediately. For example:

- **Jaundice** is a yellow discoloration of the skin and the whites of the eyes. The skin of a person with jaundice may appear yellow or golden, or it may be as orange as a Halloween pumpkin. Jaundice is usually associated with liver disorders.
- **Pallor** is paleness, and **flushing** is redness. Some people appear pale or flushed most of the time. In these people, pallor or flushing would be considered "normal." However, if you notice pallor or flushing in a person who is not normally pale or flushed, you should report this finding to the nurse.
- **Cyanosis** is a blue or gray discoloration of the skin, lips, and nail beds. Cyanosis develops when the skin does not receive enough oxygen. Cyanosis is a sign of a respiratory or circulatory disorder.

As you learned in Chapter 18, the condition of a person's hair and nails can also provide clues to

the person's overall health. The hair should be shiny and soft, not brittle and dry, and the scalp should not be flaky or crusty. The nail beds of healthy nails are pink. The nails are flush with the nail bed and, when viewed from the side, the nails are slightly rounded.

STRUCTURE OF THE INTEGUMENTARY SYSTEM

SKIN

The skin is made up of two layers, the epidermis and the dermis (Fig. 24-1).

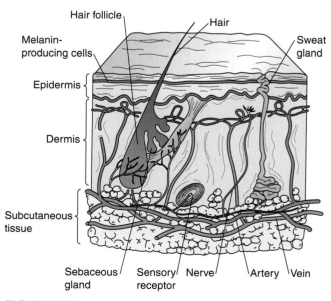

FIGURE 24-1

The skin has two layers, the dermis and epidermis. The skin rests on a layer of subcutaneous tissue.

Epidermis

The **epidermis** is the outer layer of the skin. The epidermis is thickest on the soles of the feet and the palms of the hands, and very thin in areas such as the eyelids.

If you look at Figure 24-1, you will notice that the epidermis contains no blood vessels. You will also notice that it has two sublayers, a deep layer and a surface layer. New cells are produced in the deep layer of the epidermis. As the cells age, they work their way up, toward the surface of the body. As the maturing cells move toward the surface, they move further away from the blood vessels, which are located in the dermis. This means that as the cells age, they move further away from their supply of oxygen and nutrients. They also make **keratin,** a substance that causes them to thicken and become resistant to water. When the cells reach the surface of the body, they die and are shed. This process takes approximately 28 days—so, each month, you get a "new skin!"

In addition to continually producing new cells, the deep layer of the epidermis produces a substance called melanin. **Melanin,** from the Greek word *melas* ("black"), is a dark pigment that gives our skin, hair, and eyes color. People with pale skin have less melanin than those with dark skin. Melanin helps to protect the skin from exposure to sunlight. In fact, continued exposure to sunlight causes the epidermis to produce more melanin, resulting in a tan. Sometimes melanin is deposited throughout the epidermis in an uneven pattern, resulting in freckles.

Dermis

The **dermis** is the deepest layer of the skin (see Fig. 24-1). The dermis consists of elastic connective tissue that allows it to stretch and move without damage. The dermis rests on a layer of fat called the **subcutaneous tissue.** Cutaneous is another word for "skin," and sub means "below." Therefore, *subcutaneous* means "below the skin." The blood vessels and nerves that supply the skin originate in the subcutaneous tissue and send branches into the dermis. Looking at Figure 24-1, you can see that the sensory receptors that allow us to feel pressure, pain, and temperature are located in the dermis. (The sense of touch will be discussed in more detail in Chapter 29.) The sebaceous glands, the sweat glands, and the hair follicles are also found in the dermis.

ACCESSORY STRUCTURES (APPENDAGES)

The skin's accessory structures include the sebaceous glands, the sweat glands, the hair, and the nails.

Sebaceous (Oil) Glands

The sebaceous glands secrete **sebum,** an oily substance that lubricates the skin and helps to prevent it from drying out. The sebum is also slightly acidic. This acidity helps to protect the skin from harmful bacteria that may be present on its surface. The sebaceous glands open into the hair follicles, and the sebum passes along the hair and onto the surface of the skin (see Fig. 24-1).

Sweat Glands

There are two types of sweat glands, eccrine glands and apocrine glands. Eccrine glands are found in the skin that covers most parts of our bodies. Eccrine glands produce a thin, watery liquid that contains salt and small amounts of other bodily wastes. The purpose of the eccrine glands is to help cool the body through the process of evaporation. As the watery sweat leaves the surface of the skin, it takes heat with it, cooling the body down. Therefore, when you "work up a sweat," what you are experiencing is your eccrine glands at work! Another time you may have experienced your eccrine glands at work is when you have noticed your palms beginning to sweat as a result of being nervous. Many people sweat when they are nervous, and the palms of the hands contain a very large number of eccrine glands—hence, "sweaty palm syndrome."

The other type of sweat gland is the apocrine gland. Apocrine glands are found mostly in the skin of the armpits (axillae) and the perineum. The apocrine glands produce a thicker substance. When the bacteria that normally reside on our skin mix with this substance, they produce what we know as "body odor." Apocrine glands become active when a person reaches puberty. As we age, the apocrine glands become less active.

Hair

Hair covers the entire body, except for the soles of the feet and the palms of the hands. Hair, especially that covering the scalp, helps to keep us warm. Most of the hair that covers the body is soft and fine, although in men, body hair tends to be thicker and more noticeable because of the action of certain hormones. In both men and women, the hair covering the scalp, armpits, and pubic area is thicker and coarser than the hair on the rest of the body.

Hair develops in the dermis of the skin from a sheath called a follicle (see Fig. 24-1). The part of the hair that we can see consists of dead cells that have been hardened by keratin. The living cells that produce new hair cells, causing the hair to grow, are found at the bottom of the follicle or hair root. Melanin gives the hair its color. Blonde hair contains a small amount of melanin, while brunette hair contains much more.

Nails

Nails are made of special skin cells that have been hardened by the presence of keratin. Nail growth occurs from the nail root, the area where the nail emerges from the skin. Nails help to protect the ends of our fingers and toes.

FUNCTION OF THE INTEGUMENTARY SYSTEM

The integumentary system helps to maintain the body's homeostasis in three important ways. First, it offers a physical form of protection against microbes, chemicals, and other agents that could harm the body, if they gained access to the delicate organs housed inside. Second, the skin, which is water resistant, helps to maintain the body's fluid balance by preventing excessive loss or absorption of water. Finally, the integumentary system helps to regulate the temperature of the body, ensuring that the temperature stays within a tolerable range.

PROTECTION

As you learned in Chapter 7, the body's first line of defense against the invasion of harmful microbes is intact skin. The skin is a physical barrier that prevents microbes from entering the body. The skin also offers us some protection against harmful substances, such as chemicals, that may be encountered in the environment.

MAINTENANCE OF FLUID BALANCE

Imagine what would happen if your skin were not resistant to water! Every time it rained or you took a shower, you would soak up the water like a sponge. And every time you went out in the sun, you would run the risk of having all of your internal organs dry out. Needless to say, without your water-resistant skin, maintaining the proper fluid balance would be a constant struggle. Fortunately, the keratin-rich cells of the epidermis, combined with the oils secreted by the sebaceous glands, work very well to form a water-resistant protective barrier between your internal organs and the outside world.

REGULATION OF BODY TEMPERATURE

The skin plays a very important role in regulating the body temperature. When a person gets warm—for example, after working outside in the sun—the blood vessels in the dermis of the skin dilate (widen), allowing more blood to flow close to the surface of the skin. As the blood passes just beneath the surface of the skin, the heat the blood contains radiates out from the body, lowering the temperature of the blood. The cooled blood then travels, carrying its coolness, back to the central areas of the body, thus lowering the body temperature. The production of sweat on the skin enhances this process by cooling the skin even more so that the blood cools more effectively. In essence, this process is the body's way of "opening the windows" to allow a cool breeze to circulate through the house (Fig. 24-2A).

The reverse is true when a person gets cold, for example, following exposure to cold air. The blood vessels in the skin constrict (become narrower), limiting the amount of blood that passes close to the surface of the skin. By keeping the blood in the warmer, central areas of the body, the amount of heat that is lost to the outside environment is kept to a minimum. You have seen how your skin becomes pale or bluish when you have been outside in the cold air. Your body is essentially "closing the windows" to stop the breeze from cooling the house too much (see Fig. 24-2B).

FIGURE 24-2

The skin plays an important role in maintaining the body's temperature within the proper range. (*A*) When the internal temperature is too high, the blood vessels in the skin dilate, causing more blood to pass near the surface of the skin and allowing heat to escape into the environment. Sweat evaporating from the surface of the skin also carries heat away from the body, contributing to the cooling process. (*B*) When the internal temperature is too low, the blood vessels in the skin constrict, causing less blood to pass near the surface of the skin and keeping the heat inside the body.

SENSATION

The skin contains millions of sensory receptors, special structures that allow us to detect pain, pressure, temperature, and touch. The sensory receptors and the role they play in sensation are discussed in detail in Chapter 29.

VITAMIN D PRODUCTION

As you remember from Chapter 19, vitamin D is a nutrient that helps our bodies absorb and use calcium, a mineral that keeps our bones healthy. The skin produces vitamin D when it is exposed to the sun. In fact, sun exposure is our main source of this important vitamin! Vitamin D is also obtained by eating foods such as milk and fish.

ELIMINATION AND ABSORPTION

The skin is an active organ that is capable of both removing substances from the body and taking substances into it. For example, sweat

contains small amounts of waste materials, which leave the body when the sweat evaporates. The skin can also absorb some substances, such as chemicals. We use the ability of the skin to absorb chemicals when we give drugs using a "patch." An adhesive patch containing the drug is stuck to the skin, and the drug is slowly absorbed through the skin and into the blood vessels. You may be familiar with patches that prevent motion sickness, provide birth control, or help a person to stop smoking. In all of these cases, the drug on the patch is absorbed through the skin.

THE EFFECTS OF AGING ON THE INTEGUMENTARY SYSTEM

As we age, changes occur in all of our organ systems. These changes are not related to illness. Rather, they are normal changes that occur in everyone who reaches a certain age. These changes may just affect the person's appearance, or they may actually affect the way the person's body functions. Because there is a good chance that many of the people you will be caring for will be elderly, it is important for you to know about the changes that normally occur in each body system with aging. This knowledge will allow you to recognize age-related changes as normal. It will also allow you to provide better care for your elderly patients or residents, because you will be aware of their special needs.

CHANGES IN PHYSICAL APPEARANCE

Perhaps because the integumentary system is the most visible organ system, we have come to associate "getting old" with many of the physical changes that occur in the integumentary system as we age. Wrinkles, gray hair, and "age spots" are all very visible signs of aging (Fig. 24-3)! Wrinkles form due to the loss of **collagen,** a protein that supports connective tissue, such as that found in the dermis. In addition, the adipose (fatty) tissue in the subcutaneous layer that supports the dermis thins with age, making the subcutaneous layer less supportive of the dermis. As a result, the skin loses elasticity, leading to the formation of wrinkles. Melanin also is

FIGURE 24-3

Wrinkles, gray hair, and "age spots" result from changes to the integumentary system that occur with aging. Many people view these normal signs of aging as signs of a life well lived! The woman on the right is pictured with her daughter (*middle*) and granddaughter (*left*). You can see how the skin changes in appearance over time.

FIGURE 24-4

As skin ages, it becomes more delicate and prone to injury.

FRAGILE, DRY SKIN

There are many changes that occur to the integumentary system with aging that affect more than just our appearance. As collagen is lost from the dermis and the subcutaneous layer thins, the skin becomes thinner, more fragile, and more prone to injury (Fig. 24-4). Blood flow to the dermis decreases, and the cells of the epidermis do not replace themselves as rapidly. The decrease in blood flow to the skin means that when an injury occurs, the skin takes longer to heal itself, and the person is more at risk for developing an infection.

The number of sebaceous glands decreases, and as a result, so does the output of sebum. This leads to drying of the skin, which increases the risk for skin tears and injuries. In addition, with less sebum on the skin, the bacteria that normally live on the surface of our skin have more of a chance to cause trouble. (Recall that the acidity of sebum helps to keep these bacteria in check.)

When caring for an elderly person, keep the delicate nature of older skin in mind. Actions that would not cause harm in a younger person, such as gripping the person's arm to help her to stand or accidentally grazing her skin with your fingernails while helping her to put on her socks, can cause injury in an older person. It is very easy to tear an older person's skin, causing it to bleed. In addition, the skin of an older person is more sensitive to the drying effects of bathing than that of a younger person. In Chapter 17, you learned about some of the things that you can do to

responsible for many of the changes typically associated with aging. Gray hair is caused by the loss of melanin from the hair. "Age spots" (sometimes called "liver spots") are caused by deposits of melanin in certain areas, such as the backs of the hands or the face. Whether or not a person's skin "shows his age" depends on many factors, such as heredity; the amount of time the person spends in the sun; the person's use of tobacco, drugs, or alcohol; and the person's overall state of health. Think about all of the people you know. Do any look much younger than their actual age, or much older? What factors do you think might be responsible for the person's remarkably youthful appearance, or unusually old appearance?

increase comfort and help to keep an older person's skin healthy, such as applying lotion after a bath to keep the skin soft and pliant.

THICKENING OF THE NAILS

As we age, our nails thicken and become yellow. This is especially true of the toenails. Because the nails are so tough, they are difficult to cut, and the person may be injured during the process. As you learned in Chapter 18, a nurse or a podiatrist is usually responsible for trimming an elderly person's toenails. The nurse or podiatrist may use a tool that looks like a sander to accomplish this task safely.

LESS EFFICIENT TEMPERATURE REGULATION

Changes to the integumentary system that occur with aging also affect the older person's ability to adjust to changes in the environmental temperature. The sweat glands decrease in number and the production of sweat decreases, making an older person more vulnerable to overheating. In addition, the decreased blood flow to the skin interferes with the skin's ability to participate in temperature regulation. These changes must be considered when an older person is outside on a hot day, because they affect the ability of the body to cool itself and put the person at increased risk for heat-related problems, such as heat stroke.

DISORDERS OF THE INTEGUMENTARY SYSTEM

Many people in your care will have a disorder of the integumentary system. Sometimes, this disorder is the reason the person is in the health care facility. For example, this might be the case for a person who has suffered severe burns or trauma. Other times, the disorder develops after the person is already in the health care facility. For example, a person might develop a rash or a pressure ulcer, or have surgery that results in a surgical wound that must heal. As a nursing assistant, you will play a very important role in observing signs and symptoms of skin disorders, preventing the development of skin disorders, and helping people with skin disorders to heal.

PRESSURE ULCERS

Pressure ulcers, also known as *decubitus ulcers* or *bed sores*, form when a part of the body presses against a surface such as a mattress or chair for a long period of time. Lying on wrinkled bed linens or an object in the bed, sitting on a bedpan for a long period of time, or wearing a splint or brace that presses against the skin can also start the process of skin breakdown that leads to the formation of pressure ulcers.

Pressure ulcers are particularly likely to form over **bony prominences,** or parts of the body where there is very little fat between the bone and the skin. The weight of the person's body squeezes the soft tissue between the bony prominence and the surface the person is resting on, disrupting the flow of blood to the tissue. Lack of blood flow to the tissue deprives the tissue of oxygen and nutrients, causing it to die. Tissue death as a result of a lack of oxygen is called **necrosis.** The necrotic (dead) skin and underlying tissues peel off or break open, creating an open sore (Fig. 24-5). The sore is very painful and

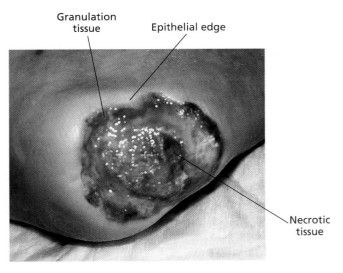

Granulation tissue

Epithelial edge

Necrotic tissue

FIGURE 24-5

Pressure ulcers are painful, difficult to treat, and potentially fatal. (Used with permission from Taylor, C., Lillis, C., & LeMone, P. [2001]. *Fundamentals of nursing: The art and science of nursing care* [4th ed., p. 935]. Philadelphia: Lippincott Williams & Wilkins.)

creates an opening for microbes to enter the body. Pressure ulcers may be very deep, extending all the way down to the bone. They are very difficult to heal once they have occurred.

You will remember from Chapter 11 that many patients and residents are not able to change position easily, due to weakness, disability, or illness. This inability to change position without help places the person at high risk for developing a pressure ulcer. The most common sites for pressure ulcers to form are on the heels, ankles, knees, hips, toes, elbows, shoulder blades, ears, and the back of the head, and along the spine (Fig. 24-6). These particular areas are referred to as **pressure points.**

The constant application of pressure on pressure points as a result of immobility is the basic cause of all pressure ulcers. Unfortunately, many people with limited mobility also have other risk factors for developing a pressure ulcer. The presence of any one of the following risk factors in a person with limited mobility makes it even more likely that the person will develop a pressure ulcer:

- **Advanced age.** As described earlier in this chapter, the normal aging process causes changes in a person's skin. The skin of an older person is fragile and thin, with less circulation. While a younger person may be able to tolerate staying in one position for 2 hours, an elderly person may need much more frequent position changes.
- **Poor nutrition and hydration.** For skin to remain healthy, good nutrition and proper hydration are essential. People who are not receiving adequate nutrition or fluids because of illness, depression, or other conditions are more likely to develop pressure ulcers. Poor nutrition will also delay the healing of any pressure ulcers that have already formed.
- **Moisture.** Prolonged contact with water, urine, feces, or sweat causes the epidermis to soften and break down. Areas where skin touches skin (such as between the thighs, the folds of the abdomen, the armpits, and under the breasts) are places where sweat or bath water may become trapped on the skin, leading to skin breakdown. In addition to moisture, sweat, urine, and feces contain irritants such as salt, ammonia, and bacteria, which further contribute to the breakdown of the skin.

Once skin breakdown begins, the door is wide open for a pressure ulcer to form.

- **Cardiovascular and respiratory problems.** A person with a heart or lung disorder often has problems getting adequate oxygen and nutrients to the tissues. In a person with a respiratory disorder, the blood that is delivered to the tissues may not contain enough oxygen. The heart of a person with a cardiovascular disorder may not be strong enough to deliver the blood to the tissues, even if it contains enough oxygen. Therefore, people with circulatory or respiratory problems are at even greater risk for developing pressure ulcers, because their tissues are already deprived of oxygen and nutrients.
- **Friction and shearing injuries.** In Chapter 11, you learned about how friction (rubbing) and shearing (pulling) forces can injure the skin and lead to skin breakdown. For example, shearing occurs when a person who is sitting up in bed slides down against the sheets. Shearing and friction injuries can also occur during repositioning.

STAGES OF PRESSURE ULCERS

Pressure ulcers develop in four stages (Fig. 24-7):

- **Stage 1.** Have you ever sat with your legs crossed for a long period of time? When you uncrossed your legs, the leg that had been on the bottom probably had a reddened area caused by the pressure of the leg that had been on top. There may even have been a slight "dent" in the skin. After a few minutes, the red area disappeared and the skin looked normal again. Every time you reposition a patient or resident, you should look carefully for reddened areas. If the person's circulation is normal, the skin will return to its normal color within a few minutes. If the skin stays red, feels hot to the touch, or is painful, you should report this finding to the nurse immediately. A reddened area that turns white means that blood flow has been compromised to the point that tissue damage has occurred. A stage 1 pressure ulcer is characterized by a reddened area of skin that does not return to the normal

FIGURE 24-6

Pressure points are areas where pressure ulcers are likely to form.

color after the pressure is removed. The reddened area may then become very pale or white and develop a shiny appearance.

- **Stage 2.** A stage 2 pressure ulcer looks like a blister, an abrasion, or a shallow crater. The epidermis peels away or cracks open, creating a portal of entry for microbes. The dermis may be partially worn away as well.
- **Stage 3.** In a stage 3 pressure ulcer, the epidermis and dermis are gone, and the subcutaneous fat may be visible in the

crater. There may be drainage from the wound.

- **Stage 4.** The crater of damaged tissue extends all the way through the tissues to the muscle or bone.

Prevention of Pressure Ulcers

As you have already learned in previous chapters, the prevention of pressure ulcers is a major concern of the nursing team. Pressure ulcers are very painful and difficult to treat. Ultimately, they

Stage 1

Stage 2

Stage 3

Stage 4

FIGURE 24-7

The four stages of pressure ulcer development. (*Stage 2 photograph © Mike Devlin/Photo Researchers, Inc. Stage 3 photograph © Science Photo Library/Photo Researchers, Inc. Stage 4 photograph © Garry Watson/ Photo Researchers, Inc.*)

can cause a person to die. For these reasons, every effort must be made to prevent a pressure ulcer from forming in the first place. As a nursing assistant, there are many things that you can do to help keep a person's skin healthy (Fig. 24-8).

- **Avoid allowing a person to remain in one position for a long period of time.** To prevent a pressure ulcer from forming, you must prevent any one part of a person's

body from being under pressure for a long period of time. This means that you should not leave a person sitting on a bedpan for a long period of time, because the bedpan places a lot of pressure on the person's lower spine, one of the pressure points. It also means that a patient or resident who must stay in bed or in a wheelchair should be repositioned at least every 2 hours. A

FIGURE 24-8

There are many things you can do to help prevent a person from getting a pressure ulcer. (*Photograph* © *Garry Watson/ Photo Researchers, Inc.*)

person who has additional risk factors for developing a pressure ulcer, as described earlier, may need to be repositioned even more often. The nursing care plan will specify how often the person should be repositioned, and the sequence of positions.

- **Use your observation skills.** Look carefully at the skin of your patients or residents each and every time you provide care. After repositioning a person, move clothing and linens aside to check for reddened areas on the side of the body that had been bearing the person's weight. When assisting a person with bathing, changing wet or soiled linens, or giving a person a back massage, take that opportunity to look carefully at the person's skin.

- **Provide good skin care.** When assisting with a bath, clean skin gently and thoroughly and rinse off the soap well. Make sure the skin is dried well and use lotion to keep the skin's surface healthy and soft. Thoroughly clean and dry areas where skin touches skin, such as under the breasts or other skin folds, and apply a light dusting of a powder containing corn starch to help keep the skin dry. Provide frequent back massage to help stimulate circulation in the skin.

- **Provide good perineal care.** Prompt removal of urine or feces from the skin is essential for the prevention of pressure ulcers. Good perineal care is especially important if a person is incontinent of urine or feces. Clean any urine or feces from the skin each time the person is incontinent. If the person is incontinent, the nurse may ask you to apply a product to the perineal area that helps to protect the skin from wetness, such as Desitin ointment, after the perineal area has been cleaned and dried.

- **Anticipate toileting needs.** Assist your patients or residents to the bathroom (or provide a bedpan or urinal) frequently, to prevent soiling of the person's clothing or bed linens. If a person is incontinent, check on him or her every hour or so. This will allow you to detect and change wet, soiled linens promptly.

- **Encourage mobility.** Some patients or residents will sit in a chair or wheelchair all day long if you do not actively encourage them to get up and move around. Ask the patient or resident to take a walk with you every 2 hours, if she is able. The exercise helps to stimulate circulation and keeps the person from sitting in the same position for long periods of time. If a person is paralyzed, remind him to change positions in his chair or have him move between the chair and the bed to prevent skin breakdown.

- **Minimize skin injury caused by friction or shearing.** Use lift devices and draw sheets when moving and repositioning people to prevent injuries caused by friction and shearing. To help prevent shearing caused by the person sliding down in bed, do not elevate the head of the bed more than 30 degrees.

- **Encourage good nutrition and hydration.** Offer refreshing drinks frequently. Encourage your patients and residents to eat well. If a patient or resident is not eating, report this observation to the nurse.

- **Use pressure-reducing devices.** Many devices are available to help reduce pressure and minimize the risk of skin breakdown. Special gel and foam pads that fit on beds or in chairs help to distribute the person's body weight more evenly, preventing any one area from bearing most of the pressure. Elbow pads and booties may help prevent friction injuries caused by the skin rubbing against the sheets (Fig. 24-9).

Some patients or residents may need a special bed to help avoid problems associated with prolonged bed rest and immobility (Fig. 24-10). Several different types of specialty beds are available:

- An **airflow bed** supports the person on a fabric-covered layer of tiny ceramic beads (see Fig. 24-10A). The beads are kept constantly in movement by a current of air. The moving beads create a fluid-like effect, much like a waterbed but without the water, that helps to prevent pressure ulcers by relieving pressure on bony prominences. In addition, the circulating air keeps the person's skin dry. If the person soils the bed, some fluids will pass through the sheet and collect in the beads. The use of a bed protector helps to greatly reduce the amount of fluid that passes through the sheet into the beads. The beads are removed from the bed and decontaminated on a regular basis by a service technician.

A

B

FIGURE 24-9

Pressure-reducing devices such as (A) elbow pads and (B) heel booties help to prevent the skin from rubbing against sheets and other surfaces.

Airflow beds are particularly useful for critically ill patients with chronic watery diarrhea or weeping wounds.

- An **alternating pressure bed** supports the person on a series of compartments that fill with air and then deflate on a rotating basis (see Fig. 24-10B). The shifting areas of inflation shift the areas of pressure from place to place, helping to improve blood flow to the skin and underlying tissues and helping to prevent pressure ulcers. These beds have protective covers, which can be wiped clean when soiled. The care of these beds is specific to type. If these beds are used in your facility, you will receive training in their care and use.

- A **wedge turning frame** (see Fig. 24-10C) or a **Circ-O-Lectric® bed** (see Fig. 24-10D) helps to prevent pressure ulcers by making it easier to reposition people who may be difficult to reposition often, such as people with spinal injuries or severe burns. These beds allow a person to be turned from front to back without changing the alignment of his or her spine. A wedge turning frame is operated by hand, whereas the Circ-O-Lectric® bed is controlled electrically. Most facilities permit only nurses to operate these beds.

WOUNDS

A **wound** is an injury that results in a break in the skin (and usually the underlying tissues as well). Although this discussion focuses on wounds that occur as a result of surgery or trauma, pressure ulcers and burns (also discussed in this chapter) are technically considered "wounds" too.

Types of Wounds

An **intentional wound** is a wound that is the result of a planned surgical or medical intervention (Fig. 24-11). For example, a woman who has delivered a baby via cesarean section or a person who is recovering from open-heart surgery will have intentional wounds caused by their surgeries. Intentional wounds also occur when intravenous (IV) lines, percutaneous endoscopic gastrostomy (PEG) tubes, or other medical devices are inserted into the body through a "man-made" opening. Intentional wounds are usually created under controlled conditions. Precautions are taken to minimize the risk of infection. The edges of the wound are usually clean and even, and held together with stitches (sutures) or staples.

An **unintentional wound** is an unexpected injury that usually results from some type of trauma. Falls, car accidents, and gun and knife violence can result in unintentional wounds (Fig. 24-12) Unintentional wounds can be *open*, which means that the surface of the skin is broken. The risk of infection is high with open wounds, because the open skin creates a portal of entry for microbes. In addition, the uneven wound edges and amount of tissue damage may make closing the wound difficult. A *closed* wound is one where the skin is not broken, but there is damage to the underlying tissues. The

A

C

D

B

FIGURE 24-10

Specialty beds help to prevent problems related to prolonged bed rest and immobility. (*A*) The Fluidair Elite® airflow bed. (*B*) The TheraPulse®ATP™ alternating pressure bed. (*C*) Wedge turning frame. (*D*) A row of Circ-O-Lectric® beds. Pictured next to the row of Circ-O-Lectric® beds is Dr. Homer Stryker, the surgeon who designed both the wedge turning frame and the Circ-O-Lectric® bed. (*Photographs A and B courtesy of Kinetic Concepts Inc. [KCI], San Antonio, Texas. Photographs C and D used with permission of Stryker Corporation.*)

deep tissue damage associated with a closed wound can be considerable, even though the only signs of injury may be redness, swelling, or bruising of the overlying skin.

Wound Healing

The human body is quite efficient at healing wounds, especially when it is otherwise healthy.

Having multiple, severe injuries; a chronic illness; or an impaired immune system can limit a person's ability to heal on his own. A person who is very young or very old may heal more slowly, or have a limited ability to heal. The same is true of a person who is malnourished.

In order for a wound to heal properly, there must be adequate blood flow to the injured area. This blood flow is responsible for the inflammation

FIGURE 24-11

A surgical incision is an example of an intentional wound. Intentional wounds are usually created under controlled conditions, minimizing the risk of infection. The edges of the wound are usually brought together and secured with stitches or staples (shown here) to promote healing and minimize scarring. (Used with permission from Craven, R.F. [2002]. *Fundamentals of nursing: Human health and function* [4th ed., p. 1017]. Philadelphia: Lippincott Williams & Wilkins.)

FIGURE 24-12

Cuts on the leg of an 80-year-old woman, who fell down the stairs. These cuts are open unintentional wounds. Open unintentional wounds carry a high risk of infection because they are often contaminated with dirt and microbes. The edges of the wound are often jagged, making it difficult to close the wound neatly. (© *Dr. P. Marazzi/ Photo Researchers, Inc.*)

that is usually observed around an injury. Inflammation is characterized by redness, swelling, heat, and pain. It is a sign that the body is working to heal itself. Healing tissues also need good hydration and nutrition. Recall from Chapter 19 that adequate protein intake is especially important when the body is trying to rebuild injured tissues.

In the health care setting, we do many things to help support the wound healing process. Some of the measures taken by the health care team to support the wound healing process include closing the wound, inserting drains, and applying dressings. As a nursing assistant, your duties related to wound care will vary, depending on your employer and the state where you work. Usually, nursing assistants are asked to assist the nurse with wound care. However, some facilities may train you to perform specific duties related to wound care on your own. As always, if you are asked to perform a task that is new to you, make sure that the task is covered by your job description and that you have received the training you will need to perform the skill properly. No matter where you work, the most important role you will play with

regard to wound care is that of "observer." As a nursing assistant, you will have the best opportunity to notice and report signs that might indicate that a wound is not healing properly or has become infected.

Wound Closure

The wound must be closed so that the body's protective covering is once again intact. If a wound is kept clean but otherwise left alone, eventually the tissue will repair itself and the wound will close on its own. However, this can take a long time, it increases the risk of infection, and it often results in a scar. To speed this process up, minimize the risk of infection, and reduce the amount of scarring, the doctor may decide to close the wound using sutures or staples. The timing for, and approach to, wound closure varies depending on the situation:

- **First-intention wound healing.** In first-intention wound healing, open wounds are closed surgically with sutures or staples. Pulling the edges of the skin and underlying tissues together and holding them closed helps speed up the healing process and minimize scarring.
- **Second-intention wound healing.** Wounds that are infected or are contaminated with dirt may be cleaned and rinsed and left open to heal from the inside out. This is called *second-intention wound healing.* Second-intention wound healing results in a wider, more noticeable scar after the wound has healed, but it prevents an unresolved infection from delaying the wound healing process.
- **Third-intention wound healing.** Sometimes it is necessary to leave a wound open, especially a traumatic wound, for a period of time to make sure that an infection is not going to occur. Then the wound edges are cleaned and closed with sutures or staples to speed the healing process. This is called *third-intention wound healing.*

Wound Drains

As part of the healing process, some wounds will produce a lot of fluid, or drainage. A wound that is infected or bleeding will also often produce a lot of drainage. Blood or fluid that is allowed to collect in a wound can promote infection, delaying the healing process. Therefore, wound drains are often used to allow blood and other fluids to flow out of the wound (Fig. 24-13).

Some drains allow fluid to collect in the wound dressing (the bandage covering the wound). Others are connected to a collection device. If a person you are caring for has a drain, take note of the characteristics of the drainage every time you check the dressing or the collection device. Is there more drainage than you expected? Does it have a foul odor that it did not have before? Has the appearance of the drainage changed? Report any unusual observations to the nurse.

FIGURE 24-13

When drainage from a wound is significant, a drain may be placed. Many types of drains are available. Here, a Hemovac drain is shown. The drainage tube is placed in the wound and attached to a suction device, which draws the fluid out of the wound.

When repositioning a person with a drain, take care not to pull on the drain tubing. Pulling on the drain tubing could pull the drain out of the wound. The loss of the drain will allow drainage to collect in the wound until the doctor can replace the drain. Drainage in the wound puts the person at risk for infection.

Wound Dressings

Sometimes dressings are applied to wounds to prevent microbes from gaining access to the body, to keep the wound dry during procedures such as bathing, or to absorb drainage from the wound. The type of dressing used depends on several factors, including:

- The type of wound
- The location of the wound
- The amount of drainage associated with the wound
- Whether or not the wound is infected
- Whether or not the wound must be kept dry
- How often the dressing must be changed

The doctor or the nurse determines which type of dressing is used.

Some dressings are made of a clear, plastic material (Fig. 24-14A). These dressings keep the wound clean and free from microbes and moisture, while allowing air to circulate freely. Some dressings are simply pieces of gauze held in place with tape (see Fig. 24-14B). Wounds that drain will have thick, absorbent dressings.

Many dressings are secured with tape. The type of tape used depends on the location of the wound and the needs of the person. For example, adhesive tape may irritate a person's skin, so a plastic or paper tape would be used instead. Elastic tape is stretchy and may be used when the wound is on a part of the body that must bend, such as the knee or elbow.

A

B

FIGURE 24-14

Various types of wound dressings and tapes are available. (*A*) Here, a wound is covered with a clear dressing that keeps moisture and microbes out of the wound, but allows air to reach the wound to promote healing. This type of dressing does not absorb drainage, but it does allow members of the health care team to look at the wound without removing the dressing. (*B*) This dressing is not waterproof, so it will need to be changed if it gets wet. The gauze prevents microbes from entering the wound, and it also absorbs drainage.

When a wound is draining heavily and the dressing must be changed often, a Montgomery tie may be used instead of tape. A Montgomery tie consists of a strip of adhesive that is attached to a cloth tie. The dressing is placed on the wound. Then, the adhesive strip of the Montgomery tie is applied to the person's skin alongside the dressing. Another Montgomery tie is placed in the same way on the other side of the dressing. Then the ties are tied together over the dressing, to hold it in place (Fig. 24-15). When it is time to change the dressing, the ties are untied, the dressing is replaced, and then the ties are retied. Because there is no need to remove the adhesive tape to change the dressing, Montgomery ties help to protect the person's skin from damage caused by the frequent removal and reapplication of tape.

You may be asked to assist the nurse with dressing changes. Procedure 24-1 explains how to help the nurse with a dressing change. Helping the nurse with a dressing change accomplishes two things. First, it minimizes the chance that the nurse's hands or other surfaces will become contaminated by the drainage on the soiled dressing. Second, it helps to ensure that the new dressing remains free of microbes that could contaminate the wound.

FIGURE 24-15

Montgomery ties can be used to secure a dressing that needs to be changed often. The adhesive is applied and then left in place. The ties secure the dressing and can be easily untied when a new dressing is needed.

BURNS

Burns are injuries to the skin and underlying tissues caused by contact with extreme heat (thermal burns), chemicals (chemical burns), or electricity (electrical burns). Burns can be minor, causing only slight redness and pain, or they can be very severe, extending down through the layers of the skin and possibly even involving the muscles and bones. Burns are classified according to the depth of the damage:

- **First-degree burns** cause injury to the outermost layer of the skin, the epidermis. Most sunburns are first-degree burns. Minor household accidents, such as touching a hot stove or leaving a heating pad that is too warm in place for too long, can also result in first-degree burns. The associated redness and pain usually goes away after a few days.
- **Second-degree burns** penetrate into the dermis of the skin. Second-degree burns are often associated with blisters. These burns are very painful and the loss of the epidermis increases the risk of infection.
- **Third-degree burns** involve the epidermis and dermis, the subcutaneous layer, and often the underlying muscles and bones as well (Fig. 24-16). People with third-degree burns need surgery and skin grafts to heal. Third-degree burns are associated with very high infection rates because the skin has been destroyed. In addition, the

scarring that results from severe burns can cause severe disfigurement and contractures of the extremities.

People who have suffered second- and third-degree burns often require months or even years of rehabilitation, and they must have multiple surgical procedures. These people need very special care. Because of the risk of infection, they may be placed in reverse (protective) isolation. Caregivers must often wear sterile gloves and gowns when providing care, and bed linens may need to be sterilized before the bed is made, to reduce the chance of infection.

LESIONS

Lesion is a general term used to describe any break in the skin. Often you will see the term *lesion* used when discussing rashes or other skin disorders. Lesions often occur in groups, forming a **rash.** Rashes can be *localized* (limited to one area) or *systemic* (occurring all over the body).

Rashes are often caused by an infection, such as chickenpox or the measles. In this case, the skin itself is not infected, but it is showing signs of an infection inside of the body. Rashes may also be caused by contact with an irritant, such as poison ivy. In people with sensitive skin, contact with substances as harmless as bath soap or laundry detergent can cause a rash called *contact dermatitis.* **Dermatitis** is a general term for

FIGURE 24-16

People with severe burns, such as the third-degree burns shown here, require special care to promote healing and prevent complications such as infection. (© *John Radcliffe Hospital/Photo Researchers, Inc.*)

inflammation of the skin. **Eczema** is a type of chronic dermatitis that is usually accompanied by severe itching, scaling, and crusting of the surface of the skin.

Itching, burning, or redness of the skin accompanies many skin lesions. The redness of the skin that often accompanies these lesions is known as **erythema.** Dermatologists (doctors who specialize in knowledge of the skin) look at the characteristics of the lesions on the skin, as well as the location of the lesions and the person's other signs and symptoms, to find clues to their cause. There are many different types of skin lesions (Fig. 24-17):

- A **macule** is a small, flat, reddened lesion. Macules often look like freckles.
- A **papule** is a small, raised, firm, lesion. Papules can be easily felt by passing your fingers lightly over the affected area.
- A **vesicle** is a small, blister-like lesion that contains watery, clear fluid.
- A **pustule** is a vesicle that contains pus, a thick, yellowish fluid that is a sign of infection.
- An **excoriation** is an abrasion, or a scraping away of the surface of the skin. Excoriations can be caused by trauma, chemicals, or burns (including friction burns from sliding a person's skin across a sheet). Urine or feces, if left on the skin for too long, can cause a chemical excoriation.
- A **fissure** is a crack in the skin. Fissures can be caused by extreme dryness. Fungal infections, such as tinea pedis (athlete's foot), can also cause fissures.
- An **ulcer** is a shallow crater that is formed when the tissue dies. The dead tissue is shed, leaving a crater behind.

Because skin lesions disrupt the skin's protective barrier, they place the person at increased risk for infection. Secondary bacterial infection of the skin is especially common when the lesion is itchy and the person scratches it excessively. *Secondary* means that the infection is occurring on top of the original problem. This is similar to what happens when you have a mosquito bite that you cannot stop scratching—eventually, you scratch it raw, it gets infected, and suddenly it takes much longer for the bite to heal than it would have if you had just left it alone.

When you are caring for a person with skin lesions, there are several things that you can do to increase the person's comfort and promote healing of the skin:

- Make sure that you are aware of any adjustments to the normal bathing and skin care routine that may be necessary. For example, you may need to use a special soap or lotion as part of the person's skin care. The nurse will be able to tell you about any necessary changes to the routine, or you can check the nursing care plan.
- Help the person to choose clothing that does not rub or irritate the skin lesion.
- Discourage the person from scratching itchy or irritated skin. Although scratching may bring temporary relief, it causes additional skin injury and puts the person at risk for infection. Soft mitt restraints or gloves may be necessary to prevent a small child or confused adult from scratching the lesions.
- Observe the lesions for changes in color, or for bleeding or drainage. Report any changes to the nurse immediately. Also note whether the lesions seem to be getting larger, or spreading to other parts of the body.

▶ *Tell the Nurse!*

The skin gives us many clues to a person's general health. In addition, if you are caring for a person who has a skin disorder, it is important to be aware of changes that might indicate that the condition is either getting better or getting worse. Tell the nurse immediately if you observe any of the following:

⟶ The person's skin looks abnormally pale or flushed, or has a bluish or yellowish hue

⟶ The person has a new rash, or changes in an existing rash

⟶ The person has a mole that has changed in appearance

⟶ The person has redness over a pressure point that does not go away within 5 minutes

⟶ An area over a pressure point that was previously red has become pale or white

⟶ A pressure ulcer has changed in size or depth

⟶ Drainage from a wound has changed in amount or appearance, or has developed a foul odor

⟶ The person has a wound that will not heal

A. Macule

B. Papule

C. Vesicle

D. Pustule

E. Excoriation

F. Fissure

G. Ulcer

FIGURE 24-17

There are many different types of skin lesions. (A) Macules are small, flat, reddened lesions. Macules are characteristic of the rash caused by measles, shown here. (B) Papules are small, raised, and firm lesions. They can be felt by lightly running your fingers over the area. (C) Vesicles are small, blister-like lesions that contain fluid. Vesicles are characteristic of the rash caused by chickenpox, shown here. (D) Pustules are vesicles that contain pus, a product of infection. Pustules are characteristic of acne vulgaris, shown here. (E) An excoriation is an abrasion, or wearing away of the surface of the skin. Irritation caused by urine or feces that has been left on the skin for too long is a type of excoriation. Excoriation can also be caused by trauma, such as the shearing and friction forces that occur when a person is dragged across a sheet. (F) A fissure is a crack in the skin, such as those associated with athlete's foot (shown here). (G) An ulcer is an open sore caused when the tissue dies. The dead tissue breaks down, leaving a crater behind. The ulcer shown here is a venous stasis ulcer. Venous stasis ulcers develop as a result of poor blood flow through the veins in the legs. (*Photo credits: A, © Dr. P. Marazzi / Science Photo Library/Custom Medical Stock Photo. B, ©Custom Medical Stock Photo. C, D, F, and G used with permission from Goodheart, H.P. [2003]. Goodheart's photoguide of common skin disorders: Diagnosis and management [2nd ed., pp. 2, 3, 154, 156]. Philadelphia: Lippincott Williams & Wilkins. E, © Logical Images/ Custom Medical Stock Photo.*)

SUMMARY

▶ The integumentary system consists of the skin and its accessory structures (hair, nails, sweat glands, and sebaceous glands).

▶ As the body's most visible organ system, the integumentary system can provide clues to a person's overall health. Changes in a person's skin tone or the development of a rash may signal an internal problem, such as liver disease, a heart or lung problem, or an infection.

▶ The integumentary system has three major functions that help maintain the body's homeostasis.

■ The skin protects us from microbes, chemicals, and other agents that could harm the body.

■ The skin helps us to maintain our internal fluid balance.

■ The integumentary system plays a major role in temperature regulation. Narrowing and widening of the blood vessels in the skin helps our bodies to maintain or release heat, respectively. The sweat glands help to cool our bodies through evaporation. Hair on our scalps and bodies helps to keep us warm.

▶ Like all organ systems, the integumentary system changes as we age.

■ Changes that affect our appearance include wrinkles, gray hair, and age spots.

■ The skin becomes more fragile and more prone to injury with age. The number and output of the sebaceous glands decrease, making the skin dry. Circulation to the skin decreases.

■ The number and output of the sweat glands decrease. This change, along with the changes in the skin, makes it harder for the older person to adjust to changes in the environmental temperature.

■ The nails become tough and yellow, making them difficult to trim.

▶ Pressure ulcers are a major concern in the health care setting.

■ Pressure ulcers develop when soft tissues are squeezed between bone and a surface, such as a mattress or chair. The weight of the body disrupts the flow of oxygen-rich blood to the tissues, causing the tissues to die and leading to the formation of a pressure ulcer.

■ Immobility is the underlying cause of all pressure ulcers. Several factors, including old age, poor nutrition, and moisture trapped in the folds of the skin, can increase an immobile person's risk of developing a pressure ulcer.

■ Warning signs of pressure ulcers include:
  • A reddened area that does not return to its normal color after the pressure is relieved
  • A previously reddened area that is hot to the touch or painful
  • An area that is pale, white, or shiny

■ Prevention of pressure ulcers is extremely important, because pressure ulcers are extremely painful, difficult to treat, and potentially fatal. The nursing assistant does many things to prevent patients and residents from developing pressure ulcers, including repositioning, observing, providing good skin and perineal care, changing wet and soiled linens promptly, and encouraging exercise.

▶ A wound is a break in the skin. The underlying tissues are usually affected as well.

■ A wound can be intentional or unintentional.

■ A break in the skin puts the person at risk for infection. Therefore, the health care team does many things to help wounds to heal quickly and with minimal complications. Sutures, dressings, and drains are commonly used to help wounds heal.

■ Nursing assistants are in an excellent position to notice and report signs and symptoms that suggest that the wound has become infected or is not healing well, such as a foul-smelling discharge or excessive drainage or bleeding.

▶ Burns are injuries caused by heat, chemicals, or electricity. People with burn wounds require special care because of the very high risk of infection.

▶ Lesions are breaks in the skin.

■ Many different types of skin lesions can form rashes.
  • The type of lesion is often a clue to the cause of the rash.
  • Rashes can be localized (limited to one area) or systemic (occurring all over the body).

■ Skin lesions can be caused by infections inside the body, infections of the skin itself, or irritation of the skin.

■ Nursing assistants are often the first to notice an unusual lesion on a patient or resident.

Chapter 24 Procedure

Getting Ready Steps

a. **W**ash your hands and observe standard precautions as necessary.

b. **G**ather needed supplies.

c. **K**nock and introduce yourself.

d. **I**dentify the person, and greet him or her by name.

e. **E**xplain the procedure.

f. **P**rovide privacy.

g. **S**ee to safety.

Finishing Up Steps

a. **C**onfirm comfort and good body alignment.

b. **L**eave the call light control within easy reach.

c. **S**ee to safety.

d. **O**pen the curtain and door.

e. **W**ash your hands.

f. **R**eport and record.

PROCEDURE 24-1

Assisting the Nurse with a Dressing Change

Getting Ready WGKIEpS

1. Complete the "Getting Ready" steps **a** through **g**.

Supplies

- gloves
- gown (if necessary)
- mask (if necessary)
- paper towels or a bed protector
- plastic bag
- tape or Montgomery ties
- dressing
- scissors

Procedure

2. Cover the over-bed table with paper towels or the bed protector. Place the dressing supplies on the over-bed table. Fold the top edges of the plastic bag down to make a cuff. Place the cuffed bag on the over-bed table.

3. Make sure that the bed is positioned at a comfortable working height (to promote good body mechanics) and that the wheels are locked. If the side rails are in use, lower the side rail on the working side of the bed. The side rail on the opposite side of the bed should remain up.

4. Help the person to a comfortable position that allows access to the wound.

5. Fanfold the top linens to the foot of the bed. Adjust the person's hospital gown or pajamas as necessary to expose the wound.

6. Put on the mask, gown, or both, if necessary. Put on the gloves.

7. The nurse will remove the old dressing. The nurse may ask you to take the old dressing and place it in the cuffed plastic bag. Be careful to keep the soiled side of the dressing out of the person's sight. Do not let the dressing touch the outside of the plastic bag.

8. Remove your gloves and dispose of them in a facility-approved waste container.

9. Wait while the nurse inspects the wound and measures it, if necessary.

10. Put on a clean pair of gloves.

11. Assist as the nurse applies a new dressing.

   a. Open the wrapper containing the dressing and hold it open so that the nurse can remove the dressing. Do not touch the dressing. Dispose of the wrapper in a facility-approved waste container.

   b. If the dressing will be secured with tape, cut four pieces of tape for securing the dressing. For a 4 ×4 dressing, each piece of

(continued)

PROCEDURE 24-1 (Continued)

Assisting the Nurse with a Dressing Change

tape should measure 8 inches long. Hang the tape from the edge of the over-bed table.

STEP 11a Hold the wrapper open so that the nurse can remove the dressing.

   c. If the nurse asks you to, use the tape strips to secure the dressing by placing one piece of tape along each side of the dressing. Center each piece of tape equally over the dressing and the person's skin.

STEP 11c The dressing is secured by placing one piece of tape along each side.

12. Remove your gloves (and gown and mask, if using) and dispose of them in a facility-approved waste container. Wash your hands.

13. Re-cover the wound with the hospital gown or pajamas. Help the person back into a comfortable position, straighten the bottom linens, and draw the top linens over the person.

14. Make sure that the bed is lowered to its lowest position and that the wheels are locked. If the side rails are in use, return the side rail to the raised position on the working side of the bed.

15. Dispose of disposable items in a facility-approved waste container. Clean equipment and return it to the storage area.

Finishing Up CLSOWR

16. Complete the "Finishing Up" steps **a** through **f**.

What did you learn?

Multiple Choice

Select the single best answer for each of the following questions.

1. Where are pressure ulcers most likely to form?
   a. On the heels, ankles, and toes
   b. On the elbows and shoulder blades
   c. On the spine
   d. All of the above

2. Why is it important to prevent pressure ulcers from forming?
   a. Pressure ulcers are disgusting to see.
   b. People who have pressure ulcers require more care than people who do not, and this is expensive for the facility.
   c. Pressure ulcers are difficult to treat and can lead to a person's death.
   d. Pressure ulcers interfere with the skin's ability to make vitamin D.

3. What is the underlying cause of all pressure ulcers?
   a. Continuous pressure applied to one area
   b. Poor nutrition
   c. Incontinence
   d. All of the above

4. Which of the following factors can increase a person's risk of getting a pressure ulcer?
   a. Advanced age
   b. Incontinence
   c. Poor nutrition
   d. All of the above

5. Mr. Underwood has developed a white, shiny area on his left hip about the size of a quarter. Yesterday, this same area was red and hot to the touch. If you were Mr. Underwood's nursing assistant, what would be your biggest concern?
   a. That Mr. Underwood has the chickenpox
   b. That Mr. Underwood has a stage 1 pressure ulcer
   c. That Mr. Underwood's wound is not healing properly
   d. That Mr. Underwood has jaundice

6. You are caring for Mrs. Kling, a 93-year-old grandmother who has limited mobility following a stroke. What should you do to minimize Mrs. Kling's chances of developing a pressure ulcer?
   a. Dry Mrs. Kling's skin thoroughly after each bath
   b. Reposition Mrs. Kling regularly, according to the nursing care plan
   c. Encourage Mrs. Kling to eat well
   d. All of the above

7. Which one of the following is an example of an intentional wound?
   a. A gunshot wound
   b. A surgical incision
   c. A lesion
   d. A burn

8. Why is it important to keep the skin healthy?
   a. The skin protects the body from microbes and helps to maintain the body's fluid balance
   b. The skin protects the body from sunburn
   c. It is easier to detect signs of disease in a person with healthy skin
   d. Keeping the skin healthy helps to prevent wrinkles in old age

Matching

Match each numbered item with its appropriate lettered description.

_____ **1.** Macules

_____ **2.** Melanin

_____ **3.** Dermatitis

_____ **4.** Vesicles

_____ **5.** Erythema

_____ **6.** Papules

_____ **7.** Pustules

_____ **8.** Excoriation

_____ **9.** Fissure

_____ **10.** Age spot

a. Redness of the skin that often accompanies rashes

b. Often seen on the backs of the hands; caused by melanin deposits

c. Cracks in the skin, such as those seen in athlete's foot

d. Abrasion or wearing away of the top layer of skin; caused by trauma, chemicals, or burns

e. Filled with pus, a thick yellow fluid associated with infection

f. Blister-like lesions that contain watery fluid, such as those seen in chickenpox

g. Flat, reddened lesions, such as those seen in measles

h. Firm, raised bumps

i. General term for inflammation of the skin

j. Gives the skin its color

Stop and think!

▶ You have been assigned to help Mrs. Sills with her morning care. While you are helping Mrs. Sills to put on her socks, you accidentally scratch Mrs. Sills' ankle, causing her to bleed. Mrs. Sills does not seem to be aware of what has happened. What should you do?

▶ Richard is providing care to Mr. O'Meara, who has just been transferred to Willow Wood Care Center. Mr. O'Meara is confined to a wheelchair. While giving Mr. O'Meara a back massage as part of evening care, Richard notices a reddened area at the base of Mr. O'Meara's spine. What are the possible explanations for this finding? What should Richard do?

CHAPTER

25

The Musculoskeletal System

What will you learn?

Think about everything you have done so far today. Before you even left the house this morning, you did a number of different tasks requiring the services of your musculoskeletal system—getting out of bed, brushing your teeth, eating breakfast, and taking the dog for a walk or feeding the cat, just to name a few. Think about all of the individual movements that each of these small tasks requires, and you will get a sense of how very important the musculoskeletal system is to our daily functioning.

The muscular system and the skeletal system work together to enable us to move. As you learned in Chapter 23, sometimes these two organ systems are referred to together as the *musculoskeletal system* because they work so closely together. In this chapter, you will learn about the structure and function of the musculoskeletal system, and about how it is affected by aging and illness. You will also learn about how the nursing assistant helps residents and patients to maintain proper function of the musculoskeletal system. When you are finished with this chapter, you will be able to:

1. List the major parts of the musculoskeletal system.
2. List and describe the four types of bones found in the skeletal system.
3. Define terms used to describe joint movement.
4. List and describe the three types of muscles found in the muscular system.
5. Discuss the main functions of the musculoskeletal system.
6. Describe how normal aging processes affect the musculoskeletal system.
7. Describe some of the disorders than can affect the musculoskeletal system.

(continued)

Photo: The musculoskeletal system allows us to move.
(© Bill Bachmann/Photo Researchers, Inc.)

8. Define normal range of motion and describe methods used to maintain joint function in the health care setting.
9. Demonstrate how to help a person to perform range-of-motion exercises.
10. Discuss the use of heat and cold applications to promote a person's comfort.
11. Demonstrate how to safely use heat and cold applications in the health care setting.
12. Discuss rehabilitation measures that are commonly used in the health care setting that are specific to the musculoskeletal system.

Vocabulary

Use the CD in the back of your book to hear these terms pronounced, defined, and used in a sentence:

Skeleton	Tendons	Arthritis	Traction
Joints	Aponeurosis	Muscular dystrophy	Trapeze bar
Range of motion	Muscle tone	Fracture	Amputation
Cartilage	Atrophy	Reduction	Stump
Ligaments	Osteoporosis	Fixation	Phantom pain

STRUCTURE OF THE MUSCULOSKELETAL SYSTEM

The musculoskeletal system consists of the skeletal system and the muscular system.

THE SKELETAL SYSTEM

The skeletal system consists of the bones. The 206 bones in the human body form a framework called the **skeleton** (Fig. 25-1). The skeleton gives structure and shape to the body, and protects key vital organs, such as the heart and the brain, from injury.

The bones of the skeleton vary in size and shape. Bones are classified according to their shape (Fig. 25-2):

- **Long bones.** When we think of a "bone," what we often picture in our mind is an example of a long bone. The long bones are found in the arms and the legs. Long bones consist of a shaft, called the *diaphysis,* and two rounded ends, called the *epiphyses.*
- **Short bones.** Short bones are round or cube-shaped. Short bones are found in the wrists and ankles.

- **Flat bones** are relatively thin and may be curved. Examples of flat bones include the ribs and the bones that form the skull.
- **Irregular bones** are oddly shaped bones that are not flat. Irregular bones are found in the spinal column and face.

Bones must be strong enough to support and protect the body, yet light enough to allow us to move. Can you imagine how heavy a large bone like the bone in your thigh would be, if it were solid? Instead, bones have two layers. The outside of the bone is hard and solid. The inside of the bone is sponge-like and airy. Thin strands of bone form a net-like structure, and the spaces in between the thin strands of bone are filled with bone marrow (Fig. 25-3). This combination of a solid, hard outside and a sponge-like inside results in bones that are very strong and able to resist a great amount of force, yet lightweight. The cells that form the bones are constantly broken down and replaced with new bone cells throughout a person's lifetime. A complex network of blood vessels supplies the bone cells with the oxygen and nutrients they need.

The areas where two bones join together are called **joints.** Joints allow us to move. The **range of motion** of a joint is the complete extent of movement that the joint is normally capable of

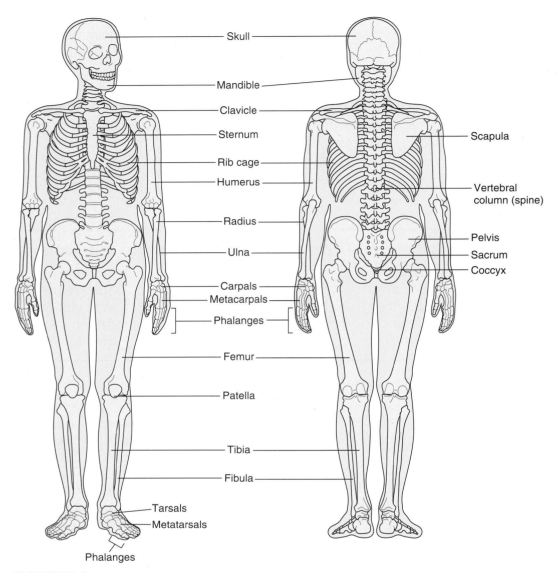

FIGURE 25-1

The human skeleton contains 206 bones. Some of the major bones are labeled here.

without causing pain. Joints can be classified according to the amount of movement they allow (Fig. 25-4):

- **Fixed joints** do not permit any movement at all. The joints between the bones of the skull are examples of fixed joints.
- **Slightly movable joints** allow for limited movement. Slightly movable joints are found between the vertebrae in the spine, and where the ribs attach to the sternum (breastbone). **Cartilage,** a tough, fibrous substance, fills in the space between the bones in the slightly movable joint. The cartilage permits limited movement and acts as a "shock absorber" between the bones.

- **Freely movable joints** allow for a wide range of movement. Examples of freely movable joints include the knees, elbows, finger and toe joints, and hip joints. Some of the ways in which freely movable joints move are shown and defined in Table 25-1. The ends of the bones that form the freely movable joint are covered with cartilage, which provides a smooth surface for the other bones to move against. A capsule formed of connective tissue encloses the ends of the bones, forming a joint cavity. The lining of the capsule secretes a thick fluid called *synovial fluid* into the joint cavity. The synovial fluid lubricates the

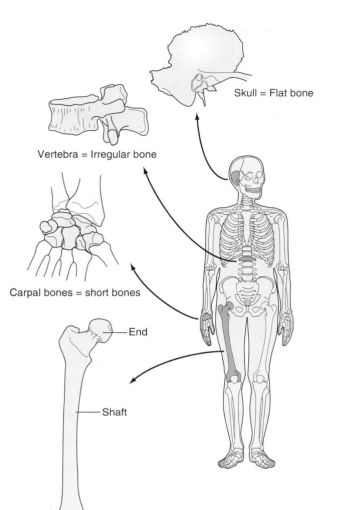

Skull = Flat bone

Vertebra = Irregular bone

Carpal bones = short bones

End

Shaft

End

Femur = long bone

FIGURE 25-2

Bones can be categorized by their shape. General types of bones include long bones, short bones, flat bones, and irregular bones.

FIGURE 25-3

An artist's drawing of healthy bone. (© *Articulate Graphics/Custom Medical Stock Photo.*)

is the type of muscle tissue found in the musculoskeletal system. Skeletal muscle is said to be *striated*, because the muscle fibers make the muscles look like they have stripes. (*Striations* is another word for "stripes.")

There are almost 700 individual skeletal muscles in the body (Fig. 25-5). These muscles account for about 40% of your total body weight. Skeletal muscles vary in shape. Some are long, thick, and band-like. Others are flat or fan-like. Muscles are named according to their location, their shape, or their function.

The skeletal muscles are attached to the bones by bands of connective tissue called **tendons.** Occasionally, skeletal muscles are attached to other muscles by a broad, flat sheet of tendon called an **aponeurosis.**

FUNCTION OF THE MUSCULOSKELTAL SYSTEM

The musculoskeletal system has several vital functions.

joint, which helps the joint to move smoothly. **Ligaments,** which are very strong bands of fibrous tissue, cross over the joint capsule, attaching one bone to another and stabilizing the joint. If the ligament is torn or weak, the joint may be able to move too much in any one direction.

THE MUSCULAR SYSTEM

The muscular system consists of the muscles. As you learned in Chapter 23, there are three types of muscle tissue found in the body (see Chapter 23, Table 23-1). Of the three types, skeletal muscle

PROTECTION

The bones of the skeletal system protect delicate internal organs. For example, the skull bones surround and protect the brain, and the rib cage surrounds and protects the lungs and heart.

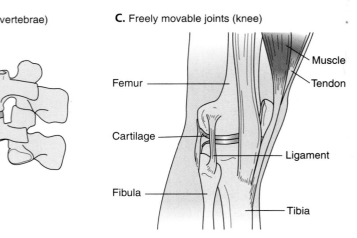

A. Fixed joints (skull)

Sutures

B. Slightly movable joints (vertebrae)

Cartilage ("shock absorber")

C. Freely movable joints (knee)

Muscle

Tendon

Femur

Cartilage

Ligament

Fibula

Tibia

FIGURE 25-4

Joints are often categorized by the amount of motion they permit. *(A)* Fixed joints, such as the joints that join the bones of the skull, do not allow for any movement. *(B)* Slightly movable joints, such as those between the vertebrae in the spinal column, permit some movement. *(C)* Freely movable joints, such as the knee joints, allow for a wide range of movement.

SUPPORT

The bones of the skeleton form a framework that supports and gives shape to the body. **Muscle tone,** or the steady contraction of the skeletal muscles, helps us to maintain an upright posture, such as sitting or standing. The muscles of the back, neck, shoulders, and abdomen are responsible for maintaining posture.

MOVEMENT

Voluntary movement occurs when a skeletal muscle contracts (shortens) or relaxes (lengthens) across a freely movable joint. In freely movable joints, each skeletal muscle attaches to the bone in two places, the origin and the insertion. The origin and the insertion points are on opposite sides of the joint. So, when the muscle contracts, the muscle shortens and the origin and insertion points are drawn closer to each other, causing the part of the body to move (Fig. 25-6).

Skeletal muscles usually work in groups to provide body movement. For example, your biceps muscle is located on the front of your upper arm. When you contract your biceps muscle, your lower arm is drawn toward your body. When you are lifting a heavy object, the brachioradialis muscle, which is also located in your upper arm, also contracts, helping to stabilize the elbow and assisting the biceps muscle with lifting. When it

is time to straighten the arm again, the biceps muscle relaxes and the triceps muscle, located on the back of the upper arm, contracts, pulling the lower arm back into a straight position.

HEAT PRODUCTION

Contraction of the skeletal muscles produces heat and helps to maintain a constant body temperature. This is why we feel warmer when we move back and forth and stamp our feet while waiting outside on a cold day for a bus or train. The movement of the muscles produces heat, which makes us feel warmer. This is also why, when it is very cold, we may start to shiver. Shivering occurs when the skeletal muscles contract rapidly in unison. The involuntary contractions help to increase the heat output of the muscles, raising the body temperature and making us feel warmer.

CALCIUM STORAGE

Calcium is an important mineral that is necessary for the proper functioning of skeletal and cardiac muscle. Calcium is also what makes the bone tissue hard and strong. Most of the calcium we need to function on a daily basis is obtained from calcium-rich foods and beverages, such as milk, cheese, yogurt, broccoli, leafy greens, tofu,

TABLE 25-1 ■ Words Used to Describe Movement

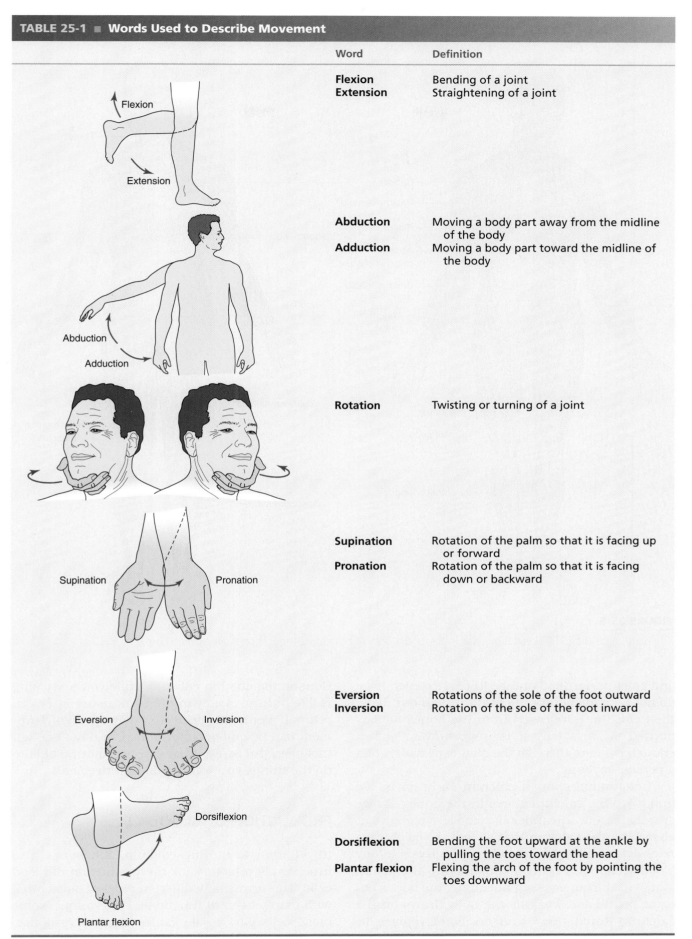

Word	Definition
Flexion	Bending of a joint
Extension	Straightening of a joint
Abduction	Moving a body part away from the midline of the body
Adduction	Moving a body part toward the midline of the body
Rotation	Twisting or turning of a joint
Supination	Rotation of the palm so that it is facing up or forward
Pronation	Rotation of the palm so that it is facing down or backward
Eversion	Rotations of the sole of the foot outward
Inversion	Rotation of the sole of the foot inward
Dorsiflexion	Bending the foot upward at the ankle by pulling the toes toward the head
Plantar flexion	Flexing the arch of the foot by pointing the toes downward

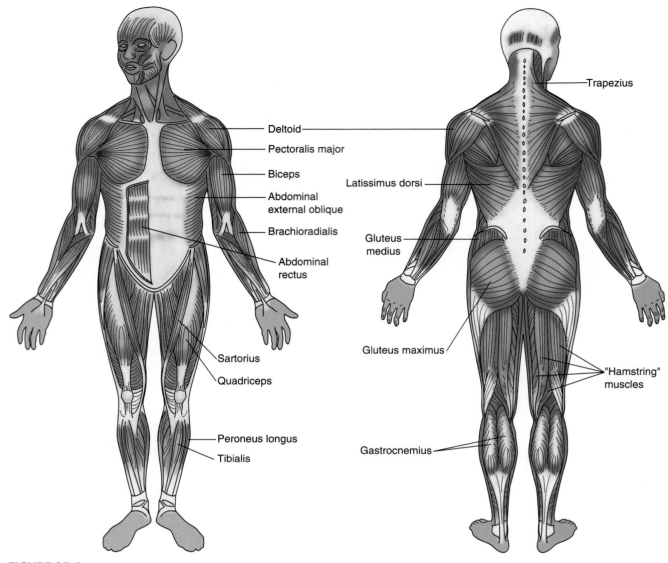

FIGURE 25-5

There are more than 700 skeletal muscles in the body! Some of the more familiar ones are labeled here.

and calcium-fortified orange juice. However, if we do not take in enough calcium through our diets, then calcium is released from the bones as it is needed. This is why it is important to obtain enough calcium through the diet, especially when a person is young.

Consuming enough calcium early on in life builds up the calcium stores in the bones. As we grow older, our intestines become less effective at absorbing the calcium that we eat, so calcium is released from the bones to keep the levels in our bloodstream constant. If the amount of calcium stored in the bones is not adequate, the bones become brittle and weak as the body draws on the calcium stored there and does not replace it.

Consuming enough calcium while you are young is like putting money in the bank to use after you retire. If plenty has been stored away, then retirement can be quite comfortable. But if not enough has been put away, then you may not be able to do the things you want to do in retirement.

PRODUCTION OF BLOOD CELLS

In addition to storing calcium, the bones also function as a factory for the production of blood cells. There are many different types of blood cells, with many different functions. For example, some blood cells play a role in the immune response,

A. Muscle relaxed

Origin of biceps

Triceps

Biceps

Insertion of biceps

B. Muscle contracted

Origin of biceps

Insertion of biceps

FIGURE 25-6

The muscular and the skeletal systems work together to produce movement. The muscle attaches to the bone in two places, the origin and the insertion. (*A*) Shown here are the attachments of the biceps muscle, the muscle in your upper arm that bulges when you "make a muscle." (*B*) When you contract your biceps muscle, the origin and insertion points are drawn closer together. As the muscle shortens, it pulls on the bone, bringing your lower arm toward your body.

and help us to fight off infection. Other blood cells carry oxygen to the tissues of the body. Blood cells form in red bone marrow, which is found in flat bones and the ends of the long bones. In young children, the shaft of the long bones also contains red bone marrow, but that red bone marrow is gradually replaced by yellow bone marrow as the person grows older. Yellow bone marrow is made up mostly of fatty tissue that can be used by the body for energy if necessary.

THE EFFECTS OF AGING ON THE MUSCULOSKELETAL SYSTEM

The normal processes of aging cause significant changes in the musculoskeletal system. It is the rare older person who does not have some degree of disability or discomfort related to the functioning of his or her musculoskeletal system! Aches, pains, and stiffness often accompany these

changes. Occasionally, the person loses the ability to move one or more parts of his or her body. Age-related changes affecting the musculoskeletal system are the leading cause of disability in older adults.

It is now known that participating in regular physical exercise and eating properly are measures that can delay or decrease the effects of aging on the musculoskeletal system. Engaging in some form of weight-bearing exercise, such as brisk walking, aerobics, or moderate weight training, has been shown to have many positive effects, even in very old people (Fig. 25-7). Weight-bearing exercise helps to maintain bone strength by stimulating the body to store extra calcium in the bones. It improves blood flow, allowing more oxygen and nutrients to be carried to the tissues of the musculoskeletal system. Continued use of the

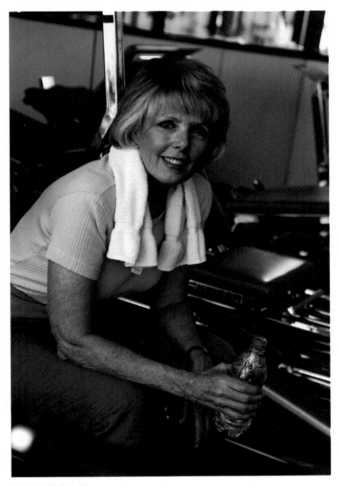

FIGURE 25-7

It is never too late to begin exercising! Regular exercise strengthens the muscles, helps to build bone mass, and lessens joint pain and stiffness.

muscles helps to retain strength. Flexibility of the joints is improved with regular exercise, which leads to fewer aches and pains.

People typically begin to experience age-related changes to the musculoskeletal system after the age of 40 years, although the onset of these changes may be significantly delayed in people who exercise regularly and are relatively healthy. The normal age-related changes that affect the musculoskeletal system include loss of bone tissue, loss of muscle mass, and wear and tear on the joints.

LOSS OF BONE TISSUE

As noted earlier in this chapter, aging decreases the body's ability to absorb calcium, a critical nutrient. When the body cannot get the amount of calcium it needs from the diet alone, it begins to draw on the calcium stored in the bones. Some people begin drawing on their calcium stores at a relatively young age, for example, when they are in their 40s. The continuous, gradual loss of calcium causes the bones to lose their strength and hardness, making them more fragile and prone to breaking. If other conditions, such as poor nutrition, poor circulation, or a lack of physical activity are present, the loss of strong bone tissue occurs much more rapidly.

LOSS OF MUSCLE MASS

The number of muscle cells also starts to gradually decrease when a person is in his or her 40s, resulting in a decrease in the size and strength of each individual muscle. The loss of muscle size and strength is called muscle **atrophy** (Fig. 25-8). If a person is poorly nourished, is not physically active, or has a chronic medical condition, muscle atrophy progresses at a much faster rate. If you have ever had a broken bone that required a cast, you probably noticed that after the cast was removed, the affected limb was smaller and weaker than the other one. What you noticed was muscle atrophy as a result of not being able to use the muscle during the time that the limb was in the cast!

Significant loss of muscle tissue can leave a person too weak to walk or carry out routine activities of daily living (ADLs). Loss of muscle

FIGURE 25-8

Muscle atrophy, or loss of muscle mass, is a normal age-related change. Immobility can make muscle atrophy much more severe.

tissue also affects the body's ability to produce heat. This is one reason why an elderly person might feel chilly in a room that a younger person would consider warm or even hot.

WEAR AND TEAR ON THE JOINTS

As we age, we lose the proteins that make the ligaments, tendons, and cartilage elastic and flexible, which can lead to stiffness and pain in the joints. The normal demands of daily life also cause a lot of wear and tear on the joints, which can, over time, lead to stiffness and pain. Overuse or injury of a joint, or being overweight, places extra strain on certain joints and will make the normal changes associated with aging more severe. Joint pain and stiffness can make simple activities, such as walking or getting out of a chair, difficult. Joint stiffness can also make a person more likely to fall.

DISORDERS OF THE MUSCULOSKELETAL SYSTEM

Depending on where you work, it is likely that many of the people in your care will have some degree of musculoskeletal disability, simply as a result of their age. You may also care for people who have musculoskeletal disability as a result of disease or trauma. Examples of diseases that affect the bones, joints, and muscles include osteoporosis, arthritis, and muscular dystrophy.

Fractures (broken bones) are usually caused by trauma. Amputation (the loss of a limb) may be necessary because of trauma or complications of a disease, such as diabetes.

OSTEOPOROSIS

Osteoporosis is the excessive loss of bone tissue. Although everyone experiences some loss of bone tissue as a normal part of aging, people with osteoporosis lose excessive amounts of bone tissue, causing the bones to become crumbly and very fragile. The bones most commonly affected by osteoporosis are the bones of the spine, the pelvis, and the long bones in the arms and legs (Fig. 25-9).

A

B

FIGURE 25-9

Osteoporosis. (*A*) A magnetic resonance imaging (MRI) scan of the spine of a 60-year-old patient with osteoporosis. This is a side view (the patient is standing , facing the left). The vertebrae (*brown*) enclose the spinal cord (*pink*). Some of the vertebrae (*orange*) have collapsed as a result of osteoporosis, causing the spine to curve. (*B*) This woman has a "dowager's hump" as a result of osteoporosis of the spine. The deformity occurs when the fragile bones of the spine crumble. (*A*, © *Zephyr/ Photo Researchers, Inc.*; *B*, © *John Radcliffe Hospital/ Photo Researchers, Inc.*)

Osteoporosis is most common in older women who have gone through menopause. This is because estrogen, a hormone that is present in the bodies of women who are still having menstrual periods, helps to prevent bone loss. However, when a woman's periods stop, her body stops producing estrogen, and this puts her more at risk for bone loss. Other risk factors for the development of osteoporosis include:

- White race
- "Small bones"
- Smoking
- Inactivity or immobility
- Diseases of the thyroid and adrenal glands
- A diet lacking in calcium, vitamin D (necessary for the absorption of calcium), and protein
- Certain drugs, such as steroids

Osteoporosis causes bones to break more easily, and physical activity becomes very difficult. Sometimes bones are so brittle that a person can break them just by bumping into a piece of furniture. Bones that have been fractured are difficult to repair and heal slowly. Crumbling of the bones of the spinal column causes the upper back to curve into the deformity known as a "dowager's hump" (see Fig. 25-9). These spinal column fractures are very painful and debilitating.

For people who have osteoporosis, some treatments are available. A drug that helps to slow the progression of osteoporosis has been developed. In addition, hormone replacement therapy and the use of calcium and vitamin D supplements can also help in the treatment of osteoporosis. Resistance training (lifting weights) slows the progression of the disease by helping to promote bone strength. However, as with most things, prevention is the best medicine! Osteoporosis can be prevented in many cases by exercising regularly and eating a diet rich in calcium, protein, and vitamin D, starting early in life.

When caring for a person with osteoporosis, remember to be gentle when helping the person with transfers. Encourage exercise by having the person take frequent walks with you. Carefully observe and document the types of foods and liquids the person eats and drinks, and encourage snacks that are high in calcium, such as milk, yogurt, ice cream, and cheese. Be especially observant of loss of function, swelling, or complaints of pain. These signs and symptoms may indicate a new fracture in a fragile bone.

ARTHRITIS

Arthritis is inflammation of the joints, usually associated with pain and stiffness. Arthritis is the most common disorder of the musculoskeletal system, affecting people of all ages. There are more than 20 different types of arthritis. Three of the most common types are osteoarthritis, rheumatoid arthritis, and gout.

Osteoarthritis

Osteoarthritis is the leading cause of physical disability among elderly people. In osteoarthritis, the cartilage that covers the ends of the bones wears away, making movement of the joint difficult and painful. Osteoarthritis appears to be the result of normal wear and tear on the joint, which is why it is seen most often in elderly people. However, obesity, previous joint injury, or a family history of the disease may increase a person's risk of developing osteoarthritis earlier in life and more severely.

Osteoarthritis usually affects weight-bearing joints, such as the knees, hips, and joints of the spinal column. Osteoarthritis begins when the smooth cartilage on the ends of the bones becomes rough, due to normal use of the joint. The rough area then becomes inflamed, and bony deposits build up. These bony deposits rub against the cartilage, causing even more damage. This cycle repeats until the cartilage has been worn down to the point where bone is actually rubbing against bone as the joint moves. The joint becomes swollen, stiff, and very painful.

A person with osteoarthritis may take medications to decrease both the pain and swelling. Heat and cold applications, discussed later in this chapter, can also increase a person's level of comfort. Mild exercise that places the affected joints through their range of motion helps to diminish stiffness and maintain joint function. People who have very severe osteoarthritis may need surgery to replace the joint. Hips and knees are the joints most commonly replaced, but replacement of shoulder, elbow, wrist, and hand joints is also possible. Joint replacement surgery, also called total joint replacement, involves removing the ends of the bones in the affected joint and replacing them with parts made from metal and plastic (Fig. 25-10).

As a nursing assistant, you may be responsible for caring for a person who is recovering from

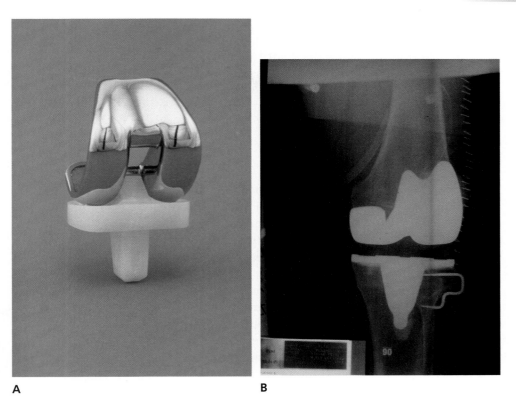

FIGURE 25-10

In joint replacement surgery, a damaged joint is replaced with an artificial (prosthetic) joint. (*A*) An artificial knee joint. (*B*) X-ray of an artificial knee joint in place. (*A, © SIU Bio Med/ Custom Medical Stock Photo; B, © R. D'Amico/Custom Medical Stock Photo.*)

A   **B**

joint replacement surgery. People who have had a joint replaced are not allowed to bear weight on the affected joint for a period of time after the surgery, so you will need to help them with transfers. In addition, people who have had a hip joint replaced have several special care requirements during the recovery period:

- Following the surgery, the muscles and ligaments that normally hold the hip joint in place are weak, making it very easy for the head of the femur (the thigh bone) to dislocate, or pop out of joint. To prevent this from happening, the person's legs must be spread apart (abducted) when the person is in the supine or lateral position. Most people who have had hip replacement surgery will have a special wedge-shaped pillow, called an *abduction pillow*, which goes between the legs and attaches to each leg with *hook-and-loop fasteners* (Fig. 25-11). The abduction pillow helps to keep the legs spread. If an abduction pillow is not available, a regular pillow can be used instead.
- When sitting, a person who has had hip replacement surgery must use a straight-backed chair. The person's hips must be flexed no more than 90 degrees, and his

feet must rest flat on the floor. This is true when the person is using the toilet or commode, as well. A special device may be used to raise the height of the toilet seat to prevent flexion in excess of 90 degrees when the person is using the toilet.

- A physical therapist will work with the person after surgery. If possible, you should be present while the therapist is working

FIGURE 25-11

When a person is recovering from hip joint replacement surgery, an abduction pillow is used to help prevent the hip joint from becoming dislocated during the recovery period.

with the person. That way, you can see the specific ambulation and transfer techniques that are being used with your patient or resident.

As always, you should ask the nurse for any specific instructions or restrictions that are specific to your patient or resident.

Rheumatoid Arthritis

Rheumatoid arthritis is a crippling condition that can cause severe joint deformities (Fig. 25-12). Unlike osteoarthritis, rheumatoid arthritis affects people much younger in life, most often between the ages of 20 and 40 years. This disease is more common in women than in men.

Researchers believe that rheumatoid arthritis is an autoimmune disorder. In autoimmune disorders, the body's immune system begins to attack the body's own tissues. So, for example, in rheumatoid arthritis, the immune system attacks and destroys the cartilage that covers the ends of the bones. Scar tissue develops within the joints, causing them to become stiff and useless. For many months, a person's rheumatoid arthritis may seem to be under control, but then the person will experience an acute flare-up of the disease. During the acute phases of the disease, the person may experience pain, swelling, redness, and heat in the joints, as well as fever and general weakness. Bed rest may be necessary, and splints can help decrease joint deformity. The gentle use of active and active-assistive range-of-motion exercises (discussed later in this chapter) helps to maintain joint mobility.

FIGURE 25-12

This woman has rheumatoid arthritis in the joints of her hands.

Gout

Gout is a type of arthritis that is caused by a disturbance in the body's metabolism. Uric acid is a waste product of metabolism that is usually eliminated from the body in the urine. If the body produces too much uric acid or the kidneys are unable to properly process the uric acid, the uric acid builds up in the body, forming crystals that are deposited within the joints. These uric acid crystals are extremely irritating to the tissues in the joint, and, as a result, the joint becomes inflamed and painful. While gout can affect any joint, the big toe is most commonly affected. Men past middle age are more commonly affected than women.

MUSCULAR DYSTROPHY

Muscular dystrophy is a general term for a group of disorders that cause the skeletal muscles to become more and more weak over time. These disorders are inherited. The types of muscular dystrophy vary according to the muscles that are affected, the age of the person typically affected, and the rate at which the disease progresses.

One type of muscular dystrophy is myasthenia gravis. In myasthenia gravis, the muscle's ability to respond to commands from the nervous system is affected. Therefore, the muscle cannot contract, and it becomes weak and atrophied. Duchenne's muscular dystrophy, another type of muscular dystrophy, usually affects children and causes death by the age of 20 years. The person dies because the muscles that allow him to breathe eventually become too weak to perform this vital function.

If one of your patients or residents has muscular dystrophy, the person will need assistance with range-of-motion exercises, walking, positioning, and ADLs. Eventually, when the disease begins to affect the muscles that control swallowing, you will also have to help the person with eating.

FRACTURES

A **fracture** is a broken bone. Fractures are usually caused by trauma, such as a fall or a car accident. However, some fractures are caused when a bone is subjected to constant and repeated stress. For example, you may have heard of a distance runner being diagnosed with a "stress fracture" in the small bones of the foot. Think about how many times a runner's foot pounds against the pavement, and the force behind each step, and you will understand how a stress fracture can occur!

Older people are especially at risk for fractures, because the bones become more fragile with age. Older people are also more likely to have diseases that put them at risk for fractures, such as osteoporosis or bone cancer. Weak, brittle bones can fracture easily, often from a seemingly minor fall or stumble. For example, hip fractures are quite common in older women who have fallen just a short distance, such as from a standing position to the floor or sidewalk. Not only do the bones of an older person fracture more easily, they take longer to heal and they may heal improperly. Delayed or improper healing may cause prolonged difficulty with mobility.

Types of Fractures

Fractures can occur in almost any bone in the body and are classified in the following manner (Fig. 25-13):

- **Closed fracture.** The bone is broken, but the broken ends do not protrude through the overlying skin.

- **Open fracture.** The bone is broken, and the sharp ends of the broken bone have broken through the skin. Because the skin is broken, open fractures carry a very high risk of infection.

- **Greenstick fracture.** Have you ever tried to snap a young, green twig? Unlike a dry, brown stick, a green twig will bend and splinter, but it will not break all the way through. In a greenstick fracture, the same thing occurs—the bone bends and splinters, but it does not break all the way through. Greenstick fractures occur most commonly in children because their bones are still quite flexible.

- **Impacted fracture.** The bone is broken all of the way through, and the broken ends of the bone are jammed into each other. These fractures are often seen in people who have jumped or fallen from a height, for example, off of a roof or ladder.

- **Comminuted fracture.** The bone is splintered into several little pieces. This type of fracture is common when a bone has been crushed under a great weight. The surrounding tissues, such as muscle and skin, may be seriously injured as well.

- **Spiral fracture.** The break circles around the bone in a winding fashion. Spiral fractures are common when the bone has been subjected to a twisting force.

| Closed fracture | Open fracture | Greenstick fracture | Impacted fracture | Comminuted fracture | Spiral fracture |

FIGURE 25-13

There are many different types of fractures.

Treatments for Fractures

Reduction and Fixation

For a fractured bone to heal properly, the broken ends of the bone must be brought together (aligned) and then held in that position until the fracture heals. **Reduction** is the word used to describe the process of bringing the broken ends of the bone into alignment. **Fixation** is the word used to describe the process of holding the bone in one position until the fracture heals. There are many ways to accomplish reduction and fixation. The method used depends on the type and location of the fracture.

In a closed reduction, the doctor lines up the broken ends of the bone by simply pushing them back into place. In a closed reduction, it is not necessary to create a surgical incision to access the broken bone. Following a closed reduction, a cast (made of fiberglass or plaster of Paris) is applied to keep the bone in the proper alignment until healing occurs (Fig. 25-14A). First, a thin layer of cotton is placed on the skin to protect it. Then, the casting material is soaked in water and wrapped around the limb. As the casting material dries, it hardens, preventing movement of the broken bone. A cast is a method of external fixation, or fixation that is achieved without surgery. General guidelines for caring for a person with a cast are given in Guidelines Box 25-1.

Sometimes it is necessary to surgically expose the bone to line up the broken ends of the bone. This is called an open reduction. Often, open reduction is followed by internal fixation. Internal fixation involves the use of metal plates, screws, rods, pins, or wires to hold the broken ends of the bone in place until the bone is healed (see Fig. 25-14B). You may see the notation "ORIF" on a person's chart. This means

A

B

FIGURE 25-14

With any fracture, the broken ends of the bone need to be brought back together (reduction) and held in place (fixation). (*A*) Fixation can be accomplished externally, with a cast, or (*B*) it can be accomplished internally, with devices such as plates, screws, pins, or wires. (*A, © L. Steinmark/Custom Medical Stock Photo.*)

GUIDELINES BOX 25-1
GUIDELINES FOR CARING FOR A PERSON WITH A CAST

What you do	Why you do it
Do not cover the cast or place it on a plastic-covered pillow until it has dried completely.	The casting material produces heat as it dries. Covering the cast can cause the person's skin underneath the cast to burn.
Do not touch the cast with your fingertips until it is totally dry. If you must handle the cast, use the palms of your hands.	Touching the cast can cause it to dent, creating pressure spots against the person's skin.
Keep the casted body part elevated on a pillow for several days.	Elevating the casted body part helps prevent and reduce swelling around the fracture site.
Because the skin underneath the cast can start to itch, the person may try to slide an object between the cast and the skin in order to scratch the itchy area. Advise the person that placing objects inside of the cast should be avoided.	Sliding an object between the cast and the skin may injure the skin, which puts the person at risk for infection.
Make sure the person's toes (or fingers, if the cast is on the arm) are pink, warm, and moving. Report any complaints of increased pain, numbness, or tingling. Report any observations of cyanosis, increased swelling, cold toes or fingers, increased drainage on the cast, or a foul odor immediately.	Cyanosis; increased swelling; increased pain, numbness, or tingling; or cold fingers or toes may indicate that swelling inside the cast is interfering with blood flow. If the tissues do not receive enough oxygen and nutrients, tissue death and skin breakdown may occur. Increased drainage or a foul odor may indicate infection.
Keep the cast clean and dry.	Plaster cast material becomes soft again when it becomes wet.
Do not allow the person to place pressure or weight on the cast unless he has been specifically instructed to do so.	Placing too much pressure or weight on the cast can cause the cast to break.

that the person has had surgery to achieve an "**O**pen **R**eduction, **I**nternal **F**ixation."

Traction

Some fractured bones cannot be repaired surgically for a period of time, especially if the person's overall medical condition is unstable. In these cases, traction is used to keep the broken ends of the bone in alignment until the fracture can be permanently repaired by surgery or casting. In **traction,** the ends of the bones are placed in the proper alignment and then weight is applied to exert a constant pull and keep the bone in alignment. In skin traction, weight is suspended from a traction unit that is attached to the person's skin (Fig. 25-15A). In skeletal traction, weight is suspended from pins that are driven through the bone (see Fig. 25-15B). A **trapeze bar** may be attached to the overhead frame

of the person's bed. The person grasps the trapeze bar to assist with movement.

A person in traction has several special care needs, many of which arise from the person's limited ability to move or change position:

- You may be asked to assist the person with range-of-motion exercises to work the unaffected joints and keep them limber.
- The person will have to use a fracture bedpan (see Chapter 20, Figure 20-3B), which is easier to slide under the buttocks.
- Pressure ulcers are always a concern, so it is important to keep the person's skin clean and dry, and to monitor for signs of skin breakdown.
- Two people usually work together to change the bed linens, and the linens are changed from the top of the bed (working

A. Skin traction   **B. Skeletal traction**

FIGURE 25-15

Traction is used to hold the broken ends of a bone in alignment until the fracture can be repaired permanently. (*A*) In skin traction, a device is attached to the person's skin, and weight is suspended from it. (*B*) In skeletal traction, pins are driven through the bone to support the weight. (*A used with permission from Smeltzer, S.C., & Bare, B.G. [2004]. Brunner & Suddarth's textbook of medical–surgical nursing [4th ed., p. 2027]. Philadelphia; Lippincott Williams & Wilkins. B used with permission from Rosdahl, C.B., & Kowalski, M. T. [2003]. Textbook of basic nursing [4th ed., p. 1195]. Philadelphia; Lippincott Williams & Wilkins.)*

down), instead of from side to side. If you need to do this, the nurse will show you how.

When you are working with a person who is in traction, be very careful not to disturb or remove the weights attached to the traction unit. When you lower the person's bed height, check to make sure the weights are not resting on the floor. They must hang freely to apply the correct amount of tension to the affected limb.

AMPUTATIONS

The removal of all or part of an arm or a leg is called an **amputation.** For example, a person may lose just a toe, or the leg from the knee down, or the entire leg. Accidents are a common cause of amputation. For example, the body part may be severed from the body during the accident. Or, the body part may be so seriously damaged during the accident that the only treatment option is to surgically remove it.

Amputation may also be necessary as a result of disease. For example, some types of cancer are treated by amputation of the affected limb. Diseases that interfere with blood flow to all or part of an extremity can also eventually result in the need for amputation. For example, as you learned in Chapter 18, people with diabetes tend to have

circulatory problems, and often, blood flow to their feet is poor. The poor blood flow to the feet is usually associated with poor sensation as well as an increased risk for infection. If a person with diabetes gets a foot infection, it may go unnoticed for a long time, and when it finally is noticed, it may be very difficult to treat. Eventually, death of the tissue (gangrene) occurs because the tissue is deprived of oxygen and nutrients (Fig. 25-16). Once gangrene develops, the only treatment option may be to remove the damaged part through amputation.

FIGURE 25-16

Impaired blood flow causes death of the tissues (gangrene). Once gangrene develops, the only treatment option may be amputation of the affected part. (© *M. English/ Custom Medical Stock Photo.*)

FIGURE 25-17

A prosthetic hand and its cover are shown here. Many times, it is hard to tell a false limb from a real one when the prosthesis is being worn. A prosthetic body part can help a person who has had an amputation regain function and mobility. (© *SIU Bio Med/ Custom Medical Stock Photo.*)

The loss of a body part, especially an arm or leg, is very emotionally traumatic for a person. The person's mobility, appearance, and sometimes even her ability to earn a living or enjoy a hobby she used to love can be affected by an amputation. For some people who have had a body part either partially or completely amputated, a prosthetic (false) part may allow the person to regain mobility, function, and a more normal appearance (Fig. 25-17).

For a prosthetic device to be fitted, the **stump,** or the end of the amputated limb that is left after surgery, must be cared for properly. Positioning is used to keep the muscles and tendons from shortening, and nearby joints are put through range-of-motion exercises to help maintain normal joint function and mobility. Wrapping the end of the stump with elastic bandages helps to shrink and shape the stump properly (Fig. 25-18). When assisting with caring for a person's stump, make sure to follow the nurse's or physical therapist's instructions exactly, as always. Finally, as you assist with the general care needs of your patient or resident, you will have numerous opportunities to observe the stump for any drainage, bleeding, or pain. These findings could be signs of poor tissue healing or infection, and must be reported to the nurse immediately.

Many people experience what is known as **phantom pain,** or the feeling that the amputated body part is still present, after an amputation. Aching, itching, and other sensations are all types

FIGURE 25-18

Wrapping the stump in bandages helps to shape it properly.

of phantom pain. The sensations are caused by the healing of the nerves that were cut when the body part was removed. Phantom pain usually goes away a short while after surgery, but some people report having these episodes for years afterward.

Tell the Nurse!

There are many signs and symptoms that may accompany disorders of the musculoskeletal system. As a nursing assistant, you have the opportunity to become very familiar with each of your patients' or residents' physical abilities and limitations. Report any of the following observations to the nurse immediately:

- The person has fallen
- An area has become swollen, red, bruised, tender, or painful to the touch
- The person complains of pain when moving a joint
- The person's usual range of motion of a joint has decreased
- The person limps or has pain while walking, or makes excuses to avoid walking

GENERAL CARE MEASURES

As a nursing assistant, you may be asked to assist a patient or resident with range-of-motion exercises, the application of heat or cold, or physical therapy. These techniques are used to prevent complications of immobility, relieve musculoskeletal discomfort, and maintain or restore musculoskeletal function.

RANGE-OF-MOTION EXERCISES

As you learned earlier, the range of motion of a joint is the complete extent of movement that the joint is normally capable of without causing pain. Normal activities—such as dressing, grooming, walking, and eating—usually put all of our joints through their complete range of motion several times throughout the day. However, some of the people you will be caring for will have conditions that prevent them from doing the activities that would normally exercise their joints and muscles.

As you know from this chapter and previous ones, immobility can have a serious impact on the musculoskeletal system. Muscle atrophy, loss of bone strength, and stiffness of the joints can quickly lead to permanent muscle weakness, brittle bones, and even contractures (Fig. 25-19). As a nursing assistant, you will play a key role in preventing these complications by helping your patients or residents with range-of-motion exercises as ordered.

Range-of-motion exercises—movements that put each joint through its complete range of motion—are done to preserve joint and muscle function in a person who has limited use of his musculoskeletal system. Range-of-motion exercises are usually performed at least twice a day, often along with other personal care activities, such as bathing or dressing. The exercises can be done while the person is in bed or sitting down. Depending on the situation, range-of-motion exercises may be performed for only one, some, or all of the joints. Sometimes, the patient or resident will be able to perform the exercises on his own, and your role will be to provide guidance and encouragement. Other times, you will need to help the person to perform the exercises.

- In **active range-of-motion exercises,** the patient or resident performs the exercises independently, with verbal guidance from the nursing assistant or nurse.
- In **passive range-of-motion exercises,** the nursing assistant or nurse moves the patient's or resident's joints through the exercises, without active involvement on the part of the person. For example, a nursing assistant might perform passive range-of-motion exercises for a person who is in a coma.
- In **active-assistive range-of-motion exercises,** the patient or resident performs the exercises with some hands-on assistance from the nursing assistant or nurse. For example, a person may be able to lift his arm out to the side, but will need help from the nursing assistant or nurse to complete the movement of bringing the arm up near the head.

Procedure 25-1 explains how to assist a patient or resident with passive range-of-motion exercises. Range-of-motion exercises can cause injury to the joints if they are not performed properly. Usually a physical therapist or nurse will evaluate a patient or resident and determine which joints should be exercised. When assisting a person with range-of-motion exercises, always follow the care plan (or the nurse's or physical therapist's instructions) exactly. This is important for two reasons:

1. There may be some exercises that the person is not allowed to do.
2. The physical therapist or nurse will most likely change the care plan as the person's condition either improves or worsens.

In addition to checking the care plan, you should make sure that helping the person with the ordered exercises is within your scope of practice. For example, in some facilities, nursing assistants are not allowed to assist people with range-of-motion exercises involving the neck. General guidelines for assisting a person with range-of-motion exercises are given in Guidelines Box 25-2.

FIGURE 25-19

Contractures can occur when a joint is not exercised regularly. Use of the joint can be permanently lost. (© *Siebert/ Custom Medical Stock Photo.*)

GUIDELINES BOX 25-2
GUIDELINES FOR ASSISTING WITH RANGE-OF-MOTION EXERCISES

What you do	Why you do it
Use good body mechanics.	Using good body mechanics saves energy and prevents muscle strain and injury.
Remove pillows and other positioning devices.	Pillows and positioning devices can prevent a person from achieving full range of motion of the joint.
Position the person so that each joint can be moved through all of the usual positions.	Positioning the person in a position that will allow each joint to be moved through all of its usual positions saves time (because the person will not have to be repositioned in between exercises) and helps to ensure that all of the exercises will be completed.
Move through the exercises in a systematic way (for example, from the head down).	Developing a routine helps to ensure that no exercise will be forgotten.
Unless instructed otherwise, perform the same exercise on each corresponding body part (for example, do the same thing for the right arm that you do for the left).	Exercising corresponding joints equally ensures that both sides of the body remain equally strong and flexible.
Support each joint as you exercise it.	Support reduces discomfort and strain on the joint.
Do not push a joint past its point of resistance.	Each joint has a limit to its range of motion. Attempting to exceed this limit can lead to joint pain and injury.
Watch the person's face for signs of pain or discomfort.	A person may not be able to tell you if what you are doing hurts. Therefore, it is important to watch the person's face for nonverbal cues, such as grimacing or wincing.
Avoid exercising a painful joint.	Exercising a painful joint can cause additional injury.
If you notice sudden, continuous contractions of the related muscles (spasticity), take a break or move the limb more slowly to allow the muscles to recover. Applying gentle pressure to the muscle can also relieve spasticity.	Spasticity is a sign that the muscles are working too hard. It may also indicate that the person is in pain, or that the joint's range of motion has been exceeded.
Expect the person's respiratory rate and heart rate to increase during the exercise. If these vital signs do not return to their normal resting rates after the activity ends, report this to the nurse immediately.	During activity, the tissues require more oxygen and nutrients, so the heart and lungs work harder to supply the tissues. However, once the activity ends, the heart rate and respiratory rate should return to normal because the tissues' demand for oxygen and nutrients will be less.
Encourage the person to help with the exercises as much as possible.	Active participation increases the person's sense of independence and improves function.

HEAT AND COLD APPLICATIONS

Disorders of the musculoskeletal system are usually painful. Pain can make it difficult for a person to relax, rest, or sleep. As a nursing assistant, many of the things you do every day are related to promoting comfort and preventing pain. For example, ensuring that a person is in proper alignment when you reposition her helps to prevent pain. Nursing assistants also play an important role in noticing and reporting pain. Many of the people you care for will be hesitant to complain about pain, even when the pain is severe or constant. Some people feel that their pain is just simply part of "growing old." Others are afraid that they will become addicted to pain medications. If you notice that a person seems to be in pain, report this to the nurse. There are many things that can be done to relieve pain, aside from the use of medications (or in addition to the use of medications). The nurse will work with the person and the other members of the health care team to find a way to lessen the person's pain.

As a nursing assistant, you may be responsible for carrying out many of the tasks on the care plan related to relieving the person's pain. For example, back massage is especially beneficial when combined with pain medication. Also, many people with musculoskeletal pain can benefit from the application of heat or cold to an affected joint or muscle. The application of heat or cold can be used to reduce or prevent tissue swelling, promote healing, ease pain, and promote comfort. Heat and cold have opposite effects on the body, which are summarized in Table 25-2. Because the application of heat or cold can be dangerous, these treatments require a doctor's order, and in some facilities, the application of heat or cold may be outside of the nursing assistant's scope of practice. However, even if you are not permitted to give these treatments, you will be involved with monitoring patients or residents who are receiving them.

Some people are at very high risk for injury from the application of heat or cold:

- **Older people, very young people, and chronically ill people.** The skin of people who are very old, very young, or chronically ill can be very fragile and sensitive.
- **People with very fair skin.** Fair skin tends to be more sensitive to temperature changes than darker skin.
- **People with impaired sensation.** People with impaired sensation, such as those

who are paralyzed or who have diabetes, are at risk for injury because they are unable to detect whether an application is too hot or too cold.

- **People who are disoriented or taking pain medications.** People with impaired levels of consciousness are also at a higher risk for injury from heat or cold applications.

People with these risk factors for injury must be monitored especially carefully during the application of heat or cold.

Cold Applications

Cold applications are often used for people who have musculoskeletal injuries resulting from trauma, such as sprains and fractures. Cold applications are also frequently used on incisions following surgical procedures. The application of cold reduces pain and swelling and decreases bleeding. It does this by cooling the skin and underlying tissues, causing the blood vessels to constrict (narrow). Because the blood vessels are constricted, less blood is carried to the tissues, resulting in less bleeding and decreased tissue swelling. The numbing effect of the cold helps to reduce pain.

Cold applications can be either moist or dry (Fig. 25-20). In moist applications, moisture comes in direct contact with the skin. Moist applications allow the cold to penetrate the tissues more quickly and deeply. A cold compress, made by soaking a gauze pad, towel, or washcloth in cold water, wringing it out, and then applying it with pressure to the affected area, is an example of a moist application (see Fig. 25-20A). Procedure 25-2 explains how to give a moist cold application.

Dry applications prevent moisture from coming in direct contact with the skin. Dry applications are usually colder than moist applications. An ice bag is an example of a dry cold application (see Fig. 25-20B). Commercially prepared ice packs that are kept frozen until the time of use are available, or a dry cold application can be made by filling an ice bag with crushed ice and wrapping it in a towel or washcloth. Procedure 25-3 explains how to give a dry cold application.

When applied directly to a person's skin, cold can cause severe burns and blisters. Dry cold applications should be wrapped in a protective cloth to prevent the icy cold plastic from coming

TABLE 25-2 ■ Uses of Heat and Cold Applications	
Heat	Cold
Reduces pain and promotes circulation to speed healing	Reduces pain and prevents swelling
Relieves muscle spasms	Numbs sensation and controls bleeding
Provides warmth	Reduces fevers

A

B

FIGURE 25-20

Cold applications are used to reduce pain and swelling. Cold applications may be either moist or dry. (*A*) A cold compress is a moist cold application. (*B*) An ice bag is a dry cold application.

in direct contact with the person's skin. If a cold application is left in place for too long, prolonged constriction of the small blood vessels can keep oxygen and nutrients from reaching the skin, resulting in tissue death and skin breakdown. For this reason, cold applications should not be left in place for longer than 20 minutes. Make sure that you check the skin underneath the cold application every 10 minutes and stop the treatment immediately if you observe any evidence of a burn or blister. Pale skin, resulting from the constriction of the blood vessels, should return to its normal color quickly after the cold application is removed. If it does not, or if you notice a burn or blister starting to develop, inform the nurse immediately. Also, if you have questions about how to apply the cold application or for how long, please ask the nurse for help.

Heat Applications

Although ice may be used initially after an injury or surgical procedure to prevent swelling and reduce pain, heat may be used a day or so later to increase blood flow to the tissues to promote healing. In addition, heat may be used on joints that are painful and stiff as a result of arthritis. Heat relaxes the muscles, relieves pain, and promotes blood flow to the area. When heat is applied to the skin, the blood vessels dilate (widen), allowing more blood to flow to the tissues. Increased blood flow speeds healing by bringing more oxygen, nutrients, and infection-fighting white blood cells to the area. In addition, heat relaxes the muscles and helps loosen stiff joints.

Like cold applications, heat applications can be either moist or dry (Fig. 25-21), and the applications may be either commercially prepared or homemade. Moist heat penetrates tissues more quickly and deeply than dry heat. Therefore, moist heat applications are used at a lower temperature to reduce the risk of burns. Examples of moist heat applications include warm compresses and hot water soaks (see Fig. 25-21A). Examples of dry heat applications include an electric heating pad or a hot water bottle wrapped in a towel. An Aquamatic pad (or K-pad) is a special type of electric heating pad (see Fig. 25-21B). The pad is connected to a heating unit that heats water to a preset temperature. The water circulates through the pad and then back into the heating device so that a constant temperature is maintained. A key is used to set the temperature, and then the key is removed, preventing anyone from accidentally turning the heat up or down. Procedure 25-4 describes how to apply a dry heat application using an Aquamatic pad.

Burns are the most common complication of heat applications. Some burns, especially on thin, delicate skin, can be very severe, resulting in blistering, tissue loss, and the need for skin grafting. It is not uncommon for a person to fall asleep with a heating pad in place and receive a

A

B

FIGURE 25-21

Heat applications are used to relax muscles, relieve pain, and promote blood flow to an area. Heat applications may be either moist or dry. (*A*) A warm soak is an example of a moist heat application. Soaks are done in either a wash basin (if the area to be soaked is small) or a tub (if the area to be soaked is large). (*B*) An Aquamatic pad is an example of a dry heat application. Water is heated in the heating unit. The heated water passes through the tubing and into a network of tubes inside the heating pad. The water never comes in contact with the person's skin.

burn from prolonged exposure to the heat. In addition to increasing the person's risk for burns, heat applications that are left in place for too long will eventually cause the blood vessels to constrict, putting the person at risk for tissue breakdown. For these reasons, heat applications should not be left in place for longer than 20 minutes. Make sure that you check the skin underneath the heat application every 5 minutes and stop the treatment immediately if you observe any evidence of burning. Warmth causes the skin to become pink or slightly reddened. Skin that is bright red or very pale could be burned. Report any observations that may indicate a burn to the nurse immediately, along with any complaints of pain, burning, or stinging.

REHABILITATION

Many of your patients or residents with musculoskeletal disorders will require physical, emotional, or vocational rehabilitation (or a combination of the three), as described in Chapter 23. Working to regain or maintain function, or learning to adjust to a loss of function, can be a long, difficult, and painful process. It is very easy for patients or residents to become frustrated and discouraged. Your reassurance and encouragement are necessary to help keep your

patients or residents focused. Be an active listener and an attentive observer. If you notice signs of skin breakdown or diminishing mobility, report these observations to the nurse. Make sure you are familiar with the supportive devices, assistive devices, and prosthetic devices used by your patients or residents so that you can assist them properly. Ask the physical therapist or nurse to explain any special procedures or rehabilitation techniques to you. As a nursing assistant, there is much you can do to help your patients or residents as they work toward regaining maximum use of their musculoskeletal system.

SUMMARY

▶ The musculoskeletal system consists of the bones, skeletal muscles, and joints.
  ■ The primary function of the musculoskeletal system is movement.
    ● Joints are the areas where two bones meet. Most movement occurs at freely movable joints.
    ● The skeletal muscles attach to the bones. When the muscle contracts (shortens), it pulls against the bone, causing the body part to move.

- Other functions of the musculoskeletal system include protection, support, heat production, calcium storage, and blood cell production.

▶ As we age, we lose bone tissue and muscle mass, and our joints begin to show the effects of a lifetime of wear and tear. Consuming a diet rich in calcium, vitamin D, and protein and exercising regularly throughout life can help to delay or decrease the effects of aging on the musculoskeletal system.

▶ Disorders of the musculoskeletal system can make mobility very difficult.

- Osteoporosis is the excessive loss of bone tissue, resulting in bones that break very easily.
- Arthritis is inflammation of the joints.
  - Osteoarthritis typically affects older people. In osteoarthritis, the cartilage that covers the ends of bones is worn away through normal use of the joint. Many people with osteoarthritis have joint replacement surgery to correct the condition.
  - Rheumatoid arthritis is a type of arthritis that affects younger people and can cause severe joint deformities. Rheumatoid arthritis is thought to be an autoimmune disorder, which means it is caused by a person's immune system attacking his or her own tissues.
  - Gout is a type of arthritis that results from the build-up of uric acid in the joints.
- Muscular dystrophy is a general term for a group of disorders that cause the skeletal muscles to become very weak over time. Muscular dystrophy is a genetic disorder, which means that it is inherited.
- Fractures are broken bones.
  - Older people are especially at risk for fractures because of the normal loss of bone tissue that is a part of aging. Fractures may take longer to heal in an older person.

- Fractures may be treated by casting or by surgical placement of plates, screws, pins, or wires. Traction may be necessary to hold the ends of the broken bone in alignment until the fracture can be permanently repaired.
- Amputation is the removal of a limb or part of a limb.
  - Amputation may be necessary because of trauma or because of complications related to a medical condition, such as diabetes.
  - Proper care of the stump increases the likelihood that a person can be fitted with a prosthetic limb.

▶ Range-of-motion exercises, the application of heat or cold, and rehabilitation are measures taken to prevent complications of immobility, relieve musculoskeletal discomfort, and maintain or restore musculoskeletal function.

- Range-of-motion exercises are used to preserve joint and muscle function in people who have conditions that limit their use of the musculoskeletal system. Range-of-motion exercises are usually performed at least twice a day.
  - Active range-of-motion exercises are performed by the patient or resident.
  - Passive range-of-motion exercises are performed by the nursing assistant or nurse on behalf of the patient or resident.
  - Active-assistive range-of-motion exercises are performed by the patient or resident with some help from the nursing assistant or nurse.
- Heat and cold applications can be beneficial for a person with disorders of the musculoskeletal system to help decrease pain and swelling and increase muscle relaxation and joint flexibility. Both heat and cold applications can cause severe injury to a person if they are used inappropriately.
- Rehabilitation is an essential part of the care needed by a person with a musculoskeletal disorder.

Chapter 25 Procedures

Getting Ready Steps

a. **W**ash your hands and observe standard precautions as necessary.

b. **G**ather needed supplies.

c. **K**nock and introduce yourself.

d. **I**dentify the person, and greet him or her by name.

e. **E**xplain the procedure.

f. **P**rovide privacy.

g. **S**ee to safety.

Finishing Up Steps

a. **Confirm comfort** and good body alignment.

b. **L**eave the call light control within easy reach.

c. **S**ee to safety.

d. **O**pen the curtain and door.

e. **W**ash your hands.

f. **R**eport and record.

PROCEDURE 25-1

Assisting a Person with Passive Range-of-Motion Exercises

OBRA ✓

Getting Ready   WGKIEPS

1. Complete the "Getting Ready" steps **a** through **g**.

Supplies

• bath blanket

Procedure

2. Make sure that the bed is positioned at a comfortable working height (to promote good body mechanics) and that the wheels are locked. If the side rails are in use, lower the side rail on the working side of the bed. The side rail on the opposite side of the bed should remain up. Raise or lower the head of the bed to a horizontal or semi-Fowler's position.

3. Assist the person into the supine position.

4. Spread the bath blanket over the top linens (and the person). If the person is able, have him hold the bath blanket. If not, tuck the corners under the person's shoulders. Fan-fold the top linens to the foot of the bed.

5. Perform each range-of-motion exercise in steps 6 through 13 according to the person's care plan, being careful to expose only the part of the body that is being exercised. Repeat each exercise 3 to 5 times, as written in the care plan.

6. If your facility permits, exercise the person's neck:

   a. **Forward and backward flexion and extension (neck).** Support the person's head by putting one hand under the person's chin and the other on the back of the head. Gently bring the head forward, as if to touch the chin to the chest, and then bring it backward, chin pointing to the sky.

STEP 6a Gently bring the head forward, then backward.

(continued)

PROCEDURE 25-1 (Continued)

Assisting a Person with Passive Range-of-Motion Exercises

b. **Side-to-side flexion (neck).** Support the person's head by putting one hand under the person's chin and the other near the opposite temple. Gently tilt the head toward the right shoulder, and then toward the left.

STEP 6b Gently tilt the head toward the right shoulder, then the left.

c. **Rotation (neck).** Support the person's head by putting one hand under the person's chin and the other on the back of the head. Gently move the head from side to side, as if the person were shaking his head "no."

Rotation to right

Rotate to left

STEP 6c Gently move the head from side to side.

STEP 7a Lift the arm up so that it is alongside the person's ear, then return it to its original position.

STEP 7b Move the arm away from the person's side, then return it to its original position.

7. Exercise the person's shoulder:

a. **Forward flexion and extension (shoulder).** Support the person's arm by putting one hand under the person's elbow and the other under the person's wrist. Keeping the person's arm straight with the palm facing up, lift the arm up so that it is alongside the person's ear, and then return it to its original position.

b. **Abduction and adduction (shoulder).** Support the person's arm by putting one hand under the person's elbow and the other under the person's wrist. Keeping the person's arm straight with the palm facing up, move the person's arm away from the side of his body, and then return it to its original position.

c. **Horizontal abduction and adduction (shoulder).** Support the person's arm by putting one hand under the person's elbow and the other under the person's wrist. Keeping the person's arm straight with the palm facing up, move the person's arm away from the side of his body. Gently bending the person's elbow, touch the person's hand to the opposite shoulder, then straighten the elbow and bring the arm back out to the side.

d. **Rotation (shoulder).** Support the person's arm by putting one hand under the person's elbow and the other under the person's wrist. Move the person's arm away from the side of his body, and bend

(continued)

PROCEDURE 25-1 (Continued)

Assisting a Person with Passive Range-of-Motion Exercises

the person's arm at the elbow. Gently move the person's forearm up, so that it forms a right angle with the mattress, and then back down. This movement is similar to the motion a police officer makes when he or she is signaling someone to stop.

STEP 7c Move the arm away from the person's side, then touch the person's hand to the opposite shoulder.

STEP 13d Move the person's forearm up, then back down.

8. Exercise the person's elbow.
   a. **Flexion and extension (elbow).** Support the person's arm by putting one hand under the person's elbow and the other under the person's wrist. Starting with the person's arm straight and with the palm facing up, bend the person's elbow so that the person's hand moves toward his shoulder. Then, straighten out the elbow, returning the person's hand to its original position.
   b. **Pronation and supination (elbow).** Support the person's arm by putting one hand under the person's elbow and the other under the person's wrist. Move the person's arm away from the side of his body,

and slightly bend the person's arm at the elbow. Gently move the person's forearm up, so that it forms a right angle with the mattress. Gently turn the person's hand so that the palm is facing the end of the bed. Then turn the hand the other way, so that the palm is facing the head of the bed.

STEP 8a Bend the arm so that the hand moves toward the shoulder, then return it to its original position.

STEP 8b Turn the hand so that the palm is facing the end of the bed, then turn the hand the other way so that the palm is facing the head of the bed.

9. Exercise the person's wrist.
   a. **Flexion and extension (wrist).** Support the person's wrist with one hand. Use the other hand to gently bend the person's hand down, and then back.

STEP 9a Gently bend the person's hand down, then back.

(continued)

PROCEDURE 25-1 (Continued)

Assisting a Person with Passive Range-of-Motion Exercises

b. **Radial and ulnar flexion (wrist).** Support the person's wrist with one hand. Use the other hand to gently turn the person's hand toward his or thumb. Then turn the hand the other way, toward the little finger.

STEP 9b Gently turn the person's hand one way, then the other.

10. Exercise the person's fingers and thumb.

a. **Flexion and extension (fingers and thumb).** Support the person's wrist with one hand. Using your other hand, flex the person's fingers to make a fist, tucking the person's thumb under the fingers. Then straighten each finger and the thumb, one by one.

STEP 10a Flex the person's fingers to make a fist, then straighten each finger and thumb, one by one.

b. **Abduction and adduction (fingers and thumb).** With one hand, hold the person's thumb and index finger together. With the other hand, move the middle finger away from the index finger. Then move the middle finger back toward the index finger, and hold the middle finger, index finger, and thumb together. Next, move the ring finger away from the other two fingers and thumb, then move it back toward the

group. Do the same with the little finger. Finally, reverse the process. Hold the little finger and the ring finger together and move the middle finger away and back. Complete with the index finger and thumb.

STEP 10b Spread the fingers away from each other, then back together again.

c. **Flexion and extension (thumb).** Bend the person's thumb into his or her palm, then return it to its original position.

STEP 10c Bend the thumb into the palm, then return it to its original position.

d. **Opposition.** Touch each fingertip to the thumb.

STEP 10d Touch each fingertip to the thumb.

(continued)

PROCEDURE 25-1 (Continued)

Assisting a Person with Passive Range-of-Motion Exercises

11. Exercise the person's hip and knee.

    a. **Forward flexion and extension (hip and knee).** Support the person's leg by putting one hand under the person's knee and the other under the person's ankle. Gently bend the person's knee, moving it toward the person's head. Then straighten the person's knee and gently lower the leg to the bed.

STEP 11a Gently bend the knee, moving it toward the head. Then straighten the leg and lower it to the bed.

STEP 11b Move the leg away from the person's side, then return it to its original position.

STEP 11c Gently turn the leg inward, then outward.

    b. **Abduction and adduction (hip).** Support the person's leg by putting one hand un-

der the person's knee and the other under the person's ankle. Keeping the person's leg straight, move the person's leg away from the side of his body, and then return it to its original position.

    c. **Rotation (hip).** Support the person's leg by putting one hand under the person's knee and the other under the person's ankle. Keeping the person's leg straight, gently turn the leg inward and then outward.

12. Exercise the person's ankle and foot.

    a. **Dorsiflexion and plantar flexion (ankle and foot).** Support the person's ankle with one hand. Use the other hand to gently bend the person's foot up toward the head, and then back.

STEP 12a Gently bend the foot toward the head, then back.

    b. **Inversion and eversion (ankle and foot).** Support the person's ankle with one hand. Use the other hand to gently turn the inside of the foot inward and then outward.

STEP 12b Gently bend the foot inward, then outward.

13. Exercise the person's toes.

    a. **Flexion and extension (toes).** Put one hand under the person's foot. Put the other hand over the person's toes. Curl the toes downward and then straighten them.

    b. **Abduction and adduction (toes).** Spread each toe the same way you spread each finger in step 10b.

(continued)

PROCEDURE 25-1 (Continued)

Assisting a Person with Passive Range-of-Motion Exercises

STEP 13a Curl the toes downward, then straighten them.

STEP 13b Spread the toes away from each other, then back together again.

14. Straighten the bed linens and make sure the person is comfortable and in good body alignment. Draw the top linens over the person and remove the bath blanket.

15. If the side rails are in use, raise the side rail on the working side of the bed. Make sure that the bed is lowered to its lowest position and that the wheels are locked.

Finishing Up

16. Complete the "Finishing Up" steps **a** through **f**.

PROCEDURE 25-2
Giving a Moist Cold Application

Getting Ready   WCKIEDS

1. Complete the "Getting Ready" steps **a** through **g**.

Supplies

- bed protector
- compress (for example, 4 ×4 gauze pad or washcloth)
- rolled gauze or ties (optional)
- bath basin
- ice
- bath towel

Procedure

2. Put the ice in the bath basin and fill the basin with cold water at the sink.

3. Make sure that the bed is positioned at a comfortable working height (to promote good body mechanics) and that the wheels are locked.

4. Help the person to a comfortable position and expose only the area to be treated.

5. Position the bed protector as necessary to keep the bed linens dry.

6. Moisten the compress with the ice water as ordered. Wring out the compress, and apply it to the treatment site.

7. Leave the compress in place for the designated amount of time, usually 15 to 20 minutes. The compress may be secured in place with ties or rolled gauze, or the patient or resident may assist by holding the compress in place.

   a. Keep the compress moistened with ice water.

   b. Check the skin beneath the compress every 10 minutes. If the skin appears pale or blue, or if the person complains of numbness or a burning sensation, discontinue treatment immediately and notify the nurse.

   c. If you must leave the room, place the call light control within easy reach and ask the person to signal if he or she experiences numbness or burning.

8. When the treatment is complete, remove the compress and carefully dry the skin.

9. Remove the bed protector. Straighten the bed linens and make sure the person is comfortable and in good body alignment. Draw the top linens over the person.

10. Make sure that the bed is lowered to its lowest position and that the wheels are locked.

11. Gather the soiled linens and place them in the linen hamper. Dispose of disposable items in a facility-approved waste container. Clean equipment and return it to the storage area.

Finishing Up   CLSOWR

12. Complete the "Finishing Up" steps **a** through **f**.

PROCEDURE 25-3

Giving a Dry Cold Application

Getting Ready WGKIEDS

1. Complete the "Getting Ready" steps **a** through **g**.

Supplies

- paper towels
- rolled gauze or ties (optional)
- crushed ice
- ice bag
- towel

Procedure

2. Fill the ice bag with water, close it, and turn it upside down to check for leaks. Empty the bag.

3. Fill the bag one-half to two-thirds full with crushed ice. Do not overfill the ice bag. Squeeze the bag to force out excess air, and close the bag.

4. Dry the outside of the bag with the paper towels and wrap it in the towel.

5. Make sure that the bed is positioned at a comfortable working height (to promote good body mechanics) and that the wheels are locked.

6. Help the person to a comfortable position and expose only the area to be treated.

7. Apply the ice bag to the treatment site.

8. Leave the compress in place for the designated amount of time, usually 15 to 20 minutes. The compress may be secured in place with ties or rolled gauze, or the patient or resident may assist by holding the compress in place.

   a. Check the skin beneath the ice bag every 10 minutes. If the skin appears pale or blue, or if the person complains of numbness or a burning sensation, discontinue treatment immediately and notify the nurse.

   b. Refill the bag with ice as necessary.

   c. If you must leave the room, place the call light control within easy reach and ask the person to signal if he or she experiences numbness or burning.

9. When the treatment is complete, remove the ice bag.

10. Straighten the bed linens and make sure the person is comfortable and in good body alignment. Draw the top linens over the person.

11. Make sure that the bed is lowered to its lowest position and that the wheels are locked.

12. Gather the soiled linens and place them in the linen hamper. Dispose of disposable items in a facility-approved waste container. Clean equipment and return it to the storage area.

Finishing Up CLSOWR

13. Complete the "Finishing Up" steps **a** through **f**.

PROCEDURE 25-4

Giving a Dry Heat Application with an Aquamatic Pad

Getting Ready   WGKIEpS

1. Complete the "Getting Ready" steps **a** through **g**.

Supplies

- aquamatic pad
- heating unit
- distilled water
- cover
- ties or tape

Procedure

2. Check the pad for leaks. Make sure the cord is not frayed and the plug is in good condition. Check the heating unit to be sure it is filled with water. If you need to fill it, use distilled water. Tap water contains minerals that can corrode the unit.

3. Place the heating unit so that the tubing and pad are level with the heating unit at all times. Make sure that the tubing is free of kinks. Plug the cord into an outlet.

4. Allow the water to warm to the desired temperature, as specified by the nurse or the care plan. If the temperature is not preset, set the temperature with the key and then remove the key.

5. Place the pad in its cover.

6. Make sure that the bed is positioned at a comfortable working height (to promote good body mechanics) and that the wheels are locked.

7. Help the person to a comfortable position and expose only the area to be treated.

8. Apply the pad to the treatment site.

9. Leave the pad in place for the designated amount of time, usually 15 to 20 minutes.

The pad may be secured in place with ties or tape, or the patient or resident may assist by holding the pad in place. (Do not use pins to secure the pad. Pins can puncture the pad, causing it to leak.)

   a. Check the skin beneath the pad every 5 minutes. If the skin appears red, swollen, or blistered, or if the person complains of pain, numbness, or discomfort, discontinue treatment immediately and notify the nurse.

   b. Refill the heating unit if the water level drops below the fill line.

   c. If you must leave the room, place the call light control within easy reach and ask the person to signal if he or she experiences numbness or burning.

10. When the treatment is complete, remove the pad.

11. Straighten the bed linens and make sure the person is comfortable and in good body alignment. Draw the top linens over the person.

12. Make sure that the bed is lowered to its lowest position and that the wheels are locked.

13. Gather the soiled linens and place them in the linen hamper. Dispose of disposable items in a facility-approved waste container. Clean equipment and return it to the storage area.

Finishing Up   CL³OⁿR

14. Complete the "Finishing Up" steps **a** through **f**.

What did you learn?

Multiple Choice

Select the single best answer for each of the following questions.

1. When a muscle atrophies, it:
   a. Becomes larger and stronger
   b. Becomes thinner and weaker
   c. Becomes stiffer
   d. Becomes more flexible

2. Which musculoskeletal disorder causes severe joint deformities and often affects younger people?
   a. Osteoarthritis
   b. Rheumatoid arthritis
   c. Multiple sclerosis
   d. Muscular dystrophy

3. What is the term for a fracture where the broken ends of the bone do not penetrate the skin?
   a. Impacted fracture
   b. Comminuted fracture
   c. Spiral fracture
   d. Closed fracture

4. Excessive loss of bone tissue is:
   a. Osteoarthritis
   b. Osteoporosis
   c. A normal effect of aging
   d. Gout

5. What does the skeletal system do?
   a. It acts as a storage site for calcium
   b. It works with the muscles to produce movement
   c. It produces blood cells
   d. All of the above

6. Ms. Vaughn broke her leg while skiing. Surgery is required to align the broken bone, and then the bone fragments are held together with wires. What is the name of the procedure Ms. Vaughn has had?
   a. Open fracture, internal fixation
   b. Open reduction, internal fixation
   c. Open reduction, external fixation
   d. Traction

7. What does the muscular system do?
   a. It produces heat
   b. It helps to maintain posture
   c. It works with the bones to produce movement
   d. All of the above

8. The purpose of cold applications is usually to:
   a. Prevent heat exhaustion
   b. Speed the flow of blood to an injured area
   c. Prevent swelling
   d. Prevent the formation of scar tissue

9. What is a heat application used for?
   a. To relieve muscle spasms
   b. To reduce pain
   c. To promote circulation and speed healing
   d. All of the above

10. Mr. Owen has severe osteoarthritis in his hips. You are caring for Mr. Owen following his hip replacement surgery. What do you need to remember?
    a. Mr. Owen's legs must always be kept together (adducted).
    b. When assisting Mr. Owen with range-of-motion exercises, make sure to flex the hips beyond 90 degrees to maintain flexibility in the joint.
    c. Mr. Owen should use an abduction pillow to keep his legs spread apart when he is in a supine or lateral position.
    d. Mr. Owen should be encouraged to get up and walk around within a day or two of the surgery.

11. Ms. Curtis has just had a cast put on her leg following a horseback riding accident. What should you remember when you are helping Ms. Curtis?
    a. Ms. Curtis's leg should not be elevated.
    b. You should check Ms. Curtis's toes frequently to make sure that the cast is not too tight.
    c. Ms. Curtis should be reminded that if the skin underneath the cast begins to itch, she can slide a tongue depressor inside the cast to scratch the itchy area.
    d. Ms. Curtis should be encouraged to get out of bed and take a shower as soon as the cast dries.

12. Mr. Jefferson is an elderly man who just came to live at your facility. Mr. Jefferson has been living on his own for several years. He has diabetes and he knows that he is not supposed to eat sweets, but he does anyway. As a result, his diabetes is not well-controlled. About 3 weeks ago, Mr. Jefferson

stubbed his toe while he was making the bed, and now gangrene has set in. What is the most likely treatment for Mr. Jefferson's toe?

a. Outside reduction, internal fixation (ORIF)
b. Amputation of the toe
c. Casting of the foot
d. Application of heat

Matching

Match each numbered item with its appropriate lettered description.

_____ **1.** Flexion/ extension

_____ **2.** Supination/ pronation

_____ **3.** Dorsiflexion/ plantar flexion

_____ **4.** Rotation

_____ **5.** Abduction/ adduction

_____ **6.** Inversion/ eversion

a.

b.

c.

d.

e.

f.

26

The Respiratory System

What will you learn?

Have you ever heard the phrase, "It's as natural as breathing?" Breathing is certainly something that many of us take for granted, because we don't have to think about it. Air enters and leaves our lungs without any conscious effort on our part. With each breath, life-giving oxygen is delivered to the body, and carbon dioxide, a waste product of cellular metabolism, is removed from the body. Breathing is the function of the respiratory system, the subject of this chapter. When you are finished with this chapter, you will be able to:

1. List and describe the main parts of the respiratory system.
2. Discuss the main functions of the respiratory system.
3. Describe how normal aging processes affect the respiratory system.
4. Describe some of the disorders that can affect the respiratory system.
5. Describe how oxygen therapy is used to assist a person with respiration.
6. Describe the guidelines that a nursing assistant should follow when caring for patients or residents receiving oxygen therapy.
7. Discuss other methods used to help a person who is having trouble with respiration.

Photo: A swimmer comes up for air. Human beings need oxygen to live.
(© Inc, MedioImages/Index Stock Imagery.)

Vocabulary

Mucous membrane	Respiration	Influenza	Flow meter
Mucus	Bronchioles	Asthma	Nasal cannula
Nasal cavity	Alveoli	Chronic obstructive	Facemask
Pharyngitis	Gas exchange	pulmonary disease	Nasopharyngeal airway
Pharynx	Pleura	(COPD)	Oropharyngeal airway
Larynx	Diaphragm	Emphysema	Mechanical ventilation
Laryngitis	Pneumonia	Chronic bronchitis	Endotracheal tube
Trachea	Sputum	Pneumothorax	Tracheostomy
Bronchi	Pleurisy	Hemothorax	Suctioning
Lungs	Bronchitis	Respiratory therapy	Hypoxic

STRUCTURE OF THE RESPIRATORY SYSTEM

The respiratory system consists of the lungs and a series of passages, collectively referred to as the *airway* (Fig. 26-1). You may hear people refer to the "upper respiratory tract" and the "lower respiratory tract." The upper respiratory tract consists of the structures located outside of the chest cavity (the nasal cavity, pharynx, and larynx). The lower respiratory tract consists of the structures located inside the chest cavity (the trachea, bronchi, bronchioles, and lungs).

AIRWAY

The purpose of the airway is to conduct air from the outside of the body to the lungs, and from the lungs to the outside of the body. The airway consists of a series of passages that become smaller in diameter as they approach the lungs. These passages are lined with a **mucous membrane,** a special type of epithelial tissue that lines many of the organ systems in the body. The surface of the membrane is kept moist by **mucus,** a slippery, sticky substance that is secreted by special cells.

Nasal Cavity

Air enters the body through the nostrils and passes into the **nasal cavity,** which is lined by a mucous membrane and coarse hairs. The coarse hairs and the mucous membrane help to trap dirt, dust, microbes, and other foreign particles, preventing these substances from entering the delicate lungs. The plentiful blood vessels in the mucous membrane transfer body heat to the air, warming it up to a comfortable temperature. In addition, the air picks up some of the moisture from the warm, moist nasal cavity. Warm, moist air is less likely than cold, dry air to damage the delicate lung tissue.

Pharynx

When you have a "sore throat," the part of your body that hurts is your pharynx. (You may have heard the term **pharyngitis,** which means inflammation of the pharynx, or a sore throat.) Both the nasal cavities and the oral cavity open into the **pharynx,** or throat region (see Fig. 26-1). This means that air passes through the pharynx on its way to the lungs, and food and fluids pass through the pharynx on their way to the stomach. This sharing of space is convenient when you have a stuffy nose, because it means that you have another way to get air into your body (that is, through your mouth). However, this sharing of space can also lead to complications, such as choking, which occurs when you try to breathe and swallow at the same time. The pharynx is divided into three sections: the nasopharynx (located right behind the nasal cavities), the oropharynx (located behind the mouth), and the laryngeal pharynx (located behind the larynx).

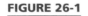

FIGURE 26-1

The respiratory system consists of the lungs and a series of passages collectively referred to as the "airway." The structures that form the airway include the nasal cavity, pharynx, larynx, trachea, bronchi, and bronchioles. Disorders of the respiratory tract are often said to affect either the "upper respiratory tract" or the "lower respiratory tract." The upper respiratory tract consists of those structures located outside the chest cavity, while the lower respiratory tract consists of those structures located inside the chest cavity.

Larynx

From the pharynx, air passes into the **larynx**. The opening of the larynx is covered by a flap of cartilage called the epiglottis, which snaps shut when you swallow, closing off the opening and preventing food from passing into the lower respiratory tract.

In addition to serving as part of the airway, the larynx is the organ responsible for speech. The larynx, often referred to as the "voice box," contains the vocal cords. When air flows over the vocal cords, it causes them to vibrate, producing sound. Humans and other animals make recognizable sounds by controlling the flow of air over the vocal cords. An inflammation of the larynx, or **laryngitis,** usually affects a person's ability to talk.

Trachea and Bronchi

The **trachea,** also called the "windpipe," is the passage that carries air from the larynx down into the chest toward the lungs. "C"-shaped rings of cartilage give the trachea its characteristic ridged appearance (see Fig. 26-1). These cartilage rings support the trachea and keep it open. At its lower end, the trachea divides into two separate passages called the **bronchi.** One

bronchus goes to the right lung and the other goes to the left lung.

The mucous membrane lining of the trachea and bronchi contains millions of tiny hair-like structures called *cilia.* The cilia constantly move in a waving or beating fashion, moving mucus upward toward the pharynx so that it can be coughed up and removed from the respiratory tract along with any trapped particles or microbes.

LUNGS

The **lungs** are the main organs of **respiration,** the process the body uses to obtain oxygen from the environment and remove carbon dioxide (a waste gas) from the body. Once inside the lungs, the bronchi divide into smaller and smaller branches called **bronchioles** (Fig. 26-2). There are more than a million bronchioles in each lung! At the end of each bronchiole, there is a grape-like cluster of tiny air sacs called **alveoli.** Each alveolus is surrounded by a network of tiny blood vessels (Fig. 26-3). The transfer of oxygen into the blood, and carbon dioxide out of it, occurs in the alveoli. This process is called **gas exchange,** and it is described in more detail later in this chapter. The tissue of healthy lungs is very elastic and sponge-like, because of all of the air-filled alveoli.

FIGURE 26-2

A resin cast of human lungs clearly shows the trachea, bronchi, and bronchioles. (© *A. Siegel/Custom Medical Stock Photo.*)

The many blood vessels that surround the alveoli give healthy lung tissue its brilliant pink color.

The lungs are divided into sections called lobes. The right lung has three lobes and the left lung has only two. The left lung is slightly smaller than the right lung because of the position of the heart in the chest cavity.

The lungs are housed in the chest cavity. The inside of the chest cavity is lined with a membrane called the **pleura,** which also covers the outside of the lungs. Because the lungs almost fill the chest cavity, the pleura on the outside of the lungs almost touches the pleura on the inside of the chest cavity. The pleura secretes a thin fluid that allows the lungs to slide easily against the chest cavity walls during the process of breathing.

FUNCTION OF THE RESPIRATORY SYSTEM

The main purpose of the respiratory system is respiration. Respiration is accomplished through the processes of ventilation and gas exchange.

VENTILATION

As you learned in Chapter 16, ventilation is the mechanical process of moving air in and out of the lungs (breathing). Ventilation has two phases: inhalation and exhalation. The **diaphragm** is a strong, dome-shaped muscle that separates the chest cavity from the abdominal cavity (see Fig. 26-1). When we inhale, the diaphragm contracts, moving downward and making the chest cavity bigger. Air flows into the lungs, filling the alveoli and causing them to expand. When we exhale, the diaphragm relaxes, moving upward and pushing the air in the alveoli out of the lungs. Another group of muscles, called the intercostal muscles, helps with the respiratory effort as well. The intercostal muscles are located between the ribs.

The rate and depth of breathing is controlled mainly by the central nervous system, in the part of the brain called the medulla. Special cells, called chemoreceptors, are located in the medulla and in some of the major arteries. The chemoreceptors monitor the amount of carbon dioxide and oxygen in the blood and adjust the rate and depth of breathing as necessary. For example, if you are resting quietly, your body does not need as much oxygen and the amount of air inhaled and exhaled is minimal. But, if you are exercising, your body's need for oxygen is greatly increased, and ventilation increases as well. Although the brain ensures that breathing occurs automatically, the individual also has some control over breathing (for example, when you hold your breath while swimming).

GAS EXCHANGE

So, we now know how air moves in and out of the lungs. But just moving air in and out of the lungs is not enough. How does oxygen get from the air into the blood? How does the carbon dioxide in the blood get into the air we exhale? This is where the second phase of respiration, gas exchange, comes into play.

FIGURE 26-3

A cluster of air sacs, called alveoli, is found at the end of each bronchiole. The alveoli are surrounded by tiny blood vessels, which make gas exchange between the blood and the lungs possible.

Gas exchange occurs in the alveoli (Fig. 26-4). The walls of the alveoli are very thin—just one cell thick. Each alveolus is surrounded by a network of tiny blood vessels. The walls of the blood vessels are very thin too. As the blood passes through the blood vessels, it is brought very close to the air in the alveolus. Because the concentration of oxygen is greater in the air than it is in the blood, the oxygen in the air moves (diffuses) across the wall of the alveolus into the blood vessel, oxygenating the blood. At the same time, carbon dioxide moves from the blood (where it is more concentrated) into the alveolus, and is removed from the body when we exhale.

THE EFFECTS OF AGING ON THE RESPIRATORY SYSTEM

There is a good chance that many of the older people you will care for will have some type of respiratory problem. When the processes of aging are

FIGURE 26-4

Gas exchange occurs in the alveoli. Oxygen moves from the alveolus into the blood vessel, and carbon dioxide moves from the blood vessel into the alveolus.

combined with chronic illness, immobility, or a lifetime of exposure to toxic chemicals (such as those in pollution and tobacco smoke), the respiratory system's ability to function properly is significantly reduced. For example, many people who are in their 60s, 70s, and 80s today began to smoke before anyone really knew about the harmful effects of tobacco smoke. In addition, many older people worked before regulations such as those resulting from the Occupational Safety and Health Act were in place to keep them safe on the job. As a result, many were exposed to substances in the workplace that we now know are very harmful to the lungs, such as asbestos and coal dust.

When we inhale toxic substances (such as those in tobacco smoke and polluted air) day after day, the delicate membranes inside the lungs and airways become inflamed and stay that way. The chronic inflammation leads to scarring and may even cause changes that lead to cancer. In addition, chemicals in tobacco smoke paralyze the tiny cilia that line the trachea and bronchi. Recall that the purpose of the cilia is to sweep mucus upward, toward the pharynx, so that it can be eliminated from the respiratory tract. When the cilia are no longer able to perform this function because they have been paralyzed by tobacco smoke, the person must work harder to keep the airway and lungs clear of mucus. These attempts to keep the airway clear are what many of us know as a "smoker's cough." Fortunately, if a person is able to stop smoking, the cilia do regain their function and the tissues of the lungs will heal if the damage is not too severe.

Regular physical exercise and avoidance of tobacco smoke and other pollutants help to keep the respiratory system functioning properly well into old age (Fig. 26-5). However, as a person ages, there are two changes that are likely to occur to the respiratory system, even if the person is otherwise healthy. These changes include less efficient ventilation and an increased risk for respiratory tract infections.

LESS EFFICIENT VENTILATION

As you have learned in other chapters, loss of tissue elasticity and loss of muscle mass occur as a person ages. In the respiratory system, these changes result in less efficient ventilation. The very elastic lung tissue loses some of its ability to

FIGURE 26-5

Exercise, especially when combined with avoidance of smoking and exposure to pollution, is a most effective way of keeping the respiratory system healthy for many years.

expand and bounce back as a person breathes, which reduces the amount of air that is taken in and let out with each breath. The diaphragm and intercostal muscles become weaker, which means that the thoracic cavity may not expand as much with each breath, so the amount of air taken in will be smaller. However, in healthy older people who do not smoke, these changes do not usually cause any problems. Often, the person will not be aware of any change, except possibly during exercise, when oxygen demands are significantly increased.

INCREASED RISK OF RESPIRATORY INFECTIONS

The immune system becomes less efficient as a result of the aging process. This change in the immune system, combined with age-related changes to the respiratory system, makes older people more likely to get infections of the respiratory tract. In addition, a respiratory tract infection is likely to be more severe in an older person than it would be in a younger person. For example, what would have been a mild respiratory infection in a younger person can easily become a life-threatening respiratory infection in an elderly person.

Immobility also puts the older adult at higher risk for developing a severe respiratory infection. Many older people are less active because of changes in other body systems or because of chronic illness. In physically active people, the lungs are "exercised" along with the body, as they fully expand to meet the person's increased oxygen needs during exercise. But in a person who is confined to bed or a chair, the lungs do not get this "workout." A person who has become weak as a result of immobility may not be able to cough forcefully enough to clear the lungs of secretions. This can lead to the development of pneumonia, a serious lung infection.

DISORDERS OF THE RESPIRATORY SYSTEM

INFECTIONS

Pneumonia

Pneumonia is inflammation of the lung tissue. It may be caused by infection with a virus or a bacterium. The infection causes the alveoli to fill with fluid and pus, which prevents air from entering the alveoli. As a result, gas exchange (the transfer of oxygen into the blood and carbon dioxide out of it) cannot occur.

Signs and symptoms of pneumonia include fever, pain when breathing, cyanosis (bluish skin as a result of decreased oxygen levels in the blood), and a productive cough. A productive cough is one in which a person coughs up sputum. **Sputum,** which is also known as "phlegm," consists of mucus and other respiratory secretions that are coughed up from the lungs, bronchi, and trachea.

Pneumonia is usually diagnosed with a chest x-ray and treated with antibiotics. Knowledge about which microbe is causing the pneumonia will allow the doctor to prescribe the most effective antibiotic therapy. You may be asked to assist by collecting a sputum specimen for analysis. Guidelines for collecting sputum specimens are given in Guidelines Box 26-1.

Pleurisy is an inflammation of the pleura, the membrane that lines the chest cavity and covers the lungs. Pleurisy often accompanies lower respiratory tract infections such as pneumonia. The inflammation of the pleura causes pain during breathing as the layers of membrane rub against each other when the lungs expand and relax. Fluid may also collect in the space between the thoracic cavity and the lung. This build-up of fluid prevents the lungs from expanding fully. The doctor may need to insert a needle into the chest cavity to drain the fluid.

Bronchitis

Bronchitis is inflammation of the bronchi. Like pneumonia, bronchitis can be caused by a viral or bacterial infection. Bronchitis may cause a dry, nonproductive cough that sounds like a "bark." Bacterial bronchitis is usually treated with antibiotics. Both bacterial and viral bronchitis can turn into pneumonia if the bronchial infection is not treated promptly.

Influenza

Influenza, commonly referred to as "the flu," is an acute respiratory infection caused by the influenza virus. Symptoms of the flu are probably familiar to you from first-hand experience: sore throat, dry cough, stuffy nose, headache, body aches, weakness, and fever. Influenza is different from the "common cold," which can be caused by many different types of viruses and usually only affects the upper respiratory tract.

The influenza virus is very contagious. Most people who get the flu will recover in about a week. However, elderly people, very young children, and people with chronic illnesses who get the flu are at risk for developing serious complications, such as an extremely severe form of pneumonia. Residents of long-term care facilities are especially at risk for contracting and spreading influenza to other residents and to the staff. An annual "flu shot" for both staff members and residents is a very effective way of preventing outbreaks of influenza in long-term care facilities (Fig. 26-6).

ASTHMA

Asthma is a condition that affects the bronchi and bronchioles. In people with asthma, triggers (such as cold weather, allergies, respiratory infections, stress, smoke, and exercise) cause the bronchi and bronchioles to constrict (become narrower). This makes breathing very difficult, because air does not flow freely through the airways. An asthma attack can be very frightening for the person experiencing it, because the airways can narrow to the point that breathing becomes almost impossible. If one of your patients or residents is having trouble breathing or is making wheezing sounds, you should call the nurse immediately.

GUIDELINES BOX 26-1
GUIDELINES FOR COLLECTING A SPUTUM SPECIMEN

What you do	Why you do it
Explain to the person that the sputum for the specimen should be coughed up from deep down in the respiratory tract.	The sputum for analysis must come from the lungs, because that is where most of the infection-causing microbes are located. Explaining this to the person helps to ensure that he produces a specimen that will result in an accurate diagnosis. If you do not explain this to the person, he may just cough up saliva, which will not result in an accurate diagnosis.
Provide privacy.	Having to spit mucus into a cup can be embarrassing and unpleasant for some people.
Have the person rinse her mouth with water before coughing up the specimen.	Rinsing with plain water helps to remove microbes that are normally present in the mouth, resulting in a "cleaner" specimen.
Do not have the person rinse with mouthwash before coughing up the specimen.	The antiseptic effects of the mouthwash might actually kill the microbes in the sputum specimen that are responsible for the infection, which will result in inaccurate test results.
Have the person spit the specimen directly into a sterile specimen container and close the lid.	Having the person spit directly into the sterile specimen container reduces the risk of contaminating the specimen and results in more accurate test results.
Make sure that the specimen container is labeled properly and that the information is correct.	Labeling errors can result in misdiagnosis or the need to repeat the test.
Take the specimen container to the laboratory immediately after collecting the specimen or ask the nurse how to store it.	Allowing a specimen to sit around or storing it the incorrect way can result in the need to repeat the test.

An acute asthma attack is usually treated with inhaled drugs called bronchodilators (Fig. 26-7). Bronchodilators stop the muscle spasms responsible for the constriction of the airways. People with chronic asthma may need to take drugs on a regular basis to prevent attacks from occurring. These drugs may be given orally, or they may be inhaled.

CHRONIC OBSTRUCTIVE PULMONARY DISEASE (COPD)

Chronic obstructive pulmonary disease (COPD) is a general term used to describe two related lung disorders, emphysema and chronic bronchitis. These disorders often occur together in the same person, which is why some health care professionals prefer the more general term, COPD. The leading cause of COPD is smoking.

Emphysema

Emphysema is a form of COPD that involves damage to the alveoli. As you learned earlier, the walls of the alveoli are very thin and delicate. When a toxin, such as tobacco smoke, is inhaled, it damages the thin walls of the alveoli. Over time, the damage causes the fragile walls of the alveoli to break. Eventually, instead of having millions of tiny alveoli where gas exchange can take place, the person has fewer, large "merged" alveoli that are no longer effective for gas exchange (Fig. 26-8). Because the lung tissue is damaged,

FIGURE 26-6

Flu shots are usually given to residents in the fall, before the start of flu season (November through April). Flu shots help to prevent infection with the influenza virus, which is very contagious and can cause serious complications in elderly people, very young children, and people with chronic illnesses.

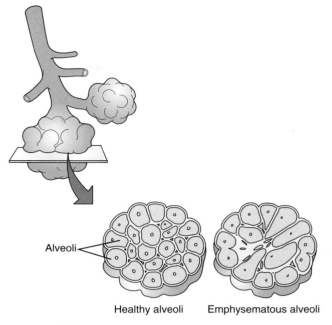

Alveoli

Healthy alveoli   Emphysematous alveoli

FIGURE 26-8

Emphysema occurs as a result of damage to the alveoli. The damage to the alveoli makes it difficult for the body to obtain oxygen and get rid of carbon dioxide. A healthy lung contains millions of tiny alveoli, where gas exchange takes place. In a person with emphysema, the walls of the alveoli break down, forming large areas where air can get trapped.

it is no longer "springy," and the air gets trapped in the large, damaged alveoli. The trapped air cannot be exhaled and exchanged for new oxygen-rich air, which limits the amount of oxygen the lungs are able to supply to the body. In addition, excess fluid can collect in the damaged alveoli, creating an excellent place for infection-causing microbes to collect and multiply.

A person with emphysema has trouble getting a "proper breath." The person's breathing is shallow and rapid, and he may have to stop to catch his breath quite frequently when talking or engaging in any type of physical activity. As the person's emphysema gets worse, he will need supplemental oxygen just to carry out even the simplest activities of daily living (ADLs). If you are caring for a person with emphysema, you may notice that his chest is enlarged and rounded. This finding is referred to as "barrel chest" and is caused by years of having extra air trapped in the lung tissue, which causes the chest cavity to enlarge over time.

Chronic Bronchitis

The other form of COPD is chronic bronchitis. **Chronic bronchitis** is caused by long-term irritation of the bronchi and bronchioles, such as that caused by inhaling tobacco smoke. The irritation leads to the production of thick mucus, which blocks the airways. Because the air cannot pass freely through the bronchi and bronchioles, breathing is impaired. In addition, infection-causing microbes can collect in the mucus and multiply, leading to infection.

A person with chronic bronchitis has a nagging, productive cough. She may complain of a

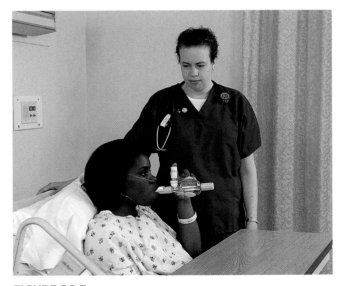

FIGURE 26-7

Asthma medications are often delivered through inhalers. (*Copyright B. Proud.*)

"tightness" in her chest, or difficulty breathing. She is likely to have frequent respiratory tract infections. Like a person with emphysema, a person with chronic bronchitis will eventually need oxygen therapy.

CANCER

In the United States, cancers involving the lungs and airway are the most common cause of cancer-related death in both men and women. The types of cancers that affect the upper respiratory tract include tumors of the mouth, tongue, and vocal cords. Cancers of the lower respiratory tract can involve the lungs or the lining of the bronchi. People who smoke cigarettes are 10 times more likely to develop lung cancer than nonsmokers are. In addition, some cancers that begin in other body parts, such as the breast or intestines, commonly spread to the lungs.

You may find yourself caring for a person who is having diagnostic tests done to determine whether or not she has cancer of the lungs or airway. It is important for you to remember that the person and her family members may be very worried about both the diagnostic test itself and the results of the test. You may notice that your patient or resident seems very quiet or distracted, or that she is having trouble concentrating on tasks.

Or, you might come into the room and find the person crying. Sometimes worrying makes a person angry, short-tempered, or agitated. Family members may show similar behaviors as they worry about their loved one.

There are several different ways that the diagnosis of cancer can be made:

- **Radiologic studies,** such as chest x-rays, computed tomography (CT) scans, and magnetic resonance imaging (MRI) scans, allow the doctor to see the tumor without actually entering the body.
- **Bronchoscopy** involves using a special instrument to look inside the airway and obtain tissue or fluids for analysis. The bronchoscope is passed through the mouth and pharynx and into the person's airway (Fig. 26-9). The person may have some discomfort during the procedure, as well as a scratchy throat afterwards.
- **Surgery** may be necessary to obtain tissue for analysis. Of all of the diagnostic methods, surgery carries the most risk for the person and is associated with the most discomfort.

You may also find yourself caring for people who are in a health care facility because they are receiving treatment for cancer of the respiratory system. There are many different ways of treating cancer, which are discussed in detail

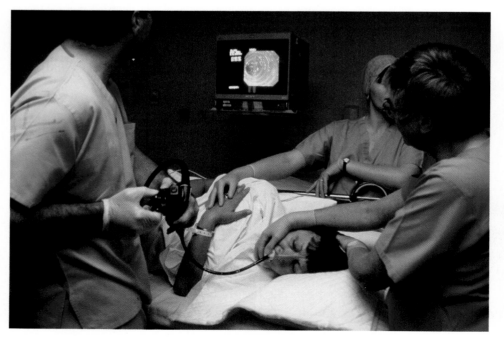

FIGURE 26-9

A doctor uses a flexible bronchoscope to examine a patient's airways. The bronchoscope is inserted in the patient's mouth, and an image of her trachea and lungs is displayed on the screen. (*© Antonia Reeve/Photo Researchers, Inc.*)

in Chapter 37. Treatment of cancer of the mouth, tongue, or vocal cords may involve surgery to remove the cancer and possibly some of the surrounding tissues as well. This type of surgery often changes the person's appearance, in very noticeable ways. For many people, coping with physical disfigurement as well as the diagnosis of cancer is very difficult. Treatment of lung cancer may involve surgical removal of all or part of the lung. A person who has had lung surgery will usually have drains inserted in the chest cavity for several days after the procedure to remove blood and fluid and to help keep the lungs expanded properly (Fig. 26-10). Make sure you have been shown how to care for a person with chest tubes if caring for a surgical patient is included in your responsibilities.

FIGURE 26-10

A chest tube drainage system is used to remove fluid (such as blood) or air that may build up in the chest cavity as a result of disease, injury, or surgery.

PNEUMOTHORAX AND HEMOTHORAX

Pneumothorax and hemothorax are often complications of chest trauma. **Pneumothorax** occurs when air builds up in the space between the lungs and the chest wall. For example, a penetrating chest wound, such as a stab wound to the chest, can lead to pneumothorax because the stab wound is a "sucking" wound. That means that because of the pressure difference between the inside and the outside of the body, air is drawn into the chest cavity through the wound. The air in the chest cavity prevents the lungs from expanding fully and makes it hard for the person to breathe. Insertion of a chest tube to remove the air is usually necessary.

Hemothorax occurs when blood builds up in the space between the lungs and the chest wall. The bleeding can be caused by an injury to the chest or a rupture in the lung tissue. As with pneumothorax, the build-up prevents the lungs from fully expanding and breathing becomes difficult. Sometimes surgery is needed to stop the bleeding, and a chest tube is inserted to remove the blood.

RESPIRATORY THERAPY

Respiratory therapy is any treatment that is used to help a person achieve satisfactory respiration. Some of these treatments are relatively simple. For example, a humidifier may be used to add moisture to the air, helping to loosen secretions during a bout of bronchitis or pneumonia. Other treatments may be quite complex and involve the use of drugs, such as oxygen, or mechanical ventilation.

Most health care facilities have a team of respiratory therapists who are specially trained to evaluate and treat problems of the respiratory system. The respiratory therapist listens to the person's breath sounds and looks at certain measurements to evaluate the person's respiratory function. For example, the respiratory therapist will measure the amount of air that is inhaled and exhaled, as well as the amount of oxygen in the person's blood. Next, the respiratory therapist helps to develop a treatment plan for the person. If you are caring for a patient or resident who needs the services of a respiratory therapist, watch the therapist and ask questions about the types of treatments he is using. This knowledge will help you to better understand the specific needs of your patient or resident. The nurse or respiratory therapist can also alert you to signs or symptoms that you should watch for and report to the nurse immediately.

OXYGEN THERAPY

The air we breathe contains only about 20% oxygen. The rest is nitrogen. People with reduced lung function (for example, people with emphysema) may have trouble getting the oxygen their bodies need from inhaled air alone. For these people, the doctor might prescribe supplemental (extra) oxygen to increase the amount of oxygen that they take in with each breath. The supplemental oxygen is pure, 100% oxygen.

Some people who are receiving supplemental oxygen will only need it for a short time. Others will need it for the rest of their lives. Oxygen can be given continuously, or it can be given on an as-needed basis. Some people only need supplemental oxygen when they are physically active.

Oxygen is considered a drug and requires a doctor's order to be used. The doctor determines the rate at which the oxygen should be delivered, and how it should be given. A nurse or respiratory therapist is responsible for setting up and adjusting the oxygen therapy. Many of the people you will care for will be receiving oxygen therapy. Therefore, you need to understand how oxygen is given and what precautions are necessary while oxygen is being used. Some states and facilities do not allow nursing assistants to adjust or assist with the administration of oxygen, but others do. Always make sure that you are familiar with your specific job responsibilities with regard to oxygen therapy. General guidelines for oxygen therapy are given in Guidelines Box 26-2. You should also review Chapter 9 for safety considerations related to oxygen therapy.

Oxygen is usually delivered to the patient or resident at a rate of 2 to 15 liters of oxygen per minute. The flow rate is set using a device called a **flow meter** (Fig. 26-11). Although you will not usually be responsible for adjusting the flow rate of oxygen, it is important for you to know what flow rate was ordered. You should make a point of checking the flow meter frequently when you are

FIGURE 26-11

A flow meter controls the rate of oxygen flow to the patient or resident. Flow meters come in a variety of styles. You should learn how the flow meters used by your patients or residents work. This will allow you to check the flow meter to make sure that the person is receiving the ordered amount of oxygen.

caring for a person who is receiving oxygen therapy to make sure that the flow rate is set properly. A patient or resident (or a visitor) might accidentally change the setting on the flow meter. If you notice that the setting on the flow meter does not match the amount of oxygen that has been ordered, notify the nurse immediately. Receiving too much oxygen is just as dangerous as receiving too little oxygen.

People who are receiving oxygen therapy may need to be monitored to make sure that enough oxygen is reaching the tissues. This monitoring may be constant for people who are critically ill. Other people will only require periodic monitoring. Monitoring of the oxygen content of the blood is done using a device called a *pulse oximeter*. The pulse oximeter is clipped to the person's fingertip or earlobe (Fig. 26-12). Infrared light is passed through the tissue to a sensor on the other side of the device. The amount of light that reaches the sensor is translated into a measurement of how much oxygen the blood is actually carrying. A normal reading is between 95% and 100%. Readings below 85% indicate that the person's tissues are not receiving enough oxygen. An alarm will usually sound if the person's blood oxygen level is too low.

Because oxygen therapy can be very drying to a person's mouth or nose, moisture is often added to the supplemental oxygen using a humidity bottle. The humidity bottle is filled with distilled water. The oxygen passes through the water before it is delivered to the patient or resident. This increases the water content of the

GUIDELINES BOX 26-2
GUIDELINES FOR OXYGEN THERAPY

What you do	Why you do it
Avoid lighting matches or cigarette lighters in the person's room. Post a "No Smoking" sign, and remind the patient or resident and any visitors not to smoke when oxygen is in use.	Use of oxygen therapy can increase the oxygen content of linens and clothing in the immediate area. If burning ashes from a cigarette should happen to drop on the bed, a fire would be more likely to start and would burn much faster as a result of the added oxygen.
Make sure that any electrical equipment is in good working order, and that cords are not frayed. Use a battery-operated razor or a blade razor when shaving a person who is receiving supplemental oxygen.	Electrical equipment that is not properly maintained can be the source of a spark, which could start a fire.
Make sure that the tubing through which the oxygen is delivered is free of kinks, and that the person is not lying on it.	If the tubing is obstructed in any way, oxygen flow will be impaired and the person will not receive the correct amount.
Do not adjust the flow rate of oxygen.	Adjusting the flow rate of oxygen is out of the nursing assistant's scope of practice. Receiving too much oxygen can be as harmful to the patient or resident as receiving too little oxygen. The doctor decides how much oxygen the patient or resident should receive.
When you are caring for a person who is receiving supplemental oxygen, be aware of the ordered flow rate, and tell the nurse if the flow rate on the flow meter does not match the ordered flow rate.	The setting on the flow meter may get changed accidentally. Checking frequently to make sure that the ordered flow rate matches the flow rate on the person's medical chart helps to keep your patient or resident safe. Receiving too much oxygen can be as harmful to the patient or resident as receiving too little oxygen.
When providing personal care, do not remove a person's facemask or nasal cannula, unless you are specifically told to do so by the nurse.	Removing the facemask or nasal cannula will deprive the person of the supplemental oxygen. Some people may not be able to tolerate a decrease in the amount of oxygen they are receiving, even for just a few minutes.
Make sure that the water level in the humidity bottle does not get too low.	Oxygen that is not humidified prior to delivery can be very drying to the mucous membrane lining of the person's nasal cavity and mouth. This dryness can be uncomfortable for the patient or resident.
Provide oral hygiene frequently, as directed by the nurse.	Frequent oral hygiene helps to relieve some of the dryness of the nose and mouth that occurs with supplemental oxygen therapy.
Watch for signs of skin irritation behind the person's ears, over his or her cheeks, or around his or her ears.	The pressure and friction from the tubing that holds the facemask or nasal cannula in place can cause skin breakdown.

FIGURE 26-12

Pulse oximetry is used to monitor the amount of oxygen that is reaching a person's tissues.

oxygen, making it less drying to the person's nose and mouth. As the oxygen flows through the water in the humidity bottle, it creates bubbles. You should check the humidity bottle frequently for the presence of bubbles, which indicate that the oxygen is flowing freely. You should also check the water level often, to make sure that it does not drop too low. Your facility policy will specify how often the humidity bottle should be changed.

Sources of Supplemental Oxygen

Supplemental oxygen can be supplied through a wall-mounted delivery system, in a pressurized tank, or through an oxygen concentrator (Fig. 26-13).

Wall-mounted Delivery Systems

In many facilities, the oxygen is piped into the patient's or resident's room from a central lo-cation. A special valve and flow meter device is inserted into the wall to access the oxygen (see Fig. 26-13A). The nurse or respiratory therapist sets the flow meter so that the oxygen is administered to the person at the correct rate.

Pressurized Tank

These tanks, which are placed in the patient's or resident's room, contain oxygen under pressure. Some of these tanks are small enough to be carried or wheeled around with the person (see Fig. 26-13B). The nurse or respiratory therapist sets the flow meter on the tank so that the oxygen is administered to the person at the correct rate.

A gauge tracks the amount of oxygen remaining in the tank. You should note when the dial shows that the supply of oxygen is getting low. If you notice that the tank is nearly empty, tell the nurse or respiratory therapist so that she can exchange the nearly empty tank for a full one.

Because the portable oxygen tanks are pressurized, they should be moved with caution. If the tank is accidentally knocked over and the valve at the top breaks, the escaping gas in the tank could propel the tank across the room with quite a bit of force. If the tank hit someone, it could cause a serious injury.

Oxygen Concentrators

Oxygen concentrators are devices that take in air and filter out the nitrogen, leaving behind pure oxygen (see Fig. 26-13C). The oxygen is then delivered to the person at the rate that has been programmed into the unit. Because the delivery amount is pre-set, the person (or caregiver) only has to turn the switch to "ON" when oxygen is needed. These units run on electricity and are often used in home and long-term care settings, especially if the person needs supplemental oxygen only once in a while.

Delivery of Supplemental Oxygen

A number of different devices are used to deliver oxygen to patients and residents. The type of delivery device used depends on several factors, including the amount of oxygen ordered, the condition being treated, and the overall physical condition of the patient or resident.

Nasal Cannulas

A nasal cannula is the most common method of administering oxygen. A **nasal cannula** is two

A. Wall-mounted delivery system

B. Pressurized tank

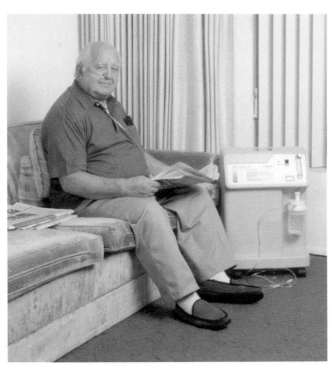

C. Oxygen concentrator

FIGURE 26-13

Supplemental oxygen can be supplied in various ways. (*A*) With a wall-mounted delivery system, the oxygen is piped into the person's room from a central location. A valve and flow meter device is inserted into the wall outlet to access the oxygen. (*B*) A pressurized tank of oxygen can go where the person goes. (*C*) An oxygen concentrator is often used in the home and long-term care settings, especially when the person only needs to use oxygen on an as-needed basis. Oxygen concentrators produce 100% oxygen by filtering the nitrogen out of room air. (*A used with permission from Taylor, C., Lillis, C., & LeMone, P. [2001].* Fundamentals of nursing *[4th ed., p. 1249]. Philadelphia: Lippincott Williams & Wilkins. C, © Custom Medical Stock Photo.*)

prongs of soft plastic tubing, which are inserted into the nostrils (Fig. 26-14A). The tubing to the cannula is connected to an oxygen source with a humidifier bottle and a flow meter. A nasal cannula is easy to apply, it does not interfere with eating or talking, and it is less likely to create a feeling of suffocation. However, the nasal cannula can dry out the mucous membranes in the nasal cavity if the oxygen is delivered at a high flow rate. The tubing can irritate the skin around the nostrils and cheeks and behind the ears. Finally, a nasal cannula may not be suitable for use in a critically ill patient, or in a person who breathes through his or her mouth, because the

concentration of oxygen delivered may not be high enough.

Facemasks

Oxygen can also be delivered through a **facemask.** A facemask is made of soft, molded plastic material that fits over the nose and mouth (see Fig. 26-14B). A facemask may be a simple device that just delivers the oxygen to the mouth and nose, or it may be quite complex, with attachments (such as bags that act as a holding place for extra oxygen). A facemask can deliver oxygen at a higher concentration than a nasal cannula can. In addition, a facemask is useful for a person who

A. Nasal cannula

B. Facemask

FIGURE 26-14

Devices used for oxygen delivery. (*A*) A nasal cannula is a two-pronged device that is inserted into the nostrils to deliver oxygen to the patient or resident. A person who has a nasal cannula in place is able to eat, drink, and speak normally. (*B*) A facemask fits over the person's nose and mouth. A facemask may be used when a person requires a high level of supplemental oxygen. Facemasks come in a variety of styles. (*A used with permission from Taylor, C., Lillis, C., & LeMone, P. [2001]. Fundamentals of nursing [4th ed., p. 1250]. Philadelphia: Lippincott Williams & Wilkins.*)

breathes through his or her mouth, instead of the nose. However, facemasks can make a person feel like he is suffocating (because they cover the person's nose and mouth), and they can interfere with the person's ability to eat, drink, and speak clearly. Sometimes a person is allowed to switch to a nasal cannula when it is time to eat or be shaved. Never remove a person's facemask without first asking the nurse. Removing the facemask, even briefly, can have serious consequences for the person.

Accessory Devices

There are some other devices that are often used in combination with nasal cannula or facemask oxygen delivery systems (Fig. 26-15). Some-

times a person is unconscious or has been sedated to the point that the muscles that keep the upper airway open relax. The lower jaw falls open and the tongue falls backwards into the throat, blocking the passage of air into the body.

To prevent this from happening, a nasopharyngeal airway (nasal trumpet) may be used. A **nasopharyngeal airway** is a soft rubber tube that is inserted into the person's nose (see Fig. 26-15A). It extends back toward the throat, providing an opening that air can flow through. Another commonly used airway device is the oropharyngeal airway. An **oropharyngeal airway** is a hard plastic device that is inserted into the person's mouth (see Fig. 26-15B). The oropharyngeal airway stops

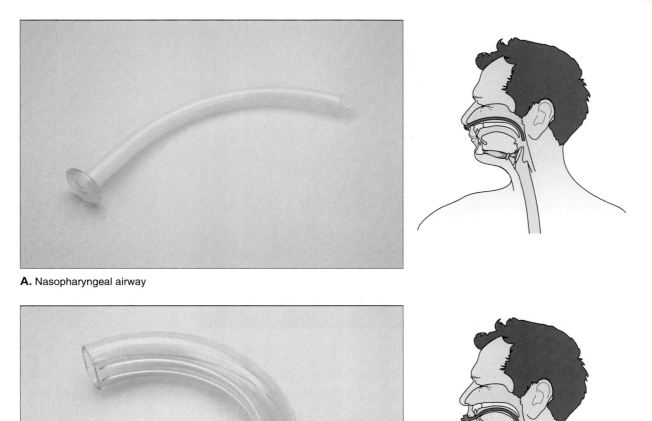

A. Nasopharyngeal airway

B. Oropharyngeal airway

FIGURE 26-15

An airway device may need to be used in a person who is unconscious or heavily sedated. The airway device keeps the airway open when the person cannot do this on his or her own. (*A*) A nasopharyngeal airway is inserted into the person's nose. (*B*) An oropharyngeal airway is inserted into the person's mouth.

the tongue from falling back into the throat, keeping the airway open. The oropharyngeal airway is used only for a person who is either heavily sedated or unconscious, because it can cause gagging and choking in a conscious person.

MECHANICAL VENTILATION

In **mechanical ventilation,** a machine called a *ventilator* breathes for a person who cannot breathe on his own (Fig. 26-16). There are many reasons that a person might need to be put on a ventilator. For example, a serious head injury, stroke, or drug overdose can affect the breathing

control centers in the brain, which means that regular breathing will no longer occur automatically. In these situations, mechanical ventilation is needed. A spinal cord injury or a neurologic disorder can interfere with the nerve impulses that cause the diaphragm to contract and relax automatically, resulting in the need for mechanical ventilation. Other conditions that may result in a person needing mechanical ventilation include acute respiratory infections and heart attacks. Mechanical ventilation is also often used both during and after surgery. Some people only need the ventilator for a short period of time, whereas others may need to be placed on a ventilator for

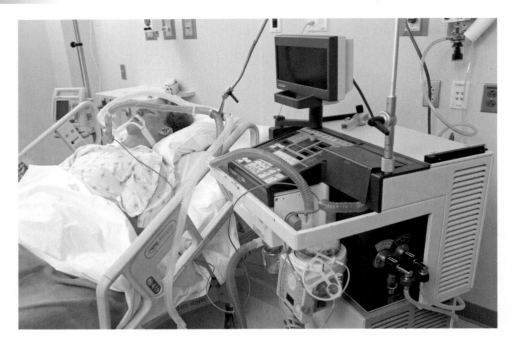

FIGURE 26-16

A mechanical ventilator performs the function of breathing for a person who cannot breathe on his own.

the rest of their lives. Not all people who require mechanical ventilation are confined to bed. Some ventilators are portable (Fig. 26-17).

A ventilator works by forcing air into the person's lungs. The air is delivered through a tube that is inserted into the airway. Depending on the situation, an endotracheal tube or a tracheostomy tube may be used (Fig. 26-18).

Endotracheal Intubation

Many people who require mechanical ventilation for only a short time will have an endotracheal

FIGURE 26-17

In 1995, actor Christopher Reeves was paralyzed by a horseback riding accident. A portable mechanical ventilator allows Mr. Reeves to lead an active life. Here, Mr. Reeves (*right*) is shown attending a conference on spinal cord injury in Australia. (© *AFP/ Corbis.*)

tube. The **endotracheal tube** is inserted into the person's nose or mouth. It extends to the trachea, where a balloon cuff on the end holds it in place and prevents secretions that drain from the mouth from entering the respiratory tract (see Fig. 26-18A). Being intubated with an endotracheal tube can be very uncomfortable and frightening for the patient or resident.

- Because the endotracheal tube travels through the larynx (voice box), a person who has an endotracheal tube in place is unable to talk, and will need to communicate using some other method, such as writing on a notepad. Imagine what it would be like to be dependent on a machine to breathe and unable to call out for help if you needed it. What would you do if the machine stopped? This is something that a person on a ventilator might worry about. Making sure that the call light control is within easy reach and checking on the person frequently are things you can do to make an intubated person feel more secure.
- The endotracheal tube makes it impossible for the person to take food or fluids through the mouth. Frequent oral care can help to relieve some of the dryness and discomfort caused by having an endotracheal tube in place.
- Wrist restraints are often used for a person who is intubated, to keep the person from reaching up and removing the endotra-

FIGURE 26-18

Mechanical ventilation requires the use of an endotracheal tube or a tracheostomy tube. (*A*) An endotracheal tube is inserted into the person's nose or mouth and passed through the pharynx and larynx to the trachea. An inflatable balloon cuff at the end of the endotracheal tube holds it in place and helps to prevent secretions from passing into the lungs. (*B*) A tracheostomy tube is inserted into a surgically created opening in the neck called a tracheostomy.

A. Endotracheal tube   **B.** Tracheostomy tube

cheal tube from the airway. The tube is uncomfortable, and it is natural for a person to try and remove it. Although the wrist restraints may be necessary, they can add to the person's anxiety. As is always the case when restraints are being used, you will need to check on the person very frequently, and the restraints will need to be removed and reapplied at regular intervals. Ensuring that a person with an endotracheal tube is as comfortable as possible and checking on the person frequently will help to relieve some of the person's worries and help him or her to feel safe.

Tracheostomy

If a person will need to be on a mechanical ventilator for more than a week or so, a tracheostomy is usually performed. A **tracheostomy** (often referred to as "a trach") is a surgically created opening in the neck that opens into the trachea. A short tube, called a tracheostomy or "trach" tube, is inserted into the opening and attached to the ventilator tubing (see Fig. 26-18B). The tracheostomy tube is usually secured around the person's neck with ties or a special collar device (Fig. 26-19). If the tube is not secured, it could be coughed out very easily.

A tracheostomy tube is much more comfortable for the person than an endotracheal tube. The person is able to eat and drink normally. The tracheostomy and tubing require special care, which is performed by the nurse. You are responsible for making sure that the tubing stays connected at all times and for observing the person for any signs that she is having trouble breathing.

Depending on the situation, a tracheostomy may be permanent or temporary. For example, a person who requires mechanical ventilation for several weeks will have a temporary tracheostomy that will be allowed to heal once the person no longer needs to be on the mechanical ventilator. However, a person who is paralyzed and will need to be on a ventilator for the rest of his or her life will have a permanent tracheostomy. A person who has had his larynx removed as a result of cancer will also have a permanent tracheostomy. The person breathes, talks, sneezes, and coughs through the tracheostomy because the airway between the pharynx and the trachea is no longer complete.

FIGURE 26-19

The tracheostomy tube is held in place with special ties or a collar.

SUCTIONING

People with respiratory disorders often need help removing secretions from the airway. Conditions such as pneumonia or chronic bronchitis can cause the production of large amounts of sputum, which builds up in the lungs and bronchi and makes it difficult to breathe. Other conditions interfere with a person's ability to cough up secretions. For example, a person who is in a coma or heavily sedated may not have an intact cough reflex. Therefore, the person does not cough and the secretions continue to build up. **Suctioning** is the process of removing fluid and mucus from a person's airway.

Suctioning is done using various types of suction catheters. The suction catheter is attached to tubing and a suction source, which works like a vacuum cleaner to remove the secretions from the airway. A Yankauer suction tip is used to remove secretions that collect in the back of the throat (Fig. 26-20). The Yankauer tip is placed in the person's mouth, and suction is applied. A long, thin, flexible catheter is used when it is necessary to suction the airways in the lower respiratory system. This soft catheter can be passed through the nose or mouth, or down an endotracheal or tracheostomy tube.

Because suctioning removes air along with the bothersome secretions, a person can easily become **hypoxic** (that is, deficient of oxygen) during the suctioning procedure. Nursing assistants are not responsible for suctioning patients and residents, but you will be responsible for letting the nurse know that suctioning may be needed, and for assisting during the procedure. Usually it is quite obvious when a person needs to have his airway suctioned. The person's breathing becomes noisy, and he may keep trying to cough up secretions, with little success.

GENERAL CARE MEASURES

Because there is little room for error when dealing with the respiratory system, many of the therapies that are used to help people with respiratory disorders can be carried out only by people who have received advanced training, such as nurses and respiratory therapists. However, many facilities and agencies offer additional training that will allow you to be more active in caring for people with special respiratory needs. For example, you may work in a facility that provides specialized care for people who depend on mechanical ventilators to breathe. In this case, your scope of practice may be widened to include procedures that are not normally part of a nursing assistant's responsibilities. Make sure that you have been adequately instructed in any special procedures that are required of you, and always be aware of what is and

FIGURE 26-20

A Yankauer suction tip is used to remove secretions from the mouth and the back of the throat. You will be able to tell when a person needs to be suctioned. Always report this observation to the nurse so that he or she can perform the procedure.

is not within your scope of practice, per your state's or facility's policy. No matter where you work, there are several general care measures related to the respiratory system that are within every nursing assistant's scope of practice.

OBSERVATION

A nursing assistant's main responsibility in caring for any patient or resident with a respiratory problem is that of observation. Because you are the one who will spend the most time with your patients or residents, you will be the one who has the best opportunity to observe signs that a person may be having problems with ventilation or gas exchange. Some of your patients or residents who have chronic respiratory problems will always have difficulty breathing when they exert themselves. It is important for you to be able to recognize what is normal for each of your patients or residents, so that you can recognize changes if they occur. You should also be aware of a person's normal skin color, so that you are able to recognize changes that may indicate that her tissues are not receiving enough oxygen.

▓▶ *Tell the Nurse!*

Not receiving adequate oxygen, even for a very short time, places a person at risk for developing severe complications, or even dying. Tell the nurse immediately if you observe any of the following:

⟫ A person experiences the sudden onset of chest pain or difficulty breathing

⟫ A person develops noisy breathing (for example, wheezing, "barking," or "crowing")

⟫ A person begins to make fluid-like, gurgling sounds (this is especially important to report if the person is very weak or comatose)

⟫ The oxygen flow rate on the oxygen flow meter does not match the ordered amount of oxygen

⟫ The gauge on a pressurized oxygen tank indicates that the oxygen level is low

⟫ The screen on a pulse oximeter shows a reading of less than 95%

⟫ A person's skin has a blue or gray tinge, either at rest or while exercising

⟫ A person coughs up sputum that is discolored (green, frothy, brown, or red-streaked)

⟫ A person's tracheostomy or endotracheal tube becomes dislodged

⟫ A person becomes short of breath during a physical activity that he or she has performed without effort in the past

⟫ A person's respirations become very slow and shallow, or they stop

PROMOTING COMFORT

There are many things that a nursing assistant can do to help a person with respiratory problems feel more comfortable. Positioning the person in the Fowler's or semi-Fowler's position is often helpful. Some people are more comfortable when they assume a forward-leaning position using pillows on the over-bed table (Fig. 26-21). If the doctor has not placed any restrictions on the person's fluid intake, encourage the patient or resident to drink plenty of fluids. Fluids help to thin respiratory secretions so that they are easier to cough up. Providing frequent oral care will also help keep the person comfortable and will reduce the number of microbes that are present in the mouth.

PROVIDING HOLISTIC CARE

Holistic care involves meeting a person's emotional needs, as well as his or her physical ones. When caring for a person with a respiratory disorder, you will have many opportunities to provide holistic care. For example, people who suffer from chronic conditions of the respiratory system, such as asthma or COPD, may be quite "needy." You may become annoyed with their frequent use of the call light control to ask for seemingly trivial things. Please stop for a moment and try to understand how frightening it would be to suddenly feel that you could not breathe! A person who is having an asthma attack or experiencing a flare-up of COPD feels that each breath might be his last. He might be afraid that in the event of another flare-up or attack, help will not arrive soon enough. Using the call light control frequently is the person's way of "testing the waters" to make sure that someone will actually come quickly if he calls. Instead of giving in to the desire to avoid a

FIGURE 26-21
Certain positions make breathing easier for people with respiratory disorders. Many people find that leaning forward helps to make breathing easier.

needy patient or resident, be patient and understanding of the underlying fears the person may have. Spend more time with the person, and get into the habit of stopping by to check on him, even when he has not called you. By addressing the person's underlying need for safety and security, you will be providing truly holistic care.

Some of the chronic disorders you have learned about in this chapter can diminish a person's quality of life significantly. Some, such as COPD and certain cancers of the respiratory system, will ultimately be the cause of the person's death. It is important to remember the stages of grief described in Chapter 21 when you are caring for a person with a chronic or terminal illness, especially when that illness is the result of a habit such as smoking. A person who has developed a smoking-related condition may have a lot of guilt or anger related to her condition. Even if the condition is not immediately terminal, the person will still grieve for the loss of health as a result of the illness.

When a person has a smoking-related illness, be careful not to be judgmental about the role the person's actions may have had in causing her disease. A person with a smoking-related illness, such as cancer or COPD, may choose to continue smoking, even though she knows doing so may significantly shorten her life. Smoking is very physically addictive and quitting can be extremely difficult, especially when the person is trying to cope with the stress of having a chronic or terminal condition. Each of your patients or residents must be allowed to make decisions concerning her own quality of life. For some people, this may mean not giving up smoking, even when it would seem to be the best thing to do.

SUMMARY

▶ "When you can't breathe, nothing else matters." (American Lung Association)
  ■ The function of the respiratory system is to provide the body with oxygen and rid the body of carbon dioxide.
  ■ The respiratory system consists of the lungs and a group of structures known collectively as the *airway*. The airway consists of the nasal cavities, pharynx, larynx, trachea, bronchi, and bronchioles.
    • The upper respiratory tract consists of those structures located outside of the chest cavity (the nasal cavity, pharynx, and larynx).
    • The lower respiratory tract consists of those structures located inside of the chest cavity (the trachea, bronchi, bronchioles, and lungs).
▶ Respiration involves two processes, ventilation and gas exchange. If one or the other of these processes is impaired, respiration will not be effective.
  ■ Ventilation is the process of physically moving air in and out of the lungs

(i.e., breathing). The diaphragm is the major muscle responsible for ventilation.

- Gas exchange is the process of transferring oxygen from the air into the blood, and transferring carbon dioxide from the blood into the air. Gas exchange occurs in the alveoli.

► Like all organ systems, the respiratory system is affected by aging.

- Loss of elasticity in the lung tissue and weakening of the muscles of respiration make breathing less efficient, because an older person is able to take in less air with each breath.

- The decreased ability of the immune system to fight infections may make an elderly person more likely to get pneumonia and other respiratory infections.

- Chronic illness, immobility, or a lifetime of exposure to pollution, chemicals, or tobacco smoke can make the effects of aging on the respiratory system much more noticeable. Regular physical exercise combined with healthy habits such as the avoidance of smoking helps to keep the respiratory system healthy throughout a person's lifetime.

► Disorders of the respiratory system can make breathing very difficult.

- Infections can be caused by bacteria or viruses and include pneumonia, bronchitis, and influenza.

- Asthma is narrowing of the bronchioles in response to certain triggers, such as allergies, cold air, exercise, smoke, or stress. An asthma attack can be very frightening for the person experiencing it.

- Chronic obstructive pulmonary disease (COPD) is a general term for two smoking-related disorders.
  - In emphysema, the alveoli are destroyed. Trapping of air in the lungs results.

Breathing is difficult and gas exchange is impaired.
  - Chronic bronchitis affects the bronchi and bronchioles. Chronic bronchitis is associated with the production of excessive amounts of secretions.

- Cancers of the lungs and airway are the most common cause of cancer-related deaths in both men and women in the United States. People who smoke are 10 times more likely to develop lung cancer than nonsmokers are.

► Respiratory therapy is used to help improve a person's processes of ventilation, gas exchange, or both.

- Oxygen therapy is the administration of supplemental oxygen.
  - Oxygen is a drug and requires a doctor's order to be used.
  - Oxygen may be supplied by way of a wall-mounted system, an individual pressurized tank, or an oxygen concentrator.
  - Oxygen can be administered through a nasal cannula or facemask.

- Mechanical ventilation is used for a person who cannot inhale and exhale on his own. A person who needs the assistance of a mechanical ventilator must be intubated with an endotracheal tube or a tracheostomy tube.

- Suctioning is often necessary to remove excessive secretions from a person's respiratory tract.

► A nursing assistant's responsibilities when caring for a person with a respiratory disorder are mainly observation and the promotion of comfort. A nursing assistant also provides holistic care by helping the person to feel safe and secure. Not being able to breathe easily can be very frightening for the patient or resident.

What did you learn?

Multiple Choice

Select the single best answer for each of the following questions.

1. Who has to write the order for oxygen to be used?
   a. The nurse
   b. The respiratory therapist
   c. The doctor
   d. No order is necessary; if someone needs oxygen, it must be given immediately.

2. The nurse asks you to obtain a sputum specimen from Mrs. Long, who has pneumonia. Which one of the following is correct to do when obtaining a sputum specimen?
   a. Have Mrs. Long rinse her mouth with mouthwash before producing the specimen.
   b. Have Mrs. Long cough the specimen into an emesis basin, and then transfer the specimen to the specimen container.
   c. Explain to Mrs. Long that the specimen must come from deep within her chest.
   d. Put the specimen container in the refrigerator after you have collected the sputum specimen and labeled the container with Mrs. Long's name and room number.

3. What color is a healthy lung?
   a. Blue
   b. Gray
   c. White
   d. Pink

4. Where does gas exchange take place?
   a. In the alveoli
   b. In the bronchioles
   c. In the pleura
   d. In the nasal cavity

5. Which of the following is true about a person who has an endotracheal tube in place?
   a. The person is able to eat and drink normally.
   b. The person is able to talk normally.
   c. The person will need frequent oral care.
   d. The person is unconscious.

6. You have been assigned to care for Mr. Fenley, who has chronic obstructive pulmonary disease (COPD). He is on continuous oxygen by a nasal cannula at a rate of 4 liters per minute. Mr. Fenley's oldest son visits daily and is very concerned about his father's condition. One morning, you enter Mr. Fenley's room to do your morning checks, and you notice that the flow rate on the flow meter is set at 8 liters per minute. What should you do?
   a. Call the nurse immediately.
   b. Decrease the flow rate back to the prescribed 4 liters per minute.
   c. Tell Mr. Fenley and his son that it is very dangerous for them to make adjustments to the flow meter on their own.
   d. Nothing. A patient or resident can adjust the flow rate of oxygen to meet his or her own needs.

7. One of your responsibilities is to assist Mr. Tang with shaving. Mr. Tang is receiving continuous oxygen via a nasal cannula. What should you do when helping Mr. Tang to shave?
   a. Remove the nasal cannula before you begin the procedure.
   b. Use a battery-operated razor or a blade razor instead of an electrical razor.
   c. Increase the flow of oxygen during the procedure.
   d. Decrease the flow of oxygen during the procedure.

8. One of your newly admitted residents, Mr. Petersen, has emphysema. You are going to meet Mr. Petersen for the first time. Thinking back on what you learned during your nurse assistant training course about people with emphysema, which one of the following would you expect to be true of Mr. Petersen?
   a. His breathing will probably be shallow and rapid.
   b. He might need supplemental oxygen.
   c. He may have to catch his breath frequently while talking.
   d. All of the above

Matching

Match each numbered item with its appropriate lettered description.

_____ 1. Respiration
_____ 2. Lungs
_____ 3. Nasoph-
           aryngeal air-
           way
_____ 4. Hemothorax
_____ 5. Pharynx
_____ 6. Trachea
_____ 7. Pneumo-
           thorax
_____ 8. Pleura
_____ 9. Hypoxic
_____ 10. Nasal cavity

a. Blood in the chest cavity

b. Also known as the "windpipe"; conducts air from the larynx to the bronchi

c. Membrane that covers the inside of the chest cavity and the outside of the lungs

d. Also known as the throat

e. A rubber tube that is inserted in a person's nose or mouth to keep the airway open

f. The process the body uses to obtain oxygen from the environment and remove carbon dioxide from the body

g. Primary organs of respiration

h. Space where air from the outside of the body is first warmed, humidified, and filtered

i. Air in the chest cavity

j. Deficient of oxygen

? Stop and think!

▶ Barbara has been assigned to care for Mrs. Nielsen, who has severe respiratory problems resulting from a long history of asthma. When she got her assignment, Barbara groaned inwardly, expecting another shift of doing nothing but answering Mrs. Nielsen's call light. Sure enough, 5 minutes into Barbara's shift, the light above Mrs. Nielsen's door is on. Barbara goes into the room to find Mrs. Nielsen gasping for breath with her nasal cannula off. Barbara replaces the cannula and tries to calm Mrs. Nielsen down. As Barbara turns to leave, Mrs. Nielsen cries, "Help me! Help me! I can't breathe!" and then she pulls out the cannula again. Barbara is getting upset and doesn't know what to do. She has several other residents to check on and she can't get out of Mrs. Nielsen's room! Do you have any advice for Barbara?

▶ Matthew is providing care for Mr. Thompson, who has smoked for more than 50 years. Mr. Thompson has advanced COPD, and requires a lot of assistance with nearly everything (including smoking, which he continues to do). One day, you and Matthew are leaving work together and you see all of the "smokers" outside having their cigarettes, shivering because it is the middle of winter. Matthew tells you that he thinks smoking is a disgusting habit, and that people who smoke are weak and lack willpower. How might Matthew's feelings about smoking affect his relationship with Mr. Thompson and other residents with smoking-related conditions?

CHAPTER

27

The Cardiovascular System

What will you learn?

The heart and the other organs that make up the cardiovascular system (also known as the *circulatory system*) are the subject of this chapter. According to the Centers for Disease Control and Prevention (CDC), about 61 million Americans live with the effects of either heart disease or stroke (a neurologic problem caused by cardiovascular disease). That's nearly 25% of the population! Given those numbers, it is highly likely that some of the people you will care for daily will have some sort of a cardiovascular problem. Not only will an understanding of how the cardiovascular system works help you to better serve your patients or residents, it will help you to keep your own cardiovascular system healthy! When you are finished with this chapter, you will be able to:

1. List and describe the major parts of the cardiovascular system.
2. Discuss the major functions of the cardiovascular system.
3. Describe how aging affects the cardiovascular system.
4. Explain how exercise and a healthy lifestyle can diminish the effects of aging on the cardiovascular system.
5. Discuss various disorders that affect the cardiovascular system.
6. List diagnostic tests that are often used to diagnose disorders of the cardiovascular system.
7. Describe rehabilitation that may be necessary for a person who has a cardiovascular disorder.

Photo: Red blood cells (erythrocytes) loaded with oxygen make their way through a capillary.
(© David M. Phillips/Photo Researchers, Inc.)

Vocabulary

Use the CD in the back of your book to hear these terms pronounced, defined, and used in a sentence:

Plasma	Venules	Pulmonary circulation	Plaques
Erythrocytes	Lymph	Systemic circulation	Arteriosclerosis
Hemoglobin	Lymph node	Systole	Peripheral vascular
Leukocytes	Endocardium	Diastole	disease
Thrombocytes	Myocardium	Cardiac cycle	Coronary artery
Coagulation	Epicardium	Varicose veins	disease
Hemostasis	Pericardium	Anemia	Angina pectoris
Arteries	Atria	Leukemia	Myocardial infarction
Veins	Ventricles	Thrombi	Heart failure
Arterioles	Ischemia	Embolus	Conduction disorders
Capillary bed	Circulation	Atherosclerosis	Cardiac rehabilitation

STRUCTURE OF THE CARDIOVASCULAR SYSTEM

The cardiovascular system, also known as the circulatory system, is made up of the blood, the blood vessels, the lymphatic system, and the heart. *Cardio* means "heart," and *vascular* means "vessels."

BLOOD

Blood is the life-giving fluid of our bodies. The blood has two main components, the plasma and the formed elements (Fig. 27-1A).

Plasma

More than half of the total blood volume is plasma. **Plasma** is the liquid part of the blood (see Fig. 27-1B). Plasma is about 90% water. The other 10% is made up of substances that are dissolved in the water (such as glucose, amino acids, fats, and salts) and proteins. Important plasma proteins include albumin, fibrinogen, and globulins. Albumin plays a role in moving fluid in and out of the bloodstream. Fibrinogen is used as part of the blood clotting process. Globulins help to fight infection.

Formed Elements

The formed elements of the blood are the blood cells.

Red Blood Cells (Erythrocytes)

Red blood cells, or **erythrocytes,** carry oxygen. The name *erythrocyte* comes from *eryth-*, which means "red," and *cyt*, which means "cell." There are approximately 5 million red blood cells per cubic millimeter of blood! Red blood cells are manufactured in the red bone marrow (see Chapter 25) and are continuously replaced as old ones wear out.

Red blood cells are tiny, disc-shaped cells that are thinner in the center than at the edges (see Fig. 27-1A). The "dent" in the center of the red blood cell contains a protein called **hemoglobin.** Oxygen molecules attach to the hemoglobin for transport to the tissues. When combined with oxygen, hemoglobin is bright red. This is what gives red blood cells their color and name.

The hemoglobin molecule on each red blood cell can carry many oxygen molecules. The hemoglobin on red blood cells that have just received a full load of oxygen from the lungs is filled to capacity with oxygen, and therefore this blood is very bright red. As the blood circulates through the body, giving off oxygen and taking on carbon dioxide, the number of oxygen molecules on the hemoglobin molecule decreases, and the blood becomes darker red in color.

White Blood Cells (Leukocytes)

White blood cells, or **leukocytes,** fight infection. The name *leukocyte* comes from *leuk*, which means "white" and *cyt*, which means "cell." The

FIGURE 27-1

(A) Blood consists of plasma and formed elements (blood cells). (B) When blood is put in a machine called a centrifuge and spun at high speeds, the formed elements (blood cells) sink to the bottom while the plasma rises to the top. Human blood is about 55% plasma. (B, © Antonia Reeve/Photo Researchers, Inc.)

name "white blood cell" is not exactly accurate because in reality, "white" blood cells are colorless. Nevertheless, "white blood cell" is a commonly accepted way of referring to leukocytes.

The blood of a healthy person contains 5,000 to 10,000 white blood cells per cubic millimeter. There are five different types of white blood cells (see Fig. 27-1A). Each type of white blood cell has a different function, related to fighting infection. As you will recall from Chapter 7, some destroy pathogens by surrounding them and "eating" them in a process called phagocytosis (see Chapter 7, Figure 7-2). Others secrete substances that cause the pathogen to die. Still others make proteins

called antibodies, which prevent us from getting some diseases twice.

White blood cells are formed in the red bone marrow and the lymphatic system (discussed later in this chapter). An infection causes white blood cell production to increase, sending more "troops" into the bloodstream to battle the invading pathogen.

Platelets (Thrombocytes)

Platelets, or **thrombocytes,** are responsible for clotting **(coagulation)** of the blood. When injury occurs, the platelets stick together to form

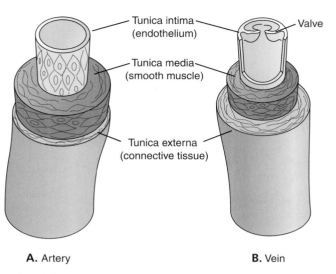

A. Artery   **B.** Vein

FIGURE 27-2

The walls of the blood vessels have three layers. (*A*) An artery. (*B*) A vein.

a temporary plug over the site of injury. They also release chemicals that react with the plasma protein fibrinogen, causing a more permanent clot (or scab) to develop. This process, known as **hemostasis,** stops the loss of blood from the circulatory system (*heme-* = "blood," *stasis* = "stop").

Platelets are not actually whole cells. They are pinched-off pieces of larger cells that are formed in the red bone marrow. There are about 150,000 to 450,000 platelets per cubic milliliter of circulating blood.

BLOOD VESSELS

The blood vessels carry blood to and from all of the tissues in the body. The walls of the blood vessels have three layers (Fig. 27-2). The layer on the inside, the *tunica intima,* is a smooth lining that helps blood to flow smoothly through the vessel. The middle layer, the *tunica media,* is formed of smooth muscle tissue. The smooth muscle in the tunica media is what allows the blood vessels to constrict or dilate according to the body's needs. Constriction (narrowing) of the vessels slows the flow of blood, whereas dilation (widening) of the vessels allows blood to flow more rapidly. The outer layer of the vessel wall, the *tunica externa,* is a tough protective layer of connective tissue.

Arteries carry blood away from the heart, and **veins** carry blood to the heart. Looking at Figure 27-2, you can see that there are two major differences between the walls of the arteries and the walls of the veins:

- The walls of the arteries contain more smooth muscle than those of the veins, because the arteries receive blood that is being pumped from the heart under great force and pressure. The smooth muscle in the walls of the arteries allows the arteries to handle the flow of blood from the heart.
- The tunica intima of the veins contains valves, which help blood to flow back to the heart. This is especially important in the arms and the legs, where blood would tend to flow away from the heart, due to the effects of gravity. The valves are assisted by contraction of nearby skeletal muscles. For example, when we walk, contraction of the leg muscles compresses the veins, pushing blood toward the heart.

Arteries carry blood away from the heart. As the arteries get further away from the heart, they branch into a network, becoming smaller and smaller in diameter (Fig. 27-3A). The smallest arteries are called **arterioles.** Arterioles send off branches called capillaries, which form a network in the tissues called the **capillary bed** (Fig. 27-4). As blood passes through the capillary bed, the oxygen and nutrients in the blood pass into the tissues, and carbon dioxide and other waste materials from the tissues pass into the blood. This transfer of substances in and out of the blood is possible because the walls of the capillaries have only one thin layer, as opposed to the three layers in the walls of the arteries and veins. After the blood passes through the capillary bed, it starts its journey back to the heart by way of very tiny veins called **venules** (see Fig. 27-4). Venules drain into small veins, which become larger in diameter as they approach the heart (see Fig. 27-3B).

LYMPHATIC SYSTEM

The pressure of the circulating blood through the tiny capillaries forces some of the blood plasma to leak out into the surrounding tissues. Approximately 10% of the circulating plasma leaks out of

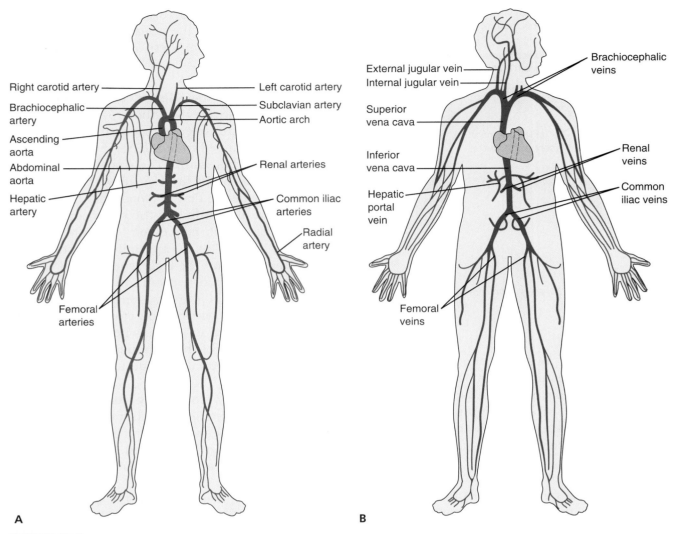

FIGURE 27-3

Blood vessels carry blood to every part of the body. (*A*) The major arteries of the body. Arteries carry blood away from the heart. Note how the arteries get smaller in diameter the further away they get from the heart. (*B*) The major veins of the body. Veins carry blood back to the heart. Note how the veins get larger in diameter the closer they get to the heart.

the capillaries in this manner. The lymphatic system helps to return the fluid that leaks into the tissues to the bloodstream. The lymphatic system also produces some of the white blood cells that fight invading pathogens.

The lymphatic system is actually a one-way, open-ended circulatory system (Fig. 27-5). Lymph capillaries absorb excess fluid from the surrounding tissues. (Once the fluid enters the lymph capillaries, it is called **lymph.**) The lymph capillaries join together to form larger vessels, called lymphatics. At certain points along the way, the lymph in the lymphatics passes through **lymph nodes,** masses of lymphatic tissue that "clean" the lymph by removing bacteria and other

large particles. Eventually, all of the lymphatics empty into the large veins in the shoulder region, returning the fluid to the general circulation.

Other parts of the lymphatic system include the thymus gland, which is located in the chest. The thymus gland secretes a chemical that stimulates the production of certain white blood cells (T cells) in the event of an infection. (Recall from Chapter 8 that T cells are the cells that the human immunodeficiency virus [HIV] virus attacks.) Another organ, the spleen, located in the abdomen, helps to filter blood and break down worn-out red blood cells. The spleen also acts as a reservoir where extra blood is stored. The body draws on this "extra" blood supply during times

FIGURE 27-4

The capillary bed is where the transfer of substances between the blood and the tissues occurs.

of massive blood loss, for example, following a major injury.

HEART

The heart is a hollow, muscular organ about the size of a fist that lies in the center of the chest, tilted a bit toward the left, behind the sternum (breastbone). Like the walls of the arteries and veins, the walls of the heart are made of three layers of tissue. The **endocardium** is the smooth inner layer of the heart. The **myocardium,** the middle layer, is formed of cardiac muscle. Coordinated contraction and relaxation of the myocardium is what causes the heart to pump. The **epicardium** is the smooth outermost layer of the heart. The epicardium forms part of the **pericardium,** a double-layered protective sac that surrounds the heart. A thin film of fluid between the epicardium and the outer layer of the pericardium allows the pericardial layers to slide smoothly against each other each time the heart pumps.

Atria and Ventricles

The hollow interior of the heart is divided into four chambers (Fig. 27-6). A thick wall of muscle, called the septum, separates the left side of the heart from the right side of the heart. Valves, flaps of tissue that help to ensure that blood flows only in one direction, separate the chambers on the top from the chambers on the bottom. The upper chambers are called the left atrium and

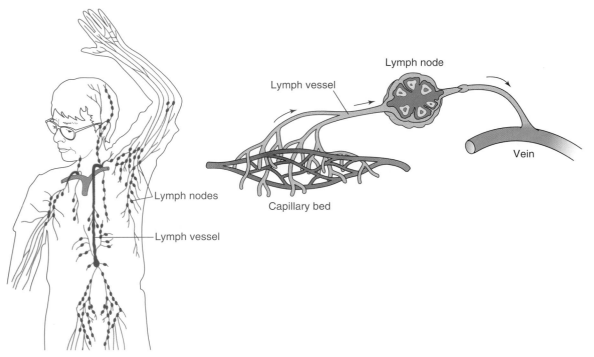

FIGURE 27-5

The lymphatic system returns fluid to the bloodstream. It is a one-way system. Lymph capillaries, located in the capillary bed, absorb fluid from the surrounding tissues. The lymph capillaries join together to form larger lymph vessels (called lymphatics). Eventually, the lymphatics empty into the subclavian veins, large veins in the shoulder region. Lymph nodes, masses of lymphatic tissue located along the lymphatics, remove bacteria and other foreign particles from the lymph before the fluid is returned to the bloodstream.

Aorta

Superior vena cava

Pulmonary valve

Right atrium

Tricuspid valve

Inferior vena cava

Right venticle

Septum

Pulmonary artery

Pulmonary veins

Left atrium

Aortic valve

Mitral (bicuspid) valve

Left ventricle

Myocardium

Descending aorta

FIGURE 27-6

The heart has four chambers. The atria receive blood that is being returned to the heart from the veins. Blood leaves the heart after passing through the ventricles.

right atrium, or the **atria.** The atria receive the blood that is being brought back to the heart from the body, and send it into the lower chambers of the heart, called the **ventricles.** When the ventricles contract, they send blood from the heart to other parts of the body. Because the ventricles must send the blood much further with each contraction, they are larger than the atria, and have thicker, more muscular walls.

Heart Valves

Blood can only flow through the heart in one direction. To keep blood flowing in the proper direction, the heart has four valves. Valves are flaps of tissue that snap shut after the blood passes through to prevent backflow.

- The tricuspid valve separates the right atrium from the right ventricle.
- The mitral (bicuspid) valve separates the left atrium from the left ventricle.
- The pulmonary valve is located where the pulmonary artery leaves the right ventricle.
- The aortic valve is located where the aorta leaves the left ventricle.

The four valves can be seen in Figure 27-6.

The valves that separate the upper and lower chambers of the heart may become diseased. For example, a type of infection called rheumatic

fever can cause the valves to become thickened and scarred. Damaged valves are unable to create a seal when they close, which allows blood to backflow into the atria when the ventricles pump. This condition is called *valvular insufficiency.* A person with valvular insufficiency may need surgery to replace the defective valve.

Conduction System

The muscle cells that make up the myocardium are very specialized, so that they contract as a unit. This unified contraction is what allows the heart to work efficiently as a pump, moving blood continuously through the body. A small mass of special tissue in the heart, called the sinoatrial node (pacemaker), sets the pace for contraction by generating an electrical impulse. The electrical impulse travels through the myocardium via a special pathway called the conduction system. As it passes through, the electrical energy causes the cardiac muscle cells in the myocardium to contract. First the atria contract, there is a pause, and then the ventricles contract.

Coronary Circulation

Like all organs, the heart needs oxygen and nutrients. In fact, the heart's demand for oxygen

FIGURE 27-7

The heart has its own blood supply, called the coronary circulation.

and nutrients is very high because it works continuously, without rest. Think about it—the normal resting heart rate of an adult is 70 beats/min, or about 100,800 beats in a 24-hour period! The heart does not have the luxury of stopping to rest when it is tired; it has to continue pumping blood through the body. All of this hard work adds up to a very high, and constant, demand for oxygen and nutrients.

The coronary circulation meets this demand (Fig. 27-7). (*Coronary* is another word for "heart.") Many people think that the cells of the heart just absorb oxygen from the blood that is passing through the chambers, but this is not the case. The tissues of the heart have their own special network of arteries and veins, just like all of the other organs in the body. Coronary arteries carry oxygen-rich blood into the heart tissue. Coronary veins remove carbon dioxide and other waste products. Any disruption in the flow of oxygen-rich blood to the tissues of the heart can cause **ischemia** (lack of oxygen to the tissues). Prolonged ischemia causes the tissue to die, resulting in permanent damage to the heart muscle.

FUNCTION OF THE CARDIOVASCULAR SYSTEM

The main function of the cardiovascular system is that of transport. However, the cardiovascular system also plays a role in regulating temperature and protecting the body from disease.

TRANSPORT

Bringing oxygen, nutrients, and other necessary substances (for example, hormones) to the cells and taking waste materials away from them is one of the most important functions of the cardiovascular system. Think of the cardiovascular system as a manufacturing company that serves customers across the nation. "Trucks" (red blood cells) are loaded up with merchandise at the "central warehouse" (the heart). The trucks set out on a huge network of "highways" (the blood vessels) to deliver their goods. When they reach their destinations, the ordered merchandise is unloaded, and the empty crates are put back on the trucks to be returned to the warehouse.

Pulmonary and Systemic Circulation

While the blood is the vehicle that transports oxygen, nutrients, wastes, and other substances to their various destinations, the heart is the organ that powers the continuous movement of the blood (known as the **circulation**). The pattern of circulation actually involves two circuits, the pulmonary circulation and the systemic circulation (Fig. 27-8). The right side of the heart pumps blood to the lungs, where it picks up oxygen and releases carbon dioxide. This is the **pulmonary circulation** (*pulmonary* is another word for "lungs.") The left side of the heart pumps the newly oxygenated blood to the body. This is the **systemic circulation.**

The pattern of circulation goes like this (follow along on Figure 27-8):

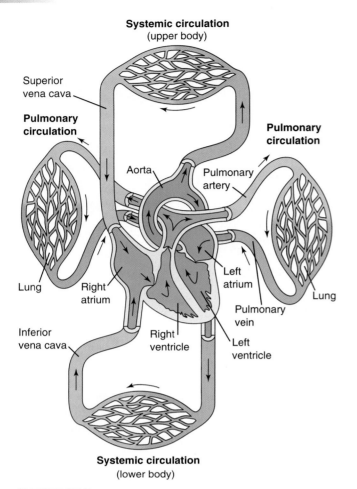

Systemic circulation
(upper body)

Superior
vena cava

**Pulmonary
circulation**

Aorta

Pulmonary
artery

**Pulmonary
circulation**

Lung

Right
atrium

Left
atrium

Lung

Inferior
vena cava

Right
ventricle

Pulmonary
vein

Left
ventricle

Systemic circulation
(lower body)

FIGURE 27-8

The pattern of circulation involves two circuits, the pulmonary circulation and the systemic circulation. In this diagram, *red* stands for oxygen-rich blood, and *blue* stands for oxygen-poor blood. Blood passes from the right ventricle into the pulmonary circulation. Once it is loaded up with oxygen, the blood returns to the left atrium, passes into the left ventricle, and is sent out to the rest of the body. This is the systemic circulation.

Pulmonary Circulation

- The largest veins in the body, the superior vena cava and the inferior vena cava, empty into the right atrium of the heart. The blood in these veins is returning from its journey to the tissues, so it has given up most of its oxygen and taken on a load of carbon dioxide.
- The right atrium pumps the oxygen-poor blood into the right ventricle.
- The right ventricle pumps the oxygen-poor blood into the pulmonary artery. The pulmonary artery branches into the right pulmonary artery, which goes to the right lung, and the left pulmonary artery, which goes to the left lung.

- Once in the lungs, the pulmonary arteries quickly branch into smaller arteries and arterioles to carry the oxygen-poor blood to the capillary beds surrounding the alveoli. As you remember from Chapter 26, gas exchange takes place in the alveoli. The oxygen in the alveolus moves into the blood, and the carbon dioxide in the blood moves into the alveolus, to be exhaled from the body.
- The blood, which now contains fresh oxygen, is carried by the network of venules, then veins, to the pulmonary veins (right and left), which empty into the left atrium of the heart.

Systemic Circulation

- The left atrium pumps the oxygen-rich blood into the left ventricle.
- The left ventricle pumps the oxygen-rich blood into the largest artery of the body, the aorta.
- The aorta branches very quickly into the coronary arteries to carry oxygen-rich blood to the heart muscle, and then into large branches of arteries that carry oxygen-rich blood to the rest of the body.
- The arteries branch into arterioles and then into capillaries, which join together to form a capillary bed. In the capillary bed, oxygen and nutrients move out of the blood and into the tissues, and carbon dioxide moves out of the tissues and into the blood.
- The blood, which now contains less oxygen, is carried by the network of venules, then veins, back to the right atrium, where the process begins again.

Cardiac Cycle

You may recall from Chapter 16 that the heart muscle contracts in two phases. During **systole,** or the active phase, the myocardium contracts, sending blood out of the heart. During **diastole,** or the resting phase, the myocardium relaxes, allowing the chambers to fill with blood. The atria are in systole when the ventricles are in diastole, and vice versa. The atria contract (atrial systole), sending the blood into the relaxed ventricles (ventricular diastole). Next, the atria relax (atrial diastole) while the ventricles contract (ventricular systole), sending the blood out to the body. This sequence is called the **cardiac cycle.**

The orderly sequence of systole and diastole is crucial for maximizing the amount of blood that is pumped throughout the body each time the heart contracts. During ventricular diastole, the ventricles are relaxed, which allows them to fill to capacity with blood. Without this rest period, the ventricles would never fill to capacity. Think about a plastic squirt bottle (the kind used at picnics to hold ketchup or mustard). If you fill the squirt bottle only partially with water, when you squeeze it, there is not enough force to push a large amount of water out. But, if you put as much water in the squirt bottle as it will hold and then squeeze, a small squeeze will cause a larger amount of water to squirt out with a lot more force. In other words, the heart is able to perform more efficiently when the ventricles are filled, because less force is required to send the maximum amount of blood out to the body.

As you may recall from Chapter 16, there are two distinct sounds that you will hear with your stethoscope when you are taking an apical pulse. The first sound, "lubb," is the sound of the tricuspid and mitral valves (the valves that separate the atria from the ventricles) snapping shut during ventricular systole. The second sound, "dupp," is the sound of the pulmonary and aortic valves closing during ventricular diastole. The two sounds heard together ("lubb–dupp") is what we know as a heartbeat.

REGULATION

Although transport is the cardiovascular system's major function, this system also plays a role in temperature regulation, as discussed in Chapter 24.

PROTECTION

The cardiovascular system helps to protect the body in two major ways. First, white blood cells, which play an important role in helping us to fight off disease, are circulated throughout the body in the blood. Second, when injury to the skin occurs, the blood has the ability to form a clot. The clot helps to protect us against excessive blood loss. It also helps to prevent microbes from gaining access to the body.

THE EFFECTS OF AGING ON THE CARIOVASCULAR SYSTEM

Cardiovascular disorders are very common in the United States, especially among older people. Perhaps more than any other organ system, the cardiovascular system is affected by the choices we make in life. For example, smoking, poor dietary habits, and a lack of exercise can all contribute to cardiovascular disease later in life. In addition, common medical problems, such as diabetes, obesity, and hypertension (high blood pressure) can cause the cardiovascular system to age faster.

Many national organizations, such as the American Heart Association, provide information and education about "healthy heart living." By following the advice of these organizations, many people are able to maintain good cardiovascular function well into old age. The keys to cardiovascular health are exercise, a diet that is low in saturated (unhealthy) fats, and avoidance of smoking (Fig. 27-9). Exercise helps to keep the heart muscle strong and working efficiently. Eating a healthy diet helps to prevent atherosclerosis, a disease of the blood vessels that is discussed later in this chapter. Finally, chemicals in tobacco smoke cause the arterioles and capillaries to constrict, depriving tissues of vital blood flow. Smoking should be avoided because it has a very negative impact on the heart, which requires a healthy supply of oxygen and nutrients to function properly. In addition to preventing problems that affect the cardiovascular system directly, exercising, eating a healthy diet, and avoidance of tobacco smoke can help to prevent or control medical conditions that can contribute to cardiovascular disease, such as obesity, diabetes, and hypertension.

There are some changes to the cardiovascular system that will take place simply as a result of the aging process. In a healthy older person, these changes do not have a major impact on day-to-day life. However, when the processes of aging are combined with a chronic illness or a lifetime of unhealthy habits, the effect on cardiovascular function can be major. Age-related changes that occur include less efficient contraction of the heart, a loss of elasticity in the arteries and veins, and decreased numbers of blood cells.

FIGURE 27-9

Regular exercise and a diet that is low in artery-clogging saturated fat are essential for maintaining a healthy heart throughout life. Raw fruits and vegetables are heart-healthy foods.

LESS EFFICIENT CONTRACTION

Changes in the tissues of the heart, such as a loss of muscle tone and a loss of elasticity, affect the ability of the heart to contract forcefully, and it takes longer for the heart to complete the cycle of filling and emptying. A healthy older person might find that she tires faster while exercising, because the heart is not able to deliver oxygen and nutrients to the body as efficiently as it once was, in times of increased demand. Medical conditions, such as obesity or hypertension, place additional strain on the heart muscle and make the effects of normal aging on the heart worse. The heart of an older person who is ill may barely be able to meet the body's needs for oxygen and nutrients when the person is at rest.

DECREASED ELASTICITY OF THE ARTERIES AND VEINS

As we age, the walls of the blood vessels lose some of their elasticity. The loss of elasticity in the muscle layer of the arteries decreases the body's ability to control blood pressure and flow, because the arteries are not able to expand and "bounce back" as easily. This means that in an older person (especially one with cardiovascular disease), the arteries lose both the ability to dilate to allow for an increase in blood flow when needed, and the ability to constrict back to a smaller size afterward. The "stretch" is gone from the vessel. The effects of this age-related change are especially noticeable when an older person gets up quickly after lying down. The arteries do not constrict quickly enough to maintain adequate blood flow to the brain, and the person feels dizzy or lightheaded as a result. In other words, the person has orthostatic hypotension (see Chapter 16).

The loss of elasticity in the walls of the veins causes them to "stretch out," slowing the flow of blood back to the heart. The valves in the walls of the veins become less effective, which also slows the return of blood to the heart. Pooling of blood in the veins just underneath the skin can cause them to become swollen and "knotty" in appearance, a condition commonly known as **varicose veins.** Immobility and bed rest can make the effects of aging on the veins worse, because the large muscles of the legs are not working to help move the blood back toward the heart.

DECREASED NUMBERS OF BLOOD CELLS

The production of blood cells slows as a person ages. A decreased number of red blood cells affects the blood's ability to deliver oxygen to the tissues. A decreased number of white blood cells puts the older person at higher risk for developing infections, because the body's ability to fight them off is reduced.

DISORDERS OF THE CARDIOVASCULAR SYSTEM

Disorders of the cardiovascular system can involve the blood, the blood vessels, or the heart.

DISORDERS OF THE BLOOD

Blood disorders are often detected through laboratory analysis of the blood. Common blood disorders include anemia, leukemia, and clotting disorders.

Anemia

Anemia is a general term for a group of disorders affecting the red blood cells. Anemia decreases the blood's ability to transport oxygen to the cells. People who have anemia may become tired very easily. Their red blood cells simply are not able to transport the extra oxygen that is needed for exertion.

Anemia can result when the number of red blood cells is decreased, either because red blood cell production is impaired or the person is losing blood. For example, a disorder that affects the bone marrow, where blood cells are made, can cause a decrease in the number of circulating red blood cells, leading to anemia. Slow chronic blood loss (for example, from heavy periods or a stomach ulcer) can also cause anemia just by decreasing the amount of circulating blood.

Sometimes the number of red blood cells is adequate, but the red blood cells do not contain enough hemoglobin. Recall that hemoglobin is the molecule that binds with oxygen, so if the red blood cells lack hemoglobin, then they are unable to carry as much oxygen, resulting in anemia. The body needs iron in order to make hemoglobin. Therefore, people who have diets that are low in iron or certain B vitamins (which help the body to absorb iron from the digestive tract) are at risk for anemia.

In disorders such as sickle cell anemia, red blood cells are produced, but they are abnormally shaped (Fig. 27-10). Because the cells lack the "dent" where the hemoglobin normally sits, they are unable to carry oxygen. Their abnormal shape also causes them to get stuck in the tiny capillaries, obstructing the flow of blood and causing pain, swelling, and fevers. Sickle cell anemia is an inherited disorder that is found mainly among people of African or Mediterranean heritage.

Leukemia

Leukemia is the excessive production of white blood cells. The white blood cells are abnormal in structure and they cannot perform their job of

FIGURE 27-10

In sickle cell anemia, the red blood cells are abnormally shaped. Here, a sickled red blood cell is shown to the left of a normal red blood cell. (© *Roseman/Custom Medical Stock Photo.*)

protecting the body from infection. Leukemia can be caused by cancer of the bone marrow or by cancer of the lymphatic tissue. Leukemia occurs in people of all ages, and can cause death if treatment is started too late or is not effective. People who have leukemia are at higher risk for developing infections. They may also have bleeding disorders, which can cause them to bruise very easily or bleed from their gums during oral care.

Bleeding Disorders

There are two types of bleeding disorders. Either the blood clots too much, or not enough.

In some people, the blood clots too easily. Clots can form in the small blood vessels, blocking the flow of blood and depriving the tissues of oxygen and nutrients. The blood clots, called **thrombi,** can also break loose and travel to other parts of the body such as the brain, lungs, or heart. A blood clot that moves from one place to another is called an **embolus.** An embolus can be life-threatening. For example, the embolus may become stuck in the pulmonary artery, the artery that receives blood in need of oxygen from the heart. If blood cannot reach the lungs, then it cannot pick up the oxygen it needs for the rest of the body. People who have blood that clots too easily may need to take drugs called anticoagulants or "blood thinners" to help keep clots from forming where they are not needed.

Other people have the opposite problem—their blood does not form clots when it is supposed to (for example, after an injury). These people may lack fibrinogen, the protein in the blood plasma that assists with clotting. Or, they may have a low platelet count. (Recall that platelets are the blood cells that participate in clot formation.) For these people, even a small bump can cause a large bruise, while a more severe injury can result in a fatal hemorrhage.

DISORDERS OF THE BLOOD VESSELS

Atherosclerosis

Atherosclerosis is blocking of the arteries. Blood is unable to flow freely through the arteries because **plaques** (fatty deposits) build up on the inside of the vessel wall (Fig. 27-11). As a result, less oxygen and nutrients are delivered to the tissues of the body. In addition, the plaques make the normally smooth inner lining of the artery rough, which can cause blood clots to form. Sometimes the clots break off and become emboli. Finally, the plaques interfere with the elasticity of the arterial walls, making them brittle and prone to breaking (a condition called **arteriosclerosis**). This "hardening of the arteries" can lead to hemorrhages (bleeding) in the small vessels.

Depending on which arteries are affected, atherosclerosis can have serious consequences. The arteries that supply the brain, heart, kidneys, and legs are affected most often.

- Atherosclerosis of the arteries that supply the brain can cause a stroke. Strokes are discussed in detail in Chapter 28.
- Atherosclerosis of the arteries that supply the heart can cause myocardial infarction ("heart attack"). Myocardial infarction is discussed later in this chapter.

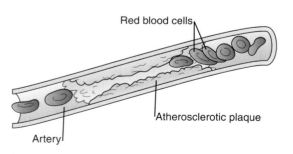

Red blood cells

Atherosclerotic plaque

Artery

FIGURE 27-11

In atherosclerosis, fatty plaques build up on the inside of the arteries, blocking the free flow of blood. This is particularly dangerous when the artery supplies a vital organ such as the heart, brain, or kidneys.

- Atherosclerosis of the arteries that supply the kidneys can cause renal failure, discussed in Chapter 32.
- Atherosclerosis of the arteries that supply the legs can cause **peripheral vascular disease.** In peripheral vascular disease, decreased blood flow to the leg muscles causes pain and cramping when the person walks. The pain and cramping, called *claudication*, occurs because the muscles are not receiving enough oxygen. In severe cases, the tissues in the leg die from lack of oxygen, and amputation may be necessary.

Although the exact cause of atherosclerosis is unknown, scientists now know that several factors contribute to the development of the disease. Diabetes, hypertension, and obesity are all medical conditions that have been associated with atherosclerosis. Heredity and stress may also play a role. Smoking, eating a diet high in cholesterol and saturated (unhealthy) fat, and a lack of physical activity can also increase a person's chances of developing atherosclerosis.

Venous Disorders

Loss of elasticity and decreased efficiency of the valves in the walls of the veins causes blood to "pool" in the legs, which can put the person at risk for several disorders:

- **Venous thrombosis.** In this disorder, blood clots form in the veins where the blood pools, because the blood is moving so slowly. These clots can block the vein, or they can become emboli. People with venous thrombosis are at risk for pulmonary embolism (an embolus that travels to the lung and blocks the pulmonary artery). Pulmonary embolism can be fatal.
- **Venous (stasis) ulcers.** As a result of pooling of the blood, plasma may leak into the tissues causing edema (swelling). The skin breaks down because of the poor circulation through the veins, resulting in sores that are slow to heal. These sores are called *venous ulcers* or *stasis ulcers*.

DISORDERS OF THE HEART

Heart disorders affect children as well as adults. Most heart disorders in children are *congenital*, which means that they were "present at birth."

Congenital heart disorders occur when the fetus' heart does not form correctly. Many babies who are born with congenital heart disorders grow up to live long and healthy lives following surgery to correct the heart defect.

In adults, heart disorders have various causes. Conditions that are known to increase a person's risk of developing a heart disorder are called *cardiac risk factors.* Some of these risk factors can be changed, while others cannot. Risk factors that cannot be changed include the following:

- **Age.** The risk of developing a heart disorder increases with age.
- **Gender.** Men are at greater risk of developing heart disease at an earlier age than women are. However, after a woman goes through menopause, her risk of developing heart disease is the same as a man's.
- **Heredity.** People who have parents or siblings with heart disease are more like to develop heart disease themselves.
- **Body build.** Some people tend to put on weight in the abdomen or chest ("apples"), while others tend to carry it in the buttocks or thighs ("pears"). "Apple"-shaped people are more likely to develop heart disease than "pear"-shaped people.

Age, gender, heredity, and body build are risk factors that cannot be changed. However, there are many risk factors for heart disease that can be changed. These risk factors include:

- Smoking
- Physical inactivity
- Obesity
- A diet high in saturated fat and cholesterol
- Poorly controlled hypertension
- Poorly controlled diabetes

Common heart disorders in adults include coronary artery disease, heart failure, and heart block.

Coronary Artery Disease

Coronary artery disease occurs when the coronary arteries narrow as a result of atherosclerosis. Recall that the coronary arteries supply the heart muscle with blood containing oxygen and nutrients. Initially, the heart muscle may receive enough oxygen to work properly when the body is at rest, but it may be unable to meet the increased needs brought on by activity. Eventually, one or more of the coronary arteries may become so narrow that no blood gets through, causing areas of the heart muscle to die.

Coronary artery disease is treated in a number of ways. Medications are available that help to keep the arteries open, permitting maximum blood flow. Balloon angioplasty is a technique that involves the insertion of a catheter into the affected artery. A balloon on the end of the catheter is inflated, squeezing the plaque to the sides of the artery and creating a larger opening for blood to flow through. As an alternative to balloon angioplasty, springs may be placed in the artery to hold the narrowed portion open. Finally, surgery can be performed to bypass the blocked arteries and reestablish blood flow.

Conditions that are closely related to coronary artery disease include angina pectoris and myocardial infarction.

Angina Pectoris

Angina pectoris is the classic chest pain that is felt as a result of the heart muscle being deprived of oxygen. Anginal pain varies among individuals. Some people describe it as a pain in the center of the chest. Others experience pain that starts in the chest and extends to the arm or neck. A person who is experiencing angina may feel as though he is suffocating, and he may become very anxious.

Many people experience angina quite frequently and know what it is. These people often keep nitroglycerin pills on hand to relieve the pain when it occurs. Nitroglycerin relaxes the arteries, increasing the flow of blood. If you have been trained to help a person with her nitroglycerin, avoid handling the pills with your bare hands. The drug can be absorbed through the skin, which can cause a decrease in your blood pressure and a pounding headache.

Myocardial Infarction

A **myocardial infarction** is a "heart attack." A myocardial infarction occurs when one or more of the coronary arteries becomes completely blocked, preventing blood from reaching the parts of the heart that are fed by the affected arteries (Fig. 27-12). The lack of blood (and vital oxygen) causes the tissue to die. The dead tissue is called an *infarct.*

The severity of the myocardial infarction depends on the extent of the tissue damaged and

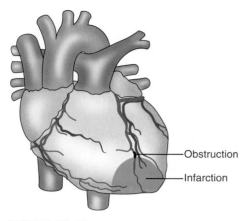

FIGURE 27-12

A heart attack occurs when one or more of the coronary arteries becomes blocked, preventing blood from reaching the myocardium. The lack of oxygen and nutrients causes the tissue that is supplied by the affected artery to die.

the part of the heart affected. Although a myocardial infarction that affects the atria may not be life threatening, one that severely damages the ventricles can reduce the heart's ability to pump blood to vital organs and cause death. Early recognition of the symptoms of a myocardial infarction (see Chapter 12) and early treatment can greatly increase a person's chances of surviving. Drugs that help to maintain a normal heart beat and restore blood flow to the affected area can greatly improve the person's outcome.

Heart Failure

Heart failure occurs when the heart is unable to pump enough blood to meet the body's needs. Heart failure has many causes. For example, disorders that cause the ventricles to lose muscle tone and become large and flabby can cause heart failure. Heart failure can also occur as a result of a myocardial infarction that leaves the ventricles unable to function properly.

Heart failure can be either "right-sided" or "left-sided." Right-sided heart failure, also called *cor pulmonale*, causes blood to back up in the venous system because the right ventricle's ability to pump the blood into the pulmonary circulation is impaired. In a person with right-sided heart failure, the veins in the legs and abdomen become swollen, and fluid may leak into the tissues, causing significant edema and skin breakdown. Left-sided heart failure, also called *congestive heart failure*, causes the blood to back up in the lungs because the left ventricle's ability to pump

the blood into the systemic circulation is impaired. The excess blood in the vessels of the lungs causes fluid to leak into the lung tissues, which causes congestion and makes breathing difficult.

For people with heart failure, drugs may be used to help increase the heart's ability to pump more effectively and to pull excess fluid from the tissues. Many people with severe heart failure may have their fluids restricted and their intake and output very carefully measured and monitored.

Conduction Disorders

Some conditions affect the pathway that the heart uses to transmit the electrical impulses that cause contraction. These disorders are called **conduction disorders.** Heart block is a common type of conduction disorder. Heart block can result from a myocardial infarction that damages the pathway, or it may occur as part of the normal aging process. A heart block causes the heart to slow down significantly, leading to dizziness or fainting episodes.

Heart block is usually treated with a pacemaker, an electrical device that stimulates the heart to contract. The pacemaker consists of a small, battery-operated device implanted under the skin below the collarbone and two wires that connect to the right side of the heart (Fig. 27-13). When the person's heart rate drops below a programmed rate, the battery-operated device sends a small electrical impulse through the wires that stimulates the heart muscle to contract.

▶ *Tell the Nurse!*

The routine taking of vital signs, especially the pulse and blood pressure, is one of the best ways to detect abnormalities in the functioning of the cardiovascular system at an early stage. In addition, there are many signs and symptoms you may observe that could indicate that a patient or resident is having a cardiovascular problem. Report any of the following observations to the nurse immediately:

⟾ Complaints of chest pain or pressure

⟾ Labored or difficult breathing

⟾ A rapid or erratic pulse

FIGURE 27-13

A pacemaker is a battery-operated device used to treat heart block. The pacemaker sends out an electrical signal that stimulates the heart to contract when the person's heart rate drops below a pre-programmed rate. In this photograph, you can see the pacemaker above the person's ribcage. A dark blue lead connects the pacemaker to the person's heart, which is the red area in the lower right of the photograph. (© *Salisbury District Hospital/Photo Researchers, Inc.*)

⇒ A slow, weak pulse

⇒ A blood pressure reading that is either much higher or much lower than the person's usual reading

⇒ Cyanosis of the face, lips, or fingers

⇒ Decreased tolerance for usual exertion

⇒ Red, painful, or swollen areas in the extremities, especially the calves of the legs

⇒ Unusual swelling of the legs, especially if it is accompanied by red, shiny skin

⇒ "Dusky" (blue or grayish) coloring of the legs, especially if it is accompanied by a diminished pulse and coldness of the skin

DIAGNOSIS OF CARDIOVASCULAR DISORDERS

Depending on where you work, you may be responsible for caring for people who are recovering from an acute cardiovascular disorder, such as a heart attack. Other people will be admitted to the hospital to have a procedure done to prevent a heart attack from occurring, such as balloon angioplasty. Often, people with cardiovascular disorders will have one or more tests done to help the doctor determine the extent of the problem, plan a course of treatment, and monitor the person after the treatment. Tests you may hear mentioned include the following:

• **Electrocardiography.** In electrocardiography, sensors are attached to the person's chest. These sensors pick up the electrical activity of the heart and record it on a piece of paper. The tracing is called an *electrocardiogram* (EKG, ECG). An EKG shows abnormalities in the conduction system of the heart. Some people have an EKG done while they are exercising. This is called a stress test (Fig. 27-14).

FIGURE 27-14

Electrocardiography is commonly used for diagnosis and monitoring of heart problems. This man is having a cardiac stress test. In a cardiac stress test, an electrocardiogram (EKG) is obtained while the person exercises. (© *Larry Mulvehill/Photo Researchers, Inc.*)

- **Echocardiography.** In echocardiography, sound waves are bounced against the body to produce an image. A computer translates the sound waves into an image. Echocardiography can provide the doctor with much helpful information, including the size and shape of the heart, its pumping strength, and the location and extent of any damage to its tissues.
- **Doppler ultrasound.** In Doppler ultrasound, sound waves are used to check the blood flow in the large arteries and veins of the arms and legs.
- **Radiography.** Radiographs, commonly known as "x-rays," are often used in the diagnosis of cardiovascular disease. A chest x-ray can show enlargement of the ventricles. Sometimes, a special dye is injected into the veins and then an x-ray is taken. The dye allows the doctor to see any abnormalities in the vessels of the heart or other parts of the body.

CARDIAC REHABILITATION

Cardiac rehabilitation is often necessary for a person who has had a heart attack or has had heart surgery. **Cardiac rehabilitation** focuses on helping a person regain strength and adopt habits that will help the cardiovascular system become healthier. A person who is in cardiac rehabilitation will begin an exercise program under the guidance of a therapist who specializes in cardiac disorders or a nurse. The exercise program is designed to strengthen the heart muscle and make it a more effective pump. As the person grows stronger, the therapist or nurse will work with the person to develop an exercise plan that will become a part of the person's daily routine. A dietitian will work with the person to teach him about dietary changes that are needed to help control obesity and blood cholesterol levels. Avoidance of unhealthy habits, such as smoking, may require the use of medications and supportive emotional therapy.

Many people with cardiovascular disease benefit greatly from cardiac rehabilitation, especially if rehabilitation is started early. Cardiac rehabilitation gives people the energy and ability to pursue things that they enjoy doing, which improves quality of life.

SUMMARY

▶ The cardiovascular system, also known as the circulatory system, is made up of the blood, the blood vessels, the lymphatic system, and the heart.
- Blood consists of plasma and formed elements (red blood cells, white blood cells, and platelets).
- Arteries carry blood away from the heart, and veins carry blood to the heart. The transfer of substances into and out of the blood occurs in the capillary bed.
- The lymphatic system is a one-way system that returns fluid that leaks into the tissues to the bloodstream.
- The heart is the muscular organ that powers circulation.
  - The heart has four chambers. The atria receive blood from the body, and the ventricles send blood to the body.
  - The heart valves make sure that blood flows through the heart in the proper direction.
  - The heart's conduction system makes and conducts the electrical impulses that cause the heart to contract regularly.
  - The coronary circulation supplies the heart with oxygen and nutrients.

▶ The main function of the cardiovascular system is to transport oxygen, nutrients, and other substances *to* the tissues, and remove carbon dioxide and other wastes *from* the tissues.
- The pattern of circulation involves two parallel circuits. The right side of the heart pumps blood into the lungs, where it picks up oxygen. The left side of the heart pumps the oxygenated blood to the rest of the body.
- During systole, the heart contracts, sending blood out of the heart. During diastole, the heart relaxes, allowing the chambers to fill. The atria are in systole when the ventricles are in diastole, and vice versa.

▶ When the effects of aging are combined with a lifetime of unhealthy habits or a chronic disease, the effect on cardiovascular function can be major.
- Exercising, eating a diet low in saturated fat and cholesterol, and avoiding tobacco smoke

help to keep the cardiovascular system healthy. Controlling chronic diseases such as diabetes and hypertension is also important.

- Risk factors for cardiovascular disease that cannot be changed include age, gender, heredity, and body build.

▶ Disorders of the cardiovascular system can affect the blood, the blood vessels, or the heart.

- Disorders of the blood include anemia, leukemia, and bleeding disorders.
- Disorders of the blood vessels include atherosclerosis, venous thrombosis, and venous (stasis) ulcers.
  - Atherosclerosis is blocking of the arteries. Depending on which arteries are affected, atherosclerosis can lead to strokes, heart attacks, kidney failure, or peripheral vascular disease.
  - Disorders that affect the veins are usually caused by widening of the veins, which allows blood to pool in the legs.

▶ Disorders of the heart include coronary artery disease, heart failure, and conduction disorders.

- Coronary artery disease is caused by a narrowing of the arteries that supply the heart muscle with oxygen and nutrients.
  - Angina pectoris is chest pain that results from the heart muscle being depleted of oxygen.
  - A myocardial infarction occurs when the blood supply to the heart muscle is completely obstructed.
- Heart failure results from the heart's inability to pump blood in sufficient amounts to supply the body.
- Conduction disorders involve the electrical pathway in the heart. A person with a conduction disorder may have a pacemaker implanted to stimulate regular contraction of the heart.

▶ The goal of cardiac rehabilitation is to help a person with heart disease to regain strength and adopt habits that will improve the health of the cardiovascular system. An exercise plan and dietary and other lifestyle changes are part of cardiac rehabilitation.

What did you learn?

Multiple Choice

Select the single best answer for each of the following questions.

1. The formation of artery-clogging plaques on the inside of the arteries is called:
   a. Atherosclerosis
   b. Arterioles
   c. Anemia
   d. Myocardial infarction
2. What is the function of the cardiovascular system?
   a. Transport of substances throughout the body
   b. Regulation of body temperature
   c. Protection of the body from blood loss and infection
   d. All of the above
3. Which circulation supplies the tissues of the heart with oxygen and nutrients?
   a. Pulmonary circulation
   b. Systemic circulation
   c. Coronary circulation
   d. Pericardial circulation
4. Which of the following is a risk factor for cardiovascular disease?
   a. Poorly controlled hypertension
   b. A diet high in cholesterol and saturated fats
   c. Lack of physical activity
   d. All of the above

Matching

Match each numbered item with its appropriate lettered description.

_____ 1. Red blood cells (erythrocytes)

_____ 2. White blood cells (leukocytes)

_____ 3. Ventricles

_____ 4. Veins

_____ 5. Atria

_____ 6. Arteries

_____ 7. Systole

_____ 8. Pulmonary circulation

_____ 9. Systemic circulation

_____ 10. Diastole

a. Upper chambers of the heart, which receive blood from the body
b. Vessels that carry blood away from the heart
c. Active phase of the cardiac cycle
d. Blood cells that help the body to fight infection
e. Circuit that sends newly oxygenated blood to the body
f. Resting phase of the cardiac cycle
g. Blood cells that contain hemoglobin and carry oxygen
h. Lower chambers of the heart, which pump blood to the body
i. Circuit that sends oxygen-poor blood to the lungs to pick up oxygen
j. Vessels that return blood to the heart

? Stop and think!

▶ You are caring for Mr. Becker, a 74-year-old gentleman with a history of heart disease. Mr. Becker keeps nitroglycerin in his bedside table to use when he has an angina attack. Lately, it seems to you that Mr. Becker's angina attacks seem to be occurring much more frequently. Just this morning, when you were changing Mr. Becker's bed, he mentions to you that he had another angina attack yesterday, and you know that he had one the day before too. Is this something you should mention to the nurse? Why or why not?

▶ Amanda has been assigned to provide morning care for Mr. Gates. While giving him a bed bath, she notices that the veins in his lower legs are swollen and very noticeable. Amanda has never seen this before and she doesn't know what to do. If you were Amanda, what would you do, and why?

28

The Nervous System

What will you learn?

Chicago's O'Hare Airport is one of the busiest airports in the United States. In 2002, 922,787 planes took off and landed at O'Hare, which averages out to around 2,500 flights a day! To ensure that air traffic flows smoothly in and out of O'Hare and other major airports in the United States, air traffic control receives information from a variety of sources, processes it, and gives instructions to the pilots to carry out. Just as an air traffic controller is in constant communication with the pilots of the planes he is monitoring, the nervous system is in constant communication with all of the other organ systems in the body. Like air traffic control at a busy airport, your nervous system receives information at a great rate, from both inside the body and outside of it. It then processes this information and issues instructions to other organ systems to carry out. "Command central" of the human body, the nervous system, is the subject of this chapter. When you are finished with this chapter, you will be able to:

1. List and describe the structures that make up the two main divisions of the nervous system.
2. Discuss the main functions of the nervous system.
3. Describe how aging affects the nervous system.
4. Discuss various disorders that affect the nervous system.
5. List common diagnostic procedures that are used to help detect nervous system disorders.
6. Describe rehabilitation measures that a person with a nervous system disorder may need.

Photo: Like air traffic control at a busy airport, your nervous system receives information at a great rate, processes it, and issues instructions.
(© Joseph Nettis/Photo Researchers, Inc.)

Vocabulary

Use the CD in the back of your book to hear these terms pronounced, defined, and used in a sentence:

Neuron	Central nervous system	Cerebrospinal fluid (CSF)	Stroke
Dendrites	(CNS)	Sensory nerves	Aphasia
Axon	Peripheral nervous	Motor nerves	Parkinson's disease
Synapse	system (PNS)	Transient ischemic	Epilepsy
Myelin	Meninges	attack (TIA)	Multiple sclerosis (MS)

STRUCTURE OF THE NERVOUS SYSTEM

Nervous tissue, which forms the organs of the nervous system, is made up of a special kind of cell, called a neuron. A **neuron** is a cell that can send and receive information. A neuron consists of dendrites, a cell body, and an axon (Fig. 28-1). **Dendrites** are short extensions from the cell body that *receive* information. The **axon** is a long

FIGURE 28-1

Neurons are special cells that have the ability to send and receive information.

extension from the cell body that *sends* information. An electrical signal, called a nerve impulse, enters the neuron at the dendrites. It passes through the cell body and travels down the axon, and then on to the dendrites of the next neuron in line. The movement of the nerve impulse is called *conduction*. The axon of one neuron does not actually connect with the dendrites of the next (see Fig. 28-1). Instead, chemicals called neurotransmitters carry the nerve impulse across the gap between the axon of one neuron and the dendrites of the next. This gap is called a **synapse.** The axons of some neurons are wrapped in **myelin,** a fatty, white substance that protects the axon. Myelin also helps to speed the conduction of nerve impulses along the axon.

The nervous system has two main divisions, the central nervous system and the peripheral nervous system (Fig. 28-2). The **central nervous system (CNS)** consists of the brain and spinal cord. The central nervous system is like the air traffic control tower for the human body, receiving information, processing it, and issuing instructions. The **peripheral nervous system (PNS)** consists of the nerves outside of the brain and spinal cord. A nerve is simply a bundle of axons, wrapped in a connective tissue sheath. The peripheral nervous system receives information from the environment, and carries commands from the brain and spinal cord to the other organs of the body, such as the muscles.

THE CENTRAL NERVOUS SYSTEM

Because it is so vital to the body's functioning, the central nervous system is well protected by three layers of connective tissue, called **meninges,** and

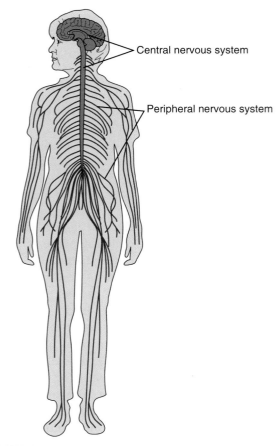

FIGURE 28-2

The nervous system has two main divisions, the central nervous system and the peripheral nervous system. "Peripheral" means "along the edge" or "away from the center."

the bony skull and vertebrae (Fig. 28-3). The three meninges are, from the inside out:

- The *pia mater,* a thin delicate layer of tissue rich in blood vessels that is attached to the surface of the brain and spinal cord
- The *arachnoid mater,* the web-like middle layer
- The *dura mater,* a thick, tough outer layer that is attached to the inside of the skull and the vertebrae

The space between the pia mater and the arachnoid mater contains **cerebrospinal fluid (CSF),** a clear fluid that circulates around the brain and spinal cord and acts as an additional "shock absorber" to protect these structures.

The Brain

The brain, a large, soft mass of nervous tissue, is where information is processed and instructions

are issued. The brain has four parts: the cerebrum, the diencephalon, the brain stem, and the cerebellum (see Fig. 28-3).

The Cerebrum

The cerebrum is the largest part of the brain, with the characteristic "folds" that we always picture when we think of a brain (see Fig. 28-3). The cerebrum:

- Controls the voluntary movement of muscles
- Gives meaning to information received from the eyes, ears, nose, taste buds, and sensory receptors in the skin
- Allows us to speak, remember, think, and feel emotions

A deep groove divides the cerebrum into two hemispheres, the left hemisphere (or "left brain") and the right hemisphere (or "right brain"). The right and left hemispheres communicate with each other and are connected by a structure called the *corpus callosum.* The right side of the brain controls the left side of the body, and vice versa. So, an injury to the tissues in the left side of the brain may result in loss of function on the right side of the body.

The Diencephalon

The diencephalon contains the thalamus and the hypothalamus (see Fig. 28-3). The thalamus is responsible for sorting out the impulses that arrive via the spinal cord from other parts of the body and sending them to the correct part of the cerebrum. The hypothalamus controls body temperature, fluid balance, appetite, sleep cycles, and some of the emotions, and regulates the pituitary gland, a gland you will learn more about in Chapter 30.

The Brain Stem

The brain stem connects the spinal cord to the brain. It has three parts: the midbrain, the pons, and the medulla (see Fig. 28-3). The medulla contains the centers that control respiration, heartbeat, and blood pressure.

The Cerebellum

The cerebellum helps to coordinate the brain's commands to the muscles so that the muscles move smoothly and in an orderly fashion. It also plays a role in balance.

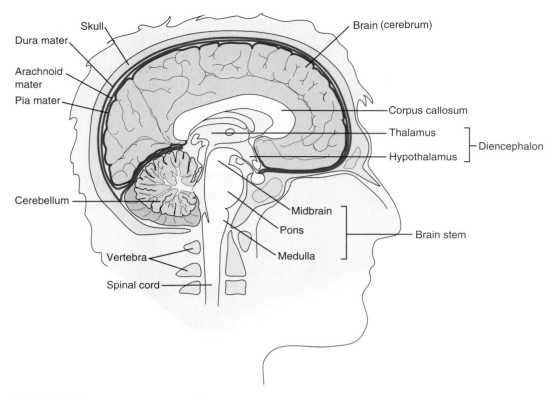

FIGURE 28-3

The brain and the spinal cord make up the central nervous system (CNS). The brain has four parts: the cerebrum, the diencephalon, the brain stem, and the cerebellum. Three layers of connective tissue, called the dura mater, the arachnoid mater, and the pia mater, help to cushion and protect the brain and spinal cord. Additional protection is provided by the bony skull and vertebrae.

The Spinal Cord

The spinal cord is a "cord" of nervous tissue that extends from the base of the brain downward, to a point approximately even with your bellybutton. The vertebrae (the bones that make up your spine) surround and protect the spinal cord.

The spinal cord is the main connection between the brain and the rest of the body. Pathways of nerve tissue in the spinal cord, also called *tracts*, carry messages to and from the brain. Ascending tracts carry information from the peripheral nervous system to the brain. Descending tracts carry information from the brain to the peripheral nervous system.

THE PERIPHERAL NERVOUS SYSTEM

The peripheral nervous system consists of the nerves, or the lines of communication between the central nervous system and the rest of the body. Every part of the body is innervated, or supplied, by nerves, which form a vast network throughout the body.

The nerves that form the peripheral nervous system are either sensory nerves or motor nerves. **Sensory nerves** carry information from the "outside in." In other words, the sensory nerves carry information from the internal organs and the outside world to the spinal cord and up into the brain so that the brain can analyze the information. **Motor nerves** carry information from the "inside out." In other words, the motor nerves carry commands from the brain down the spinal cord and out to the muscles and organs of the body. Motor nerves allow the brain to control voluntary muscle movement and the involuntary functions of the internal organs.

Thirty-one pairs of nerves, called spinal nerves, connect to the spinal cord. Each spinal nerve consists of one sensory nerve and one motor nerve. The spinal nerves that innervate the arms and the upper part of the body are located in the neck region, whereas the spinal nerves that innervate the legs and the lower part of the body are located in the back.

Some nerves are connected directly to the brain. These nerves are called cranial nerves. There are 12 pairs of cranial nerves.

FUNCTION OF THE NERVOUS SYSTEM

The nervous system receives, processes, and responds to information.

REGULATION OF THE INTERNAL ENVIRONMENT

By now, you are familiar with the concept of homeostasis, or balance. For the body to function well, a state of homeostasis must be maintained. The nervous system regulates what is going on within the body and makes adjustments as necessary to keep things within the range of normal. For example, control centers in the hypothalamus monitor the body temperature, and control centers in the medulla monitor heart beat and respirations.

When the central nervous system detects an imbalance, a special part of the peripheral nervous system, called the autonomic system, is activated. The autonomic system has two lower divisions, the sympathetic nervous system and the parasympathetic nervous system. Generally speaking, the sympathetic nervous system speeds things up, and the parasympathetic nervous system slows them back down. Perhaps you have heard of the "fight or flight" response. When we are put in a dangerous situation, our heart rate and breathing increase, and the adrenal glands release adrenaline, a chemical that helps us to cope with stress. These changes allow us to run faster or be stronger in a fight, and they are caused by activation of the sympathetic nervous system. Once the danger has passed, the parasympathetic nervous system slows things back down.

INTERACTION WITH THE EXTERNAL ENVIRONMENT

The nervous system allows us to interact with the world around us. The special senses—touch, taste, smell, sight, and hearing—provide the brain with information about the outside world. The brain responds to this information. The ability to receive information about the outside world and respond to it not only makes life more pleasurable, it helps to protect us from harm. (The special senses are discussed in detail in Chapter 29.)

THE EFFECTS OF AGING ON THE NERVOUS SYSTEM

Neurons cannot divide and reproduce as other body cells do. That means that we keep the same 100 billion neurons our whole lives, give or take a few! Despite the fact that neurons are not replaced, they experience relatively little wear and tear over the course of a lifetime. Still, some structural changes occur as a result of aging, which can result in slowed conduction times and slight memory changes.

SLOWED CONDUCTION TIMES

You may notice that some of your elderly patients or residents are not as quick to react to things as they used to be. This is a normal age-related change that is caused by changes in the myelin sheath and the amount of neurotransmitters. As we age, the amount of myelin surrounding the axons decreases, reducing the speed of nerve conduction by approximately 10 percent. In addition, neurotransmitter imbalances can interfere with the ability of a nerve impulse to travel across a synapse, slowing conduction. These changes are a normal part of the aging process, and they occur gradually over time.

Slowed conduction times can increase an elderly person's risk for falling and other household accidents. For example, it will take an older person longer to regain his balance if he starts to fall, or to avoid an obstacle (such as a pet or small child) that suddenly darts into his path. For this reason, it is especially important to remember the general safety guidelines from Chapter 10 when caring for an older person. For example, when helping an older person to walk, you will want to make sure that the pathway is well-lit and clear, that the person's clothes and shoes fit properly, and, if the person wears glasses, that she is wearing them.

MEMORY CHANGES

Memory and thought processes usually remain intact with normal aging. It may take an older person slightly longer to remember names, dates, or other information from the past, but given enough time, the person will eventually remember. Many older people experience a mild loss of memory for recent events, while still having excellent long-term memory. Engaging in activities that stimulate the mind (such as reading, traveling, working crossword puzzles, and doing crafts and other handiwork) throughout life helps to keep thought processes sharp and active well into old age (Fig. 28-4).

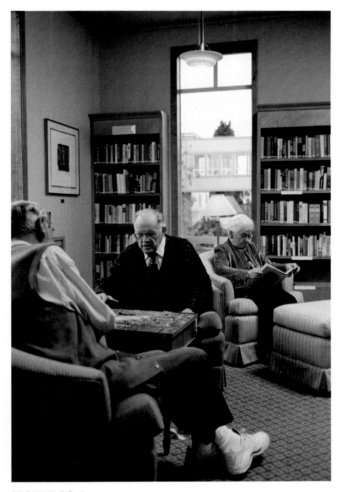

FIGURE 28-4

Use it or lose it! Studies have shown that actively exercising your mind throughout life helps to preserve mental function.

Dementia is a significant loss of mental capabilities. Dementia is a disorder, not a normal age-related change. If you work in a long-term care facility, it may seem to you that dementia is common, because approximately 66% of the residents in long-term care facilities have some degree of dementia. However, in the United States, only about 15% of people 65 years or older have dementia, and of these 15%, only 5% have severe dementia. Dementia is discussed in detail in Chapter 36.

DISORDERS OF THE NERVOUS SYSTEM

There are many types of nervous system disorders. Some disorders affect a person's ability to control movement, or experience sensation. Other disorders may affect a person's ability to speak. Still other disorders affect a person's memory or behavior. Disorders can be the result of a disease process, such as Parkinson's disease, or the result of an injury that damages the brain, spinal cord, or peripheral nerve pathways. Disorders of the nervous system are one of the most common causes of disability among elderly people. Approximately 50 percent of the disabilities seen in people older than 65 years are caused by a disorder of the nervous system.

TRANSIENT ISCHEMIC ATTACKS (TIAs)

Ischemia is decreased blood flow to the tissues. The tissue that is not getting enough blood is said to be *ischemic*. **Transient ischemic attacks (TIAs)** are temporary (transient) episodes of dysfunction that are caused by decreased blood flow (ischemia) to the brain. Any condition or situation that decreases blood flow to the brain can cause a TIA. For example, small blood clots can form in the heart or the arteries that supply the brain. These clots can break off and travel into the narrow arterioles of the brain, where they temporarily block the blood flow. Low blood pressure, certain medications, cigarette smoking, or standing up suddenly after lying down can also lead to a TIA.

Symptoms of a TIA vary according to the part of the brain affected by the decreased blood supply. Common symptoms may include dizziness, nausea, blurring or loss of vision, double vision, paralysis on one side of the body or face (with or without loss of sensation), or the inability to speak or swallow. The symptoms of a TIA may only last a few minutes, or they may last for several hours. The person usually recovers completely within 24 hours.

If you suspect that one of your patients or residents is having or has just had a TIA, please report this to the nurse immediately. TIAs are usually a warning that the person could have a stroke in the near future. A TIA may also be a sign of an underlying medical condition that needs to be addressed.

STROKE

A **stroke,** also known as a "brain attack" or cerebrovascular accident (CVA), occurs when blood flow to a part of the brain is completely blocked, causing the tissue to die. Unlike a TIA, a stroke causes permanent effects, because the obstruction of blood flow lasts long enough for the brain tissue to die or become damaged. Stroke is the third leading cause of death in people older than 65 years. Even if death does not occur, the person may be left with significant disabilities following a stroke. A very high number of the residents in long-term care facilities are survivors of a stroke.

A stroke can occur suddenly, in a person who was previously healthy. Signs and symptoms vary, depending on the area of the brain that is affected. Personality changes, drooping of the eyelid or corner of the mouth, slurring of speech, paralysis, severe headache, and loss of consciousness can all be signs of a stroke. If you notice a difference in a patient's or resident's usual behavior, appearance, or medical condition, you should report your observations to a nurse immediately (Fig. 28-5).

▶ *Tell the Nurse!*

Signs and symptoms of stroke can vary. Observations that should be reported to the nurse immediately include the following:

⮕ The person is unconscious or difficult to arouse from sleep

⮕ The person suddenly seems confused or disoriented

⮕ The person slurs his or her speech or is unable to speak clearly

⮕ The person is drooling

⮕ One of the person's eyelids or the corner of the mouth is drooping

⮕ The person complains of the sudden onset of a severe headache

⮕ The person complains of paralysis, tingling, or numbness of an arm or leg or the side of the face

⮕ There is a change in the person's vital signs, especially the blood pressure or pulse

Causes of Stroke

The most common cause of a stroke is a blood clot that blocks the flow of blood to a part of the brain. Therefore, people who smoke, have atherosclerosis, or have poorly controlled hypertension or diabetes are at high risk for having a stroke. Another, less common, cause of a stroke is cerebral hemorrhage. A cerebral hemorrhage occurs when a small artery in the brain bursts. The bleeding into the surrounding brain tissue puts pressure on the delicate tissue, damaging it. A cerebral hemorrhage is more likely in people with chronic hypertension, arteriosclerosis ("hardening of the arteries"), or certain deformities of the blood vessels in the brain.

FIGURE 28-5

A severe headache, personality changes, slurring of speech, paralysis, or loss of consciousness may all signal the onset of a stroke.

Effects of Stroke

The lasting effects of a stroke depend on the area of the brain that is affected and the amount of tissue that is damaged. For example, a stroke that affects the vital control centers of the brain stem will result in death, whereas a stroke that affects part of the cerebrum may result only in disability. The most common disabilities resulting from a stroke are hemiplegia and aphasia.

Hemiplegia, you will recall from Chapter 10, is paralysis on one side of the body. (Remember that the right side of the brain controls the left side of the body, and the left side of the brain controls the right side of the body—so a stroke that damages the right side of the brain will affect the left side of the body, and vice versa.) Depending on the amount of tissue damage, the hemiplegia may be mild or severe. A person with mild hemiplegia may have slight muscle weakness or shaking on the affected side, whereas a person with severe hemiplegia may not be able to move or feel any type of sensation at all on that side of the body. A person with severe hemiplegia who has lost sensation on one side of the body will need frequent repositioning to prevent pressure ulcers from forming (Fig. 28-6). Care must also be taken to prevent other injuries, such as burns, because the person will not have the ability to detect extreme heat, cold, or pain on the affected side.

Another common disability caused by a stroke is aphasia. **Aphasia** is a general term for a group of disorders that affect the ability of the person to communicate with others.

- **Expressive aphasia** is caused by damage to the motor centers of the brain that control the ability to speak or form sounds into meaningful words. A person with expressive aphasia may also have trouble swallowing, increasing her risk of choking.
- **Receptive aphasia** is caused by damage to the area of the brain that allows the person to understand words. The person can speak clearly, but he no longer knows the meaning of the words. For example, a person with receptive aphasia may say "no" when he means "yes."

Treatment of Stroke

In the past, the treatment of stroke focused on stabilizing the person's medical condition and then using aggressive physical therapy to help retrain disabled muscles to perform simple tasks. However, now new treatments are available that can help to minimize the permanent damage caused by the stroke. For example, medications that dissolve blood clots are sometimes used to reestablish blood flow to the brain before permanent damage can occur. To work, these drugs must be given very soon after the onset of the stroke.

Treatment immediately following a stroke depends on the severity of the damage to the brain, and on whether the person or family members want life-support measures to be taken. A person who has had a stroke may be very critically ill initially and need intensive care nursing. Respiratory support, oxygen, medications to support the heart rate and blood pressure, and continuous monitoring of vital signs may be necessary.

During this crisis period, the person's family members face uncertainty and difficult decisions. For example, they may need to decide whether or not to prolong life-support measures. If the person survives the stroke, family members may need to make some decisions about where the person will live in the future. For example, the person may need to move to a long-term care facility, or a home health care agency may need to be hired. During this difficult time, family members will appreciate a nursing assistant who demonstrates empathy, patience, and understanding.

FIGURE 28-6

A person who has had a stroke may lose the ability to detect sensations on one side of the body. With these people, extra care must be taken to prevent pressure ulcers and other injuries, because the person will be unable to sense warnings of impending injury, such as pain, cold, or heat.

A person who suddenly experiences a stroke and regains consciousness only to find that she is paralyzed or unable to communicate can be totally devastated. Rehabilitation, which is started as soon as the person's medical condition stabilizes, can be physically and emotionally difficult. Depression, frustration, anger, and major behavioral and personality changes can be expected. As a nursing assistant, you will be responsible for supporting the person both physically and emotionally during this difficult phase of his or her life.

PARKINSON'S DISEASE

As you learned earlier, neurotransmitters are chemicals that carry nerve impulses across the gap between the axon of one neuron and the dendrites of the next. There are many different types of neurotransmitters. In **Parkinson's disease,** one of these neurotransmitters, called *dopamine,* is not produced in sufficient amounts. Dopamine is necessary for proper functioning of the motor neurons. In a person with Parkinson's disease, the brain's instructions regarding muscle movement never reach the muscle, because of the lack of dopamine. Without enough dopamine, the impulse cannot be passed on to the next neuron in line. Because of this nervous system "short circuit," the brain loses its ability to properly control body movement.

Parkinson's disease is a progressive disease, which means that it gets worse with time. The average age for the onset of Parkinson's disease is 55 years. Men are affected more often than women. We do not know exactly what causes the neurons to stop producing dopamine, but some studies have linked this disorder to a history of metal poisoning, encephalitis (infection or inflammation of the brain tissues), and arteriosclerosis of the vessels of the brain.

Parkinson's disease usually starts with a faint tremor that gets worse over a long period of time. The tremor is most apparent when the person is resting and decreases when the person attempts purposeful movement. As the disorder progresses, muscles become weaker and rigid. The person may walk with a shuffling, leaning gait (Fig. 28-7), and it may be hard for the person to stop suddenly, once he has begun walking. A person with Parkinson's disease may speak very slowly, in a voice that does not vary

FIGURE 28-7

People with Parkinson's disease often develop a characteristic shuffling gait with a forward lean.

in tone. The person may lose the ability to move the small muscles of the face that are responsible for facial expression, giving the face a "mask-like" appearance. Eventually, the person's ability to chew and swallow is affected, and drooling may occur.

Although a person with Parkinson's disease may have difficulty speaking, he will have no problem understanding what you are saying. Picture boards and asking simple questions that can be answered with a nod or shake of the head can help improve the person's ability to express himself.

EPILEPSY

Epilepsy is a disorder characterized by chronic seizure activity. As you recall from Chapter 12, seizures are caused by interruptions of the normal electrical activity in the brain. A person with epilepsy experiences seizures periodically. The seizures may be grand mal seizures, which are characterized by generalized and violent contraction and relaxation of the body's muscles, or they may be petit mal (absence) seizures, which can be very mild and hardly noticeable. Because the seizures often occur without any warning, a person with epilepsy may not be able to participate in certain activities, such as driving or swimming. Care for a person who is having a grand mal seizure is described in Chapter 12.

There are many possible causes of epilepsy. For example, a person may develop epilepsy following a head injury, brain infection, or stroke. A difficult delivery that results in the infant not getting enough oxygen during the birth process can also lead to epilepsy. Many times, the exact cause of a person's epilepsy is never determined.

Drugs are available that help to reduce the frequency of seizures. For some people with epilepsy, these drugs do not work, but for others, they are very successful. A person whose epilepsy can be well controlled with drugs may have very few restrictions as far as activities are concerned.

MULTIPLE SCLEROSIS (MS)

It is thought that **multiple sclerosis (MS)** is an autoimmune disorder—the immune system attacks and destroys the myelin sheaths that protect the nerves, resulting in faulty transmission of nerve impulses. MS usually affects the nerves in the hands, feet, and eyes first, and then moves inward toward the central nervous system. Muscle weakness, tingling sensations, twitching of the eyes, and visual disturbances may be early signs of MS.

MS usually strikes people early in life, between the ages of 20 and 40 years. The disorder progresses at different rates, depending on the individual. Some people may have a period of remission (mild or no symptoms) followed by a relapse (the symptoms return and are much worse). In the late stages of the disease, the person may become totally paralyzed. At this time, there is no cure for MS, although some drugs have been shown to slow the progression of the disease.

AMYOTROPHIC LATERAL SCLEROSIS (ALS, LOU GEHRIG'S DISEASE)

Amyotrophic lateral sclerosis (ALS), like MS, is a nervous system disorder that causes progressive muscle weakness. In ALS, the nerves that transmit impulses between the spinal cord and the muscles are totally destroyed. People in the

late stages of the disease are totally paralyzed, yet their minds remain sharp. Death occurs when a person loses the ability to breathe and swallow.

ALS usually affects people later in life, between the ages of 40 and 60 years. Men are affected more often than women. Most people who have ALS die within 10 years of the diagnosis.

HEAD INJURIES

Head injuries leading to brain damage can be caused by falls, car and motorcycle accidents, bicycle accidents, and gunshot wounds (Fig. 28-8). Brain damage can also occur from events that cause a person to stop breathing for a long period of time, such as near-drowning, drug overdose, or choking.

Because neurons are not able to repair themselves or "grow back," traumatic injuries to the brain often result in physical disability, loss of mental function, or both. The type of disability will depend on the area and extent of the brain tissue damaged. Some people with head injuries will have paralysis similar to that seen in people who have had a stroke. Others will develop epilepsy, memory problems, or behavioral problems. Still others will be comatose and will need ventilator assistance to live. The type of care and rehabilitation that a person with a head injury needs is very individualized, according to the person's specific needs. Many of the younger people who live in

FIGURE 28-8

Taking standard safety precautions, such as wearing a helmet while riding a bike, can dramatically reduce the likelihood of a head injury should an accident occur. (© *Comstock IMAGES*.)

long-term care facilities are there because of a head injury that resulted in severe disability.

SPINAL CORD INJURIES

Injuries to the spinal cord are usually caused by trauma, but they can also be caused by birth defects or tumors of the spine. Trauma can cause the vertebrae to break, and the sharp fragments of bone can cut the soft tissue of the spinal cord, causing damage. Permanent damage can also result from the swelling that occurs inside the spinal canal after an injury. Following an injury, the soft tissue of the spinal cord swells. The bones that surround the spinal cord do not "give." As a result, the spinal cord is squeezed, cutting off blood flow and resulting in tissue death from lack of oxygen.

The disability that results from a spinal cord injury depends on the severity of the injury and the level of the spine where the injury occurred. Remember that the spinal cord is the line of communication between the brain and the rest of the body. If this line is broken at any point, then nerve impulses cannot travel beyond the break in the line. So, an injury to the spinal cord in the neck area can result in quadriplegia (paralysis from the neck down) because nerve impulses are not able to travel past the neck. An injury further down the spinal cord may result in paraplegia (paralysis from the waist down). The paralysis may be partial or complete, depending on the severity of the injury.

As with other types of disorders of the nervous system, the care and rehabilitation needed by a person with a spinal cord injury will depend on the severity and extent of the injury. A person with quadriplegia will usually need total assistance with his activities of daily living (ADLs), whereas a person with paraplegia may require little or no assistance following rehabilitation. For some people, the emotional effects of a spinal cord injury may be harder to overcome than the physical disabilities. Loss of control over one's body, and the accompanying loss of independence, can be very devastating. Some people may not be able to return to their jobs, which can cause financial problems. Others may never be able to enjoy a favorite hobby again. When you care for a person with a spinal cord injury, it is very important to encourage the person to do as

much as possible for herself. Doing so helps the person to maintain a sense of independence.

DIAGNOSIS OF NEUROLOGIC DISORDERS

When a person is showing signs or symptoms that suggest a neurologic disorder, the doctor may order one of several diagnostic tests to help determine the exact cause of the person's signs and symptoms. Improved diagnostic tools have led to the earlier detection of many neurologic disorders. Diagnostic tests that are often ordered for people with signs and symptoms of a neurologic disorder include the following:

- **Imaging studies.** Tumors of the nervous system can occur in the brain, the spinal cord, or along the peripheral nerve tracts. Many of these tumors are not cancerous, but they may cause problems as they grow and invade healthy brain tissue or nerves. Imaging studies such as radiography ("x-rays"), computed tomography (CT), and magnetic resonance imaging (MRI) are used to help locate tumors of the brain, spinal cord, or surrounding bony structures (Fig. 28-9). Imaging studies are also useful for detecting fractures of the skull

FIGURE 28-9

Imaging studies, such as computed tomography (CT) scans, allow doctors to see physical abnormalities of the brain, spinal cord, and surrounding bony structures. Here, a doctor looks at a CT scan of a patient's brain. (© *Simon Fraser/Photo Researchers, Inc.*)

or vertebrae. When used with special dyes (injected into a vein), imaging studies can help to reveal abnormalities in the blood vessels that supply the brain.

- **Electroencephalography.** An electroencephalogram (EEG) records the electrical activity of the brain (Fig. 28-10). EEGs are used to pinpoint seizure activity within the brain. Also, as you will recall from Chapter 22, a doctor can declare a person dead when there is a permanent loss of brain function. Therefore, when there is a possibility that someone is "brain dead" (for example, following a severe head injury), electroencephalography is used to monitor the person's brain activity. If

there is no electrical activity for the period of time specified by the law (usually 24 hours or more), the person may be declared dead.

REHABILITATION

For people with neurologic disorders or injuries, rehabilitation is started as soon as possible after the person's medical condition stabilizes. One very important aspect of the rehabilitation effort is the prevention of complications of immobility, such as contractures, muscle atrophy, and pressure ulcers. These complications can lead to failure of the rehabilitation effort and permanent disability. The use of splints, supportive devices, and assistive devices can help prevent complications and promote independence.

There are facilities that specialize in providing care and rehabilitation for people who are recovering from a brain or spinal cord injury. Perhaps working in a facility that specializes in helping people with neurologic disorders is a special interest of yours. However, even if you do not work in a facility that is dedicated to helping people with neurologic disorders, you may still find yourself caring for a person who requires restorative care as a result of a neurologic disorder or injury.

For a person with a neurologic disorder, rehabilitation can be a very long, frustrating experience. Although the brain has an incredible capacity for relearning basic functions, this process can be very slow. Therefore, all successes, no matter how small, should be celebrated. As a nursing assistant, you will be responsible for helping to prevent complications of immobility, and for reinforcing the rehabilitation efforts and techniques that are being used with your patient or resident (Fig. 28-11). Make sure you ask the nurse or physical therapist how to properly use any special equipment. Also make an effort to learn about any specific techniques that the patient or resident should be practicing. And above all else, be patient and empathetic with the person. Do not let the person's frustration and anger affect your ability to provide the best care possible. After all, how would you feel if you were suddenly put into a similar situation?

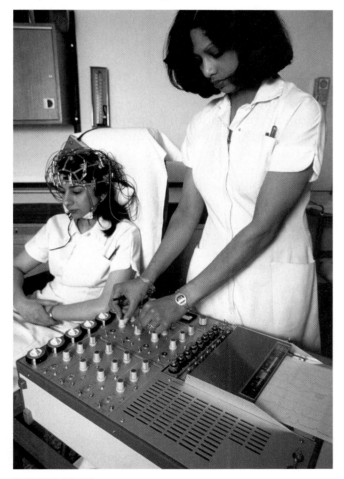

FIGURE 28-10

Electroencephalograms (EEGs) are used to monitor the electrical activity of the brain. (*Electro-* = "electric," *cephalo-* = "head," *-gram* = "tracing.") Here, a young woman is pictured having an EEG. The printout of her brain activity is visible in the lower right corner of the photograph. (© *Jerry Mason/Photo Researchers, Inc.*)

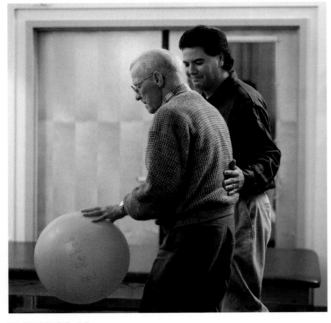

FIGURE 28-11

Learning about special equipment used by your patient or resident, as well as the rehabilitation techniques that the physical therapist is using with the person, can help you to provide better care.

SUMMARY

▶ Neurons are the basic cell of the nervous system.
- A neuron can send and receive information.
- Information, in the form of a nerve impulse, enters the neuron at the dendrites, travels through the cell body and down the axon, and then across the synapse and onto the dendrites of the next neuron in line.

▶ The nervous system consists of the central nervous system (CNS) and the peripheral nervous system (PNS).
- The central nervous system consists of the brain and the spinal cord. The central nervous system receives information, processes it, and issues commands. These delicate organs are protected by three layers of tissue (called meninges) and the cerebrospinal fluid (CSF).
  - The brain processes information and issues commands. The brain has four parts: the cerebrum, the diencephalon, the brain stem, and the cerebellum.
  - The spinal cord carries information to and from the brain.

- The peripheral nervous system consists of the nerves. The nerves carry information to and from the central nervous system.
  - Sensory nerves carry information from the "outside in." Sensory nerves give the brain information about other organ systems or the outside world.
  - Motor nerves carry information from the "inside out." Motor nerves allow the brain to control the movement of muscles.

▶ The nervous system receives, processes, and responds to information.
- The nervous system receives information from other organ systems and reacts to it, helping the body to maintain a state of homeostasis.
- The nervous system allows us to experience the world around us. Without our nervous systems, we would not be able to enjoy the taste and smell of a ripe peach, a beautiful piece of music, the sight of a loved one, or the soft fur of a favorite pet. We would not be able to move, think, or create.

▶ The changes in the nervous system that result from normal aging are relatively few.
- Older people are not as quick to react to things as younger people, which increases the older person's risk for falling and other household accidents.
- Some older people find it harder to remember recent events, even though they remember events that happened long ago quite clearly. Extreme memory loss, such as that seen in people with dementia, is not a normal age-related change.

▶ Disorders of the nervous system can affect the brain, spinal cord, or nerves.
- Transient ischemic attacks (TIAs) are caused by decreased blood flow to the brain. Once blood flow returns, the person's symptoms go away. Although the effects of a TIA are not lasting, a person who has had or is having a TIA needs medical attention because TIAs are often warnings that the person could have a stroke in the near future.
- A stroke, also known as a cerebrovascular accident (CVA) or "brain attack," can be caused by a blood clot or hemorrhage that disrupts blood flow to the brain. The part of the brain that does not receive enough blood dies, due to lack of oxygen and

nutrients. The effects of a stroke are permanent and can be mild or severe.

- Parkinson's disease affects the brain's ability to conduct motor impulses to the muscles because of a lack of the neurotransmitter dopamine.
- Epilepsy is a seizure disorder caused by abnormal electrical activity in the brain.
- Multiple sclerosis (MS) is a nervous system disorder that affects the motor neurons, resulting in muscle weakness that gets worse over time.
- Head injuries that result in brain damage and spinal cord injuries are a major reason why many younger people come to live in long-term care facilities or require the services of a home health care agency.

▶ Diagnostic procedures used to detect disorders of the nervous system include imaging studies—such as x-rays, computed tomography (CT) scans, and magnetic resonance imaging (MRI) scans—and electroencephalograms (EEGs).

▶ Rehabilitation can be a long, frustrating experience for the patient or resident, his or her family members, and the health care team. As a nursing assistant, you will play an important role in helping people with disabilities caused by nervous system disorders or injuries to live the most satisfying lives possible.

What did you learn?

Multiple Choice

Select the single best answer for each of the following questions.

1. Any condition that temporarily decreases blood flow to the brain can cause what to occur?
   a. A "senior moment"
   b. A transient ischemic attack (TIA)
   c. A heart attack
   d. A cerebral hemorrhage

2. Mrs. Romanelli has had a stroke and has a lot of trouble forming words. What term is used to describe Mrs. Romanelli's difficulty with language?
   a. Aphasia
   b. Dysphasia
   c. Paraplegia
   d. Hemiplegia

3. Mr. Owens had a stroke that left him paralyzed on the left side of his body. Which one of the following statements is true?
   a. The stroke occurred in the left side of Mr. Owens' brain.
   b. The stroke occurred in the right side of Mr. Owens' brain.
   c. The stroke affected Mr. Owens' brain stem.
   d. Mr. Owens has paraplegia.

4. What are the major goals of rehabilitation for a person who has a nervous system disorder or injury?
   a. To protect the person's self-esteem by not letting the person struggle with tasks he cannot do easily
   b. To get the person out of a wheelchair and back on his feet as soon as possible
   c. To prevent complications of immobility and help the person learn to do as much for herself as possible

   d. Because nervous system disorders and injuries often cause permanent damage, rehabilitation is of little use

5. Which of the following can increase a person's risk for a transient ischemic attack (TIA)?
   a. Low blood pressure
   b. Certain drugs
   c. Smoking
   d. All of the above

6. Which nervous system disorder is characterized by a lack of the neurotransmitter dopamine?
   a. Multiple sclerosis (MS)
   b. Epilepsy
   c. Parkinson's disease
   d. Dementia

7. What neurologic disorder is characterized by chronic seizure activity?
   a. Multiple sclerosis (MS)
   b. Epilepsy
   c. Parkinson's disease
   d. Stroke

8. What diagnostic test is used to monitor electrical activity of the brain?
   a. Electrocardiogram (EKG)
   b. Imaging studies, such as computed tomography (CT)
   c. Electroencephalogram (EEG)
   d. There is no test available to monitor the electrical activity of the brain

9. How does aging affect the nervous system?
   a. Older people usually become "senile" and forgetful.
   b. Older people lose the ability to form or understand words.
   c. Older people may take slightly longer to react to things.
   d. Aging does not affect the nervous system because old neurons are constantly replaced.

Matching

Match each numbered item with its appropriate lettered description.

_____ 1. Meninges

_____ 2. Cerebrospinal fluid (CSF)

_____ 3. Central nervous system

_____ 4. Peripheral nervous system

_____ 5. Axon

_____ 6. Myelin

_____ 7. Dendrite

_____ 8. Neuron

_____ 9. Synapse

a. Sends a nervous impulse

b. Consists of the brain and spinal cord

c. Fatty white substance that speeds the conduction of nerve impulses

d. A cell that can send and receive information

e. Receives a nervous impulse

f. The gap between the axon of one neuron and the dendrites of the next

g. Three layers of connective tissue that protect the brain and spinal cord

h. Consists of the nerves

i. Clear fluid that cushions the brain and spinal cord

? Stop and think!

▶ You have been caring for Mr. Elkins, a resident in the long-term care facility where you work, for about 6 months now. Normally, you and Mr. Elkins have quite a lively chat while you help him get ready for breakfast in the mornings. However, this morning, while you were helping Mr. Elkins with his morning care, you noticed that he seemed to be slurring his speech and saying things that didn't really make sense. What do you think might be going on?

▶ Ken works in a facility that specializes in providing rehabilitation services to people with nervous system disorders. One of Ken's new residents is a 17-year-old named Mike, who was recently injured while "body surfing." After spending several weeks in the hospital, recovering from surgery to repair his fractured vertebrae and the pneumonia he developed when he aspirated sea water during the accident, Mike has come to the facility where Ken works. Because Mike broke his neck during the accident and the spinal cord was damaged, there is a very good chance that Mike will be confined to a wheelchair for the rest of his life. Ken is not much older than Mike, and he has made a few attempts at friendly conversation, only to be snubbed every time. What might Mike be feeling that would make him act this way toward Ken? If you were Ken, how would you act going forward?

29 The Sensory System

What will you learn?

Have you ever heard the story of Helen Keller (1880–1968)? It is a famous story about a little girl who lived in a dark, silent, lonely world for nearly the first 7 years of her life, and how a young teacher, named Annie Sullivan, helped her to escape from that world. Helen was nearly 2 years old when she became ill and developed a very high fever. She survived the illness, but was left blind and deaf. For the next 5 years, Helen lived in her own world, unable to talk, hear, or see. Then one day, Annie Sullivan, a teacher from the Perkins Institute for the Blind in Massachusetts, came to live with Helen and her family in Alabama. Miss Sullivan started working with Helen by spelling words into the palm of Helen's hand, even though Helen didn't know what a word was. One day, after several months had passed, Helen and Miss Sullivan walked to the outdoor pump together. Miss Sullivan spelled the word "W-A-T-E-R" onto Helen's palm, while holding her hand under the running water. Suddenly, Helen understood what Miss Sullivan was doing. Words had meaning, and every "thing" had a word attached to it! Miss Sullivan was teaching her words! From that moment on, Helen was no longer alone in a dark, silent world. Although she still could not see or hear, she now had a way of communicating with others. Eventually, she learned to read Braille, to write, and to talk. In 1904, she graduated with honors from college, a truly remarkable accomplishment for a young woman who started out with so many odds against her.

From this story, you can see how much we rely on our special senses—sight, hearing, taste, smell, and touch—to understand and interact with the world around us. Our sensory system allows us to experience the beauty and joy of the world we live in. It also helps to protect us from harm. Many of the people you will care for will have disorders or disabilities involving the sensory system. In this chapter, you will learn about how the sensory system works and about some of the disorders that can affect the sensory system. You will also learn how you can help to meet the

(continued)

Photo: Helen Keller, around the time that Miss Sullivan came to live with Helen and her family. (Courtesy of the American Foundation for the Blind, Helen Keller Archives.)

needs of people who cannot see or hear well. When you are finished with this chapter, you will be able to:

1. Describe the main function of the sensory system.
2. List and define the two main divisions of the sensory system.
3. Understand the different types of pain that a patient or resident may experience.
4. Describe methods used to help control pain.
5. Describe how we experience taste and smell.
6. Discuss how aging affects a person's senses of taste and smell.
7. Describe how we experience sight.
8. Discuss the effects of aging on the eye.
9. List and describe disorders that can affect the eye.
10. Describe how to care for eyeglasses, contact lenses, and artificial eyes.
11. Describe special considerations that are taken when caring for a blind person.
12. Describe how we experience sound.
13. Discuss the effects of aging on the ear.
14. List and describe disorders that can affect the ear.
15. Describe techniques for communicating with a hearing-impaired person.
16. Demonstrate proper technique for inserting and removing an in-the-ear hearing aid.

Vocabulary

Use the CD in the back of your book to hear these terms pronounced, defined, and used in a sentence:

Sensory receptors	Myopia	Diabetic retinopathy	Vertigo
Sense organs	Hyperopia	Macular degeneration	Tinnitus
Tactile receptors	Astigmatism	Braille	Conductive hearing
Referred (radiating)	Presbyopia	Cerumen	loss
pain	Conjunctivitis	Presbycusis	Otosclerosis
Acute pain	Cataract	Otitis media	Sensorineural hearing
Chronic pain	Glaucoma	Otitis externa	loss

STRUCTURE OF THE SENSORY SYSTEM

The sensory system is part of the nervous system. The sensory system consists of **sensory receptors,** specialized cells or groups of cells associated with a sensory nerve. The sensory receptor picks up information, called a *stimulus,* and translates it into a nerve impulse, which is then sent to the brain for interpretation, via the sensory nerve. Sensory receptors are found throughout the body. Some are found in the **sense organs,** which you probably can name already—the eyes, the ears, the nose, and the taste buds. Other sensory receptors are found throughout the skin, and even in the tissues of internal organs.

The sensory system is sometimes divided into two major parts. This division is based on the location of the sensory receptors. The first part is called *general sense.* The sensory receptors that are responsible for general sense are found everywhere throughout the body. The second part is called *special sense.* The sensory receptors that are responsible for special sense are located in the specific sense organs (the eyes, the ears, the nose, and the taste buds).

GENERAL SENSE

General sense is responsible for our sense of touch, position, and pain.

TOUCH

Our sense of touch allows us to feel textures (such as the plush velvet of a party dress or the hot sand between our toes at the beach) and the shapes of objects. The sense of touch is made possible by tactile receptors found in the skin (Fig. 29-1). (*Tactile* is another word for "touch.") The **tactile receptors** are stimulated when something comes in contact with the surface of the body and presses on them, causing them to change shape. Some areas of the skin have more tactile receptors than others, and are therefore considered more sensitive to touch. For example, the tips of the fingers and toes and the lips contain many tactile receptors and are more sensitive to touch than other parts of the body.

Some of the tactile receptors in the skin allow us to sense pressure, also known as *deep touch.* Intolerance to prolonged pressure is what makes us shift our position when we have been sitting in one position for a long time. A person who is unable to sense pressure (for example, a person who is paralyzed) does not become uncomfortable from being in one position for a long time. Therefore, the person is not motivated to change positions. What effect do you think this has on the person's risk for developing skin breakdown and pressure ulcers?

POSITION

Position receptors, found in the muscles, tendons, and joints, keep the brain informed about the position of various body parts in relation to each other. For example, you can tell if your leg is bent or straight without actually looking down to check its position. These same receptors also relay information to the brain about the degree of muscle contraction, especially when the muscle is contracting against resistance (for example, when you are lifting weights). Position sense provides us with muscle tone and the ability to move our muscles in a smooth, coordinated way.

PAIN

Pain is the body's distress signal. Pain tells us that we have been injured, that we have overworked a muscle group, that an organ is not working properly, or that we are ill.

Free nerve endings (dendrites) in the skin and the tissues of our internal organs allow us to detect pain. Your brain is usually pretty good at identifying what hurts when the cause of the pain is on the surface of your body (for example, when you burn your finger while removing a hot dish from the oven). But your brain may have more trouble pinpointing the exact location of pain that is coming from an internal organ. This results in the phenomenon known as **referred (radiating) pain.** For example, a person who is having a heart attack may complain of pain in the shoulder, neck, arm, or jaw. Gallbladder disease may cause pain in the back and shoulder on the person's right side. A back injury may cause pain to radiate down the leg and into a person's foot. Figure 29-2 shows how pain from certain internal organs can be referred to other areas of the body.

Many of the people you will care for will be experiencing some type of pain. There are two types of pain. **Acute pain** is sharp, sudden pain, such as that which occurs with an injury. Acute pain

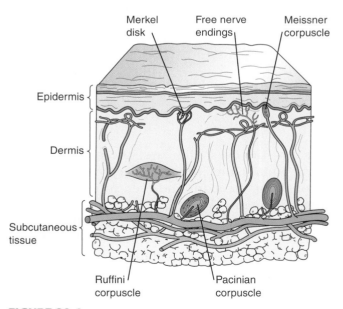

Merkel disk   Free nerve endings   Meissner corpuscle

Epidermis

Dermis

Subcutaneous tissue

Ruffini corpuscle   Pacinian corpuscle

FIGURE 29-1

Tactile receptors and free nerve endings in the dermis of the skin allow us to feel things that come in contact with our bodies. There are four main types of tactile receptors: Ruffini corpuscles, Meissner corpuscles, Pacinian corpuscles, and Merkel disks.

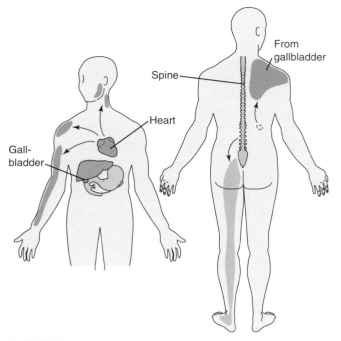

FIGURE 29-2

Pain may not always be felt at its exact source. Pain from the heart may be felt in the arm, shoulder, neck, or jaw (*red shading*). Pain from the gallbladder may be felt in the back and shoulder on the person's right side (*green shading*). A back injury can cause pain to radiate down the leg and into the foot (*yellow shading*).

lasts a short period of time and decreases as the body's tissues repair themselves and heal. **Chronic pain** is widespread, constant pain that continues even after tissue healing has taken place. Chronic pain may be caused by conditions such as arthritis or certain cancers.

There are many factors that affect a person's response to pain. Culture and upbringing play a very large role in how people perceive and manage pain. For example, in some families, admitting to pain may be considered a sign of weakness. People who were raised in families that took a stoic approach to pain may feel that it is better to "work through" the pain than to complain about it or ask for relief. Other people, however, may come from families where family members discussed every little ache and pain loudly and in great detail. People with a background like this might not hesitate to discuss or ask for relief from their own pain. Other factors that can influence a person's response to pain include the person's age and past experience with pain, and the person's sense of responsibility toward others. For example, it is quite common for women with young children to ignore their own pain because

they are so caught up in meeting the needs of their children.

As a nursing assistant, you may be the first to notice that one of your patients or residents is in pain. Sometimes the person will tell you about his discomfort. Other times, your observation skills will tip you off. For example, facial expressions (such as grimacing or gritting the teeth) can be a clue that someone is uncomfortable. A person may try to avoid using a certain body part, or an area may be red and swollen. Profuse sweating or changes in the person's vital signs may also be signs that a person is in pain.

Once you determine that someone is in pain, you will need to get some details so that you can accurately report what the person is experiencing to the nurse. Pain is a totally subjective experience. Only the person feeling the pain can describe what she is feeling. The pain may feel sharp or dull. The person may describe it as "throbbing," or it may be more like a constant ache. If a person says that she is in pain, ask her the following questions, and report the answers to the nurse:

- Where is the pain?
- How does the pain feel (for example, is it throbbing, aching, sharp, dull)?
- How long have you been feeling this pain?
- Does anything make the pain feel better (or worse)?
- How intense is the pain? (To help the person answer this question, you could ask her to rate the pain on a scale of 1 to 10, with 10 being the worst pain imaginable and 1 being slight discomfort.)

It is important for the nurse to know if a patient or resident is in pain. If the pain is new, the nurse will need to take steps to find out what is causing the pain. Even if the pain is familiar and the cause of it is known, there may still be something the nurse can do to help make the person more comfortable.

There are many ways of relieving and controlling pain. You have already learned about heat and cold applications, which are often used to treat musculoskeletal pain (see Chapter 25). Another common way of addressing pain is through the use of pain-relieving drugs. Over-the-counter drugs—such as aspirin, acetaminophen (Tylenol), and ibuprofen (Advil)—can be very effective for relieving mild to moderate pain. Severe pain, such as that which often accompanies traumatic injury, surgery, an acute illness, or some types of cancer, may only be controlled by the use of narcotics, such as morphine or Demerol. People who need narcotics to control their pain should be encouraged to ask for drugs before the pain becomes too intense. Giving a small dose of a narcotic early on can help to stop the pain before it gets too bad. If left untreated, the pain will only get worse and a higher dose of the medication will be needed to relieve it. Many people hesitate to ask for pain medications because they have heard horror stories about people becoming addicted to painkillers. Although this can happen, it is rare.

Although giving heat and cold applications may be beyond your scope of practice, and most nursing assistants are not permitted to dispense medications to patients and residents, there are many things that you can do to help a person who is experiencing pain and discomfort:

- Report any observations that suggest that a patient or resident is in pain, or any complaints that the person may have of pain, to a nurse promptly. Prompt and accurate reporting will help to ensure that measures are taken to make the person more comfortable, sooner.
- Help the person to relax. Anxiety causes the body to become tense, which increases pain. Simple care procedures, such as straightening the bed linens and positioning the person comfortably, can help the person to relax. Dim lights, a quiet environment, and a back massage can also be very comforting to a person who is in pain.
- Some people like to be distracted from their pain by listening to music, watching television, reading, or just talking.

Remember that each person's response to pain, and the methods that he is most comfortable using to address it, will vary.

TASTE AND SMELL

The sense organs of taste and smell are the taste buds and the roof of the nasal cavity, respectively. Special cells in these areas, called chemoreceptors, detect chemicals in the food we eat, the beverages we drink, and the air we breathe. The chemical signal is changed to an electric one and carried by sensory neurons to the brain, which tells us what we are tasting or smelling.

Taste buds cover the surface of the tongue. We have thousands of taste buds, and each taste bud consists of about 100 chemoreceptors, plus some supporting cells. The taste buds are bathed in fluid (either saliva or the liquids that we drink). The fluid contains dissolved chemicals, which stimulate the taste buds.

There are four basic tastes: sweet, salty, sour, and bitter. The taste buds that detect these four basic tastes are arranged in a particular pattern on the tongue. The "sweets" are found on the tip of the tongue. The "salties" are found on each side of the tongue, toward the front. The "sours" are located on each side of the tongue, toward the back. And the "bitters" are located across the back of the tongue.

The receptors that allow us to smell are located on the roof of the nasal cavity. Like the taste buds, these receptors are stimulated by chemicals that have been dissolved in fluid. However, in this case, the "fluid" is the moist mucous membrane lining of the nasal cavity. The sense of smell is easily fatigued, or worn out. This explains why an odor that is very strong at first becomes less noticeable over time.

Together, taste and smell have a very powerful effect on the appetite (Fig. 29-3). Under normal circumstances, a person will not eat something that tastes or smells bad, even if he is hungry. But, how often have you found yourself eating too much of something just because it tastes or smells so good? Similarly, how often have you noticed that when you have a head cold and a stuffy nose, food seems to lose appeal? This

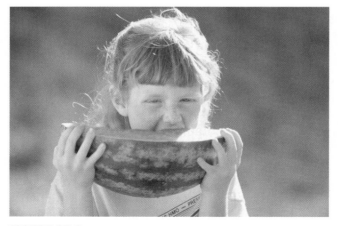

FIGURE 29-3

The senses of taste and smell are closely related. Eating a ripe piece of fruit is a treat for the tongue and the nose!

happens in large part because you can't smell the food!

As we get older, the number of chemoreceptors on the tongue and on the roof of the nasal cavity decreases. In addition, we produce less saliva, which makes it harder to dissolve the chemicals that stimulate the taste buds. As a result of these changes, the senses of taste and smell become less intense, leading to an overall decrease in appetite. To make up for a diminished sense of taste and smell, older people often season their food more heavily than younger people.

There are many dangers associated with a diminished ability to taste or smell. For example, an older person may not be able to tell that food has spoiled, and become ill from eating it. Or, he may not be able to detect the smell of smoke or a gas leak. It is surprising how much we rely on our senses of taste and smell to keep us safe.

SIGHT

Our sense of sight allows us to detect light, color, and shape.

STRUCTURE OF THE EYE

The sense organ of sight is the eye. Each eye is protected by the bones of the skull, which form a protective cavity ("orbit," "eye socket") around the eye. Only the very front of the eyeball lacks the bony protection of the skull. To protect the front of the eye, we have eyelids that close and eyelashes and eyebrows that serve as "dust catchers" (Fig. 29-4A). Lacrimal glands, located above the eye in the orbit, form tears that help to keep the eye moist and free of dust and bacteria. Skeletal muscles located around the eyeball allow us to move our eyes.

It may be helpful to look at Figure 29-4B as we go through the internal structure of the eyeball. The eyeball itself is made up of three layers of tissue—the sclera, the choroid, and the retina:

- The *sclera* is the tough outer layer. The sclera is made of connective tissue. Although most of the sclera is white (hence the term, "white of the eye"), the front of the sclera, which is called the *cornea*, is clear. Light passes through the cornea to the inside of the eye.

A. External structure of the eye

B. Internal structure of the eye

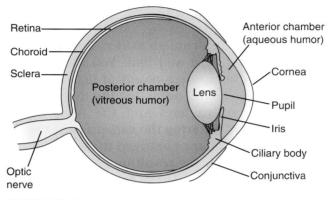

FIGURE 29-4

The eye. (*A*) External view of the eye. (*B*) Internal structures of the eye.

- The *choroid* is the middle layer. This layer contains the blood vessels that supply the retina and other parts of the eye. At the front of the eye, the *choroid* also forms the ciliary body and the iris. The *ciliary body* is a muscular structure that attaches to the *lens*, a flexible, transparent, curved structure that adjusts to focus light rays onto the retina. The ciliary body changes the shape of the lens, allowing the eye to focus. The other structure formed by the choroid, the *iris*, is the colored part of the eye. The iris is actually a round muscle with an opening in the center (the *pupil*). The iris controls the amount of light that enters the eye through the pupil.
- The *retina* is the innermost layer. The retina contains receptors, called *rods* and *cones*, which turn light into nerve impulses. The nerve impulses travel through the *optic nerve* to the brain for interpretation.

The eyeball also has two fluid-filled chambers (see Fig. 29-4B):

- The *anterior chamber* is located between the cornea and the lens. Special cells in

the ciliary body secrete *aqueous humor*, a watery fluid that fills the anterior chamber. The aqueous humor passes through the anterior chamber and is reabsorbed back into the bloodstream.
- The posterior chamber is located between the lens and the retina. The posterior chamber is filled with *vitreous humor*, a jelly-like substance that gives the eyeball its shape.

FUNCTION OF THE EYE

Think about how a camera works. To take a picture, you need light and film. You also need a way of controlling the amount of light that enters the camera, and adjusting the distance between the camera lens and the film. If the amount of light entering the camera is not sufficient, or if the distance between the lens and the film is not correct, the resulting photograph will be out of focus.

The human eye works much like a camera:
- The retina is the "film."
- The iris and pupil control the amount of light that enters the eye. In bright sunlight, the iris constricts, making the pupil smaller so that less light is allowed into the inner part of the eye. In low light, the iris dilates, making the pupil bigger so that more light can enter the eye.
- The cornea and lens work to focus light rays onto the retina, resulting in a clear image. First, the curve of the cornea focuses the light rays as they enter the eye. Next, the light rays pass through the lens, where the focus is refined (Fig. 29-5A). If the object the person is looking at is close, then the ciliary body contracts, causing the lens to become shorter and rounder. If the object is far away, then the ciliary body relaxes, causing the lens to become longer and flatter. The curved lens bends the light rays and brings them into focus on the retina, forming an image.

Clear, sharp vision is indeed a true gift. Many people need some help (in the form of corrective lenses, such as glasses or contact lenses) to achieve this goal! People who wear corrective lenses need help focusing the image properly on the retina. Some people need help focusing because of the shape of their eyeball. For example,

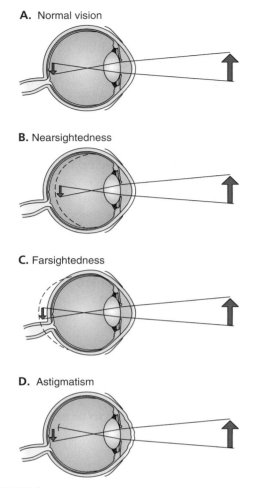

A. Normal vision

B. Nearsightedness

C. Farsightedness

D. Astigmatism

FIGURE 29-5

Many people need corrective lenses, such as glasses or contact lenses, to achieve clear vision. Three common problems that require the use of corrective lenses are nearsightedness (myopia), farsightedness (hyperopia), and astigmatism. (*A*) Normal vision. Light rays pass through the cornea and the lens and are focused on the retina. (*B*) Nearsightedness (myopia). The eyeball of a person who is nearsighted is more oval in shape than normal, which increases the distance between the lens and the retina. As a result, the image comes into focus before the retina. (*C*) Farsightedness (hyperopia). The eyeball of a person who is farsighted is more round in shape than normal, which decreases the distance between the lens and the retina. As a result, the image is not yet focused when it hits the retina. (*D*) Astigmatism. In astigmatism, the cornea is not perfectly curved. Some of the light rays that pass through the cornea are focused on the retina, but others are not, resulting in blurred vision.

the eyeball may be a little more oval than normal, causing the distance between the lens and the retina to be greater than usual. This results in nearsightedness, or **myopia** (Fig. 29-5B). People who are nearsighted are able to see fairly well close up, but they have trouble seeing images that are far away. This is because the distance between the person's lens and retina is longer than usual, which means that the image actually comes into focus before it hits the retina. This is a very common problem—20% of the people in the United States have some degree of nearsightedness!

Some people have the opposite problem, called farsightedness, or **hyperopia** (Fig. 29-5C). People who are farsighted are able to see objects in the distance fairly well, but they have trouble seeing objects that are close. In people who are farsighted, the eyeball is rounder than normal, causing the distance between the lens and the retina to be shorter than usual. Therefore, when the image hits the retina, it is not yet in focus.

Other people have trouble focusing images properly because the cornea is not perfectly curved. This condition is called **astigmatism** (Fig. 29-5D). The irregular curve of the cornea bends the light rays in funny ways, which results in a blurred, distorted image.

THE EFFECTS OF AGING ON THE EYE

As we age, many changes occur in the eye that can affect vision:

- The number of receptors in the retina decreases, and the lens becomes more opaque (cloudy). As a result, images are not focused as sharply as in younger days, and colors may not be as bright.
- The iris becomes more rigid, which means that it takes longer for an older person's eyes to adjust when she moves from a bright area to a dim one, or vice versa.
- The lens becomes less flexible, which affects the older person's ability to focus on objects that are close, a condition known as **presbyopia.** Presbyopia is why many people start using reading glasses in their 40s (Fig. 29-6).
- There is a decrease in tear production, which leads to dryness and irritation of the eyes. Many older people use lubricating eye drops to help keep the eyes moist and comfortable.

DISORDERS OF THE EYE

Conjunctivitis ("Pink Eye")

Conjunctivitis is infection and inflammation of the conjunctiva, a clear membrane that lines the inside of the eyelids and covers most of the surface

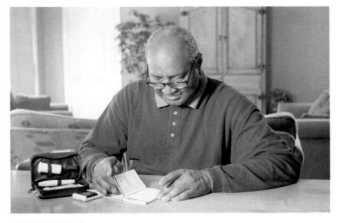

FIGURE 29-6

Presbyopia, which occurs when the lens becomes less elastic with age, is a common age-related change. People with presbyopia often need to use reading glasses to help them focus on things that are close.

of the eye (see Fig. 29-4B). In conjunctivitis, the white of the eye appears red. The eye may itch or burn, and it tears excessively (Fig. 29-7). There may be a sticky white or yellow discharge.

There are many different causes of conjunctivitis. Microbes that cause bad colds and sinus infections can travel through the tear ducts and onto the surface of the eye, causing an infection. Or, microbes from an infection somewhere else in the body can be transferred into the eye when the person touches the infected area and then rubs his eyes. For example, methicillin-resistant *Staphylococcus aureus* (MRSA) and herpes virus can cause conjunctivitis in this way.

Conjunctivitis is highly contagious. Rubbing the eyes and then touching something transfers the microbes to that surface, where they can easily be picked up by someone else. All that person has to do is touch her own eyes, and she could find herself with her own case of conjunctivitis! Conjunctivitis is usually treated with eye drops or an eye ointment prescribed by a doctor.

Cataracts

Cataracts are very common in older people, but they can occur in younger people as well. It is thought that excessive exposure to sunlight increases a person's chances of developing cataracts. A **cataract** is the gradual yellowing and hardening of the lens of the eye. The lens becomes opaque and eventually prevents light from passing though to the retina. The person's vision becomes

FIGURE 29-7

Conjunctivitis, or "pink eye," is a very contagious infection of the conjunctiva, the clear membrane that covers most of the surface of the eye and lines the inside of the eyelids. The affected eye is red, itchy, and teary, and there may be a sticky white or yellow discharge. (© *Science Photo Library/Photo Researchers, Inc.*)

A. Normal vision

B. Cataract

FIGURE 29-8

Cataracts occur when the lens of the eye becomes yellow and hard over time, resulting in cloudy vision. This is what the world looks like to (*A*) a person with normal vision and (*B*) a person with cataracts. (*Courtesy of the National Eye Institute, National Institutes of Health.*)

more and more cloudy as the cataract worsens (Fig. 29-8). It is like looking through a sheer curtain panel. When you look through one thickness of the sheer panel, your vision is only slightly cloudy. If you fold the panel to make a double thickness, your vision gets cloudier. And if you fold the panel again to make a triple thickness, your vision becomes cloudier still. This is what a person with a cataract experiences. Total blindness can result as a cataract becomes more opaque.

Many people with cataracts have surgery to remove the opaque lens and replace it with an artificial one. Improvements in equipment and surgical techniques have made this procedure simple and routine. Surgery is often performed on an outpatient basis using only a local anesthetic. The person usually can return home a few hours after the procedure. Cataract surgery enables people with cataracts to once again enjoy activities such as needlework and reading that would have been nearly impossible before.

Glaucoma

Glaucoma is a disorder of the eye that occurs when the pressure within the eye is increased to dangerous levels. This occurs when the aqueous humor in the anterior chamber is not reabsorbed into the bloodstream. As more and more aqueous humor is formed, it creates pressure, which builds up in the eye. The pressure squeezes the nerves and the blood vessels in the retina. Eventually, the nerves are destroyed and vision is lost.

People who are older than 40 years and have a family history of glaucoma are at high risk for developing glaucoma themselves. Glaucoma also seems to be more common in people with dark irises (brown eyes), as opposed to light ones (blue or green eyes). The most common type of glaucoma occurs gradually, over a long period of time. However, in some people, the onset of glaucoma happens suddenly, and is accompanied by a great deal of pain. Both chronic and acute glaucoma can lead to blindness if left untreated.

Early detection and treatment of glaucoma can help to save the person's vision. Therefore, routine eye examinations are essential. If a person is found to have glaucoma, medicated eye drops are usually used to help control the pressure within the eye. Some people may need surgery if the eye drops are not effective.

Diabetic Retinopathy

Diabetic retinopathy is a complication of diabetes that can lead to blindness. In the early stages, the tiny blood vessels that supply the retina burst, leading to hemorrhages and damaging the retina. As the retina tries to heal, new blood vessels start to grow along the retina and in the vitreous humor. These new vessels are very fragile and they often burst as well, damaging the retina even more.

The number of cases of blindness caused by diabetic retinopathy in the United States is rapidly increasing. Early detection during an eye examination is essential for preserving the person's vision. Laser treatment is often necessary to help seal off hemorrhages in the retina.

Macular Degeneration

The macula is the small area in the middle of the retina where images are sharpest. In **macular degeneration,** deposits build up in the macula. The receptors in the area become damaged, and the person's ability to see is impaired. Factors that can increase a person's risk of developing macular degeneration are smoking, excessive exposure to sunlight, a diet high in cholesterol, and an inherited tendency for the disorder.

Blindness

Blindness has many different causes and takes many different forms. Many people are considered blind but have partial sight. Some people see nothing but darkness, but many others can see light, movement, shapes, and even colors, just not clearly enough to distinguish between them. Some people who are blind have been blind since birth and have never seen anything, whereas others may have lost their sight later in life. With time, most people who are blind adapt very well and are very independent. People who have recently lost their sight, however, may be very frightened, especially of walking or moving around on their own. Rehabilitation for a person who has recently lost his sight focuses on safety and the person's return to independence. Ambulation and navigation

skills are taught so that the blind person can be independent again. During rehabilitation, a blind person may learn to work with a companion animal that has been specially trained to guide the person as she walks (Fig. 29-9). The person may learn **Braille,** a system that uses letters made from combinations of raised dots (Fig. 29-10). The person runs her fingers over words written in Braille to read them. In addition, many books are available on tape for the person to listen to.

As a nursing assistant, treating a person who is blind with respect and allowing the person to be as independent as possible are the best things you can do to help the rehabilitation effort. Learn the techniques that your patient or resident is being taught and reinforce them by helping the person to practice them continuously. Guidelines for caring for a person who is blind are given in Guidelines Box 29-1.

CARING FOR EYEGLASSES, CONTACT LENSES, AND PROSTHETIC EYES

Many of your patients or residents will wear glasses or contact lenses. Some may even have a prosthetic (artificial) eye. Most people are able to

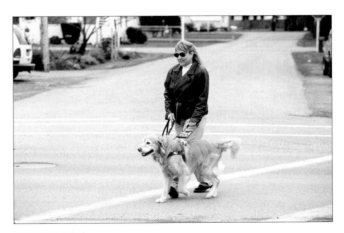

FIGURE 29-9

Many people who are blind have specially trained companion animals that help to keep them safe. For example, when preparing to cross a busy intersection, the blind person will listen to the traffic and tell the dog to move "forward" when she believes that the intersection is clear. If the dog judges that it is unsafe to move forward (for example, there is a car passing through the intersection that the person did not hear), the dog will refuse the command. This is called *intelligent disobedience*. Most companion animals require almost 2 years of training in order to do their jobs! (© *Peter Skinner/Photo Researchers, Inc.*)

A	B	C	D	E	F	G	H	I	J

K	L	M	N	O	P	Q	R	S	T

U	V	W	X	Y	Z

FIGURE 29-10

Braille, invented by Louis Braille in 1853, uses a system of letters formed from raised dots to enable a blind person to read.

care for their own vision accessories, but others may need your help.

Eyeglasses

Eyeglasses are commonly used to correct vision. Some people wear eyeglasses only for reading or close work, whereas others may need to wear them all the time when they are awake. Always make sure that your patients or residents who need glasses wear them, especially if the person is confused or disoriented. Being unable to see clearly can make confusion and disorientation worse and adversely affect the person's quality of life.

Eyeglasses are very expensive to replace if broken or lost. As with all of your patients' or residents' personal belongings, you should be careful when handling a person's eyeglasses.

Clean eyeglasses with cloths or a special solution made specifically for that purpose, or with warm water (Fig. 29-11). If water or a special cleaning solution is used to clean the lenses, finish by drying them with a soft cloth or tissue. Paper towels or napkins may scratch the lenses and should not be used. When not in use, the person's eyeglasses should be stored in their case within easy reach.

Contact Lenses

Contact lenses are also commonly worn to help make vision sharp. Contact lenses are made of molded plastic and fit directly on the eyeball. Contacts may be soft or hard. How long they can be worn before taking them out depends on the type of lens. Some lenses are removed and cleaned daily, whereas others can be left in for several days at a time.

Contact lenses must be cared for carefully to prevent infection and irritation of the eyes (Fig.

29-12). Special cleaning and soaking solutions are used to clean and store the lenses. The types of solutions that are used vary according to the type of lens. Each lens is kept in its own case ("left" and "right") because the correction and size for the left and right eyes may be different. If one of your patients or residents wears contact lenses, make sure you are familiar with the proper technique for helping the person to care for them. Report any complaints of eye irritation or discharge to the nurse immediately.

Prosthetic Eyes

Sometimes a person's eye must be surgically removed, either because of injury or disease. A person who has had an eye removed may choose to wear a patch to cover the missing eye, or he may wear a prosthetic (artificial) eye. Prosthetic eyes are made of ceramic or plastic and are usually designed to be very close in appearance to the person's own eye, in terms of color and shape (Fig. 29-13). When the person's natural eye is removed, a supporting structure is often inserted into the empty socket and the tissues inside the eyelids (the conjunctiva) are closed over it. Many times, the muscles that move the eyeball are attached to the supporting structure. This allows the prosthetic eye, if the person chooses to wear one, to move with the other eye.

A prosthetic eye is usually a curved disc (not a ball) that fits underneath the person's eyelids. Some prosthetic eyes are removable and others are permanent. If your patient's or resident's prosthetic eye is removable, you may need to help him with cleaning and storing it. Like eyeglasses, a prosthetic eye is very expensive to replace and should be cared for carefully. Improper handling can cause scratches or nicks on the prosthetic eye that can injure or irritate the person's eyelids. Handling the prosthetic eye with dirty hands or not cleaning it properly can result in an infection. If one of your patients or residents wears a prosthetic eye, make sure you have been instructed in the proper way to care for it.

HEARING AND BALANCE

The sense organ of hearing and balance is the ear.

GUIDELINES BOX 29-1
GUIDELINES FOR CARING FOR A PERSON WHO IS BLIND

What you do	Why you do it
Speak in a normal tone of voice.	Unless the person is hearing impaired as well as blind, there is no need to raise your voice.
Do not try to avoid using words such as "see," "look," and "watch." Do be descriptive in the things you see around you. For example, tell the person that the sky is a beautiful shade of blue or that there are lovely yellow flowers blooming right outside the window.	There is no need to be self-conscious about your ability to see, as compared with the blind person's inability to see. Most people who are blind are comfortable with that fact. Many appreciate your ability to share what you see with them through your descriptions.
Ask the person about the extent of her blindness, and do not hesitate to ask the person what type of help she needs from you.	Asking the person about her blindness will help you to better plan the person's care. You might be surprised at what the person is able to do for herself, with little or no assistance from you!
When you enter the person's room, knock and tell the person who you are and why you are there. Similarly, when you leave, tell the person that you are leaving.	If you do not announce yourself when you enter the room, you could startle the person. Imagine how frightening it would be to hear someone walking around in your room and not know who they are or what they are doing! Similarly, if you do not tell the person that you are leaving, he may not be aware that you have left. How would you feel if you started talking to someone who was no longer in the room and were left to figure it out on your own that the other person had left?
Make sure you explain procedures completely and descriptively. Throughout the procedure, tell the person what type of equipment you are using, what you are doing, and what you are going to do next.	With all patients and residents, you should take care to explain procedures thoroughly. However, with a blind person, you may have to modify your approach a bit. For example, instead of just showing the person a piece of equipment, you will need to describe it to him, or let him touch it. Also, you should tell the person what is happening as it happens so that the person is not left wondering where you are in the procedure, or what is coming next.
Do not rearrange the furniture in the person's room, unless the person asks you to.	The person is used to moving around the room on her own. If you move the furniture, the person could injure herself by running into something that has been moved and is now in an unfamiliar location.

(continued)

GUIDELINES BOX 29-1 (*continued*)
GUIDELINES FOR CARING FOR A PERSON WHO IS BLIND

What you do	*Why you do it*
Leave the door either completely open or completely closed.	If the door is partially open, the person may feel for the door, think that it is all the way open, and walk into the edge of the door.
When helping a blind person to walk, do not propel the person in front of you. Instead, let the person walk beside you and slightly behind you as she rests a hand on your elbow. Walk at a normal pace. Let the person know when you are about to turn a corner, or when a curb or step is approaching (and whether or not you will be stepping up or down).	In this way, you guide the person and reduce the risk of stumbles over unforeseen obstacles.

STRUCTURE OF THE EAR

The ear has three main sections: the outer ear, the middle ear, and the inner ear (Fig. 29-14).

The Outer Ear

The outer ear consists of the part of the ear that you can see (called the *pinna* or the *auricle*), plus a short canal called the *external auditory canal* (see Fig. 29-14). The shape of the pinna allows it to collect sound waves and direct them down the external auditory canal toward the *tympanic membrane* (also called the eardrum). The external auditory canal is lined with small hairs and special glands that secrete **cerumen** (ear wax). Cerumen helps to protect the ear canal by trapping dirt and other particles.

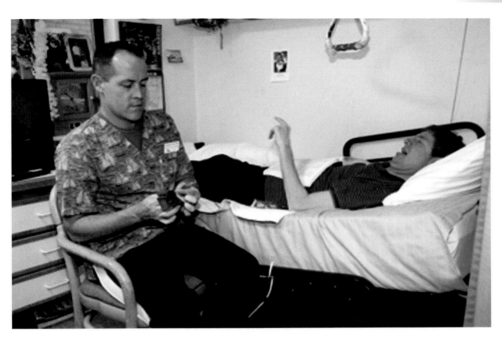

FIGURE 29-11

Take special care when handling a person's eyeglasses. They are expensive to replace.

The Middle Ear

The middle ear consists of an air space containing three very small bones (called *ossicles*) and the opening of the *eustachian tube*. The eustachian tube connects the middle ear to the pharynx (throat) and serves to equalize the pressure in the middle ear. If you have ever gone up or down a mountain or flown in an airplane, then you have probably felt your eustachian tube at work. As you change altitudes, your ears feel funny and you yawn to open them. The yawn allows air to travel through the eustachian tube, making the air pressure in the middle ear equal to the air pressure outside of your body. Equalizing the air pressures prevents the tympanic membrane from rupturing.

The three small bones (ossicles) in the middle ear are connected to the tympanic membrane. These bones, individually called the *malleus*, the *incus*, and the *stapes*, form a tiny bridge between the tympanic membrane and the inner ear (see Fig. 29-14).

The Inner Ear

The most complex part of the ear is the inner ear, which contains the receptors that make hearing and balance possible. The part of the inner ear

FIGURE 29-12

Contact lenses must be cleaned and stored properly in order to prevent infection and irritation of the eyes.

FIGURE 29-13

Artificial eyes are custom-made to look very similar to the person's other eye. (© *Lawrence Lawry/National Artificial Eye Service/Photo Researchers, Inc.*)

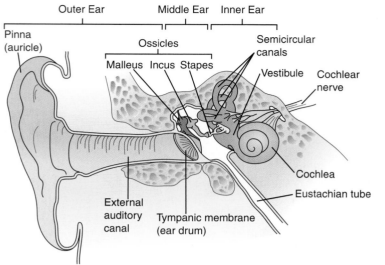

FIGURE 29-14

The ear.

that is responsible for hearing is called the *cochlea*. The cochlea looks like a snail's shell and is filled with fluid (see Fig. 29-14). Receptors for hearing are found within the cochlea.

The other part of the inner ear consists of two sac-like structures, called the *vestibule*, and three *semicircular canals* (see Fig. 29-14). Like the cochlea, the semicircular canals are filled with fluid. The vestibule and the semicircular canals, which are referred to together as the *vestibular apparatus*, help us to keep our balance.

FUNCTION OF THE EAR

Hearing

Sounds travel in the form of sound waves. Sound waves are captured by the pinna and sent down the external auditory canal. As the sound waves travel down the external auditory canal, they come in contact with the tympanic membrane, causing it to vibrate. The tympanic membrane vibrations are then passed to the first bone of the inner ear, the malleus, which sends the vibrations to the second bone, the incus, and then to the last bone, the stapes. The stapes rests against the oval window, a membrane at the opening of the cochlea. When the stapes vibrates, it causes the oval window to vibrate, sending the vibrations through the fluid inside the cochlea. The moving fluid stimulates the receptors inside the cochlea, which then send nerve impulses via the cochlear nerve to the brain. The brain interprets these nerve impulses as sound.

Balance

When your body position changes, receptors in the vestibular apparatus are stimulated. These receptors then send nerve impulses via the vestibular nerve to the brain. These nerve impulses tell the brain what the body's position is, relative to the ground. Have you ever gotten sick on an amusement park ride, in a car, or on a boat? Motion sickness occurs when the messages your ears are sending to your brain about your body's position do not match the messages your eyes are sending to your brain about your body's position!

THE EFFECTS OF AGING ON THE EAR

Like other organs, the ear is prone to age-related changes. The tympanic membrane and ossicles become stiffer, and the number of sensory receptors decreases. As a result, many older people gradually lose the ability to hear high-pitched sounds. This type of hearing loss is called **presbycusis.**

A person with presbycusis has trouble telling the difference between similar-sounding high-pitched sounds like *th* and *s*, which can lead to frequent misunderstandings. Conversations can be difficult to follow, especially when many people are talking at once or there is a lot of background noise. As a result, an older person with presbycusis may start to avoid social situations, because she cannot hear well and is embarrassed to have to keep asking others to repeat themselves. Avoiding social gatherings can lead to a feeling of isolation and a decreased quality of life for the older person.

Many older people with presbycusis are mistakenly labeled "confused" or "disoriented" by family members, friends, or health care professionals. But think about it—how can a person answer a question correctly if she cannot hear it clearly in the first place? When speaking with an elderly person with presbycusis, it is helpful to speak slowly using a lower tone of voice. This may make it easier for the person to understand what you are saying.

DISORDERS OF THE EAR

Ear Infections

Otitis media is an infection of the middle ear that is common in young children. It occurs when fluid builds up in the middle ear. Bacteria from the throat find their way into the middle ear through the eustachian tube. Once there, they start to grow and multiply in the trapped fluid.

Otitis media is usually accompanied by ear pain, fever, and difficulty hearing. If untreated, otitis media can cause scarring of the tympanic membrane and a permanent loss of hearing. If the infection is bacterial, antibiotics are usually given to treat it. Children who have frequent middle ear infections may need to have "tubes put in their ears." During this surgical procedure, called a *myringotomy*, the doctor makes a small slit in the eardrum and inserts a tube to equalize the pressure and prevent the build-up of fluid in the middle ear.

Another infection commonly seen in the ear involves the external auditory canal. **Otitis externa,** commonly referred to as "swimmer's ear," is an infection of the lining of the external auditory canal. Otitis externa is common in people who swim frequently or get the insides of their ears wet during showering or bathing. The ear becomes very painful to the touch. Antibiotic ear drops are usually needed to treat the infection.

Ménière's Disease

Ménière's disease, named after the French doctor who first described it, is a disease of the inner ear. Doctors do not know exactly what causes Ménière's disease. People with this disorder periodically experience episodes of dizziness (**vertigo**), ringing in the ear (**tinnitus**), temporary hearing

loss, and a feeling of pressure or fullness in the ear. One or both ears may be affected, and with time, many people begin to experience permanent hearing loss in the affected ear or ears. There is usually no cure for this disorder.

Although Ménière's disease is not fatal, it can be very difficult to live with. Each attack can last between 2 and 4 hours, and is often accompanied by nausea, vomiting, or both. A person who is having an attack should lie down and keep his eyes fixed on an object that is not moving. This helps to reduce the nausea and lowers the risk of falling as a result of the dizziness. After a severe attack, the person may be very tired. A person with Ménière's disease may need to take more time when getting up from a sitting or lying position, to prevent an attack from occurring.

Deafness

Like blindness, deafness has many different causes and takes many different forms. Some people have been deaf since birth, whereas others may have lost their hearing gradually later in life. Deafness can be partial or complete. The two main types of deafness are conductive hearing loss and sensorineural hearing loss:

- **Conductive hearing loss** occurs when something prevents sound waves from reaching the receptors in the cochlea. For example, the external auditory canal may be blocked by built-up cerumen, or by a tumor. The tympanic membrane may be damaged and not vibrate well, or the ossicles might not move freely. **Otosclerosis** is a disorder that causes a change in the stapes, preventing it from moving properly. Often, surgical removal and replacement of the stapes with a wire prosthesis can help to restore some hearing in people with otosclerosis.
- **Sensorineural hearing loss** occurs when the receptors are unable to receive stimuli or transmit nerve impulses. Presbycusis, or age-related hearing loss, is sensorineural. However, there are many other causes of sensorineural hearing loss that are not necessarily the result of aging. For example, prolonged exposure to loud noise (especially industrial noise), recurrent ear infections, trauma to the ear, and some types of medications can all cause sensorineural hearing loss.

A person with hearing loss may work with a speech therapist to learn how to speak more clearly. In addition, many adaptive devices are available to help a person with hearing loss maintain his independence. For example, telephone devices for the deaf (TDD) systems can be used in combination with a standard phone to allow a hearing-impaired person to communicate using the telephone. Television shows are available with "closed captioning," a system that prints the words that are being spoken at the bottom of the screen so that the person can read them. The person's doorbell, alarm clock, telephone, and smoke alarms may flash instead of ring. Like a blind person, a deaf person may have a companion animal that is trained to act as the person's "ears."

Communicating with a Person Who Is Hearing-Impaired

When caring for a person with hearing loss, there are a few easy things you can do to ensure good communication:

- **Face the person when you are speaking to him or her.** Many people who lose their hearing gradually develop the ability to partially lip-read what people are saying to them. Therefore, you should always face the person as you speak so that the person has a clear view of your mouth (Fig. 29-15). Avoid chewing gum or speaking unusually fast. Doing so can hinder the person's ability to lip-read.
- **Use a notepad to write down important questions or directions so that the person can read them.** This helps to elimi-

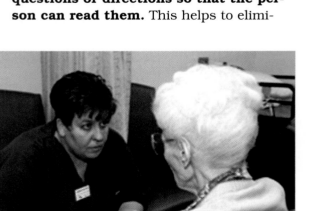

FIGURE 29-15

Always give a person who is hearing impaired an unobstructed view of your mouth. This will help the person to lip-read.

nate misunderstandings. If the person cannot read or reads in a language that is unfamiliar to you, a picture board (see Chapter 5, Fig. 5-4) may be quite helpful.
- **Make sure that the person fully understands what you said.** Some people, especially if the hearing loss is recent, are very reluctant to ask other people to repeat themselves. They may feel embarrassed by their hearing loss. Therefore, you need to make sure that the person has indeed gotten the message you were trying to send. If you are not sure that a person has understood what you have said to her, simply ask the person to repeat what you said back to you. For example, say, "If you could please repeat back to me what I said, I can make sure I told you everything I needed to." When the question is phrased in this way, the person feels as though she is helping you to do your job by repeating back the information. This helps to preserve the person's self-esteem and is a much better approach than just saying, "Now what did I say?"
- **Let the person know if you cannot understand what he is saying to you.** Many people with hearing impairments have difficulty speaking clearly. If you cannot understand what the person is saying to you, please do not pretend that you did to spare the person's feelings. The person may be trying to tell you something that is vitally important to his care or health. Tell the person that you did not understand and look for another way for him to get his message across. For example, you might offer him a notepad so that he can write down what he needs to tell you.
- **Consider learning sign language.** Many people who have significant hearing loss use sign language to communicate (Fig. 29-16). Knowing how to communicate in this manner can be a very useful skill for a nursing assistant to have.

Hearing Aids

Many people who are hearing-impaired use a hearing aid. A hearing aid is a battery-powered device that amplifies sound (makes it louder) before it enters the external auditory canal. There are many different styles of hearing aids (Fig. 29-17). Some styles fit entirely

"Thirsty"   "Pain"

FIGURE 29-16

Some people who are deaf use sign language to communicate. (*Photo © Will & Deni McIntyre/Photo Researchers, Inc.*)

A

B

C

FIGURE 29-17

Hearing aids come in a variety of styles. (*A*) This type of hearing aid fits entirely inside the external auditory canal. (*B*) This type of hearing aid fits behind the person's ear. (*C*) This type of hearing aid is carried in a pocket. (*A © L. Steinmark/ Custom Medical Stock Photo; B © Bishop/Custom Medical Stock Photo; C © SPL/Custom Medical Stock Photo.*)

GUIDELINES BOX 29-2
GUIDELINES FOR CARING FOR HEARING AIDS

What you do	*Why you do it*
Clean the hearing aid daily, according to the manufacturer's instructions.	If the hearing aid is not cleaned daily, the sound passages can become blocked with cerumen. The cerumen build-up can cause the hearing aid to stop working properly.
Make sure that the person has a spare set of batteries on hand at all times, and replace dead batteries immediately.	The hearing aid is battery-operated and will not work if the batteries are dead. It is very inconvenient for a person who uses a hearing aid to be without it for any length of time.
Keep hearing aids away from heat and moisture.	Heat and moisture can damage the plastic ear mold.
Do not use hairspray or other hair care products on a person who wears a hearing aid while the hearing aid is in place.	The chemicals in many hair care products can damage the plastic ear mold.
Store hearing aids at room temperature when they are not being worn.	Hearing aids are delicate instruments. Exposure to very hot or very cold temperatures is not good for them.
Keep replacement batteries and small hearing aids away from children and pets.	These small objects can pose a choking hazard to children and pets. In addition, hearing aids are expensive to replace.

within the external auditory canal. Others attach behind the ear or to the person's eyeglasses. Others take the form of a small box that the person carries in his pocket.

Not all people with hearing loss can benefit from the use of a hearing aid. It depends on the type of hearing loss the person has. An otologist (ear specialist) evaluates the person's hearing deficit to determine whether a hearing aid will be useful, and to determine what type of hearing aid should be used.

Hearing aids amplify all sounds, not just the voice of the person who is speaking. Noises from the environment, such as traffic noise or background music in a restaurant, are also amplified. This can be very distracting to a person wearing a hearing aid, and as a result, the person may choose to keep his hearing aid turned off most of the time.

Hearing aids are expensive and must be cared for carefully. General guidelines for caring for hearing aids are given in Guidelines Box 29-2. If one of your patients or residents uses a hearing aid, make sure that you know how to care for it and operate it. If a person who uses a hearing aid seems unable to hear you, make sure the hearing aid is turned on, and that the volume is turned up high enough. If the hearing aid still does not seem to be working, check the batteries to see if they need to be replaced and make sure the sound passageway is not blocked with cerumen. As with eyeglasses, it may be your responsibility to make sure that your patients or residents have their hearing aids in place because they may forget them or be physically unable to put them in and turn them on. Procedures 29-1 and 29-2 explain how to help a person to insert and remove an in-the-ear hearing aid.

SUMMARY

▶ Our sensory system protects us from harm and lets us experience the world that we live in. The sensory system has two main divisions: general sense and special sense.

■ The receptors for general sense are spread throughout the body.

- The receptors for special sense are located in special sense organs (the eyes, the ears, the nose, and the taste buds).
▶ General sense is responsible for our sense of touch, position, and pain.
  - Tactile receptors in our skin allow us to feel textures and the shapes of objects.
  - Position receptors in our muscles, tendons, and joints let us know where our body parts are in relation to each other.
  - Pain receptors (free nerve endings) in our skin and internal organs let us know when we are injured or ill.
    - Pain can be referred, which means that the part of the body that hurts is not actually the part of the body that is injured. Referred pain is especially common when the pain is coming from an internal organ.
    - Pain can be acute or chronic.
    - The way a person responds to pain depends on several factors, including the person's culture and the person's previous experience with pain.
    - As a nursing assistant, one of the most important things you can do for your patients or residents is notice and report pain.
    - There are many ways of controlling and relieving pain, including medications, massage, and heat and cold applications.
▶ Chemoreceptors in the taste buds and the roof of the nasal cavity give us our senses of taste and smell. Together, taste and smell play a very large role in stimulating the appetite. These senses also help to keep us safe by alerting us to signs of danger (such as spoiled food, a gas leak, or smoke from a fire).
▶ The eye is a complex organ that gives us our sense of sight.
  - Many people need corrective lenses (eyeglasses or contact lenses) to see clearly. Common problems with focusing include myopia (nearsightedness), hyperopia (farsightedness), and astigmatism.

- Changes in the eye as a result of aging can lead to presbyopia (an inability to focus on objects that are close), cataracts, and dry eyes. In addition, older people need more time to adjust when moving from a brightly lit area to a dim one, or vice versa.
- Some eye disorders, such as glaucoma and diabetic retinopathy, can lead to permanent vision loss if they are not treated.
- There are many different degrees of blindness.
  - Most people who are blind manage quite well on their own.
  - When caring for a person who is blind, you may have to make a few changes in the way you normally do things, to make up for the person's inability to see.
- Always handle your patients' or residents' eyeglasses, contact lenses, and prosthetic (artificial) eyes with care. These items are expensive and difficult to replace. In addition, improper handling of contact lenses or prosthetic eyes can lead to infection of the eye.
▶ The ear is responsible for our senses of hearing and balance.
- Sensory receptors for sound are located in the cochlea.
  - Presbycusis is age-related hearing loss caused by a gradual decrease in the number of sensory receptors for sound.
  - There are many different degrees of hearing loss. Hearing loss may be conductive or sensorineural in origin.
  - When talking to a person with hearing loss, be sure that the person can see your face, take care to speak clearly, and clarify information as necessary. Sometimes, it may be necessary to write information down or use a picture board to ensure complete understanding.
- Sensory receptors for balance are located in the vestibular apparatus, which consists of the vestibule and the semicircular canals. These receptors tell the brain where the body is in relation to the ground.

Chapter 29 Procedures

Getting Ready Steps

a. **W**ash your hands and observe standard precautions as necessary.

b. **G**ather needed supplies.

c. **K**nock and introduce yourself.

d. **I**dentify the person, and greet him or her by name.

e. **E**xplain the procedure.

f. **P**rovide privacy.

g. **S**ee to safety.

Finishing Up Steps

a. **C**onfirm **comfort** and good body alignment.

b. **L**eave the call light control within easy reach.

c. **S**ee to safety.

d. **O**pen the curtain and door.

e. **W**ash your hands.

f. **R**eport and record.

PROCEDURE 29-1

Inserting an In-the-Ear Hearing Aid

Getting Ready WGKIEPS

1. Complete the "Getting Ready" steps **a** through **g**.

Procedure

2. Check the hearing aid to make sure the volume is down and the hearing aid is turned off.

3. Help the person to a comfortable position, with his head turned so that the ear needing the hearing aid is closest to you.

4. Inspect the ear canal for excessive cerumen (ear wax). If you see excessive wax build-up in the ear canal, gently wipe the ear canal with a warm, moist washcloth.

5. Gently insert the tapered end of the hearing aid into the external auditory canal. Gently rotate the hearing aid so that it fits into the curve of the ear. With one hand, push up and in. Use your other hand to pull gently down on the person's earlobe. The hearing aid should fit snugly but comfortably, flush with the ear.

6. Turn on the control switch. Adjust the volume by talking to the person as you increase the volume. Stop increasing the volume when the person can hear you.

Finishing Up CLSOWR

7. Complete the "Finishing Up" steps **a** through **f**.

PROCEDURE 29-2

Removing an In-the-Ear Hearing Aid

Getting Ready WGKIEpS

1. Complete the "Getting Ready" steps **a** through **g**.

Procedure

2. Turn off the hearing aid.

3. Gently pull up on the person's ear. This will allow you to lift the hearing aid up and out of the person's ear.

4. Remove the batteries before storing the hearing aid in its case. Make sure the case is labeled with the person's name.

Finishing Up CLSOWR

5. Complete the "Finishing Up" steps **a** through **f**.

What did you learn?

Multiple Choice

Select the single best answer for each of the following questions.

1. Where are sensory receptors that are responsible for "special sense" located?
   a. In the muscles, tendons, and joints
   b. In the eyes, ears, nose, and taste buds
   c. In the brain and spinal cord
   d. In all of the organs of the body

2. Mrs. Knight is having a heart attack. She complains to the nurse of pain in her arm and jaw. What type of pain is Mrs. Knight experiencing?
   a. Chronic pain
   b. Referred (radiating) pain
   c. Imagined pain
   d. Musculoskeletal pain

3. Which one of the following can be used to treat and control pain?
   a. Medications, such as aspirin and morphine
   b. Back massage
   c. Heat and cold applications
   d. All of the above

4. One of the residents in the facility where you work, Mr. Hepberg, is 85 years old and in fairly good overall health. Mr. Hepberg always says to you, "Don't ever get old, honey! When you get old, even the food doesn't taste good anymore." Why might Mr. Hepberg feel this way?
   a. The meals at the facility are very bland for dietetic reasons.
   b. Mr. Hepberg is depressed.
   c. As we get older, our sense of taste and smell decreases, making food less appealing.
   d. Mr. Hepberg has a head cold.

5. Which one of the following symptoms of conjunctivitis should be reported to the nurse?
   a. Itching and burning of the eye
   b. Redness of the eye
   c. A sticky white or yellow discharge from the eye
   d. All of the above

6. Jessica is assigned to take care of Mr. Golden, who has recently become blind. What should Jessica remember when caring for Mr. Golden?

   a. Jessica should greet Mr. Golden and state her name when she enters his room.
   b. Jessica can help Mr. Golden to feel more secure when walking by walking a step or two ahead of Mr. Golden and letting Mr. Golden rest his hand lightly on her elbow.
   c. During procedures, Jessica should explain each step of the procedure to Mr. Golden as she does it so that he knows what is happening.
   d. All of the above

7. Which one of the following is true about cataracts?
   a. Many elderly people develop cataracts, but young people can develop them too.
   b. Cataracts are very painful.
   c. There is no cure for cataracts.
   d. Cataracts are a complication of diabetes.

8. Michael is taking care of Miss Jordan, who has a hearing loss. Miss Jordan is wearing her hearing aid, but it does not seem to be working. What should Michael do first?
   a. He should raise his voice.
   b. He should make sure that the hearing aid is turned on, and that the volume is high enough.
   c. He should remove the hearing aid and replace its batteries.
   d. He should report the problem to the nurse immediately.

9. Mr. Campi, one of your elderly residents, is very hard of hearing. What should you remember when you are talking to Mr. Campi?
   a. You should sit or stand so that Mr. Campi has a clear view of your face, and you should avoid chewing gum or speaking quickly.
   b. If you think that Mr. Campi has not completely understood what you are saying, you should demand that he repeat it back to you so that you can correct his mistakes.
   c. If you do not understand what Mr. Campi has said, you should just let it pass. Letting him know that you did not understand might embarrass or frustrate him.
   d. There is no point in talking to Mr. Campi. He cannot hear you anyway. It is better to just write everything down.

Matching

Match each numbered item with its appropriate lettered description.

_____ **1.** Iris

_____ **2.** Cornea

_____ **3.** Lens

_____ **4.** Myopia

_____ **5.** Astigmatism

_____ **6.** Retina

_____ **7.** Hyperopia

_____ **8.** Pupil

_____ **9.** Vitreous humor

_____ **10.** Ciliary body

a. Nearsightedness

b. Clear portion of the sclera, through which light passes to the inside of the eye

c. A round muscle; the colored portion of the eye

d. Farsightedness

e. A disorder of the cornea that results in blurred vision

f. The hole in the center of the iris

g. A flexible, transparent, curved structure that helps to focus images on the retina

h. Contains rods and cones, the sensory receptors responsible for vision

i. The jelly-like substance contained in the posterior chamber that helps to give the eyeball its shape

j. The muscle that allows the lens to either become shorter and rounder or longer and flatter

? *Stop and think!*

▶ You work in an assisted-living facility and have known one of the residents, Mrs. Zinner, for almost 6 years now. Mrs. Zinner is in her 70s and enjoys very good health. She moved to the facility with her husband, who is several years older and requires some assistance with his activities of daily living (ADLs). You have always liked Mrs. Zinner. She is very outgoing, and is always organizing outings and parties for the other residents in the community. Lately, though, you have noticed that Mrs. Zinner seems to be making a lot of excuses to avoid doing things with her friends. You've also noticed that sometimes Mrs. Zinner seems startled when she finds you in the apartment, even though you made sure to knock and call out your name before entering. What might be going on with Mrs. Zinner? Is there anything you can do to help?

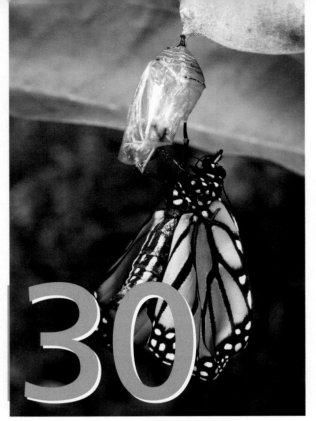

30

The Endocrine System

What will you learn?

The endocrine system produces hormones, chemicals that act on cells to produce a response. The word "hormone" comes from the Greek word *hormaein,* "to set in motion." This is, in fact, exactly what hormones do—set things in motion. Sometimes, the effects of the hormone occur over a long period of time. For example, hormones allow us to grow to our adult height, and they cause the physical changes that turn boys and girls into men and women. Other times, the effects of hormones are more immediate. Hormones with short-term effects help the body to maintain homeostasis. For example, insulin is a hormone that regulates blood sugar levels.

The hormones produced by the endocrine system control many of the body's functions. In this chapter, you will learn about the glands of the endocrine system, some of the hormones they produce, and how these hormones act to "set things in motion." You will also learn about some of the disorders that occur when the body produces too much or too little of a certain hormone. When you are finished with this chapter, you will be able to:

1. State the main function of the endocrine system.
2. Identify the various glands that make up the endocrine system.
3. Describe the negative-feedback mechanism that controls the endocrine system.
4. List the hormones produced by the different glands of the endocrine system.
5. Explain how the aging process affects the endocrine system.
6. Discuss how too little or too much of the various hormones can affect homeostasis.
7. Discuss the special care needs of people who have endocrine system disorders.

Photo: Hormones, which are produced by the endocrine system, set processes in motion. For example, hormones help to turn caterpillars into butterflies and children into adults!
(© E. R. Degginger/Photo Researchers, Inc.)

Vocabulary

Use the CD in the back of your book to hear these terms pronounced, defined, and used in a sentence:

Hormones	Hyperthyroidism	Type I diabetes mellitus	Hyperglycemia
Negative-feedback	(Graves' disease)	(insulin-dependent	Type II diabetes mellitus
system	Hypothyroidism	diabetes mellitus,	(non–insulin-
Goiter	Diabetes	IDDM)	dependent diabetes
Tetany	mellitus	Hypoglycemia	mellitus, NIDDM)

STRUCTURE OF THE ENDOCRINE SYSTEM

A group of glands, called the endocrine glands, make up the endocrine system. Be careful not to confuse endocrine glands and exocrine glands! Endocrine glands produce hormones and release them directly into the bloodstream. Exocrine glands produce substances that are not hormones and release them into a hollow organ or onto a surface. Examples of exocrine glands include the salivary glands in the mouth, which produce saliva, and the sweat glands in the skin, which produce sweat. Exocrine glands are not part of the endocrine system.

The endocrine glands are found throughout the body (Fig. 30-1):

- The *pituitary gland* is about the size of a cherry and lies underneath the brain. It is connected by a stalk, called the infundibulum, to the hypothalamus.
- The *pineal gland* is also located underneath the brain.
- The *thyroid gland* is located in the neck. It is butterfly-shaped, with two oval lobes located on either side of the larynx. The lobes are connected by a narrow band of tissue called the isthmus.
- The *parathyroid glands* are four tiny glands that are embedded in the back of the thyroid gland.
- The *thymus gland* is located in the upper part of the chest above the heart.
- The *adrenal glands* are located on top of the kidneys.
- The *pancreas* is located in the abdomen.
- The *sex glands (gonads)* are the ovaries in women and the testes in men. These

glands are also considered part of the reproductive system and are discussed in detail in Chapter 33.

FUNCTION OF THE ENDOCRINE SYSTEM

The endocrine system controls many of the body's processes, such as growth and development, reproduction, and metabolism. It does this by

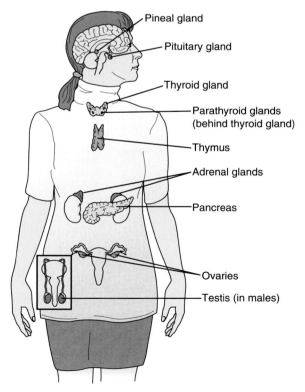

Pineal gland
Pituitary gland
Thyroid gland
Parathyroid glands (behind thyroid gland)
Thymus
Adrenal glands
Pancreas
Ovaries
Testis (in males)

FIGURE 30-1

The endocrine system is made up of the endocrine glands, which are spread throughout the body.

producing **hormones,** chemicals that act on cells to produce a response. The hormones are released into the bloodstream, which means that they can affect cells far from the gland that produced them. The hormone travels in the blood until it reaches its target cell. Once there, it attaches to a special receptor in the cell wall. Just as turning a key in a lock causes a door to open, attaching a hormone to a receptor causes a specific reaction in the cell. Some hormones have receptors in all of the body's cells, whereas other hormones have receptors in only certain types of cells.

Perhaps you are wondering what causes an endocrine gland to secrete (release) its hormone into the bloodstream. The secretion of many hormones is regulated by a **negative-feedback system.** In a negative-feedback system, some change in the internal environment causes the gland to begin producing its hormone. The gland continues to produce the hormone until the amount of hormone (or some other related substance) reaches a certain level in the body. At that point, the gland stops producing the hormone. The negative-feedback system works very much like a central heating unit in a house. The thermostat is pre-set to keep the temperature inside the house within a certain range. When the thermostat detects that the temperature has dropped below this pre-set range, the thermostat signals the furnace to turn on to heat the air. After the furnace creates heat and the temperature in the house rises to the desired range, the thermostat turns the furnace unit off.

In the rest of this section, we will explore the individual glands of the endocrine system, the hormones they secrete, and the effects of these hormones on the body.

PITUITARY GLAND

The pituitary gland, which is controlled by the hypothalamus, releases hormones that affect the function of other glands in the endocrine system. In this sense, the pituitary gland is like the "master gland." The pituitary gland has two parts, the posterior lobe and the anterior lobe.

Posterior Lobe Hormones

The posterior lobe of the pituitary gland stores and releases hormones that are produced by the hypothalamus. Two hormones are released by the posterior lobe (Fig. 30-2).

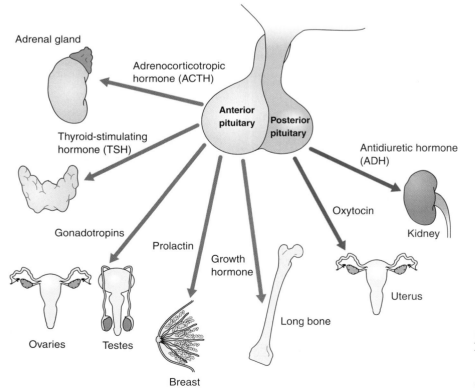

FIGURE 30-2

The pituitary gland, or "master gland," releases hormones that affect other glands in the endocrine system.

- *Antidiuretic hormone (ADH)* acts on the kidneys. ADH limits the amount of water that is lost from the body in the form of urine. When a person does not take in enough fluid or loses too much fluid through sweating, vomiting, or diarrhea, the hypothalamus detects a lower fluid level in the blood and signals the pituitary gland to release more ADH. The ADH causes the kidneys to save body fluid by decreasing the amount of urine produced. Similarly, when the hypothalamus detects that fluid levels are too high, it signals the pituitary gland to secrete less ADH. The lack of ADH causes the kidneys to produce more urine, eliminating the excess fluid from the body.
- *Oxytocin* is the hormone that causes labor to begin and is responsible for the let-down of milk in the breasts of a nursing mother.

Anterior Lobe Hormones

The anterior lobe of the pituitary gland makes and releases several different hormones (see Fig. 30-2).

- *Growth hormone* is what causes our bodies to get bigger and taller as we move from infancy into adulthood. Growth hormone is usually released in greater amounts during short periods of time, resulting in a child's "growth spurts." Although the output of growth hormone is highest during childhood, the anterior lobe continues to release growth hormone long after the growing phase of development is finished. Cells continue to need to be replaced throughout a person's lifetime, and growth hormone is necessary for that to occur.
- *Thyroid-stimulating hormone (TSH)* stimulates the thyroid gland to produce thyroid hormones, which affect the rate of metabolism in the body's tissues.
- *Adrenocorticotropic hormone (ACTH)* stimulates the adrenal glands to produce their hormones, which help the body to deal with stress.
- *Prolactin* stimulates the milk glands of the breast to produce milk when a baby is born.
- *Gonadotropins* regulate the functioning of the sex glands (gonads) in both males and females. There are two gonadotropins, *follicle-stimulating hormone (FSH)* and *luteinizing hormone (LH)*. The action of the gonadotropins is discussed in more detail in Chapter 33.

PINEAL GLAND

The pineal gland secretes *melatonin,* which helps to regulate the body's sleep–awake cycles. The pineal gland is stimulated by light and darkness and secretes melatonin during the dark part of the day.

THYROID GLAND

The thyroid gland produces two hormones that help to regulate the body's metabolism, the main one being *thyroxine.* In addition, the thyroid gland produces *calcitonin,* a hormone that helps to regulate the amount of calcium in the bloodstream.

Thyroxine

The hormone thyroxine sets the rate of metabolism for the cells of the body. How quickly body cells and tissues use nutrients (especially protein) and produce energy is determined by the amount of thyroxine present in the bloodstream. If the thyroid gland releases more thyroxine, the metabolic rate of the cells increases, and if the thyroid gland releases less thyroxine, the metabolic rate of the cells decreases.

The thyroid gland needs iodine to produce thyroxine. Iodine is found naturally in fish and shellfish and is added to salt and other commercial products. When a person does not get enough iodine in her diet, the thyroid gland is not able to produce adequate amounts of thyroxine. The sensors in the hypothalamus and pituitary gland detect a decrease in the level of thyroxine in the bloodstream and release TSH to stimulate the thyroid gland to produce more. However, because the thyroid gland has no iodine, it cannot respond to the request for more thyroxine, and the cycle repeats itself. The constant stimulation of the thyroid gland causes it to enlarge. An enlargement of the thyroid gland is called a **goiter** (Fig. 30-3). Iodine deficiency is just one cause of goiter. Goiter can also occur when the thyroid

FIGURE 30-3

The swelling in this woman's neck is a goiter, or an enlarged thyroid gland. Goiter can be caused by a lack of iodine in the diet or by a tumor or disease that affects the thyroid gland's ability to produce thyroid hormone. (© *Marka/Custom Medical Stock Photo.*)

gland does not produce enough hormone because of disease or tumors.

Calcitonin

Another important hormone produced by the thyroid gland is calcitonin. Calcitonin is one of the hormones that helps to maintain calcium levels in the bloodstream. As you learned in Chapter 25, calcium is very important for proper functioning of the skeletal and cardiac muscle. Calcium helps transmit nerve impulses into and out of the muscle fibers, allowing for the smooth contraction and relaxation of the muscles. Too little calcium makes the muscle fibers irritable and unable to relax after they contract, causing cramping. A condition called tetany (not to be confused with a tetanus infection)

may result if the calcium level drops too low. **Tetany** is characterized by cramping of the skeletal muscles and an irregular heart beat. Too much calcium in the bloodstream causes muscles to become weak and slow to respond.

Calcitonin lowers the amount of calcium in the bloodstream by allowing the calcium to be deposited in the bones and eliminated by the kidneys. For example, if a person drinks a lot of milk or takes calcium supplements, the level of calcium in the bloodstream increases as the calcium is absorbed from the intestines. The high calcium level in the blood stimulates the thyroid gland to produce calcitonin. Calcitonin transports the extra calcium to the bones. Any calcium that cannot be stored in the bones is excreted by the kidneys in the urine.

PARATHYROID GLANDS

The parathyroid glands produce *parathyroid hormone (PTH)*, which has the opposite effect of calcitonin. PTH causes calcium to be released from the bones into the bloodstream, increasing the amount of calcium in the bloodstream. In addition, PTH helps the kidneys to keep calcium, instead of excrete it in the urine. As you learned in Chapter 25, a calcium-rich diet is important to build up stores of calcium in the bones. PTH is what allows us to draw on these stores later in life, when our bodies become less efficient at absorbing the calcium that we eat. The actions of calcitonin and PTH balance each other and help to keep the levels of calcium in the bloodstream constant.

If the parathyroid glands are surgically removed or become damaged by disease, PTH is not produced in adequate amounts and the calcium levels may drop, causing tetany. Some tumors of the parathyroid gland can cause an overproduction of PTH that results in too much calcium being removed from the bones. The bones then become very fragile and fracture easily. Because the kidneys are responsible for excreting the excess calcium, kidney stones are likely to form.

THYMUS GLAND

The thymus gland secretes *thymosin*, a hormone that helps infection-fighting T cells to mature. An increase in the secretion of thymosin stimulates

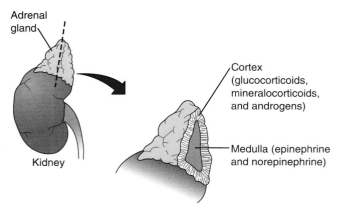

FIGURE 30-4

The adrenal gland consists of an inner part (the adrenal medulla) and an outer part (the adrenal cortex). Each part produces and secretes different hormones. Many of these hormones help us to deal with stressful situations.

the body to produce more T cells during an infection or illness.

ADRENAL GLANDS

Each adrenal gland has two separate parts: the *medulla,* or inner portion, and the *cortex,* or outer portion (Fig. 30-4). Each part secretes distinct hormones.

Medullary Hormones

The medulla of the adrenal glands secretes two hormones that are responsible for the "fight-or-flight" response of the body in emergency situations. Those hormones are *epinephrine* (also known as adrenaline) and *norepinephrine.* Epinephrine and norepinephrine help the heart and lungs deliver more oxygen and nutrients to the muscles, preparing the body to "stand up and fight or turn tail and run." A "side effect" of these hormones is the dry-mouthed, heart-pounding reaction that occurs when you are frightened!

Cortical Hormones

The outer portion of the adrenal glands secretes three main groups of hormones:

- *Glucocorticoids* play a role in the metabolism of fats and proteins, and help the body to maintain a reserve of glucose (sugar) that can be used in times of stress. They are also able to suppress the body's inflammatory response. For this reason, glucocorticoids are often given in the form of drugs for severe inflammatory disorders such as asthma, rheumatoid arthritis, or severe allergic reactions. Hydrocortisone is a common medication that is a glucocorticoid.
- *Mineralocorticoids,* as the name implies, help to regulate the level of certain minerals in the body, particularly sodium and potassium. *Aldosterone* is the primary hormone in this group. Aldosterone helps the kidneys to reabsorb sodium and secrete potassium.
- *Androgens* are secreted in small amounts by the adrenal cortex. Androgens are converted by the body into the sex hormones *testosterone* (in men) and *estradiol* (in women).

PANCREAS

The pancreas is both an exocrine gland and an endocrine gland. It functions as an exocrine gland by producing and secreting enzymes into the small intestine that help to digest food. It functions as an endocrine gland by producing two hormones, *insulin* and *glucagon.*

Insulin

Special cells within the pancreas, called the *islets of Langerhans,* produce and secrete the hormone insulin. Insulin, which affects all of the body's cells, allows glucose (sugar) to be transported from the bloodstream into the individual cells, where it is used for energy. In this way, insulin lowers the blood glucose level.

When a person eats, food is digested and absorbed by the bloodstream in the form of glucose. The blood glucose levels determine how much insulin is released by the pancreas. After eating, a person's blood glucose is elevated, and the pancreas releases insulin. The insulin causes the glucose to move from the bloodstream into the cells, where it can be used for energy. Any extra glucose is converted to glycogen. Glycogen is stored in the liver for later use, or it is converted to fat and deposited in various places on the body.

Glucagon

Glucagon has the opposite effect of insulin. While insulin is responsible for lowering blood glucose levels, glucagon is responsible for raising them. When the glucose levels in the bloodstream drop, as they normally do when a person has not eaten for some time, the pancreas secretes glucagon. The glucagon stimulates the liver to release the glucose that has been stored as glycogen into the bloodstream, to supply the cells of the body with fuel for energy. Insulin and glucagon work together to keep the body's blood glucose levels stable.

SEX GLANDS

The sex glands (or gonads) secrete the hormones that result in the onset of puberty and that regulate reproduction. Because the ovaries and testes are also considered a part of the reproductive system, these glands are discussed in greater detail in Chapter 33.

THE EFFECTS OF AGING ON THE ENDOCRINE SYSTEM

The normal processes of aging decrease the amount of hormones produced and slow their secretion by the glands of the endocrine system. Many of the physical changes that are part of aging are directly related to the smaller amounts of hormone released. For example, decreases in growth hormone levels slow the rate at which the body's cells and tissues divide and replace themselves, and decreases in thyroid hormone levels slow the body's metabolism.

In women, menopause (the end of menstruation, which signals the end of a woman's ability to bear children) occurs as a result of decreased hormone production by the ovaries. In men, secretion of hormones by the testes decreases, affecting sexual drive and function.

DISORDERS OF THE ENDOCRINE SYSTEM

Disorders of the endocrine system occur when the body produces too much or too little of a certain hormone. Imbalances in hormone secretion can be caused by disorders of the hypothalamus, the pituitary gland, the specific endocrine gland

responsible for the hormone, or as a result of poor nutrition. Corrective measures may be needed to restore the body's homeostasis and prevent the imbalances from causing health problems. There are many different types of endocrine disorders. Some of the ones you will be most likely to encounter in the health care setting are described here.

PITUITARY GLAND DISORDERS

Pituitary Dwarfism and Pituitary Gigantism

A deficiency in the amount of growth hormone secreted during the growing years results in a condition known as *pituitary dwarfism*. A person with pituitary dwarfism is much smaller than average, but still well proportioned. If the condition is diagnosed while the person is still a child, growth hormone may be given to help stimulate growth. Similarly, an excess in the amount of growth hormone secreted during the growing years results in a condition known as *pituitary gigantism* (Fig. 30-5). A person with

FIGURE 30-5

A condition known as pituitary gigantism occurs when the pituitary gland produces too much growth hormone during a person's growing years. These men are identical twins, but the man on the left is much taller than his average-sized brother because his body produced an excess amount of growth hormone. (*Photo courtesy of Gagel, R.F., & McCutcheon, I.E. [1999]. Images in clinical medicine. New England Journal of Medicine, 340, 524. Copyright © 2003, Massachusetts Medical Society.*)

abnormalities of the pituitary gland or by abnormalities of the thyroid gland itself. Thyroid disorders can also result from nutrient deficiencies, such as a lack of iodine. A simple blood test can be used to detect imbalances in thyroid hormones. Once detected, these imbalances can usually be treated.

Hyperthyroidism

Hyperthyroidism (sometimes called **Graves' disease**) is caused by the excessive secretion of thyroxine (*hyper* = "above"). In a person with hyperthyroidism, the metabolic rate of the body's cells is increased. Signs and symptoms of hyperthyroidism include increased hunger accompanied by weight loss, an irregular heart beat, an inability to sleep, irritability, confusion, increased perspiration, and intolerance to heat. Hyperthyroidism may be treated by surgically removing part of the thyroid gland, or by destroying part of the gland with radiation.

Hypothyroidism

Hypothyroidism results when thyroxine secretion is too low (*hypo* = "below"). Some babies are born with hypothyroidism, which, if left untreated, can result in a condition known as *cretinism*. Because thyroxine's control of the body's metabolism is essential for growth and development, cretinism is characterized by a lack of physical growth and mental development. However, if the hypothyroidism is detected and treated soon after birth, cretinism is prevented and the child will go on to develop normally. Hypothyroidism is treated by administering thyroxine in the form of a pill.

Most cases of hypothyroidism develop later in life, as a result of a disorder of the hypothalamus, pituitary gland, or thyroid gland. In adults, hypothyroidism is more common among women and the elderly. Hypothyroidism causes signs and symptoms that are opposite those of hyperthyroidism. Signs and symptoms of hypothyroidism include fatigue, weakness, depression, anorexia, weight gain, constipation, and intolerance to cold. The administration of oral thyroxine helps to restore the body's metabolism to a normal rate and relieve the signs and symptoms of hypothyroidism.

FIGURE 30-6

Secretion of too much growth hormone in an adult causes acromegaly, excessive growth of the bones of the hands, feet, and face. (© *Custom Medical Stock Photo*.)

pituitary gigantism is much larger than average, but still well proportioned.

Acromegaly

The secretion of too much growth hormone after a person has reached adulthood causes excessive growth of the bones of the hands, feet, and face. This condition is called acromegaly (Fig. 30-6). The person does not grow taller, but he does have a disproportioned appearance, especially in the face and hands.

THYROID GLAND DISORDERS

Remember that the secretion of the thyroid hormones is controlled by the pituitary gland. Therefore, thyroid disorders can be caused by

ADRENAL GLAND DISORDERS

Two of the most common adrenal gland disorders, Addison's disease and Cushing's syndrome, result from imbalances of the adrenal cortical hormones.

Addison's Disease

In Addison's disease, the adrenal cortex is destroyed, resulting in low levels of the adrenal cortical hormones. Because the glucocorticoids play a role in protein metabolism, a person with Addison's disease experiences muscle weakness and atrophy. Dark discoloration of the skin and disturbances in the body's salt and water balance are also seen. The person may have hypertension as a result of the Addison's disease. A person with Addison's disease may need assistance with walking and range-of-motion exercises.

Cushing's Syndrome

Cushing's syndrome results from excessive secretion of glucocorticoids. Cushing's syndrome can be caused by disorders of the pituitary gland that affect ACTH secretion or by disorders of the adrenal gland itself. Some people develop Cushing's syndrome after taking high doses of steroid medications, such as hydrocortisone, for a long period of time. Because glucocorticoids help us to metabolize fat, people with Cushing's syndrome tend to develop pockets of fat in the abdomen, on the back, and in the face. Increased facial hair is also common (Fig. 30-7). A person with Cushing's syndrome will have high blood glucose levels because one of the effects of glucocorticoids is to decrease the use of glucose by the tissues. Easy bruising of the skin and muscle weakness are also seen.

DIABETES

Diabetes mellitus results when the pancreas is unable to produce enough insulin. Diabetes mellitus can occur in people of all ages and races, but people between the ages of 65 and 74 years and people of African descent are affected most often. Diabetes mellitus is the most common of all endocrine gland disorders and is the seventh leading cause of death among the elderly. There are two types of diabetes mellitus, type I and type II.

Type I Diabetes Mellitus (Insulin-Dependent Diabetes Mellitus, IDDM)

Type I diabetes mellitus is less common but much more severe than type II diabetes mellitus. **Type I diabetes mellitus** is caused by destruction of the insulin-producing cells of the pancreas. Also called juvenile diabetes, type I diabetes mellitus is the form of diabetes that most often affects children. Most people who have type I diabetes are diagnosed while they are children or young adults.

Insulin

Because the pancreas is unable to produce adequate amounts of insulin, a person with type I diabetes mellitus must receive daily injections of insulin. The insulin is injected into the subcutaneous layer of the skin, where it is absorbed by the bloodstream. Several types of insulin are available. The types of insulin differ in the speed at which they start working and how long they last in the body. Some of your patients or residents will receive only one injection of insulin each day, while others may receive two or three.

FIGURE 30-7

Cushing's syndrome results from excessive amounts of the adrenal cortical hormones. The excessive secretion of androgens, which are converted into sex hormones, is what caused this woman to develop facial hair. The accumulation of fat on the woman's back and face is the result of excess glucocorticoids. (*Reprinted with permission from Rubin, E., & Farber, J.L. [1999].* Pathology *[3rd ed., p. 1193]. Philadelphia: Lippincott Williams & Wilkins.*)

A

B

FIGURE 30-8

People with type I diabetes mellitus must inject insulin into their bodies daily. (*A*) A syringe is used to administer insulin at regular intervals throughout the day. (*B*) A portable insulin pump allows for the continuous infusion of insulin. (*B courtesy of Animas.*)

Insulin can also be delivered continuously by a pump device (Fig. 30-8).

Monitoring Blood Glucose Levels

People who are receiving insulin injections need to have their blood glucose levels monitored closely. Too much insulin causes **hypoglycemia,** a dangerous drop in blood glucose levels. Hypoglycemia robs the brain of the glucose that is essential for it to function. Too little insulin results in **hyperglycemia,** or too much glucose in the bloodstream. If a person's blood glucose level increases too much, he can enter a state called diabetic coma. If not treated, diabetic coma can lead to death.

Many devices are available to monitor blood glucose levels, and new ones are constantly entering the market as new technology is developed. Older models use a drop of blood obtained from the person's finger to determine the blood glucose level (Fig. 30-9A). The "finger stick" method of monitoring blood glucose levels is painful for the person and can also expose the health care worker to bloodborne diseases. Make sure to wear gloves any time you are checking a person's glucose level using this method. Newer devices are clipped on the end of the finger and use infrared light to measure the amount of glucose present in the blood (see Fig. 30-9B).

Many people with diabetes monitor their own glucose levels and have been taught to adjust their insulin intake as needed, but some residents or patients may need help with monitoring their blood glucose levels. Different facilities will have different policies about who is responsible for blood glucose monitoring. You may work in a facility that allows nursing assistants to perform the glucose monitoring. Make sure that you have been adequately trained in how to use the equipment and record your findings. Be aware of which glucose levels need to be reported to the nurse immediately.

Diet

It is very important for a person with diabetes to eat an adequate amount of nutritious food, especially if the person is taking insulin. In addition to regular meals, snacks are served to help regulate the person's blood glucose levels. A person with type I diabetes must eat a diet with specific amounts of carbohydrates, sugars, fats, and proteins to react with the amount of injected insulin. If a person does not eat at the recommended time

A   **B**

FIGURE 30-9

Several different devices are available to monitor a person's glucose level. (*A*) Some devices determine the glucose level using a drop of the person's blood. (*B*) Many of the newer devices clip to the end of the person's finger and use infrared light to determine the blood glucose level. Cygnus, Inc.'s GlucoWatch G2® Biographer is shown here. (*A* © *T. Bannor/Custom Medical Stock Photo; B* © *2004 Cygnus, Inc., Redwood City, California.*)

after receiving her insulin, her blood glucose level can drop too low, resulting in a condition known as insulin shock. This is why it is important to serve meals and snacks at the scheduled time, especially when your patient or resident is taking insulin (Fig. 30-10). Also, if one of your patients or residents with diabetes refuses to eat or only partially finishes his meal or snack, you should report this to the nurse immediately.

Many people with diabetes understand how a balanced, nutritious diet can help them to manage their blood glucose levels and prevent complications from developing. However, some

FIGURE 30-10

It is very important for a person with diabetes to eat regular, nutritionally sound meals and snacks. If one of your patients or residents with diabetes refuses to eat or only eats part of a meal or snack, report this to a nurse immediately.

people may not follow their diet as closely as they should. For a person with diabetes, consuming too many sweets can result in hyperglycemia and lead to complications, both short-term and long-term. Some of your patients or residents, especially the older ones, may keep stashes of candy. If you notice that a patient or resident is hoarding sweets, you should report this to the nurse.

Type II Diabetes (Non–Insulin-Dependent Diabetes Mellitus, NIDDM)

Type II diabetes mellitus, sometimes referred to as glucose intolerance, commonly occurs in overweight adults. In people with **type II diabetes mellitus,** the pancreas still produces some insulin, but the cells of the body are unable to respond to the insulin. This results in higher blood glucose levels because the body is unable to transport the glucose into the cells. Symptoms of type II diabetes mellitus may occur gradually and go undetected for a long time.

Type II diabetes is treated through diet, exercise, and the use of oral medications to increase the effectiveness of insulin. People with severe type II diabetes may need to be treated with insulin injections, especially during times of illness or stress. Controlling the diet may be quite difficult, especially for the person who enjoys sweets. When caring for a person with type II diabetes, be sure to watch closely the amounts and types of food the person eats, just as you would for a person with type I diabetes.

 ## *Tell the Nurse!*

People with diabetes are very prone to developing both hyperglycemia (having too much sugar in the blood) and hypoglycemia (not having enough sugar in the blood). Hyperglycemia can be caused by eating too much food, not receiving enough insulin, being ill or under stress, being immobile or lacking exercise, or having diabetes mellitus that has not been diagnosed. Hypoglycemia can be caused by not having enough food, getting too much insulin, vomiting, or exercising more than usual.

Signs and symptoms of hyperglycemia and hypoglycemia are often very similar and should be reported to the nurse immediately. These signs include:

- Excessive hunger
- Excessive thirst
- Weakness, dizziness, or both
- Drowsiness and confusion
- Shaking and increased perspiration
- Rapid pulse and low blood pressure
- Headache
- Nausea and vomiting
- Slow, labored respirations with sweet-smelling breath
- Frequent urination
- Convulsions
- Loss of consciousness

Complications of Diabetes

Many organ systems can be affected by uncontrolled diabetes mellitus of either type. Low insulin levels increase the release of lipids (fats) into the bloodstream. The lipids then build up in the linings of the arteries, damaging them. Atherosclerosis, high blood pressure, heart disease, kidney disease, and blindness (diabetic retinopathy; see Chapter 29) can result from the damaged blood vessels. In addition, peripheral nerve damage results from reduced blood flow to the neurons, causing diminished sensation in the arms and legs. Poor circulation to the feet and lower legs also increases the risk of infection and poor tissue healing in the event of injury.

Early detection of diabetes mellitus is essential for preventing complications. Once diabetes mellitus is diagnosed, there are many measures that can be taken to keep the disease under control and minimize the person's risk of developing complications. People who are overweight should try to lose the excess weight. In addition, exercising regularly, following the recommended diet closely, and taking prescribed medications correctly are also very important.

SUMMARY

▶ The endocrine system is made up of glands throughout the body that produce hormones. Hormones are chemical messengers that allow the body to reproduce, grow, develop, metabolize energy, respond to stress and injury, and maintain homeostasis.

- The pituitary gland is considered the master gland of the endocrine system because it secretes hormones that affect other glands. The pituitary gland is controlled by the hypothalamus.
  - The posterior lobe of the pituitary gland stores and releases antidiuretic hormone (ADH) and oxytocin.
  - The anterior lobe of the pituitary gland produces and releases growth hormone, thyroid-stimulating hormone (TSH), adrenocorticotropic hormone (ACTH), prolactin, and the gonadotropins [luteinizing hormone (LH) and follicle-stimulating hormone (FSH)].

- The thyroid gland produces thyroxine, which helps to regulate metabolism, and calcitonin, which helps to maintain calcium levels in the bloodstream.

- The parathyroid glands secrete parathyroid hormone (PTH), which helps to move calcium from the bones into the bloodstream.

- The adrenal glands produce hormones that help us to deal with stress.
  - The adrenal medulla secretes epinephrine and norepinephrine, which play a role in the "fight or flight" response.

- The adrenal cortex secretes glucocorticoids, mineralocorticoids, and androgens.
- The pancreas secretes insulin and glucagon, which play a role in regulating blood glucose (sugar) levels.

▶ Disorders of the endocrine system result from either too much hormone or too little hormone.

- The most common of all endocrine disorders is diabetes mellitus.
  - There are two forms of diabetes mellitus.
  - Type I diabetes mellitus (insulin-dependent diabetes mellitus, IDDM) is the more severe form of diabetes. People with type I diabetes need daily insulin injections.
  - Type II diabetes mellitus (non–insulin-dependent diabetes mellitus, NIDDM) is also called glucose intolerance because the cells and tissues of the body no longer respond to the action of insulin. Type II diabetes mellitus can usually be managed with diet, exercise, and oral medications.

- A person with diabetes mellitus is prone to hyperglycemia (blood glucose levels that are too high) and hypoglycemia (blood glucose levels that are too low). As a result, careful monitoring of the blood glucose level is necessary because both hyperglycemia and hypoglycemia can cause complications, some of which are life-threatening.
  - A person with diabetes needs to eat regular, nutritionally balanced meals and snacks.

- Hypothyroidism (secretion of too little thyroid hormone) and hyperthyroidism (secretion of too much thyroid hormone) are also common endocrine disorders. Thyroid hormone imbalances alter the body's metabolic rate, causing many uncomfortable symptoms. Fortunately, hypothyroidism and hyperthyroidism can usually be treated.

What did you learn?

Multiple Choice

Select the single best answer for each of the following questions.

1. Hormones are chemical messengers that allow the body to:
   a. Metabolize energy
   b. Grow
   c. Reproduce
   d. All of the above

2. Which endocrine disorder causes an increased metabolic rate, increased hunger, weight loss, an irregular heart beat, an inability to sleep, irritability, and intolerance to heat?
   a. Hyperthyroidism
   b. Diabetes
   c. Acromegaly
   d. Pituitary gigantism

3. Mrs. Snow has type I diabetes mellitus. What special care considerations might a nursing assistant who is caring for Mrs. Snow need to keep in mind?
   a. Mrs. Snow will be unable to tolerate cold, and therefore, will often need a sweater.
   b. Mrs. Snow will need to eat meals and snacks on a regular schedule.
   c. Mrs. Snow may grow tired very easily.
   d. Mrs. Snow is likely to be irritable.

4. Why must a person with type I diabetes receive regular doses of insulin?
   a. The cells of the body do not respond to the insulin produced by the pancreas.
   b. The person's pancreas does not produce insulin on its own.
   c. The person's pancreas produces too much glucagon.
   d. People with type I diabetes do not need to take insulin; their disease can be controlled through diet, exercise, and oral medications.

5. Mr. Byron has type II diabetes mellitus. Although he knows that he should limit the amount of sweets that he eats, he has a real "sweet tooth" and often eats candy. In addition, he only monitors his blood glucose on days when he does not feel well. What complications is Mr. Byron at risk for developing if he does not make more of an effort to control his blood glucose levels?
   a. Kidney failure
   b. Blindness
   c. Heart disease
   d. All of the above

6. Mrs. Barney takes oral thyroxine to control her hypothyroidism. Without this medication, what sort of signs and symptoms do you think Mrs. Barney would have?
   a. Loss of appetite, weight gain, and constipation
   b. Frequent urination and excessive thirst
   c. Fat deposits on her back, abdomen, and face
   d. Excessive growth of the bones of the hands, feet, and face

Matching

Match each numbered item with its appropriate lettered description.

_____ 1. Parathyroid hormone (PTH)

_____ 2. Antidiuretic hormone (ADH)

_____ 3. Growth hormone

_____ 4. Thyroid-stimulating hormone (TSH)

_____ 5. Calcitonin

_____ 6. Adrenocorticotropic hormone (ACTH)

_____ 7. Thyroxine

_____ 8. Norepinephrine and epinephrine

_____ 9. Glucocorticoids

_____ 10. Insulin

a. Secreted by the adrenal cortex; helps the body to deal with stress

b. Secreted by the posterior pituitary gland; acts on the kidneys to limit the amount of water lost in the urine

c. Secreted by the anterior pituitary gland; causes our bodies to get bigger and taller

d. Secreted by the pancreas; helps the body to manage blood glucose levels

e. Secreted by the thyroid gland; lowers the amount of calcium in the bloodstream

f. Secreted by the anterior pituitary gland; stimulates the adrenal glands to produce their hormones

g. Secreted by the thyroid gland; sets the metabolic rate for the cells of the body

h. Secreted by the parathyroid glands; stimulates the release of calcium from the bones into the bloodstream

i. Secreted by the anterior pituitary gland; stimulates the thyroid glands to produce their hormones

j. Secreted by the adrenal medulla; participates in the "fight-or-flight" response

Stop and think!

▶ You are a home health aide. One of your clients, Mr. Singer, has type I diabetes mellitus. This morning, while you are helping Mr. Singer to the bathroom for his morning shower, you notice that he is shaky and that his breath seems to have a sweet, fruity odor. Mr. Singer tells you that something he had for dinner last night "just didn't agree with him" and that he got up during the night to vomit. What would you ask Mr. Singer next?

31

The Digestive System

What will you learn?

Did you know that over the course of a lifetime, you will eat about 50 *tons* (100,000 pounds) of food? As you already know from Chapters 19 and 20, it is your digestive system's job to process that food so that your body can use it, and to rid the body of the solid waste that is created as part of the food processing process. In this chapter, you will learn more about the individual organs of the digestive system and how they work. You will also learn about some common disorders of the digestive system. When you are finished with this chapter, you will be able to:

1. List the organs that are part of the digestive system.
2. Describe the function of the organs of the digestive system.
3. Discuss the effects of aging on the digestive system.
4. Discuss common digestive disorders and their symptoms.
5. Describe some of the tools used to diagnose digestive disorders.
6. Demonstrate how to provide routine stoma care.

Photo: Down the hatch! The digestive system processes the food that we eat.
(© Oscar Burriel/Photo Researchers, Inc.)

Vocabulary

Esophagus	Salivary glands	Mechanical	Hernia
Stomach	Liver	digestion	Barium
Esophageal (cardiac)	Bile	Enzymes	Ostomy
sphincter	Gallbladder	Chemical	Ileostomy
Pyloric sphincter	Pancreas	digestion	Colostomy
Rugae	Mastication	Villi	

STRUCTURE OF THE DIGESTIVE SYSTEM

Essentially, the digestive system is a long tube, or *tract*, consisting of the mouth, pharynx, esophagus, stomach, small intestine, and large intestine (Fig. 31-1). In addition, several accessory organs (appendages) along the way assist in the process of breaking down food so that our bodies can use it. These accessory organs include the teeth, tongue, salivary glands, liver, gallbladder, and pancreas.

THE DIGESTIVE TRACT

The walls of the "tube" that forms the digestive tract are made up of four layers of tissue (Fig. 31-2). The layers are basically the same throughout the digestive tract, although there is some variation from region to region. The four basic layers are the mucosa, the submucosa, the muscle layer, and the serosa:

- The *mucosa*, a mucous membrane, lines the digestive tract. The mucosa helps to trap disease-causing microbes. This is important because the digestive tract is open to the outside world at both ends (that is, the mouth and the anus). In addition to trapping microbes, the mucosa helps to protect the delicate tissues of the digestive tract from stomach acid, a very harsh fluid produced by the stomach to help digest food.
- The *submucosa* contains blood vessels and nerves.
- The *muscle layer* contains smooth muscle. Recall from Chapter 23 that smooth muscle

is not under voluntary control—it contracts and relaxes automatically. Peristalsis (contraction of the smooth muscle in the walls of the digestive tract) moves food through the system.

- The *serosa* is a tough outer layer of connective tissue.

Let's take a look now at the individual organs that form the digestive tract.

The Mouth, Pharynx, and Esophagus

Food begins its journey through the digestive tract at the mouth, or oral cavity. The mouth is lined with a mucous membrane and houses the teeth and tongue, accessory organs that assist with chewing and swallowing food. From the mouth, food moves into the pharynx (throat), and then into the esophagus.

The **esophagus**, a long narrow tube, serves mainly as a passageway for food to get from the pharynx to the stomach. The esophagus passes through the chest cavity, behind the heart (see Fig. 31-1). It enters the abdominal cavity at the *hiatus*, an opening in the diaphragm (the large, flat muscle that separates the abdominal and chest cavities). After entering the abdominal cavity, the esophagus connects with the upper part of the stomach. The mucus secreted by the esophageal mucosa, as well as the action of the muscle layer, helps to move food downward and into the stomach.

The Stomach

The **stomach** is a hollow, muscular holding pouch for food. The stomach has three main regions (Fig. 31-3):

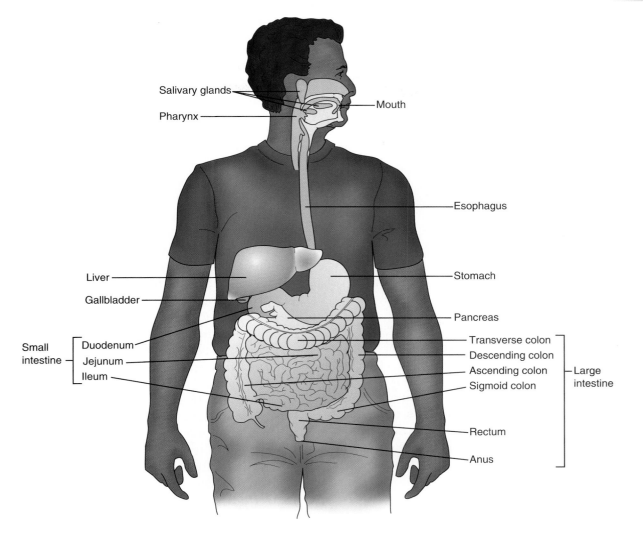

FIGURE 31-1

The digestive system breaks down food, absorbs nutrients, and gets rid of waste.

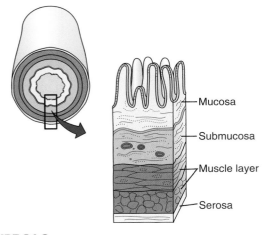

FIGURE 31-2

The walls of the digestive tract consist of four basic layers.

- The *fundus* is the upper region.
- The *body* is the main region. The esophagus enters the stomach here. The **esophageal (cardiac) sphincter,** a circle of muscular tissue, surrounds the place where the esophagus enters the stomach and keeps food from going back up the esophagus after it has entered the stomach.
- The *pylorus* is the bottom region. Food leaves the stomach through the **pyloric sphincter,** a circle of muscular tissue that surrounds the place where the stomach empties into the small intestine. The pyloric sphincter helps to prevent food from returning to the stomach once it enters the small intestine.

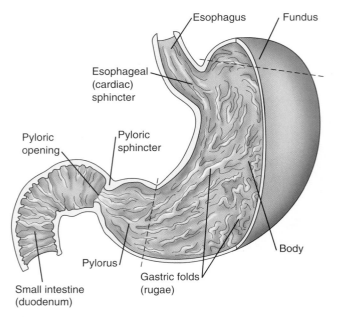

FIGURE 31-3

The stomach is a hollow holding pouch for food.

As most of us have experienced after eating a large holiday dinner, the stomach is capable of stretching and holding a large amount of food. Folds of the mucosa, called **rugae,** flatten out as food enters the stomach, almost doubling the stomach's holding capacity.

The Small Intestine

The small intestine, which is about 20 feet long, is so named because its diameter is much smaller than that of the large intestine. The small intestine has three regions, called the *duodenum*, the *jejunum*, and the *ileum* (Fig. 31-4).

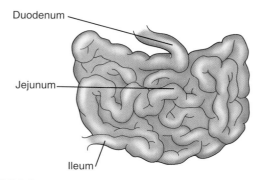

FIGURE 31-4

The small intestine has three regions: the duodenum, the jejunum, and the ilium.

The Large Intestine

The large intestine (also called the *colon*) is 4½ feet long and is much larger in diameter than the small intestine. Like the small intestine, the large intestine has several distinct regions (Fig. 31-5):

- The *cecum* is like a waiting room for food that is leaving the small intestine through the ileocecal valve and entering the large intestine. Food moves through the large intestine much more slowly than it moves through the small intestine. Therefore, incoming deliveries from the small intestine need a place to wait until the next segment of the large intestine, the ascending colon, is able to accept more food for processing.
- The *ascending colon* travels upward from the cecum.
- The *transverse colon* travels across.
- The *descending colon* travels down.
- The *sigmoid colon* is an S-shaped curve at the end of the descending colon.
- The *rectum* is the last segment of the colon. The place where the rectum opens to the outside of the body is the *anus*.

The *appendix*, a tiny, closed pouch that dangles from the cecum, has no known function. Scientists think that in our ancient ancestors, the

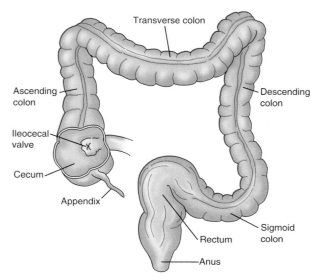

FIGURE 31-5

The large intestine has several regions: the cecum, the ascending colon, the transverse colon, the descending colon, the sigmoid colon, and the rectum. The appendix is a small pouch attached to the end of the cecum.

appendix may have played a role in digesting food, but that role has since been lost. Still, the appendix has a way of making its presence known. Inflammation or infection of the appendix causes *appendicitis*, a painful condition that is life-threatening if not treated. Treatment is surgical removal of the appendix.

THE ACCESSORY ORGANS

Several organs—the salivary glands, liver, gallbladder, and pancreas—play a role in digestion but are not actually part of the digestive tract (see Fig. 31-1).

- The **salivary glands** are located near the mouth. They produce and secrete saliva, a substance that helps with chewing and swallowing by moistening the food.
- The **liver** is a large organ located just underneath the diaphragm (see Fig. 31-1). The liver produces and secretes bile into the duodenum. **Bile** is a substance that helps with the digestion of fats. The liver also has several other important functions that are not related to digestion. For example, it produces clotting factors (chemicals that help our blood to clot) and it helps to clear our blood of toxins, such as alcohol and drugs.
- The **gallbladder,** a small pouch that is attached to the liver, stores bile produced by the liver that is not secreted directly into the duodenum.
- The **pancreas** is located behind the stomach, in the curve of the duodenum (see Fig. 31-1). The pancreas produces substances that aid in digestion and secretes them into the duodenum. The pancreas also produces insulin and glucagon, hormones that are secreted directly into the bloodstream. (Recall from Chapter 30 that insulin and glucagon regulate glucose levels in the blood.)

FUNCTION OF THE DIGESTIVE SYSTEM

The digestive system breaks down the food we eat into nutrients, which are then absorbed into the bloodstream for use by the body's cells. In addition, the digestive system removes unusable digested food from the body, in the form of feces.

DIGESTION

Digestion, or the breaking down of food into simple elements (nutrients), begins in the mouth. First, we physically break the food into smaller pieces by chewing it. Another word for chewing is **mastication.** This physical breaking up of the food, such as occurs when we chew, is called **mechanical digestion.** Next, chemical substances in our saliva start to work on the smaller pieces of food, breaking them down even more by breaking the bonds that hold the food molecules together. Substances that have the ability to break chemical bonds are called **enzymes.** The human body produces many different types of enzymes, each with a specific function. The process of breaking down food through the use of chemical substances such as enzymes is called **chemical digestion.**

After passing through the esophagus, the food we eat stays in the stomach for 3 to 4 hours, where digestion continues to take place. Special glands in the stomach lining produce hydrochloric acid (sometimes called "stomach acid") and enzymes. The stomach acid and enzymes act on the pieces of food to break them down even further. The peristaltic action of the stomach helps to mix the food with the acid and enzymes, creating a liquid substance called *chyme.*

The chyme passes into the duodenum, the first segment of the small intestine. Once in the duodenum, the chyme mixes with bile (secreted by the liver) and digestive enzymes secreted by the pancreas. These substances cause further breakdown of the food. From the duodenum, the chyme passes into the jejunum.

ABSORPTION

Once the chyme reaches the jejunum, absorption of nutrients begins. At this point, the food is fairly well digested. Now, it is time to start moving the nutrients from the digestive tract into the bloodstream. To reach the bloodstream, the nutrients pass through the mucosa and into the blood vessels in the next layer, the submucosa. The mucosa

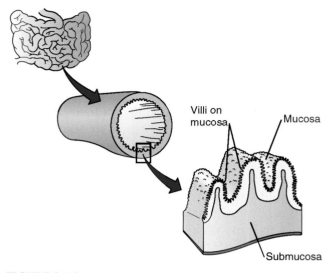

Villi on mucosa — Mucosa — Submucosa

FIGURE 31-6

Villi are finger-like projections that increase the small intestine's ability to absorb nutrients.

of the small intestine has millions of tiny finger-like structures called **villi** (Fig. 31-6). The villi increase the small intestine's ability to absorb nutrients by increasing the surface area of the mucosa.

Although most of the absorption of nutrients takes place in the small intestine, the large intestine also plays a role in absorption. Bacteria that live in the large intestine act on the chyme to produce vitamin K and some B vitamins, which are absorbed by the body. The action of these bacteria on the chyme can also produce gas as a by-product, especially when high-fiber foods such as beans, onions, and broccoli are part of the diet. As the chyme passes slowly through the large intestine, water is absorbed into the bloodstream. By the time the chyme reaches the end of the long intestine, all nutrients and most of the water have been removed, and the chyme has taken on the soft, moist, semi-solid consistency of normal feces.

EXCRETION

The feces (waste products of digestion) collect in the rectum, the last segment of the large intestine. The walls of the rectum gradually expand as the feces build up. At a certain point, the brain senses that the rectum is "full" and the urge to defecate (have a bowel movement) occurs.

EFFECTS OF AGING ON THE DIGESTIVE SYSTEM

Like all of the body's organ systems, the digestive system is affected by the process of aging.

LESS EFFICIENT CHEWING AND SWALLOWING

In older people, the production of saliva decreases, which may make chewing and swallowing more difficult. In addition, many older people have dental problems, such as missing or painful teeth. An older person may choke as a result of trying to swallow food that has not been chewed properly. Remember this when you are helping an older person to eat. Create a relaxed, social environment for eating and help the person to cut food up into small, easy-to-chew pieces. Also, report complaints of poorly fitting dentures, sores in the mouth or on the tongue, or a toothache to the nurse immediately.

LESS EFFICIENT DIGESTION

Food is most easily digested when it has been thoroughly chewed. Mechanical digestion increases the effectiveness of chemical digestion by making the pieces of food smaller. In an older person, the production of saliva, stomach acid, and digestive enzymes slows, making chemical digestion less efficient. Digestion is less efficient because not only are fewer chemicals available for chemical digestion, but the pieces of food that the chemicals must work on may be larger, due to inefficient chewing.

INCREASED RISK FOR CONSTIPATION

In an older person, the movement of food through the digestive tract may be slower. This can put the older person at risk for constipation. The chyme spends more time in the large intestine, which allows more water to be reabsorbed into the bloodstream. As a result, by the time the chyme reaches the end of the large intestine, almost all of the water has been removed and the resulting feces are hard, dry, and difficult to pass. Certain medications (such as prescription pain relievers) and immobility can also increase a person's risk for constipation. Measures that you can take to help your patients and residents avoid constipation are described in Chapter 20.

DISORDERS OF THE DIGESTIVE SYSTEM

Many of the people you will care for will have a digestive disorder of some sort, or will be recovering from one. Because the digestive system contains so many different organs, there are many different disorders that can occur. Four of the most common digestive disorders that you are likely to see in the health care setting are ulcers, hernias, gallbladder disorders, and cancer.

ULCERS

Ulcers (sores caused by wearing away of the protective mucosa that lines the digestive tract) can occur anywhere along the digestive tract. The most common sites are the stomach (*gastric ulcer*) and the duodenum (*duodenal ulcer*). Ulcers occur when the stomach produces too much hydrochloric acid. Factors such as smoking, frequent use of over-the-counter pain drugs, and infection with a bacterium called *Helicobacter pylori* can increase a person's chances of developing ulcers. In severe cases, the ulcer may affect all of the layers of the stomach or duodenum wall, not just the mucosa. This condition, called a *penetrating ulcer*, is life-threatening.

A person with an ulcer may feel uncomfortably full or nauseous after eating. Stomach pain is common, especially within 3 hours of eating (or when the person does not eat). Most ulcers are chronic. The person will have periods of feeling well, interrupted by flare-ups of symptoms.

Most ulcers can be treated with medication. People with severe ulcers may need surgery.

HERNIAS

The abdominal cavity (the space in the body where most of the digestive organs are found) is bounded by muscular walls. The muscular walls

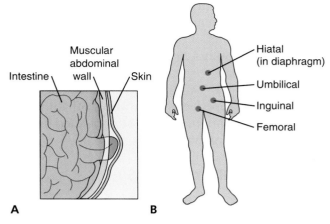

FIGURE 31-7

(*A*) A hernia occurs when an internal organ bulges through a weakness in the abdominal wall. (*B*) Hernias can occur in a number of different places.

of the abdominal cavity give structure to the body and help to keep the internal organs where they belong. A **hernia** occurs when an internal organ bulges through a weakness in the muscular wall of the abdominal cavity (Fig. 31-7). Sometimes the weakness occurs at the site of an old surgical incision. Other times, the muscle is just weak in spots. If there is a weak spot in the muscular wall, and the person does something that requires a lot of physical effort (such as lifting a heavy object), a hernia may occur. Hernias can occur in a number of different places:

- *Inguinal hernias* and *femoral hernias* occur when a loop of intestine bulges through the abdominal wall in the groin area. Inguinal hernias are more common in men, and femoral hernias are more common in women. These types of hernias are repaired surgically.

- *Umbilical hernias* occur around the navel (belly button). If the umbilical hernia is very small, no treatment may be needed. However, surgery may be required to repair a larger umbilical hernia.

- *Hiatal hernias* occur when part of the stomach passes through the hiatus, the opening in the diaphragm that allows the esophagus to pass into the abdominal cavity. People with hiatal hernias often have heartburn because the stomach acid moves back up into the esophagus. A person with a hiatal hernia may find that eating small, frequent meals and sitting up for at least 2 hours after every meal helps to relieve the heartburn. Medication can also provide relief of symptoms. People with severe symptoms may need surgery to repair the hernia.

Complications occur if the muscle tightens around the trapped tissue, cutting off its blood supply. This situation, called a *strangulated hernia*, is a surgical emergency.

GALLBLADDER DISORDERS

Gallstones can form and block the flow of bile from the gallbladder into the duodenum (Fig. 31-8). This can lead to inflammation and infection of the gallbladder. A person with a gallbladder disorder has episodes of severe pain. The pain may stay in the upper abdominal region, or it may radiate to the back and shoulder on the person's right side. The person may also have indigestion, especially after eating foods that are high in fat. Because bile gives feces their characteristic brown color, in a person with a gallbladder disorder, the feces may be pale and "clay-colored" due to their low bile content. Remember also that bile helps the body to digest fat. Therefore, in a person with

FIGURE 31-8

A gallbladder that has been removed and cut open to reveal the many gallstones inside. Gallstones can block the flow of bile into the duodenum, causing indigestion and severe pain. *(Rubin, E., & Farber, J. L. [1999]. Pathology [3rd ed., p. 791]. Philadelphia: Lippincott Williams & Wilkins.)*

gallbladder disease, the feces may float because they contain a great deal of undigested fat.

Medication or laser treatment may be used to dissolve the gallstones. In some cases, surgical removal of the gallbladder is needed.

CANCER

Any of the organs in the digestive system can be affected by cancer. The person's signs and symptoms will vary, depending on the location of the tumor. A person with cancer involving the digestive system may have one or more of the following signs and symptoms: loss of appetite, indigestion, pain, vomiting, constipation, changes in bowel movements, or blood in the stool. Depending on the location and type of cancer, it may be treated with surgery, radiation, chemotherapy, or a combination of these.

DIAGNOSIS OF DIGESTIVE DISORDERS

Digestive complaints—such as heartburn, indigestion, nausea, vomiting, stomachache, gas, diarrhea, and constipation—are common. Often, these symptoms are not a sign of anything more serious than eating too much! Sometimes, however, they may signal a serious disorder. Always report a new symptom, or a change in the person's symptoms, to the nurse immediately.

Sometimes, the doctor will order one or more tests to evaluate a person's symptoms. Some of these tests are simple, such as laboratory analysis of a stool sample. Others are more involved. Tests you may hear mentioned include the following:

- **Endoscopy** involves using a special instrument to look inside the digestive tract and obtain tissue or fluids for analysis. Endoscopy allows the doctor to look inside the digestive tract for tumors or other abnormal growths. The type of endoscope used depends on whether the instrument will be passed through the person's mouth (to view the upper digestive tract) or anus (to view the lower digestive tract).
- **Imaging studies,** such as x-rays, computed tomography (CT) scans, and magnetic resonance imaging (MRI) scans allow

the doctor to view the organs of the digestive system without actually entering the body. Sometimes, the person is asked to swallow barium or have a barium enema prior to the procedure. **Barium** is a liquid substance that coats the mucosa of the digestive tract and makes the organs appear on an x-ray (Fig. 31-9).

You may find yourself caring for a person who is about to have one of these diagnostic procedures. The person may have a special diet in the days leading up to the procedure, or be placed on NPO status. Sometimes, an enema is ordered to clean out the large intestine prior to the procedure. The nurse will let you know of any special care needs for a person who is having one of these procedures.

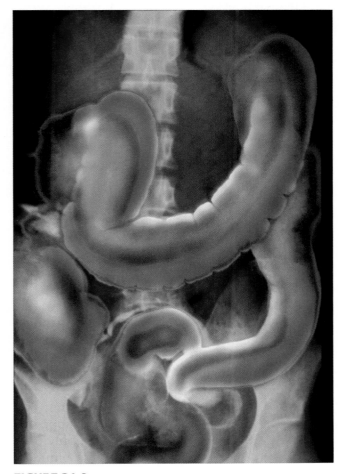

FIGURE 31-9

A person may be given a barium enema or asked to drink barium prior to having an x-ray taken. The barium helps to enhance the x-ray image. This is a false-color barium x-ray of a person's digestive tract. (© *BSIP/Custom Medical Stock Photo.*)

CARING FOR A PERSON WITH AN OSTOMY

As a nursing assistant, you may care for people with ostomies. For example, a person with a tumor in the large intestine may have surgery to remove the diseased part of the intestine. Depending on the location of the tumor and the length of the segment of the intestine that had to be removed, the person may need an alternate way of eliminating feces from the body following the surgery. In this case, the person may have an **ostomy.** An artificial opening, called a stoma, is made in the abdominal wall and the remaining portion of the intestine is connected to it (Fig. 31-10). Feces pass through the stoma and into a pouch (called an *ostomy appliance*) that is worn over the stoma (Fig. 31-11).

- An **ileostomy** is created if the entire large intestine must be removed. The end of the small intestine (that is, the ileum) is attached to the abdominal wall. Because the chyme does not have the chance to travel through the large intestine (where water is reabsorbed), the person's feces are very liquid and may flow fairly continuously. For this reason, a person with an ileostomy is quite prone to dehydration.

- A **colostomy** is created if part of the large intestine is still present. After the diseased part of the large intestine is removed, the healthy end is attached to the abdominal wall. Among people with colostomies, the feces vary in consistency. If the portion of the intestine that was removed was near the beginning of the large intestine, then the feces will be more liquid because the chyme will spend less time in the large intestine. On the other hand, if the portion of the intestine that was removed was near the end of the large intestine, then the feces will be more solid and formed.

Cancer is not the only reason a person might have to have an ostomy procedure. Bowel trauma and diseases such as diverticulitis (an inflammatory disease of the bowel) are other common reasons that ostomies are performed. Sometimes, a temporary ostomy is done to allow a portion of the bowel to "rest." Later, the ends of the bowel are sewn back together and normal bowel elimination resumes.

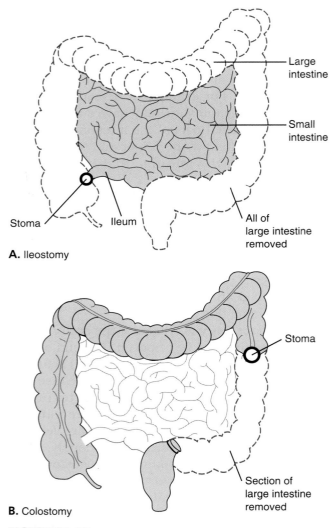

A. Ileostomy

B. Colostomy

FIGURE 31-10

Some of the people you will care for may have had surgery to remove all or part of the large intestine. Such a surgery may be necessary because of cancer, a bowel obstruction, or trauma. (*A*) Ileostomy. The entire large intestine is removed. A stoma is made in the abdominal wall, and the end of the small intestine (the ileum) is sewn into place. (*B*) Colostomy. Part of the large intestine is removed. A colostomy can be done at any point along the large intestine; here, a section of the descending colon was removed. A stoma is made in the abdominal wall, and the healthy end of the remaining large intestine is sewn into place.

For many people, having an ostomy is very difficult, emotionally. First, the person must cope with having an illness or injury serious enough to require major surgery. Second, as you learned in Chapter 20, many people consider elimination, especially bowel elimination, a very private activity. Having to wear a bag to collect feces on the outside of the body is very embarrassing for many people.

FIGURE 31-11

An ostomy appliance is worn over the stoma to collect the feces. (© *Dr. P. Marazzi/Science Photo Library/Custom Medical Stock Photo.*)

Especially in the beginning, it may be very hard for a person to accept the ostomy. If you are caring for someone who is getting used to the idea of having an ostomy, take the time to listen carefully if the person wants to talk about his fears or uncertainties. Be careful not to brush off the person's concerns with a comment such as "Oh, everything will be OK now; don't worry." Instead, put yourself in the person's shoes and think about how you would feel if you were in the same situation. Report the person's comments and questions to the nurse. Once the nurse knows that the person is having trouble adjusting to the ostomy, there are many things he or she can do to help the person adjust.

In some states and facilities, helping patients or residents to care for an ostomy is within the scope of the nursing assistant. Ostomies, like the people who have them, are very individual. Ostomies can be located in many different places on the abdomen. In addition, abdomens vary from person to person. For these reasons, the supplies used for ostomies vary greatly. Some ostomy appliances consist of a bag with an adhesive opening that adheres to the skin around the stoma. Other ostomy appliances have two pieces—a ring of flexible rubber that is applied to the skin around the stoma, and a bag that is snapped on to the ring. Some appliances are used only once and then discarded, while others are emptied, cleaned, and used again. If you are permitted to provide ostomy care, make sure that you are familiar with the different types of ostomy appliances used in your facility and ask the nurse for help with any that are new to you.

No matter what type of ostomy appliance is used, certain principles of ostomy care remain the same for every patient or resident with an ostomy. Because the skin around the ostomy comes into contact with feces, it must be kept clean to prevent irritation. The ostomy appliance can be changed with the person sitting or standing in the bathroom, or while the person is in bed. If the ostomy appliance is being changed while the person is in bed, the person should either sit upright or lie flat. The procedure for providing routine stoma care is given in Procedure 31-1.

SUMMARY

▶ The digestive system consists of the digestive tract and several accessory organs.
  ■ The digestive tract consists of the mouth, pharynx, esophagus, stomach, small intestine, and large intestine.
    • The walls of the digestive tract are lined with a mucous membrane (called the mucosa).
    • The walls of the digestive tract contain smooth muscle, which contracts to help move food through the tube (peristalsis).
  ■ Accessory organs include the teeth, tongue, salivary glands, liver, gallbladder, and pancreas.
▶ The digestive system breaks down the food we eat into nutrients that can be used by the cells of the body. The digestive system also removes waste from the body in the form of feces.
  ■ Most digestion takes place in the mouth and stomach. There are two types of digestion: mechanical and chemical.
    • Mechanical digestion is the physical breaking down of food. Chewing is an example of mechanical digestion.
    • Chemical digestion is the breaking down of food through chemical means, such as digestive enzymes.
  ■ Most absorption takes place in the small and large intestines.
    • Most absorption of nutrients takes place in the jejunum and ileum, the last two segments of the small intestine.
    • Water is reabsorbed into the bloodstream as the chyme passes through the large intestine.
  ■ Feces are what are left after all of the nutrients and most of the water are removed from the chyme, during its passage through the small and large intestines. Feces collect in the rectum, the last segment of the large intestine, until the urge to defecate occurs.
▶ As a person gets older, he may have more trouble chewing and swallowing food. Digestion is less efficient. In addition, the older person may be at higher risk for becoming constipated.
▶ Common disorders of the digestive system include ulcers, hernias, gallbladder disorders, and cancer. Always report a new gastrointestinal complaint, or a change in a person's usual symptoms, to the nurse immediately.
▶ A person who is about to have a diagnostic procedure to evaluate her digestive system may have special care needs prior to the test. The nurse will let you know of any special instructions, which should be followed carefully.
▶ An ostomy is an alternate way of removing feces from the body.
  ■ For many people, having an ostomy is difficult, emotionally.
  ■ Proper care of the ostomy site is necessary to keep the skin clean and healthy.

Chapter 31 Procedures

Getting Ready Steps

a. **W**ash your hands and observe standard precautions as necessary.

b. **G**ather needed supplies.

c. **K**nock and introduce yourself.

d. **I**dentify the person, and greet him or her by name.

e. **E**xplain the procedure.

f. **P**rovide privacy.

g. **S**ee to safety.

Finishing Up Steps

a. **C**onfirm comfort and good body alignment.

b. **L**eave the call light control within easy reach.

c. **S**ee to safety.

d. **O**pen the curtain and door.

e. **W**ash your hands.

f. **R**eport and record.

PROCEDURE 31-1

Providing Routine Stoma Care

Getting Ready

1. Complete the "Getting Ready" steps **a** through **g**.

- gloves
- paper towels
- bed protector
- toilet paper
- 4 × 4 gauze pad
- clean ostomy appliance
- clean ostomy belt (if one is used)
- skin barrier (if not part of the ostomy appliance)
- bedpan

- bedpan cover (or paper towels)
- wash basin
- soap (or other cleansing agent, per facility policy)
- adhesive remover (optional)
- deodorant for ostomy appliance (optional)
- washcloths
- towel

Procedure

2. Cover the over-bed table with paper towels. Place the ostomy supplies and clean linens on the over-bed table.

3. Make sure that the bed is positioned at a comfortable working height (to promote good body mechanics) and that the wheels are locked.

4. If the side rails are in use, lower the side rail on the working side of the bed. The side rail on the opposite side of the bed should remain up. If necessary, lower the head of the bed so that the bed is flat (as tolerated).

5. Fanfold the top linens to below the person's waist.

6. Position the bed protector on the bed, alongside the person, to keep the bed linens dry. Adjust the person's clothing as necessary to expose the person's stoma.

7. Put on the gloves.

8. Disconnect the ostomy appliance from the ostomy belt, if one is used. Remove the belt. If the ostomy belt is soiled, dispose of it in a facility-approved waste container (if it is disposable) or place it in the linen hamper or linen bag (if it is not disposable).

9. Remove the ostomy appliance by holding the skin taut and gently pulling the appliance away, starting at the top. If the adhesive is making removal difficult, use warm water or the adhesive solvent to soften the adhesive. Place the ostomy appliance in the bedpan.

(continued)

PROCEDURE 31-1 (Continued)

Providing Routine Stoma Care

STEP 9 Hold the skin taut and gently pull the ostomy appliance away.

10. Gently wipe the stoma with toilet paper to remove any feces or drainage. Place the toilet paper in the bedpan. Cover the stoma with the gauze pad to absorb any drainage that may occur until the new appliance is in place.

STEP 10 Gently wipe the stoma with toilet tissue to remove drainage.

11. Cover the bedpan with the bedpan cover or paper towels. Take the bedpan to the bathroom. (If the side rails are in use, raise them before leaving the bedside.)

12. Note the color, amount, and quality of the feces before emptying the contents of the ostomy appliance and the bedpan into the toilet. (If anything unusual is observed, do not empty the ostomy appliance until a nurse has had a chance to look at its contents.)

13. Dispose of the ostomy appliance in a facility-approved waste container.

14. Remove your gloves and dispose of them in a facility-approved waste container. Wash your hands.

15. Fill the wash basin with warm water (110°F [43.3°C] to 115°F [46.1°C] on the bath thermometer). Return to the bedside. Place the basin on the over-bed table. If the side rails are in use, lower the side rail on the working side of the bed.

16. Put on gloves.

17. Form a mitt around your hand with one of the washcloths. Wet the mitt with warm, clean water and apply soap (or other cleansing agent, per facility policy). Remove the gauze pad from the stoma and dispose of it in a facility-approved waste container. Clean the skin around the stoma. Rinse and dry the skin around the stoma thoroughly.

18. Apply the skin barrier, if needed, according to the manufacturer's directions.

19. Place the deodorant in the ostomy appliance, if deodorant is used.

20. Put the clean ostomy belt on the person, if an ostomy belt is used.

21. Make sure that the opening on the ostomy appliance is the correct size. Remove the adhesive backing on the ostomy appliance.

STEP 21 Make sure the opening on the ostomy appliance is the correct size.

22. Center the appliance over the stoma, making sure that the drain or the end of the bag is pointed down. Gently press around the edges to seal the ostomy appliance to the skin.

(continued)

OCEDURE 31-1 (Continued)

Providing Routine Stoma Care

STEP 22 Gently press the edges to seal the ostomy appliance to the skin.

23. Connect the ostomy appliance to the ostomy belt, if one is used.

24. Remove the bed protector.

25. Remove your gloves and dispose of them in a facility-approved waste container.

26. Adjust the person's clothing as necessary to cover the ostomy appliance. If the bedding is wet or soiled, change the bed linens. Help the person back into a comfortable position, straighten the bottom linens, and draw the top linens over the person. Raise the head of the bed, as the person requests.

27. If the side rails are in use, return the side rail to the raised position. Make sure that the bed is lowered to its lowest position and that the wheels are locked.

28. Gather the soiled linens and place them in the linen hamper or linen bag. Dispose of disposable items in a facility-approved waste container. Clean equipment and return it to the storage area.

Finishing Up CLSOWR

29. Complete the "Finishing Up" steps **a** through **f**.

What did you learn?

Multiple Choice

*Select the single best answer for each of the
following questions.*

1. Where does the process of digestion begin?
   a. In the stomach
   b. In the large intestine
   c. In the mouth
   d. In the esophagus

2. What is a hollow, muscular pouch for holding
food?
   a. The appendix
   b. The gallbladder
   c. The duodenum
   d. The stomach

3. What is another term for the large intestine?
   a. Stomach
   b. Duodenum
   c. Colon
   d. Appendix

4. Where does most absorption of nutrients take
place?
   a. In the jejunum and ileum of the small intestine
   b. In the rectum of the large intestine
   c. In the stomach
   d. In the liver

5. Where is most of the water absorbed from the
chyme, resulting in the formation of formed,
semi-moist feces?
   a. In the large intestine
   b. In the small intestine
   c. In the stomach
   d. In the gallbladder

6. Normal changes in the digestive system
related to aging include:
   a. Less efficient chewing and swallowing
   b. Less efficient digestion
   c. Increased risk for constipation
   d. All of the above

7. Mr. Pak has an ileostomy, and you assist him
with stoma care. What would you expect his
feces to be like?
   a. Very liquid, continuously flowing
   b. Hard, dry, pellets
   c. Soft, brown, moist, and formed
   d. None of the above

8. What is the artificial opening for a colostomy
called?
   a. A stoma
   b. A rectum
   c. An anus
   d. None of the above

9. You have been caring for Mrs. Zimmerman for
several months. Mrs. Zimmerman has always
had a "sensitive stomach," which she complains about loudly and often. She often tells
you that she is "queasy" or that something
she ate "didn't agree with her." Although she
always complains about the food at the facility, she usually cleans her plate. Today, however, you noticed that not only did Mrs. Zimmerman not eat her lunch, she has seemed
particularly listless all afternoon. What
should you do?
   a. Nothing; Mrs. Zimmerman always has
   "stomach issues"
   b. Record Mrs. Zimmerman's lack of appetite
   in her chart; the nurse will follow up later
   c. Report this change in Mrs. Zimmerman's
   behavior to the nurse immediately
   d. Wait and see if Mrs. Zimmerman has any
   appetite for dinner

? Stop and think!

▶ Mr. Scott is a 42-year-old executive
at an advertising agency who was recently diagnosed with colon cancer. Mr. Scott is married,
with three young children. He is an avid golfer
and swimmer. Following surgery to remove the
cancer, Mr. Scott will have a colostomy. You are
the nursing assistant who will be caring for Mr.
Scott in the hospital in the days following the
surgery. Describe some of the emotions Mr. Scott
may be feeling after the surgery, and how you
would respond if Mr. Scott decided to share
some of these feelings with you.

32

The Urinary System

What will you learn?

As you learned in Chapter 20, the urinary system rids the body of waste products that have been filtered from the bloodstream, along with excess fluid, in the form of urine. In Chapter 20, you also learned how to assist patients and residents with urinary elimination. In this chapter, you will learn a little bit more about the organs that make up the urinary system and how they work. As a nursing assistant, many of your daily responsibilities will allow you to observe changes in the functioning of a patient's or resident's urinary system that could indicate a serious problem. This is why it is important for you to know about the effects of aging on the urinary system, and about some of the disorders that can affect this very important organ system. When you are finished with this chapter, you will be able to:

1. List the organs that make up the urinary system.
2. Describe the primary function of each organ of the urinary system.
3. Discuss the effects of aging on the urinary system.
4. Describe various disorders that can affect the urinary system.
5. List common diagnostic procedures that may be used to detect and diagnose urinary system disorders.

Photo: Drinking plenty of fluids helps to keep the urinary system healthy.
(© Mitch Diamond/Index Stock Imagery.)

Vocabulary

Use the CD in the back of your book to hear these terms pronounced, defined, and used in a sentence:

Renal
Nephrons
Glomerulus
Filtrate
Urine
Urethritis
Cystitis

Pyelonephritis
Kidney stones
   (renal calculi)
Dialysis
Ureterostomy
Urostomy

STRUCTURE OF THE URINARY SYSTEM

The urinary system consists of the kidneys, the ureters, the urinary bladder, and the urethra (Fig. 32-1).

THE KIDNEYS

We have two kidneys, which are like kidney beans in shape and color (only much larger!). The kidneys are located toward the back of the upper abdominal cavity, one on either side of the spinal column. The bottom of the rib cage and a layer of fat help to protect the kidneys.

Because the job of the kidneys is to filter the blood to remove waste products, the kidneys are supplied by two large arteries, called the left and right renal arteries. (**Renal** is a word meaning "related to, involving, or located in the region of the kidneys.") The renal arteries are branches of the aorta, the largest artery in the body. The blood flow through the renal arteries is so efficient that the kidneys are able to filter all of the body's blood every half-hour.

Inside each kidney are approximately 1 million tiny **nephrons,** the basic functional units of the kidney (Fig. 32-2). The nephrons are responsible for actually filtering the blood that passes through the kidney. Each nephron consists of a glomerulus and a series of tubules (see Fig. 32-2). The **glomerulus** is a capillary bed, enclosed within a structure called *Bowman's capsule.* The blood entering the kidneys through the renal arteries is

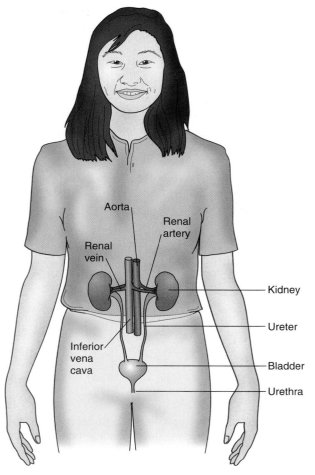

FIGURE 32-1

The urinary system consists of the kidneys, ureters, bladder, and urethra. Each kidney is supplied by a renal artery, which branches off of the aorta. After the kidneys filter the blood, the filtrate (urine) passes into the ureters and the blood passes into the renal veins, which empty into the inferior vena cava.

under great pressure. Once inside the kidneys, the blood passes through a series of arteries that get smaller and smaller, until it reaches the capillary bed of the glomerulus. The blood enters the glomerulus through a vessel called the afferent arteriole (*afferent* means "enter") (see Fig. 32-2). At this point, the blood is under a lot of pressure because the capillaries are very small. The walls of the capillaries in the glomerulus are semi-permeable, which means that they have tiny openings in them. Because the blood is under a lot of pressure, a lot of the liquid in the blood squeezes through the walls, taking the wastes and nutrients that are dissolved in it with it. This liquid, known as the **filtrate,** forms the

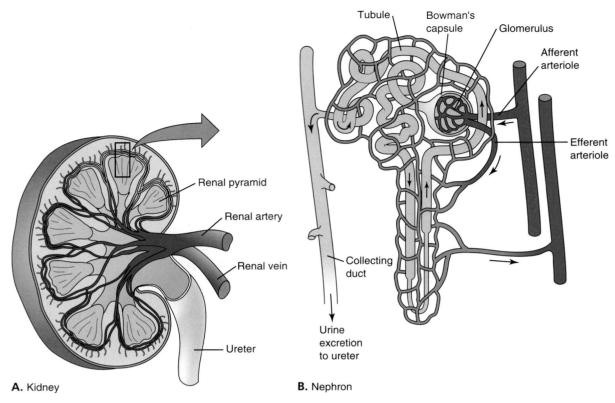

A. Kidney   **B.** Nephron

FIGURE 32-2

The kidney. (*A*) If you were to cut open the kidney and look at the tissue through a microscope, you would see nephrons, the functional units where filtration actually takes place. Each kidney contains about 1 million nephrons, arranged in a radiating pattern. (*B*) Each nephron consists of a glomerulus and a series of tubules. Blood (*red*) is filtered in the glomerulus, producing filtrate, the basis of urine (*yellow*). Filtered blood (*purple*) leaves the glomerulus through the efferent arteriole and is returned to the circulation through the renal veins.

basis of the urine. Next, two things happen (see Fig. 32-2B):

- The filtered blood leaves the glomerulus through the efferent arteriole (*efferent* means "exit"). It is returned to circulation through the renal veins, which empty into the inferior vena cava (the largest vein in the body).
- Meanwhile, the filtrate enters Bowman's capsule, and from there, flows into the tubules that make up the rest of the nephron. Small capillaries surround the tubules of the nephron. As the filtrate passes slowly through the tubules, these small capillaries reabsorb useful substances such as water, nutrients, and minerals from the filtrate. By the time the filtrate reaches the end of the tubules, only excess fluid and waste substances remain.

This is **urine.** The kidneys produce 160 to 180 liters of filtrate each day, but only about 1 to 1.5 liters are excreted from the body in the form of urine. (One liter is equal to about one quart.)

Urine from each nephron is emptied into a collecting area, called the *renal pelvis.* From the renal pelvis, the urine flows into the ureters.

THE URETERS

Two ureters, slender, muscular tubes approximately 10 to 13 inches (25 to 32 cm) long, carry urine from the kidneys to the bladder (see Fig. 32-1). The ureters are wider at the top where they connect to the renal pelvis, but they quickly become very narrow. Where the two ureters enter the bladder, a small triangular fold of tissue called the *trigone* keeps urine from flowing back into the ureters after it has emptied into the bladder.

The ureters are lined with a mucous membrane, which helps to protect against infection. Smooth muscle in the walls of the ureters contracts rhythmically, moving urine away from the kidney and toward the urinary bladder. The peristaltic movements that help move urine through the ureters are similar to the peristaltic movements that help move food through the digestive tract.

THE BLADDER

The bladder is a hollow sac that is a holding place (reservoir) for urine. Urine is constantly produced by the kidneys and transported through the ureters to the bladder, where it is stored until urination occurs. The bladder is very small when empty but can become quite large as it fills with urine. Like the ureters, the inside of the bladder is lined with a mucous membrane. The walls of the bladder contain three layers of smooth muscle. When the walls of the bladder contract, urination occurs. Where the bladder and the urethra join (the *bladder outlet*), the internal sphincter (a ring of involuntary muscle) keeps the bladder closed while it fills.

THE URETHRA

The urethra is a tube that carries urine from the bladder to the outside of the body. The urethra begins at the bladder outlet, just below the internal sphincter, and ends at the external urinary opening (called the *urinary meatus* or *urethral orifice*). Below the internal sphincter, the external urethral sphincter, a ring of voluntary muscle, relaxes to allow urine to pass during urination.

Male and female urethras are very different in size and function (Fig. 32-3). In women, the urethra measures about 1½ to 2½ inches and is used only as a passageway for urine to leave the body. In men, the urethra measures about 6 to 8 inches and serves as a passageway for both urine and semen. In men, the urethra passes through the prostate gland soon after leaving the bladder outlet. The prostate gland produces seminal fluid, the fluid that, along with sperm cells, makes up semen.

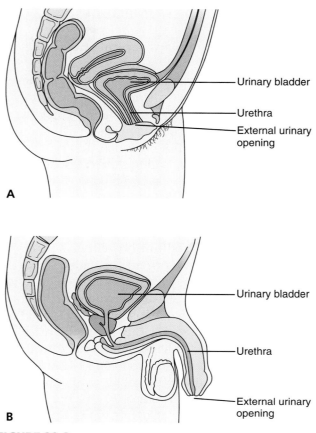

FIGURE 32-3

While a woman's urethra (*A*) is straight and only about 2 inches long, a man's urethra (*B*) is curved in an "S" shape and is about 6 inches long. Because of the differences in anatomy, women are more prone to urinary tract infections than men, but men are harder to catheterize than women.

FUNCTION OF THE URINARY SYSTEM

REMOVAL OF LIQUID WASTES

The main function of the urinary system is to filter the blood and remove waste products and excess fluid from the body. A moderately full bladder usually contains about 1 pint (470 mL) of urine. When about 200 to 300 mL of urine collect in the bladder, the internal sphincter opens and allows urine to flood the upper segment of the urethra. At this point, the urge to urinate occurs. The person voluntarily relaxes the external urethral sphincter and the muscles of the bladder contract, allowing urine to pass out of the body through the urethra. Although it is possible to delay urination for some time, the bladder continues to fill with urine and eventually, the bladder will empty itself automatically.

MAINTENANCE OF HOMEOSTASIS

The urinary system plays several important roles in maintaining the body's homeostasis:

- The urinary system helps to keep fluid levels within the body constant. As the filtrate passes through the tubules in the nephrons, water is reabsorbed as necessary to maintain the body's fluid balance. Too much fluid in the blood can lead to fluid overload, causing swelling in parts of the body. Too little fluid can lead to dehydration.
- The urinary system regulates the levels of essential minerals—such as potassium, calcium, and sodium—by either saving them or releasing them through urine.
- The urinary system regulates the acidity of the blood. The pH scale, which you might remember from chemistry class, is used to rate the degree of acidity of a substance. Human blood is slightly above a 7 on the scale, which ranges from 1 to 14. Anything above 7 is said to be basic, or alkaline. Anything below 7 is acidic. Our blood cannot be either too acidic or too basic. When there is even a slight change in the blood's pH, damage to the cells can occur. Acid is a normal by-product of cellular metabolism. So, to maintain the blood at a constant pH level, the kidneys excrete the excess acids produced by cellular metabolism.

THE EFFECTS OF AGING ON THE URINARY SYSTEM

The normal processes of aging affect the urinary system:

- **Less efficient filtration.** After a person reaches 40 years of age or so, the number of functioning nephrons in the kidneys starts to decrease, decreasing the kidneys' ability to filter waste products from the bloodstream.
- **Decreased muscle tone.** Loss of muscle tone as a result of aging can reduce bladder capacity and may contribute to stress incontinence. This type of urinary incontinence, which is most common in older women who have had children or are obese, can often be corrected with exercises or surgery.

- **Enlargement of the prostate gland (in men).** In older men, enlargement of the prostate gland is common. The enlargement may be benign (a normal effect of aging) or it may be due to cancer of the gland. As the prostate gland enlarges, it pushes against the urethra, causing it to narrow. Total emptying of the bladder of urine becomes difficult, and the man may experience episodes of overflow incontinence. As you recall from Chapter 20, overflow incontinence can occur when urine is retained in the bladder. Because the bladder does not empty completely when the man voids, it refills with urine quickly, and the urine simply overflows. As a result, the man may "dribble" urine in between visits to the bathroom. An enlarged prostate is treated with medications, surgery, or both.
- **Increased risk for urinary tract infections.** Older people are also more likely to get urinary tract infections. Incomplete emptying of the bladder can contribute to the development of infections, as can a decrease in immune system functioning.

Although it is important for everyone to drink plenty of water and other fluids, it is especially important for older people. Drinking plenty of fluids helps the kidneys to work properly, and regular urination flushes harmful bacteria from the bladder, helping to prevent urinary tract infections (Fig. 32-4).

DISORDERS OF THE URINARY SYSTEM

Illness or injury to any part of the urinary system affects the whole system, and, eventually, the whole body. Common disorders of the urinary system include infections, kidney stones, renal failure, and tumors.

INFECTIONS

Infections can affect any part of the urinary system:

- **Infection of the urethra (urethritis).** Urethritis is especially common in men, because the urethra is longer and curved.

FIGURE 32-4
Encourage your patients or residents to drink plenty of fluids, unless a person has a medical condition that requires fluid restriction.

FIGURE 32-5
Urine that is cloudy, is an abnormal color, or has an abnormal odor may be a sign of a urinary tract infection. Always look at the urine before discarding it. If you notice anything unusual, get the nurse before discarding the urine.

Microbes responsible for sexually transmitted diseases (STDs) such as gonorrhea, herpes, and chlamydia are common causes of urethritis in men. STDs are discussed in more detail in Chapter 33.

- **Infection of the bladder (cystitis).** Bladder infections are more common among women than men for two reasons. First, the urethral opening in women is located close to the anus. Because feces, which contain bacteria from the digestive tract, exit the body at the anus, this area is often contaminated with microbes that could cause a bladder infection. (This is why it is important to wipe from the front to the back when providing perineal care for a woman.) Second, a woman's urethra is short and straight, which means that once microbes gain access to the urinary tract, they do not have far to travel to infect the bladder.
- **Kidney infections (pyelonephritis).** If a bladder infection is not treated promptly with appropriate drugs, the pathogens can travel up the ureters and infect the kidneys. A kidney infection can cause severe illness. If untreated, the infection might result in permanent damage to the nephrons.

In younger people, symptoms of urinary tract infections include urinary frequency, burning, and cramping. However, many older people do not have these symptoms. The nursing assistant may be the first to notice a change in the appearance or odor of the urine or a change in a person's voiding habits that would indicate that a urinary tract infection may be present (Fig. 32-5).

KIDNEY STONES (RENAL CALCULI)

As you have learned, the main function of the kidney is to filter and remove waste products from the bloodstream. Many of these waste products are in the form of mineral salts, such as calcium salts and uric acid. If waste products become very concentrated, they can start to group together, forming tiny crystals that continue to grow in size as more of the mineral is deposited around them. These clumps of minerals are called **kidney stones,** or renal calculi (Fig. 32-6). Kidney stones are most common in middle-aged adults. Factors that may increase an older person's risk of developing kidney stones include immobility, not drinking enough fluids (which causes urine to be more concentrated with the waste salts), and infections of the urinary system.

Stones most often form in the collecting area (renal pelvis) of the kidney, but they can also form in the bladder. Kidney stones usually cause severe pain as they move downward through the ureter, and then through the urethra. The rough

FIGURE 32-6

This is a kidney, cut open to reveal the kidney stones inside. Kidney stones can grow to be quite large, with sharp edges. They may cause obstruction of the ureters or urethra. Once the stone is passed, it is usually sent to the laboratory for analysis to determine which waste salt is causing the stones to form. (© *Dr. E. Walker/Photo Researchers, Inc.*)

edges of the stone can damage the mucosal lining of the ureter or urethra, causing it to bleed, resulting in hematuria (blood in the urine).

A person with a kidney stone usually needs to drink plenty of fluids to help flush the stone through the urinary tract. Medication may be necessary to help control the pain. You may be asked to collect all of the person's urine after each voiding and strain it to retrieve the stone. To strain the urine, place a piece of filter paper or a 4 × 4 gauze pad in a graduate, and then pour the urine into the graduate (Fig. 32-7). The urine will pass through the filter paper or gauze pad, leaving any stones behind. It is important to retrieve the kidney stones because then they can be sent to the laboratory for chemical analysis. Once the doctor knows which waste salt is causing the stones to form, he may be able to prevent future stones from developing.

If a stone becomes lodged in the narrow ureter, it can block the flow of urine to the bladder. The urine builds up, placing pressure on the delicate nephrons of the kidney. In this case, the person will need to have the stone removed surgically. Often, the stones are removed using a procedure called *lithotripsy*. In lithotripsy, high-frequency sound waves are directed at the stone, causing it to break into smaller pieces that can then be passed through the urinary tract. Sometimes, a surgical incision needs to be made for stone removal.

FIGURE 32-7

You may be asked to strain a person's urine to retrieve kidney stones. To strain urine, put a piece of filter paper or a 4" × 4" gauze pad in a graduate, and then pour the urine into the graduate. The urine will pass through the paper or gauze pad, leaving any stones behind. The stones are then transferred to a specimen container and sent to the laboratory for analysis.

KIDNEY (RENAL) FAILURE

Kidney (renal) failure is the inability of the kidneys to filter blood effectively. As a result of kidney failure, waste products and fluid build up in the body, straining the heart and other organs. The person becomes very ill and can easily die if treatment is delayed.

Causes of Kidney Failure

Kidney failure can be either acute or chronic:
- Acute renal failure can result from a medical or surgical emergency that causes a decrease in the amount of blood flow through the kidneys. It can also be caused by poisoning, a severe infection, or a severe allergic reaction.
- Chronic renal failure results from a gradual loss of functioning nephrons. Because the kidneys lose their ability to function gradually, the person usually does not show signs of kidney failure until approximately

80%–90% of kidney function is lost. The most common causes of chronic renal failure are hypertension and diabetes, chronic conditions that damage the blood vessels in the glomerulus. Other causes are related to chronic infections, blockage of the urinary system by stones or growths, and cancer.

Signs of Renal Failure

Signs of renal failure may include:

- Dehydration from excessive loss of fluid (usually early in acute renal failure because the kidneys cannot reabsorb filtrate back into the bloodstream)
- Swelling from the build-up of fluid in the tissues of the body (later in chronic renal failure when the kidneys are unable to eliminate excess fluid)
- Hypertension from fluid overload in the circulation
- Oliguria (scant amounts of urine, less than 400 mL in 24 hours), followed by anuria (the absence of urine)

Care of the Person with Kidney Failure

People with kidney failure often need to have dialysis. **Dialysis** does the job of the kidneys by removing waste products and fluids from the body. A person with acute renal failure may need dialysis treatment only for a short period of time, until kidney function returns. A person with chronic renal failure must remain on dialysis for the rest of her life, or until a donor kidney becomes available for transplant. There are two types of dialysis:

- In *hemodialysis,* the person's blood is drawn intravenously, passed through a machine with filters and solutions that clean the blood of waste, and then returned to the person's body through another vessel (Fig. 32-8A).
- In *peritoneal dialysis,* solutions that absorb waste products are instilled (placed) into a person's abdominal cavity through a tube that has been surgically inserted for this purpose (see Fig. 32-8B). The solution remains in the abdominal cavity for a specified period of time so that waste products can be absorbed into the solution through the membrane lining the abdominal cavity.

The used solution is then drained into a collecting bag and is discarded according to facility policy.

Dialysis takes several hours and must be performed several times a week to keep the blood cleaned of waste products. Dialysis is performed by specially trained nurses. Most patients and residents who need dialysis travel to a health care center specifically designed to perform this service. Sometimes a patient or resident is too ill to be taken to a dialysis center, so nurses and technicians may bring portable equipment to the facility where you work. You may be asked to monitor vital signs quite frequently after your patient or resident has had a dialysis treatment.

When caring for a person with renal failure, you must carefully measure the amounts of urine produced and document the amounts accurately. As you recall from Chapter 20, the amount of urine produced is an indication of how well the kidneys are functioning. In addition to monitoring urine output, you may be frequently asked to obtain urine samples so that the urine can be tested for the presence of excessive waste products. Fluid restrictions and special diets that are very low in salt and protein may be ordered and should be followed strictly. Vital signs may need to be monitored frequently and any changes reported to the nurse immediately. People in renal failure may be on bed rest and need care measures to help prevent the complications of immobility. Frequent skin care is necessary to help prevent the skin irritation and itching that accompanies renal failure.

TUMORS

Tumors, which may or may not be malignant (cancerous), can affect all of the organs of the urinary system. Tumors can obstruct the flow of urine through the urinary system, resulting in kidney damage. Kidney damage may also result from tumors of the kidney that invade the healthy tissue, damaging the nephrons. Surgical removal of the affected kidney is usually necessary, but as long as the remaining kidney is functioning properly, it should be able to handle removal of waste and fluid.

Tumors of the bladder are common among people who have smoked cigarettes. The risk of bladder cancer increases with age, with older men twice as likely to develop bladder cancer as

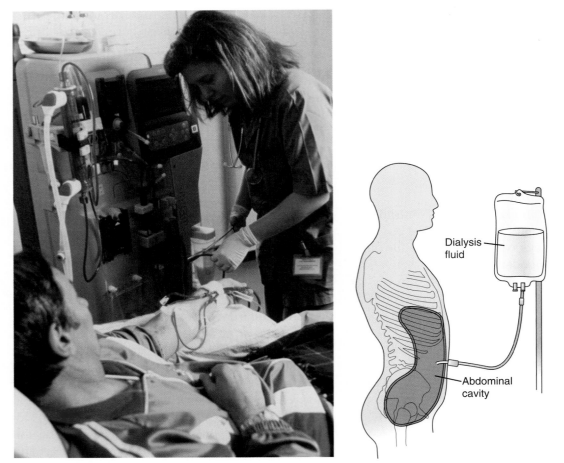

A. Hemodialysis

B. Peritoneal dialysis

FIGURE 32-8

Dialysis machines perform the job of the kidneys for people who have kidney failure. (*A*) Hemodialysis. The dialysis machine (*upper left*) receives blood drawn from an artery in the person's arm. The blood is filtered and then returned to the body. (*B*) Peritoneal dialysis. A special solution is placed in the person's abdominal cavity to absorb wastes, and then the solution is drained. (*A* © *Mauro Fermariello/Photo Researchers, Inc.*)

older women. Bladder tumors are usually malignant and may spread to other organs. Tumors may be treated with medication, radiation, or surgery, depending on the type of tumor and whether or not it has spread to other parts of the body. In some cases, it is necessary to remove the bladder, disrupting normal flow of urine out of the body. Because the urine needs a new pathway to leave the body, a *urinary diversion* is created. A surgeon can divert (redirect) the urine's flow out of the body in several ways:

- In a **ureterostomy,** the ureters are brought through the abdominal wall by way of small incisions, and sutured in place (Fig. 32-9A). The ureters then drain freely into an ostomy appliance designed to collect urine.

- In a **urostomy,** the ureters are attached to a small portion of the small intestine (usually the ileum) (see Fig. 32-9B). When the ileum is used, the person is said to have an *ileal conduit.* One end of the segment of intestine is sealed off, and the other end is brought through the abdominal wall and sutured into place to create a stoma. The urine then drains freely into an ostomy appliance designed to collect urine (see Fig. 32-9C).

Bladder cancer is a common reason for a person to have a ureterostomy or urostomy. However, injuries (for example, to the bladder or spinal cord) and birth defects (such as spina bifida) can also result in a person having a urinary diversion procedure done. Regardless of the reason for the procedure, good skin care around

A. Ureterostomy   **B.** Urostomy (ileal conduit)

FIGURE 32-9

Urinary diversion procedures are necessary when part of the urinary system must be removed. (*A*) In a ureterostomy, the ureters are brought through the abdominal wall and sutured into place. (*B*) In a urostomy, the ureters are joined to a small segment of the small intestine, and then the intestine is brought to the surface of the body and sutured into place. (*C*) An ostomy pouch is worn to collect the urine, in both cases. The man shown here had a urostomy following removal of his bladder to treat cancer. (*C © Dr. P. Marazzi/Photo Researchers, Inc.*) **C**

the ostomy site is essential. If urine is allowed to leak around the appliance, skin irritation and breakdown are very likely. The urostomy bags need to be emptied regularly and the urine may need to be measured and recorded. As always, the urine needs to be observed for any changes that might indicate infection or other urinary disorders.

 Tell the Nurse!

Observations that may be a sign of a urinary system disorder and should be reported to the nurse immediately include:

⟫ Complaints of sharp, sudden pain of the abdomen, side, or back

⟫ The presence of blood in the urine

⟫ A significant increase or decrease in the amount of urine voided in a period of time

⟫ Changes in a person's voiding habits, especially increased or decreased frequency, or a new onset of incontinence

⟫ Pain or burning when urinating

⟫ Urine that appears cloudy or has a strong ammonia smell

DIAGNOSIS OF URINARY DISORDERS

Observations that indicate problems affecting the urinary system are often nonspecific. For example, kidney stones or urinary tract infections can cause abdominal pain, a common symptom of many digestive disorders as well. Usually, additional testing is needed to find out what the real problem is. Many types of tests are used to diagnose disorders of the urinary system:

- **Urinalysis.** In urinalysis, the urine is examined under a microscope and by chemical means.
- **Imaging studies.** Computed tomography (CT) scans, magnetic resonance imaging (MRI) scans, and radiographs (x-rays) can allow a doctor to see tumors and other abnormalities of the urinary system. With x-rays, a special dye may be injected into the veins before the x-ray is taken to highlight the kidneys, ureters, and bladder (Fig. 32-10).
- **Ultrasound.** Ultrasound may be used to detect tumors of the urinary system.
- **Cytoscopy and ureteroscopy.** A small, lighted scope is inserted through the urethra and used to view the inside of the bladder (cytoscopy) or ureters (ureteroscopy).

You may be asked to collect and measure urine for testing or to help prepare a patient or resident for other diagnostic tests or procedures. Make sure that you are informed about any specific procedures that you will be responsible for, such as keeping the person on NPO status, restricting or encouraging fluids, or straining urine.

FIGURE 32-10

In intravenous pyelography (IVP), a type of radiographic (x-ray) procedure, a special dye is injected intravenously to allow visualization of the kidneys, ureter, and bladder. (© *Scott Camazine/Photo Researchers, Inc.*)

SUMMARY

▶ The organs of the urinary system are the kidneys, the ureters, the urinary bladder, and the urethra.
- The two kidneys filter the blood to remove waste products and excess fluid.
- The ureters carry urine from the kidneys to the bladder.
- The bladder is a holding place for urine.
- The urethra carries urine from the bladder to the outside of the body.

▶ The main function of the urinary system is to remove waste products and excess fluid from the body. The urinary system also plays a key role in homeostasis by maintaining fluid balance and regulating the pH of the blood.

▶ Aging affects the urinary system just as it affects the other organ systems.
- In an older person, loss of muscle tone affects the bladder's ability to hold urine and empty properly.
- Older men may experience difficulty voiding as a result of an enlarged prostate gland.
- An older person is more likely to develop urinary tract infections, because of decreased immune function and incomplete emptying of the bladder.
- As we age, the number of nephrons decreases, reducing the kidney's efficiency at filtering blood.

▶ Disorders of the urinary system include infections, kidney stones (renal calculi), renal failure, and tumors.
- As a nursing assistant, you may be the first to notice signs and symptoms of a urinary problem that a patient or resident is having.
- You may also be involved in helping a patient or resident to prepare for a diagnostic test used to evaluate the urinary system.

What did you learn?

Multiple Choice

Select the single best answer for each of the following questions.

1. Urine leaves the body through the:
   a. Nephrons
   b. Urethra
   c. Ureters
   d. Bladder
2. How does aging affect the urinary system?
   a. The number of nephrons is decreased, reducing the kidney's ability to filter blood efficiently
   b. The ability to empty the bladder completely is decreased
   c. Bladder capacity is decreased
   d. All of the above
3. How much urine does an average adult pass each day?
   a. 200 mL of urine per day
   b. 500 mL of urine per day
   c. 1 to 1.5 liters of urine per day
   d. 160 to 180 liters of urine per day
4. Why are urinary tract infections more common in women than in men?
   a. A woman's urethra is short, and the opening of the urethra is located close to the anus
   b. A woman's urethra is long and curved
   c. Women tend to be more careless with perineal care
   d. Women do not drink as much water as men
5. Which of the following might be a sign of a urinary tract infection?
   a. Pain or burning while urinating
   b. Extreme thirst
   c. Anuria (absence of urine)
   d. Kidney failure
6. Which procedure uses high-frequency sound waves to break up kidney stones?
   a. Lithotripsy
   b. Dialysis
   c. Filtration
   d. Urostomy

7. How is the male urethra different from the female urethra?
   a. It is longer
   b. It serves as a passageway for urine and for semen
   c. The opening is further away from the anus
   d. All of the above
8. Mr. Loyd has a urostomy, which was done to treat his bladder cancer. What do you need to remember when caring for Mr. Loyd?
   a. He may develop renal failure at any time
   b. He will require good skin care around the ostomy site to prevent skin irritation and breakdown
   c. He is more at risk for kidney stones
   d. He will not require any special care
9. Sally is caring for Mrs. Brady, who has been going to the bathroom more frequently than usual. Now, Mrs. Brady is complaining of a burning sensation when she urinates. Why is it important for Sally to report what she has observed to the nurse?
   a. Mrs. Brady may be in kidney failure
   b. Mrs. Brady may have a urinary tract infection
   c. The nurse will assign another nursing assistant to help with Mrs. Brady's care
   d. It is not necessary for Sally to report these observations to the nurse

Matching

Match each numbered item with its appropriate lettered description.

_____ 1. Cystitis
_____ 2. Renal calculi
_____ 3. Pyelonephritis
_____ 4. Glomerulus
_____ 5. Urethritis

a. Infection of the kidneys
b. Capillary bed in the nephron; surrounded by Bowman's capsule
c. Infection of the urethra
d. Kidney stones
e. Infection of the bladder

? Stop and think!

▶ Janice works in a hospital and is assigned to care for Mr. Roberts, who is in the hospital because of kidney stones. This morning, while helping Mr. Roberts with his A.M. care, she noticed that the urinal hanging on his side rail was full, so she emptied the urinal into the toilet, cleaned it, and returned it to Mr. Roberts' bedside table. If you were Janice, what (if anything) would you have done differently?

▶ Laura is taking care of Mr. George, who has a history of diabetes and hypertension. He is on a low-sodium diet because of his high blood pressure, but he cannot seem to resist salty snacks, especially when the football game is on. Today, Laura is taking Mr. George's blood pressure when she notes that it is unusually high for him. She has emptied his urinal at the start of her shift and now, near the end of her shift, there is only about 50 mL of urine in the urinal. She also notices that Mr. George's hands and feet are getting puffy. If you were Laura, what questions would you ask Mr. George? What would you report to the nurse?

▶ Steve has just received his report and learns that he is going to care for Mr. Sarandis, who is in renal failure. Steve has just completed orientation and is not quite sure what Mr. Sarandis's needs may be. What would you tell Steve about the care needs of a person with renal failure?

▶ Kelly has been assigned to care for Mrs. Ralph, who has a urostomy. She is unfamiliar with this term and doesn't know what to expect. If you were on Kelly's team, what would you tell Kelly to expect? What things would you tell Kelly to look for in caring for Mrs. Ralph?

33

The Reproductive System

What will you learn?

Of all of the systems that make up the human body, perhaps none is as fascinating and miraculous as the reproductive system. **Reproduction** is the process by which a living thing makes more living things like itself. Because all living things eventually die, the ability to reproduce is essential for the survival of any species. Without the ability to reproduce, the species would slowly die off and cease to exist.

In this chapter, you will learn about the male and female reproductive systems, which are very different from each other. You will learn about their structure and function, the effects of aging on each, and common disorders that can affect each. In addition, you will learn about sexually transmitted diseases (STDs), which can affect both men and women. When you are finished with this chapter, you will be able to:

1. Describe the main function of the reproductive system.
2. List the organs that make up the female reproductive system.
3. Discuss the normal function of the female reproductive system.
4. Explain the effects of aging on the female reproductive system.
5. Describe the disorders that may affect the female reproductive system.
6. List diagnostic tests commonly used to detect disorders of the female reproductive system.
7. List the organs that make up the male reproductive system.
8. Discuss the normal function of the male reproductive system.
9. Explain the effects of aging on the male reproductive system.
10. Describe the disorders that may affect the male reproductive system.
11. List diagnostic tests commonly used to detect disorders of the male reproductive system.
12. Discuss sexually transmitted diseases (STDs) that may affect the male or female reproductive systems.

Photo: A fetus develops from a single fertilized egg.
(© Petit Format/Photo Researchers, Inc.)

Vocabulary

Reproduction
Sex cell (gamete)
Sperm cell
Egg (ovum, ova)
Conception
  (fertilization)

Ovulation
Lactation
Menstrual period
Amenorrhea
Dysmenorrhea
Menorrhagia

Infertility
Postmenopausal
  bleeding
Mastectomy
Hysterectomy
Ejaculation

Impotence (erectile
  dysfunction)
Sexually transmitted
  disease (STD)
Pelvic inflammatory
  disease (PID)

Has anyone ever told you that you have "your mother's eyes" or "the family nose"? Do you look very much like your brothers or sisters, or not much like them at all? Each of us receives our genes, the bundles of DNA that determine how we develop and what we look like physically, from our parents. Your mother gave you half of your genes and your father gave you the other half, to make a full set. This is why you may look a lot like either one of your parents, or like a blend of the two. Or why you may look very much like one of your siblings, and not much like another one. It all depends on the combination of genes that you received.

Each species has a set number of genes, or chromosomes. For example, human beings have 46 chromosomes. This means that to keep the number of chromosomes the same from generation to generation, the father contributes 23 chromosomes and the mother contributes 23 chromosomes. The special cells contributed by each parent that contain half of the normal number of chromosomes are called **sex cells,** or **gametes.** The male sex cell is called a **sperm cell.** The female sex cell is called an **egg,** or **ovum** (*ova,* plural). When the sperm joins the egg, forming a cell that contains the complete number of chromosomes, **conception (fertilization)** occurs. During the 9 months leading up to the birth of a baby, the single original cell that formed at conception copies itself over and over again, forming all of the baby's tissues and organs.

One of the main functions of the reproductive system in both males and females is to produce and transport sex cells. However, unlike other organ systems in the body, the organs that make up the reproductive system are very different in men and women. The male reproductive system is designed to produce sperm and deposit it inside the female's body. The female reproductive system is designed to produce eggs, receive sperm cells, contain and nourish a developing baby, give birth, and provide nourishment after the baby's birth by producing breast milk. Because of the physical and functional differences between the male and female reproductive systems, we will look at each system separately in the sections that follow.

THE FEMALE REPRODUCTION SYSTEM

STRUCTURE OF THE FEMALE REPRODUCTIVE SYSTEM

The organs and structures of the female reproductive system are located both inside and outside of the body. The internal organs are the ovaries, fallopian tubes, uterus, and vagina (Fig. 33-1A). The outer structures are the labia, the clitoris, and the vaginal opening (see Fig. 33-1B). These outer structures are sometimes referred to collectively as the *vulva.* In addition, the breasts (mammary glands) are considered accessory organs of the female reproductive system, because they play a role in nourishing a newborn baby.

The Ovaries

The ovaries are two small, almond-shaped organs located deep inside the abdomen on either side of the uterus (see Fig. 33-1A). The ovaries store the ova, or eggs. When a baby girl is born, her ovaries contain all of the eggs that she will ever have. The

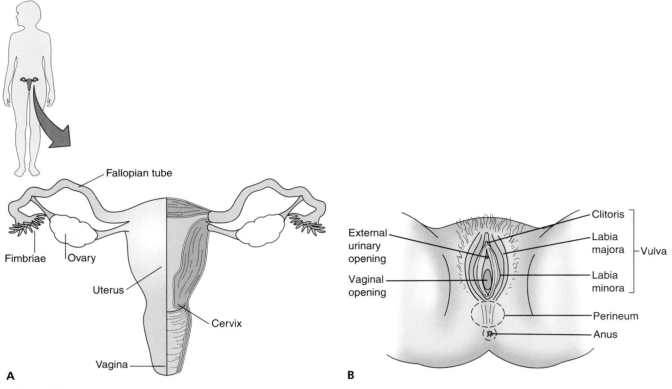

FIGURE 33-1

The female reproductive system. (*A*) Internal structures include the ovaries, fallopian tubes, uterus, and vagina. (*B*) External structures, collectively known as "the vulva," include the vaginal opening, labia, and clitoris.

stored eggs are kept in a "holding pattern" until they are needed. Once a girl passes through puberty and reaches reproductive age, she begins to ovulate. **Ovulation** is the release of a ripe, mature egg from the ovaries each month.

The Fallopian Tubes

The fallopian tubes, also called *uterine tubes* or *oviducts,* are slender tubes about 4 to 5 inches long that transport the egg from the ovary to the uterus. After leaving the ovary, the egg moves through the fluid in the abdomen to the entrance of the nearest fallopian tube. The open ends of the fallopian tubes nearest the ovaries have small, fringe-like projections called *fimbriae* (see Fig. 33-1A). The fimbriae beat in a wave-like motion, helping to move the egg into the tube. Once in the fallopian tube, the egg moves toward the uterus, helped along by the peristaltic contractions of the smooth muscle layer in the walls of the fallopian tube and the tiny, hair-like cilia on the lining of the fallopian tube. Like the cilia in the airways of the lungs, the cilia in the fallopian

tubes move gently back and forth, creating a sweeping motion that helps to move the egg along the length of the tube. Conception, if it occurs, occurs in the fallopian tubes.

The Uterus

The uterus, sometimes referred to as the *womb,* is a hollow, pear-shaped organ (see Fig. 33-1). The uterus has three sections:

- The *fundus* is the upper, rounded portion of the uterus.
- The *body* is the mid-portion of the uterus.
- The *cervix* is the lower, narrow portion of the uterus. Normally, the cervix is closed, except for a very tiny opening. This opening, which is no larger than a pinpoint, allows sperm to enter the uterus, and menstrual blood to pass out of it. When a woman is about to give birth, the cervix dilates (opens), becoming as large as 10 centimeters in diameter. Dilation of the cervix creates an opening wide enough for the baby to pass through into the vagina.

The walls of the uterus are made of thick, smooth muscle tissue. The muscular walls of the uterus expand to accommodate a growing baby and then contract during labor to push the baby out. The inner cavity of the uterus is shaped like a capital "T" and is lined with tissue called *endometrium.*

The Vagina

The vagina is a muscular tube about 3 inches long that connects the uterus to the outside of the body (see Fig. 33-1A). The vagina is the receiving organ for sperm. It also serves as the birth canal, through which a baby passes during birth. The mucous membrane lining of the vagina helps to lubricate the vagina during sexual intercourse and protect the body from infection. It contains many folds, which allow the vagina to expand enough to allow a baby to pass through.

The Vulva

The vulva consists of the vaginal opening, the labia, and the clitoris (see Fig. 31-B).

- The vaginal opening, also called the *vaginal orifice,* is where the vagina opens to the outside of the body. The vaginal opening is located between the external urinary opening (the urinary meatus or urethral orifice) and the anus. The area between the vaginal opening and the anus is often called the *perineum.* However, the term *perineum* can also be used to describe the entire external genital area of both men and women.
- The labia, or "lips," are folds of tissue that surround the vaginal opening. The many folds of the external female reproductive system can create difficulties with hygiene, especially if a woman is injured, ill, or otherwise unable to provide for her own cleanliness needs. Perineal care and hygiene assistance is discussed in Chapter 17.
- The clitoris is located at the upper folds of the internal labia. This tissue, which is very sensitive to touch, helps to initiate a woman's sexual arousal.

The Breasts (Mammary Glands)

In women, the breasts are considered accessory organs of the reproductive system because they play a role in nourishing the newborn. Although

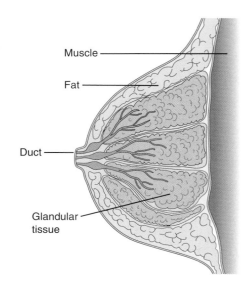

FIGURE 33-2

The breasts consist of glandular tissue and fat.

the female breasts develop during puberty, they do not become functional until the end of pregnancy. The breasts are made up of lobes, or sections, that contain glandular tissue and fat (Fig. 33-2). When it is stimulated by the hormone prolactin (which is secreted by the pituitary gland at the end of pregnancy), the glandular tissue of the breasts produces milk, a process known as **lactation.** In response to an infant's suckling, the glandular tissue contracts, sending the milk through the ducts to the nipple.

FUNCTION OF THE FEMALE REPRODUCTIVE SYSTEM

Each month during a woman's reproductive years (from puberty to menopause), her body prepares itself to become pregnant. If pregnancy does not occur, the woman has a menstrual period and the cycle begins again.

The cycle begins when the pituitary gland releases follicle-stimulating hormone (FSH), a hormone that causes about 20 eggs in the ovaries to begin to grow and mature (Fig. 33-3). Each egg grows within its own "shell," called a follicle. FSH also stimulates the follicles to produce estrogen, another hormone. As the estrogen level increases, it "turns off" FSH production. This biofeedback mechanism limits the number of follicles that mature each month. One egg-containing follicle continues to grow and mature, and the others die off.

FIGURE 33-3

Each month during a woman's reproductive years, her body prepares itself for pregnancy. In response to hormones, an egg develops and is released, and the lining of the uterus prepares itself to receive the fertilized egg, should fertilization occur. If fertilization does not occur, the egg and the lining of the uterus are shed during the woman's menstrual period, and the cycle begins again.

When the egg has matured, luteinizing hormone (LH), another hormone released by the pituitary gland, causes the follicle to burst, releasing the egg from the ovary (ovulation) (see Fig. 33-3). Following ovulation, the empty follicle becomes

known as the *corpus luteum.* The corpus luteum continues to produce estrogen, and it also begins to produce progesterone. Estrogen and progesterone cause the uterus to begin to prepare itself to receive a fertilized egg.

In response to estrogen and progesterone, the lining of the uterus (the endometrium) thickens, creating a soft, nourishing environment for a fertilized egg, should one arrive (see Fig. 33-3). Estrogen and progesterone allow the fertilized egg to attach itself to the endometrium (a process called *implantation*). Once the fertilized egg implants, it begins to divide, forming the cells and tissues that will eventually become a new human being (Fig. 33-4). If fertilization does not occur, the egg passes into the uterus, where it usually dissolves. The levels of hormones decrease, causing the endometrial lining to break down and pass through the vagina as the **menstrual period.**

This cycle of hormone secretion and egg development occurs in a regular pattern throughout a woman's reproductive years. The cycle from the first day of one menstrual period until the start of another one averages from 22 to 45 days.

THE EFFECTS OF AGING ON THE FEMALE REPRODUCTIVE SYSTEM

Unlike the age-related changes that affect other organ systems, the age-related changes that affect the female reproductive system are usually very noticeable.

Increased Difficulty Becoming Pregnant

Many women in their late 30s and early 40s have difficulty becoming pregnant. This is because each month, the number of healthy eggs remaining in a woman's ovaries decreases. (Remember that at birth, a woman's ovaries contain all of the eggs that she will ever have.) Becoming pregnant is often still possible at this age, just more difficult. Fertility treatments, such as the use of drugs to cause more eggs to ripen each month or in-vitro fertilization (IVF), are often very helpful for women in this age group who wish to become pregnant.

Decreased Sex Hormone Production

As a woman ages, her body produces lower amounts of sex hormones, especially estrogen and

A

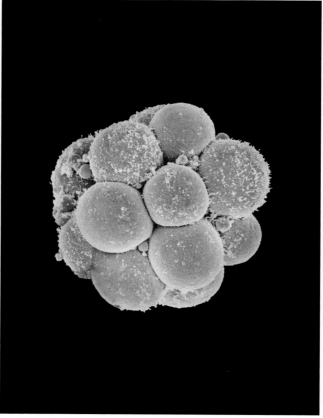

B

FIGURE 33-4

If the egg is fertilized, it travels to the uterus and attaches itself to the endometrium, which thickens in preparation for pregnancy. (*A*) The male sperm cell fertilizes the egg. (*B*) The fertilized egg then attaches itself to the soft, thick endometrium (the lining of the uterus) and begins to divide, forming the cells and tissues that will eventually become a new human being. Here, a human embryo is shown 4 days after fertilization. It now consists of 16 cells. (*A © David M. Phillips/Photo Researchers, Inc. B © Dr. Yorgos Nikas/Photo Researchers, Inc.*)

progesterone. Eventually, this decreased hormone production results in menopause, the complete ending of a woman's menstrual cycles. Menopause occurs in most women sometime between the ages of 45 and 55 years and is caused by the loss of ovary function due to age. After the onset of menopause, the reproductive organs do not function and shrink to the size they were before puberty. Menopause can cause many bothersome symptoms, including "hot flashes," irritability, a loss of energy, and an inability to sleep. Decreased production of estrogen and progesterone, which are "feminizing" hormones, may also cause some women to develop facial hair and a coarse ("scratchy") voice. Some women experience vaginal dryness and irritation and may need to use a lubricant during sexual intercourse.

Many women who have gone through menopause choose to replace the hormones their bodies no longer produce by taking estrogen and progesterone orally. This is called hormone replacement therapy (HRT). HRT helps to minimize some of the more annoying "side effects" of menopause, such as hot flashes. In addition, some research shows that taking estrogen and progesterone after menopause can help keep bones strong and prevent heart disease and some types of dementia. However, other research indicates that HRT may actually increase a woman's chances of developing certain types of cancer. Each woman must work with her health care provider to determine whether HRT is right for her, given her unique situation and health history.

DISORDERS OF THE FEMALE REPRODUCTIVE SYSTEM

Many types of disorders can affect the female reproductive system. For example, many factors, such as hormone imbalances, can cause a woman to have problems with her menstrual cycle. Cysts (fluid-filled sacs) and noncancerous tumors can interfere with the functioning of the reproductive system, or cause pain or excessive bleeding. Finally, cancer can occur in almost any organ of the female reproductive system.

Menstrual Disorders

A woman may have problems with her menstrual cycle, such as irregular periods, excessive pain, or excessive bleeding. Common disorders associated with the menstrual cycle include the following.

- **Amenorrhea** is the absence of menstrual flow. Primary amenorrhea occurs when a girl has not begun to menstruate by the age of 16 years. Abnormalities in the reproductive organs, a hormone disorder, or malnutrition may be the cause. Secondary amenorrhea is the absence of menstrual flow in a woman who has had previous menstrual periods. Secondary amenorrhea can result from hormone imbalances or tumors, and is usually the first sign of pregnancy.
- **Dysmenorrhea** is painful menstruation. Many women experience cramps in the lower abdomen during menstrual periods, but for some women the pain is severe enough to interfere with daily activities. Extremely painful periods that prevent a woman from doing what she normally does should be brought to the attention of a health care provider.
- **Menorrhagia** is excessive bleeding during a menstrual period, either in terms of the amount of blood lost or the number of days that bleeding lasts. Hormonal disturbances, infections, and growths inside the uterus can cause menorrhagia. Excessive bleeding for an extended period of time can cause a woman to become anemic from the chronic blood loss.

Infertility

Infertility is the inability to become pregnant or to carry a pregnancy to full term. Although the cause of a couple's infertility may be related to the man's inability to produce the amount of sperm needed to fertilize the egg, in many cases, it is related to a problem with the woman's reproductive system. Hormone imbalances, deformities of the reproductive organs, or scar tissue can lead to infertility.

Cysts and Noncancerous Growths or Tumors

Many organs in the female reproductive system can be affected by cysts or other noncancerous growths. Although these cysts and growths are not cancerous, they can still cause problems.

- **Cysts** can form on the ovaries after ovulation, causing intense pain. Although not malignant, ovarian cysts may need to be surgically removed if they occur frequently and are painful. Cysts may also form in the lubricating glands located inside the vagina, creating a painful, infected lump that may have to be surgically drained.
- **Fibroids (myomas)** sometimes form in the muscle wall of the uterus. Fibroids can cause problems during pregnancy if they are large enough to crowd a developing baby inside the uterus. They may also cause severe menorrhagia if they grow toward the inside of the uterine cavity.

Cancer

Common cancers affecting the female reproductive system include cervical cancer, endometrial cancer, ovarian cancer, and breast cancer.

- **Cervical cancer** (cancer of the cervix, the lower region of the uterus) is more common among women between the ages of 30 and 50 years and can be caused by a sexually transmitted viral infection. Other factors that can increase a woman's risk of developing cervical cancer include having sexual intercourse at an early age and having multiple sexual partners. If diagnosed early enough, cervical cancer can be effectively treated without putting a woman's ability to have children at risk.
- **Endometrial cancer** (cancer of the lining of the uterus) is the most common type of cancer that affects the female reproductive tract. It is most common in women after menopause. The first sign of this type of cancer is **postmenopausal bleeding,** uterine bleeding that occurs after a woman has completed menopause. Postmenopausal bleeding can also result from hormone imbalances.
- **Ovarian cancer** (cancer of the ovary) most commonly occurs in women between the ages of 40 and 65 years. Ovarian cancer is a leading cause of cancer death for women. This cancer is associated with a high rate of death because it grows quickly and

spreads easily to other organs. Early diagnosis and treatment can improve a woman's chances of survival.

- **Breast cancer** is the most commonly occurring cancer in women. Breast cancer can develop in women with relatives with breast cancer, especially a mother or sister. But it can also develop in women who have no family history of the disease. Women are encouraged to get into the habit of examining their breasts at the same time each month. During the self-exam, the woman looks and feels for any changes in the breast tissue (Fig. 33-5). Monthly breast self-exams can help a woman to become familiar with the way her breast tissue normally looks and feels. This knowledge may allow her to recognize lumps or other problems that need to be reported to the nurse or doctor for further evaluation. Many breast lumps are not cancer, but the only way to be sure is to have them checked. Early detection and new treatment methods for breast cancer allow many women to be completely cured of this disease.

Tell the Nurse!

Your duties will include assisting your female patients or residents with their personal hygiene and toileting needs. Because of this, you may be the first to observe signs of a problem involving the reproductive organs. In addition, a female patient or resident may tell you about a problem that she is experiencing. Report any of the following observations or complaints to the nurse immediately:

- The woman has an unusual vaginal discharge
- The woman has vaginal bleeding, but she has already gone through menopause
- The woman has very heavy vaginal bleeding during her menstrual period
- The woman has pain or cramping in her lower abdomen
- The woman reports itching or burning around the vulva
- The skin around the vulva is inflamed or irritated
- There are changes in skin coloring, sores that do not heal, lumps, unusual swelling, or thickened areas around the vulva
- There is a lump or thickened area in the breast
- There is a discharge from the nipples or puckering of the skin of the breasts

Rows   Circles

A. Feeling for abnormalities

B. Looking for abnormalities

FIGURE 33-5

Women are encouraged to examine their breasts monthly, so that they become familiar with the way their breast tissue normally looks and feels. A breast self-exam involves (A) feeling the breasts for abnormalities and then (B) looking at the breasts for abnormalities. There are many different ways to do a breast self-exam. For example, the exam can be performed while lying down or standing up, and the fingers can be moved across the breast in circles or in rows. The important thing is to do the exam the same way each time, at the same time each month, and to report any unusual findings to a health care provider immediately.

COMMON DIAGNOSTIC PROCEDURES

As a nursing assistant, you may be required to help prepare a female patient or resident for a procedure used to diagnose problems with the reproductive system. Many women are hesitant or embarrassed to discuss problems involving the reproductive organs. You must be especially careful to help maintain a woman's modesty and privacy when she is being prepared for a diagnostic procedure involving the reproductive system. Make sure that the privacy curtains and the door are closed, and keep sensitive body parts (such as the breasts or vulva) covered as much as possible. Also be aware that your patient or resident may be fearful or anxious about the test results. Be careful not to give advice or tell the person what you would do if you were in her situation. Instead, listen, give competent and compassionate care, and report your observations to the nurse.

Routine physical examinations are very effective for detecting disorders of the female reproductive system while they are in the early stages and easier to treat. In addition to routine physical examinations, several diagnostic procedures are used to screen for female reproductive disorders:

- **Pap test.** A Pap test (named after the doctor who invented the test, George Papanicolaou) is routinely performed to detect changes in the cervix that may indicate early cervical cancer. The doctor uses a swab to gather a sample of cells from the cervix, and then the cells are examined under a microscope to make sure they are healthy.
- **Biopsy.** In a biopsy, a tissue sample is obtained and examined under a microscope for cancerous cells. A biopsy may be used to detect endometrial, cervical, or breast cancer.
- **Dilation and curettage (D&C).** A D&C is a surgical procedure. The cervix is dilated (made wider) and tissue is curetted (scraped) from the inside of the cervix and the uterus. This tissue is then examined to determine the cause of abnormal bleeding.
- **Imaging studies.** Radiographic imaging studies can allow a doctor to see tumors or scar tissue that may be blocking the fallopian tubes, a common cause of infertility.
- **Ultrasonography.** During an ultrasound study, sound waves are "bounced off" an organ and then translated into a three-dimensional image. Ultrasound can reveal tumors or cysts on the ovaries and in other structures of the female reproductive tract. Ultrasound can also be used to check breast cysts. In addition, ultrasound is used when a woman is pregnant to check on the fetus and make sure that it is developing properly (Fig. 33-6).

FIGURE 33-6

Ultrasound, a common diagnostic procedure, is used to view a developing baby inside the uterus. It can also be used to detect tumors or cysts on reproductive structures. (© *Laurent/Dr. Gaillard/ Photo Researchers, Inc.*)

- **Mammography.** A mammogram is an x-ray of breast tissue (Fig. 33-7). Mammography can detect breast lumps at a very early stage, before they become large enough to be seen or felt. For this reason, many doctors recommend that women receive routine mammograms, in addition to performing monthly breast self-exams.

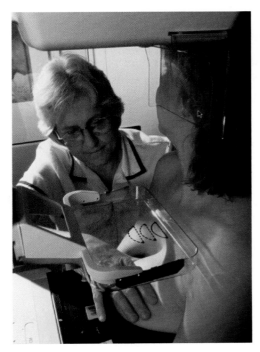

FIGURE 33-7

Mammograms can detect early forms of breast cancer. Many doctors recommend that women older than 40 years have a mammogram done annually. (© *Geoff Tompkinson/Photo Researchers, Inc.*)

COMMON SURGICAL PROCEDURES

Many of your patients or residents may be preparing for, or recovering from, surgery involving the reproductive organs. Common surgical procedures involving the female reproductive system include mastectomy and hysterectomy.

Mastectomy

A **mastectomy** (surgical removal of a breast) may be performed on a woman who has been diagnosed with certain types of breast cancer. For some women with breast cancer, the cancer can be treated by removing only the cancerous lump and some of the surrounding tissue. But for many women, the entire breast must be removed to treat the cancer effectively. When this is the case, many women choose to follow the mastectomy with reconstructive surgery. A new breast is created either by inserting a prosthesis (implant) under the skin and muscle, or by grafting tissue from another part of the body. For many women, removal of a breast is very difficult to handle emotionally. This means that in addition to healing physically from the procedure, the woman will need to heal emotionally.

Hysterectomy

A **hysterectomy** (surgical removal of the uterus) is a very common procedure. It may be used to treat uterine cancer, excessive bleeding, or other disorders of the female reproductive tract. When a hysterectomy is performed through an incision in the abdomen, it is called a *total abdominal hysterectomy (TAH)*. When it is performed through the vagina by cutting around the cervix, it is called a *total vaginal hysterectomy (TVH)*. The woman's fallopian tubes and ovaries may or may not be removed, depending on the reason for the surgery.

THE MALE REPRODUCTIVE SYSTEM

STRUCTURE OF THE MALE REPRODUCTIVE SYSTEM

The organs and structures of the male reproductive system include the testicles (testes), the epididymis, the vas deferens, and the penis (Fig. 33-8). Accessory organs include the seminal vesicles and prostate gland, which play a role in producing semen (the fluid that carries sperm cells out of the body).

The Testicles (Testes)

The testicles are two walnut-like organs located in the *scrotum,* a loose, bag-like sac of skin that is suspended outside of the body, between the thighs. The testicles have two important functions: they secrete testosterone, the hormone that is responsible for the development of male secondary sex characteristics and for the proper

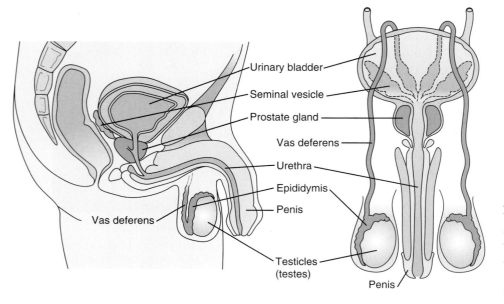

Urinary bladder
Seminal vesicle
Prostate gland
Vas deferens
Urethra
Epididymis
Penis
Vas deferens
Testicles (testes)
Penis

FIGURE 33-8

The male reproductive system consists of the testicles (testes), the epididymis, the vas deferens, and the penis. Accessory organs include the seminal vesicles and prostate gland.

functioning of the male reproductive system, and they produce sperm cells. The testicles are located outside of a man's body because the temperature necessary for the proper development of sperm is lower than the temperature inside the body.

The Epididymis

After the sperm cells leave the testes, they move into the epididymis, a series of coiled tubes where the sperm cells mature and gain the ability to "swim." A sperm cell's ability to swim comes from its flagellum, a whip-like "tail" (Fig. 33-9). The whip-like motion of the flagellum moves the sperm cell forward, allowing it to "swim" through the female reproductive tract in search of an egg to fertilize. The sperm cell is the only human body cell that has a flagellum.

The Vas Deferens

From the epididymis, the sperm cell moves into the vas deferens, a passageway that transports the sperm cell to the urethra (see Fig. 33-8). While in the vas deferens, the sperm cells are mixed with the secretions from the seminal vesicles and the prostate gland. These secretions, which nourish and protect the sperm cells, form the fluid portion

FIGURE 33-9

Each sperm cell has a whip-like "tail," called a flagellum, that allows it to move. The ability to move is important for sperm cells. After leaving the man's body, the sperm cells need to travel through the woman's vagina, into the uterus, and then into the fallopian tubes to meet the egg. (*CNRI/Photo Researchers, Inc.*)

of semen. In the prostate gland, the vas deferens joins with the urethra, which is the final passageway through which the sperm cells leave the man's body.

The Penis

The male urethra, described in Chapter 32, is contained in the penis. Semen (and urine) leave the man's body by way of the external urinary opening, which is located at the tip of the *glans penis*, the enlarged portion at the end of the penis. If a male has not been circumcised, a loose fold of skin called the *foreskin* covers the glans penis.

The urethra is surrounded by "spongy" tissue. Stimulation by the nervous system causes this spongy tissue to fill with blood. This, in turn, causes the penis to become hard and erect. When erect, the penis can be inserted into a woman's vagina, allowing sperm cells to be deposited into the woman's reproductive tract.

FUNCTION OF THE MALE REPRODUCTIVE SYSTEM

The function of the male reproductive system is to produce and nourish male sex cells (sperm), and to deposit these cells inside the female's body so that fertilization can occur. The mature female reproductive system usually produces only one egg each month. In contrast, the mature male reproductive system produces sperm cells constantly. Many millions of sperm cells are needed to fertilize one egg because so many sperm cells die during their journey through the woman's reproductive tract. After puberty, sperm cells are produced in the testicles in response to the release of FSH by the pituitary gland. The pituitary gland also secretes interstitial cell-stimulating hormone (ICSH), which stimulates the testicles to produce testosterone. Testosterone is needed for the continued development and growth of the sperm cells.

Sperm cells are deposited in the female reproductive tract through the process of **ejaculation.** During sexual intercourse, stimulation of the erect penis causes the forceful release of semen from the body. Ejaculation is how sperm cells leave the man's body and enter the woman's vagina so that the process of fertilization and reproduction can begin.

THE EFFECTS OF AGING ON THE MALE REPRODUCTIVE SYSTEM

As they get older, many men find that the frequency and duration of their erections decreases. Many men also develop enlargement of the prostate gland.

Decreased Frequency and Duration of Erections

Beginning at around the age of 20 years, production of testosterone and sperm begins to gradually decline. A man can remain fertile until late in life, even as late as 80 years of age, but most men find that as they get older, erections occur less frequently and last for shorter periods of time. This is a result of decreased production of testosterone. The ability to have and maintain an erection is also affected by the effects of aging on the cardiovascular system, which can result in decreased blood flow to the penis. Finally, medications taken for hypertension and other common disorders can also affect sexual abilities.

Enlargement of the Prostate Gland

As a man ages, the prostate gland tends to enlarge. Because the prostate gland surrounds the urethra, this enlargement can make urination difficult. Prostate problems associated with aging are discussed in Chapter 32.

DISORDERS OF THE MALE REPRODUCTIVE SYSTEM

Common disorders of the male reproductive system include impotence (erectile dysfunction) and cancer.

Impotence (Erectile Dysfunction)

Impotence (erectile dysfunction) is the inability to achieve or maintain an erection long enough to engage in sexual activity. A patient or resident may experience erectile dysfunction for several reasons. Lowered levels of male hormones, circulatory problems that restrict blood flow to the penis, medications, or emotional disturbances can all affect a man's ability to have an erection, either temporarily or permanently. In many cultures, the ability to have an erection and father children is often considered a mark of "manliness." Because of this, many men who have erectile dysfunction are embarrassed to tell a health care provider about this problem. However, once the cause has been discovered, many effective methods of treatment can allow a man to remain sexually active throughout his life span.

Cancer

Cancers affecting the male reproductive system include testicular cancer, prostate cancer, and penile cancer. In addition, men may get breast cancer, although this cancer is much less common in men than in women.

- **Testicular cancer** usually affects young to middle-aged adult men and can easily spread to other parts of the body through the lymphatic system before it is detected. Men of all ages are encouraged to examine their testicles regularly. Testicular self-examination can help detect lumps and other abnormalities at an early stage. Early detection and treatment of cancer leads to a better survival outcome.
- **Prostate cancer.** Cancer of the prostate gland most commonly occurs in men older than 50 years. Rectal examination, during which a doctor inserts a finger into the man's rectum to feel for enlargement of the gland, can lead to early detection. Prostate cancer typically grows slowly and has a good cure rate with early detection.
- **Penile cancer.** Occasionally, lesions that appear on the penis may be cancerous. As always, it is important for you to report any changes in the skin of patients or residents, no matter what part of the body they appear on.

▶ *Tell the Nurse!*

A conscientious nursing assistant always observes a patient or resident for changes that indicate that something is "not quite right" and reports those observations to the nurse immediately. Listed below are some observations that may indicate disorders of the male reproductive system. Please report to the nurse immediately if you observe:

➡ Any unusual discharge from the penis, especially if it contains blood or other discolored secretions

➡ Pain or burning when urinating

➡ Lumps or thickening of the testes

➡ Changes in the skin surrounding the scrotum or penis

➡ Reddened or irritated skin in the genital area

➡ Complaints of pain or aching in the scrotum or rectal area

COMMON DIAGNOSTIC PROCEDURES

Many of the diagnostic procedures that are used to detect disorders of the urinary system (see Chapter 32) are also used to detect disorders of the male reproductive system. You may care for a male patient or resident who is scheduled for one of these tests, or for one of the following tests:

- **Bloodwork.** A blood sample can be used to determine hormone levels (for example, in a man with erectile dysfunction). A blood sample can also be analyzed for prostate-specific antigen (PSA), a substance that is found in the blood of men with prostate problems.
- **Biopsy.** A biopsy may be necessary to test tissue for the presence of cancer in the prostate gland or the testes.

As always, be sensitive to how your patient or resident might be feeling. The person may be afraid of finding out that he has cancer, or worried that problems with sexual functioning will be permanent.

SEXUALLY TRANSMITTED DISEASES

A **sexually transmitted disease (STD)** is an infection that is most often transmitted by sexual contact. These infections, also known as *venereal diseases*, can be caused by bacteria or viruses. The pathogens are transmitted through semen and vaginal secretions. Infection of the organs of the reproductive system is most common, although the mucous membranes of the eyes, mouth, or anus may also become infected following contact with infected semen or vaginal secretions. Some STDs, such as acquired immunodeficiency syndrome (AIDS), involve the entire body.

TYPES OF SEXUALLY TRANSMITTED DISEASES

There are many different types of STDs. Some of the most common include the following:

- **Herpes simplex** is a viral infection. There are two forms of herpes simplex. Herpes simplex type I causes the common "cold sore" or "fever blister" on the lip. Herpes simplex type II, or genital herpes, causes painful blisters to form around the vaginal opening and perineum (in women) or the external urinary opening (in men) (Fig. 33-10). There is no cure for genital herpes and the blisters may return over and over again throughout the lifetime of the person who is infected.
- **Gonorrhea** is a bacterial infection. In men, the bacterium that causes gonorrhea infects the urethra. The man may experience a burning sensation during urination and notice a greenish discharge from the urethra, or he may have no symptoms at all. Women who are infected with the bacterium that causes gonorrhea also may not have any symptoms. Because the infection may not be detected and treated for some time, the bacterium can travel to the fallopian tubes and into the abdominal cavity, resulting in a condition called **pelvic inflammatory disease (PID).** PID often results in severe pain and scar tissue that can lead to infertility. If detected, gonorrhea can be treated with antibiotics.
- **Chlamydia,** the most commonly occurring STD, is caused by a type of bacteria. Like gonorrhea, chlamydia often is not associated with any noticeable symptoms. Chlamydia can cause infertility in both men and women and is treated with an antibiotic.
- **Genital (venereal) warts** are caused by a virus. In men infected with the virus, small, wart-like growths may occur inside the urethra. In women, the warts may be

A   **B**

FIGURE 33-10

Genital herpes is a viral infection that causes blisters to form (*A*) on the penis (in men) and (*B*) on the vulva (in women). There is no cure for genital herpes. The sexual partner of a person with genital herpes is at risk for infection even when blisters are not seen, if a condom is not used.

seen around the vaginal opening, inside the vagina, or on the cervix. Infection with genital warts increases a woman's risk of developing cervical cancer. Treatment may involve removal of the growths with a laser.

- **Syphilis** is a bacterial infection. The signs and symptoms of syphilis occur in three stages. During the first stage, a painless lesion is seen on the genitals. This lesion heals, and 2 to 4 weeks later, the person develops a skin rash and a fever. This is the second stage. If not detected and treated, the infection becomes latent. This means that the pathogen that is causing the infection is still in the person's body, but it is not active. As many as 20 or more years later, the pathogen can become active again, resulting in the third stage. The third stage usually involves damage to the cardiovascular and nervous systems, which can result in confusion, dementia, and paralysis.

- **AIDS** is caused by human immunodeficiency virus (HIV). The HIV virus can be transmitted in semen, vaginal secretions, or blood. To date, there is no cure for AIDS, and most people with AIDS die as a result of the disease. AIDS is discussed in detail in Chapters 8 and 38.

PREVENTION OF SEXUALLY TRANSMITTED DISEASES

People who begin having sexual relations at a young age (for example, in their early teens) and people who have many sexual partners are at increased risk for getting an STD. Women are also at greater risk than men for STDs. Although some STDs can be effectively treated and cured with antibiotics, the best treatment still remains prevention. The following methods are useful in the prevention of STDs.

- When having sexual relations, use a barrier, such as a condom. Condoms help to prevent the transmission of infected secretions from one person to another. Some contraceptive creams, when used with a condom, help to increase the condom's effectiveness against both pregnancy and STDs.

- If you or your partner has signs or symptoms of an STD, do not have sexual relations until treatment has been sought. Remember that you both must be treated. If you are not both treated, then reinfection can occur.

Knowing about STDs can help to keep you safe and healthy. In addition, this knowledge will help you to care for your patients or residents. Even if you work in a health care setting where you care mostly for elderly people, information about STDs is still useful. Some of the residents of long-term care facilities may continue to be sexually active and can still get an STD if they have relations with an infected partner. Also, symptoms of the third stage of syphilis may not appear until late in a person's life. To provide quality care to the people who depend on you for assistance, you need to be aware of the many different types of disorders that require the services of the health care industry.

SUMMARY

► Reproduction is the process by which a living thing makes more living things like itself. Although in both men and women, the reproductive system produces the cells and hormones that are necessary to create a new life, the organs that make up the reproductive system are very different in men and women.

► The female reproductive system consists of internal structures (the ovaries, the fallopian tubes, the uterus, and the vagina), external structures (the labia, the clitoris, and the vaginal opening, referred to collectively as the vulva), and the accessory organs (the breasts).

■ The female reproductive system is designed to produce eggs, receive sperm cells, contain and nourish a developing baby, give birth, and provide nourishment after the baby's birth by producing breast milk.

■ Each month during a woman's reproductive years (from puberty to menopause), her body prepares itself to become pregnant. If pregnancy does not occur, the woman has a menstrual period and the cycle begins again.

■ Aging affects the female reproductive system by causing a decline in the amount of hormones produced and the number of eggs that mature.

■ Many disorders may affect a woman's reproductive system throughout her lifetime, including menstrual disorders, cancer, infertility, and infections.

► The male reproductive system consists of the testicles (testes), the epididymis, the vas deferens, and the penis. Accessory organs include the seminal vesicles and prostate gland, which play a role in producing semen (the fluid that carries sperm cells out of the body). Sperm cells leave the body through the urethra.

■ The male reproductive system is designed to produce sperm and deposit it inside the female's body.

■ After puberty, the male reproductive system produces sperm cells continuously. Sperm cells are produced in the testes and mature in the epididymis. From the epididymis, they pass through the vas deferens and urethra to reach the outside of the body. Before leaving the body, the sperm cells are mixed with secretions from the seminal vesicles and the prostate gland, forming semen.

■ As they get older, many men find that the frequency and duration of their erections decreases. Many men also develop enlargement of the prostate gland.

■ Disorders of the male reproductive system include impotence (erectile dysfunction), cancer, and infection.

► Sexually transmitted diseases (STDs) are infections of the reproductive system that are commonly transmitted by sexual contact.

■ Some STDs do not cause signs or symptoms. Because they may not be diagnosed for a long time, the infected person can spread the infection to his or her sexual partners without knowing it. In addition, the untreated infection can damage the passageways that carry the sperm or eggs, causing infertility.

■ Common STDs include herpes simplex, gonorrhea, chlamydia, genital (venereal) warts, syphilis, and AIDS. Although some STDs can be treated, there is no known cure for herpes simplex or AIDS.

■ The best treatment for STDs is prevention. The risk of getting an STD can be lowered by using a barrier (such as a condom) when engaging in sexual activity and avoiding sexual activity with infected partners.

What did you learn?

Multiple Choice

Select the single best answer for each of the following questions.

1. What occurs when a male sex cell joins the female sex cell, forming a cell that contains the complete number of chromosomes?
   a. Ovulation
   b. Menstruation
   c. Menopause
   d. Conception (fertilization)

2. Which one of the following is a sexually transmitted disease (STD)?
   a. Breast cancer
   b. Herpes simplex
   c. Hepatitis A
   d. Tuberculosis (TB)

3. Which sexually transmitted disease (STD) is caused by a bacterium and may cause a man to have a burning sensation during urination and a greenish discharge from the urethra?
   a. Gonorrhea
   b. Syphilis
   c. Pelvic inflammatory disease (PID)
   d. Acquired immunodeficiency syndrome (AIDS)

4. Where does conception (fertilization) usually occur?
   a. In the uterus
   b. In the vagina
   c. In the fallopian tube
   d. In the vas deferens

Matching

Match each numbered item with its appropriate lettered description.

_____ 1. Sperm

_____ 2. Estrogen and progesterone

_____ 3. Amenorrhea

_____ 4. Egg (ovum)

_____ 5. Hysterectomy

_____ 6. Menopause

_____ 7. Menorrhagia

_____ 8. Mastectomy

_____ 9. Impotence (erectile dysfunction)

_____ 10. Infertility

a. Surgical removal of the uterus
b. Excessive menstrual bleeding
c. Male sex cell
d. Surgical removal of the breast
e. Female sex hormones
f. Absence of menstruation
g. The complete ending of a woman's menstrual cycles
h. Female sex cell
i. Inability to become pregnant or to carry a pregnancy to full term
j. Inability to achieve an erection

? Stop and think!

▶ You work in a hospital. One of your patients is Mrs. Dyer, a 38-year-old mother of two young children. Mrs. Dyer will be having a mastectomy tomorrow, to remove one of her breasts. The doctors believe that with the mastectomy and follow-up chemotherapy and radiation, there is a good chance that Mrs. Dyer's breast cancer will not return or spread to other parts of her body. You know from things that Mrs. Dyer has said that she is worried not only about her health in the future, but also about whether or not her husband will still find her attractive after the surgery. What could you do or say that might reassure Mrs. Dyer? After the surgery, what could you do to help Mrs. Dyer adjust to the loss of her breast?

Nursing Assistants Make a Difference!

"When the accident first happened, I didn't think I would even live through the night, much less be here to tell my story now. I'm Mike Lewis. Two years ago, I was out walking my dog when I got hit by a drunk driver. The dog was smart enough to jump out of the way, but I ended up with a broken back and some serious spinal cord injuries. When I regained consciousness, the pain was so intense, I didn't really want to live. Although the doctors determined that I would be paralyzed from the waist down for the rest of my life, the nurses, nursing assistants, and therapists insisted that I allow them to exercise my lifeless legs several times a day. I asked them what the purpose of this was, since my legs were paralyzed. They explained that the exercises would allow my legs to keep their mobility and flexibility, which was important, even if I would never walk again.

After a while, I was sent to the Western Spinal Rehabilitation Center for intensive rehabilitative therapy. The staff there kept trying to teach me how to use my arms to move myself out of the wheelchair. I can't count the number of times I fell on the floor. Mark, one of the nursing assistants at the center, would always help me back up. Each time, he'd encourage me to try again. Instead of telling me how wonderful I was doing (which I wasn't) he would ask me what I eventually wanted to be able to do after I was released from the center. Well, duh, that was easy. I wanted to go back home to my dog and be a normal, independent person again. Some days, I would get so depressed or frustrated. That's when Mark would remind me of the goal I had set for myself. Then he would tell me to focus on what I could do, and use that focus to help me to achieve my ultimate goal. Mark's good advice and encouragement really kept me going.

Eventually, I learned how to transfer myself and how to get around some pretty tight places in that wheelchair. I was able to return to my job with only a few minor modifications to my desk height and keyboard position. And my dog still goes on walks with me, only he walks and I wheel. Now I'm healthy and independent, thanks to the caring efforts of people like Mark."

You can listen to more stories about how nursing assistants make a difference on the CD in the back of your book.

Special Care Concerns

Because nursing assistants are employed in so many different health care settings, you may be involved with the care of patients, residents, or clients who have developmental disabilities, mental illness, dementia, cancer, or AIDS. Along with the normal assistance needed for feeding, bathing, and toileting, these groups have other unique needs. The purpose of this unit is to introduce you to these groups and help you to recognize, and assist with meeting, their special needs.

Photo: An athlete competes in the Special Olympics.
(© Lawrence Migdale/Photo Researchers, Inc.)

Caring for People With Developmental Disabilities

What will you learn?

In this chapter, you will learn about caring for people with developmental disabilities. Permanent disabilities that affect a person before adulthood are called *developmental disabilities* because they interfere with normal physical or mental development. As a nursing assistant, you will be primarily responsible for providing the assistance that people with developmental disabilities need to meet their physical and emotional needs on a daily basis. When you are finished with this chapter, you will be able to:

1. Define the term *developmental disabilities* and discuss various causes.
2. List common developmental disabilities and describe characteristics of each one.
3. Describe the special needs of people with developmental disabilities.
4. Discuss physical problems that people with developmental disabilities may have.
5. Discuss types of rehabilitation that may be used to help people with developmental disabilities.

Photo: Participating in events such as the Special Olympics provides physical as well as emotional benefits for people with developmental disabilities.
(Richard Hutchings/Photo Researchers, Inc.)

Vocabulary

Developmental disability	Cerebral palsy
Congenital	Fragile X syndrome
Mental retardation	Fetal alcohol syndrome
Down syndrome	Spina bifida
Autism	Hydrocephalus

WHAT IS A DEVELOPMENTAL DISABILITY?

A **developmental disability** is a permanent disability that affects a person before he reaches adulthood (that is, before 19–22 years of age) and interferes with the person's ability to achieve developmental milestones. A developmental disability may be **congenital** (something a child is born with) or acquired (occurring after birth, as a result of trauma or illness). Common causes of developmental disabilities are shown in Box 34-1. A developmental disability may affect mental function, physical function, or both. Developmental disabilities vary in severity. Some people with developmental disabilities are very independent, whereas others require total care.

BOX 34-1 Common Causes of Developmental Disabilities

Congenital (present at birth)
Genetic (inherited) disorders
Consumption of alcohol, drugs, or other toxic substances during pregnancy
Infections during pregnancy, such as German measles (rubella) or human immunodeficiency virus (HIV)
Poor nutrition during pregnancy
Conditions that deprive the baby of oxygen

Acquired (occurring after birth)
Birth trauma
Head injury
Near-drowning
Poisoning

SPECIAL NEEDS OF PEOPLE WITH DEVELOPMENTAL DISABILITIES

People with developmental disabilities have the same physical and emotional needs as everyone else. For example, they need good nutrition, plenty of exercise, and the sense of well-being that comes from feeling loved and cared for. However, many people with disabilities have additional special needs.

SPECIAL EDUCATION

Many children with developmental disabilities go to public school alongside friends and classmates who have no disabilities. This is called *mainstreaming.* Mainstreaming benefits children with developmental disabilities by making them feel less isolated. Children with disabilities who are "mainstreamed" have higher self-esteem and better social skills, because they have the opportunity to interact with other children who are not disabled (Fig. 34-1). Mainstreaming also benefits children who are not disabled by making them aware that people with disabilities are just like they are, except that they need extra help to do certain things.

FIGURE 34-1

"Mainstreaming" benefits everyone. Here, a teenager with Down syndrome participates in a pottery class at his high school. (*Richard Hutchings/Photo Researchers, Inc.*)

FIGURE 34-2

Vocational training helps to prepare people with disabilities for the work force. (*Courtesy of the Wood County Board of Mental Retardation and Developmental Disabilities, Bowling Green, OH.*)

Children with developmental disabilities may also take part in special educational programs. Special educational programs are focused on the individual's needs and cover a wide range of topics, such as self-care skills (for example, eating or dressing), life skills (for example, counting money), and social skills (for example, understanding appropriate behavior and "limits"). Vocational training focuses on teaching work skills that help people with disabilities become less dependent on others for their care (Fig. 34-2).

PROTECTION OF RIGHTS

Government agencies and organizations help protect the rights of people with developmental disabilities. The Americans with Disabilities Act ensures that people who have disabilities are treated the same as those without disabilities, by guaranteeing people with disabilities access to public education, employment, and public places such as parks, restaurants, and transportation. The Arc of the United States is an organization that promotes the rights of people with mental disabilities, very similar to how the Omnibus Budget Reconciliation Act (OBRA) helps to protect the rights of the elderly.

EMOTIONAL NEEDS

Reassurance, love, and acceptance are vital for everyone's well-being, and especially for those with disabilities that can make them appear or feel "different." One notable way in which people with developmental disabilities gain self-esteem is through the Special Olympics, a sporting event established to promote the physical and emotional health of people with developmental disabilities. The participants are matched for their competitions according to their level of physical and mental ability. The athletes compete against their own personal best performance. The Special Olympics emphasizes the joy that comes with physical activity, recognizing each athlete as a winner. Their motto is: "Let me win, but if I cannot win, let me be brave in my attempt." Participating in events such as the Special Olympics benefits athletes with disabilities emotionally as well as physically.

TYPES OF DEVELOPMENTAL DISABILITIES

MENTAL RETARDATION

A person with **mental retardation** has below-average intellectual functioning and problems with adaptive skills. *Intellectual functioning* is the ability to reason, think, and understand. *Adaptive skills* are skills needed to live and work, such as communication skills, social skills, and self-care skills. A mentally retarded person has an intelligence quotient (IQ) score of less than 70 points and limited adaptive skills in two or more areas.

Mental retardation can be caused by abnormalities in the brain that are present at birth. It can also be caused by problems that interfere with oxygen getting to the brain before, during, or after birth. The severity of mental retardation, like that of other disabilities, varies:

- **Mild mental retardation.** Most people with mental retardation fall into this category. Mild mental retardation may go unnoticed until a child begins school and starts having trouble with reading or solving math problems. With special education, a person with mild mental retardation is usually able to achieve a third- to sixth-grade learning level and master the skills needed for socially appropriate behavior. Vocational (job) training is useful.

- **Moderate mental retardation.** People with moderate mental retardation have delays in both motor (manual) skills and speech development. With special education, a person with moderate mental retardation is usually able to learn self-care skills, communication skills, and safety habits. However, academically, she will probably not progress beyond a second-grade learning level. The person may also have trouble learning socially appropriate behavior.

- **Severe mental retardation.** With special education, people with severe mental retardation are able to learn some communication and basic self-care skills, such as how to feed themselves. A person with severe mental retardation can usually learn to walk, if he does not have other physical disabilities.

- **Profound mental retardation.** *Profound* means "deep." People with profound mental retardation have minimal function in all developmental areas, physical and mental. These people need complete assistance with their activities of daily living (ADLs), and constant supervision to provide for their safety.

One of the great rewards that you will experience as a nursing assistant is the satisfaction of helping a person with mental retardation to feel loved, and allowing her to express love back to you (Fig. 34-3). Many people with mental retardation need guidance with "appropriate" methods of displaying their love and affection to other people. In the same manner that a child learns that hugging a kitty too hard will lead to being scratched, people with mental retardation may need gentle reminders that a hug may sometimes be too tight and that not everyone appreciates physical affection.

Adults with mental retardation may function mentally at the level of a seven- or eight-year-old, with child-like curiosity and innocence. However, they are adults and will experience the same hormonal changes and sexual drives as everyone else. Because the person may not un-

FIGURE 34-3

One of the great rewards that you will have as a nursing assistant is the satisfaction of helping a person with mental retardation to feel loved, and allowing him to express love back to you. (© *Stephanie Maze/CORBIS.*)

derstand what is happening, these physical drives may be very confusing. Education and guidance from caregivers is very important to help a person with mental retardation learn about appropriate touch and sexual behavior. In addition, caregivers must protect the person from sexual abuse. Because people with mental retardation tend to be very trusting, and because they are not able to understand what is happening to them, they are often targets of sexual abuse. As a nursing assistant, you must be especially observant for signs of sexual abuse when caring for a person with mental retardation. Any observations you make or suspicions that you have should be reported to the nurse immediately.

DOWN SYNDROME

Down syndrome is a developmental disability that is the result of a genetic disorder. Normally, each of our body's cells contains 23 pairs of chromosomes, for a total of 46. A person with Down syndrome has one extra chromosome. Down syndrome is the most common chromosome-related disorder, affecting 1 in every 1000 children born. Although the exact cause of Down syndrome is unknown, studies have shown that babies with Down syndrome are born more often to women who have children later in life.

People with Down syndrome have some degree of mental retardation and muscle weakness. In

FIGURE 34-4

Certain physical characteristics are typical of Down syndrome, such as almond-shaped eyes. (© *LWA-Dann Tardif/CORBIS.*)

addition, they have certain characteristic physical features (Fig. 34-4):

- Eyelid folds that give the eyes an almond-shaped appearance
- A large tongue in a small mouth
- Square hands with short, stubby fingers
- A small, wide nose and small ears
- Short stature and a wide, short neck

Many people with Down syndrome are also born with heart defects that require corrective surgery or medication. Frequent respiratory tract infections are also common among people with Down syndrome, due to muscle weakness (which affects the muscles used for breathing) and a compromised immune system.

Many people with Down syndrome live independently and hold down jobs. Children with Down syndrome are usually raised in their own homes with their families. Once a person with Down syndrome reaches adulthood, the person may continue to live with family members, or he may choose to move to a group home. Group homes allow a person with Down syndrome to live independently within a supervised and supportive environment.

AUTISM

A person with **autism** has extreme difficulty communicating and relating to other people and surroundings. Although the specific cause of autism is unknown, experts suspect a genetic link. Like Down syndrome, autism affects about 1 in every 1000 children born. Boys are affected more often than girls.

Autism affects a person's reasoning skills, language skills, ability to socialize, ability to perform self-care activities, and response to touch and pain. A person with autism may seem very withdrawn, like he is in his "own world" (*auto-* means "self"). The person may have lengthy or extreme tantrums, or show aggressive or violent behavior that can result in self-injury. Other disorders, such as mental retardation and seizure disorders, may accompany autism. However, many people with autism have average or above-average intelligence. Therapy focusing on communication and social skills can be very useful for a person with autism.

CEREBRAL PALSY

Cerebral palsy is caused by damage to the cerebrum, the part of the brain involved with motor control. Cerebral palsy has many possible causes, including physical brain deformity and conditions that interfere with the flow of oxygen to the baby's brain before, during, or shortly after birth. Babies who are born prematurely or have a low birth weight are at higher risk for cerebral palsy. Accidents in early childhood can also cause cerebral palsy. For example, head trauma that causes swelling or bleeding in the brain and events that interfere with the flow of oxygen to the brain (such as choking, near-drowning, or poisoning) can all cause this disability. The degree of disability depends on the extent of the damage to the brain.

Recall that the cerebrum plays a role in motor activity. This is why cerebral palsy typically affects the person's ability to voluntarily move parts of her body. Cerebral palsy can affect body movements in two different ways. One type of cerebral palsy causes spasms and shortening of the muscles. The affected joints may develop contractures. If the hands and arms are affected, the person may be unable to perform self-care skills such as feeding, bathing, or dressing. If the feet and legs are affected, the person may be unable to walk (Fig. 34-5). The second type of cerebral palsy causes involuntary movements of the arms, legs, and upper body. Facial and tongue muscles may also be involved, making the person appear to be chewing constantly. Varying degrees of mental retardation may also accompany the physical disabilities associated with cerebral palsy.

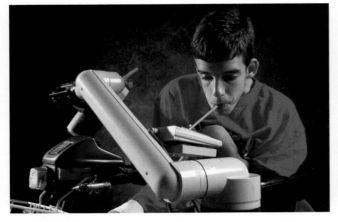

FIGURE 34-5

Cerebral palsy affects a person's motor function. Here, a child with cerebral palsy is using a pencil held in his mouth to operate a computer. (© *Richard T. Nowitz/Photo Researchers, Inc.*)

FIGURE 34-6

Children with fetal alcohol syndrome are usually smaller than other children their age. They may have mental retardation and behavioral problems. (© *David H. Wells/CORBIS.*)

FRAGILE X SYNDROME

Fragile X syndrome is an inherited type of mental retardation caused by a defect in the X chromosome. Fragile X syndrome is more common and usually more severe in boys, as compared with girls. People who have fragile X syndrome are usually moderately to severely mentally retarded and may have physical characteristics such as large, cupped ears; a slim build; wide-set, somewhat squinting eyes; and velvet-like skin. They usually have delayed speech and communication skills. They may be hyperactive, and prone to "mood swings." Autism may also accompany fragile X syndrome.

Special education helps people with fragile X syndrome learn self-care and behavior skills. A calm, structured environment that keeps distractions and disturbances to a minimum is useful when caring for a person with fragile X syndrome. Unfortunately, because the syndrome has only recently been identified as a developmental disorder, more research is still needed to determine the most effective methods of caring for people with this disability.

FETAL ALCOHOL SYNDROME

Fetal alcohol syndrome is a combination of physical and mental problems that affect a child whose mother consumed alcohol during pregnancy. The degree of disability seems to depend on the amount of alcohol the mother drank during her pregnancy, as well as on how frequently she drank. Babies born with fetal alcohol syndrome are usually smaller than normal and have mental retardation, behavioral problems, learning difficulties, and facial deformities (Fig. 34-6). Although the disabilities caused by fetal alcohol syndrome are permanent, special education and therapy can help to maximize the person's abilities.

SPINA BIFIDA

Spina bifida is a congenital defect of the spinal column. Normally, the vertebrae enclose the spinal cord, protecting it from harm. In a person with spina bifida, the vertebrae do not close properly during development, leaving the spinal cord exposed. As with other developmental disabilities, spina bifida varies in severity. Some people with spina bifida have only a slight bone deformity that is not even visible on the outside of the body, except for possibly a dimple or tuft of hair on the back. Other people have more severe deformities that result in the meninges, the spinal cord, or both bulging through a large opening on the back (Fig. 34-7). The person may just have weakness in the legs, or she may be totally paralyzed below the waist. Problems with bowel and bladder control are common. Sometimes, people with spina bifida also have mental retardation.

HYDROCEPHALUS

Hydrocephalus, sometimes called "water on the brain," results from a build-up of cerebrospinal fluid (CSF). Recall from Chapter 28

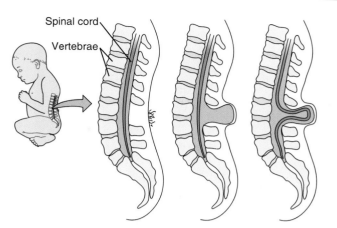

A. Spina bifida occulta   **B.** Meningocele   **C.** Myelomeningocele

FIGURE 34-7

Spina bifida occurs when the vertebrae do not close properly during development. (A) Spina bifida occulta. There is an opening in one or more of the vertebrae, but the spinal cord is not injured. A tuft of hair or a dimple on the back may be the only external sign. (*Occult* means "hidden.") (*B*) Meningocele. The meninges bulge through an opening in the back, but the spinal cord is unharmed. (*C*) Myelomeningocele. The meninges and the spinal cord bulge through an opening in the back.

that the ventricles of the brain constantly produce CSF, which circulates around the brain and spinal cord. Normally, the CSF is reabsorbed into the bloodstream after it makes its circuit through the central nervous system (CNS). In hydrocephalus, either too much CSF is produced, or the CSF cannot drain properly. Eventually, the fluid builds up, placing pressure on the delicate tissues of the brain and putting the person at risk for permanent brain damage.

Many cases of hydrocephalus are congenital. For example, babies with spina bifida often have hydrocephalus as well. When hydrocephalus occurs in a child younger than 2 years, the child's head often enlarges, because the bones of the skull have not yet fused together (Fig. 34-8A). Hydrocephalus may also occur later in life, as a result of a tumor, head trauma, or infection. Whether the hydrocephalus is congenital or acquired, it is often treated by surgically inserting a tube (called a *shunt*) that allows the fluid to drain from the brain to another part of the person's body (see Fig. 34-8B).

CARING FOR A PERSON WITH A DEVELOPMENTAL DISABILITY

During your career as a nursing assistant, you may have many opportunities to care for people with developmental disabilities, in many different types of health care settings:

- If you work in a hospital, you may care for a person with a developmental disability while he is receiving treatment for an acute health problem, such as a heart problem, a respiratory tract infection, a nutritional deficiency, or seizures.

- If you work for a home health care agency, you may have the opportunity to form a longer-lasting relationship with a person with a developmental disability. Many parents who have children with disabilities choose to raise them at home, with their brothers and sisters. The parents of a child with severe disabilities may need the assistance of a home health care aide to provide the best care to the child at home.

- If you work in a long-term care facility, you may also have the opportunity to form a long-lasting relationship with a person with a developmental disability. People with developmental disabilities become residents of long-term care facilities for many reasons. A young person may become a resident of a long-term care facility because her disabilities are simply too difficult or too numerous for the family to manage at home. Older people with disabilities often become residents of long-term care facilities because their parents or other caregivers die or become too old to physically care for them. If you work in a long-term care facility, be aware that the adjustment of having to leave home—where the person felt comfortable and safe—and move into a health care facility can be incredibly traumatic for a person with developmental disabilities, just as for any other resident or patient. These new residents may feel angry, isolated, or deserted, and will need your compassion and understanding to help them

A

B

FIGURE 34-8

Hydrocephalus results from a build-up of cerebrospinal fluid (CSF). (*A*) In children younger than 2 years, the accumulation of cerebrospinal fluid can cause the head to grow larger because the bones of the skull have not yet fused together. (*B*) To prevent additional brain damage from occurring, a shunt is inserted to drain the cerebrospinal fluid. (*A* © *A. Ansary/Custom Medical Stock Photo.*)

become comfortable in their new surroundings. It is important that you understand the frustrations that may accompany a change like this for a developmentally disabled person so that you avoid taking actions personally.

The degree to which a person is disabled varies greatly from person to person. Some physical disabilities are very mild and may only cause minor muscle weakness and coordination problems. Others are more severe and may leave the person without any control over her muscles at all. The severity of mental disabilities also varies from person to person. People with mild mental retardation are able to function independently, holding down jobs and raising families with minimal support from others. Severely mentally disabled people, however, require constant care and supervision just to keep them safe.

When working with a person who has a developmental disability, the care that you provide must be specific to the person's abilities and disabilities. Learn as much as you can about each person in your care. Focusing on each person's abilities, whether developmentally disabled or not, will help you to provide the standard of care that each of your patients or residents needs from you.

COMMUNICATING WITH A PERSON WITH A DEVELOPMENTAL DISABILITY

Many people with developmental disabilities have difficulty communicating with other people. Some are unable to speak or to learn language skills due to a lack of motor skills, mental capabilities, or both. Vision or hearing problems can also make communication difficult. However, many people with developmental disabilities find other ways of communicating. For example, they may rely heavily on nonverbal communication techniques, such as facial expressions, nods, and body language. When caring for a person with a developmental disability:

- Ask family members what communication techniques work best with the person. Family members are often glad to share with you what they have learned about which communication methods work best.
- If the person has a mental disability, use simple words and short phrases. This allows the person to comprehend ideas or tasks, one at a time.
- Perhaps the most useful communication method is that of a touch, a smile, or a kind word, all of which transmit the message of your care and compassion for the person (Fig. 34-9).

Because many people with severe developmental disabilities have difficulty communicating, they may be unable to tell you if they are experiencing pain or discomfort. Learn to watch for small, subtle changes in your patients or residents, such as changes in behavior, eating habits, or sleeping habits. Changes like these may be a sign that the person is ill. Because you will most likely be the member of the health care team who spends the most time with the person, you will likely be the first to notice that "something is not quite right." Always be sure to report your observations to the nurse.

➤ Tell the Nurse!

A person with a mental disability may not be able to tell you when something is wrong. Use your observation skills and be sure to report any of the following to the nurse immediately:

➤ There is a change in the person's vital signs, especially body temperature or pulse rhythm

➤ There is a change in the person's appetite

➤ There is a change in the person's level of activity

➤ There is a change in the person's level of mental functioning (for example, the person seems confused or disoriented)

➤ There is a change in the person's behavior (for example, a normally gentle person becomes aggressive)

➤ The person complains of pain or discomfort

➤ The person's skin is red or swollen in areas

➤ The person shows signs of physical or mental abuse

MEETING THE PHYSICAL NEEDS OF A PERSON WITH A DEVELOPMENTAL DISABILITY

A person with a developmental disability has the same physical needs as everyone else. Because of the person's disability, however, he may need some help in meeting those needs. As always, you will need to consider the specific needs of each person. Nursing assistants often are involved with assisting people with disabilities with their ADLs, and with activities related to rehabilitation.

Assisting the Person with Activities of Daily Living (ADLs)

Depending on the severity and type of disability, the person may need assistance with ADLs. Some types of disability, such as cerebral palsy, can cause muscle weakness on one or both sides of the body, making dressing and grooming difficult. The short fingers of a person with Down syndrome may make it hard for the person to manage buttons or zippers on clothing. Assistive devices, many of which you have learned about in previous chapters, allow many people with physical disabilities to manage their ADLs independently or with minimal assistance. A person with mental disabilities may simply need supervision and reminders (for example, about which step comes next) to complete his ADLs. As with any

FIGURE 34-9

Good communication skills are especially important when working with people with developmental disabilities. (*Sacramento Bee/Jose Luis Villegas.*)

patient or resident, helping a person achieve the greatest possible level of independence is the best type of assistance that you can give.

Assisting with Rehabilitation

Physical therapy or respiratory therapy may be needed to help the person maintain levels of function or to treat accompanying illnesses. For example, a person who has physical limitations may need assistance with passive range-of-motion exercises to keep the affected parts of her body functional. As a nursing assistant, you may play a very important role in helping the person with physical rehabilitation.

SUMMARY

▶ Permanent disabilities that affect a person before she becomes an adult are called *developmental disabilities* because they interfere with that person's normal physical or mental development.
  - Developmental disabilities can be due to congenital abnormalities, traumatic injury, infection, disease, deprivation of oxygen or nutrition, or the result of poisoning or drug use.
  - Developmental disabilities can affect a person physically or mentally.
  - The severity of the disability varies greatly with each individual.
  - Special education, assistive devices, and rehabilitation can help a person with a developmental disability maximize his abilities and become more independent.
▶ Many developmentally disabled people have special needs.
  - Educational opportunities designed specifically for people with developmental disabilities help teach self-care, communication and social and vocational skills.
  - Legislation (such as the Americans with Disabilities Act) and organizations (such as The Arc of the United States) help to protect the rights of people with disabilities.
  - The Special Olympics was established to promote the physical and emotional health of people with developmental disabilities.
▶ There are many different types of developmental disabilities. The degree to which a person's abilities are affected varies considerably, even among people who have the same type of disability.
  - Mental retardation affects a person's general intellectual functioning. A person with mental retardation has an IQ score of less than 70 and limited adaptive skills in two or more areas.
  - Down syndrome is a developmental disability that is the result of an extra chromosome. People with Down syndrome have some degree of mental retardation as well as certain physical characteristics.
  - Autism is a congenital disorder. People with autism have extreme difficulty communicating with and relating to other people and their surroundings.
  - Cerebral palsy affects the motor region of the brain (the cerebrum) and causes varying degrees of paralysis in the body. Some people with cerebral palsy also have some degree of mental retardation.
  - Fragile X syndrome is an inherited type of mental retardation that is more common in boys.
  - Fetal alcohol syndrome is a combination of physical and mental abnormalities that affect a child whose mother consumed alcohol during pregnancy.
  - Spina bifida is a defect of the spinal column that can cause paralysis of the lower extremities.
  - Hydrocephalus occurs when the ventricles of the brain produce too much cerebrospinal fluid (CSF), or when the fluid is not able to drain properly. Hydrocephalus can result in brain damage.
▶ Nursing assistants care for people with developmental disabilities in a variety of health care settings.
  - Because people with developmental disabilities may have trouble communicating with others, nursing assistants often must rely on their observation skills to tell when something is wrong.
  - Nursing assistants often must provide some or complete assistance with activities of daily living (ADLs). However, many people with developmental disabilities are able to manage their ADLs quite independently by using assistive devices.
  - Nursing assistants are often very involved in assisting people with developmental disabilities with tasks related to rehabilitation.

What did you learn?

Multiple Choice

Select the single best answer for each of the following questions.

1. Which one of the following statements about mental retardation is correct?
   a. It affects the motor region of the brain
   b. It can occur before, during, or after birth
   c. It is always severe
   d. None of the above

2. What physical characteristics does a person with Down syndrome have?
   a. Large, cupped ears; a slim build; wide-set, somewhat squinting eyes; and velvet-like skin
   b. Almond-shaped eyes, square hands with short fingers, large tongue in a small mouth
   c. A large head
   d. Facial deformities and small stature

3. What do scientists think is a cause of autism?
   a. Genetics
   b. Oxygen deprivation at birth
   c. Drugs
   d. Trauma at birth

4. Cerebral palsy can be caused by:
   a. Infection during pregnancy
   b. A lack of oxygen to the brain
   c. An extra chromosome
   d. A high fever

5. A person with autism may have:
   a. Mental retardation
   b. Hearing and vision problems
   c. Problems with social relations
   d. Muscle weakness

6. A person with Down syndrome always has some degree of:
   a. Mental retardation
   b. Spastic movements
   c. Cerebral palsy
   d. Autism

7. Which one of the following statements about fetal alcohol syndrome is correct?
   a. It occurs when a woman smokes during pregnancy
   b. A newborn with fetal alcohol syndrome is larger than normal
   c. It occurs when a woman drinks alcohol during pregnancy
   d. It is caused by oxygen deprivation at birth

8. What is spina bifida?
   a. A seizure disorder
   b. A defect of the spinal canal
   c. A shunt
   d. Another name for fragile X syndrome

9. What is common in a person with spina bifida?
   a. Autism
   b. Bowel and bladder incontinence
   c. Drooling
   d. Seizures

10. Hydrocephalus occurs when:
    a. Cerebrospinal fluid (CSF) collects in the brain
    b. The person has a seizure
    c. A person is born with an extra chromosome
    d. A person has nerve damage

? Stop and think!

▶ Today a new resident has been admitted to the long-term care facility where you work. Mr. Theodore has severe cerebral palsy. He is an only child. His parents, who are in their 80s, are experiencing health problems of their own and are no longer able to provide the physical care that Mr. Theodore needs. Mr. Theodore is very upset. He is crying, and he keeps asking why his family doesn't want him anymore. What can you do in the coming days and weeks to help Mr. Theodore make the adjustment to his new home?

35

Caring for People With Mental Illness

What will you learn?

A **mental illness** is a disorder that affects a person's mind, causing the person to act in unusual ways, experience emotional difficulties, or both. (*Mental* means "mind.") In many societies and cultures, mental illness is viewed as something to be ashamed of. A mentally ill person's odd behavior may be frightening to those who do not understand it. In addition, movies, television, and books have contributed to the popular image of mentally ill people as crazy, violent, and out of control. Although some people who are mentally ill may behave in violent or dangerous ways, most do not. There are many different types of mental illness, and mental illness varies in severity from person to person.

As a nursing assistant, you will care for many people with different types and degrees of mental illness. You may find the idea of caring for a mentally ill person frightening. Learning about common mental illnesses can help you to overcome this fear. In this chapter, you will learn about several common mental illnesses, and how they affect the people who suffer from them. When you are finished with this chapter, you will be able to:

1. Define the term *mental illness*.
2. Describe some of the qualities that define good mental health.
3. Discuss methods that people use to cope with stress effectively.
4. List possible causes of mental illness.
5. Discuss the different treatments that are available for people with mental illness.

(continued)

Photo: Mental illnesses are disorders that affect the mind and emotions.
(© Piko/Photo Researchers, Inc.)

6. Describe common mental illnesses that you may encounter in the health care setting.

7. Discuss special concerns related to the health care setting and aging that may affect a person's mental health.

8. Describe the responsibilities of the nursing assistant when caring for mentally ill patients and residents.

Vocabulary

Use the CD in the back of your book to hear these terms pronounced, defined, and used in a sentence.

Mental illness	Suicide	Depression	Anorexia nervosa
Stress	Anxiety	Bipolar disorder	Bulimia nervosa
Coping mechanisms	Panic disorder	(manic depression)	
Defense mechanisms	Obsessive-compulsive	Schizophrenia	
Psychiatrist	disorder	Delusions	
Psychologist	Phobia	Hallucinations	

MENTAL HEALTH

To better understand mental illness, it is often useful to start by understanding mental health. Simply put, mental health is the absence of mental illness. One of the main qualities of mental health is a state of emotional balance. In Unit 5, you learned how physical health is related to the body's ability to make adjustments to maintain a state of physical balance, or homeostasis. Similarly, mental health is characterized by a person's ability to make adjustments to maintain a state of emotional balance.

Stress, which results from any change from the normal routine, affects a person's ability to maintain a state of balance. Changes that affect us physically, such as illness or disability, cause physical stress. Life events, such as getting married, getting divorced, starting a new job, having a baby, or losing a loved one cause a great deal of mental stress. For most of us, stress is a constant in our lives. Even day-to-day activities, such as reading the newspaper, raising children, or performing our jobs, are sources of stress (Fig. 35-1). Stress that is not managed properly can affect a person's physical health, as well as his mental health. For example, not being able to manage stress can put a person at risk for cardiovascular problems, such as a heart attack, and digestive disorders, such as ulcers.

Each person has a limit to the amount of stress that she can effectively deal with at any given time. Fatigue, illness, and everyday stress sometimes affect our ability to cope well with change. Many times, stress does not come from a single source. For example, a person may be able to cope fairly well with one type of stress, such as the loss of a job. But when other stresses, such as a sick child, are added, the person may reach his "breaking point." When this happens, the person may cry, sleep excessively, be unable to sleep, have difficulty concentrating, or feel depressed for a time. Most people with good mental health are able to eventually overcome these feelings and regain their emotional balance (Fig. 35-2). People who are mentally ill cannot cope effectively with stress and may become unable to work, care for their children, make simple decisions, think clearly, or even provide their own self-care. A mentally ill person may need medication, counseling, or support groups to help regain emotional balance.

COPING MECHANISMS

What do you do when you start to feel overwhelmed or "stressed out"? Maybe you exercise, practice a hobby, get together with friends, meditate or pray, or just find a quiet place to relax (Fig. 35-3). Over time, many people come to know

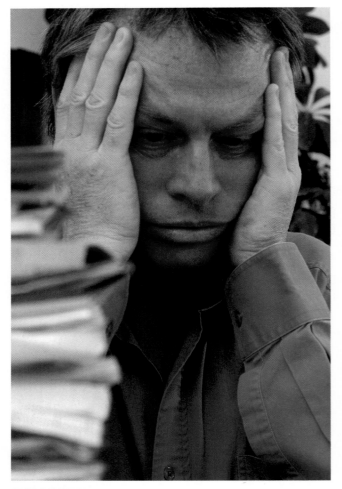

FIGURE 35-1

Stress is a constant in most people's lives. Work, family, and world events are common sources of stress. (© *Jean-Paul Chassenet/Photo Researchers, Inc.*)

what they can do to make themselves feel better when they start to feel overwhelmed by life's pressures. These conscious and deliberate ways of dealing with stress are called **coping mechanisms.**

Many people rely on positive coping mechanisms, such as exercise, prayer and meditation, getting together with friends, or engaging in a hobby. Other people rely on less effective coping mechanisms. These people seek short-term relief through behaviors such as nail biting, pacing, overeating or not eating enough, smoking, or abusing drugs or alcohol (Fig. 35-4). Initially, these behaviors may help the person to reduce stress. But over time, they place the person at risk for serious physical problems, mental problems, or both.

DEFENSE MECHANISMS

As you know, our bodies are "programmed" to try and return to a state of balance. Therefore, when a person is under stress, the mind may try to return the person to a state of emotional balance by using defense mechanisms. **Defense mechanisms** are methods of dealing with stress that "just happen." Usually the person is not even aware that he is using them. Defense mechanisms help to protect us from emotionally traumatic events. The behaviors associated with defense mechanisms occur when the mind attempts to restore or maintain emotional balance

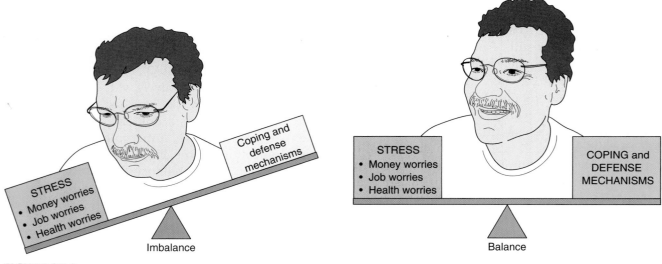

FIGURE 35-2

A person who is mentally healthy is able to maintain a state of emotional balance on most days. Stress can drag us down, causing the scale to tip out of balance, but a person who is mentally healthy is able to adjust to the stress and return to a state of emotional balance.

FIGURE 35-3

Our physical and mental health depends on our ability to manage everyday stress. Enjoying a hobby (*A*), laughing with friends (*B*), and taking a long walk (*C*) are just some of many positive approaches people take to relieve stress! (*B © Christopher Briscoe/Photo Researchers, Inc.; C © Jeff Greenberg/Photo Researchers, Inc.*)

in response to stress. Common defense mechanisms include the following.

- **Compensation** means to make up for a loss by "filling in" or "substituting" something else. For example, a person who feels lonely may eat too much. This person is substituting food for affection.
- **Conversion** means "to change." For example, a person who is depressed (an emotional problem) may develop a stomach ache (a physical problem), and then use the physical problem as a reason to avoid participating in an activity.
- **Denial** is refusing to believe something that is true, especially if the truth is unpleasant. For example, a person who has been diagnosed with cancer may truly believe that the doctor has made the wrong diagnosis, and that she does not have cancer.

- **Displacement** is shifting an emotion from one person to another who is less threatening. For example, a resident who is angry with her daughter for moving her to a long-term care facility—and who is afraid of expressing this anger because she fears the daughter will abandon her—may take her anger out on the nursing assistant instead.
- **Projection** is blaming someone else for your own uncomfortable or unacceptable actions or feelings. For example, a resident may accuse a nursing assistant of breaking a vase when in fact, the resident actually broke the treasured vase herself.
- **Rationalization** is making excuses or creating acceptable reasons for poor behaviors or actions. For instance, a student who does not study for a test and then fails it

FIGURE 35-4

Many people drink alcohol excessively, use illegal ("street") drugs, or abuse legally prescribed drugs to deal with stress. This is called substance abuse. Although substance abuse may provide short-term relief from the pressures of daily life, in the long run it is not an effective coping mechanism.

may tell herself that the reason she failed is because the teacher is "too hard."

- **Regression** means to turn back to a former or earlier state. For example, many older children who experience stress as a result of being hospitalized begin demonstrating behaviors from when they were younger, such as thumb-sucking or bedwetting.
- **Repression (suppression)** is the refusal to remember or think about a frightening or painful memory. A person may repress memories of an automobile accident or childhood abuse.

CAUSES AND TREATMENT OF MENTAL ILLNESS

There are many different types of mental illness, and many different causes. Some types of mental illness run in families (that is, they are inherited). Others result from chemical imbalances in the brain. In Chapter 28, you learned about chemicals called *neurotransmitters*. An imbalance in these chemicals can lead to some forms of mental illness. Finally, some mental illnesses may be caused by a person's environment. For example,

a person who is abused by a family member may develop ineffective coping or defense mechanisms that lead to mental illness.

Fortunately, many mental illnesses, just like many physical illnesses, can be successfully managed and treated with medications, psychiatric counseling, or both. The word *psychiatric* comes from the Greek words *psyche* (the soul) and *iatreia* (healing). A **psychiatrist** is a medical doctor trained in diagnosing and treating mental illness. A psychiatrist is allowed to prescribe medications. A **psychologist,** while not a medical doctor, has education and training that allows him to provide counseling services to help people with mental illness. A psychologist is not allowed to prescribe medications. Depending on the person's situation, he may need the services of a psychiatrist, a psychologist, or both. With treatment, many people with mental illnesses are able to lead happy, productive lives. Because many people with mental illnesses are at risk for committing **suicide** (taking their own lives, intentionally and voluntarily), diagnosis and treatment of mental illness is very important.

Treatment for mental illness has changed dramatically over the last 50 years. In the past, mentally ill people were usually sent to special hospitals ("mental institutions"), where they were given large doses of medications to keep them quiet and sedated. Techniques such as electro-shock therapy (passing electricity through the brain to cause a seizure) and lobotomy (surgical removal of part of the brain) were used frequently, often with little success. Now we know more about why mental illnesses occur and how they should be treated. For example, now that we know that moods and behaviors can be affected by chemical imbalances, we have developed new medications that help to restore the brain's chemical balance. Rather than simply sedating the person into submission, these new medications help the person to act and think more "normally." And electro-shock therapy, while still used in some cases, is used much more effectively.

TYPES OF MENTAL ILLNESS

Some of the more common mental illnesses include anxiety disorders, depression, bipolar disorder (manic depression), schizophrenia, and eating disorders. In this chapter, we will give you only a brief overview of these disorders. As you care for patients or residents who suffer from these mental illnesses (or others not discussed here), make an effort to learn more about their conditions. For example, you might ask the nurse if she can explain the person's condition to you more fully. The nurse may also be able to recommend articles or books for you to read to learn more about the person's condition. Increasing your knowledge about your patients' or residents' specific conditions allows you to better understand and care for them.

ANXIETY DISORDERS

Anxiety is a feeling of uneasiness, dread, apprehension, or worry. Anxiety is a normal feeling that we have in response to situations that are threatening to our body, lifestyle, values, or loved ones. A certain level of anxiety is normal and may actually lead us to do something positive about a bad or potentially dangerous situation. But too much anxiety or prolonged periods of anxiety can make it hard for us to function or cope with everyday situations. Feelings of anxiety can cause many physical signs and symptoms, such as sleeplessness, restlessness, fatigue, changes in appetite, or an increased heart rate and blood pressure. It is also common for an anxious person to be irritable and to have difficulty thinking clearly.

Although we all have experienced periods of increased anxiety, some people have periods of anxiety that continue to build until they can no longer function. Anxiety is a typical symptom in many common mental illnesses. However, in some mental illnesses, overwhelming anxiety is the key feature of the disorder. These mental illnesses are grouped under the general term *anxiety disorders*. Common anxiety disorders include panic disorder, obsessive-compulsive disorder, and phobias.

Panic Disorder

Panic is a sudden, overpowering fright. A person with a **panic disorder** has terrifying episodes or "panic attacks," during which she experiences sudden increases in anxiety and feelings of intense fear. A person who is having a "panic

FIGURE 35-5

People with panic disorder suffer from "panic attacks," which are characterized by feelings of intense fear and anxiety, accompanied by physical signs and symptoms such as chest pain and a rapid heart beat. (© *Chris Priest & Mark Clarke/Photo Researchers, Inc.*)

attack" usually also has physical signs and symptoms, such as chest or abdominal pain, a rapid heart beat, shortness of breath, and dizziness (Fig. 35-5). These symptoms may be very similar to those of a heart attack or other severe physical illness. Panic attacks can be very brief, or they may last for some time. Some people will experience these attacks rarely while others will have them quite often. It is important to remember that even though the physical symptoms may not be a sign of a serious physical condition, they are no less real and frightening to the person who is experiencing them.

Obsessive-Compulsive Disorder

Obsessive-compulsive disorder is an anxiety disorder that causes a person to suffer intensely from recurrent unwanted thoughts (*obsessions*). The obsessions are usually associated with rituals that the person cannot control (*compulsions*). The rituals may include actions such as hand-washing, counting, or checking, and are repeated over and over again in hopes that the obsessive thoughts will go away. Not performing the rituals increases a person's level of anxiety. When it is severe, obsessive-compulsive disorder takes over the person's life. The person becomes unable to perform the tasks that are associated with normal daily activities, because of his obsessions and compulsions.

Phobias

A **phobia** is an excessive, abnormal fear of an object or situation. Phobias can be incredibly disabling for the person affected by them. The person will do anything to avoid the thing she is afraid of, to the point where she may be unable to do something as simple as leaving the house. There are three main groups of phobias:

- *Simple phobias* are the most common type. A person with a simple phobia is abnormally afraid of a specific thing (for example, dogs, cats, insects, heights, water, or flying in an airplane).
- *Social phobias* involve a fear of being humiliated or embarrassed in front of other people. Social phobias may be related to feelings of inferiority and low self-esteem and may cause a person to drop out of school, avoid making friends, or remain unemployed.
- *Agoraphobia* is the fear of having a panic attack in a place from which there is no easy escape, or in a place where help is not available. For example, a person may be intensely afraid of having a panic attack in an elevator or on a crowded bus.

DEPRESSION

Depression is a feeling of excessive sadness or hopelessness. Many events in life, such as the loss of a loved one, can cause temporary feelings of intense sadness and hopelessness. In a person with good mental health, the painful emotions of an event-related depression (such as the loss of a loved one) go away over time. Sometimes, short-term treatment with medication or counseling may be needed to help the person through the crisis.

Some people, however, experience intense feelings of sadness and hopelessness that do not go away, even with time. These feelings may or may not be brought on by a sad event, such as the

FIGURE 35-6

Depression is common among older people. If you think that one of your patients or residents is depressed, you should report your suspicions to the nurse. (© *Conor Caffrey/Photo Researchers, Inc.*)

death of a loved one. When depression is severe and persistent, it is called *clinical depression*.

Clinical depression is one of the most common mental illnesses. It affects more than 19 million Americans each year. Some research indicates that a family history of clinical depression increases a person's risk of developing this mental illness. Women seem to experience clinical depression about twice as much as men do. Clinical depression is also the most frequently treated mental illness among elderly people (Fig. 35-6).

Several factors can lead to the development of clinical depression, including:

- Chemical imbalances in the brain
- Low self-esteem and poor coping skills
- Hormonal changes, such as those that affect women during pregnancy, menstruation, childbirth, and menopause
- Medications

A person who is depressed loses interest in activities that she usually finds pleasurable or fulfilling, such as eating, working, socializing with friends, and pursuing hobbies. The person may feel sad or anxious, and she may cry frequently. Many people who are depressed have problems with sleeping. The person may sleep too much, or not enough. The person may be restless or irritable. Instead of being grateful when someone tries to help, the person may become angry and defensive. The person may have feelings of guilt and worthlessness and struggle with thoughts of death or suicide. Physical complaints (for example, of pain or a digestive disorder) are also common among people who are depressed. Prompt treatment is needed to help a clinically depressed person return to an enjoyable, productive life.

The incidence of depression increases with age. Unfortunately, elderly people are less likely to seek treatment for this disorder. Many older people who are depressed feel that their depression is just part of getting older, and must be accepted. However, this is not the case. If you will be working with older patients or residents, pay attention to changes in their behaviors or moods that may indicate clinical depression. By reporting these observations to the nurse, you play an important role in helping to ensure that the person receives treatment that will help him feel better.

BIPOLAR DISORDER (MANIC DEPRESSION)

Bipolar disorder (manic depression) is a mental health disorder that causes mood swings. Periods of excessive happiness and excitement that may cause the person to engage in impulsive or reckless behavior (*mania*) are followed by periods of excessive sadness and hopelessness (*depression*). Experts believe that bipolar disorder is caused by chemical imbalances in the brain that affect a person's moods.

A person with bipolar disorder may have mood swings several times a day, or less frequently, with days or even weeks passing between episodes. Between mood swings, a person with bipolar disorder may have periods of "normal" mood. Bipolar disorder can be difficult to recognize and properly diagnose.

SCHIZOPHRENIA

Schizophrenia is a very disabling form of mental illness. It tends to run in families and may have a genetic basis. As with other mental illnesses, schizophrenia may be mild or severe. A person with severe schizophrenia that is untreated may be a danger to himself, or to others.

A person with schizophrenia has trouble determining what is real and what is imaginary. He may suffer from **delusions,** or false ideas. For example, the person may believe that he is someone famous or that someone is spying on him or trying to take his belongings. He may also experience **hallucinations,** or episodes where he sees, feels, hears, smells, or tastes something that does not really exist. For example, the person may hear voices in his head telling him to perform a certain act. The person's thinking and speech become disordered. He may switch from one topic to another during a conversation, or make up new words or patterns of speech. As a result of these symptoms, the person may say or do very strange things, making it hard for him to function normally in social situations. A schizophrenic person's behavior is often very frightening and confusing to others.

EATING DISORDERS

There are many different types of eating disorders. Two of the most commonly known types are anorexia nervosa and bulimia nervosa. No matter what the type, all eating disorders involve serious (and potentially fatal) changes in eating behavior, such as reducing the amount of food eaten to almost nothing, or severe overeating. Eating disorders cause many physical problems, including kidney failure and serious heart problems that can lead to death. Like people with other mental illnesses, people with eating disorders cannot voluntarily control their impulses, and they need treatment to help them learn to eat normally again.

Eating disorders usually start during adolescence or early adulthood. Women are at higher risk than men for developing an eating disorder. Many people who suffer from depression or anxiety disorders also suffer from eating disorders.

Anorexia Nervosa

People with **anorexia nervosa** see themselves as very overweight, even though they are excessively thin (Fig. 35-7). Anorexia (loss of appetite) is a key feature of this disorder. The person simply does not eat enough food. She will skip meals, take tiny portions at meal times, or make excuses for why she cannot eat. She may only allow herself to eat small amounts of very "safe" low-calorie foods. Many people with anorexia nervosa exercise excessively, in addition to severely reducing their food intake.

FIGURE 35-7

A person with anorexia nervosa has an intense and irrational fear of being overweight. Without treatment, many people with anorexia nervosa die. (© Oscar Burriel/Photo Researchers, Inc.)

Bulimia Nervosa

A person with **bulimia nervosa** regularly eats huge amounts of food (*binging*) and then induces vomiting or uses laxatives to rid the body of the food before it is digested (*purging*). A person with bulimia nervosa often is of normal weight for her age and height. However, like a person who suffers from anorexia nervosa, a person with bulimia nervosa is extremely focused on her body weight and shape, and believes that she is excessively overweight.

CARING FOR A PERSON WITH MENTAL ILLNESS

You may choose to work in a facility that specializes in the care of people with mental illnesses. Treatment facilities for people with mental health disorders differ in purpose. Some facilities care for mentally ill people who cannot function on their own and need assistance with activities of daily living (ADLs) and safety. These facilities provide a form of long-term care specifically for people with mental illnesses. Other facilities specialize in acute care services. These facilities provide care to a person who is experiencing a mental crisis that may result in attempted suicide, drug overdose, or danger to others. After the crisis phase has passed, the person may be able to return home and receive treatment on an outpatient basis. Outpatient mental health clinics see people on a regular basis and offer services such as counseling, medication, and support groups. They may even help the person to obtain education, job training, or employment.

Even if you do not choose to work in a facility that specializes in the care of people with mental illnesses, it is very likely that some of the patients or residents at the facility where you work will have or develop mental illnesses. The additional stress of illness or injury that brings a person to a health care facility could become the person's "breaking point," causing a mild mental illness to worsen. Remember all the new challenges that your patients or residents face when they enter a health care facility. They may have fears of being disabled or disfigured from illness or injury. The people you care for have been separated from loved ones and are now in unfamiliar surroundings. A lengthy illness can mean the loss of a job and income. Many people will have worries related to their current and future health. Any of these additional emotional stresses can push a person toward mental illness if he has poor or ineffective coping mechanisms.

In addition, many of the people cared for in health care facilities are elderly. Approximately 25% of elderly people in the United States have serious mental health problems. Of this 25%, approximately half are living in long-term care facilities, and approximately 10% have turned to alcohol abuse as a way of dealing with their stress. Most elderly people have successfully lived through many struggles and stresses during their lives and have developed excellent abilities to cope. However, some of the unique losses and challenges that an elderly person faces may overwhelm the person emotionally and promote mental illness (Fig. 35-8). For example:

- Elderly people face the loss of spouses, friends, and sometimes even adult children. Often, an elderly person has to face the death of several loved ones within a short period of time.
- Elderly people face retirement. Although many people view retiring from a job as an event to be celebrated, some people miss the structure, routine, and sense of identity that their jobs gave them. Retirement also

Death of a Husband/Wife
- Loss of companion
- Loss of sexual partner
- Emptiness, loneliness, grief
- Changes in responsibility
- Dependency on others

Retirement
- Loss of income
- Loss of purpose in life
- Loss of identity
- Loss of contact with others
- Loss of structure or schedule

Loss of Physical or Mental Ability
- Loss of independence
- Worries about "being a burden"
- Worries about future

Moving to a Long-Term Care Facility
- Loss of independence
- Loss of space
- Moving away from friends/ a familiar neighborhood

Death of Friend/Other Loved One
- Loss of companion
- Emptiness, loneliness, grief
- Worries about own health

FIGURE 35-8

As we age, we face very challenging life events. These additional stresses can put an elderly person at risk for clinical depression and other mental illnesses.

means that a person's income becomes fixed, which can lead to money worries.
- Elderly people face the loss of physical abilities and independence, either as a result of illness or the normal process of aging. As a result, many elderly people feel that they are a burden to their families. Others fear the need to move to a long-term care facility, because of the associated loss of independence.

LISTENING AND OBSERVING

Listening and observation skills are very important when you care for a person with mental illness. In some cases, your observations may lead to the diagnosis of a mental illness in one of your patients or residents. As noted earlier, the diagnosis and treatment of mental illness is very important. Not only might the person be suffering needlessly, she may be at high risk for committing suicide. The rate of suicide increases as a person ages and is highest among elderly white men, especially those who have lost their wives. Nearly 25% of all people who commit suicide are 65 years of age or older. As a nursing assistant, you may hear a person speak of "ending it all," or the person may wonder aloud "if anyone would

miss me if I were gone." Take comments like these seriously and tell the nurse immediately.

Sometimes a physical problem can cause a person to appear to be mentally ill. This is especially common in older people. Nervous system disorders, kidney disorders, and the effects of other chronic illnesses such as hypertension and diabetes may cause a person to seem depressed or anxious. The symptoms that accompany hypothyroidism and anemia are often mistaken for clinical depression. Early signs of dementia (see Chapter 36) can also be very similar to some types of mental illness. Infections, dehydration, and the side effects of many medications can also affect an elderly person's behavior. When you notice a change in a patient's or resident's behavior or mental status and report this change to the nurse, you are taking the first step toward making sure the person gets the help he needs. The health care team will work to determine the cause of the person's change in behavior, which will lead to prompt treatment. Never assume that your elderly patient or resident is just "entering his second childhood" or becoming senile. The person may have a serious mental or physical problem that needs to be treated.

If you work in a facility that specializes in caring for mentally ill people, special methods of recording and reporting may be used. Know what is expected of you and how to report and record according to facility policy. When reporting and recording subjective information about patients and residents with mental illnesses, be very careful to use the person's own words, and avoid adding your own opinions or judgments. This is especially important when caring for a person with mental illness because certain phrases or words may have special meaning for the person. To accurately gauge the person's mental status, the health care team will need to know exactly what the person said.

▶ *Tell the Nurse!*

There are many signs and symptoms of mental illness. Sometimes a physical problem or a medication will make a person show signs of mental illness. As a nursing assistant, you must know what types of behaviors and moods are "normal" for each patient or resident who is in your care. Watch for the subtle signs that something is not quite right and make sure to tell the nurse immediately if you notice any of the following in your patients or residents:

➡ Changes in appetite, such as eating too much, or not eating enough

➡ Changes in sleep patterns, such as sleeping too much, or not being able to sleep

➡ Restlessness, pacing, or unusual "handling" of objects such as bed linens

➡ Crying for long periods of time or crying frequently

➡ Loss of interest in daily activities that were previously enjoyed

➡ An inability to focus during a conversation, or an unwillingness to make conversation

➡ Fatigue or irritability

➡ Expressions of feelings of hopelessness or helplessness

ASSISTING WITH ACTIVITIES OF DAILY LIVING (ADLs)

Mental illness may affect a person's ability to eat, sleep, rest, or manage routine grooming and hygiene. People with mental illnesses will need different levels of assistance with their ADLs,

depending on the severity of their disorders. As always, help to promote the person's independence by allowing the person to provide as much of his self-care as possible. Because some mental illnesses affect a person's ability to think through the steps of routine care, you may need to gently remind the person of what step comes next. For instance, you may need to say, "OK, you're all dressed now . . . you just need to brush your teeth before we take our walk."

SUMMARY

▶ One of the main qualities of mental health is a state of emotional balance.
- Life causes stress, which can threaten our ability to maintain emotional balance.
- People who are mentally healthy are able to manage stress effectively. People who are mentally ill have trouble effectively coping with stress.
- Coping mechanisms and defense mechanisms help us to deal with stress.
  - Coping mechanisms are actions that a person does deliberately to manage stress, such as going to an exercise class or engaging in a hobby.
  - Defense mechanisms occur when the mind attempts to restore or maintain emotional balance in response to stress. Defense mechanisms often occur automatically, without conscious effort.

▶ A mental illness is a disorder that affects a person's mind, causing the person to act in unusual ways, experience emotional difficulties, or both.
- Mental illnesses may be temporary or permanent, and of varying severity.
- Mental illnesses may be caused by genetics, chemical imbalances in the brain, or a person's environment.
- Mental illnesses are typically treated using a combination of medication and psychiatric therapy.
- Mental illness places a person at risk for committing suicide. Therefore, diagnosis and treatment of mental illness is extremely important.

▶ Common mental illnesses include anxiety disorders, depression, bipolar disorder (manic depression), schizophrenia, and eating disorders.

- Anxiety disorders are characterized by overwhelming feelings of uneasiness, dread, apprehension, or worry. Specific anxiety disorders include panic disorder, obsessive-compulsive disorder, and phobias.
- Clinical depression is characterized by feelings of excessive sadness and hopelessness that do not go away with time.
- Bipolar disorder (manic depression) is a mental illness that causes mood swings. The person's mood varies between periods of mania (extreme highs) and depression (extreme lows).
- Schizophrenia is a mental illness that causes a person to have trouble determining what is real and what is imaginary. The person may have delusions and hallucinations.
- Eating disorders such as anorexia nervosa and bulimia nervosa are characterized by serious (and potentially fatal) changes in eating behavior, such as reducing the amount of food eaten to almost nothing, or severe overeating.

▶ Nursing assistants care for people with varying degrees of mental illness in all types of health care settings.

- The additional stress of illness or injury that brings a person to a health care facility may trigger the onset of mental illness, or make an existing mental illness worse.
- The unique losses and challenges that face the elderly may trigger a mental illness. For example, clinical depression is very common among elderly people.
- By using their observation and listening skills, nursing assistants are able to give the health care team important information about subtle changes in a person's behavior or mood. These observations help to ensure that the person receives prompt treatment.
- Learning more about specific mental illnesses and special ways of caring for people with these illnesses enables the nursing assistant to provide better care to affected patients and residents.

What did you learn?

Multiple Choice

Select the single best answer for each of the following questions.

1. Which physical sign or symptom can be caused by anxiety?
   a. Sleeplessness
   b. Fatigue
   c. Increased heart rate and blood pressure
   d. All of the above

2. What is depression?
   a. An overwhelming feeling of uneasiness, dread, apprehension, or worry
   b. An overwhelming feeling of sadness and hopelessness
   c. A sudden, overpowering fright
   d. Recurrent, unwanted thoughts

3. One of your residents insists that she is the Blessed Virgin Mary. What is your resident experiencing?
   a. A manic episode
   b. A hallucination
   c. A delusion
   d. A religious vision

4. You are caring for a resident who has schizophrenia. You know that when you are recording or reporting subjective information about this resident, you should:
   a. Report or record what the resident has said, using his own exact words
   b. Report or record your interpretation of what the resident has said, since the resident often says things that do not make much sense
   c. Report or record your own opinion about what the resident has said, in addition to reporting or recording the subjective information in the resident's own words
   d. Avoid reporting or recording any subjective information about this resident at all

5. One of your elderly residents, Mrs. Sigfried, has been acting strangely the last few days. She is refusing to eat, and she insists on sleeping all of the time. Why is it important for you to report your observations to the nurse immediately?
   a. Refusing to eat and extreme sleepiness are signs that death is approaching.
   b. Mrs. Sigfried's change in behavior could be caused by a physical or mental problem, and sharing your observations with the nurse will help Mrs. Sigfried to get the help she needs, sooner.
   c. Mrs. Sigfried is in violation of facility policy.
   d. Mrs. Siegfried is a danger to the other residents.

6. One of your residents tells you that he hears voices inside his head, telling him to contact aliens on another planet. What is this resident experiencing?
   a. The effects of doing too many drugs in the '70s
   b. Hallucinations
   c. Delusions
   d. Mania

7. Which one of the following is a negative way to manage stress?
   a. Smoking in moderation
   b. Taking an exercise class
   c. Taking a bubble bath
   d. Getting together with friends

Matching

Match each numbered item with its appropriate lettered description.

_____ **1.** Panic disorder

_____ **2.** Phobia

_____ **3.** Obsessive-compulsive disorder

_____ **4.** Schizophrenia

_____ **5.** Bipolar disorder (manic depression)

_____ **6.** Anorexia nervosa

_____ **7.** Bulimia nervosa

a. An eating disorder characterized by eating excessive amounts of food, and then vomiting it up or taking laxatives to remove the food from the body before it can be digested

b. An anxiety disorder characterized by an extreme, abnormal fear of an object or situation

c. A mental illness characterized by an inability to tell what is real from what is imaginary

d. An anxiety disorder characterized by recurrent unwanted thoughts and rituals that the person cannot control

e. An anxiety disorder characterized by sudden increases in anxiety, often accompanied by physical signs and symptoms such as a rapid heart beat and chest pain

f. An eating disorder characterized by an extremely reduced food intake

g. A mental illness characterized by mood swings, from extreme highs to extreme lows

Stop and think!

▶ Think about an elderly person whom you know well. What major life events has this person experienced in recent years? How did these events affect the person? What coping mechanisms did the person use to deal with the stress caused by these life events?

▶ You are a home health aide and you have been caring for a fairly new client, Mrs. Watkins, for the past 2 weeks. Mrs. Watkins has had a stroke, and needs assistance with many of her activities of daily living (ADLs). You are scheduled to visit the Watkins home daily. Lately, you have noticed that Mrs. Watkins' husband, Ralph, does not seem to be doing too well. He barely speaks to you any more. Most of the time, he just lies on the sofa, staring at the television set, drinking beer. You decide to share your concerns about Ralph with your supervisor at the agency. Why was this a smart thing to do?

▶ You work in a hospital. One patient on your floor is a 36-year-old woman named Anne who is receiving treatment and evaluation following her second failed suicide attempt. In your opinion, Anne has everything anyone could possibly want—a loving husband, two young children, and a comfortable lifestyle. You are finding it hard to understand why Anne wants to kill herself, and as a result, you are having a hard time feeling empathetic toward her. What are you forgetting?

36

Caring for People With Dementia

What will you learn?

Can you imagine what it would be like to know that there is something terribly wrong with your ability to remember or to think? For example, you are out to lunch with friends and when the check comes, you can't remember how to figure out the tip. Or you leave your house to go to the grocery store, a place you have been a thousand times before, and you can't remember how to get home. Or you can't remember the middle name of the person you have been married to for the last 40 years. For a person with dementia, a frightening experience like this is often the first sign that something is wrong. Dementia, which is caused by changes in the brain tissue, affects a person's ability to remember and think. As the disorder progresses, the person loses the ability to perform even the most basic tasks related to self-care. Dementia is devastating, both for the person who has it and for his or her family members.

More than 50% of the residents in long-term care facilities are there because they have dementia and are no longer able to care for themselves. In this chapter, you will learn about some of the types of dementia, and about the special care needs of people with dementia. When you are finished with this chapter, you will be able to:

1. Explain the difference between dementia and delirium.
2. Describe two major types and causes of dementia.
3. List and describe the stages of Alzheimer's disease, a common form of dementia.
4. Describe behaviors that are common in people with dementia.
5. Describe strategies for managing difficult behaviors in people with dementia.

(continued)

Photo: Dementia robs a person of her identity and sense of self.
(© Benelux Press/Index Stock Imagery.)

6. Describe special considerations that the nursing assistant must keep in mind while helping a person with dementia with activities of daily living (ADLs), such as bathing, eating, and toileting.

7. Describe special care measures that are taken to help maintain quality of life for a person with dementia.

8. Describe the effects of caring for a person with dementia on the caregiver, and strategies for coping.

Vocabulary

Use the CD in the back of your book to hear these terms pronounced, defined, and used in a sentence:

Dementia	Vascular (multi-infarct)	Catastrophic reaction	Reminiscence
Delirium	dementia	Sundowning	therapy
Alzheimer's disease	Perseveration	Validation therapy	

WHAT IS DEMENTIA?

Dementia is the permanent and progressive loss of the ability to think and remember, caused by damage to the brain tissue (Fig. 36-1). A person with dementia experiences the following:

- Problems with memory, especially short-term memory
- Difficulty putting thoughts together and understanding concepts
- Problems with judgment (the person is not able to make good decisions)
- Disorientation (the person is not oriented to person, place, or time)
- An inability to manage activities of daily living (ADLs)

In the early stages of dementia, the person is aware that his memory is lacking, and may take action to make up for, or cover, the memory loss. Disorientation becomes more evident as the disease progresses. The person may develop problems with language, and may act "out of character" or in socially inappropriate ways. The person loses the ability to recognize others and, eventually, the ability to remember his own identity. In the final stage of the disease, the person dies.

Dementia must not be confused with **delirium,** which is a temporary state of confusion. Delirium is a symptom of an underlying disorder, such as an infection. It may also be a side effect of medication.

Once the underlying disorder is treated or the medication is stopped, the delirium goes away. In some cases, the person may die if the underlying cause of the delirium is not identified and treated.

▶ *Tell the Nurse!*

As a nursing assistant, you may be the first to notice changes in a resident's behavior that may suggest delirium. If you notice any of the following in a person who is normally alert and oriented, report your observations to a nurse immediately:

▶ The person is hallucinating (seeing or hearing something that you know cannot possibly be true, such as mice crawling all over the bed)

▶ The person does not recognize someone familiar, or mistakes a stranger for a family member or close friend

▶ The person is very restless, especially at night

▶ The person seems confused

▶ The person talks frequently about events from the past, but cannot remember events that occurred recently (such as a meal eaten 2 hours ago)

▶ The person gets lost and wanders the halls aimlessly, even though the person knows his or her way around the facility

A   B

FIGURE 36-1

Dementia is the permanent and progressive loss of the ability to think and remember. (*A*) Brain scan of a healthy person. (*B*) Brain scan of a person with Alzheimer's disease, the most common type of dementia. The blue areas indicate areas where brain activity is lost. (*Alzheimer's Disease Education Referral Center, a service of the National Institute on Aging.*)

TYPES OF DEMENTIA

There are many different types of dementia (Table 36-1). In a person with advanced dementia, it is usually hard to tell exactly what type of dementia the person has, because people with all types of dementia show similar behaviors and have similar disabilities in the late stages of the disease. In many cases, the type of dementia is not known for sure until after the person dies and an autopsy is done. Two of the most common types of dementia are Alzheimer's disease and vascular (multi-infarct) dementia.

ALZHEIMER'S DISEASE

Alzheimer's disease is the most common type of dementia, accounting for more than 50% of cases of dementia. Approximately 4 million people in the United States have Alzheimer's disease. If no

TABLE 36-1 ■ Causes of Dementia		
Cause	Source of Damage to Brain Tissue	Course of Disease
Alzheimer's disease	Plaques and tangles (abnormal protein deposits in brain)	Slow, steady decline; death occurs 3 to 20+ years after diagnosis
Vascular (multi-infarct) dementia	Lack of blood flow to brain results in tissue death	Variable
Pick's disease	Atrophy (shrinking) of the neurons in the brain	Relatively rapid decline; death occurs within 4 years of diagnosis
Cruetzfeldt-Jacob disease ("mad cow disease")	Viral infection of brain tissue	Rapid decline; death occurs within 2 years of diagnosis
Huntington's chorea	Genetic defect	Slow, steady decline; death occurs (on average) 25 years after diagnosis
Parkinson's disease*	Neurotransmitter (dopamine) deficiency	Slow, steady decline
AIDS dementia (HIV encephalopathy)	AIDS-related infections and tumors	Onset variable, but may be abrupt; decline is rapid
Syphilitic dementia	Infection with the bacterium *Treponema pallidum* (tertiary syphilis)	Onset occurs many years after the initial infection; decline is slow

*Only about 20% of people with Parkinson's disease develop dementia, and then only during the later stages of the disease.

cure is found, it is estimated that around 14 million people will have the disease by the year 2050.

Alzheimer's disease occurs in 10% of people older than 65 years, and nearly 50% of people older than 85 years. However, people as young as 40 years may also get the disease. Alzheimer's disease is the fourth most common cause of death, after heart disease, cancer, and stroke. However, a person can live anywhere from 3 to 20 years or more after the disease is diagnosed.

Alzheimer's disease is named after Alois Alzheimer (1864–1915), a German doctor who discovered the disease in 1906. One of Dr. Alzheimer's patients, a 51-year-old woman, died after showing unusual mental changes and behaviors. To learn why these changes occurred, Dr. Alzheimer performed an autopsy on her brain. He found that certain areas of her brain seemed soft and shrunken. In addition, he saw abnormal deposits of protein, especially in the parts of the brain that function in memory. He called these abnormal deposits *plaques* and *tangles* (Fig. 36-2).

Although we do not know exactly what causes Alzheimer's disease, scientists have a number of theories. One of the leading theories is that Alzheimer's disease can be caused by an abnormality in a person's genes. The abnormal gene causes the body to start producing the abnormal protein that forms plaques and tangles. The plaques and tangles interfere with the way that nerves inside of the brain communicate with each other. Another theory is that exposure to toxins, such as aluminum and mercury, may play a role in the development of Alzheimer's disease.

A person with Alzheimer's disease passes through a number of stages (Table 36-2). Most people with Alzheimer's disease are cared for by family members during the early stages of the disease. However, as the disease progresses, many people with Alzheimer's disease must move to a long-term care facility because they become very difficult to care for. The person needs more and more assistance with basic activities, such as bathing and toileting. In addition, the disease can cause the person to behave in disruptive or annoying ways, which can place a great deal of emotional stress on the caregiver. The emotional pain suffered by a person with Alzheimer's disease, as well as her family members, is immeasurable (Fig. 36-3).

VASCULAR (MULTI-INFARCT) DEMENTIA

Damage to the blood vessels that supply the brain can affect the delivery of oxygen to the brain tissue, and may contribute to the onset of vascular (multi-infarct) dementia. In **vascular (multi-infarct) dementia,** mental functions are lost because multiple areas of the brain tissue die due to lack of adequate oxygen and nutrients. (Recall that an infarction is death of tissue due to lack of oxygen and nutrients.) Vascular dementia is thought to be the cause of dementia in approximately 20%–25% of people with dementia.

Vascular dementia most often affects people between the ages of 55 and 75 years, most commonly occurring in people who are about 70 years old. It is more common in men than in women. Conditions that put a person at risk for developing vascular dementia include:

- A history of myocardial infarction (heart attack)
- Hypertension (high blood pressure)
- Diabetes mellitus
- Peripheral vascular disease
- Transient ischemic attacks (TIAs)
- Obesity
- Smoking
- High blood cholesterol levels

Symptoms may appear suddenly and they may vary from person to person, depending on which areas of the brain are affected. Like

Normal brain neuron   Plaques and tangles
                           of Alzheimer's disease

FIGURE 36-2

Protein deposits, called plaques and tangles, are found in the brains of people with Alzheimer's disease.

TABLE 36-2 ■ Stages of Alzheimer's Disease	
Stage	Description
1	The person's ability to think and remember is normal.
2	The person is forgetful, but not abnormally so. For example, the person may forget where she has put common objects, such as car keys.
3	The person begins to have trouble doing complex tasks, especially in social settings or at work (for example, calculating the tip on a restaurant check). Other people may begin to notice that the person is having trouble with memory or mental tasks.
4	The person's ability to do complex tasks, such as manage bills or travel alone, continues to decline. The person's confusion increases, and he is less aware of current events.
5	The person now needs help with dressing, although she can manage eating and toileting without help. The person is often disoriented to time and place, and has trouble remembering the names of familiar people.
6	The person's short-term memory is gone. The person is unaware of her surroundings, and cannot tell you what year it is, or even what season of the year it is. The person may forget the name of close family members, such as a spouse or children. The person's personality may change, and she may begin to behave differently, often in challenging ways. The person loses the ability to manage bathing and toileting independently, and may become incontinent of urine or feces.
7	The person loses the ability to walk and sit independently. He is no longer able to speak, swallow, or smile. The person becomes totally incontinent of urine and feces. The person dies.

Alzheimer's disease, vascular dementia is irreversible and incurable. Keeping the person's blood pressure, blood glucose, and blood cholesterol levels within normal limits can help to slow the progression of the dementia.

BEHAVIORS ASSOCIATED WITH DEMENTIA

People with dementia often show a wide range of behaviors, especially as the dementia progresses. Some of these behaviors can be dangerous for the person, such as the tendency to wander. Others are not dangerous, but they can be very annoying to caregivers or other residents. Many of these behaviors occur because of changes in the brain caused by the disease. When you are caring for a person with dementia, you will come to know the behaviors that are "normal" for that person. A change in a person's "normal" behavior is a cause for concern. Remember that as the dementia progresses, the person loses the ability to communicate effectively. A change in the person's behavior may be a sign that the person is trying to tell you something. For example, the person may have an acute physical problem, such as a bladder infection, pain, dehydration, or constipation.

FIGURE 36-3

The emotional pain suffered by a person with dementia, as well as his or her family members, is immeasurable.

TYPES OF BEHAVIORS

Common behaviors in people with dementia include the following.

Wandering

People with dementia may stray away from home. When this occurs, it is very dangerous because the person is confused and disoriented. The person might get lost, walk into the path of an oncoming car, or drown in a body of water, such as a lake or river. Depending on the weather and climate, the person may not be dressed appropriately to be outside. For example, if it is raining or cold, the person may not have a coat.

Because this tendency to wander cannot be stopped, many long-term care facilities have developed ways to allow residents to wander safely. Many facilities have outside courtyards with high fencing, which allow the resident to wander outside while still keeping her within the safe environment of the facility (Fig. 36-4). A resident who tends to wander may also wear a bracelet or an anklet that will set off an alarm if the resident tries to leave the facility through a doorway that leads to an unsafe area. When the alarm sounds, staff members are alerted and can guide the person back to safety.

Pacing

A person with dementia may pace back and forth. Often, the person is pacing because he has a physical need that is not being met. For example, the person may be hungry or need to use the bathroom. A person might also pace in response to a noisy, overstimulating environment, or because he is feeling scared or lost. If one of your residents is pacing, try to figure out what is causing the behavior, and take steps to relieve the cause of the behavior. Sometimes there is nothing to do but to let the person pace. In this case, you might take the person to a safe place (for example, a fenced-in garden) and walk alongside him or her until the behavior has run its course.

FIGURE 36-4

Wandering and pacing are two very common behaviors in people with dementia. Many long-term care facilities that specialize in the care of people with dementia have enclosed areas outdoors where people can wander and pace safely.

Repetition

A person with dementia may do the same thing over and over again. This is called **perseveration.** For example, the person might repeat the same phrase or question constantly. Or she might constantly move a piece of cloth around on a coffee table, as if dusting. Although these behaviors are usually not physically harmful to the person, they can be a sign that the person is bored. These behaviors can also be very annoying to caregivers and other residents. Distracting the person by offering to take her for a walk, or by getting her involved in an activity such as looking through a magazine, may help to break the cycle.

Rummaging

A person with dementia may go through drawers or closets, searching for an item that he is never able to find. If you notice that a resident is rummaging, ask the person what he is trying to find, and offer help in finding it. If the person tends to rummage through other residents' belongings or every single drawer in his own dresser, it may be necessary to make certain areas "off-limits" by locking them. You can then show the person a special drawer or a box filled with small personal items that he can rummage through.

Delusions and Hallucinations

A person with dementia may think that she is someone she is not, such as the Queen of England. Thoughts like these are called *delusions.* If one of your residents is delusional, do not try to correct the person. This will only upset her, because she honestly does believe that she is the Queen of England. It would be like someone telling you that you are not who you think you are! Instead, just try to redirect the conversation. For example, you might say, "Tell me about your day" or "Would you like to take a walk now?"

Hallucinations are also common in people with dementia. A *hallucination* is seeing, hearing, tasting, or smelling something that is not really there. For example, a person with dementia may tell you that there is a cat in the hallway or insects on the bed. If a person is hallucinating, reassure the person. For example, you might tell the person that you will ask the cat to leave, or go through the motion of sweeping the bugs off the bed. Then, gently redirect the person's attention.

Agitation

People with dementia often become very upset and excited. When a person with dementia is agitated, he may pace, shout, or strike out at caregivers or other residents. Remember that people with dementia often lose the ability to communicate effectively with others, so they express themselves through behavior (Fig. 36-5). Many things can cause agitation, including pain or an infection, an unmet physical need (for example, hunger, a full bladder, or lack of sleep), or a noisy environment.

Catastrophic Reactions

A person with dementia may over-react to something that would cause a healthy person minimal or no stress. This is called a **catastrophic reaction.** For example, a person with dementia may become very agitated or begin to scream or sob loudly when you try to give him a bath. Catastrophic reactions often occur when the person feels threatened. For example, the person may feel that his privacy is being threatened when you attempt to give him a bath. Feeling overwhelmed can also cause a person to have a catastrophic reaction. For example, a ringing telephone in a room where the television is on and people are talking might be too much for a person with dementia to handle.

Sundowning

Sundowning is the worsening of a person's behavioral symptoms in the late afternoon and evening, as the sun goes down. For example, the person may become more agitated, restless, and confused in the evening hours, and may have trouble getting to sleep.

No one knows for sure exactly why sundowning behavior occurs. Some people think that it might be brought on by fatigue, especially if the person frequently wanders, paces, or engages in other repetitive behavior of a physical nature. Helping to ensure periods of quiet and rest during the day might help to reduce fatigue, in turn reducing sundowning. Another theory is that sundowning occurs because the person cannot see as well in the evening hours, when the sun starts to go down. Not being able to see well can increase the person's confusion and agitation. Turning on lights earlier in the evening may help to prevent or reduce sundowning behavior.

Inappropriate Sexual Behaviors

A person with dementia may attempt to get into bed with a resident who is not her spouse. Sometimes the person will begin to masturbate or undress in a public area, such as the dining room. These behaviors occur because the person is disoriented to person, place, and time.

You must take measures to stop inappropriate sexual behaviors, especially if the person is making unwelcome sexual advances toward another person. Gently, but firmly, lead the person back to her room and redirect the person's attention by introducing another activity. Although OBRA specifically says that a resident of a long-term care facility must be allowed to fulfill her sexual needs with another consenting resident, another resident with dementia is not able to give that consent. Therefore, you have a responsibility to protect all of the residents of the facility from unwelcome sexual advances.

FIGURE 36-5

People with dementia often lose the ability to communicate effectively with others, so they express themselves through behavior. Agitation is often a sign that a physical or emotional need is not being met.

MANAGING DIFFICULT BEHAVIORS

Many of the behaviors demonstrated by people with dementia can be very trying to deal with on an ongoing basis. Try to remember that the person with dementia does not want to act this way and cannot help it. He is not behaving this way to be difficult or annoying. Often, there is some physical or emotional reason for the behavior (Box 36-1).

In many cases, finding the underlying cause of the behavior and addressing it causes the behavior to stop, providing relief to you and the person. Also, remember, in a person with dementia, a change in the person's behavior might be the first and only sign of a medical problem. For example, a problem such as a urinary tract infection can cause a person with dementia who is normally pleasant and calm to become agitated and strike out at a caregiver. Therefore, it is important to try and determine the cause of the behavior, rather than just accepting it as a normal part of the person's disease process.

When caring for a person with dementia who is demonstrating a particular behavior, you must use your observation skills to try and answer the following questions:

- **What** is the behavior? Describe the behavior in as much detail as possible.
- **Whom** is the behavior associated with? For example, does the person act this way only in the presence of certain people?
- **When** does the behavior occur?
- **Where** does the behavior occur?

BOX 36-1 Situations That Can Cause Dementia-Related Behaviors

- The person is in a room that is too large or too small.
- The person is in a room that is overstimulating (cluttered, noisy, or decorated with fabrics and wallpapers with "busy" patterns).
- The person is in a place that is new or unfamiliar (for example, the person is hospitalized for treatment of an acute problem).
- The person is being asked to do something that is too complicated, has too many steps, or is unfamiliar.
- The person is trying to express a physical or emotional need.

Having answers to these questions can help you to answer the biggest question of all: "Why is the behavior happening?" Once you have a few ideas about what is causing the behavior, you can try doing different things to see if the person's behavior improves. For example, if you suspect that the person is acting a certain way because she is hungry or needs to use the bathroom, you can try offering a snack or taking the person to the restroom. If you observe that the room is noisy and there is a lot of activity, you might try taking the person to a quieter place. If you suspect that the person is behaving in a certain way because he has a medical problem or is in pain, report your suspicions to the nurse so that the nurse can investigate further. Knowing your resident is the key to stopping (and sometimes preventing) difficult behaviors.

The way that you interact with a person with dementia can also affect the person's behavior. Many years ago, caregivers used a technique called *reality orientation* with people with dementia. Reality orientation was based on the idea that it is important to bring the person back to the "here and now" by constantly orienting the person to time, place, people, and things. If the person was given enough information to stay on track, then he could be brought back to the present. We now know that although reality orientation is useful for people who are experiencing temporary confusion that is reversible and treatable (that is, delirium), it is not an effective technique to use with a person who has dementia. People with dementia often cannot remember what they have been told just a few minutes earlier. Because of this, attempting to orient the person to reality can embarrass the person and increase her irritation and agitation.

Now, caregivers use a technique called **validation therapy** with people with dementia (Table 36-3). Validation therapy stresses the importance of acknowledging the person's reality. Rather than correcting the person, you attempt to distract the person and redirect the conversation whenever possible. For example, you might change the course of the conversation by encouraging the person to talk about things from her past. Pay special attention to the words, phrases, and body language that the person uses, so that you can better understand what the person is trying to communicate. What the person is saying may seem like nonsense to you, but there may be

TABLE 36-3 ■ Reality Orientation Versus Validation Therapy

Example	Reality Orientation Approach	Validation Therapy Approach
Mrs. Rivera is trying to leave the facility. She is very agitated. She keeps repeating that she needs to go home to take care of her mother.	Nursing assistant: "Don't you remember? Your mother died 20 years ago. You are staying here with us." Mrs. Rivera's agitation increases. She may continue to insist on going home, or begin to grieve her mother's death.	Nursing assistant: "You want to go home to see your mother. Aren't mothers wonderful? Here, sit down and tell me about your mother." Mrs. Rivera is diverted from wanting to go home. She happily sits down with the nursing assistant to discuss mothers.
Dr. Carroll, a retired family doctor, believes that he needs to leave the facility and go to the hospital to deliver babies and make rounds on his patients.	Nursing assistant: "I'm sorry. Don't you remember that you are retired? You live here in the nursing home with us now. We can't let you leave because you might get lost or hurt." Dr. Carroll becomes agitated because what the nursing assistant is saying does not match his current reality.	Nursing assistant (leading Dr. Carroll to the nurse's station): "I bet we can find you a nurse who would love to have you make rounds with her and see the patients here." Dr. Carroll is diverted while still thinking that he has some value as a doctor.

important meaning behind the words. Validation therapy protects the feelings of the person with dementia. It also helps the caregiver to understand what the person with dementia is experiencing.

CARING FOR A PERSON WITH DEMENTIA

As a person's dementia progresses, he will need more and more help with all activities of daily living (ADLs). In addition to physical needs, the person will have emotional needs that must be met as well. General guidelines for caring for a person with dementia are given in Guidelines Box 36-1.

MEETING THE PHYSICAL NEEDS OF A PERSON WITH DEMENTIA

For a person with dementia, everyday activities such as bathing, dressing, eating, and using the bathroom can be very challenging. The person cannot remember how to do these things, and as a result, may become very frustrated. Sometimes the person will resist doing what you need her to do.

When you are helping a person with dementia with her ADLs, there are several general things you can do to make the task at hand go more smoothly:

- **Speak clearly, in a calm tone of voice.** Also, consider gently resting one of your hands on the person's arm or hand. Many people with dementia respond positively to touch (Fig. 36-6).
- **Remind the person at each step what she needs to do next.** The person may be able to complete tasks such as dressing, shaving, or brushing the teeth with your guidance. Allowing a person to complete tasks independently for as long as possible is important for the person's self-esteem.
- **Use hand gestures in addition to spoken instructions.** For example, if you are trying to get the person to sit down at the table and eat, pat the seat of the chair as you ask the person to come sit down.
- **Plan for the procedure in advance.** "Getting ready" steps are always important, but especially so when you are caring for a person with dementia. Many routine procedures, such as bathing, are very stressful for a person with dementia. Being prepared and having everything you need before you begin a procedure will allow you to accomplish the task as quickly as possible, which can help to reduce the amount of stress the person feels.

GUIDELINES BOX 36-1
GUIDELINES FOR CARING FOR A PERSON WITH DEMENTIA

What you do	Why you do it
Maintain a calm, structured environment.	A person with dementia can become overwhelmed very easily. When the person becomes overwhelmed, difficult or dangerous behaviors such as wandering, agitation, or a catastrophic reaction are likely to increase.
Approach the person with dementia slowly, announcing yourself before touching him.	Many people with dementia also have hearing problems, vision problems, or both. If you approach quickly without warning, you may startle the person, triggering a catastrophic reaction.
Avoid arguing or disagreeing with the person.	A person with dementia exists in a different reality from the rest of the world. Trying to force the person with dementia to understand or acknowledge anything other than her own reality will increase the person's agitation.
When asking a person with dementia to do something, use short words and short sentences. Avoid negatively worded instructions (such as, "Don't put that there!"). Avoid instructions that require the person to remember more than one action at a time.	Because a person with dementia has problems with short-term memory, he will not be able to remember or process long words and sentences. A positively worded command ("Please put that here") is easier to understand than a negative one. Failing at a task increases the person's frustration. When you give the person instructions in a way that she can understand, you increase the person's chances of successfully completing the task.
Give a person with dementia enough time to respond to questions and directions.	It may take the person a while to think of the word or words he needs to answer your question, or the actions he must take to follow your directions. Feeling rushed can cause the person to become agitated or upset.
"Listen" to the person by paying attention to body language. Make good use of your observation skills.	As a person's dementia gets worse, she loses the ability to communicate effectively. Often, body language and behaviors become the person's main way of expressing herself.
When managing difficult behaviors, be aware that solutions that work today may not work tomorrow. Be creative, and do not give up.	Dementia is a progressive disease. Therefore, the person's abilities, disabilities, and needs change over time, and your approaches to managing difficult behaviors may also need to change.
Help the person with dementia to feel secure and loved by showing affection (kind words, a gentle touch) and smiling.	Like all people, people with dementia have emotional needs that must be met.
Allow the person with dementia to do as much as he can for himself, for as long as possible.	This is important for maintaining the person's dignity and self-esteem. No one likes to feel helpless or useless.
Help the person to maintain independence for as long as possible by using visual cues to orient the person to place and time. For example, place	Using visual cues can help the person to maintain his independence longer, which is important for the person's self-esteem.

(continued)

GUIDELINES BOX 36-1 (Continued)
GUIDELINES FOR CARING FOR A PERSON WITH DEMENTIA

What you do	*Why you do it*
a large-faced clock in the person's room, decorate for the holidays, and post names and other reminder signs in prominent, meaningful places. (For example, if a person keeps trying to walk out the front door, apply a big, red and white "stop" sign to the inside of the door.)	
Help the person to exercise her mind by getting the person involved in activities that relate to the person's former interests and experiences.	Participating in activities helps to prevent boredom and increases the person's sense of purpose and accomplishment.
Protect the person from physical injury.	People with dementia often become clumsy as a result of their disease, which increases their risk of falling. In addition, they lose the ability to make good decisions related to their well-being. For example, a person with dementia might walk in front of an oncoming car, leave the house without a coat in the middle of a snowstorm, or drink the contents of a bottle found under the sink.
Maintain the person's hygiene and good grooming habits.	This is important for the person's health as well as for her self-esteem.
Be as tolerant as possible of the person.	The person's behaviors are a result of his dementia, and are beyond the person's control. The person is not purposely trying to frustrate or annoy you.
When you become tired and frustrated, take time out, be good to yourself, and share your feelings with the nurse. Know that these emotions and thoughts are normal.	Caring for a person with dementia is emotionally draining and physically difficult. If you do not take measures to protect your own mental health, you run the risk of "burn-out." In addition, you place the resident at risk for abuse, should you lose your temper.

- **Keep to a regular schedule.** A person with dementia responds best to a very structured environment. To a person with dementia, the world is very confusing. Structuring the person's world as much as possible, by following an established routine, can reduce the person's confusion and fear.

Assisting with Bathing

Bath time can be a very frightening time for a person with dementia. The person may not remember what a bath or shower is, or why he needs to take one. The sound of running water, the bright lights, and the shiny surfaces in the tub room can be very upsetting. Being naked makes the person feel exposed and vulnerable. The person may be very afraid of falling.

As a result, the person may become agitated when you tell him that it is "time to take a bath." If this is the case, try to avoid the word "bath." Instead, say "Let's go freshen up" or "It's time for an activity you will enjoy." If the person seems very agitated, you might try singing to the person. Singing can have a very calming effect on people with dementia.

Bath time will generally go more smoothly if you prepare the tub room in advance. Make sure

FIGURE 36-6
Many people with dementia respond well to touch.

that the room is warm, and fill the tub ahead of time so that the person does not become frightened by the sound of the running water. Put a folded towel on the shower chair for comfort. Allow the person to wear his robe as long as possible, and consider draping a bath blanket or towel over the person's shoulders while he is bathing (Fig. 36-7). The bath blanket or towel will make the person feel less exposed and it will also provide some warmth. Hand the person a washcloth and let the person assist as much as possible.

Assisting with Dressing

Many people with dementia have trouble selecting an outfit to wear. They often want to wear the same clothes every day. Limiting the number of outfits the person has to choose from and asking family members to purchase several identical outfits for the person can help to solve these problems.

For a person with dementia, putting on and fastening clothing can also be very difficult. To help make dressing less frustrating for the person, select articles of clothing that are simple, rather than complex. For example, a shirt that pulls over the head is easier to manage than a shirt that buttons up the front. Pants with elastic waistbands are easier to manage than pants with zippers and buttons.

Assisting with Eating

You might find that it is difficult to get a person with dementia to focus on eating at meal times. The person may forget why she is at the table, or become distracted by others at the table. A quiet setting and limited food choices can help. Many times, the person will not recognize eating utensils, or she will forget how to use them. You may have to remind the person how to eat by placing your hand over the person's hand. Together, you bring the fork or spoon with the bite of food to the person's mouth (Fig. 36-8). Make sure that the person is swallowing the food after chewing it. People with dementia often have a tendency to chew and then pack the food in the cheeks, increasing the risk of choking. If the person cannot focus long enough to eat a proper meal, try offering the person "finger foods" such as sandwiches, cut-up vegetables or fruit, or a stuffed baked potato. A plastic cup with a lid and a straw or a spout can help to ensure that the person drinks enough fluids.

FIGURE 36-7
Bath time can be very frightening for a person with dementia. Making every effort to maintain the person's modesty is important.

FIGURE 36-8
You may have to remind a person with dementia how to eat.

People in the advanced stages of dementia eventually lose the ability to eat independently. When we eat, the tongue pushes the food to the back of the throat so that we can swallow it. People with advanced dementia often "forget" how to do this. Most of the food placed in the mouth of a person with advanced dementia just comes right back out again. Because a person with advanced dementia loses the ability to use his tongue to move food to the back of the throat, sometimes a special syringe with a nozzle-shaped tip is used for feeding instead of a spoon (Fig. 36-9). The food is semi-liquid and the syringe is used to place the food further back in the mouth so that the person can swallow it more easily. The food is given slowly in small amounts to prevent choking. Using a feeding syringe may allow the person with advanced dementia to continue taking food by mouth for a longer period of time, instead of through a feeding tube. Feeding tubes can be very uncomfortable. Some facilities consider this feeding technique to be outside the nursing assistant's scope of practice, so before using a syringe to feed a person, check with the nurse.

Assisting with Elimination

Elimination can present many problems for the person with dementia. The person may forget where the bathroom is, or fail to recognize the toilet. Sometimes, the person will have an accident because he is unable to move the necessary clothing out of the way fast enough. Taking the person to the bathroom on a regular schedule (for example, every 2 hours) can help, as can helping the person to select clothing with fasteners that are easy to manage. If a person suddenly seems to be having a lot of accidents, report this to the nurse. The person may have a medical problem, such as a urinary tract infection, that needs to be addressed.

MEETING THE EMOTIONAL NEEDS OF A PERSON WITH DEMENTIA

Helping a person with dementia to meet his emotional needs is just as important as helping the person to meet his physical needs. Just like everyone else, a person with dementia needs to feel loved and needed. Several approaches are taken to help meet the emotional needs of a person with dementia, including reminiscence therapy and activity therapy.

Reminiscence Therapy

To *reminisce* means to remember. In **reminiscence therapy,** the person with dementia is encouraged to remember and share experiences from his past with others (Fig. 36-10). For example, if a person with dementia insists that she

FIGURE 36-9

A feeding syringe is sometimes used instead of a spoon to feed people in the advanced stages of dementia.

FIGURE 36-10

Reminiscence therapy increases a person's self-esteem and happiness by encouraging him to remember the past. (*Courtesy of Copper Ridge.*)

needs to go see her mother (who has been dead for years), you might say, "What does your mother look like?" or "Tell me about a favorite food that your mother used to make when you were growing up." Talking about the past diverts the person's attention and increases her self-esteem. Reminiscence therapy can be used in a "one-on-one" setting, or in a group setting. When done in a group setting, reminiscence therapy gives the person a chance to socialize with other residents.

Activity Therapy

People with dementia, like all people, need to exercise their minds. Even though a person with dementia is confused, he still can become bored. In fact, boredom may be an underlying cause of some difficult behaviors, such as wandering or rummaging. Activities are so important to a resident's well-being that many facilities display a large calendar with daily planned activities on the wall (Fig. 36-11A). Engaging in activities helps the person to feel useful and gives him a sense of purpose and accomplishment.

Activities may be planned for a group of residents, or just for one resident (see Fig. 36-11B). There are many different types of activities that a person with dementia can enjoy:

- Creative activities (flower arranging, painting, baking)
- Intellectual activities (looking at a book of photographs, reading the newspaper aloud together, attending a play)
- Social activities (hosting a tea party, going on a picnic)
- Physical activities (taking a walk, participating in a group exercise class)

When planning an activity, take care to choose one that relates to the former interests and abilities of the person or people who will be participating in it. For a group activity, assign tasks according to each resident's abilities and interests. For example:

Debra, a nursing assistant, works in a facility that specializes in providing care to people with dementia. Debra is responsible for planning one special activity a week for a group of residents. This week, she decides that she, Mr. Pitt, Mrs. Winger, and Mrs. Kemp will make fruit smoothies and then share them with some of the other residents. Debra knows that both Mrs. Winger and Mrs. Kemp used to enjoy baking for their families, so she asks Mrs. Winger to peel the bananas and Mrs. Kemp to measure the orange juice. Mr. Pitt worked for years as a bartender, so once all of the ingredients are in the blender, Debra asks Mr. Pitt to turn the blender on, and then to help her pour the drinks into cups to serve to the other residents.

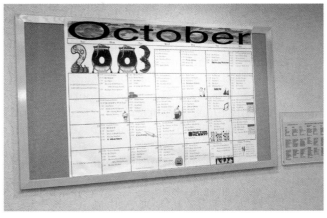

A

FIGURE 36-11

Activity therapy is an important part of caring for people with dementia. (*A*) Many facilities keep a large calendar so that residents can see the activities that are planned for each day. (*B*) Activities can be planned for an individual or for a group of residents. (*B courtesy of Copper Ridge.*)

B

Debra's activity was successful because she considered the special interests and talents of each of the residents who would be participating in it. Planning the activity in advance, gathering all necessary supplies, and having a back-up plan "just in case" are other things that a nursing assistant can do to help ensure success when planning an activity for residents.

Incorporating music into a planned activity can be very beneficial for people with dementia. Research has shown that when we listen to music we enjoy, our heart and respiratory rates slow, and our blood pressure becomes lower. In this way, music can calm an agitated person. Activities that involve holiday music, religious music, or music from a certain time period (for example, 1940s big band music) may be particularly appealing to residents with dementia.

EFFECTS ON THE CAREGIVER OF CARING FOR THE PERSON WITH DEMENTIA

Caring for people with dementia is very important work. The difference you make in the life of the person with dementia, as well as those of her family members, is significant. However, caring for a person with dementia can take its toll on you, physically and emotionally.

- A person with dementia is prone to outbursts of anger, and can become agitated very easily. Therefore, it is likely that on any given day, you may be cursed at, spit on, slapped, hit, scratched, or pinched. Because you will most likely develop a fondness for the residents in your care, it can be very difficult when a resident has a "bad day" and that affection is not returned!
- Many of the behaviors of people with dementia can be very annoying, because they are repetitious. It is not always easy to figure out what you can do to make the behavior stop, and until a solution is found, the behavior can really try your patience.
- Caring for a person is hard physical work. As the dementia progresses, the person becomes completely dependent. Exhaustion and fatigue can put you on edge, making it difficult for you to keep your emotions in check.

If you feel yourself becoming overwhelmed by your responsibilities or a particular situation, take a deep breath and remind yourself that a person with dementia cannot be held responsible for her actions. If you still feel angry, make sure that the person is safe and walk away. Ask a coworker or the nurse for help with the person. Sometimes you may need to ask to be assigned to another resident for a while. If your frustration or anger moves you to the point of actually causing a resident physical harm, you will lose your job (as well as all chances of future employment in the health care field). You may even be punished by a court of law for abuse. Remember, a member of the health care team is particularly at risk for becoming abusive when the resident is "difficult" or hard to manage, and the relationship is a long-term relationship. When you become tired and frustrated, take time out, be good to yourself, and share your feelings with the nurse. To provide the best care to your residents, you need to care for yourself.

SUMMARY

▶ Dementia is the permanent and progressive loss of the ability to think and remember, caused by damage to the brain tissue.
  - There are several types and causes of dementia. Two of the most common types are Alzheimer's disease and vascular (multi-infarct) dementia. Currently, there is no cure for dementia.
  - Dementia must not be confused with delirium, which is confusion in a person who is normally alert and oriented. Delirium goes away when the underlying cause is treated.
▶ A person with dementia often shows a wide range of behaviors, especially as the dementia progresses.
  - A change in a person's behavior is often a sign that the person has a physical or emotional need that is not being met.
  - Nursing assistants use their observation skills to try and figure out the underlying cause of the person's behavior. If the cause can be determined, then actions can be taken to stop the behavior.

■ The way that you interact with a person with dementia can affect the person's behavior. Try to understand what is "real" for the person with dementia, and do not try to correct the person. This technique of communicating is called *validation therapy.*

▶ A person with dementia has physical and emotional needs that must be met.

■ As the person's dementia gets worse, he needs more and more help with activities such as eating, bathing, dressing, and toileting.

■ Reminiscence therapy and activity therapy are used to help meet the emotional needs of the person with dementia.

▶ Caring for a person with dementia is very demanding, yet very important, work. Dementia is a terrible disease that is devastating both to the person who has it, as well as his family members.

What did you learn?

Multiple Choice

Select the single best answer for each of the following questions.

1. Which one of the following is experienced by a person with dementia?
   a. Problems with memory, especially short-term memory
   b. Confusion and disorientation
   c. An inability to manage activities of daily living (ADLs)
   d. All of the above

2. When caring for a person with dementia, it is helpful to:
   a. Be understanding and see the person's behaviors as part of the disease
   b. Take the same approach with every resident
   c. Correct the person to bring him or her back to the "here and now"
   d. Avoid acknowledging your own feelings

3. When communicating with a person with dementia, what is the best approach to take?
   a. Speak loudly and quickly to get the person's attention
   b. Speak clearly, in a calm tone of voice
   c. Avoid touching the person or using hand gestures
   d. Avoid talking about the past

4. Which statement about validation therapy is true?
   a. Validation therapy stresses the importance of bringing the person with dementia back to the "here and now."
   b. Validation therapy is based on the belief that people with dementia are able to return to the present, if given enough information to do so.
   c. Validation therapy stresses the importance of acknowledging the person's reality.
   d. Validation therapy encourages the caregiver to correct the person, to help the person to stay on track.

5. A person with dementia may show which one of the following behaviors?
   a. Pacing and wandering
   b. Hallucinations
   c. Agitation
   d. All of the above

6. Which statement about reality orientation is true?
   a. Reality orientation helps a person with dementia to remember the past, which might be less painful than thinking about the "here and now."
   b. Reality orientation suggests that when we interact with someone with dementia, we pay special attention to the words, phrases, and statements that the person uses to understand what the person is trying to express.
   c. Reality orientation ties past memories to the present and helps bring the person back to the current time.
   d. Reality orientation is useful for people who are temporarily confused but not permanently impaired.

7. What is sundowning?
   a. Increased confusion, restlessness, and insecurity that occurs late in the day, as it becomes darker outside
   b. Aimless wandering after dark
   c. Worry and increased suspicion
   d. Crying inconsolably for a long time

8. Mr. Greene, one of the residents in your care, has Alzheimer's disease. For the last hour, Mr. Greene has been folding and unfolding a piece of paper, and he is showing no signs of stopping. What should you do?
   a. Let him keep doing it; perseveration is a normal behavior in a person with dementia.
   b. Try to distract Mr. Greene by starting a new activity with him, such as reading the newspaper together or going for a walk.
   c. Tell the nurse; she will be able to give Mr. Greene a sedative to make the behavior stop.
   d. Tell Mr. Greene firmly that the behavior is unacceptable and it must stop, immediately.

9. What is a catastrophic reaction?
   a. A response to a situation that is more extreme than would normally be expected
   b. An abnormal protein deposit that is found in the brains of people with Alzheimer's disease

c. The belief that you are someone you are not (for example, the President of the United States)

d. The reaction family members have on learning that a loved one has Alzheimer's disease

10. When helping a person with dementia with her activities of daily living (ADLs), such as bathing, eating, and dressing, what should you remember?

a. Keep to an established routine as much as possible

b. Prepare for the procedure ahead of time

c. Many ADLs are very frightening or frustrating for the person with dementia

d. All of the above

Stop and think!

▶ You work in a nursing home. Mrs. Wallingford, one of your residents, has Alzheimer's disease. As a younger woman, Mrs. Wallingford was a concert pianist. She came from a well-to-do family and always was a proper lady. Now, Mrs. Wallingford is missing from the facility! You find her in the corner bar, playing pool with the guys in her nightgown. Her safety is at risk and her dignity is being compromised. You need to get her back to the nursing home. What approach would you take with Mrs. Wallingford? What would you say or do to get Mrs. Wallingford to come back to the facility with you?

▶ You work in a facility that specializes in providing care to people with dementia. Each nursing assistant is responsible for planning one special group activity a week for a small group of residents. This week, the residents who will be in your group are Mrs. Darden, Mrs. Stahl, Mr. Roberts, and Mrs. Holly. You know that both Mrs. Darden and Mr. Roberts used to be avid gardeners. Mrs. Holly used to run a catering service with her husband. And Mrs. Stahl always took great pleasure in hosting parties for friends and family. What sort of activity might you plan that would appeal to the residents in your group? What steps would you take to make sure that the activity was a success?

▶ You work in a long-term care facility. One day, you go to the room of one of your residents, Mrs. Craven, to answer her call light. When you enter the room, Mrs. Craven cries out to you in a frightened voice, "Get them out of here! Get them out of here now!" You don't know what she is talking about—you don't see anybody or anything in the room. You ask Mrs. Craven to explain what she means, and she tells you that there are spiders crawling all over the walls. Normally, Mrs. Craven is alert and oriented, but today, she definitely seems "out of it." What do you think is wrong with Mrs. Craven? What should you do?

▶ Mrs. Rowan has Alzheimer's disease. You have cared for Mrs. Rowan for a long time and know pretty much what to expect from her in terms of behavior. Although she does tend to pace and to rummage quite frequently, she is usually calm and pleasant. Today in the dining room, however, when you are trying to help Mrs. Rowan eat lunch, she becomes angry and strikes out at you. What might be the explanation for this behavior?

37

Caring for People With Cancer

What will you learn?

Cancer is the second leading cause of death in the United States. Only heart disease kills more people in this country each year. However, it is important to remember that many people who are diagnosed with cancer survive it, especially when the cancer is diagnosed and treated early. As a nursing assistant, you will play an important role in making sure that changes in a patient or resident that might be early signs of cancer are reported to the nurse promptly. In addition, you will almost certainly care for people who have already been diagnosed with cancer and are receiving treatment for it, or who are waiting to find out if they have cancer. In this chapter, you will learn more about cancer, how it is diagnosed, and how it is treated. You will also learn about the special physical and emotional needs of people with cancer. When you are finished with this chapter, you will be able to:

1. Describe the difference between benign and malignant tumors.
2. List the common causes of cancer.
3. Describe the seven warning signs of cancer.
4. List some common types of cancer.
5. Describe how early detection and treatment affects the outcome of a cancer diagnosis.
6. List and explain the types of treatment used for people with cancer.
7. Describe some of the side effects of cancer treatment, and discuss how a nursing assistant can help a person who is experiencing these side effects feel more comfortable.
8. Discuss how cancer affects a person emotionally and how a nursing assistant can provide holistic care.

Photo: A nursing assistant talks with a patient who is receiving chemotherapy to treat cancer. A common side effect of chemotherapy is hair loss.
(© M. Moreland/Custom Medical Stock Photo.)

Vocabulary

Use the CD in the back of your book to hear these terms pronounced, defined, and used in a sentence:

Tumor	Chemotherapy
Benign	Radiation therapy
Malignant	Stomatitis
Metastasis	Prognosis
Biopsy	

WHAT IS CANCER?

The word *cancer* comes from the Greek word *karkinos,* or "crab." Indeed, cancers are "crab-like," with a central body and arms that reach out into the surrounding tissues (Fig. 37-1). The central body is a mass of abnormal cells, called a tumor. A **tumor** is simply an abnormal growth of tissue. All tumors are not necessarily cancer.

Tumors that are not cancerous are called benign. (*Benign* means "kind.") A **benign** tumor is made of abnormal cells that tend to stay together, without spreading into surrounding tissues. In addition, benign tumors tend to grow slowly, because their cells do not divide rapidly. Many benign tumors are easily treated, because they are slow-growing and their cells tend to stay together.

However, an untreated benign tumor can enlarge and press on vital organs, which can cause serious problems (or even death), depending on the organs that are affected.

Cancerous tumors are called malignant. (*Malignant* means "evil.") A **malignant** tumor is made up of abnormal cells that do not function properly. Malignant cells divide rapidly and invade nearby healthy tissue. Malignant cells can also travel through the bloodstream to other parts of the body, where they "take root" and start a new cancerous tumor. The process by which cancer cells spread from their original location in the body to a new location (which may be quite distant from the first) is called **metastasis** (Fig. 37-2). Death from cancer almost always results from metastasis. The cancer simply takes over the body.

TYPES OF CANCER

It is estimated that 200 different types of cancer can affect the human body. All organ systems can be affected by cancer. Some cancers are very rare, while others are quite common. Common cancers that you may have heard of include skin cancer, lung cancer, breast cancer, brain cancer, colon cancer, ovarian cancer, prostate cancer, leukemia, and lymphoma. Cancer can occur at any age, but 67% of cancer deaths occur in people older than

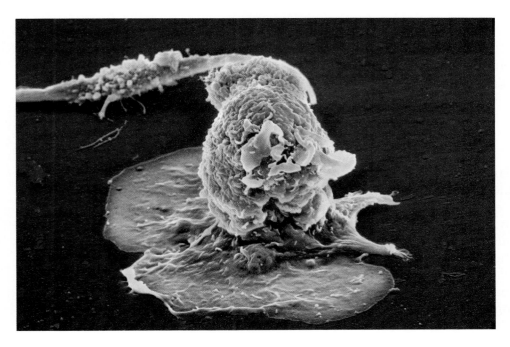

FIGURE 37-1

Cancerous tumors have the ability to send crab-like arms of cancerous cells into the surrounding tissue. This is a scanning electron micrograph (SEM) of a breast cancer cell. Color has been added to the photograph to make the cancer cell stand out. (© *Biophoto Associates/Photo Researchers, Inc.*)

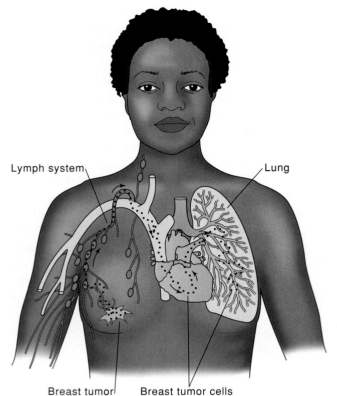

FIGURE 37-2

Metastasis is the process by which malignant cells spread to other parts of the body, or metastasize. A common example of metastasis is when a woman with breast cancer also develops lung cancer. First, the malignant cells of the breast tissue gain access to the lymphatic system, which empties into the bloodstream. The malignant cells are pumped, along with the blood, through the right side of the heart. Some of the malignant cells are deposited in the tiny blood vessels in the lungs, where they begin to multiply and grow, forming a new tumor.

65 years. The most common cancers seen in elderly people are breast, lung, prostate, and colon cancer.

CAUSES OF CANCER

There has been much research into what causes cancer and why some people get cancer and others do not. At present, the exact cause of cancer is still unknown. Currently, researchers believe that whether or not a person develops cancer may be related to a combination of many factors, including:

- **Inheritance.** Some cancers seem to "run in families." For example, a woman with a mother or sister who has breast cancer is more likely to develop breast cancer herself. This suggests that genetics may play a role in whether or not a person develops cancer.
- **Environmental factors.** What we are exposed to on a daily basis also seems to play a role in the development of cancer. For example, a person who smokes or spends a lot of time around people who smoke is more likely to develop lung cancer than a person who is not exposed to tobacco smoke. Some people work in jobs or live in places that expose them to cancer-causing agents (*carcinogens*), such as radiation, asbestos, chemicals, and pollution.
- **Lifestyle.** Factors such as a person's diet and the amount of time he or she spends exercising have been shown to play a role in the person's risk for developing cancer. For example, diets that contain lots of fruit and vegetables are known to lower a person's risk for many cancers, whereas diets that are high in fat increase a person's risk for some cancers. Similarly, exercising on a regular basis can lower a person's risk for developing cancer, while not exercising can increase the person's cancer risk.

The American Cancer Society (ACS) reports that approximately one third of the deaths caused by cancer in the United States are the result of smoking, and another third are related to dietary habits. Eating a healthy diet, exercising, and avoiding smoking and job-related carcinogens are important steps that people can take to lower their risk of developing cancer.

DETECTION OF CANCER

Early detection of cancer can lead to early treatment, which greatly improves a person's chances of surviving the disease. Many cancers are caught in their early stages when a person notices alarming signs and symptoms and makes an appointment with a health care provider to "get checked out." For example, a person may feel an odd lump, or notice blood in the stool. Other cancers are caught in their early stages through routine physical examinations and screening tests.

WARNING SIGNS OF CANCER

Our bodies are very good at letting us know when something is not quite right. A person who has cancer may experience one or more of the following early warning signs. These warning signs can be remembered by thinking of the word **CAUTION:**

Change in bowel or bladder habits. A person with colon cancer may have diarrhea or constipation, or he may notice that the stool has become smaller in diameter. A person with bladder or kidney cancer may have urinary frequency and urgency.

A sore that does not heal. Small, scaly patches on the skin that bleed or do not heal may be a sign of skin cancer. A sore in the mouth that does not heal can indicate oral cancer.

Unusual bleeding or discharge. Blood in the stool is often the first sign of colon cancer. Similarly, blood in the urine is usually the first sign of bladder or kidney cancer. Postmenopausal bleeding (bleeding after menopause) may be a sign of uterine cancer.

Thickenings or lumps. Enlargement of the lymph nodes or glands (such as the thyroid gland) can be an early sign of cancer. Breast and testicular cancers may also present as a lump.

Indigestion or difficulty in swallowing. Cancers of the digestive system, including those of the esophagus, stomach, pancreas, and biliary system, may cause indigestion, heartburn, or difficulty swallowing.

Obvious change in a wart or mole. Moles or other skin lesions that change in shape, size, or color should be reported (Fig. 37-3).

Nagging or persistent cough or hoarseness. Cancers of the respiratory tract, including lung cancer and laryngeal cancer, may cause a cough that does not go away or a hoarse (rough) voice.

A sudden, unexplained weight loss can also be a sign of cancer. Unfortunately, many people recognize these early warning signs of cancer but put off making an appointment with a health care provider because they are embarrassed or scared. As a nursing assistant, you may be the first to notice that a patient or resident has an early warning sign of cancer. Reporting your concerns to the nurse immediately can lead to early detection and treatment. Early detection and treatment plays a very important role in preventing deaths due to cancer.

ROUTINE PHYSICAL EXAMINATIONS AND SCREENING TESTS

Many cancers are detected during routine physical examinations, or by screening tests that are done on a regular basis. Examples of screening tests include mammograms (used to detect breast cancer), Pap smears (used to detect cervical cancer), and fecal occult blood tests (used to detect colon cancer). These tests can help to

A   B   C

FIGURE 37-3

Moles that change in appearance or bleed, have jagged borders, display two or more colors (for example, brown, black, pink, gray, or white), or are larger than a pencil eraser may be malignant melanoma. Malignant melanoma is the most lethal type of skin cancer, accounting for 4% of deaths from cancer overall. (*Photographs courtesy of Goodheart, H. P. [2003]. Goodheart's photoguide of common skin disorders: Diagnosis and management [pp. 325, 354]. Philadelphia: Lippincott Williams & Wilkins.*)

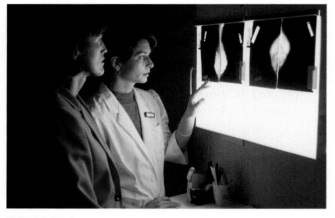

FIGURE 37-4

A doctor reviews the results of a routine mammogram with a patient. Routine screening tests, such as mammograms, are helpful for detecting cancer in its very early stages. (© *K. Beebe/ Custom Medical Stock Photo.*)

detect cancer long before the person develops noticeable signs or symptoms of the disease (Fig. 37-4). The early detection of cancer allows the tumor to be removed before it has time to spread (metastasize) to nearby tissues or other organs.

If physical examination or screening tests reveal that a person might have cancer, the doctor may order additional studies or exploratory surgery (surgery that is performed when a person is thought to have a significant medical problem but the doctors do not know exactly how bad the problem is or exactly what is causing it). As a nursing assistant, you may need to help prepare a patient or resident for surgery or other diagnostic tests that will be performed to determine if cancer is present. Examples of additional studies that may be ordered for a person who might have cancer include the following (Fig. 37-5).

- **Imaging studies,** such as x-rays, computed tomography (CT) scans, and magnetic resonance imaging (MRI) scans, allow the doctor to see the tumor without actually entering the body (see Fig. 37-5A).
- **Endoscopic studies** involve using a special lighted instrument to look inside the body and obtain tissue or fluids for analysis (see Fig. 37-5B). Examples of endoscopic studies that you read about in Unit 5 include

A

B

C

FIGURE 37-5

As a nursing assistant, you may need to help prepare a patient or resident for studies that are done to diagnose cancer. (*A*) Radiologic imaging studies, such as magnetic resonance imaging (MRI) scans, allow the doctor to see the tumor without actually entering the person's body. (*B*) Endoscopic studies, such as colonoscopy, involve passing a lighted instrument through an opening in the body to view the inside of a structure. (*C*) In a needle biopsy, cells are removed from the body so that they can be examined under a microscope for abnormalities. Here, a surgeon is performing a needle biopsy to check for breast cancer. (*A* © *R. Gould/Custom Medical Stock Photo; B* © *Antonia Reeve/Photo Researchers, Inc.; C* © *Daiwei/Custom Medical Stock Photo.*)

bronchoscopy (when a scope is passed into the lungs through the mouth), gastroscopy (when a scope is passed into the stomach through the mouth), and colonoscopy (when a scope is passed into the large intestine through the anus).

- **Biopsy** is the surgical removal of cells or a small piece of tissue for microscopic examination (see Fig. 37-5C). Biopsy is done to determine if cells are cancerous, and to determine exactly what type of cancer is present.

TREATMENT OF CANCER

There are three main approaches to treating cancer (Fig. 37-6). The approach used depends on the type of cancer and the extent to which the cancer has spread to other tissues and organs. Treatment methods may be used alone or in combination with each other, depending on the type and extent of the cancer.

- **Surgery** involves cutting away the tumor and surrounding tissue to remove the cancer and stop the spread of the disease (see Fig. 37-6A). Many cancer surgeries alter the person's physical appearance significantly. For example, a woman with breast cancer may lose one or both breasts. A person with bone cancer may lose all or part of an arm or leg. A person with colon cancer may need to use an ostomy appliance for the rest of his life. Although it is a relief to have the cancer gone, the person must still deal emotionally with the change in his or her appearance.
- **Chemotherapy** involves the use of medications (chemical agents) to destroy the cancer cells (see Fig. 37-6B). There are many different chemotherapy drugs available now, each for specific types of cancer. Chemotherapy is often used in

A

B

C

FIGURE 37-6

The three main approaches to treating cancer are (*A*) surgery, (*B*) chemotherapy, and (*C*) radiation therapy. Doctors may choose to use these methods alone or in combination, depending on the type and extent of the cancer. (*A* © *St. Bartholomew's Hospital/ Photo Researchers, Inc.; B and C © Bradford/Custom Medical Stock Photo.*)

FIGURE 37-7

Hair loss (alopecia) is a common side effect of cancer chemotherapy. Many people who have lost their hair temporarily as a result of chemotherapy find that wearing an attractive hat or scarf helps them to feel more confident about their appearance. (© *Colin Cuthbert/Photo Researchers, Inc.*)

combination with surgery to help destroy any malignant cells that the surgery may not have removed completely. Alopecia (the loss of hair) may accompany chemotherapy. Chemotherapy works by killing cells that divide rapidly, such as cancer cells. Unfortunately, some types of normal cells in the body also divide rapidly, such as the cells in the hair follicles. This is why people who are receiving chemotherapy often lose their hair. Many people, especially women, may be very self-conscious about their hair loss. These people may find that wearing a hat or a scarf helps them to feel more confident about their appearance (Fig. 37-7).

- **Radiation therapy** involves the use of powerful x-ray beams to destroy the cancer cells (see Fig. 37-6C). The beams are directed at the tumor to destroy the cells. Sometimes tiny pellets that contain radiation are placed inside the tumor so that the cells are destroyed from the inside. This is a common method of treating prostate cancer—radioactive pellets are placed inside the prostate gland with a needle-like instrument to destroy the cancerous cells.

Surgery, chemotherapy, and radiation may be either *curative* or *palliative*. When a treatment is performed with the goal of curing the person of cancer by completely removing the cancerous cells from the body, the treatment is said to be *curative*. However, sometimes the cancer cannot be cured. When this is the case, the goal of treatment is to make the person as comfortable as possible until death occurs. This sort of treatment is referred to as *palliative* (see Chapter 21, Figure 21-4). Examples of palliative cancer treatments include surgery to bypass an obstruction caused by a tumor and chemotherapy or radiation to shrink a large tumor that is pressing on an organ and causing pain.

CARING FOR A PERSON WITH CANCER

Many of us know someone who has had cancer. In fact, the experience of losing someone to cancer, or of witnessing someone's recovery from cancer, may be what inspired you to become a nursing assistant in the first place. Like all patients and residents, those with cancer have special physical and emotional needs that must be met.

MEETING THE PHYSICAL NEEDS OF A PERSON WITH CANCER

People with cancer have special physical needs that are directly related to the cancer, the treatment, or both. Cancer can be very painful. The pain may be temporary, related to surgery or radiation treatment. Or it may be chronic, related to the cancer itself. In addition, many of the treatments used for cancer have unpleasant side effects. As a nursing assistant, you will play an important role in helping your patients or residents who have cancer to manage their pain and deal with the unpleasant side effects of treatment.

Managing Pain

Pain control is an essential part of the treatment for a person with cancer. Advanced cancerous tumors often cause severe pain that can only be relieved by the regular use of strong pain medications. Report any observations that suggest that a patient or resident is in pain, or any complaints that the person may have of pain, to a nurse promptly. (See Chapter 29 for a complete discussion of pain, and the nursing assistant's role in detecting it and helping to control it.) As a nursing assistant, you will also need to be aware of and look for side effects of pain medication, such as constipation. The discomfort from the constipation alone may be as bad as the tumor pain. Recall what you learned in Chapter 20 about the measures you can take to help prevent your patients or residents from becoming constipated. And if one of your patients or residents does become constipated, do not hesitate to tell the nurse.

Managing Side Effects of Treatment

The treatments used for cancer, especially chemotherapy and radiation therapy, may have severe side effects:

- **Digestive problems.** Nausea, vomiting, anorexia (loss of appetite), and diarrhea are common with chemotherapy and radiation treatments. Patients or residents who are having digestive problems as a result of cancer treatment will appreciate frequent mouth care. In addition, you can offer ice chips to prevent the person from becoming dehydrated. Many people are able to tolerate ice chips when nothing else will stay down. If a person is able to tolerate some foods or liquids and has an appetite for something special, try to accommodate the person's request.
- **Skin problems.** People who are receiving radiation therapy may develop irritation and burning where the skin is exposed to the treatment rays. Skin breakdown can be prevented with gentle, thorough skin care.
- **Mouth problems.** People who are having chemotherapy may develop **stomatitis** (inflammation of the mouth). Sores in the mouth may be very painful and cause discomfort during eating. Offering the person drinks that are blended with ice, ice cream, yogurt, and fruit may be very soothing and provide much-needed nutrition at the same time. Frequent, gentle oral care is necessary to prevent infection. A special mouthwash or spray may be used to numb the inside of the person's mouth before providing oral care.
- **Fatigue.** People who are receiving cancer treatment may be very tired, all of the time. Mild exercise combined with periods of rest is necessary to maintain muscle strength.
- **Increased risk for infection.** Some cancer treatments temporarily interfere with the body's ability to fight off infections. People who are having these treatments will be at high risk for getting contagious illnesses, such as colds or the flu. In addition, if they do get a cold or the flu, it is very likely that it could turn into something more serious, such as pneumonia. For this reason, you must be very careful to protect patients or residents with lowered immunity from contact with other people who have a contagious illness.

➧ *Tell the Nurse!*

When caring for a person who has cancer, be sure to report any of the following observations to the nurse immediately:

➧ The person has severe nausea, vomiting, or both

➧ The person has pain or sores in the mouth

➧ The person's skin is red or irritated in areas

➧ The person has an unusual discharge or bleeding from the vagina, urethra, or rectum

➧ The person complains of pain, or shows body language that suggests he is in pain

➧ The person has diarrhea or is constipated

➧ The person has redness, swelling, or pain around an intravenous (IV) or venous access site

➧ The person has a fever or other signs of infection

MEETING THE EMOTIONAL NEEDS OF A PERSON WITH CANCER

A person who is awaiting test results or who has just been diagnosed with cancer will have many emotional needs. The word *cancer* is very frightening to many people, because the disease is so often associated with death. However, a diagnosis of cancer is not necessarily a "death sentence."

Many types of cancer can be successfully treated. Still, many people are very anxious about their prognosis, especially right after the cancer is diagnosed. A **prognosis** is the doctor's prediction of the course of a disease, and his estimation of the person's chances of recovering from it.

A person who has cancer may have many other fears as well. For example, the person may fear the side effects of treatment. Or he may worry about how his body will look during treatment or following surgery. The person may be afraid of experiencing a great deal of pain as a result of the cancer or treatment. The person may worry that even if the cancer is treated successfully now, it may return later in life.

If one of your patients or residents has been diagnosed with cancer, be sure to check in on the person as often as you check in on your other patients or residents. Spend time with the person. Many nursing assistants are uncomfortable with the subject of cancer, and as a result may avoid a person with cancer without even being aware that they are doing so. You might be afraid that you "won't know what to say." Remember, caring for a person with cancer does not require you to say anything—the person will be comforted just by the fact that you are there and willing to listen.

Often, people with cancer find comfort in their spiritual beliefs and practices. The person may request visits from clergy members. Time spent in prayer, reading religious texts, meditation, and listening to spiritual music may be very comforting to the person. Provide privacy for the person during these times, and make sure you relay any requests for clergy visits to the nurse so that the appropriate calls can be made, according to facility policy.

A person who has cancer may need to decide among several different treatment options. Sometimes, the person will have to decide whether she even wants to go ahead with treatment. Some people may choose to have every type of treatment available. Others may choose to skip treatment, even if it means a chance for longer survival. You must always remember that each patient or resident has the right to choose. The reasons behind treatment choices are unique and specific for each individual person. Although one choice may be right for one person, a different choice will be the right one for another. To truly provide holistic care to a person with cancer, you must respect the person's decisions and choices concerning treatment. You do not have to necessarily agree with your patients' or residents' choices, but you must respect what they have decided to do. Use your listening skills to show the person that you care. Allow the person to verbalize his fears and feelings without adding your own opinion as to whether you think the person is doing the right thing or not. When you respect the decisions of the people you provide care for and support them emotionally, you demonstrate true compassion and caring.

SUMMARY

▶ A tumor, or mass of abnormal cells, may be *malignant* (cancerous) or *benign* (not cancerous). The cells that make up malignant tumors divide rapidly and spread into nearby tissues. They can also enter the bloodstream and spread to distant organs, a process called *metastasis.*

▶ Early detection of cancer can lead to early treatment, which greatly improves a person's chances of surviving the disease.
  ■ The nature of your duties as a nursing assistant will put you in an ideal position to observe changes in a patient or resident that may be early warning signs of cancer.
  ■ Many cancers are detected at an early stage through routine physical examinations or screening tests. If the doctor suspects cancer, he or she might recommend follow-up tests (such as radiologic studies, endoscopic studies, or biopsy).

▶ The three main approaches to treating cancer are surgery, chemotherapy, and radiation therapy.
  ■ These approaches may be used alone or in combination, depending on the type of cancer and whether it has spread.
  ■ Treatment may be curative or palliative. The goal of curative treatment is to rid the body of the disease. The goal of palliative treatment is to keep the person comfortable when the disease cannot be cured.
  ■ Cancer treatment can be associated with unpleasant side effects, including hair loss (alopecia), nausea, vomiting, diarrhea, loss of appetite (anorexia), mouth sores

(stomatitis), skin breakdown, lowered immunity, and fatigue.

- A person with cancer often faces many treatment choices, including the choice of not having treatment at all. It is important to respect the person's choice, even if you do not agree with it.

▶ A patient or resident with cancer requires holistic care, just as any other patient or resident does. Nursing assistants must take steps to prevent their own discomfort with the subject of cancer from compromising their ability to care for their patients or residents with the disease.

- A person with cancer has many physical needs that are directly related to the cancer, or to its treatment. Nursing assistants play an important role in helping the person with cancer to manage pain and deal with unpleasant side effects of cancer therapy.

- A person with cancer will need assistance to meet emotional and spiritual needs as well. Often, the best thing a nursing assistant can do is listen if the person wants to talk, or spend quiet time with the person if he or she does not want to talk.

What did you learn?

Multiple Choice

Select the single best answer for each of the following questions.

1. Which one of the following statements best describes a malignant (cancerous) tumor?
   a. It consists of abnormal cells that divide rapidly and are capable of spreading to nearby tissues and distant organs.
   b. It consists of abnormal cells that divide slowly and tend to stay together.
   c. All tumors are malignant.
   d. All malignant tumors are fatal.

2. Which one of the following factors plays a role in whether or not a person develops cancer?
   a. Inheritance (genes)
   b. Lifestyle choices, such as diet and exercise
   c. Environment
   d. All of the above

3. Mrs. Worthington is receiving chemotherapy following surgery to remove a malignant tumor. Following each treatment, she is very nauseous, and often she vomits. What could you do to help Mrs. Worthington feel better?
   a. Offer her strong pain medications
   b. Offer her ice chips, and sit with her and hold her hand
   c. Enter her room only when necessary to avoid disturbing her
   d. Serve her meal tray as usual, in hopes that the smell of the food will increase her appetite

Matching

Match each numbered item with its appropriate lettered description.

_____ 1. Alopecia

_____ 2. Stomatitis

_____ 3. Biopsy

_____ 4. Metastasis

_____ 5. Palliative

_____ 6. Tumor

_____ 7. Prognosis

a. Surgical removal of cells or tissue for examination under a microscope
b. Treatment done with the goal of reducing pain and discomfort, not curing the disease
c. Loss of hair
d. The doctor's prediction of the course of a person's disease, and the person's chance of recovering from it
e. Inflammation of the mouth
f. The spread of malignant cells to other parts of the body
g. Abnormal growth of tissue

? Stop and think!

▶ You are caring for Mr. Lukens, a resident who was recently diagnosed with cancer. The doctors have presented Mr. Lukens and his family with a number of different treatment options, and for the last few days, Mr. Lukens has been weighing the pros and cons of each. In addition, he is still trying to adjust to the diagnosis he has just been given, and what it means for his future. One morning, while you are making Mr. Lukens' bed, he starts to talk to you about his father, who died of cancer after going through several months of agonizing treatments. He tells you that he is scared that he, too, will go through the treatments and in the end, all of his suffering might be for nothing. "Maybe it would just be easier to give up now and die peacefully," he says. How would you react to what Mr. Lukens is telling you? Is there anything you can do or say that might help Mr. Lukens with the difficult choices he needs to make?

38

Caring for People With AIDS

What will you learn?

In 1981, two doctors in Los Angeles noticed something strange. Five young men, all previously healthy, had been treated for a rare form of pneumonia that was usually only seen in people whose immune systems were severely damaged. Because this was so strange, the doctors reported what they had found to the Centers for Disease Control and Prevention (CDC) in Atlanta, which ran a brief article in its newsletter that summer about their findings. Soon, the CDC started to receive reports of other strange occurrences from doctors around the country. For example, doctors began to report seeing more cases of a rare skin cancer called Kaposi's sarcoma. The patients who were being diagnosed with Kaposi's sarcoma tended to be young men, instead of older men, and their form of the disease seemed much more severe than any previously seen. Doctors began to suspect that maybe these unusual cases of Kaposi's sarcoma and pneumonia were related in some way, especially when they noticed that most of the patients with these rare disorders were either homosexual men, intravenous drug users, or people who had required frequent blood transfusions in the past. This is how the disease that came to be known as acquired immunodeficiency syndrome (AIDS) was "discovered" in the early 1980s.

In Chapter 8, you learned how human immunodeficiency virus (HIV), the virus that causes AIDS, is transmitted. You also learned about measures you can take to protect yourself from HIV infection in the workplace, and about how HIV takes over the body's immune system, eventually leading to the condition known as AIDS. In this chapter, you will learn more about AIDS, and how it affects the

(continued)

Photo: The AIDS memorial quilt contains more than 44,000 panels. Each panel memorializes a person who died from AIDS. (© Jeff Greenberg/Index Stock Imagery.)

people who have it, physically and emotionally. When you are finished with this chapter, you will be able to:

1. List common symptoms of HIV infection.
2. Describe how AIDS affects a person physically.
3. Discuss who is at risk for HIV infection and AIDS.
4. Discuss legal concerns related to caring for people with HIV and AIDS.
5. Describe how AIDS affects a person emotionally.
6. Recognize the importance of the nursing assistant's responsibility to provide for the physical and emotional needs of the person with HIV and AIDS.

Vocabulary

Use the CD in the back of your book to hear this term pronounced, defined, and used in a sentence:

HIV-positive

WHAT IS AIDS?

Currently, more than 800,000 people in the United States are infected with HIV. A person who is infected with HIV is said to be **HIV-positive,** because he or she has tested positive on the blood test for HIV antibodies. HIV invades a person's white blood cells. In doing so, the virus destroys the very cells that are responsible for protecting the body. As HIV takes over the body's immune system, the infected person begins to have more and more health problems, such as severe infections and aggressive cancers. Most HIV-positive people eventually develop AIDS, an advanced stage of HIV infection. AIDS is said to occur when the person's battered immune system is no longer able to fight off infections and malignancies. People with AIDS do not die from the virus that has infected their bodies. Rather, they die from infections and malignancies that the body is no longer able to fight.

Most people who become infected with HIV experience a brief, flu-like illness about 2 to 4 weeks after they are first exposed to the virus. During this brief illness, the person may have a fever, swollen lymph nodes, a sore throat, a rash, or any combination of these signs and symptoms. These signs and symptoms eventually go away, and may be forgotten. In many cases, if the person is tested for the virus within the next 3 to 6 months, the test will not be positive, even though the person is infected with the virus. A person can be infected with HIV for many years before developing AIDS, or he may never develop AIDS. The amount of time that it takes before AIDS develops and death occurs varies greatly from person to person. For example, in children and people in poor health, HIV infection is likely to progress to AIDS more quickly. As HIV infection progresses, the person is likely to experience:

- Loss of appetite, nausea, vomiting, or diarrhea
- Weight loss
- Fever (with or without night sweats)
- Pain or difficulty swallowing (dysphagia)
- Fatigue
- Swollen lymph nodes in the neck, armpits, and groin
- A cough or recurrent episodes of pneumonia
- Sores or white patches in the mouth
- Bruises or dark bumps on the skin that do not heal (Kaposi's sarcoma; Fig. 38-1)
- Forgetfulness and confusion
- Dementia

To date, there is no cure for AIDS, although medications have been developed that can delay the onset of AIDS in HIV-positive people. These medications can cost more than $10,000 per year and are not always successful. In addition, they often have severe and disabling side effects, such as headache, dizziness, nausea, diarrhea, fever, skin rash, severe anemia, and extreme fatigue. Currently, no medication can kill HIV and offer a complete cure for AIDS.

▶ *Tell the Nurse!*

When caring for a person who is HIV-positive, it is very important for you to immediately

FIGURE 38-1

As a result of their weakened immune systems, people with AIDS often develop malignancies, such as Kaposi's sarcoma. The lesions of Kaposi's sarcoma are often seen on the skin and mucous membranes of people with advanced HIV infection (AIDS). (*Photograph courtesy of Goodheart, H. P. [2003]. Goodheart's photoguide of common skin disorders: Diagnosis and management [p.374]. Philadelphia: Lippincott Williams & Wilkins.*)

report any of the following observations to the nurse:

➠ The person has a fever

➠ The person has sores or white patches in the mouth

➠ The person has diarrhea, nausea, or vomiting

➠ The person is coughing

➠ The person has a skin rash or bruises

➠ The person's mental status has changed (for example, he or she has become confused or disoriented)

➠ The person seems depressed or talks of suicide

➠ The person is bleeding from any body opening

WHO IS AT RISK FOR AIDS?

Although the first cases of AIDS were reported in homosexual men, we now know that *anyone* can get AIDS—young, old, homosexual, heterosexual, male, or female. In Chapter 8, you learned that HIV is transmitted from one person to another through body fluids, such as blood, semen, and vaginal secretions. Exposure to HIV can also occur either before or during birth, or through breast milk. Behaviors and situations that

increase a person's risk for becoming infected with HIV include the following:

- **Having unprotected sex.** Unprotected sexual intercourse, both homosexual and heterosexual, is the most common method of HIV transmission.
- **Sharing of needles.** Sharing of needles among people who abuse intravenous drugs is the second most common method of transmission.
- **Receiving tissue transplants or transfusions of blood or blood products.** Before 1985, people who received blood transfusions may have been exposed to HIV. This method of transmission is less common now in developed nations with more advanced health care systems, because donated blood is screened for the virus. However, some developing countries still fail to screen their blood supplies.

In the United States, the highest rate of HIV infection is among adults between the ages of 30 and 39 years. However, this is not the only at-risk age group. Although many people do not consider the elderly population to be at risk for becoming infected with HIV, the CDC reports that people 50 years and older make up approximately 10% of the total number of AIDS cases nationwide. In addition, HIV infection in older adults is increasing at an alarming rate.

A GLOBAL HEALTH CRISIS

Today, AIDS is considered a global health crisis. The rate of infection continues to increase around the world, and there is no cure for this devastating disease. At the end of 2002, the CDC reported that an estimated 42 million people worldwide were HIV-positive or already had AIDS. AIDS awareness programs, which teach people about AIDS and how to lower their risk of becoming infected with HIV, have helped to lower the rate of infection in developed countries, such as the United States and many European nations (Fig. 38-2). In addition, people who live in developed countries often have better access to health care if they do become infected with HIV.

But in developing nations, such as India and many countries in Africa and Southeast Asia, the rate of HIV infection is increasing, and the

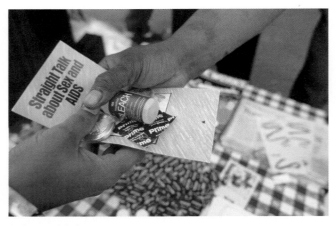

FIGURE 38-2

AIDS awareness programs provide information about HIV infection and AIDS to the general public. These programs provide free advice about the disease, how it can be prevented, and where a person can go to get tested for HIV. (© *Allen Russell/Index Stock Imagery.*)

number of people dying from AIDS is doubling and even tripling (Fig. 38-3). In these countries, access to health care services and information about the prevention of HIV infection may be extremely limited, especially to women. Women in these countries often have a low social or economic status. As a result, they may not be able to insist on safe sex practices, or afford treatment. These women may become pregnant without knowing that they are HIV-positive. Even if they do know that they are infected with HIV, they may

FIGURE 38-3

AIDS is a global health crisis. Some developing countries report HIV infection in as many as 70% of adults. This woman, who lives in Africa, discovered that she was HIV-positive when her daughter was born HIV-positive. Developing nations are hit hardest by the AIDS epidemic because they lack money for education and health care. (© *Gideon Mendel/CORBIS.*)

not be able to afford treatments to reduce the chance that the virus will be transmitted to their unborn children during pregnancy. As a result, more and more babies in developing nations are being born with HIV.

PROTECTION OF RIGHTS

In many cultures, being HIV-positive or having AIDS is considered shameful. As a result, a person who is HIV-positive or who has AIDS may experience discrimination and poor treatment by others. There are many factors that contribute to the negative attitude many people have toward those who are HIV-positive or have AIDS:

- Because HIV infection is associated with many behaviors that people can control (such as whether or not they practice safe sex), some people may feel that the person with HIV or AIDS "has only himself to blame."
- Many of the behaviors associated with HIV infection are behaviors that many people do not approve of for moral or religious reasons (such as abusing street drugs or being homosexual).
- Many people lack information about how HIV is transmitted, and as a result, fear becoming infected with HIV through casual contact with an infected person.

Because a person who is HIV-positive or who has AIDS is at risk for discrimination, many states have laws designed specifically to protect the rights of people who are HIV-positive or who have AIDS. These laws ensure the person's right to employment, education, privacy, and health care. It would be difficult to detail all of the laws here, because they vary from state to state and they change frequently, as lawmakers write and introduce new laws. However, as an example, in most states, people with AIDS are protected under the Americans with Disabilities Act.

As with all of your patients or residents, protecting the person's privacy and right to confidentiality is very important. This is especially true when a person has a condition, such as being infected with HIV or having AIDS, that could cause him to experience discrimination. For example, if a person is known to be HIV-positive, he may have trouble getting a job, obtaining health insurance, or renting an apartment. Although laws are in place to protect the person from discrimination, discrimination can still occur.

As a nursing assistant, you are responsible for maintaining absolute confidentiality about a person's HIV status. You need to know the HIV status of a person to whom you are providing care. However—no one else needs to know. Know your facility's or agency's policies related to keeping health information private, and follow these policies carefully at all times, with all patients and residents.

CARING FOR A PERSON WITH AIDS

HIV-positive people and people with AIDS often require the services of the health care industry throughout the course of their illness. In many communities, organizations exist for the sole purpose of serving people with AIDS. These organizations can help the person with transportation, housing, employment, mental health counseling, financial aid, and medical services. As the disease progresses, the person may be hospitalized several times for the treatment of severe infections and other problems. In the advanced stage of AIDS, pain and weakness cause the person to become almost completely dependent on others for assistance with activities of daily living (ADLs) (Fig. 38-4). As a result, the person may need the

FIGURE 38-4
Toward the end of their lives, most people with AIDS require almost complete assistance with activities of daily living (ADLs). As a result, many seek care from home health care or hospice agencies, or in long-term care facilities. (© *Joel Steffenheim/ CORBIS.*)

services of a home health care agency, or she may need to move to a long-term care facility. Most people with AIDS also eventually require the service of hospice agencies.

MEETING THE PHYSICAL NEEDS OF A PERSON WITH AIDS

A person with AIDS becomes more dependent on others for basic physical care as the disease progresses. Fatigue and disability will make it difficult for the person to perform basic activities, such as those related to personal hygiene and grooming. As a result, you will need to help the person with any ADLs that he can no longer manage. As always, encourage the person to do as much for himself as possible, for as long as possible. Special considerations with regard to physical care for the person with AIDS include the following:

- People with AIDS often develop painful sores on the inside of the mouth. These sores can make eating difficult, putting the person at risk for poor nutrition. In addition, people with AIDS often suffer from chronic diarrhea, which puts them at risk for dehydration. As a result, you may be required to measure and record intake and output. You should also offer the person fluids, as ordered.
- As a result of sores on the inside of the mouth, oral hygiene can be painful for a person with AIDS. A special mouthwash or spray to numb the inside of the person's mouth may be used before providing oral care. Rashes and other skin disorders may require the use of special cleansing agents, special bathing techniques, or both.
- Because people with AIDS are at high risk for opportunistic infections, you will need to ask visitors who have colds or other contagious illnesses to delay their visit until after they have recovered from their illness. In addition, the person with AIDS needs to avoid other potential sources of infection, such as undercooked meat and eggs. Always practice proper infection control measures, especially good handwashing. Avoid coming to work if you have a contagious illness. This is important with

FIGURE 38-5

Practicing standard precautions is essential with all patients and residents, not just those who are known to have an illness caused by a bloodborne pathogen (such as AIDS).

all patients and residents, but especially so when you are caring for people with weak immune systems.

As you already know, your job responsibilities place you at risk for contacting body fluids that are known to transmit HIV and other bloodborne pathogens. For this reason, you must use standard precautions (see Chapter 8) with every patient or resident, not just those who are known to be infected with HIV (Fig. 38-5). Remember that a person can be infected with HIV and not know it. You may find it frightening to provide physical care for a person who is known to have a communicable, potentially fatal illness. Know that with the proper and consistent use of standard precautions, your risk of exposure to HIV and other bloodborne pathogens in the workplace is actually quite low.

MEETING THE EMOTIONAL NEEDS OF A PERSON WITH AIDS

People who are HIV-positive or who have AIDS can face a great deal of emotional stress. Because of increasing levels of stress, people with HIV may lose their ability to cope. As a result, clinical depression and an increased risk for suicide are very common among people who are HIV-positive or who have AIDS. Sources of emotional stress include the following:

- Fear, shame, or disapproval can cause friends and even family members to abandon a person when they find out that she is HIV-positive. They may avoid the person because they fear that they, too, could get the disease from casual contact or conversation. Or they may just be ashamed to know a person who is HIV-positive or who has AIDS. Can you imagine how you would feel if your friends or family members could not give you emotional support when you needed it most?

- People who are HIV-positive or who have AIDS may lose their jobs as a result of their disease. Health care and the medications used to slow the progression of HIV are very expensive, and the loss of employment usually means the loss of health care benefits. For these reasons, the person with HIV or AIDS may have many worries about money.

- A person who is infected with HIV may suffer from a lot of guilt, especially if the cause of infection was due to risky behavior. For example, a man who finds out that he is HIV-positive must face the fact that he may have transmitted a deadly disease to his sexual partner.

- A person who is HIV-positive may have many fears related to his declining health and how this will affect his ability to care for himself. The person may also have fears about pain related to the disease, or about death itself.

Providing emotional care for the person with AIDS is an essential responsibility of the nursing assistant. When caring for a person who is HIV-positive or has AIDS, you can use touch to comfort the person, spend time listening and talking, or share a simple hug. None of these activities will transmit the virus to you. Many times, the only human touch a person with HIV or AIDS will experience will come from the person providing care within the health care setting (Fig. 38-6). How would you feel if people were afraid to touch you? Would you feel dirty, unloved, and alone? Instead of being afraid to care for people who are HIV-positive or who have AIDS, learn how to protect yourself from infection and practice what you have learned consistently. Knowledge is the best way to overcome fear.

Remember that it does not really matter how a person became infected with HIV. Even if you do not approve of the person's lifestyle, you must not

FIGURE 38-6

A hospice volunteer visits with a man who has AIDS. HIV cannot be transmitted from one person to another through touching or hugging. Lack of human touch can make a person feel unloved and alone. When caring for a person who is HIV positive or who has AIDS, try not to let fear get in the way of your ability to provide compassionate care. (© *Frank Pedrick/Index Stock Imagery.*)

let your personal beliefs affect the care that you give the person. Instead of focusing on *how* the person got HIV, focus on *who* the person is. What does she enjoy about life? Whom does she admire? Try to remember that a person is defined by a lot more than just her HIV status. A patient or resident with HIV infection or AIDS needs your care and support, perhaps more than anything else she has ever needed before. Your ability to provide supportive and compassionate care to your patients or residents with HIV infection or AIDS will make a significant difference in their quality of life.

SUMMARY

▶ Acquired immunodeficiency syndrome (AIDS) is caused by infection with the human immunodeficiency virus (HIV). HIV invades the body's immune system, leaving it unable to do its job. As a result, the person eventually dies from infections or cancers that take over the body.
  ■ A person who has tested positive for having antibodies to HIV in his or her blood is said to be *HIV-positive.*
  ■ Most HIV-positive people eventually develop AIDS, an advanced stage of HIV infection. A person who is infected with HIV may live for many years before AIDS develops. AIDS is a terminal illness.
▶ AIDS is a global health crisis. Since it was first identified in the early 1980s, AIDS has spread rapidly, killing a large number of people throughout the world in a short period of time.
  ■ In developed countries, such as the United States, Canada, and England, rates of HIV infection and death from AIDS are decreasing due to the efforts of AIDS-awareness programs and the availability of funding for research and health care.
  ■ Rates of HIV infection and death from AIDS continue to soar in developing countries, such as India and many nations in Africa and Southeast Asia, where money and access to health care and education about HIV infection are limited.
▶ Anyone can get HIV, regardless of race, gender, sexual orientation, or age.
  ■ Behaviors that increase a person's risk of getting HIV include having unprotected sexual intercourse and using dirty needles to inject street drugs.
  ■ The virus can also be transmitted through tissue transplants or transfusions of blood or blood products, and from a mother to a child during birth or through breast milk.
▶ A person who is HIV-positive or who has AIDS may experience discrimination and poor treatment by others. It is important for the nursing assistant to keep information about a person's HIV status, or any other medical condition, private and confidential.

▶ HIV-positive people and people with AIDS often require the services of the health care industry throughout the course of their illness.

- Infections that cause pneumonia, diarrhea, and malignancies such as Kaposi's sarcoma are common in people who are infected with HIV, causing them to be hospitalized repeatedly.

- As the disease progresses, the person becomes unable to care for himself, and he may need the services of a home health care agency or long-term care facility.

- In the final months of their lives, people with AIDS may require the services of a hospice agency.

▶ In addition to providing physical care, the nursing assistant plays an important role in providing emotional care to the person with HIV infection or AIDS.

- With the proper and consistent use of standard precautions, your risk of exposure to HIV and other bloodborne pathogens in the workplace is actually quite low.

- Human touch is a very effective way of comforting a person and communicating care and concern. You cannot get HIV from holding a person's hand or giving a person a hug.

- Remember that it is not important how a person became infected with HIV. Try not to let your personal beliefs or fears get in the way of your ability to provide compassionate, competent care.

What did you learn?

Multiple Choice

Select the single best answer for each of the following questions.

1. When are standard precautions used?
   a. When a person who is HIV-positive develops AIDS
   b. When a person is HIV-positive or has AIDS
   c. When caring for a patient or resident who is homosexual
   d. When caring for any patient or resident and contact with blood or body fluids is possible

2. Which one of the following statements about HIV infection and AIDS is true?
   a. Anyone can become infected with HIV, regardless of age, gender, sexual orientation, or race.
   b. People who become infected with HIV and get AIDS are only drug abusers or homosexuals.
   c. HIV infection and AIDS are not a problem among the elderly.
   d. AIDS usually develops soon after a person is first exposed to HIV.

3. When caring for a person who is HIV-positive, which one of the following observations should be reported to the nurse?
   a. The person has diarrhea
   b. The person seems depressed
   c. The person seems disoriented
   d. All of the above

4. Why is it especially important for nursing assistants to keep information about a person's HIV status private and confidential?
   a. AIDS is a shameful disease and should not be discussed in public.
   b. Many states have laws to protect the rights of HIV-positive people and people with AIDS, including their right to privacy and confidentiality of medical information.
   c. Nursing assistants have a responsibility to make sure that everyone who might come in contact with the person knows the person's HIV status, so that others can protect themselves.
   d. AIDS is a global health crisis.

5. Which one of the following physical problems is a person with AIDS at risk for?
   a. Alopecia (loss of hair), due to the medications used to slow the progression of HIV to AIDS
   b. Dehydration, due to chronic diarrhea
   c. Blindness, due to nerve damage as a result of HIV infection
   d. Heart failure, due to myocardial infarction

? Stop and think!

► You work in a hospital. One of the patients you will be caring for today, Camilla, is a 34-year-old woman who has been admitted for the treatment of AIDS-related pneumonia. Although Camilla has been admitted to the hospital for AIDS-related infections and complications several times in the past, you have never had her as a patient because you are a relatively new employee. In fact, you have never cared for any patient with AIDS. Frankly, you are a little bit nervous about meeting Camilla and about providing hands-on physical care to a person who is known to be HIV-positive. What will be your approach to Camilla, and to your responsibilities as a nursing assistant?

Nursing Assistants Make a Difference!

"I am Clarence Wright and I live in the Sunny Shores Nursing facility. I came here about a year ago after my dear wife Callie passed away. We had been married for 53 years and I thought my heart was broken forever the day they lowered her into the grave. I didn't want to eat, get out of bed, or even take a bath; heck, I didn't want to go on living without her! A good friend visited me a week or so after the funeral and I guess I frightened him so much that he called the ambulance for me.

I went to the hospital and stayed a few days to be evaluated. After a thorough physical, they called in a mental health specialist and diagnosed me with severe depression. They decided that I probably shouldn't live by myself any longer, so I came here to Sunny Shores. They prescribed some medication to help me feel more "normal" and arranged for me to have counseling to help me come to terms with losing Callie.

After moving here, I was still pretty depressed. But, there was this really nice woman named Celia who helped care for me each day. She was my nursing assistant. At first she would help me get dressed and shaved and out for breakfast. Then she would ask me to go walk around the grounds with her. We didn't talk much at first. She didn't pry; instead, we just walked quietly. After I started feeling like talking, she let me talk about my life with Callie, and would sit and look at pictures of her with me. One day I broke down and just cried like a baby and Celia just sat quietly with me and held my hand. That day, I knew I would be able to make it.

Yes, I still get sad when I think of Callie's death. But I've learned to make use of what I have left of my life. I help Celia out with some of the residents who aren't as fortunate as I am. I read to one fellow who is blind and we have some of the most wonderful conversations. I help some of the little ladies get up for exercise, and we play cards every Thursday evening in the activities room. I have regained the feeling that my life has meaning and I know that Celia had a major part in that. Medicine is great for helping people with depression, but no medicine ever created can take the place of knowing that a person cares about you. And Celia shows that she cares about me and all the other residents down this hall. We love her and think that she's our angel in disguise."

You can listen to more stories about how nursing assistants make a difference on the CD in the back of your book.

Acute Care

The acute care setting can be an exciting place to work. If you choose to work in an acute care setting, such as a hospital, you will have the opportunity to meet and care for many different people. In this unit, you will learn about how to care for three special groups of patients who often receive treatment in hospitals: surgical patients; women who are about to deliver, or have just delivered, babies; and children.

Photo: The acute care setting can be an exciting place to work.
(© George Mattei/Photo Researchers, Inc.)

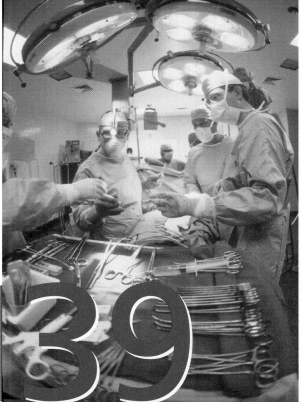

39 Caring for Surgical Patients

What will you learn?

Surgery is a branch of medicine that involves treating diseases and disorders by entering the body and physically removing or repairing damaged organs or tissues. Advances in surgical tools and techniques have made many surgeries safer and have opened up treatment options for many diseases and disorders that were considered fatal in the past. Surgeries that once made headlines, such as kidney transplants, are now done fairly routinely.

The longer a person lives, the greater the chance that the person will need surgery sometime during her lifetime, simply because the person will have more of a chance to develop a disease or disorder that is treated surgically. As a nursing assistant, you may have many opportunities to help prepare people for surgery and care for them afterwards. When you are finished with this chapter, you will be able to:

1. Discuss the various reasons surgery is done.
2. Define the term *anesthesia* and describe the three main types of anesthesia.
3. Describe changes in the health care field that affect the care of the surgical patient.
4. Understand the fears and concerns that a person who is about to have surgery may have, and describe actions the nursing assistant can take to help relieve some of these worries.
5. Describe what needs to be done to physically prepare a person for surgery, and explain the nursing assistant's role in these preparations.
6. Describe potential complications of surgery, and the measures taken to prevent them.
7. Discuss observations that would be important to report to the nurse, relevant to the care of a patient who is recovering from surgery.
8. Demonstrate the proper way to apply anti-embolism (TED) stockings.

Photo: A surgical team performs an operation.
(© K. Beebe/Custom Medical Stock Photo.)

Vocabulary

Exploratory surgery	General anesthesia	Post-operative phase	Atelectasis
Definitive surgery	Regional anesthesia	Peri-operative period	Thrombophlebitis
Elective	Local anesthesia	Pre-operative teaching	Pulmonary embolism
Urgent	Pre-operative phase	Post-anesthesia care	Sequential compression
Emergent	Intra-operative phase	unit (PACU)	device (SCD)

A person may need surgery for many different reasons. **Exploratory surgery** may be performed when a person has a significant medical problem but the doctors do not know exactly how bad the problem is or exactly what is causing it. For example, doctors might want to do exploratory surgery following an accident when the extent of the damage to the person's internal organs is unknown, or when cancer is suspected but cannot be confirmed by other means. Often times, the problem is not only discovered but solved during the same surgery. **Definitive surgery** is performed when the person's medical problem is known and the best way to address it is through surgery. For example, surgeries are performed to repair organ defects or injuries, as in a hernia repair or surgical repair of a fractured bone. Surgeries are also performed to remove diseased body parts, as when the cancerous part of the colon is removed as treatment for colon cancer.

Surgeries may be elective, urgent, or emergent. Surgeries are performed on an **elective** basis when the procedure is planned for and scheduled ahead of time. An example of an elective procedure would be cataract surgery or a plastic surgery procedure, such as a face-lift. **Urgent** surgeries are planned and scheduled ahead of time, but usually an effort is made to schedule the procedure as soon as possible to prevent the person's condition from getting worse. Examples of urgent procedures would include a mastectomy (in a person with breast cancer) or cardiac bypass surgery (in a person with coronary artery disease). An **emergent** surgery is one that must be performed immediately to prevent the person from dying or becoming disabled. Emergent surgeries are unplanned and unscheduled and are usually the result of an acute illness or injury, such as a ruptured appendix.

Most surgical procedures are done under anesthesia. Anesthesia prevents the person from feeling pain during the surgery, and is accomplished through the use of medications. Depending on the situation, the doctor may choose to use a general anesthetic, a regional anesthetic, or a local anesthetic:

- **General anesthesia** causes a loss of consciousness. Usually, a combination of inhaled drugs (in the form of a gas) and injected drugs are given to cause general anesthesia. The person is "put to sleep" for the duration of the surgical procedure. When the procedure is completed, the drugs are stopped and the person "wakes up." The person will be sleepy for several hours after the procedure and may experience some nausea or vomiting during the recovery period.

- **Regional anesthesia** causes a loss of sensation in part, but not all, of the body. The person remains conscious throughout the procedure. A sedative drug may be given in addition to the anesthetic to help the person relax. The anesthetic drug is injected near a nerve pathway, causing the part of the body beyond the injection site to become numb. After surgery, the sensation returns gradually. The person may experience temporary paralysis and weakness of the anesthetized body part until the anesthetic has worn completely off. An example of regional anesthesia is "an epidural block," which numbs the body from the waist down and is often given to women during childbirth.

- **Local anesthesia** causes a loss of sensation in only a very small part of the body (the surgical site). As with regional anesthesia, the drug is injected near a nerve pathway, the person remains conscious throughout the procedure, and a sedative may be given to help the person relax. The surgical site remains without sensation until the local anesthetic wears off. Eye surgeries, breast biopsies, and hernia repairs are examples of surgeries that are often performed under local anesthesia.

In the past, people who were having a planned surgical procedure were admitted to the hospital the day before the scheduled surgery. The tests required prior to surgery were done, the surgical site was shaved and cleaned, the person and his family members were told what to expect during and after the surgery, and the person was given a sleeping pill to ensure a restful night's sleep. Following the surgery, the person usually stayed in the hospital for several days to recover under the watchful eyes of the hospital staff.

Now, changes in how we pay for health care have led to changes in the lengths of hospital stays. People are discharged from the hospital "quicker and sicker." For the surgical patient who is having elective or urgent surgery, this means that most of the tasks that used to be done in the hospital the day before surgery are now done in the surgeon's office or on an outpatient basis in the days leading up to the surgery. The person remains home until the morning of surgery and goes to the hospital or surgical center an hour or two before the surgery is scheduled. The surgical site is shaved and cleaned in the operating room or in a preparation area next to the operating room just prior to the procedure. After the surgery, the person is often discharged from the hospital within a few hours to recover at home, in an extended care facility, or in a long-term care facility. Even though surgery is performed in a hospital or surgical center, these changes mean that as a nursing assistant, you can expect to care for people who are either preparing for surgery or recovering from it, no matter where you work.

There are three phases of care for the person having surgery (Fig. 39-1). These phases are:
- The **pre-operative phase,** or before surgery
- The **intra-operative phase,** or during surgery
- The **post-operative phase,** or after surgery

The term **peri-operative period** is used to describe all three phases of the surgical process as a whole.

CARE OF THE PRE-OPERATIVE PATIENT

The pre-operative phase begins when the person is first informed about the need for surgery, and ends when the person actually enters the operating room. The pre-operative period can be as long as several weeks (for an elective, scheduled procedure) or as short as a few minutes (for an emergent procedure). During the pre-operative period, the person who is having surgery is prepared both emotionally and physically for the procedure.

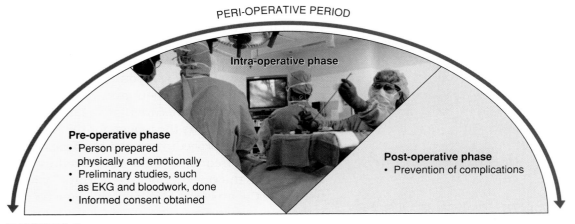

FIGURE 39-1

There are three phases of care for the person having surgery. As a nursing assistant, you will provide care during the pre-operative and post-operative phases.

EMOTIONAL PREPARATION

A person facing surgery usually has many fears, concerns, and worries. For example, the person may be afraid of not waking up from the anesthesia, dying as a result of the surgery, or experiencing pain during or after the procedure. He may worry that the doctor will make a mistake, and remove the wrong organ or limb. If the person is having exploratory surgery, the person may be very worried about what the doctor will find (for example, a malignant tumor). Many people worry about how long it will take to recover from the surgery, and what this will mean in terms of time missed from work and lost income needed to support a family.

To help reduce a person's anxiety about the upcoming surgery, the health care team spends time talking with the person and his family members about the procedure, its benefits and possible risks, and what can be expected during the post-operative recovery period. These conversations, which occur during the pre-operative phase, are commonly called **pre-operative teaching**. Pre-operative teaching begins with the doctor's explanation of why she feels the procedure is the best treatment option for the person. The doctor tells the person what complications can occur as a result of the procedure, what will actually occur during the procedure, and what other treatment options, if any, are available (Fig. 39-2).

FIGURE 39-2

During the pre-operative period, the doctor tells the person why he or she feels surgery is the best treatment option, explains the surgical procedure and any associated risks to the person, and obtains informed consent to perform the surgery. (© *Custom Medical Stock Photo*.)

The doctor must explain these things in a way that is understandable to the person, so that the person can make an informed decision about whether he wants to have the surgery. To go ahead with the procedure, informed consent must be given by the person and documented in the person's medical record. If the person is not able to make an informed decision on his own, informed consent must be obtained from the person's family members. The nurse is responsible for making sure that informed consent has been obtained and that the person signs a form giving permission for the procedure to take place (Fig. 39-3). As a nursing assistant, you will not be responsible for either explaining the procedure to the person or obtaining the person's signed consent for it.

Once informed consent for the procedure is obtained, the nurse continues the pre-operative teaching by explaining what will need to be done both before and after the surgery. The nurse explains the pre-operative procedures that are done to physically prepare the person for surgery, as well as the purpose of any medications or tests that are required during the pre-operative period. The nurse also explains what will happen during the post-operative period, and teaches the person how to do any exercises that may be necessary to prevent complications following the surgery.

Although as a nursing assistant you will not participate directly in pre-operative teaching, you will still play a very important supporting role. You will reinforce what the nurse has told the person, and keep the nurse informed of any questions the person may ask you about the procedure. Anxiety can make the person forget to ask important questions when the doctor or nurse is explaining the surgery. Often, the person will remember questions she wanted to ask later, when the doctor or nurse is no longer in the room. As a result, the person may ask you the questions instead. If the question is about an aspect of preoperative or post-operative care that you are directly involved with, such as the reason for the NPO status prior to the procedure or the purpose of taking vital signs frequently after the procedure, you can answer the question yourself. But if you do not know the answer to the person's question, or if the question is about the surgical procedure itself, please tell the nurse immediately that the person has a question. The nurse will see to it that the person's question is answered.

Davis Hospital and Medical Center

Acknowledgement of Informed Consent for Procedures / Invasive Procedures

1. My treating Physician,_____, has explained my medical condition to my satisfaction and I have had an opportunity to have my questions answered.

2. My proposed treatment, its purpose, risks and alternatives, have been explained to me. I accept this treatment in hopes of obtaining the desired beneficial result of such care.

3. I recognize that, during the procedure(s), unforeseen conditions may require additional or different procedures than those explained. I request that my physician(s) and associates perform those procedures as, in their professional judgment, are desirable.

4. I agree to observation by medical personnel in training during my procedure in order to advance medical education.

Check all that apply:

- ❏ I agree to the administration of anesthesia or intravenous sedation.
- ❏ I agree to the administration of intravenous therapy to include blood products, chemotherapy, or antibiotics as ordered by my physician.
- ❏ I understand that any tissues removed from my body may be examined and then disposed of by hospital personnel.
- ❏ I agree to the presence of a medical product representative, as required and requested by the physician, for consultation purposes only.
- ❏ I agree to photography/video, during the procedure for the purposes of advancing medical education.
- ❏ As a <u>cardiac patient,</u> I acknowledge that the risks of no on-site surgical back-up have been explained to me by my physician.
- ❏ As a <u>cardiac patient,</u> I agree to be transferred to another facility in the event that surgical intervention becomes necessary.
- ❏ I understand that the procedure that is being done to me results in <u>sterilization.</u> I understand that the word "sterility" means that I may forever and irrevocably be unable to conceive or bear children, and in giving my consent to the operation have in mind the possibility, (probability) of such a result.
- ❏ I certify that I have had nothing to eat or drink, including water, since_____AM / PM.
- ❏ I have been given patient information sheets on_____and have had my questions answered.

Proposed Medical Procedure (in layman's terms) _____

_____

_____

_____   _____
Patient's Signature   Signature Witnessed By:

_____
Signature of Next of Kin or Legal Guardian

Time_____   Date_____

FIGURE 39-3

A signed informed consent form is necessary before any surgical procedure can be done. By signing the informed consent form, the person indicates that he or she understands what is going to be done, why it is being done, and what the possible risks are. *(Courtesy of Davis Hospital and Medical Center, Layton, Utah.)*

It is very easy to tell a person that a procedure is "minor" or "just routine." Many surgical procedures are, indeed, relatively low risk, and considered "routine" by health care professionals who see these procedures done every day. But no matter how simple or low-risk a surgical procedure is, there is nothing minor or routine about it to the person who is having it! Recognizing the person's fears, listening to his questions and concerns, and taking action to get those questions or concerns addressed are all very important things that you can do to help a person to prepare emotionally for the upcoming surgery.

PHYSICAL PREPARATION

Several things are done to physically prepare the person for surgery.

In the Days Leading Up to the Surgery

Typically, a person who is having surgery will need to have several tests done before the surgery to assess her level of health. Tests to assess the functioning of the person's cardiovascular, respiratory, and urinary systems are typically done. In addition, the doctor may request bloodwork.

The Evening Before Surgery

A person who is scheduled for surgery will usually be on NPO status for 6 to 8 hours before surgery (Fig. 39-4). This is necessary to ensure that the person's stomach is empty during and after the procedure. It is common for a person who has had general anesthesia to vomit as the anesthesia is given or starts to wear off. Vomiting while in a semi-conscious state puts the person at risk for aspiration (the inhalation of foreign material into the lungs). Aspiration puts the person at risk for developing pneumonia. Going into the procedure with an empty stomach helps to reduce the risk of aspiration and pneumonia.

You will need to tell the person, as well as any visitors, that NPO means that the person may not have anything by mouth, including water, ice, gum, and mints. It can be difficult for a person who is on NPO status to be around other people who are eating and drinking. For this

FIGURE 39-4

Many people will not be allowed to have anything by mouth for 6 to 8 hours before the surgery. When a person is on NPO status, the water pitcher and drinking glass are removed from the person's room.

reason, it may be helpful to show visitors to an area outside of the person's room where they can enjoy their snacks and beverages, away from the person who is on NPO status. Remember to remove the water pitcher and the drinking glass from the bedside table. Frequent mouth care helps to keep the person on NPO status comfortable. The person is usually allowed to brush her own teeth as long as no water is swallowed.

The Morning of Surgery

Many things are done the day of surgery to prepare the patient. You should arrange your schedule as necessary, allowing enough time to help the person get ready for surgery. This is especially important if you work in a long-term care facility or for a home health care agency, to ensure that the person arrives at the hospital or surgical center at the appointed time. The nurse will tell you what you need to do to help to prepare the person for surgery. Tasks that you may be involved with include the following:

- **Administering an enema or vaginal douche.** A cleansing enema is given before many procedures to empty the bowel. For example, an enema may be given if the person is scheduled for intestinal surgery, to prevent feces from contaminating the abdominal cavity during the surgery. If a woman is having a vaginal procedure, the doctor may order vaginal irrigation (a douche) prior to the surgery to clean the vagina. When vaginal irrigation is ordered, a special solution is placed in the vagina and then allowed to drain out.

- **Bathing.** You may need to help the person to bathe and wash his hair prior to the surgery. Bathing and shampooing reduces the number of microbes on the skin. In some cases, the doctor may order a special antimicrobial soap to be used.
- **Grooming.** Make-up, including nail polish, is not permitted during surgery. Prosthetic devices, glasses, contact lenses, hearing aids, dentures, wigs, jewelry, and hair ornaments may also be removed prior to the surgery. Although the person may want or need to wear some of these items up until the very last minute, you should let the person know about these restrictions and encourage him to leave all but the most necessary items at home.
- **Dressing.** If the person will be going to the hospital or surgical center the day of the surgery, have him wear clothing that is loose and comfortable. This will make changing into a hospital gown before the procedure easier, and it will also ensure that when the person goes home, the clothing will fit over any bulky dressings or casts that may have been applied during the procedure.

Immediately Before the Surgery

Outpatients

Once the person arrives at the hospital or surgical center, she will go to a preparation area next to the operating room. The person will be shown to a private area and asked to undress and put on a clean hospital gown and surgical cap.

A nurse will check that all paperwork has been properly completed, and will answer any questions that the person has. The person will then be asked to void, and may be given an anti-emetic drug (to prevent nausea) and a sedative (to help relieve anxiety). After these drugs have been given, the side rails must remain up on the bed or stretcher and the person must not get up without assistance, because the sedative may make the person drowsy and weak (Fig. 39-5).

Make sure the call light control is within easy reach, and that the person is comfortable and warm.

If the surgery will be performed under general anesthesia, the person's glasses or contact lenses, hearing aids, dentures, prosthetic devices, jewelry, and hair ornaments may be removed at this time. If the surgery will be performed under regional or local anesthesia, the doctor may request that the person wear hearing aids or dentures during the surgery, to make communication easier. Items that are removed from the person are documented and given to the person's family or placed in the facility safe.

The surgical site may be prepared at this time, or this may be done in the operating room. The surgical site is the area of the body that will be operated on. Preparation of the surgical site may or may not involve removal of body hair. If hair removal is ordered, there are several ways to remove hair from the surgical site. The hair may be shaved, clipped with an electric clipper, or removed with a chemical depilatory (hair-removing) lotion. If one of your duties is to perform pre-operative hair removal, make sure you have been instructed in the proper technique.

Last, a pre-operative checklist is completed (Fig. 39-6). The checklist is used to confirm that all pre-operative tests and procedures have been completed. The nursing assistant is often responsible for completing and recording many of the tasks on the checklist.

FIGURE 39-5

Last-minute preparations for surgery take place in the preparation area next to the operating room. Once drugs have been given to prevent nausea and reduce anxiety, the person must remain in bed with the side rails up to reduce the risk of falling.

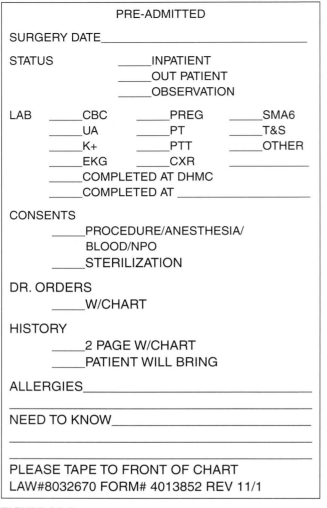

```
              PRE-ADMITTED

SURGERY DATE_____

STATUS           _____INPATIENT
                 _____OUT PATIENT
                 _____OBSERVATION

LAB    _____CBC      _____PREG    _____SMA6
       _____UA       _____PT      _____T&S
       _____K+       _____PTT     _____OTHER
       _____EKG      _____CXR     _____
       _____COMPLETED AT DHMC
       _____COMPLETED AT _____

CONSENTS
       _____PROCEDURE/ANESTHESIA/
            BLOOD/NPO
       _____STERILIZATION

DR. ORDERS
       _____W/CHART

HISTORY
       _____2 PAGE W/CHART
       _____PATIENT WILL BRING

ALLERGIES_____
_____

NEED TO KNOW_____
_____
_____

PLEASE TAPE TO FRONT OF CHART
LAW#8032670 FORM# 4013852 REV 11/1
```

FIGURE 39-6

A pre-operative checklist documents that all of the tasks that must be completed during the pre-operative period have been completed. The pre-operative checklist goes in the person's medical record and must be completed before the person goes into surgery. (*Courtesy of Davis Hospital and Medical Center, Layton, Utah.*)

Inpatients

If the person was admitted to the hospital prior to the surgery, the tasks that are completed immediately before the surgery may be completed in the person's room, before taking her to the operating room. In addition, you may need to help your patient from the bed onto the stretcher when it is time to go to the operating room. Let the person's family members know where they can wait while the person is in surgery. Some facilities have surgical waiting rooms, whereas others allow the family to wait in the person's room. Please remember that family members are often anxious and nervous about the surgery. Refer any questions family members may have about the procedure or the person's condition to the nurse.

CARE OF THE POST-OPERATIVE PATIENT

Immediately after surgery, the person is taken to the **post-anesthesia care unit (PACU),** also known as the recovery room (Fig. 39-7). While in the PACU, the person is closely monitored by the health care team to make sure that he is recovering without complications from the surgery or the anesthesia. The person is usually groggy, but can be awakened. Once awake, the person will usually be oriented to person and place. The person will remain in the PACU until his condition is stable. While in the PACU, the person usually receives supplemental oxygen. Suctioning is also available, in case the person vomits or has secretions that interfere with respiration.

While the person is in surgery, you will most likely be responsible for preparing the person's room for his arrival post-operatively (Fig. 39-8). The bed linens are usually changed and a surgical bed is prepared (see Chapter 15). The bed is raised to make transferring the person from the stretcher to the bed easier. Furniture is moved, if necessary, to ensure a clear pathway for the stretcher. Finally, items that may be needed at the time of the person's arrival are gathered and placed in the room. Items that may be needed include:

FIGURE 39-7

Following surgery, the person is taken to a post-anesthesia care unit (PACU), also known as a recovery room. The person remains here and is monitored closely until the anesthesia has worn off.

FIGURE 39-8

The nursing assistant prepares the person's room for her return while the person is in surgery. The linens are changed and a surgical bed is made. The bed is raised to a height that will make transferring the person from the stretcher to the bed easier. The equipment that may be needed during the post-operative period is gathered and placed in the room. Before the occupant of this room arrives, the over-bed table will need to be moved out of the way to ensure a clear pathway from the door to the bed.

- Equipment for taking vital signs and a flow sheet for recording the vital signs
- An intravenous (IV) pole
- A towel and washcloth
- An emesis basin
- A bed protector
- Suction to connect to drainage devices
- Supplemental oxygen
- Pillows or other positioning aids to elevate the extremities
- Warmed blankets

When the person is returned to his room, you will need to assist in transferring the person from the stretcher to the bed. The nurse assesses the person's overall condition, checks for blood on the dressing and for the presence of drains and catheters, and adjusts the IV flow rate. While the nurse is doing this, you may be asked to take the person's vital signs. Vital signs are taken as ordered and recorded on the flow sheet. Post-operatively, routine vital sign measurements, including temperature, are usually taken every 15 minutes for the first hour, every 30 minutes for the next 1 to 2 hours, every hour for the next 4 hours, and then every 4 hours as ordered (Fig. 39-9). As always, any changes in vital signs must be reported to the nurse immediately. In a person who is recovering from surgery, a change in a vital sign could be the first sign that the person is developing a post-operative complication.

FIGURE 39-9

Vital signs are taken frequently during the immediate postoperative period because a change in vital signs could signal a complication of the surgery or the anesthesia.

The person may need to be positioned in a particular way post-operatively. For example, if the person is recovering from an anesthetic that was injected into the spinal canal, she may need to remain in the supine position for a period of time. Children may be positioned laterally or in Sims' position to help prevent aspiration in the event of vomiting. If the person had surgery on an arm or leg, the arm or leg is usually elevated on a pillow or folded blanket to help prevent swelling and pain. Make sure you check with the nurse for any specific instructions or restrictions regarding the person's position. In all cases, the person should be positioned comfortably and in a way that will prevent stress on the surgical incision.

In the hours and days that follow surgery, the health care team focuses on preventing complications and assisting the person with routine tasks, such as grooming and elimination, as necessary. As a nursing assistant, you will play a large role in helping the person to make a good recovery.

PREVENTING COMPLICATIONS

People who have had surgery are at risk for developing complications, especially related to breathing and circulation. In addition, the surgical site may become infected or the wound may not stay closed. As a nursing assistant, there are several things that you will do to prevent complications from developing. Also, if one of your patients develops a complication from surgery, you may be the first one to notice. Reporting your observations to the nurse promptly helps to ensure that action will be taken quickly to prevent the person's condition from getting worse.

Respiratory Complications

The combined effects of general anesthesia, the drugs given to relieve post-operative pain, and a painful incision make it difficult for a person who is recovering from surgery to clear the lungs and airways of fluid and mucus. The person is drowsy from the anesthesia and painkillers, and it hurts to cough! If the person also has a chronic respiratory disorder, such as asthma or chronic obstructive pulmonary disease (COPD), or if the person smokes, then her risk of developing a respiratory complication increases even more.

Common respiratory complications of surgery include pneumonia (fluid fills the alveoli) and **atelectasis** (the alveoli collapse). Both atelectasis and pneumonia make it difficult for oxygen to pass into the blood, and carbon dioxide to pass out of it.

To prevent fluid and mucus from collecting in the person's lungs, you may need to assist the person with frequent repositioning and with performing respiratory exercises. Commonly used respiratory exercises include coughing and deep breathing, and incentive spirometry (Fig. 39-10).

- **Coughing and deep breathing.** The person is helped into a comfortable position and then instructed to take a few deep breaths and cough forcefully. If the person has had abdominal or chest surgery, you may need to support the incision site with a small pillow or folded towel while the person coughs (see Fig. 39-10A). Supporting the incision site helps to minimize pain.
- **Incentive spirometry.** The person forcefully inhales through a special device called an incentive spirometer (see Fig. 39-10B). The device consists of a tube and a chamber that contains balls. The goal is for the person to inhale hard enough through the tube to raise the balls in the chamber.

If your patient has orders to perform respiratory exercises, these exercises will need to be done every few hours, or as directed. Elevating the head of the bed while the person is supine will also make it easier for the person to breathe.

Cardiovascular Complications

Anesthetic agents, pain medications, and general immobility after surgery can cause the body's circulation to slow down, leading to pooling of the blood in the legs. When blood flow slows and blood pools, a thrombus, or blood clot, may form. Surgical patients who are elderly or have a history of circulatory problems are at the most risk for developing thrombi. Certain conditions (such as fractures of the femur, or thigh bone) and certain surgeries (such as joint replacement surgery) also carry a high risk of thrombus formation.

A

B

FIGURE 39-10

Respiratory exercises may be ordered during the post-operative period to prevent the person from developing respiratory complications such as pneumonia and atelectasis. (*A*) Coughing and deep breathing exercises. The person takes a few deep breaths and then coughs forcefully. (*B*) Incentive spirometry. The person inhales through an incentive spirometer with the goal of causing the balls to rise in the chamber.

A thrombus in one of the veins of the legs causes inflammation and pain, a condition known as **thrombophlebitis.** Sometimes the blood clot will break loose and travel through the bloodstream. This puts the person at great risk. A blood clot that breaks loose and moves through the bloodstream is known as an *embolus.* The embolus can travel to the brain and get stuck in one of the blood vessels there, causing a stroke. Or, the embolus can travel to the pulmonary artery, the artery that carries blood from the heart to the lungs so that it can receive oxygen. Blocking of the pulmonary artery by an embolus is called a **pulmonary embolism** and it is often fatal. Restlessness and shortness of breath may be signs of pulmonary embolism and should be reported to the nurse immediately.

A number of different measures are taken to lower the person's risk of cardiovascular complications.

Sequential Compression Device (SCD)

A **sequential compression device (SCD)** is a device that is applied to the calves to help prevent pooling of blood in the lower legs (Fig. 39-11). Disposable plastic sleeves are wrapped around the person's lower legs. The sleeves, which have several different compartments, are connected to an air pump via tubing. Air is pumped into the first compartment (the one closest to the foot) to inflate it. Then the next compartment inflates, then the next, helping to move the blood from the lower legs toward the heart. When the top-most compartment has been inflated, all the compartments deflate and the cycle begins again at the bottom. The inflating and deflating action massages the veins, pushing the blood through the veins and back to the heart. Many of your patients will return from the PACU with SCDs in place.

Anti-embolism (TED) Stockings

Anti-embolism (TED) stockings are made of a tight-fitting elastic fabric. The stockings, which may be knee-high or thigh-high, are specially fitted for the person by the nurse or the physical therapist. The elastic fabric applies pressure, compressing the veins and helping to return blood to the heart. This helps to prevent pooling of blood in the legs.

Anti-embolism (TED) stockings may be applied before surgery, or ordered afterward. If the stockings are allowed to be removed at night, they should be reapplied before the person gets out of bed for the day. Once the person stands up, gravity increases blood flow to the veins in the lower legs, causing the veins to widen and the blood to pool. Procedure 39-1 describes how to apply anti-embolism (TED) stockings.

Leg Exercises

The doctor may also order leg exercises for the person following surgery, to help reduce the risk of embolism. If the person is weak or unconscious, you may need to help her with these exercises (Fig. 39-12). The person usually must do these exercises every 1 to 2 hours while he or she is awake.

FIGURE 39-11

A sequential compression device (SCD) helps to prevent pooling of blood in the lower extremities. The plastic sleeves around the person's lower legs contain multiple chambers, which alternately inflate and deflate, pushing blood through the veins.

FIGURE 39-12

If your patient is weak or unconscious, you may have to help him or her to perform leg exercises. Leg exercises help to prevent blood from pooling in the veins of the legs.

The exercises are done while the person is in the supine position. One leg is exercised at a time. The person rotates the ankle, flexes and points the foot, flexes and extends the knee, and finishes by raising the leg off the bed and lowering it again. Each movement is repeated five times, and then the movements are repeated with the other leg, unless the person had leg surgery. In this case, the exercises might only be done on the "well" leg. A doctor's order is required to exercise the leg that was operated on. You should check with the nurse to see if there are any specific instructions for your patient.

Tell the Nurse!

During the post-operative period, you may be the first person to notice signs of a post-operative complication. Report any of the following observations to the nurse immediately:

⟶ There is an increased amount of bright red drainage (blood) on the person's wound dressing or in the drainage device

⟶ There is a significant change in the person's vital signs (blood pressure, pulse, respirations, temperature)

⟶ The person is having trouble breathing, or is making wheezing or gurgling sounds

⟶ The person is restless, confused, or disoriented

⟶ The person's lips or nailbeds are very pale or have a bluish tinge

⟶ The person's skin is cool and clammy

⟶ The person complains of increased pain, tingling, or numbness of an extremity with a cast or bandage

⟶ The person complains of pain or swelling at the IV site, or the IV is not dripping

⟶ The person complains of abdominal pain, nausea, or vomiting

ASSISTING WITH POSITIONING

During the post-operative period, most people will need assistance with repositioning themselves every 1 to 2 hours. Frequent repositioning is necessary for the person's comfort. In addition, it helps to prevent the post-operative complications of pneumonia and embolism. Depending on where the incision is, moving may be very painful for the person. Use a lift sheet to help reposition the person, and move him gently and slowly.

ASSISTING WITH NUTRITION

A person who is recovering from surgery usually needs intravenous (IV) therapy until she is able to take fluids orally and is no longer nauseated. If the person has had surgery involving the digestive system, she may have a nasogastric tube. The nasogastric tube is connected to suction to keep the stomach empty. These patients may need to remain on IV fluids for several days.

Once the person is able to take fluids orally and is no longer nauseated, she will usually be started on a clear liquid diet. The diet is progressed as the person's condition improves. From a clear liquid diet, the person usually progresses to a full liquid diet and then gradually to a regular diet. Good hydration and a proper diet help with the healing process.

ASSISTING WITH ELIMINATION

Following surgery, the person may have difficulties related to elimination. Some people may need to use a bedpan or a urinal after surgery. The person's NPO status, pain medications, and immobility can lead to constipation. A full bladder can increase pain from an abdominal incision, making voiding difficult. As a result, some people may need to be catheterized. Your responsibilities will include reporting the person's first voiding after surgery. Often, you will also need to measure and record the person's intake and output (I&O) for a period of time following surgery as well.

ASSISTING WITH HYGIENE

People who are recovering from surgery may need help with personal hygiene. Assisting with frequent oral care, helping the person to wash his face and hands, and changing soiled gowns promptly are all things you can do to help promote comfort. Many people will not be able to take a bath or a shower for a few days following surgery, because the incision cannot get wet.

These people will need your help in the form of either partial or complete bed baths.

ASSISTING WITH WALKING (AMBULATION)

Early and frequent ambulation is helpful in preventing many of the complications that can result from surgery. Many times, a person who has had surgery is able to get out of bed within a few hours of returning to his room. Because the person will be weak and unsteady, he will need your help when ambulating. Allow the person time to sit on the edge of the bed ("dangle") before getting out of bed. If the person complains of feeling dizzy or lightheaded while he is dangling, help the person to lie back down and call the nurse. Otherwise, check the person's pulse and blood pressure and then help the person to stand. Usually, you and the person will walk only a short distance to begin with. As the person's strength returns, you can go for longer walks.

SUMMARY

▶ Surgery is a branch of medicine that involves treating diseases and disorders by removing or repairing damaged organs or tissues.
  ■ Surgery may be exploratory or definitive. It may be elective, urgent, or emergent.
  ■ Surgery is performed under anesthesia. A general, regional, or local anesthetic may be used.
  ■ Because many surgeries are now done on an outpatient basis, you may be responsible for helping a person to prepare and recover from surgery, even if you do not work in a hospital or other acute care setting.

▶ There are three phases of care for a person who is having surgery. The term *peri-operative period* is used to describe all three phases of the surgical process as a whole.
  ■ During the pre-operative period, the patient is prepared emotionally and physically for the procedure.
    • People who are about to have surgery often have many fears and concerns. Pre-operative teaching helps to relieve some of the person's fears. By listening to your patients and promptly relaying any questions they may have to the nurse, you can make an important contribution to the pre-operative teaching process.
    • A pre-operative checklist is completed to verify that the tasks needed to prepare the person physically for surgery have been accomplished, and that informed consent has been obtained.
  ■ During the intra-operative period, surgery is performed.
  ■ During the post-operative period, the nursing team's efforts focus on preventing complications and helping the person to recover.
    • Coughing and deep breathing exercises, along with incentive spirometry, may help to reduce the person's risk of developing respiratory complications, such as pneumonia and atelectasis.
    • Application of sequential compression devices (SCDs) or anti-embolism (TED) stockings may help to prevent cardiovascular complications, such as thrombophlebitis or embolism. Leg exercises and frequent ambulation are also helpful.
    • In addition to performing tasks related to preventing complications, nursing assistants may need to assist surgical patients with activities of daily living (ADLs), such as bathing and elimination, during the post-operative period.

Chapter 39 Procedures

Getting Ready Steps

a. **W**ash your hands and observe standard precautions as necessary.

b. **G**ather needed supplies.

c. **K**nock and introduce yourself.

d. **I**dentify the person and greet him or her by name.

e. **E**xplain the procedure.

f. **P**rovide privacy.

g. **S**ee to safety.

Finishing Up Steps

a. **C**onfirm comfort and good body alignment.

b. **L**eave the call light control within easy reach.

c. **S**ee to safety.

d. **O**pen the curtain and door.

e. **W**ash your hands.

f. **R**eport and record.

PROCEDURE 39-1

Applying Anti-embolism (TED) Stockings

Getting Ready

1. Complete the "Getting Ready" steps **a** through **g**.

Supplies

- anti-embolism (TED) stockings in the correct size

Procedure

2. Make sure that the bed is positioned at a comfortable working height (to promote good body mechanics) and that the wheels are locked. If the side rails are in use, lower the side rail on the working side of the bed. The side rail on the opposite side of the bed should remain up.

3. Help the person into the supine position.

4. Fanfold the top linens to the foot of the bed. Adjust the person's hospital gown or pajama bottoms as necessary to expose one leg at a time.

5. Turn the stocking inside out down to the heel.

STEP 5 Turn the stocking inside out down to the heel.

6. Slip the foot of the stocking over the person's toes, foot, and heel. The stocking has an opening in the toe area, which allows the health care team to assess the person's toes to make sure they are receiving enough blood. Depending on the manufacturer, this opening may be on the top or on the bottom of the stocking.

(continued)

PROCEDURE 39-1 (Continued)

Applying Anti-embolism (TED) Stockings

STEP 6 Slip the foot of the stocking over the person's toes, foot, and heel.

7. Grasp the top of the stocking and pull it up the person's leg. The stocking will turn itself right-side out as you pull it up the person's leg.

STEP 7 Grasp the top of the stocking and pull it up the person's leg.

8. Check to make sure that the stocking is not twisted and that it fits snugly against the person's leg, with no wrinkles. Also make sure that the stocking fits smoothly over the heel, and that the opening in the toe area is correctly located in the toe region.

9. Cover that leg, expose the other leg, and repeat steps 5 through 8.

10. Help the person back into a comfortable position, straighten the bottom linens, and draw the top linens over the person. Raise the head of the bed as the person requests. Make sure that the bed is lowered to its lowest position and that the wheels are locked.

Finishing Up C L S O W R

11. Complete the "Finishing Up" steps **a** through **f**.

What did you learn?

Multiple Choice

Select the single best answer for each of the following questions.

1. Mrs. Jones is recovering from surgery. How often will she need assistance with repositioning?
   a. Every shift
   b. Every 1 to 2 hours
   c. Every 3 to 4 hours
   d. Every 15 minutes

2. Which one of the following patients is at high risk for an embolism?
   a. Mr. Smith, who is 75 years old and has just had cardiac bypass surgery
   b. Mrs. Greene, who is 60 years old and has just had a hip joint replaced
   c. Ms. Kirkpatrick, who is 40 years old and has just had surgery to repair a fractured leg
   d. All of the above

3. Which one of the following may be a sign of pulmonary embolism?
   a. Fever
   b. Fatigue
   c. Profuse sweating
   d. Restlessness and shortness of breath

4. The nurse asks you to help Mr. Huang in Room 340 with coughing and deep breathing exercises. What is the purpose of these exercises?
   a. To help Mr. Huang build up his strength following the surgery
   b. To lower Mr. Huang's risk of pulmonary embolism
   c. To lower Mr. Huang's risk of pneumonia or atelectasis
   d. All of the above

5. Why might emergent surgery be necessary?
   a. The person has been in a car accident and is bleeding internally
   b. The person needs to have a cataract removed
   c. The person needs to have a hip joint replaced
   d. The person needs to have a tumor in the breast removed

6. During which type of anesthesia is the person unconscious?
   a. Regional anesthesia
   b. Local anesthesia
   c. General anesthesia
   d. All of the above

7. Which one of the following activities takes place before surgery?
   a. Frequent ambulation
   b. Completion of the pre-operative checklist
   c. Performance of coughing and deep breathing exercises
   d. Careful monitoring in the post-anesthesia care unit (PACU)

8. Why must a person who is having surgery avoid taking food or fluids by mouth for 6 to 8 hours before the surgery?
   a. If the person vomits as a result of the anesthesia, he or she could be at risk for aspiration
   b. An empty stomach is necessary to prevent infection of the abdominal cavity
   c. The anesthesia is more effective if the person's stomach is empty
   d. An empty stomach helps to prevent problems with elimination after the surgery

Stop and think!

▶ You are a nursing assistant in an assisted-living facility. One of your residents, Mrs. Wight, is scheduled to have a surgical procedure done on an outpatient basis at the local hospital. Mrs. Wight is a very stylish woman who takes a lot of pride in her appearance. Her nails are always done, she always accessorizes her outfits, and she always makes sure to apply a fresh coat of lipstick before leaving her room. Mrs. Wight knows that she is not permitted to wear make-up during the surgery, but when you arrive in her room to help her get ready the day of the surgery, you find that she is looking like her usual self—nails done, jewelry on, lipstick applied. What would you do, and why?

▶ You work as a nursing assistant in a hospital. One of your patients, Mr. Newman, is scheduled for exploratory surgery to determine whether a tumor in his brain is cancerous. Mr. Newman is married, with three children ranging in age from 8 to 14 years. He has a very large extended family, many of whom have been staying at the hospital day and night since Mr. Newman was admitted. How might Mr. Newman and his family members be feeling right now? Is there anything you could do to help them?

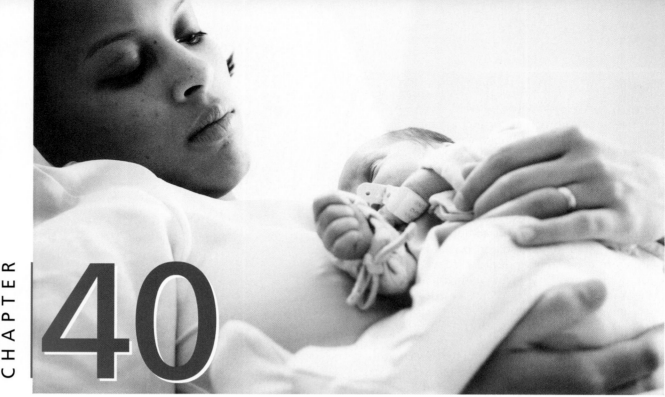

40

Caring for Mothers and Newborns

What will you learn?

Every day, thousands of babies are born in the United States. Many are born in hospitals or birthing centers. Some are born at home. A very few choose to make a dramatic entrance, by being born in the car on the way to the hospital or birthing center! No matter where the birth occurs, few events are met with as much excitement as the birth of a baby.

In this chapter, you will learn how to care for a newborn baby. You will also learn about the care required by the mother in the months leading up to the birth, during the birth, and following the birth. Although many states and health care facilities do not allow nursing assistants to participate in the care of an expectant mother or a newborn, others do. You may work in a hospital, providing care for mothers and newborns before, during, and after delivery. Or you may be employed by a home health care agency that provides home care to expectant and new mothers and their newborns. When you are finished with this chapter, you will be able to:

1. Describe physical changes that occur in the female reproductive system during pregnancy.
2. List reasons that an expectant mother may need home care or hospitalization during her pregnancy.
3. Describe the two ways of delivering a baby.
4. Describe the responsibilities a nursing assistant would have when caring for a new mother.
5. List observations you might make while caring for a new mother that should be reported to the nurse immediately.
6. Explain how to bottle-feed a baby.

(continued)

Photo: Few events are met with as much excitement as the birth of a baby.
(© Laurent/Ravonison/Photo Researchers, Inc.)

7. Explain how to care for the umbilical cord stump.
8. Explain how to care for a baby boy who has been circumcised.
9. Explain how to bathe a baby.
10. Discuss important security and safety issues related to caring for a newborn.

Vocabulary

Use the CD in the back of your book to hear these terms pronounced, defined, and used in a sentence:

Antepartum (prenatal) period
Placenta
Prenatal care
Pre-term labor

Preeclampsia/ eclampsia
Labor
Cesarean section
Epidural block

Vernix
Bonding period
Postpartum period
Lochia
Episiotomy

Sitz bath
Colostrum
Umbilical cord

THE ANTEPARTUM (PRENATAL) PERIOD

When a woman is pregnant, the period of time from conception until the baby is born is called the **antepartum (prenatal) period.** (The prefixes *ante-* and *pre-* both mean "before," and the roots *partum* and *natal* both mean "birth.") The antepartum period lasts approximately 9 months and is divided into three trimesters of 3 months each.

PHYSICAL CHANGES IN PREGNANCY

Very soon after conception, the pregnant woman's body undergoes dramatic changes that allow for the growth and development of the new life she carries inside. The changes are the result of hormones secreted by the woman's pituitary gland and the **placenta,** the structure that develops from the inside lining of the uterus during pregnancy and participates in the exchange of gas and nutrients between the mother and the developing baby (called a *fetus*). Prolactin, a hormone secreted by the pituitary gland, causes the woman's breasts to enlarge and prepare for the production of milk to nourish the baby after birth. The uterus enlarges to make room for the growing fetus. More blood is formed to manage the extra demand created by the fetus's need for

oxygen and nutrients. The extra blood also helps to remove the extra waste products created by the fetus.

These physical changes can result in many "signs and symptoms" of pregnancy. For example, changes in hormone levels may be responsible for the morning sickness that many women have during the first trimester of pregnancy. In a pregnancy that is progressing normally, certain "signs and symptoms" are expected at certain times (Fig. 40-1).

ROUTINE PRENATAL CARE

Prenatal care, or the health care given to a woman in the months leading up to the birth of her baby, helps to ensure the health of both the mother and the fetus during the pregnancy. Routine prenatal care involves screening tests and regular check-ups. The woman is also given advice about how to care for herself and her developing fetus:

- **Nutrition.** A pregnant woman should eat a healthy diet, containing a variety of nutritious foods. Because a pregnant woman must meet her own body's nutritional needs, plus those of the developing fetus, her nutritional needs are increased. For example, because she has an increased need for calcium, a pregnant woman should consume 3 to 4 servings of dairy foods each

First trimester
- First missed menstrual period
- Morning sickness
- Swollen, tender breasts

Second trimester
- Visibly enlarged uterus
- Weight gain
- Breast enlargement
- Will feel baby move

Third trimester
- Indigestion and shortness of breath (caused by enlarged uterus pressing on stomach and lungs)
- Difficulty sleeping
- Swollen ankles

FIGURE 40-1

The antepartum period is divided into three trimesters. In a pregnancy that is progressing normally, certain signs and symptoms are expected at certain times.

day (versus 2 to 3 servings for a woman who is not pregnant). Most doctors also suggest that pregnant women take a special prenatal vitamin supplement daily to ensure that their nutritional needs are met.

- **Avoidance of toxins.** A pregnant woman should avoid smoking, drinking alcohol, or taking any medications that have not been specifically approved by her doctor. Many of these substances are known to harm the growth and development of the fetus.
- **Exercise.** Moderate exercise throughout pregnancy has been shown to have benefits for both the mother and the fetus. If a woman is interested in either starting an exercise program or continuing one during her pregnancy, the health care team will provide information about how to safely do this.

COMPLICATIONS DURING PREGNANCY

Prenatal care helps to prevent complications from developing during the pregnancy. It also helps to detect complications at an early stage,

should any develop. If a complication develops, the pregnant woman may be hospitalized or placed on partial or complete bed rest at home for the rest of her pregnancy to help protect her own health, as well as that of the fetus. Examples of complications that can develop during pregnancy include **pre-term labor** (labor begins too early, before the fetus is capable of surviving on its own) and **preeclampsia/eclampsia** (the woman develops dangerously high blood pressure). Some pregnancies are "high risk" right from the start—for example, the woman has had trouble carrying a baby to term in the past, she is carrying more than one baby, or she has a chronic health condition, such as diabetes. These women may also be hospitalized or put on bed rest at some point during their pregnancies.

A pregnant woman who is having, or is at risk for, complications may be hospitalized for weeks or even months prior to the birth of the baby. Depending on the situation, she may be permitted to stay at home, but with extreme limitations on activity. In this case, she will often need the services of a home health care aide.

MEETING THE PREGNANT WOMAN'S PHYSICAL NEEDS

A nursing assistant who is caring for a pregnant woman in the hospital or home health care setting may have the following responsibilities:

- **Measuring and recording vital signs.** Any change in the woman's vital signs must be reported to the nurse immediately.
- **Obtaining urine samples.** Depending on the situation, the woman may need to provide urine samples on a regular basis. The urine is tested for glucose and protein. You may be responsible for obtaining these samples.
- **Helping with personal care.** Many women who are on bed rest are allowed to get up for short periods of time to go to the bathroom, but they will need assistance with bathing in bed and grooming. If the woman is not allowed to get out of bed at all, then she will also need assistance with toileting.

Make sure you follow all directions that are given to you regarding the woman's care, and ask the nurse for help if you are unsure about how to complete any of your assigned duties.

▶ Tell the Nurse!

Complications during a pregnancy can endanger the life of the mother and the baby if they are not reported promptly. When caring for a pregnant woman, report the following observations to the nurse immediately:

- There is a change in the woman's vital signs (especially an elevated blood pressure or body temperature)
- The woman complains of a headache or of seeing "spots" or "bright flashes" in front of her eyes
- The woman faints or is dizzy
- The woman has nausea, vomiting, or diarrhea
- The woman complains of abdominal pain
- The woman is experiencing uterine contractions that are frequent or severe and are not relieved by resting
- The woman has vaginal bleeding or there is fluid leaking from the vagina

MEETING THE PREGNANT WOMAN'S EMOTIONAL NEEDS

When caring for a pregnant woman, be aware that the woman's feelings may differ from what you consider "normal." Some women have mixed emotions when they find out that they are pregnant. The pregnancy may be unplanned, or another child may cause financial hardship for the family. Sometimes there are health concerns associated with the pregnancy. All of these are reasons that an expectant mother may not behave in a "typical" way. It is important to respect your patient's feelings, even if they differ from what yours would be in a similar situation. Also, avoid being judgmental about a woman's marital situation or other lifestyle choices. Remember that not all pregnant women have (or necessarily want) husbands.

A pregnant woman who is experiencing complications and has been placed on partial or complete bed rest prior to the birth of her child may have many emotional needs. The woman may feel lonely and bored—imagine what it would be like to be stuck in the same bed, in the same room, for weeks, or even months. Making pleasant conversation as you complete your duties can help to ease the woman's loneliness. The woman may also have lots of worries. She may be worried about her own health, as well as that of her unborn child. She may worry about children she already has, and how they are being cared for in her absence. She may worry about how she will pay her bills during the time that she cannot work. Taking the time to listen to the woman's concerns, and reporting these concerns to the nurse, is important (Fig. 40-2).

Pregnancy can be a time of great joy and anticipation. It can also be a time of great stress, especially if complications develop that jeopardize the mother's health and that of the baby.

Sometimes pregnancy does not end with the birth of a healthy baby. Many pregnancies result in miscarriage. Some babies are born too early to survive on their own, and die. Some babies are stillborn (born dead). The loss of a child is an emotional time for the family. Loss affects each person differently. Be respectful of the family's feelings. Acknowledge the loss, and simply say "I'm sorry."

FIGURE 40-2

A pregnant woman who is having complications is likely to be lonely, bored, scared, or all three. Making yourself available to listen is part of providing holistic care.

LABOR AND DELIVERY

LABOR

When it is time for a baby to be born, the mother's pituitary gland releases oxytocin, a hormone that stimulates the uterus to contract. The contractions of the uterus squeeze the baby downward, forcing his head against the cervix so that it opens, or *dilates.* This process is known as **labor.** The length of time a woman is in labor varies greatly from person to person. Some women have very short labors, while other labors may last as long as 36 hours or so. When caring for a woman who is in labor, your responsibilities are to provide the support and care required by your facility. In many cases, your only responsibility will be to measure and record vital signs and other observations. However, some facilities or birth centers provide additional training, which will allow you to perform more specialized tasks when assisting a woman who is in labor.

DELIVERY

A woman may deliver (give birth to) the baby vaginally or by cesarean section (Fig. 40-3). Delivery of the baby through the vagina (a vaginal delivery) is usually preferred, unless there are complications. A **cesarean section** (delivery of the baby through a surgical incision made in the mother's abdomen) is done when a vaginal delivery is not possible or safe for the mother or the baby. For example, many doctors choose to do a cesarean section when labor has gone on for too long, when the baby is not positioned correctly for a vaginal delivery, or when the mother has a serious health problem (such as heart disease) that would make a prolonged labor dangerous. Because a cesarean section is a surgical procedure, the recovery time following a cesarean delivery is generally longer than the recovery time following a vaginal delivery.

Women who give birth vaginally may choose to deliver with or without pain medications. Many women choose to have an **epidural block,** anesthesia given through a catheter that is placed in the spinal canal. The catheter is placed in the lower back, so that the anesthetic affects only the

A. Vaginal delivery

B. Cesarean delivery

FIGURE 40-3

A baby may be delivered (A) vaginally or (B) by cesarean section. (A © B. Proud; B © Constantino Margiotta/Photo Researchers, Inc.)

FIGURE 40-4

The baby is (A) weighed and (B) measured.

A   B

pelvis and legs. This allows the woman to be awake and participate fully in the birth of her child, while numbing the pain of labor.

Woman who give birth by cesarean section are having major abdominal surgery, and therefore require an anesthetic of some sort. The woman may be given an epidural block, or in some cases, general anesthesia. An incision is then made in the woman's abdomen, and the baby is lifted out of the uterus. After delivery, the incision is closed and the mother is recovered in the same manner as with any other type of operation (see Chapter 39).

IMMEDIATELY FOLLOWING DELIVERY

Immediately following the birth of the baby, if the baby is breathing well and otherwise stable, she may be handed directly to her mother for a few moments. Then, the baby is weighed and measured and evaluated by the nurse or doctor (Fig. 40-4). The baby's footprints are taken, and identification bracelets are applied to her wrists and ankles. Because it takes a while for a newborn's body to adjust to life outside of the mother's body, especially with regard to regulation of body temperature, the baby may be placed for a short period of time in a special bed to help keep her warm. A temperature monitor may be taped to the baby's skin, or you may need to measure the baby's axillary temperature as often as ordered or until the baby's temperature has stabilized. Once the baby's temperature has stabilized, she is given a bath to remove the **vernix,** a protective, cheese-like substance that is present on the skin of newborns (Fig. 40-5). Finally, the baby is wrapped snugly in a blanket; a soft, stretchy cap is put on the baby's head to prevent heat loss; and the baby is placed in the waiting arms of her mother.

FIGURE 40-5

Vernix is a white, cheese-like, water-resistant substance that helps to protect the fetus' skin from constant exposure to the watery amniotic fluid. After birth, any vernix that is present on the skin is washed off. (© *Educational Images/Custom Medical Stock Photo.*)

FIGURE 40-6

The first 1 to 2 hours following birth is a critical time for parents to bond with their newborn, and vice versa.

The first hour or two immediately following delivery is important for mother–infant bonding. This **bonding period** helps to develop the emotional and physical attachment between the mother and the infant. It is important to remember the importance of the bonding process for the father also (Fig. 40-6).

THE POSTPARTUM PERIOD

During the **postpartum period** (the 6-week period of time following the birth), you may be involved in the care of both the new mother and the new baby.

CARE OF THE MOTHER

Birth is a stressful, difficult activity affecting the entire body. After delivery, the mother will likely be tired, hungry, and thirsty. She may want to sleep, especially if the labor was long and difficult. She may only want privacy, to cuddle and get to know her new baby.

When you are caring for a woman who has just delivered a baby, you will have several general responsibilities related to her care, including:

- **Taking vital signs as ordered.** You will need to take the woman's vital signs as often as ordered. As always, any change in vital signs should be reported immediately.
- **Assisting with transferring and walking.** If the woman has had an epidural block, she may be unsteady on her feet for some time after delivery, and she will need help with transferring and walking.
- **Assisting with toileting.** Assist the new mother to the bathroom, or provide a bedpan if needed. Measure and record the amount of urine voided. Many women experience swelling after delivery and may not be able to void. If this is the case with your patient, tell the nurse. The woman may need to be catheterized.
- **Observing.** A complication that develops during the immediate postpartum period can become life-threatening very quickly. Being observant can make the difference between life and death for the new mother.

Tell the Nurse!

When caring for a woman who has just given birth, report any of the following observations to the nurse immediately:

⮕ There is an increased amount of vaginal bleeding

⮕ There is a change in the woman's vital signs, especially an increase in pulse rate and a decrease in blood pressure, or an increase in temperature

⮕ The woman complains of dizziness or excessive thirst

⮕ The woman has trouble breathing or complains of pain in the chest

⮕ A woman who has had an epidural block complains of increased numbness in her legs and pelvic region, or a headache

⮕ The woman is having trouble urinating or is unable to urinate

You may also have additional responsibilities, as described in the sections that follow.

Managing Vaginal Discharge

Following delivery, the mother will have vaginal discharge, called **lochia**:

- *Rubra lochia.* Initially, the discharge is bright red and is called *rubra lochia* (*rubra* means "red"). The woman will wear special sanitary napkins to collect this flow, which may last for 2 to 3 days. If she is recovering from a cesarean section or is on bed rest for other reasons, you may have to assist her with changing these napkins. Note the amount and color of the discharge and report your observations to the nurse. Remember that vaginal secretions should be handled according to standard precautions. Always wear gloves anytime you might come into contact with soiled sanitary napkins, bed linens, or bed protectors.

- *Lochia serosa* follows for approximately 3 to 10 days longer. Serosa is pink- or brown-tinged fluid. Any large clots are abnormal and should be reported immediately.
- *Lochia alba* follows for another week or two and is mostly creamy white to yellowish in color.

Assisting with Perineal Care

If the woman delivered her baby vaginally, she may have perineal tears, caused by the baby's head as it exited the birth canal. Sometimes, doctors perform an episiotomy to prevent the perineum from tearing so much. An **episiotomy** is an incision made in the perineum to enlarge the vaginal opening, making delivery of the baby's head easier. If the perineum was torn during the delivery, or if an episiotomy was done, the perineum will be sore and tender for several days and the new mother may find sitting uncomfortable.

Ice may be applied to the perineum for a period of time immediately following delivery to help prevent swelling. Afterwards, the use of Sitz baths may help ease the discomfort. A **Sitz bath** is a hot water soak for the perineal area. The basin, which usually fits over the toilet seat, is filled with hot water [105°F to 110°F (40.5°C to 43.4°C)] and the woman sits in it for the prescribed amount of time. Depending on facility policy, new mothers may also be instructed to cleanse the perineal area after each trip to the bathroom by spraying warm water over the area using a small plastic sprayer. Increased pain, swelling, or drainage from the episiotomy site could indicate an infection and should be reported to the nurse immediately.

Assisting with Breastfeeding

Many women choose to breastfeed their babies. Immediately following delivery of the baby, the new mother's breasts produce **colostrum,** a thin yellowish fluid that contains extra calories and protein, as well as important antibodies. Colostrum is usually secreted for 2 to 3 days after birth and is then replaced by the mother's breast milk. Breastfeeding requires the mother to take in extra calories and fluids. Therefore, you should offer the mother fresh water frequently, as directed by the nurse.

The woman's breasts may become swollen and painful when the milk comes in. Frequent nursing of the infant will help to ease the discomfort, which usually only lasts for a couple of days. The appearance of a painful lump, reddened areas, or an elevated temperature could indicate a breast infection and should be reported to the nurse immediately.

If a woman chooses to breastfeed her baby, the nurse will teach her how. You may need to help the new mother get in a comfortable position, especially if she has had a cesarean section or a painful episiotomy. Help her to first wash her hands and then gently clean the nipple of the breast with warm water. Next, hand the mother the baby. There are several different ways to hold a baby during breastfeeding. With time, the mother will usually find the way of holding the baby that works best for her. Have the mother stroke the baby's cheek with her nipple to stimulate the baby's rooting reflex. The baby will turn his head toward the breast and open his mouth. The mother needs to place all of the nipple and part of the *areola* (the colored portion of the breast surrounding the nipple) into the baby's mouth. She may need to use her finger to help keep her breast from blocking the baby's nose while he nurses (Fig. 40-7). As the baby sucks on the breast, the mother may experience cramping pains in her lower abdomen. This is normal. After the baby has finished feeding from the first breast, the mother inserts her finger gently into his mouth to break the suction before removing him from the breast. After burping the baby, the process is repeated with the other breast.

After the baby has finished nursing, have the mother clean her breasts with warm water. Soap should not be used, because it can cause dryness or irritation of the nipples. Some

FIGURE 40-7

When breastfeeding, the mother may need to use a finger to hold the breast away from the baby's nose. Note that the baby's mouth covers both the nipple and the areola.

women use special creams or ointments when they first start breastfeeding to help keep the nipples from cracking and becoming sore. Some women find that a supportive nursing bra is more comfortable than a regular bra, while others do not.

CARE OF THE BABY

A newborn is considered a neonate for the first 28 days of his or her life. You may help to care for a neonate in the hospital or birth center, or in the home as a home health aide. You may also find yourself caring for older babies, especially if you work in the home health care setting or in the pediatrics unit of a hospital.

 Tell the Nurse!

A baby can become very sick very quickly. When caring for an infant, report any of the following observations to the nurse immediately:

▶ The baby appears weak or "floppy"

▶ The baby is pale

▶ The baby cries, and nothing you try makes him stop

▶ The baby's temperature is abnormal (either high or low)

▶ The baby's heart rate is abnormal (either fast or slow)

▶ The baby is breathing rapidly and shallowly

▶ The baby cannot be wakened

▶ The baby has a rash

▶ The baby will not eat

▶ The baby's eyes are red or discolored

▶ The baby has vomited

Taking Vital Signs

You may be responsible for taking vital signs on the newborn infant. If the baby is in the room with the mother, make sure you explain what you are going to do before beginning.

- A newborn's temperature may be measured either by the axillary or tympanic method (Fig. 40-8). Rectal temperatures are not routinely taken on newborns. The range of normal is the same as that for an adult.

- A newborn's apical pulse is taken for a full minute by listening (auscultating) with a stethoscope over the heart. The normal heart rate in a newborn is 100–180 beats/min. A newborn's respirations are also counted for a full minute by watching the abdomen rise and fall. The normal respiratory rate in a newborn is 30–60 breaths/min. Vital signs taken on a crying baby are not going to be accurate, so it is best to measure the baby's pulse and respirations while the baby is sleeping, if possible.

FIGURE 40-8

A newborn's temperature is measured using either the axillary or tympanic method. The axillary method is shown here.

FIGURE 40-9

A newborn's blood pressure may be measured manually or using an electronic measuring device. Here, an electronic measuring device is being used. Note the very small cuff, which is sized according to the baby's weight.

- A newborn's blood pressure is measured in the baby's arm using a cuff specifically sized according to the baby's weight (Fig. 40-9). Most facilities use electronic blood pressure devices for taking a newborn's blood pressure. These devices inflate the cuff and measure the blood pressure automatically. The range of normal for a newborn is 73–92 mm Hg systolic, 52–65 mm Hg diastolic.

Ensuring Security

If you work in the postpartum unit of a hospital or in a birthing center, there will be many policies and procedures in place to ensure the security of the newborn (Fig. 40-10). These security measures are taken to prevent newborns from being kidnapped from the facility by people posing as relatives or health care workers. Always follow the security procedures in place at your facility. These procedures usually require visitors to sign in. The baby is brought from, and returned to, the nursery by a member of the health care team. A member of the health care team must also accompany the baby if a family member wishes to take him to another part of the hospital. Finally, the identification bands on the baby's wrist and ankle are always checked against the parent's identification band before the baby is handed to the parent. The identification bands cannot be removed until after the baby goes home with his parents.

FIGURE 40-10

Protecting the security of the newborn is very important. In some health care facilities, a security device like the one pictured here is attached to the newborn. If someone tries to remove the baby from the nursery, the device sounds an alarm.

Caring for the Umbilical Cord Stump

The **umbilical cord** supplies the growing fetus with nutrients and oxygen, and removes waste. When the baby is born, the umbilical cord is clamped and cut. Eventually, the "stump" (the part of the cord that remains) dries up and falls off, leaving behind the navel (or belly button). Until the stump dries up and falls off, it must be cared for properly to prevent infection (Fig. 40-11). At each diaper change, rub an alcohol swab over the entire stump. The purpose of this is to clean and to dry the stump. If the stump or surrounding area is red, bleeding, or has any drainage,

FIGURE 40-11

The umbilical cord stump is wiped with an alcohol swab at each diaper change to keep it clean and promote drying. The stump will dry up and fall off in about 10 days.

tell the nurse. The baby should not be given a complete bath (in a bath basin) until the umbilical cord stump has dried up and fallen off. This usually occurs within about 10 days of the birth.

Providing Circumcision Care

Circumcision is the surgical removal of the foreskin from the head of the penis. Many studies have been done regarding the long-term benefits and risks associated with circumcision. To date, whether to circumcise remains largely a matter of parental choice. Circumcision is also a rite of the Jewish religion.

The circumcision is done using local anesthetic. The procedure can be performed at the hospital before the baby is discharged home, or it may be done at the doctor's office. Following circumcision, the penis should be kept clean and dry. A petrolatum dressing may be applied to keep the penis from sticking to the diaper. Triple antibiotic ointment may also be applied, as an added precaution against infection. Be sure to follow any specific instructions that are given to you regarding care of the circumcision.

The baby's penis will be red and sore (Fig. 40-12). If you notice bleeding, drainage, or odor when you are changing the baby's diaper, tell the nurse. The circumcision should heal within 10 to 14 days. After the circumcision has healed, the baby can be given a complete bath in a bath basin.

FIGURE 40-12

Following circumcision, the penis will be red and sore, but there should not be any bleeding, discharge, or odor. Report any of these observations to the nurse immediately.

Feeding

Babies who are not being breastfed are fed with a bottle. The bottle may contain the mother's breast milk, or a prepared formula. Infants who are younger than 1 year should not be fed cow's milk. Cow's milk can cause the baby to develop food allergies. In addition, it does not contain many of the nutrients that are essential for the baby's growth.

Many commercial formula preparations are available. Some formulas come prepared and ready to feed to the baby, while others are in the form of a powder or a concentrated liquid that must be mixed with water prior to feeding (Fig. 40-13A). Make sure you follow the label instructions carefully when preparing infant formula, so that the prepared formula is neither too strong nor too weak. Often, several bottles are prepared at once and stored in the refrigerator (see Fig. 40-13B). Before preparing the bottles, wash your hands.

Prepared bottles that have been stored in the refrigerator will need to be brought to room temperature before feeding the baby. To warm the bottle, place the prepared bottle in a container of warm water. Check the temperature of the bottle by shaking a few drops of the formula onto your wrist before feeding the baby. Never use a microwave oven to warm the bottle. Microwaving can cause the formula inside the bottle to become very hot in some spots, while remaining cool in others. When you test the formula on your wrist, the "hot spots" might go undetected. The hot formula will then burn the baby's mouth when she swallows it.

Hold the baby upright while feeding her (Fig. 40-14). Never prop the bottle up during feeding, or lay the baby down to take the bottle. After every few ounces of formula, stop feeding the baby so that she can burp. Burping gets rid of the excess air that is swallowed during feeding. The baby can be burped in several ways (Fig. 40-15). Hold the baby upright on your knee, or place the baby over your shoulder, and gently rub or pat her back. Be patient—some infants burp easily, while others may need more time.

Bottles, nipples, and rings should be cleaned in the dishwasher. They can also be washed by hand in hot, soapy water and rinsed well. Bottles do not need to be boiled for sterility, unless the doctor specifies that this should be done. In a hospital setting, disposable bottles are usually used.

A

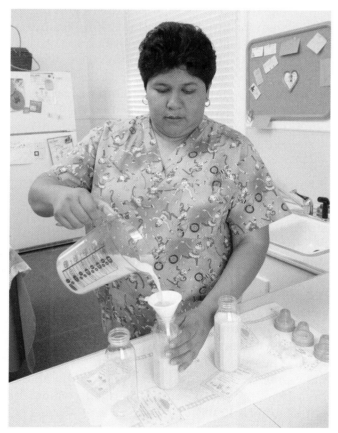

B

FIGURE 40-13

Babies who are not breastfed are bottle fed. (*A*) Many types of prepared formulas for bottle feeding are available. (*B*) When preparing bottles, always be sure to mix the formula according to the label instructions, if the formula is not "ready-to-feed."

Diapering

Infants are diapered, using disposable or cloth diapers. To prevent diaper rash and skin break-down, change the baby's diaper every time the baby has a bowel movement or urinates:

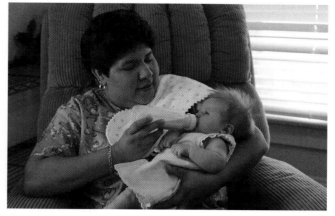

FIGURE 40-14

Always hold a baby upright to feed her.

1. Wash your hands and gather your supplies. It is important to gather all of your supplies first because you must never leave a baby alone, even for a moment. Even very small infants can easily roll off the changing table or other surface, leading to serious injury.
2. Put on the gloves, and remove the soiled diaper. Clean the perineal area, wiping from front to back if the baby is a girl. The perineal area can be cleansed with baby wipes (soft disposable wet cloths that contain a cleansing agent) or with a warm, wet washcloth. A mild baby soap may be used in addition to a warm, wet washcloth if the baby had a bowel movement. Be sure to rinse and dry the area thoroughly. Apply diaper rash ointment or a light dusting of cornstarch powder, if used.
3. Position the clean diaper, fastening it with the provided tabs (or diaper pins, if you are using a cloth diaper). Place the baby in an infant carrier or some other secure place.
4. Dispose of the soiled diaper in an appropriate waste container. Before placing a cloth diaper that is soiled with stool in the diaper pail, rinse it in cool water to prevent the stool from drying in the diaper.
5. Remove your gloves and wash your hands.

Bathing

A newborn infant is given a complete bath at birth. Once the umbilical cord stump has fallen

A

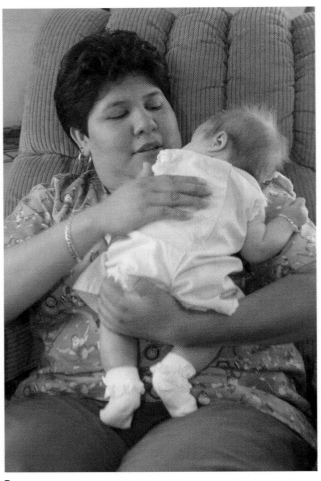

B

FIGURE 40-15

To burp the baby, (A) hold her upright on your knee, or (B) place her over your shoulder.

off and the circumcision has healed (if the baby was circumcised), the baby may be given a complete bath in a bath basin on a routine basis. Until that time, partial baths (sponge baths) are given as needed.

To bathe a baby in a bath basin:

1. Gather all of the supplies you will need before beginning the bath. This is important because you must never leave a baby alone in a bath.
2. Fill the bath basin with only 1 to 2 inches of warm water. Check the water temperature with a bath thermometer before putting the baby in the bath basin (Fig. 40-16A). The temperature should be between 100°F and 105°F (37.8°C to 40.5°C).
3. Place the baby in the bath basin and put on your gloves. Lather the baby's hair with a baby shampoo and rinse well (see Fig. 40-16B). Next, use a washcloth and soap formulated for infant skin. Wash the baby's face first. Then move on to the rest of the body, making sure to rinse all soap from the skin (see Fig. 40-16C). Keep a firm grip on the baby at all times and work quickly, to avoid chilling the baby.
4. After the bath, dry the baby thoroughly. Baby lotion may be applied as desired.

Putting a Baby Down to Sleep

A baby should be placed on his back or side to sleep. Research has shown that positioning babies on their backs or sides is safer than positioning them on their stomachs (Fig. 40-17). When placing a baby on his side to sleep, roll a receiving blanket or towel and tuck it securely next to the baby's back. This will help the baby to stay in the side-lying position. Remove all fluffy blankets, pillows, and toys from the sleeping area. These items pose a suffocation risk (the baby may get tangled in them and not be able to breathe). Instead of using blankets, place the baby in a blanket sleeper to keep him warm.

A baby can also be placed in an infant carrier to sleep. After putting the baby in the carrier, make sure that the carrier straps are properly secured (Fig. 40-18). Place the carrier on a low, level surface (such as the floor) so that it does not tip. Make sure that the carrier is out of the reach of pets or other small children who could accidentally knock the carrier over. Never place an infant carrier on a table or counter.

Transporting a Baby

A baby's first ride in a car seat occurs when the parents leave the hospital or birthing center.

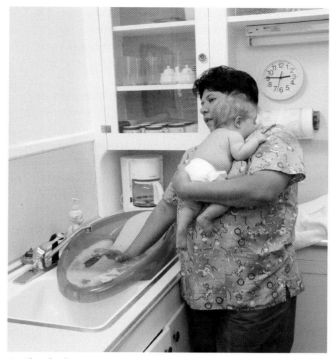

A. Check the water temperature.

B. Wash the baby's hair.

C. Wash the baby's body.

FIGURE 40-16

Bathing a baby. (*A*) The bath basin is only filled to a depth of 1 to 2 inches. Always check the temperature of the bath water before you put the baby in it. (*B*) Wash the baby's hair first. (*C*) Then wash the baby's body.

A   **B**

FIGURE 40-17

A baby is placed on his back or side to sleep, never on his stomach. (*A*) Positioning on the back. (*B*) Positioning on the side. Note the rolled receiving blanket bolstering the baby's back.

FIGURE 40-18

A baby may also sleep in her carrier. Always make sure to secure the baby in the carrier.

In all states, it is against the law to transport a baby in a car without first properly securing her in a car seat. You may need to help the parents install the car seat correctly, and show them how to place the baby in it. Written instructions for installation are provided with the car seat packaging. Instructions for installation can also be found on many manufacturers' websites.

An infant car seat is placed in the back seat. The baby faces the back of the car, not the front. This is safer in the event of an accident. An infant car seat is required until the child reaches the age of 1 year and weighs more than 20 pounds. The use of car seats for older babies and children is discussed in Chapter 41.

SUMMARY

▶ Nursing assistants often are involved in the care of pregnant women, women who are in labor or have just given birth, and newborns.

■ Complications during pregnancy can require a woman to be on complete or partial bed rest, either at home or in the hospital, for weeks or even months before delivery. When this occurs, the nursing assistant is usually responsible for measuring and recording vital signs and assisting with personal care for the expectant mother. In addition, the nursing assistant provides companionship and emotional support.

■ When assisting a woman who is in labor, the nursing assistant is usually only responsible for measuring and recording vital signs and other observations, unless he or she has received advanced training from the facility.

■ Following the delivery of the baby, the nursing assistant cares for both the new mother and the baby. The immediate post-delivery period is a critical time physically for both the mother and the

infant. The nursing assistant plays an important role during this time by reporting any unusual observations or vital sign measurements to the nurse promptly.

▶ During the postpartum period, the nursing assistant helps the new mother recover from the birth. The nursing assistant may also assist the new mother with breastfeeding her baby.

▶ A nursing assistant may care for a baby in the hospital, birthing center, or home setting.

■ Neonates require special care.

● The umbilical cord stump is wiped with an alcohol swab after each diaper change to prevent infection. The umbilical cord stump falls off after about 10 days.

● If a baby boy has been circumcised, the circumcision will also require special care for about the first 2 weeks.

● The neonate should not be submerged in bath water until the umbilical cord stump (and circumcision, if applicable) have completely healed, approximately 10–14 days.

■ Nursing assistants also assist with feeding, diapering, and bathing babies.

■ Following procedures and policies designed to keep the infant safe and secure is very important.

● Procedures and policies related to security in the postpartum units of facilities such as hospitals and birthing centers are designed to prevent babies from being kidnapped.

● When bathing or diapering a baby, never leave the baby alone, not even for a minute.

● Babies are placed on their backs or sides to sleep, never their stomachs.

● A baby must never be taken anywhere in a car without first placing him or her in a car seat. The car seat must be properly installed, and the baby must be properly positioned in it and strapped in.

What did you learn?

Multiple Choice

Select the single best answer for each of the following questions.

1. Mrs. Gutierrez had an episiotomy during the birth of her son. What might the nursing assistant do to help relieve the soreness and tenderness at the episiotomy site?
   a. Apply triple antibiotic ointment to the perineum
   b. Give Mrs. Gutierrez a bed bath
   c. Assist Mrs. Gutierrez with a Sitz bath
   d. Avoid washing the area until the episiotomy has healed

2. What is the period of time after delivery during which the parents and the new baby develop an emotional and physical attachment called?
   a. The epidural period
   b. The prenatal period
   c. The bonding period
   d. The antepartum period

3. You are caring for Ms. Bergen, who just had a baby. Which one of the following observations should you report immediately to the nurse?
   a. Ms. Bergen has what you think is an abnormal amount of vaginal discharge
   b. Ms. Bergen's pulse rate is elevated
   c. Ms. Bergen's blood pressure is low
   d. All of the above

4. Mrs. Ling has just delivered a daughter by cesarean section. You are helping her to breastfeed her baby, and she complains of cramping in her lower abdomen while the baby nurses. What is this a sign of?
   a. Mrs. Ling may be hemorrhaging
   b. The baby is kicking her in the stomach
   c. Cramping in the abdomen is a normal response during breastfeeding
   d. Mrs. Ling is not holding the baby correctly for breastfeeding

5. What position should an infant be placed in to sleep?
   a. On his back
   b. On his stomach
   c. On his side
   d. Either on his back or on his side

6. Which one of the following observations would be a cause for alarm when caring for a baby?
   a. The baby is pale
   b. The baby cries all the time, no matter what you do
   c. The baby will not eat
   d. All of the above

7. Mr. and Mrs. Saccamundi are going home from the hospital today with their new baby. How should the car seat be placed?
   a. In the front seat, facing the back of the car
   b. In the back seat, facing the back of the car
   c. In the back seat, facing the front of the car
   d. It makes no difference, as long as the baby is secure

8. You are checking vital signs on a newborn. Which one of the following measurements would you report to the nurse immediately?
   a. Heart rate 90 beats/min, respiratory rate 20 breaths/min
   b. Heart rate 160 beats/min, respiratory rate 34 breaths/min
   c. Heart rate 152 beats/min, respiratory rate 58 breaths/min
   d. None of the above

Matching

Match each numbered item with its appropriate lettered description.

_____ 1. Lochia

_____ 2. Colostrum

_____ 3. Vernix

a. Whitish, cheese-like protective coating on the skin of newborns
b. Vaginal discharge following the birth of a baby
c. Thin, yellowish fluid produced by the breasts before the milk comes in; rich in calories, protein, and antibodies

? Stop and think!

▶ You work in the newborn nursery at your local hospital. The other nursing assistant who works in the nursery with you, Shelly, has just left to take a baby to his mother for his noon feeding. You are attending to the other babies, when a pleasant-looking woman approaches and asks to see the new Sitko baby. She explains that she is the baby's grandmother, and she has just arrived from out of town to visit her son, daughter-in-law, and new grandchild. How would your respond to this request?

▶ Donna is a home health care aide who has been assigned to care for Mrs. Upchurch and her new baby, David. David was born very prematurely and spent several months in the hospital, but now the doctors have allowed him to come home. David still has numerous problems related to his premature birth, but coming home is a big milestone. Donna cannot help but notice that Mrs. Upchurch does not seem to be as thrilled about David's homecoming as Donna herself would be. Mrs. Upchurch seems very high-strung and almost frightened of the baby. In addition, she cries frequently. Why might Mrs. Upchurch be feeling this way? If you were Donna, how would you behave around Mrs. Upchurch?

41

Caring for Pediatric Patients

What will you learn?

Children receive health care in many different types of health care settings. For example, children who have acute illnesses or injuries are often cared for in a hospital setting. Children who need regular therapy or medical treatment for congenital or chronic health conditions may receive this care in a hospital, clinic, or home health care setting. Other children are residents of long-term care facilities because of developmental disabilities, injuries, or illnesses. Although many of the procedures used to provide physical care to a child are very similar to those used with adults, it is very important to remember that children are not simply "little adults." In this chapter, you will learn about the unique physical and emotional needs of children of different ages. You will also learn about your role in reporting suspected cases of child abuse. When you have finished with this chapter, you will be able to:

1. Discuss the specific physical needs that children in health care settings have, according to their ages and abilities.
2. Understand how the stages of development affect the emotional needs of children in health care settings.
3. Describe measures that the nursing assistant can use to assist a child in a health care setting.
4. List safety considerations that are specific for a child's age and developmental level.
5. Discuss the signs of abuse of a child and the nursing assistant's role in reporting suspected abuse.

Photo: Children who have acute illnesses or injuries are often cared for in a hospital setting.

Vocabulary

Use the CD in the back of your book to hear these terms pronounced, defined, and used in a sentence:

Failure to thrive
Regress
Magical thinking
Egocentric

Shaken baby
syndrome
Munchausen
syndrome by proxy

In Chapter 6, you learned about the stages of growth and development that we all pass through as we live our lives. Childhood is a time of rapid growth and development. A child's physical and emotional needs change constantly as he grows. Although only a few years separate a 3-year-old from an 8-year-old, there is a huge difference between these two age groups in terms of growth and development. A child's ability to understand and cooperate with the health care team depends on his particular stage of development. While a 3-year-old will need to be cuddled and sung to for comfort during a treatment or procedure, an 8-year-old will need answers to specific questions before he will feel comfortable. For example, an 8-year-old might ask *"What exactly is going to happen?" "What are you going to use to do that?" "Can I see it/touch it/hold it?"* and *"How will it feel?"* An understanding of the basic stages of growth and development will better prepare you to provide the type of care that each child requires.

In Chapter 6, you also learned how illness, injury, or disability affects people and their needs. You learned that although providing physical assistance to a person in a health care setting is a vital responsibility of the nursing assistant, recognizing and providing for the person's emotional needs is just as important. Think about what a frightening place a health care setting must be to a child. A child, especially a very young child, does not understand illness and pain. She has been taken from the comfort of her home and is now surrounded by people she does not know. Her room may be filled with strange, frightening machines, and "getting better" might mean having to have painful treatments or therapies first.

Think also about the effect a child's illness has on the family as a whole. Family members will worry that the child is suffering or uncomfortable. If the child's injury or illness is severe or acute, family members may wonder whether the child will survive the event, and if he does, what effects the illness or injury will have on his future growth and development. Sometimes, a child's illness requires one family member to travel to a distant health care facility to be with the child, while the rest of the family stays at home. When this is the case, the family member who is away may worry about the rest of the family at home, and how they are managing on their own. Families may worry about how they will pay for the health care that the child is receiving. The other children in the family may feel "left out" while most of the family's attention is being focused on the child who is sick or injured. Or they may feel guilty that they are healthy while their brother or sister is sick. Including the child's family members in his or her care whenever possible is one thing you can do to help the family cope with a child's illness (Fig. 41-1). The family members will feel like they are actively doing something to help the child, and the child will be happier being cared for by familiar people.

When working with children and families, remember that families come in all different shapes and sizes. Many families are "traditional," in the sense that they consist of two parents and one or more children. However, many families consist of only one parent and the children. Or, the children may be raised by grandparents, guardians, foster parents, or other caregivers. Regardless of the family structure, the effects of a child's illness on the people who care about the child are the same.

FIGURE 41-1

A child's illness can be very stressful for the family.

CARING FOR INFANTS

Infancy is the period of time from a child's birth to his first birthday. Infants grow and develop very rapidly during the first year of life. They progress from being totally helpless—unable to roll over, sit up, or move about without help—to being able to crawl, walk, and feed themselves small pieces of food by the time they reach the age of 1 year.

MEETING THE INFANT'S PHYSICAL NEEDS

An infant is totally dependent on her caregiver to help her meet her most basic physical needs. The procedures for feeding, diapering, bathing, and positioning a newborn that you learned in Chapter 40 apply for older infants as well. In addition, you may be responsible for monitoring food and fluid intake and output, and for monitoring the infant's temperature:

- **Monitoring food and fluid intake and output.** An infant who is ill or unable to drink or eat properly can quickly become dehydrated. An infant who is receiving adequate food and fluid will urinate regularly and have regular bowel movements. Since it is not possible to know exactly how much breast milk a nursing infant is taking at each feeding, keeping track of the number of wet diapers or actually weighing the wet diapers may be necessary to ensure that the baby is not dehydrated. Observing and recording the number, consistency, and amount of bowel movements may also be one of your responsibilities.
- **Monitoring body temperature.** An infant, especially one who is ill or very young, must be kept warm. A very small infant can be wrapped securely in a blanket. An older, more mobile infant can be clothed in snuggly one-piece pajamas if the weather is cold. A change in body temperature (either above or below the normal range) is cause for concern and should be reported immediately.

Because an infant's medical condition can change very quickly, you must report any unusual signs or symptoms (see Chapter 40) to the nurse immediately.

MEETING THE INFANT'S EMOTIONAL NEEDS

Aside from being clean, warm, and fed, an infant's greatest need is to feel secure. Infants need to be spoken to or sung to softly (Fig. 41-2). They need to be rocked gently, touched, and held. Human contact is essential for an infant to develop physically and emotionally. Many studies have shown that infants, even those who are well cared for physically, fail to grow and develop both physically and emotionally if they are not held and talked to. This is called **failure to thrive.**

To help meet an infant's emotional needs, you must take the time to touch, cuddle, stroke, and talk soothingly to him. Encourage family members to hold the baby, if the baby's condition allows. The nurse can show family members how to hold the baby without disturbing medical devices, such

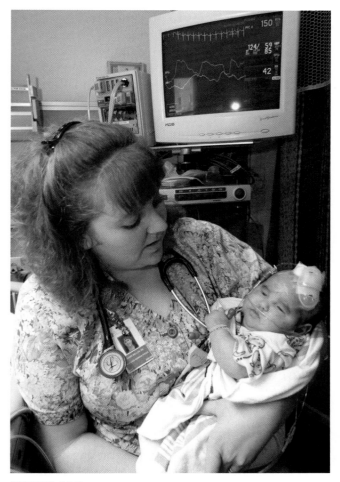

FIGURE 41-2

The infant's greatest emotional need is to feel safe and secure. Infants need to be held, cuddled, rocked, and spoken or sung to.

as monitors and tubes. Provide music and infant-appropriate toys. If possible, position the infant's bed so that he can watch activity out a window or through a doorway.

MEETING THE INFANT'S NEED FOR SAFETY

Safety and the prevention of accidents is essential for children of all ages, but especially for the youngest. As helpless as they may seem, infants can wriggle, roll, and twist themselves into dangerous situations very quickly.

- Never leave an infant on a surface unattended, even for a moment. Even very young infants can easily roll off of a bed, changing table, or examination table. An infant who falls to the floor could receive severe or fatal head injuries. If you are changing diapers, taking vital signs, or bathing an infant, keep one hand on the child at all times to prevent a fall.
- As the infant grows and is placed in an infant carrier, swing, or high chair, make sure that safety straps are securely fastened both across the infant's waist and between his legs to prevent him from falling out of, or sliding down in, the carrier, swing, or chair.
- Always secure the infant in a car seat when traveling in a car or other vehicle. An infant car seat is placed in the back seat. The baby faces the back of the car, not the front.
- An infant explores her world by placing everything she can get her hands on in her mouth. Therefore, make sure that toys are appropriate for the age of the infant and that they have no small, removable parts that she could choke on. Keep the toys clean by washing them frequently in warm, soapy water. As the infant learns to crawl and move about, make sure that the floor or play area is free of small objects or plants that the infant could place in her mouth.
- Keep plastic bags and balloons away from infants. With regard to plastic bags, a young infant could roll over and become tangled in the plastic. An older infant could put the bag over his head. The infant is unable to breathe through the plastic,

and suffocates. Balloons also pose a suffocation risk. The infant may put the balloon (or a piece of a broken balloon) in his mouth. When the infant inhales, the rubber balloon gets sucked into the airway, blocking air flow and leading to suffocation.
- Do not leave an infant unattended, even for a moment, in water of any depth. Babies who can stand up have drowned in a mop bucket!
- Make sure that electrical cords and window blind cords are out of the reach of the infant. The infant could become tangled in the cord and strangle himself. Or, he could put the electrical cord in his mouth, which could result in electrocution.

These are just a few of the many safety concerns that you must be aware of when caring for very small children. A primary rule of thumb is that if a child can reach an object, he will grab it and try to put it in his mouth. Child-proofing everything, whether in the home or the health care setting, is very critical for the safety of the infant.

CARING FOR TODDLERS

A toddler is a child between the ages of 1 and 3 years. Toddlers are mobile, curious, independent spirits who are into everything. Toddlers can feed themselves, and are busy learning how to communicate, how to use the potty, and how to dress themselves. Because of their newfound independence, toddlers may be very uncooperative with treatment and therapy related to health care.

Toddlers who need health care services are also likely to be very, very frightened little children. It is not uncommon for a child of this age to **regress,** or return to an earlier stage of development. For instance, a child who has been potty trained for some time may suddenly start wetting her pants, or she may ask for a bottle or pacifier after being previously weaned from these items. While frustrating, especially for the child's caregivers, regression is just a normal way for a young child to cope with stress. A toddler is still too young to verbalize her fears or even understand what exactly she is afraid of, so she just returns to an earlier, more comfortable stage of development temporarily until the stress passes. When caring for a toddler, it is important to recognize regression for what it is and ignore it. For example, rather than scolding a potty-trained child who has had an accident and telling her to "stop acting like a baby," clean her up and comfort her, without drawing a lot of attention to the accident.

MEETING THE TODDLER'S PHYSICAL NEEDS

A toddler will rely on you for assistance with meeting many of his physical needs, according to his abilities. Ask the toddler's regular caregiver how much help the child usually needs with eating, toileting, and dressing. Find out what words the child uses for urination and bowel movements. It is important for you to allow the toddler to remain as independent as possible. One way to do this is to offer choices that are realistic. For example, instead of asking the child what he wants to wear, limit his choices to those that are actually possible ("Do you want to wear your red pajamas, or your blue ones?").

Because a toddler's physical growth slows during this stage, his appetite may also be small. Being scared (for example, because he is in a health care setting) can also affect the toddler's appetite. Ask the child's caregiver what he likes to eat and drink. Many children in this age group have very clear, and very limited, food preferences. Most toddlers enjoy finger foods such as crackers, fruit (for example, an apple or banana) cut into small pieces, and dry cereal. They can drink from a cup and may enjoy a variety of juices and milk. Toddlers are usually on an "eat and run" type of dietary schedule and need to have small amounts of food provided throughout the day. You may be responsible for monitoring and recording the toddler's food and fluid intake. If the toddler's fluid intake is low, try offering foods such as popsicles, ice cream, or gelatin. These foods count toward the fluid intake and may be more enticing than a cup of water.

Older toddlers who sleep in a regular bed at home may be offered a small adjustable bed in the health care facility if their condition allows. However, a toddler who is at risk for falling out of bed may need a crib with side rails and a top cover. The use of restraints is common among children in this age group, because toddlers are simply too young to understand that intravenous lines, drains, catheters, and other medical devices are a necessary part of their treatment and should not be pulled out. If restraints are being used, be sure to check on the toddler very frequently (at least every 10 minutes). The best alternative to using a restraint is to keep the toddler occupied by offering distracting activities and toys, and by having someone stay with the toddler at all times.

MEETING THE TODDLER'S EMOTIONAL NEEDS

Most toddlers are afraid of strangers and therefore will prefer to be with their usual caregivers. Remember that you are a stranger to the toddler. Speak softly and get down on the toddler's level when you are talking with him. That way you will not appear quite so tall and scary. Many toddlers are more cooperative during procedures and therapy if they are allowed to sit in their usual caregiver's lap (Fig. 41-3). They also like to touch and explore any equipment that is being used in the procedure. Allow the child to handle your stethoscope and blood pressure cuff before attempting to measure vital signs.

Toddlers love to play with brightly colored toys such as blocks, simple puzzles, and stuffed toys. They also love to clap, move, and sing along with children's songs. Because their attention spans are very short, toddlers become bored and

FIGURE 41-3

Most toddlers enjoy handling the equipment that will be used in a procedure. Procedures will usually go more smoothly if it is possible for the toddler's usual caretaker to be present. (© *B. Proud.*)

fretful very quickly. Make sure that the toddler has access to activities that can help keep him entertained. Toddlers also may need to nap in the middle of the day, especially if they are sick or injured. Provide quiet time, soothing music, and a comforting touch to help the child fall asleep.

MEETING THE TODDLER'S NEED FOR SAFETY

Toddlers are sometimes referred to as "tornadoes in training pants" because of their boundless energy, mobility, and natural curiosity. They learn to open locked doors quickly and can wander away from the facility or home. They run, climb, and reach for things without any thought to safety. They love to explore cabinets and will not hesitate to taste the contents of any containers they find there. As a result, accidental poisonings are very common among this age group. Toddlers must be observed at all times to help prevent accidents, and safety locks on doors, cabinets, and drawers are essential.

When a child reaches 1 year of age and 20 pounds in weight, she moves from an infant car seat to a toddler car seat. Toddler car seats, like infant car seats, are placed in the back seat of the car. However, the toddler sits facing forward. As with infants, it is illegal in all states to transport a toddler in a car without first properly securing him in a car seat.

CARING FOR PRESCHOOLERS

Preschoolers are children between the ages of 3 and 5 years. Like toddlers, preschoolers are very physically active and love to run, jump, ride on toys, and swing. However, because the preschooler's attention span is now a bit longer, she may also enjoy activities that require her to sit still for a period of time, such as arts and crafts projects using paper, scissors, crayons, beads, and glue. Because the preschooler enjoys being physically active, being confined to bed or indoors because of an injury or illness can become quite a challenge. Books, art supplies, games, movies, and television can be good entertainment for a child of this age. Preschoolers also love to have stories read to them and many are learning to read simple books on their own.

MEETING THE PRESCHOOLER'S PHYSICAL NEEDS

At this age, a child has developed most of his or her self-care skills. A healthy preschooler can dress himself, go to the bathroom unassisted, and brush his own teeth. However, a sick or injured preschooler may need help with these daily tasks.

Most preschoolers are picky eaters and eat only a small variety of foods, in small amounts. You may find it frustrating when your attempts to get a preschooler to eat foods that are high in nutritional value are met with failure. A preschooler who is not feeling well is even less likely to have an appetite for foods that are "good for her." Offering a variety of nutritious foods in small amounts throughout the day is often more effective than insisting that the preschooler eat regular meals.

You may be required to help hold or restrain a preschooler during a procedure. Make sure you plan ahead and have been shown how to hold a child gently but securely, so that the procedure can be performed as efficiently as possible. Remember that a frightened child can be very strong if he feels cornered and may strike out to protect himself in any way possible. He may kick, pinch, hit, or bite to get away. You will have to protect both the child and yourself from injury in this situation.

MEETING THE PRESCHOOLER'S EMOTIONAL NEEDS

Preschoolers have vivid imaginations and enjoy pretend play. As a result, preschoolers may have a lot of anxiety about being in a health care facility. A young preschooler may fear that a procedure will involve "cutting off" body parts or other drastic measures. An older preschooler has begun to understand the concept of death and may think that the hospital is "where people go to die." Because children of this age have learned to understand that discipline or punishment is the consequence of bad behavior, they may think that the reason they have to have a painful treatment or stay in bed is because they were "bad."

"Magical thinking" is a thought process that is common among preschoolers. Preschoolers believe that if they wish for something hard enough, it will happen. As a result, a preschooler may think that because she wished for something bad to happen to a parent or a sibling, her current medical condition is punishment for having those bad thoughts. Or she may think that her bad thoughts actually made something bad happen (for example, if several members of a family are now hospitalized because of an accident or fire).

Preschoolers need their questions answered simply and honestly. They are very interested in whether a procedure will "hurt." If the procedure will hurt, please do not tell a child that it will not. Not being honest about the procedure and what it will feel like will destroy the child's ability to trust you and the other members of the health care team. Instead, be truthful and describe what the procedure will feel like in words that the child can understand. For example, you might tell the child that the procedure will "pinch," "squeeze," or "pull."

Using a stuffed animal or doll to demonstrate the procedure helps the child to understand what is expected of her and will help to relieve the child's fears (Fig. 41-4). For example, you could use a doll to demonstrate how you do range-of-motion exercises. Similarly, the preschooler will enjoy being able to listen to her own heart through the stethoscope, or seeing a demonstration of how the blood pressure cuff "squeezes her arm to check her muscles."

MEETING THE PRESCHOOLER'S NEEDS FOR SAFETY

A preschooler is beginning to learn the difference between right and wrong behavior. As a result, he is more able to "follow the rules of safety," if these rules are explained to him in a way that he understands. Some preschoolers are still prone to placing items in their mouths and are therefore at risk for choking. As in younger children, balloons and inflated gloves pose a choking risk and should be used with caution. Scissors used for crafts projects should be blunt-tipped, and markers, crayons, glue, and other art supplies should be nontoxic and approved for use for children between the ages of 3 and 5.

The toddler car seat is used until the child weighs 40 pounds. At that point, the child will have outgrown the toddler car seat and will need a booster seat. The booster seat raises the child

FIGURE 41-4

A preschooler who needs to have a medical procedure often finds it comforting to have the procedure explained using a toy or stuffed animal as a model. Here, a nurse uses an educational toy to explain a procedure to a preschooler.

up so that the lap and shoulder belts in the car fit properly. The booster seat is placed in the back seat of the car, facing forward. As with younger children, it is illegal to drive with a child in the car who is not properly restrained.

CARING FOR SCHOOL-AGE CHILDREN

School-age children are children between the ages of 5 and 12 years. This is a period of relative tranquility, compared with the rapid growth and development of earlier years, and the yet-to-come rapid growth and development of adolescence. School-age children are developing many interests outside of their own families. They are learning to socialize and spend a lot of time playing with their friends. They enjoy physical activities, such as riding bicycles, swimming, skating, skiing, and climbing. Unfortunately, these activities often result in injury and a stay in a health care facility. "Fitting in" socially is very important to the school-age child, and children who are physically or mentally disabled may be excluded from play or teased by their peers.

Caring for a child of this age in a health care setting involves answering lots of questions. School-age children are typically very cooperative if their questions are answered in a manner that they can understand. These children like to be included as active participants in their own care and are very good at following directions.

MEETING THE SCHOOL-AGE CHILD'S PHYSICAL NEEDS

School-age children are very independent and are quite proud that they no longer have to rely on anyone else for self-care, although they do need to be reminded that the purpose of a bath or shower is to clean their bodies. If a child is not able to bathe, dress, or go to the bathroom by himself as a result of injury or illness, he will need the assistance of others, and this is likely to make him very unhappy. He simply does not want to be "treated like a baby." Allow the child to do as much as he is able to by himself. Sometimes, taking the approach that the child is helping you because you simply cannot do the task without his assistance is helpful.

When caring for a school-age child, you must check on her frequently. Although the child may be badly injured and in pain, she may not pay attention to your directions to call for help if she needs to get out of bed. She will want to do it herself. A reward system for following the rules may be necessary. For example, you might tell the child that if she uses the call light control to ask for your assistance each time she needs to get out of bed, then you will allow her to choose a small treat or privilege. Rewards and praise work very well for children of this age.

MEETING THE SCHOOL-AGE CHILD'S EMOTIONAL NEEDS

School-age children expect to receive direct, although simple, answers to their questions. If a school-age child asks you a question that you cannot answer, be sure to relay the question to the nurse, so that she can answer it for the child. Never make promises or assurances about a school-age child's condition or treatment that are not certain. Children of this age are usually very aware of when they are being told the truth, and when they are not. A school-age child usually has developed a very strong moral conscience and feels very strongly about what is right and what is wrong.

FIGURE 41-5

School-age children who must be confined to bed due to injury or illness will miss socializing with their friends. Phone calls, greeting cards, and visits from peers are thoroughly enjoyed. Here, a patient uses a computer to instant-message her friends.

A school-age child will enjoy reading, doing arts and crafts projects, playing video games, and talking with caregivers (Fig. 41-5). If possible, allow the child to accompany you throughout the health care facility in a wheelchair for company, or take her to a common area where there may be other children her age to socialize or play games with. For a child of this age who is confined due to accident or illness, staying in touch with friends is a huge emotional boost. Phone calls, visits (if possible), and cards from friends and classmates are thoroughly enjoyed. Make sure you help the child to place cards and notes safely on a table or bulletin board so they can be looked at often.

MEETING THE SCHOOL-AGE CHILD'S NEED FOR SAFETY

The school-age child is less vulnerable to certain dangers than younger children are. For example, school-age children know not to drink poisonous liquids or stick objects into an electrical socket. However, their curiosity and habit of pushing their physical abilities to the limit bring new dangers. School-age children are often interested in fire. They may dart into the path of oncoming traffic on bicycles and skateboards or when chasing a ball. They climb trees and buildings, and then fall. Burns, broken bones, and head injuries are the reason many children in this age group require hospitalization and rehabilitation.

When transporting a school-age child in a car, use a booster seat until the car's lap and shoulder restraints fit the child properly. This usually occurs when the child reaches a height of 4 feet, 9 inches, and a weight of about 80 pounds. Children should continue to ride in the backseat until the age of 12 years.

CARING FOR ADOLESCENTS

Adolescents are children between the ages of 12 and 20 years. Adolescence is a time of tremendous growth and development. We enter adolescence as children and exit as young adults. During adolescence, logical thinking skills develop. Adolescents have the ability to understand possibilities and make judgments. As a result, it is essential that children of this age be included in plans and decisions regarding their medical care.

MEETING THE ADOLESCENT'S PHYSICAL NEEDS

Allow the child to be as independent as possible with his daily care. An adolescent may hesitate to ask for help or for pain medication if he is trying to seem "tough," mature, or grown up. He may act angry or aloof when in reality he is really just frightened. Adolescence is a very difficult time of life to require health care. The physical changes that occur during adolescence can make adolescents self-conscious about their bodies. As a result, they are often very embarrassed by care or treatments that expose their bodies to others. Remember this when caring for an adolescent, and make a special effort to provide privacy. Also be aware that an adolescent girl may need your assistance with obtaining or changing sanitary napkins or tampons, if she is too ill to manage this task on her own. Be sensitive to the embarrassment she may feel at having to ask for your help.

To help adolescents meet their nutritional needs, offer the types of foods that they like to eat. A teenager may totally refuse the types of meals served in a health care facility, but will eat pizza, milkshakes, or other nutritional alternatives. Because of the increased need for extra calories during periods of growth spurts, an adolescent may need nutritious snacks in between meals. Peanut butter and crackers, cheese, fruit, yogurt, and ice cream are good nutritious alternatives for chips and soda and should be readily available for the teenager if her dietary orders allow.

MEETING THE ADOLESCENT'S EMOTIONAL NEEDS

Psychologically, the period of adolescence is stormy. Adolescents are **egocentric,** meaning that they place themselves at the center of the world and often overestimate their importance to others. They begin to question the moral teachings of authority figures and parents. As a result, experimentation with alcohol, drugs, and sex may occur during this stage.

Adolescents are torn between wanting to be treated as grown-ups and being afraid to make their own decisions. They need adults to respect their individuality. When caring for an adolescent, listen to what she is saying. Try not to lecture her on morals or proper behavior. Include the adolescent in discussions and decisions regarding her care and treatment. Adolescents need to feel that their opinions count (Fig. 41-6).

Many adolescents require care in a health care facility because of complications related to mental illnesses, such as depression, attempted suicide, or eating disorders. Others may have had accidents related to drug or alcohol abuse. An adolescent girl may need health care as a result of a pregnancy, which may not be planned or wanted. Sexually transmitted diseases (STDs) are common among this age group. All of these situations require tact and sensitivity on the part of caregivers. Be very observant for any changes in the adolescent's emotional behavior or mood and report anything unusual to the nurse immediately.

MEETING THE ADOLESCENT'S NEED FOR SAFETY

In the health care setting, most adolescents are fairly safe. However, an adolescent who has a history of abusing drugs or other substances may

FIGURE 41-6

Adolescents need to be included in plans and decisions regarding their medical care. It is important to listen to what the adolescent is telling you. Avoid lecturing her on morals or proper behavior.

try to obtain pain medication that is not needed. Depressed adolescents will need to be observed closely for suicide attempts or other types of self-injury. Make sure that the adolescent knows you are available if he needs assistance, and answer the call light promptly.

CHILD ABUSE

Children, like the elderly, are often targets of abuse.

FORMS OF ABUSE

Like elder abuse, child abuse can be physical, psychological (emotional), or sexual in nature.

Physical Abuse

Neglect is a common form of physical abuse in children. The child's caregiver simply fails to provide for the child's basic physical human needs. For example, the child may be malnourished from lack of nutritious food, dirty from lack of proper hygiene, or ill from a lack of medical care.

Physical abuse can also take the form of striking, biting, slapping, shaking, or handling a child roughly. Violently shaking an infant or toddler can cause the child's brain to hit the inside of his skull repeatedly, leading to severe brain damage or death. This is called **shaken baby syndrome.** Shaken baby syndrome is most often seen in children younger than 1 year. About 25% of children with shaken baby syndrome die, and the rest suffer from permanent disabilities. Many cases of shaken baby syndrome occur accidentally, when a frustrated caregiver shakes a child to get him to stop crying. Because of the risk of head injury, it is never acceptable to shake an infant or toddler.

In **Munchausen syndrome by proxy,** another form of physical abuse seen in children, the child's caregiver (usually the mother) deliberately does things to make the child appear ill. For example, the caregiver may feed the child soap or other substances to make her vomit. Or she might smother the child for a period of time to deprive her of oxygen, leading to neurological symptoms. Often, the child is forced to have painful diagnostic procedures or surgery as health care providers try to discover the cause of the child's strange signs and symptoms. Munchausen syndrome by proxy is often very difficult to detect and to prove, because nearly constant observation is needed to determine the cause of the child's health problems. In some cases, it becomes necessary to hide a camera in the child's hospital room to observe what happens when the caregiver is alone with the child.

Psychological (Emotional) Abuse

A caregiver can inflict psychological (emotional) abuse on a child in many ways. A caregiver might make a child fearful by threatening him with physical harm or abandonment. Or he might say cruel things to the child, such as "You're no good," "You're stupid," or "I wish you had never been born." Isolating a child by preventing him from seeing friends or other family members (an act called *involuntary seclusion*) is another form of psychological abuse. Involuntary seclusion can involve keeping a child in a room alone with the door closed. In extreme cases, it may involve locking a child in a closet or attic for years. Children who are the victims of psychological abuse can struggle for the rest of their lives with emotional pain, depression, thoughts of suicide, and lack of self-esteem.

Sexual Abuse

Sexual abuse occurs when a parent or caregiver:
- Touches or fondles a child's sexual organs
- Shows his or her sexual organs to a child, or asks the child to touch or otherwise stimulate them
- Forces a child to have sexual intercourse with him or her (rape)
- Forces a child to engage in a sexual act and then films or photographs it (pornography)
- Forces a child to engage in a sexual act for money, often with many different people (prostitution)

When a stranger sexually abuses a child, it is called *sexual assault.*

RISK FACTORS FOR CHILD ABUSE

Child abuse can occur in all levels of society and in all ethnic groups. However, there are certain situations that seem to increase the risk that abuse will occur. Risk factors for child abuse include the following:
- Caregivers who are very stressed by situations such as unemployment, depression, marital or relationship problems, substance abuse, or health problems of their own
- Caregivers who are very young, lack parenting skills, or lack knowledge about the normal behaviors and developmental stages of children
- Caregivers who have no family or social support and feel "trapped" by their parenting responsibilities
- Children who are "difficult" to care for, such as those who cry frequently, do not sleep well, are hyperactive or aggressive, wet the bed, or suffer from physical or mental disabilities

ROLE OF THE NURSING ASSISTANT IN REPORTING ABUSE

As a nursing assistant, you may find yourself in a situation where you suspect that one of your pediatric patients is being abused (Box 41-1). You may see physical signs that suggest abuse, or the child's behavior or play-acting may raise your suspicions. In some cases, the child might tell you something that makes you suspicious. Make sure to listen carefully to what the child is telling you. Report the child's words exactly as you heard them. Be very careful not to influence the child's ideas or "put words in her mouth." In the event of an abuse investigation, a young child may repeat what she has been

---

BOX 41-1 Signs of Child Abuse

- Unclean or unsafe living conditions, as evidenced by rotting food, unchanged sheets, or a lack of heat or water services
- Poor personal hygiene, as evidenced by an unclean body, clothes, or both; uncombed hair; skin irritation (from wearing urine-soaked undergarments for long periods of time); dried stool on buttocks; or a lack of oral hygiene
- Loss of weight or dehydration
- Multiple, unexplained fractures or bruises in various stages of healing; explanations of injuries that are not consistent with the location of the injury
- Burn marks (for example, from cigarettes or stove burners) or scalds (for example, from having a hand or foot held in hot water)
- Abrasions from ropes or other bindings
- Patches of missing hair
- Vaginal bleeding or discharge; urinary tract infection; or pain, itching, redness, or bruising around the genitals or anus
- Excessive sexual curiosity or play
- Sleeping problems or nightmares
- An anxious, fearful or withdrawn demeanor, especially in the presence of the abuser
- Uncontrolled medical conditions (possibly the result of a lack of prescribed medication or treatment)
- A history of requiring health care for similar injuries

told, rather than describe what actually happened. If you are suspicious about something a child has told you, do not question the child further yourself. Report your suspicions to the nurse and allow a person who has experience and training in detecting child abuse to continue the questioning.

It may be very difficult to work with parents or caregivers if you suspect that they have abused their child. You may feel angry toward the parents or caregivers, or disgusted by their behavior. Remember that it is not your place to pass judgment on a parent or caregiver. Your responsibility is to simply report your suspicions, and to let the state agencies that handle abuse reports determine if abuse has occurred and, if so, who did it. The agencies will also determine how the child will be protected going forward. Your top priority is to meet the child's physical and emotional needs as best you can while the child is in your care. If you feel that your emotions about a particular situation may affect your ability to provide care, talk with your supervisor and ask for help or to be assigned to another area.

SUMMARY

▶ Children receive health care in many different types of health care settings, for many different reasons. To provide holistic care for children, you must first understand that children are not simply "little adults." An understanding of the basic stages of growth and development will better prepare you to provide the type of care that each child requires.

▶ Pediatric patients range in age from newborn through 20 years.

- Infants are children younger than 1 year. Infants are totally dependent on others for their physical care. Their greatest emotional need is to feel secure and to develop trust.

- A toddler is a child between the ages of 1 and 3 years. Toddlers may have a fear of strangers that could affect their response to health care providers. In addition, they commonly regress to an earlier stage of development in response to the stress of being in a health care setting.

- Preschoolers are children between the ages of 3 and 5 years. Preschoolers have vivid imaginations and enjoy pretend play. Preschoolers may indulge in magical thinking. The preschooler's questions must be answered simply and honestly.

- School-age children are children between the ages of 5 and 12 years. School-age children like to be included as active participants in their own care and are very good at following directions. However, they may resist asking for help when they need it.

- Adolescents are children between the ages of 12 and 20 years. Adolescents have a great need for privacy, and for control over what is happening to them.

▶ Children are frequently the helpless victims of many types of abuse. All members of the health care team are legally obligated to report any type of suspected abuse.

- Physical abuse can take the form of neglect or deliberate injury.

- Psychological (emotional) abuse can involve threatening a child, saying demeaning or cruel things to a child, or isolating the child from others.

- Sexual abuse occurs when an adult touches a child inappropriately or forces the child to perform sexual acts.

What did you learn?

Multiple Choice

Select the single best answer for each of the following questions.

1. When is a pediatric patient most likely to co-operate with the health care team?
   a. When members of the health care team treated him like a "little adult"
   b. When members of the health care team recognize the child's particular stage of development and provide age-appropriate care
   c. When members of the health care team always give the child choices
   d. When the child is restrained

2. To help determine whether a breast-fed infant is receiving an adequate amount of milk, the nursing assistant may need to:
   a. Supplement the breastfeeding with extra formula
   b. Monitor the baby's intravenous (IV) line
   c. Have the mother pump her breasts and measure the amount of milk she produces
   d. Weigh the infant's wet diapers

3. A behavior that could indicate regression in a toddler might be
   a. Asking for a bottle or pacifier
   b. Becoming potty trained
   c. Feeding herself
   d. Fearing strangers

4. Which one of the following is an example of magical thinking?
   a. Believing in Santa Claus
   b. Fearing strangers
   c. Thinking that an accident occurred because you were mad at your sister
   d. Pretending to be a princess

5. A child in which one of the following age groups is likely to be experiencing a period of "relative tranquility," as far as growth and development is concerned?
   a. Preschooler
   b. School-age child
   c. Adolescent
   d. Infant

Matching

Match each numbered item with its appropriate lettered description.

_____ 1. Infant

_____ 2. Toddler

_____ 3. Preschooler

_____ 4. School-age child

_____ 5. Adolescent

a. This child has developed a very strong moral conscience and will expect truthful answers to his many questions.

b. This child may be very self-conscious and become embarrassed if she is exposed during a medical procedure.

c. This child needs to be touched, cuddled, stroked, and spoken to soothingly to thrive.

d. This child has a vivid imagination and may fear monsters under the bed and doctors who will "cut off" body parts.

e. This child is at the highest risk for accidental poisoning.

Stop and think!

▶ You are the nursing assistant on a pediatric floor of a hospital. One of your small patients, Sarah, is 5. As you walk into her room, you notice that she is playing with a doll and a teddy bear. As you listen, you hear her talking to the toys. Sarah is pretending that the bear is asking the doll to touch him between the legs. When the doll refuses, the bear becomes very angry and demands that the doll touch him. What is happening in this room? What should be your response?

▶ You are caring for a 2-year-old child who has a fractured arm. You notice that the mother seems very fearful of talking about what happened and her version of the story changes frequently. As you are helping to bathe the child you notice small burn marks on his buttocks and some bruises on his back. How do you feel? Is the mother protecting herself or some one else? What do you report and to whom?

Nursing Assistants Make a Difference!

"My husband, Fred, and I have been fortunate enough to enjoy relatively good health all of our lives. Although we are both in our early 70s, we are active and travel to many places. A few months ago, the arthritis in Fred's right knee really started giving him trouble. When our doctor learned that the arthritis had gotten so bad as to cause Fred to cut his weekly golf outings to one (down from three), he suggested that Fred have a joint replacement so he could continue to be active.

One of the first people we met when we went to the hospital was a nursing assistant named Patrick. Patrick showed us to Fred's hospital room took his vital signs, and got him into a hospital gown. The surgery went well and Fred was back in his room before lunchtime. Patrick was there as well, taking his vital signs fairly frequently. He explained that this was normal procedure after surgery.

Early that afternoon, Patrick took Fred's pulse and blood pressure, but instead of writing them down, he took them again. He reassured me that it was probably nothing, but that he had noticed something that he wanted the nurse to take a look at. Well, Fred had had a minor heart attack after the surgery, and Patrick had noticed a bit of an irregularity in his pulse rhythm. Because he had noticed it and reported the change to the nurse, they were able to start treating Fred's heart soon enough to prevent any permanent damage from occurring.

Now, 8 months later, Fred's golf swing is as bad as it always was. Fred has started taking a medication to regulate his heart rate, but he feels great and we're loving life. Thank goodness for Patrick and his attention to detail!"

You can listen to more stories about how nursing assistants make a difference on the CD in the back of your book.

Home Health Care

Home health care—skilled nursing care that is given to a person in his or her home—is a rapidly growing part of the health care industry. Currently, more than 2.2 million Americans use the services of home health care agencies, and that number is expected to keep growing each year. The purpose of this unit is to introduce you to the home health care setting.

Photo: Home health aides care for clients in their homes.
(© John Henley/CORBIS.)

815

42

Introduction to Home Health Care

What will you learn?

Many nursing assistants choose to work in home health care. A nursing assistant who works in home health care is often called a **home health aide.** Perhaps becoming a home health aide is something you have thought about. The basic skills and concepts that you have learned will apply no matter where you decide to work. But some aspects of providing care to a person in his or her own home are unique. In this chapter, you will learn about why a person might need the services of a home health care agency, and how these services are paid for. You will also learn about some of the key responsibilities you would have, if you decided to work in the home health care setting. Finally, we will discuss the personal qualities that a person must have to succeed as a home health aide. When you are finished with this chapter, you will be able to:

1. Describe why a person might need home health care.
2. Discuss how home health care is paid for.
3. Describe how the home health care team works together to provide client care.
4. Describe the major duties of a home health aide.
5. List personal qualities that a home health aide must have to be successful.

Photo: A home health aide interacts with a client.
(© Frank Siteman/Index Stock Imagery.)

Vocabulary

Use the CD in the back of your book to hear these terms pronounced, defined, and used in a sentence:

Home health aide	Case manager
Respite care	Nurse's bag
Homebound	Abandonment

WHAT IS HOME HEALTH CARE?

If you were ill, where would you rather be? In your own home, surrounded by the people, pets, and things that you love? Or in a hospital or long-term care facility? Given a choice, most people would prefer to stay in the comfort of their own homes when they are sick. Home health care, also known as *home care*, makes it possible for people who are not critically ill to receive health care in the comfort of their own homes. A person who is receiving the services of a home health care agency is called a *client*, instead of a "patient" or a "resident." There are many reasons why a person might become a client of a home health care agency:

- **The person may have just been discharged from the hospital following an acute illness or injury.** The care provided in a hospital is costly, and the number of beds in the hospital is limited. For these reasons, a person may be discharged from the hospital as soon as she is out of danger, but before she is fully recovered. In this situation, a home health aide may be needed to help care for the person at home until she has made a full recovery.
- **The person may have a chronic illness or disability that makes it hard for him to manage some tasks independently.** For example, a person who is paralyzed might need a home health aide to help him get out of bed and ready for work each morning.
- **The person may have an illness, such as dementia, that makes it dangerous for the person to be left alone in the house.** In this case, a home health aide might come to the home on a regular basis to provide care and companionship for the person and to relieve the primary caregiver. Care that allows the primary

caregiver to rest or leave the house for a short period of time is called **respite care** (Fig. 42-1). Being able to "take a break" and leave the house is critical for managing the stress that can be caused by providing constant care for a family member who is ill.
- **The person may be terminally ill.** Hospice care is often provided in the person's home. A home health aide who works for a hospice agency will receive special training in providing end-of-life care.

PAYING FOR HOME HEALTH CARE

Home health care is paid for in many different ways. A client may pay for home health care entirely from his own income or savings. Or, he

FIGURE 42-1

Part of a home health aide's duties may be to provide respite care. Respite care allows the family member who has primary responsibility for caring for the client to have time to herself. (© *Sally Moskol/Index Stock Imagery.*)

might have insurance coverage that covers all or part of the costs. Insurance coverage is provided by insurance companies and by government agencies, such as Medicare or state Medicaid.

Insurance companies and government agencies often have strict rules regarding what type of care is covered, and under what circumstances. For example, many times the client must be completely homebound before the insurance company will pay for the costs of home care. **Homebound** means that the person is unable to leave the house without a lot of help from another person. Insurance companies and government agencies may also control the length of each visit and the number of visits a person may have each week. For example, a client who needs minimal assistance with bathing may be allowed three visits per week, whereas a client who cannot get out of bed and is at risk for developing pressure ulcers may be allowed two visits each day. One client may be allowed a 1-hour visit, while another client is allowed a 2-hour visit. Proper documentation (recording) of the care provided to the client during each visit is necessary to justify continued payment for home care services and to determine the frequency and length of future visits.

THE HEALTH CARE TEAM

Just as in any other health care setting, health care that is provided in the home is provided by a health care team. The health care team consists of the client, the client's family members, the home health aide, a nurse, a doctor, a case manager, and other specialists (such as a physical therapist or social worker). As always, the client is the focus of the health care team's efforts, and the goal of the health care team is to provide holistic care. Each team member provides a specific aspect of care for the client. For example, the home health aide may be responsible for monitoring vital signs and helping the client with routine activities of daily living (ADLs), whereas the nurse may be responsible for giving medications or providing wound care (Fig. 42-2). The health care team provides care in the home as directed by the client's care plan. The care plan is a set of instructions for the client's care, created by the case manager with input from all members of the health care team. The **case manager,** usually a registered nurse, is responsible for overseeing all

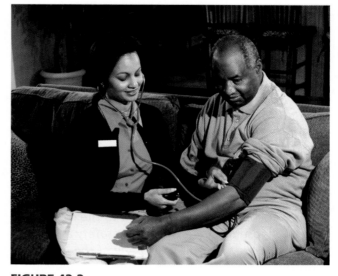

FIGURE 42-2
Home health aides are often responsible for monitoring the vital signs of their clients.

of the client's care, from admission through discharge.

The home health aide is a very important member of the health care team. Because the home health aide is often scheduled to visit the client on a frequent, routine basis, he has the best chance to observe changes that could indicate a change in the client's health. In addition, the client may feel most comfortable with the home health aide, and as a result, may tell him things she might not tell other members of the health care team. By communicating his observations to the rest of the health care team, the home health aide becomes the "eyes and ears" of the members of the team who do not see the client as frequently. For this reason, communicating with the case manager and other members of the health care team is an essential part of the home health aide's responsibilities.

In the hospital and long-term care settings, team members often have the chance to communicate face-to-face, because everyone is together in the same building. This is not true in the home health care setting. Team members travel to the client's home according to their own individual schedules. As a result, they may rarely see each other. In the home health care setting, most communication among team members takes place through documentation. As always, you must accurately document the care you provide on the appropriate paperwork, including the date, time, and duration of the visit. Proper documentation is necessary to ensure that all members of the home health care team are kept "in-the-know."

▶ *Tell the Nurse!*

As a home health aide, you will play a very important role in reporting changes in a client's medical condition that could indicate a serious problem. Your agency will have written guidelines about observations that should be reported. Make sure you are familiar with these guidelines, and if you are ever in doubt about whether an observation should be immediately reported to the case manager, choose to err on the side of safety and report it. Make sure you report any of the following observations to the case manager immediately:

▶ One or more of the client's vital signs is above or below the standards set by the agency

▶ The client has a fever or other signs of infection

▶ There is a change in the client's mental alertness or orientation

▶ The client has signs of skin breakdown or pressure sores

▶ The client has signs or symptoms that could indicate a medical emergency

▶ You suspect that the client is being abused (physically, sexually, or psychologically)

▶ There are unsafe or unsanitary conditions in the home

RESPONSIBILITIES OF THE HOME HEALTH AIDE

The home health aide usually assists clients with tasks related to personal care, such as bathing, grooming, and repositioning. Depending on the client's needs, the home health aide may also be assigned light housekeeping duties, such as cleaning, preparing meals, and doing laundry. The home health aide's responsibilities are clearly outlined in the client's care plan. You must follow the care plan exactly. Any changes to the care plan must first be approved by the case manager.

As noted earlier, it is very important for you to keep accurate records of the care that you provide

and the observations that you make. Proper documentation of the care that you provide helps to ensure that the client's insurance will continue to pay for the services. In addition, good documentation is necessary to ensure that all of the members of the health care team are kept informed of the client's status. Each home health care agency has specific policies related to documentation. Your supervisor will review these policies with you.

In addition to documenting the care that you provide to the client, you may be required to keep a daily record of your activities. For example, you might be asked to keep a *time and travel log*, which details how much time you spent at each client's house, how much time you spent traveling between houses, and your mileage for the day. Always record information in a timely manner. If you must wait until the end of the day to record something, keep accurate notes so that the information you record will be accurate.

You will provide care for many different clients. Some of your clients may have limited income and live in very small homes or apartments. Others may be quite wealthy and live in large homes with many modern conveniences. Some homes will be very clean, while others will not live up to your personal standards. Each home, and each family, is different. Remember that you are a guest in the client's home. You must be careful not to allow your opinions about how a person lives to affect the care that you provide. If you feel that something about a client's home environment puts the client at risk for injury (such as extremely dirty conditions, an abusive relationship with a family member, or a potential fire hazard), report your concerns to the case manager.

PERSONAL CARE

As a home health aide, many of your responsibilities will be related to helping your clients with activities such as bathing, eating, getting dressed, exercising, toileting, repositioning, and transferring (Fig. 42-3). As always, the amount of help you will need to provide will vary from client to client, and you should encourage the client to do as much as possible for himself.

The skills you will use to assist with personal care are the same no matter where you work. However, in the home setting, some of the equipment may be different. Medical equipment, such as

FIGURE 42-3

Home health aides assist with all types of personal care. Here, a home health aide helps a client to transfer out of bed.

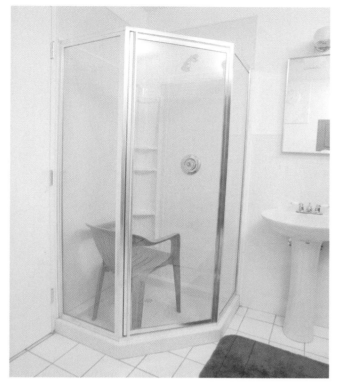

FIGURE 42-4

Sometimes common household items can be used in place of expensive medical equipment. Here, a plastic lawn chair is used as a shower chair.

shower chairs, bedside commodes, or adjustable beds, can be purchased or rented from a medical supply store for use in the home, but this can be expensive. Many clients will not be able to afford this expense. Therefore, many times you must be resourceful and use items that are readily available in the home. For example, if the person's bed is not adjustable, you can use extra pillows or a back rest to position the person in Fowler's position. A sturdy webbed or plastic lawn chair may substitute for a shower chair (Fig. 42-4). However, as with the use of any type of equipment, safety is a top priority. If you think that a client is at risk for injury because he or she does not have a certain piece of medical equipment, ask the case manager for advice. The case manager may be able to work with outside resources to get the equipment the client needs at low cost, or no cost.

HOMEMAKING

Depending on the client's needs, part of your responsibilities as a home health aide may include preparing and serving meals, cleaning, and doing laundry. Homemaking duties are outlined on the client's care plan. You will document the homemaking duties that you perform on a *homemaker flow sheet*, according to your agency's policies. The homemaker flow sheet becomes part of the client's medical record. As always, you must accurately document your work.

Meal Preparation

Preparing meals is a duty frequently assigned to the home health aide (Fig. 42-5). Some states require home health aides who will be preparing and serving food to have a food handler's permit. Because requirements may differ from state to state, it is important for you to know your agency's policies and to check with the nurse aide registry in the state where you work.

FIGURE 42-5

Meal preparation is often part of the home health care aide's routine duties.

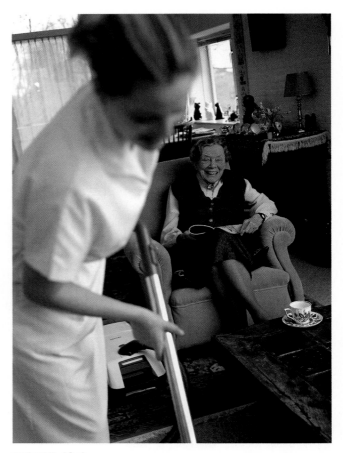

FIGURE 42-6

Light housekeeping might also be part of the home health aide's responsibilities. (© *Benelux Press/Index Stock Imagery.*)

When preparing a meal, consider the special needs and individual preferences of the client. The meal should be nutritious. If the person is on a special diet, such as a restricted-sodium diet, then you must make sure that the meal you prepare meets the diet's requirements. For some clients, you will have to cut the food into very small pieces or puree it in a blender before serving it.

Serve the meal or snack at the time specified in the care plan. As always, make an effort to make meal time as pleasant as possible. Present the meal in an attractive way, and sit down and talk with the person as she is eating. The amount of assistance with eating that your client will need will vary. For example, some clients will be able to feed themselves if you assist with opening cartons or peeling a piece of fruit. Others will need more help. Involve the person in the process of eating by allowing her to do as much as she can for herself.

Housekeeping

Many times, the home health aide is also responsible for providing some cleaning services (Fig. 42-6). These tasks may be done on a weekly basis, or as scheduled on the care plan. Depending on the client's needs, you may be responsible for:

- Dusting
- Vacuuming carpets
- Mopping floors
- Disinfecting kitchen and bathroom surfaces
- Changing the client's bed linens
- Washing and drying the client's bed linens and clothing

When providing housekeeping services, care for the client's home as if it were your own. Be careful not to damage decorative items on tables and shelves. Pay attention to details. For example, when vacuuming a room, be thorough. Don't just vacuum the center of the room—make sure the edges and baseboards are clean too. When using cleaning solutions, make sure that the product you are using is approved for use on the surface you are cleaning, to avoid causing

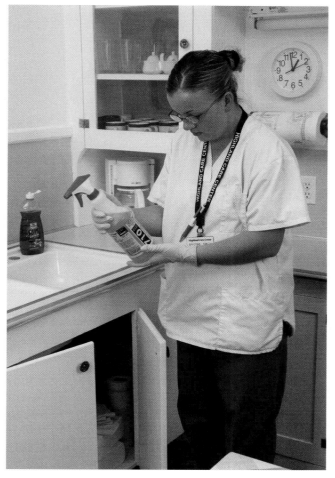

FIGURE 42-7

When using cleaning solutions, make sure the product you are using is approved for use on the surface you are cleaning. Cleaning solutions should always be kept in properly labeled containers.

permanent damage (Fig. 42-7). It is important to be respectful of the client's home and its contents. When you show respect for a client's home and personal belongings, you are letting the person know that you truly care for him or her.

QUALITIES OF THE SUCCESSFUL HOME HEALTH AIDE

So maybe you are thinking that you would like to work in the home health setting. Of course, just as in any health care setting, a strong work ethic is important. For example, being honest, compassionate, courteous, conscientious, and reliable will serve you well, no matter where you work.

However, the people who make the best home health aides also have other qualities that help them to succeed in the home health care setting. The most successful home health aides:

- Enjoy working independently and are self-motivated
- Are organized and able to manage their time well
- Are reliable
- Are able to set professional boundaries

Let's look at each of these qualities in more detail.

ABILITY TO WORK INDEPENDENTLY

As a home health aide, you will be working in a client's home without direct supervision most of the time. If you like a lot of feedback and guidance as you complete your assignments, then working in the home health care setting might not be right for you. To work in the home health care setting, you need to be very comfortable with your own caregiving and problem-solving skills. You also need to be self-motivated. No one will be there to help you, or to tell you what to do next.

ABILITY TO BE ORGANIZED AND MANAGE TIME

Because you will be working independently, you will be responsible for making sure that you complete your assigned duties as scheduled. You will be given a list of the clients you must care for each day and you will be told the length of each client visit. However, it will be up to you to determine how to best provide the required care, complete the necessary documentation, and travel between clients during the workday. You must work efficiently and safely.

Organization is one key to working efficiently and safely. When preparing to visit a client's home, gather all of the supplies you will need before you enter the person's home. Having the necessary supplies on hand allows you to work more efficiently, because you will not have to interrupt care to search for something you need. Some supplies and equipment may be kept at the client's home in a designated place (Fig. 42-8). Others, you will have to carry with you to each client's home in your **nurse's bag** (Fig. 42-9). For

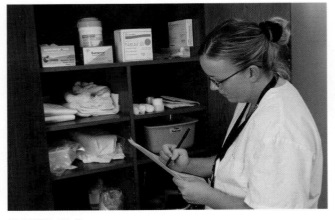

FIGURE 42-8

Some of the supplies and equipment you will need to care for your client will be kept in a special place in the client's home. Here, a home health aide is checking to see if any of the supplies are getting low.

FIGURE 42-9

A nurse's bag is used to carry supplies that will be used with every client, such as equipment for taking vital signs and personal protective equipment. The many compartments help you to keep the bag organized and clean. (*Courtesy of Hopkins Medical Products, Baltimore, MD/ (800) 835-1995, www.hmponline.com.*)

example, some of the things you might carry in your nurse's bag include:

- Forms needed for documentation, and a pen
- Personal protective equipment (PPE)
- Equipment used for taking vital signs
- Supplies for cleaning your equipment
- Alcohol-based hand rub

The nurse's bag has many compartments, which makes it easy for you to organize and find your supplies and equipment. Keeping each item in a special place makes it easy for you to see if you need to restock your nurse's bag. It also makes it easy for you to check that you have everything you need before you leave for the day. Organizing the paperwork needed for documentation in the order of your visits for the day is also very helpful.

Planning is the other key to working efficiently and safely. If possible, you should plan your day so that you visit clients in an order that allows for the most efficient use of travel time. For example, it would not be the best use of your time to spend all day traveling back and forth across town, when you could see all of your clients on the east side in the morning and all of your clients on the west side in the afternoon. When planning your day's work, map out your client's addresses and try to limit your travel time as much as possible. However, keep in mind that your clients' preferences and needs must also be taken into account when arranging care sched-

ules. For example, a client with paraplegia may need your help to get ready for work in the morning, whereas another client with diabetes might need you at his house at a certain time to prepare and serve lunch. It takes planning to make sure that your clients' needs are met while minimizing your travel time between homes.

RELIABILITY

Clients who receive home care depend on the home health aide to arrive and provide the appropriate care. For example, how would you feel if you depended on someone to help you get out of bed, shower, and get ready for work in the morning, and that person did not come to help you when she said she would come? Failing to keep appointments is not only inconsiderate, it can cause the client harm. For example, if you are responsible for preparing lunch for a client with diabetes, then you must do that at the scheduled time, or else the person is at risk for an adverse insulin reaction due to low blood glucose levels. Being reliable is a critical quality for a home health aide to have.

The term **abandonment** means to withdraw one's support or help from another person, in spite of duty or responsibility. A home health aide who fails to show up at a client's home to provide scheduled care is guilty of abandonment (Fig. 42-10). Similarly, a home health aide who leaves a client's home without completing the scheduled tasks may also be guilty of abandonment. As with any job, there may be situations beyond your control that will cause you to be unable to keep your appointments. If you are running late, it is your responsibility to notify the home health care agency. You must also try to contact the clients who are expecting you and let them know that you will be late. If you are unable to report to work at all, you must notify the home health care agency so that another aide can be sent to care for your scheduled clients. Also make sure you notify your agency if a personal emergency arises during your work day that would make it necessary for you to leave before completing your scheduled visits and care duties.

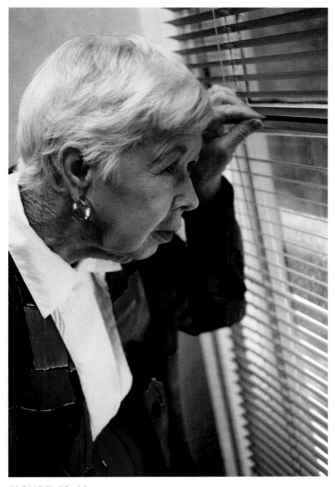

FIGURE 42-10

Your clients depend on you to arrive and provide the appropriate care, as scheduled. Leaving a client alone and without proper assistance is called *abandonment*.

Follow your agency's policies regarding situations of this nature so that the care needed by your clients is provided without delay.

ABILITY TO SET PROFESSIONAL BOUNDARIES

Many of your clients and their family members will come to regard you as a friend, or maybe even part of the family. You may also become close to clients and their family members. As a result, the line between your professional life and your personal life might become blurry. To succeed as a home health aide, you must be able to maintain a professional relationship with both clients and their family members at all times. Although it may be tempting to "drop in" on a client, or to go to the client's home after working hours to visit socially, this is not appropriate. Also, you should refuse any gift (including gifts of food or money) that may be offered to you by a client or family member. Your employer will have very specific policies regarding personal relationships between health care professionals and clients, and the acceptance of gifts. Make sure that you always follow these policies, and if you are in doubt about any type of relationship or gift, ask your supervisor for clarification.

Professional boundaries are also necessary to prevent clients or their family members from taking advantage of you. You will have a helping relationship with the client and family members that can easily be taken advantage of in many different ways. For example, a family member might ask you to provide care that has not been listed in the care plan. If you ever have any question about whether or not it is acceptable to perform additional duties or "favors" for a client or family member, make sure you ask your supervisor first.

SUMMARY

▶ Home health care is skilled nursing care that is given to a person in his or her home.
- People of all ages, and with all types of illnesses and disabilities, use the services of home health care agencies. Home care may be needed for a short time to help a person

recover from an acute illness or injury, or it may be needed for the rest of the person's life.

■ Home health care can be paid for privately by the client, by insurance, or by Medicaid or Medicare. Proper documentation of the care that you provide helps to ensure that the client's insurance will continue to pay for the services. The information that you record is also used to plan the client's future care.

■ Home health care is provided by a health care team. At minimum, the home health care team consists of a client, the client's family members, the home health aide, a nurse, a doctor, and a case manager. Other specialists may be included as well, depending on the client's needs.

   • The home health aide is the "eyes and ears" of the health care team. Most communication with other health care team members takes place through recording.

   • The home health aide's major responsibilities include tasks related to personal care and light housekeeping.

▶ To succeed as a home health aide, a person must have several qualities.

■ The home health aide must be resourceful. All of the standard equipment that is available in other health care settings may not be available in a person's home.

■ The home health aide must be able to work independently, without a lot of supervision or help from others.

■ The home health aide must be organized, with good time management skills.

■ The home health aide must be reliable. Leaving a client alone and without proper assistance is called *abandonment*.

■ The home health aide must have the ability to set appropriate professional boundaries with the client and family.

What did you learn?

Multiple Choice

Select the single best answer for each of the following questions.

1. Which one of the following is a routine responsibility of a home health aide?
   a. Providing respite care for the wife of a client with dementia
   b. Picking up a client's prescription at the drugstore
   c. Grocery shopping for the family
   d. Washing the windows of the home

2. One of your clients is turning 90 next week, and his family has invited you to attend his birthday party. What should you do?
   a. Accept the invitation, and take a card or a gift to the party
   b. Decline the invitation, but give the client a card or gift during your next scheduled visit
   c. Decline the invitation after thanking the family for inviting you
   d. Accept the invitation, but avoid bringing a card or a gift to the party

3. You are scheduled to work today, but the weather is beautiful and your best friend is begging you to take the day off and go to the beach with her. What should you do?
   a. Ask your friend if she would be willing to go with you in the afternoon. You will take care of all of your scheduled clients in the morning, and then you will be free to go.
   b. Call the case manager on your way to the beach and tell her that you will not be able to visit your clients today. This will allow the case manager to find another aide to cover for you.
   c. Tell your friend that you are sorry, but you cannot go to the beach today.
   d. Call each of the clients who you are scheduled to visit and ask them if it would be okay if you came tomorrow instead.

4. Why is documentation a very important responsibility of the home health aide?
   a. Documentation is the main way that the members of the home health care team communicate with each other about the care given to the client and the client's condition, and the home health aide has the most frequent contact with the client.
   b. Documentation provides information that is used to determine if a client is recovering, or getting worse.
   c. Documentation of all care provided is needed to justify continued payment for home care services.
   d. All of the above

5. Peggy is a home health aide. Today, while Peggy is helping a client, her son's teacher calls Peggy on her cell phone to tell her that her son has had an accident on the playground, and he needs to be picked up. What should Peggy do?
   a. Tell the client that she has a family emergency and she has to leave
   b. Tell the teacher that she will be there to pick up her son after her shift ends, in another 2 hours
   c. Call her supervisor and ask if there is another aide who could cover for her while she goes to pick up her son at school
   d. Take the client in the car with her to pick up her son

6. Elizabeth has been caring for Mrs. Robinson for several months and has become friendly with her bachelor son, Richard. One day, Richard asks Elizabeth out for a cup of coffee after she is finished working. What should Elizabeth do?
   a. Decline Richard's invitation because dating family members of clients is against the home health care agency's policy
   b. Accept Richard's invitation—after all, she is single and she likes to date
   c. Ask Mrs. Robinson if it is all right if she dates her son
   d. Ask Richard if he would be willing to go for a cup of coffee on a day when she is not scheduled to work

Matching

Match each numbered item with its appropriate lettered description.

_____ 1. Case manager

_____ 2. Care plan

_____ 3. Respite care

_____ 4. Hospice care

_____ 5. Time and travel log

_____ 6. Homemaker flow sheet

a. End-of-life care provided to a person who is terminally ill

b. Member of the health care team responsible for overseeing a client's care, from admission through discharge

c. Form the home health aide uses to record how much time he spent at each client's house, how much time he spent traveling between houses, and his mileage for the day

d. Form used to document housework that is done

e. A set of instructions for the client's care

f. Care that allows the primary caregiver to rest or leave the house for a short period of time

? Stop and think!

▶ You are thinking about becoming a home health aide, and you decide to talk to your friend Darlene, who has worked in both the long-term care setting and as a home health aide. What do you think Darlene will tell is different about working in the home health care setting? What will she tell you is the same?

▶ You work for the Home-Aid Home Health Care Agency, which is located in a city called Evergreen. You have received your assignments for the day and are trying to plan your day's work. Look at the assignment list and the map of Evergreen on the next page, and decide how you will organize your day. You know that it will take you 15 minutes to travel between each client's home.

Client	Assignment	Length of visit	Address
Mr. Diaz, a 93-year-old man who is confined to bed	Assist client with toileting and repositioning	45 minutes, twice daily	13th & Chestnut
Miss Louise, an 84-year-old woman who is blind and has diabetes	Assist client with eating snack, change bed linens	45 minutes	7th & Spruce
Ms. Lindgren, a 65-year-old woman with advanced dementia	Assist client with activities of daily living (ADLs) and provide respite care for client's daughter	3 hours	16th & Walnut
Ms. Chang, a 26-year-old woman with paraplegia	Assist client with morning care and breakfast so that she can leave for work by 8:30 A.M.	90 minutes	14th & Arch

43

Safety and Infection Control in the Home Health Care Setting

What will you learn?

Keeping yourself and your clients safe, from both physical hazards and infection, is a priority in the home health care setting, just as it is in other health care settings. As a home health aide, you must be aware of unsafe situations that could put your client at risk for injury in his own home. In addition, working as a home health aide poses unique risks to your safety and well-being. In this chapter, you will learn how to adapt the principles of safety and infection control that you learned earlier to meet the unique needs of the home health care setting. When you are finished with this chapter, you will be able to:

1. List safety concerns that are unique to the home health care environment.
2. Understand ways that home health aides can spread infection.
3. Identify ways to reduce the spread of infection within the home.
4. Identify ways to properly prepare and store food.
5. Describe measures that the home health aide can take to protect herself from personal harm while carrying out her duties.

Photo: A home health aide checks to make sure a client is comfortable using her walker. This is just one of many ways that home health aides help to keep their clients safe.

Vocabulary

Use the CD in the back of your book to hear this term pronounced, defined, and used in a sentence:

Bag technique

WORKPLACE SAFETY

Many of us consider our homes places of safety and security. However, the home environment can actually be quite dangerous. As a home health aide, you need to be aware of conditions in the home that put the client at risk. You also need to know how to react in the event of an emergency.

ACCIDENTS AND MEDICAL EMERGENCIES

Health care settings, such as long-term care facilities and hospitals, are built with safety in mind. The hallways are wide and well lit; there are no throw rugs to trip over; and the bathrooms come equipped with handrails and other safety devices. A person's private home is a different story, however. Many factors in the home can put a person at risk for falling, especially if the person has limited mobility or poor eyesight:

- Many homes are old, with worn carpets or uneven floors.
- Hallways, rooms, and staircases might be dimly lit, or not lit at all.
- The bathroom may be small, or not located in a place that is easy for a person with poor mobility to reach.
- The home may be filled with a lifetime of collected objects and furniture, which can lead to crowding and clutter.
- Many people have pets, which can run underfoot.

Remember from Chapter 10 that falling is the most common type of accident that occurs in the health care setting, and the number one cause of accidental death among elderly people.

Fire is also a concern in the home:

- The wiring in the house may be old.
- Outlets may be overloaded. Overload can be caused by plugging too many cords into a single outlet, or by using extension cords.
- Electrical cords may be covered by carpet. This is a fire hazard as well as a tripping hazard.
- The family may rely on a space heater to provide heat. Space heaters can be dangerous if they are not used properly.
- Many people do not have functioning smoke detectors in their homes.

Guidelines for helping to maintain a safe home environment are given in Guidelines Box 43-1. It is not your responsibility to change the client's home to ensure safe conditions. However, your observations about the overall safety of the home are important and should be reported to the case manager. For example, based on your observations, the case manager might decide that the client needs better lighting and a smoke detector installed in the hallway, handrails installed on the staircase, and grab bars installed in the bathroom. The client may also need assistive devices, such as an elevated toilet seat or a bedside commode (to make toileting easier) or a side rail (for help with getting into and out of bed). The case manager will arrange for the necessary modifications and equipment. Your job is to make the case manager aware of the client's needs.

It is quite possible that despite your efforts to maintain a safe home environment, an accident, fire, or medical emergency will occur. For example, you may arrive at the home to find that your client has fallen and hurt himself. You may smell smoke or gas when you enter the client's home. The client may have a medical emergency, such as a heart attack or stroke, while you are there, or she may choke on food. Remember what you learned in Chapters 9 and 12 about reacting to fire and medical emergencies. Remain calm, and use good judgment. Call the fire department or activate the emergency medical services (EMS) system by calling "911" or the emergency telephone number specified by your agency. Then provide appropriate care until help arrives. After the situation has been resolved, you will need to report and record according to your agency's policy. For example, if an accident occurred while you were working, most agencies will require you to complete an incident (occurrence) report (see Chapter 10, Fig. 10-3).

GUIDELINES BOX 43-1
GUIDELINES FOR MAINTAINING A SAFE HOME ENVIRONMENT

What you do	Why you do it
Make sure that the furniture is arranged to allow for wide walkways. Chairs and small tables should be placed around the edges of the room, rather than in the center.	A cluttered, narrow walkway increases a person's risk of tripping and falling.
Remove any clutter or obstacles from indoor and outdoor walkways and steps. Provide adequate lighting.	Proper lighting enhances the ability to see, which helps to prevent falls. Removal of obstructions is an easy way to minimize falls.
Place a small lamp and a telephone on the person's bedside table.	Having these items close at hand can help to prevent falls. If the phone rings, the person can answer it without getting out of bed. If the person needs to get out of bed in the middle of the night, he can turn on the light first. The ability to see helps to prevent falls.
Install night-lights as needed.	Some people may hesitate to turn on the light when they get up in the middle of the night. Night-lights can help the person to see the route to the bathroom or kitchen without turning on the lights in the room or hallway. The ability to see helps to prevent falls.
Avoid running cords across walkways. Instead, move the furniture so that the electrical cords for lamps and other appliances are close to the outlet.	A person could trip over a cord that is stretched across a room or walkway.
In wintry climates, make arrangements for snow and ice to be removed from outdoor walkways and steps.	A person could easily slip and fall on icy or snowy walkways and steps.
Clean up spills on the bathroom or kitchen floor promptly.	Tile or linoleum floors become very slippery when wet, increasing the person's risk of falling.
Use a no-slip rubber bath mat on the floor of the bathtub.	A no-slip rubber bath mat helps to provide traction, reducing the person's risk of falling while getting into or out of the bathtub.
Provide a bath bench or a shower chair for the person to use while showering.	An unsteady person will be more stable and at less risk for falling if he can sit down during the shower.
Be aware of potential fire hazards (for example, frayed wires and overloaded outlets) and report these immediately.	A house fire can have tragic consequences, especially when the people who live in the home are relatively unable to help themselves should a fire break out.
Keep chemicals, cleaning solutions, and other poisonous substances in a locked storage area.	Poor eyesight, confusion, or a decreased sense of taste or smell can cause an elderly person to eat or drink something that will cause her harm. Children are also at risk for accidental poisonings because they are curious.
Program emergency telephone numbers into the telephone (for example, for the person's doctor, a family member, and emergency services), or keep a written list next to the telephone.	Having emergency phone numbers handy will make it easier for the person to call for help in the event of an emergency.

ABUSIVE SITUATIONS

In Chapter 4, you learned about abuse. Abuse can be physical, psychological (emotional), or sexual. Anyone can be a target for abuse. Families are complex, and many things go on "behind closed doors." As a home health aide, you may witness some of these things. For example, one of the family members may be the target of abuse, either by another family member or a friend of the family. A disabled or elderly person is more likely to be abused in the privacy of his or her own home because the abuser may feel that the abuse will go undiscovered. Children are also often targets of abuse.

As a home health aide, you may find yourself in a situation where you suspect that one of your patients is being abused (see Chapter 4, Box 4-1). Laws require that any health care worker who suspects the abuse of a child or elderly person must report his or her suspicions to the proper authorities. Your agency will have specific policies regarding the chain of reporting. It is not your responsibility to investigate whether or not abuse has actually occurred, or who has caused it. The state agencies that handle abuse reports will proceed through the proper channels. Your responsibility is to simply report your suspicions.

If a family situation turns violent while you are in the client's home, and you feel unsafe, you should leave the home after doing your best to make sure that the client is also safe. Activate the EMS system by calling "911" or the emergency telephone number specified by your agency if you feel that someone in the house is in immediate danger, and then report the situation to the case manager.

INFECTION CONTROL

Just as in any other health care setting, infection control is a top priority. Many of the people you will care for as a home health aide will have risk factors for infection. Your clients will be sick, recovering from surgery, elderly, or have a chronic illness or conditions that will increase their risk of getting an infectious disease. A major part of your responsibility in caring for other people involves protecting them from infection.

As a home health aide, you will visit several clients' homes each day. Improper or careless use of infection control methods can result in pathogens being carried from the home of one client to the home of another one. You can transmit pathogens on your hands, clothes, or equipment. By maintaining a sanitary environment and using standard precautions, you can protect your clients and yourself from communicable disease.

MAINTAINING A SANITARY ENVIRONMENT

No matter where you work, you will do many things to help maintain a sanitary work environment (see Chapter 7, Guidelines Box 7-1). When working in a client's home, you will have additional responsibilities related to maintaining a sanitary environment and preventing the spread of infection.

Using Proper Bag Technique

Bag technique is a procedure that is used to keep your nurse's bag free from contamination. Using proper bag technique helps to prevent the transmission of microbes from one client's home to another client's home. To practice proper bag technique:

1. When you arrive at the client's home, place your nurse's bag on a clean surface, such as the kitchen table, after laying down a newspaper, plastic bag, or other clean barrier object (Fig. 43-1). Placing a barrier between your nurse's bag and the surface helps to prevent contamination of the nurse's bag.
2. After washing your hands, remove the equipment you will need from your nurse's bag.
3. After you use the equipment, clean it and disinfect it according to agency policy and return it to its proper location in your nurse's bag (Fig. 43-2). Equipment that is used with all clients, such as your stethoscope, is not to be transported to another client's home until it has been properly cleaned and disinfected. Equipment that has been cleaned and disinfected is stored in the "clean" area of the nurse's bag.
4. Some items that are used for a client's care must be returned to the agency for

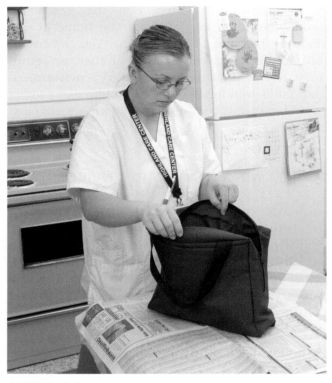

FIGURE 43-1

The nurse's bag is placed on a barrier, such as a clean sheet of newspaper, to help prevent the bag from becoming contaminated.

FIGURE 43-2

Equipment that is used for each client, such as equipment for measuring vital signs, is cleaned after each use and before placing it back in the nurse's bag. Alcohol wipes are usually used to clean the ear pieces, bell, and diaphragm of a stethoscope.

proper cleaning and disinfection before they are used again. You may also be required to transport specimens, such as urine or sputum samples, to the agency or laboratory. Dirty equipment and specimens are considered contaminated and are stored in the "dirty" area of the nurse's bag. (If equipment is too large to fit in the nurse's bag, then it can be stored in the "dirty" area of your car trunk, which may be divided in a way similar to the way the nurse's bag is divided.)

Cleaning Equipment and Household Surfaces

You will use many pieces of equipment as you care for your clients. Some of this equipment will be kept in the client's home, such as a bedside commode or equipment used for bathing. As always, this equipment must be properly cleaned and disinfected after each use. A commercial disinfectant solution or a solution of bleach and water mixed 1:10 (1 cup of bleach to 10 cups of water) may be used, according to

your agency's policy. Use gloves when cleaning any equipment.

Many of your duties as a home health aide will be related to keeping clean areas where food is prepared or personal care is given. A disinfectant solution is used to clean floors, kitchen counters, bathroom fixtures (including the toilet, bathtub, sink, and counters), and surfaces that are frequently touched by many people (such as doorknobs, telephone receivers, and refrigerator handles). These areas should be cleaned according to agency policy to decrease the spread of pathogens in the home. When cleaning floors and other household surfaces, remember the following:

- Empty dirty mop water into the toilet, *not* into sinks where food will be prepared.
- Disinfect mop heads and sponges after use by soaking them in a 1:10 bleach and water solution.
- Clean up blood or body fluid spills immediately. Wearing gloves, use paper towels to soak up as much fluid as possible. Place the soiled towels in a plastic bag and seal it. Then place that plastic bag in a second plastic bag. Seal the second bag, write "biohazard" on the outside of it, and dispose of it in the trash, or according to your agency's policies. Then clean the area where the spill occurred with a disinfectant solution.
- Pregnant women and people who have weak immune systems should not clean

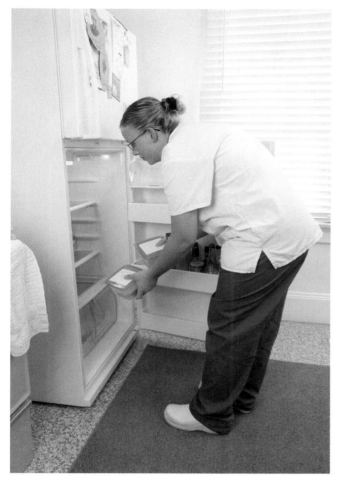

FIGURE 43-3

Leftovers should be placed in appropriate sealed containers, labeled (contents and date), and stored in the refrigerator.

litter boxes, bird cages, or other pet-related items. Cat feces, bird droppings, and other animal wastes can contain microbes that can cause harm to a developing fetus, or to a person with a weak immune system.

Handling Food Properly

You may be responsible for preparing meals for clients. Before preparing any food, always wash your hands using proper handwashing technique, and make sure that the surface where you will be preparing the food is clean. When preparing foods, remember to:

- Take note of expiration dates on packaged foods
- Avoid using eggs that are cracked
- Thoroughly wash and dry fresh fruits and vegetables before serving them

- Wash your hands after handling raw meat or poultry, and before touching anything else
- Wash cutting boards, utensils, and dishes used to prepare raw meat or poultry in hot, soapy water immediately after use
- Cook meat and poultry thoroughly, according to the United States Department of Agriculture (USDA) safe food handling labels that are attached to all supermarket meat packages
- Use a clean spoon each time if you must taste the food to check for seasonings

Raw or cooked food that is not stored properly can easily spoil and cause food poisoning. Leftovers should be placed in appropriate sealed containers, labeled, and refrigerated (Fig. 43-3). Food in the refrigerator should be inspected and disposed of before it is outdated or spoiled. The refrigerator itself should be cleaned with hot, soapy water periodically.

After each use, clean kitchen counters and stovetops with a disinfectant solution. If the house has a dishwasher, rinse the dishes and utensils and place them in the dishwasher. When the dishwasher is full, run it using the hot water cycle and dishwasher detergent. Pots, pans, and other items that are not "dishwasher safe" should be washed by hand using hot, soapy water. If possible, allow these items to air dry in a rack. Otherwise, use a clean dishtowel or paper towels to dry them. If no dishwasher is available, the dishes and utensils will also need to be washed by hand and dried. Be sure to wear gloves when washing dishes.

Assisting Clients with Personal Hygiene

Helping your clients to maintain good personal hygiene is essential to maintaining a sanitary environment. Bathing, washing hair, brushing teeth, and wearing clean clothing are all grooming practices that help prevent the spread of infection. Change the client's bed linens frequently, and encourage the client to wear clean clothing each day. (As always, soiled bed linens and clothing should be changed immediately.) Wash soiled linens and clothing in the washing machine, using the warmest water temperature available. Use a lengthy wash cycle and laundry soap. Add bleach if fabrics are colorfast. Dry the laundry on the high heat setting in a dryer. If a dryer is unavailable, hang laundry in the sun to dry.

FIGURE 43-4

Handwashing is the single most important method of preventing the spread of infection, no matter where you work. Here, a home health aide washes her hands at the kitchen sink.

▶ *Tell the Nurse!*

As a home health aide, you will have the unique opportunity to observe the home for conditions and situations that may increase a client's risk of spreading or getting an infection. You must be very diligent about observing your client for signs or symptoms of a developing infection. You must also be aware of practices of the client or family members that may spread an infection. Report any of the following observations to the case manager immediately:

⟾ The client has signs of an infection, such as fever, pain, reddened skin, coughing, a thick nasal discharge, vomiting, or diarrhea

⟾ A family member has signs of infection, especially if the client is at high risk for catching a communicable infection (because of a weakened immune system)

⟾ Members of the household have poor sanitation practices (for example, there is spoiled food, accumulated trash, or soiled linens lying around the house)

⟾ The house lacks running water or toilet facilities

USING STANDARD PRECAUTIONS

Maintaining a sanitary workplace is one important way to limit the spread of pathogens. In addition, you must always use standard precautions when providing client care. Standard precautions, covered in detail in Chapter 8, are used to reduce your risk of getting a communicable disease from a client. Proper use of standard precautions also helps to prevent the transmission of an infection to family members or other clients.

Handwashing

Handwashing is the single most important method of preventing the spread of infection in any type of health care setting (see Chapter 7). Always wash your hands:

- When you first arrive at a client's home
- Whenever your hands become visibly soiled with blood or other body fluids or substances
- Whenever you remove your gloves
- After each task or procedure that you perform

Wash your hands with soap and warm water, using the technique you learned in Chapter 7 (Fig. 43-4; see also Procedure 7-1). If paper towels are not available, use a *clean* cloth towel to dry your hands.

If handwashing facilities are not available or are inadequate, and your hands are not visibly soiled with dirt, blood, or other body fluids or substances, you can use an alcohol-based hand rub to decontaminate your hands (Fig. 43-5). If your hands are visibly soiled, then you should seek proper handwashing facilities as soon as possible.

Using Personal Protective Equipment (PPE)

As in other health care settings, gloves, gowns, masks, and goggles are worn as necessary to control the spread of pathogens. Your agency is required by the Occupational Safety and Health Administration (OSHA) to provide you with adequate personal protective equipment (PPE). You may carry PPE in your nurse's bag, or store it on site, depending on the situation. It is your responsibility to make sure that you have the PPE that you need before you leave for work, and to

A

B

FIGURE 43-5

An alcohol-based hand rub can be used for routine hand decontamination. Alcohol-based hand rubs are easy to use. (*A*) Apply the recommended amount of product to one of your palms. (*B*) Rub your hands together, covering your hands and fingers (front and back) with the product. Keep rubbing your hands together until your skin is dry.

use the PPE consistently, conscientiously, and correctly (see Chapter 7). Eye protection that is not disposable must be cleaned and disinfected after each use.

Disposing of Sharps

Many clients will use needles, lancets, or other sharp instruments or devices on a routine basis. For example, a client who has diabetes may routinely prick his finger with a lancet to check his blood sugar, and then use a syringe and needle to inject his daily doses of insulin. Clients who routinely use needles and lancets should be instructed to dispose of these items properly to prevent accidental needlesticks. If a commercial sharps container is not available, one can be made by cutting a small slit in the plastic lid of an empty coffee can or in the side of a heavy plastic bottle. When it is two-thirds full, seal the container with wide tape and write "biohazard" on the side. The container should be disposed of according to the guidelines set by the client's waste management company or according to agency policy.

PERSONAL SAFETY

As a home health aide, you will use standard methods to keep yourself safe on the job. For example, you will use proper body mechanics to minimize your risk of physical injury when lifting or transferring clients, and you will use standard precautions to protect yourself from infection. But some aspects of the home health aide's job pose unique safety risks. Instead of working in one building, you will be required to travel from one client's home to another. This puts you at increased risk for traffic accidents, flat tires, and other hazards of driving. In addition, some of your clients may live in unsafe neighborhoods, which could put you at risk for being attacked. Protecting yourself while traveling to and from your clients' homes is a top priority. Here are some things you can do to keep yourself safe while traveling between clients' homes:

- Keep your car in good repair, and always start out with a full tank of fuel.
- Choose the safest route of travel. Avoid driving or walking through unknown areas and alleys.
- Take a defensive driving course.
- Keep an emergency kit in the trunk of your car. Include flares, a blanket, a shovel, food, drinking water, a flashlight and batteries, jumper cables, and a tire jack.
- Be aware of the dangers of driving in ice and snow. When the weather is bad, be prepared with snow tires, a bag of sand or kitty litter (for weight and traction), antifreeze, and windshield washer fluid.
- Always keep your car doors locked and stay alert for strangers who may wish to cause you harm.
- Leave excessive amounts of cash and expensive personal items (such as jewelry or electronics) at home. Do not leave items in plain view on the car seat. Instead, take them with you or put them in the trunk or

under the seat before leaving the car. Always lock your car.
- Visit clients who live in unsafe neighborhoods during the day, preferably during the morning hours. Or, speak with the case manager about arranging an escort to help ensure your safety.
- Park your car in a safe, well-lighted area as close to the client's home as possible.
- Choose the safest walking route to reach the home. When walking between your car and the client's home, be aware of other people, strange animals, and your surroundings in general.
- Wear a name badge identifying yourself as a home health care provider according to your agency policy. If you are attacked, let the attacker know that you do not carry syringes, needles, or medication.
- Consider taking a self-defense course. If you are attacked, use your bag, arms, and hands to protect your face, neck, and throat. Kick the attacker with your legs. Use your car keys to slash the attacker's face. Scream or yell loudly to attract attention.
- Make sure that someone else (your case manager, a friend, or family member) knows your planned schedule. Follow your schedule and check in with the office frequently.
- Carry a fully charged cell phone with you at all times.

SUMMARY

▶ Home health aides are responsible for protecting themselves and those in their care from physical harm and infection.
▶ The home environment poses many safety risks. Home health aides are responsible for noting dangerous situations in the home and reporting their observations to the case manager, and for knowing how to react should an emergency occur.
  ■ Worn carpets or uneven floors, poor lighting, and clutter increase a person's risk of falling, especially if the person has poor mobility or eyesight.
  ■ Fire is always a risk in the home.
  ■ Abuse can take place in the home.

▶ Infection control is a priority in the home health care setting, just as it is in any other health care setting. The home health aide helps to prevent the spread of infection by maintaining a sanitary environment and using standard precautions.

- Using proper bag technique helps to prevent the spread of microbes from one client's home to another client's home.
- Disinfecting household surfaces, especially those where food is prepared or personal care is given, is essential to maintaining a sanitary environment.

- Handling and storing food properly is important for preventing food poisoning and other illnesses.
- Practicing good personal hygiene, and helping clients to do the same, is an important part of infection control.

▶ Home health aides must be concerned with keeping themselves safe while traveling between clients' houses. Keeping your car in good repair, being prepared for roadside and weather emergencies, using common sense, and being aware of your surroundings are important safety measures to take when traveling.

What did you learn?

Multiple Choice

Select the single best answer for each of the following questions.

1. You have just entered a client's home and are preparing to wash your hands at the kitchen sink, when you notice that there is no soap. How else could you accomplish the task of decontaminating your hands?
   a. You could wipe your hands with moisturizing hand lotion and a tissue
   b. You could use an alcohol-based hand rub
   c. You could run your hands under hot water and dry them with a dishtowel
   d. You could skip washing your hands at this time because you have just arrived in the home, and you have not done anything yet

2. Where are laboratory specimens stored for transport?
   a. In the "dirty" section of the nurse's bag
   b. In the "clean" section of the nurse's bag
   c. In the home health aide's uniform pocket
   d. In a cooler on the front seat of the car

3. You have just finished mopping a client's kitchen floor. Where do you dispose of the dirty water?
   a. Out the back door
   b. Down the kitchen sink
   c. Down the toilet
   d. Down the bathroom sink

4. You arrive at a client's home, only to find the client tied down in bed. The client's daughter tells you that her mother keeps falling out of bed, so she has tied her to the bed for her own protection. What should you do about this situation?
   a. Ignore it. The client's daughter obviously knows what is best for her mother.
   b. Report your observations to the case manager immediately.
   c. Call the police.
   d. Untie the client and tell the daughter that she is guilty of abusing her mother.

5. You are at the DiTomo home, caring for Mrs. DiTomo who has advanced emphysema. Suddenly, Mr. DiTomo, who also has health problems, complains of chest pain and slumps to the floor. What should you do first?
   a. Call the case manager.
   b. Dial "911" to activate the emergency medical services (EMS) system.
   c. Call the DiTomos' daughter and ask her to come over right away.
   d. Leave for your next assignment. You owe it to your next client to be on time, and caring for Mr. DiTomo is not your responsibility.

6. Which one of the following observations about a client's home should be reported to the client's case manager?
   a. The client has all of the most modern kitchen appliances
   b. The client has newspapers and magazines stacked 3 feet high lining both sides of a hallway
   c. The client has a large collection of dishes, which she stores in a sideboard in the dining room
   d. The client has very poor taste in decorating

Stop and think!

▶ Janis has been assigned a new client, Mrs. Peterson. Mrs. Peterson is a widow who lives alone in a small home on a limited income. She is recovering from a stroke, so her ability to get around independently is limited. Janis is expected to assist Mrs. Peterson with her activities of daily living (ADLs) and to do some light housekeeping. When Janis arrives at Mrs. Peterson's home for her first visit, she notices the garbage cans outside of the house are overflowing, and there are a lot of flies. On entering the kitchen she notices the kitchen sink is full of dirty dishes, there are dirty dishes all over the counter, and there is a strange odor coming from the refrigerator. After Janis finishes helping Mrs. Peterson to bathe and she has cleaned up the bathroom, she starts to wonder what to do about Mrs. Peterson's breakfast. Mrs. Peterson needs breakfast, but the kitchen is too filthy to do any cooking. In addition, Janis only has another half hour before she must leave for her next appointment. If you were Janis, what would you do?

▶ You have been assigned to provide home health care for Mrs. Abrams. Mrs. Abrams is pregnant with her third child and on complete bed rest because of pregnancy-related complications. During your visits, you are assigned to help Mrs. Abrams with personal care, as well as look after her twin two-year-old boys, Sammy and Alex. When you arrive at the Abrams home today, you learn that both Sammy and Alex have had diarrhea and have been vomiting since the middle of the previous night, as the result of a virus. You really do not want to take this virus home to your own kids, or get it yourself. Nor do you want Mrs. Abrams to get it, since being sick will only make her more uncomfortable than she already is. And you definitely do not want the client you will be visiting next, Mrs. Jefferson, to get it. Mrs. Jefferson has been receiving chemotherapy as part of her treatment for cancer and as a result, her immune system is weak. What measures will you take to try to contain the virus and prevent anyone else from getting it?

Nursing Assistants Make a Difference!

"Oh, I certainly had my doubts about having someone come to my home to help me care for my husband. I'm Sally Richards, and my husband Carl suffered a severe stroke about 4 months ago. The stroke left him totally paralyzed on his right side and I was terrified that I would have to place him in a nursing home. I mean, there's no way that I would have been able to lift him and care for him, as he needed. Carl was a big man.

The social worker at the hospital suggested that we use the services of a local home health care agency. The agency sent a nurse to our home to evaluate our needs even before Carl was discharged from the hospital. When we got home, a hospital bed, wheelchair, and specialized bathroom equipment had already been delivered and set up for his arrival. That day, we also met Angie, our home health aide.

The home health nurse explained that in addition to helping with Carl's personal care, Angie would be responsible for handling some housekeeping duties. For instance, Angie would be responsible for cleaning the bathroom after bathing Carl, and for changing and laundering his bed linens. I must admit that this caused me some concern. I have always taken great pride in making sure that my home was as neat as a pin. I figured that I would have to go back and re-do everything Angie did to my own standards.

Well, that Angie really surprised me! She was always personally clean and neat, and she took great care to avoid bringing germs from other clients' homes into ours. For example, as soon as she came into the house, she would spread out a clean piece of newspaper to put her nurse's bag on, and then she would wash her hands. She was always very conscientious about wearing gloves when she provided personal care to Carl and she washed her hands frequently during her visit. And, I hate to admit it, but I think my bathroom was cleaner after she finished with it than I ever kept it!

My Carl lived for 3 months after his first stroke. He then had another one that ended his life, but I feel very comforted that I was able to have him at home for those last months. Angie really made a difference in our lives."

You can listen to more stories about how nursing assistants make a difference on the CD in the back of your book.

Answers to the *What Did You Learn?* Exercises

Chapter 1: The Health Care System
Matching: 1-e, 2-b, 3-j, 4-h, 5-a, 6-k, 7-d, 8-f, 9-g, 10-c, 11-i, 12-l

Chapter 2: The Nursing Assistant
Multiple choice: 1-c, 2-b, 3-c, 4-b, 5-b, 6-d

Chapter 3: Professionalism and Job-Seeking Skills
Multiple choice: 1-b, 2-c, 3-b, 4-d, 5-a, 6-d, 7-b, 8-c, 9-c, 10-d, 11-a, 12-b, 13-c

Chapter 4: Legal and Ethical Issues
Multiple choice: 1-b, 2-a, 3-b, 4-b, 5-d, 6-d, 7-c, 8-a, 9-b, 10-a
Matching: 1-e, 2-a, 3-d, 4-b, 5-c

Chapter 5: Communication Skills
Multiple choice: 1-b, 2-a, 3-d, 4-b, 5-c, 6-a, 7-b, 8-c, 9-b, 10-b
Matching: 1-e, 2-a, 3-d, 4-c, 5-b

Chapter 6: Those We Care For
Multiple choice: 1-d, 2-a, 3-a, 4-b, 5-c, 6-a, 7-d, 8-b
Matching: 1-e, 2-f, 3-b, 4-a, 5-g, 6-c, 7-d

Chapter 7: Communicable Disease and Infection Control
Multiple choice: 1-d, 2-b, 3-b, 4-a, 5-d, 6-c, 7-d, 8-d, 9-a, 10-c
Matching: 1-c, 2-d, 3-f, 4-g, 5-e, 6-a, 7-h, 8-i, 9-j, 10-b

Chapter 8: Bloodborne and Airborne Pathogens
Multiple choice: 1-d, 2-b, 3-d, 4-d, 5-b, 6-b, 7-c

Chapter 9: Workplace Safety
Multiple choice: 1-a, 2-b, 3-d, 4-a, 5-c, 6-c, 7-c, 8-a, 9-a, 10-c, 11-b

Chapter 10: Patient and Resident Safety and Restraints
Multiple choice: 1-d, 2-b, 3-c, 4-b, 5-b, 6-c, 7-c, 8-b

Chapter 11: Postioning, Lifting, and Transferring Patients and Residents
Multiple choice: 1-a, 2-a, 3-d, 4-c, 5-d, 6-d, 7-d, 8-c, 9-b, 10-c, 11-d, 12-b, 13-d, 14-b, 15-d, 16-a

Chapter 12: Basic First Aid and Emergency Care

Multiple choice: 1-d, 2-b, 3-c, 4-c, 5-b, 6-d, 7-d, 8-d

Matching: 1-g, 2-f, 3-i, 4-b, 5-c, 6-e, 7-j, 8-h, 9-d, 10-a

Chapter 13: The Patient or Resident Environment

Multiple choice: 1-c, 2-d, 3-c, 4-b, 5-a, 6-c, 7-d

Matching: 1-c, 2-b, 3-a

Chapter 14: Admissions, Transfers, and Discharges

Multiple choice: 1-c, 2-b, 3-a, 4-d, 5-b, 6-c, 7-c, 8-c, 9-c, 10-d

Chapter 15: Bedmaking

Multiple choice: 1-b, 2-d, 3-c, 4-b, 5-c, 6-c, 7-a, 8-d

Chapter 16: Vital Signs, Height, and Weight

Multiple choice: 1-c, 2-a, 3-b, 4-c, 5-d, 6-d, 7-a, 8-c, 9-d, 10-d, 11-b, 12-c

Chapter 17: Cleanliness and Hygiene

Multiple choice: 1-a, 2-c, 3-d, 4-d, 5-c, 6-d, 7-b, 8-a, 9-d, 10-d, 11-d, 12-c

Matching: 1-g, 2-b, 3-f, 4-d, 5-c, 6-e, 7-a

Chapter 18: Grooming

Multiple choice: 1-c, 2-a, 3-a, 4-c, 5-b, 6-d, 7-d, 8-c, 9-d, 10-c, 11-a, 12-d

Matching: 1-d, 2-b, 3-e, 4-c, 5-a

Chapter 19: Basic Nutrition

Multiple choice: 1-c, 2-b, 3-c, 4-b, 5-b, 6-a, 7-c, 8-c, 9-b, 10-c, 11-b, 12-d

Matching: 1-c, 2-f, 3-a, 4-e, 5-d, 6-b

Chapter 20: Assisting with Urinary and Bowel Elimination

Multiple choice: 1-b, 2-a, 3-a, 4-a, 5-c, 6-d, 7-b, 8-d, 9-a, 10-c

Matching: 1-i, 2-j, 3-e, 4-f, 5-b, 6-c, 7-g, 8-d, 9-h, 10-a

Chapter 21: Caring for People Who Are Terminally Ill

Multiple choice: 1-d, 2-d, 3-d, 4-a, 5-c, 6-d, 7-d, 8-b

True or false: 1-T, 2-F, 3-T

Chapter 22: Caring for People Who Are Dying

Multiple choice: 1-c, 2-c, 3-b, 4-b, 5-a, 6-d, 7-b, 8-a

Matching: 1-d, 2-e, 3-b, 4-c, 5-a

Chapter 23: Basic Body Structure and Function

Multiple choice: 1-d, 2-d, 3-c, 4-d

Matching: 1-f, 2-j, 3-a, 4-d, 5-e, 6-c, 7-k, 8-b, 9-h, 10-g, 11-i

Chapter 24: The Integumentary System

Multiple choice: 1-d, 2-c, 3-a, 4-d, 5-b, 6-d, 7-b, 8-a

Matching: 1-g, 2-j, 3-i, 4-f, 5-a, 6-h, 7-e, 8-d, 9-c, 10-b

Chapter 25: The Musculoskeletal System

Multiple choice: 1-b, 2-b, 3-d, 4-b, 5-d, 6-b, 7-d, 8-c, 9-d, 10-c, 11-b, 12-b

Matching: 1-f, 2-c, 3-d, 4-e, 5-b, 6-a

Chapter 26: The Respiratory System

Multiple choice: 1-c, 2-c, 3-d, 4-a, 5-c, 6-a, 7-b, 8-d

Matching: 1-f, 2-g, 3-e, 4-a, 5-d, 6-b, 7-i, 8-c, 9-j, 10-h

Chapter 27: The Cardiovascular System

Multiple choice: 1-a, 2-d, 3-c, 4-d

Matching: 1-g, 2-d, 3-h, 4-j, 5-a, 6-b, 7-c, 8-i, 9-e, 10-f

Chapter 28: The Nervous System

Multiple choice: 1-b, 2-a, 3-b, 4-c, 5-d, 6-c, 7-b, 8-c, 9-c

Matching: 1-g, 2-i, 3-b, 4-h, 5-a, 6-c, 7-e, 8-d, 9-f

Chapter 29: The Sensory System

Multiple choice: 1-b, 2-b, 3-d, 4-c, 5-d, 6-d, 7-a, 8-b, 9-a

Matching: 1-c, 2-b, 3-g, 4-a, 5-e, 6-h, 7-d, 8-f, 9-i, 10-j

Chapter 30: The Endocrine System

Multiple choice: 1-d, 2-a, 3-b, 4-b, 5-d, 6-a

Matching: 1-h, 2-b, 3-c, 4-i, 5-e, 6-f, 7-g, 8-j, 9-a, 10-d

Chapter 31: The Digestive System

Multiple choice: 1-c, 2-d, 3-c, 4-a, 5-a, 6-d, 7-a, 8-a, 9-c

Chapter 32: The Urinary System

Multiple choice: 1-b, 2-d, 3-c, 4-a, 5-a, 6-a, 7-d, 8-b, 9-b

Matching: 1-e, 2-d, 3-a, 4-b, 5-c

Chapter 33: The Reproductive System

Multiple choice: 1-d, 2-b, 3-a, 4-c

Matching: 1-c, 2-e, 3-f, 4-h, 5-a, 6-g, 7-b, 8-d, 9-j, 10-i

Chapter 34: Caring for People with Developmental Disabilities
Multiple choice: 1-b, 2-b, 3-a, 4-b, 5-c, 6-a, 7-c, 8-b, 9-b, 10-a

Chapter 35: Caring for People with Mental Illness
Multiple choice: 1-c, 2-b, 3-c, 4-a, 5-b, 6-b, 7-a
Matching: 1-e, 2-b, 3-d, 4-c, 5-g, 6-f, 7-a

Chapter 36: Caring for People with Dementia
Multiple choice: 1-d, 2-a, 3-b, 4-c, 5-d, 6-d, 7-a, 8-b, 9-a, 10-d

Chapter 37: Caring for People with Cancer
Multiple choice: 1-a, 2-d, 3-b
Matching: 1-c, 2-e, 3-a, 4-f, 5-b, 6-g, 7-d

Chapter 38: Caring for People with AIDS
Multiple choice: 1-d, 2-a, 3-d, 4-b, 5-b

Chapter 39: Caring for Surgical Patients
Multiple choice: 1-b, 2-d, 3-d, 4-c, 5-a, 6-c, 7-b, 8-a

Chapter 40: Caring for Mothers and Newborns
Multiple choice: 1-c, 2-c, 3-d, 4-c, 5-d, 6-d, 7-b, 8-a
Matching: 1-b, 2-c, 3-a

Chapter 41: Caring for Pediatric Patients
Multiple choice: 1-b, 2-d, 3-a, 4-c, 5-b
Matching: 1-c, 2-e, 3-d, 4-a, 5-b

Chapter 42: Introduction to Home Health Care
Multiple choice: 1-a, 2-c, 3-c, 4-d, 5-c, 6-a
Matching: 1-b, 2-e, 3-f, 4-a, 5-c, 6-d

Chapter 43: Safety and Infection Control in the Home Health Care Setting
Multiple choice: 1-b, 2-a, 3-c, 4-b, 5-b, 6-b

State Hourly Training Requirements and Registry Information

State	Total Required Hours of Training	Classroom Hours	Laboratory Hours	Clinical Hours	Comments	Registry Contact Information
Alabama	75	35	20	20	The breakdown of hours is not state-mandated, but this is the usual breakdown.	Department of Public Health Nursing Assistant Registry PO Box 303017 Montgomery, AL 36130-3017 (334) 206-5169
Alaska	80	—	—	—	—	Division of Occupational Licensing Department of Commerce and Economic Development 3601 C Street #722 Anchorage, AK 99503 (907) 269-8169
Arizona	120	—	—	—	The state does not specify the number of hours by clinical and classroom, but programs do need to meet the federal minimum for clinical hours (16 hours).	Arizona Board of Nursing 1651 East Morten Suite 210 Phoenix, AZ 85020 (602) 331-8111
Arkansas	75	59	—	16	—	Office of Long-Term Care PO Box 8059 #402 Little Rock, AR 72203 (501) 682-8484
California	150	50	—	100	—	California Dept of Health Services Div of Licensing and Certification PO Box 942732 Sacramento, CA 94234-7320 (916) 327-2445
Colorado	75	16	—	16	Although 75 hours is the required minimum, most programs are at least 80 hours.	Colorado Board of Nursing 1560 Broadway #670 Denver, CO 80202 (303) 894-2816 1-888-274-5050 CNA test
Connecticut	75	—	—	—	—	Dept of Health 410 Capitol MS #12M QA PO Box 340308 Hartford, CT 06134-0308 (860) 509-7596
Delaware	150	75	—	75	—	Division of Long-Term Care Health Facilities Lic & Cert 3 Mill Road, Suite 308 Wilmington, DE 19806 (302) 577-6666

(continued)

State	Total Required Hours of Training	Classroom Hours	Laboratory Hours	Clinical Hours	Comments	Registry Contact Information
District of Columbia	120	45	30	45	—	Dept of Consumer & Regulatory Affairs 614 H Street NW #1003 Washington, DC 20001 (202) 727-7200 or 442-4727
Florida	120	40	40	40	—	Dept of Health/CNA 4052 Bald Cypress Way Bin #13 Tallahassee, FL 32399-3263 (850) 245-4567
Georgia	85	—	—	—	—	Office Reg Serv-NA Registry Dept Human Resources 2 Peachtree Street NW 32-415 Atlanta, GA 30303-3167 (404) 657-5730
Hawaii	75	—	—	—	—	Prof & Voc Licensing Dept of Comm & Cons Affairs PO Box 3469 Honolulu, HI 96801 (808) 739-8122
Idaho	120	80	—	40	—	Idaho Board of Nursing PO Box 83720 Boise, ID 83720-0061 (208) 364-1953
Illinois	120	80	—	40	—	Dept of Health/Education Sect 525 W Jefferson Springfield, IL 62761 (217) 782-3070
Indiana	105	30	—	75	The 30 classroom hours also include laboratory hours.	State Dept of Health Div of Long-Term Care PO Box 1964 Indianapolis, IN 46204-1964 (317) 233-7612
Iowa	75	30	15	30	—	Dept of Inspections & Appeals Health Facilities Division Lucas State Office Building Des Moines, IA 50319-0083 (515) 281-4963
Kansas	90	45	20	25	Part I consists of 40 hours (20 classroom and 20 laboratory). Part II consists of 50 hours (25 classroom and 25 clinical).	Health Occupations Credential 900 SW Jackson LSOB 1051 South Topeka, KS 66612-2218 (785) 296-6877

(continued)

State						Description	Registry Information
Kentucky	75	—	—	—	—	—	Kentucky Board of Nursing NA Registry 312 Whittington Pkwy #300A Louisville, KY 40222-5172 (502) 329-7047
Louisiana	80	40	—	40	—	—	State Bd Examiners for NFA NA Registry 5615 Corporate Blvd Suite 8D Baton Rouge, LA 70808 (504) 925-4591
Maine	150	80	20	50	—	—	Maine Registry NA State House Station II 35 Anthony Ave Augusta, ME 04333 (207) 624-5205
Maryland	100	60	—	40	—	—	Licensing & Certif Admin 4201 Patterson Avenue Baltimore, MD 21215 (410) 764-2770
Massachusetts	75	54	—	21	—	There is no specific breakdown for classroom and laboratory hours. However, the 21 clinical hours are a mandatory minimum.	Dept of Public Health Division of Health Care Quality 10 W Street 5th Floor Boston, MA 02111 (617) 753-8143
Michigan	75	—	—	—	—	—	Bureau of Health Services Div of Federal Support Serv PO Box 30664 Lansing, MI 48909 (800) 752-4724 or (571) 241-0554
Minnesota	75	—	—	16	—	Programs must include at least 16 hours of classroom instruction prior to a trainee's direct contact with a resident. Skills training, which includes laboratory and classroom hours, must be no less than 50% of the total program hours.	Facility & Provider Compliance NA Registry PO Box 64501 St Paul, MN 55164-0501 (651) 215-8705
Mississippi	75	16	—	8 to 16	—	The balance of the hours are divided between the classroom and the laboratory.	Dept of Health Lic/ Cert PO Box 1700 Jackson, MS 39215-1700 (888) 204-6213

State	Total Required Hours of Training	Classroom Hours	Laboratory Hours	Clinical Hours	Comments	Registry Contact Information
Missouri	175	75	—	100	—	Health Education Unit Division of Aging PO Box 1337 Jefferson City, MO 65102 (573) 751-3082
Montana	—	45 to 55	—	25 to 30	—	DOH/QAD NA Registry PO Box 202953 Helena, MT 59620-2953 (406) 444-4980
Nebraska	75	—	—	—	—	Dept of Health Bureau of Health Facility Standards PO Box 95007 Lincoln, NE 68509-5007 (402) 471-0537
Nevada	75	—	—	—	State law does not differentiate between classroom and clinical hours.	State Board of Nursing PO Box 46886 Las Vegas, NV 89114 (702) 486-5800
New Hampshire	100	40	—	60	—	New Hampshire Board of Nursing PO Box 3898 Concord, NH 03002-3938 (603) 271-6282 or (603) 271-6599
New Jersey	90	50	—	40	—	Assessment Systems Inc Processing Center Suite 300 3 Bala Plaza West Bala Cynwyd, PA 19004-3481 (610) 617-9300
New Mexico	75	51	—	24	Although 75 hours is the required minimum, most programs are longer.	New Mexico Dept of Health Nurse Aide Registry 1421 Luisa Street, Suite R Santa Fe, NM 87505 (505) 827-1453
New York	100	—	—	30	—	NY Dept of Health Office of Continuing Care 161 Delaware Avenue Delmar, NY 12054-1393 1-800-274-7181 verification (518) 478-1060
North Carolina	75	—	—	—	Programs must include at least 16 hours of classroom instruction prior to a trainee's direct contact with a resident. Although 75 hours is the required minimum, most programs average 120 hours.	Dept of Health and Human Services Division of Facility Services Nurse Aide Training 2709 Mail Service Center Raleigh, NC 27699-2709 (919) 715-0562

State				Notes	Registry Information
North Dakota	75	—	—	—	North Dakota Dept of Health Div of Emergency Health Serv 600 E Boulevard Avenue Bismarck, ND 58505-0200 (701) 328-2675
Ohio	75	—	16	—	Department of Health Nurse Aide Registry PO Box 118 Columbus, OH 43266-0118 (614) 752-9500
Oklahoma	75	—	—	Vocational–technical programs are 120 hours.	OK Department of Health/CNA 1000 NE 10th Street Oklahoma City, OK 73117-1299 (800) 695-2197
Oregon	150	75	75	—	Oregon Board of Nursing 800 NE Oregon Street Suite 25 Portland, OR 97232 (503) 731-4745
Pennsylvania	75	37.5	37.5	Programs range from 75 to 144 hours. Although 75 hours is the required minimum, most approved programs are longer.	Dept of Health Division of Long Term Care PO Box 90, Room #526 Harrisburg, PA 17108 (800) 852-0518
Rhode Island	100	80	20	Although 100 hours is the required minimum, most programs are 120 hours.	Dept of Health Division of Professional Regulation 3 Capitol Hill, Room 104 Providence, RI 02098 (401) 277-2827
South Carolina	80	40	40	—	Dept of Health and Environment 2600 Bull Street Columbia, SC 29201 (803) 737-7207
South Dakota	75	—	—	Programs must include at least 16 hours of classroom instruction and 16 hours of clinical instruction prior to a trainee's direct contact with a resident. Programs typically include 40 classroom hours (including 16 laboratory hours) and 35 clinical hours.	Board of Nursing 4300 S Louise Sioux Falls, SD 57106-3124 (605) 362-2760

(continued)

State	Total Required Hours of Training	Classroom Hours	Laboratory Hours	Clinical Hours	Comments	Registry Contact Information
Tennessee	75	—	—	—	—	Board of Nursing/CAN 424 Fifth Avenue N 1st Floor Nashville, TN 37247 (888) 310-4650
Texas	75	51	—	24	—	Department of Human Services NA Registry PO Box 149030 MC Y979 Austin, TX 78714-9030 (800) 452-3934
Utah	80	—	16	—	Programs must include at least 16 hours of laboratory instruction prior to a trainee's direct contact with a resident. The division of the remaining program hours is up to the discretion of the individual program, but 16 hours must be clinical.	Utah Health Technology Certification Center 550 E 300 S Kaysville, UT 84037 (801) 547-9947
Vermont	75	—	—	—	—	Vermont Board of Nursing NA Registry 109 State Street Montpelier, VT 05609-1106 (802) 828-2819 or (802) 828-2453
Virginia	120	—	—	40	The minimum requirement for clinical training is 40 hours, 35 of which must be spent in a long-term care facility. The division of the remaining program hours is up to the discretion of the individual program. Most approved programs have 60 hours of clinical time and 60 hours of combined classroom/laboratory time.	Dept of Health Profession 6606 W Broad Street 4th Floor Richmond, VA 23230-1717 (804) 662-7310
Washington	85	35	—	50	—	Aging & Adult Services Admin OBRA NA Registry PO Box 45600 Olympia, WA 98504-5600 (360) 725-2570

West Virginia	120	—	—	55	Bureau of Public Health OHFLAC/WV NA Registry 350 Capitol St Room 206 Charleston, WV 25301-3718 (304) 558-0688
Wisconsin	75	—	—	—	Dept of Health & Family Serv Bureau of Quality-NA Registry PO Box 309 Madison, WI 53701-0309 (877) 329-8760
Wyoming	75	—	—	—	Board of Nursing 2020 Carey Street Suite 110 Cheyenne, WY 82002 (307) 777-7601

C

Introduction to the Language of Health Care

All professions have their own sets of words and abbreviations that are used to describe objects and situations that are specific to that particular profession. The health care profession is no different. In fact, the health care profession has so many unique words and abbreviations, you might think that health care professionals are speaking a different language from everyone else!

Understanding the terms and abbreviations that are unique to the health care profession is essential if you expect to be able to communicate effectively with the other members of the health care team. Not knowing these terms and abbreviations will make it difficult for you to read and follow orders for patient or resident care. In addition, you will need to know these terms and abbreviations to accurately record and report.

In this appendix, you will learn some tricks that will allow you to figure out the meaning of many unfamiliar words you may hear or read. We will also introduce you to some commonly used medical terms and abbreviations. Finally, you should always make it a point to look up new words or abbreviations in a medical dictionary as soon as you hear or read them. Or, you can ask the nurse to explain the meaning of the word or abbreviation to you. Before long, you will become very comfortable using and understanding the language of the health care profession!

MEDICAL TERMINOLOGY

Although the strange-sounding language of the health care profession may seem overwhelming at first, it is really quite easy to pick up. Some medical terms come from the names of people (for example, Down syndrome, Alzheimer's disease, Parkinson's disease, Papanicolaou smear). Other terms come from Greek or Latin words, just as many everyday English, Spanish, French,

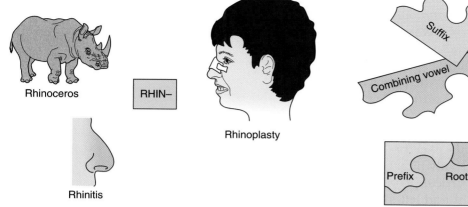

FIGURE C-1

Many of the words you use in everyday conversation have the same Greek or Latin origins as medical words that you may be less familiar with. For example, the Greek word *rhin-* means "nose." You see *rhin-* in words such as *rhinoceros, rhinitis,* and *rhinoplasty.* When you are trying to figure out the meaning of a new medical word, think about similar-sounding words that you may already know!

FIGURE C-2

Big words can be broken down into smaller parts, and if you know the meaning of the individual parts, then you can figure out the meaning of the entire word.

and Italian words do. For example, you know what a rhinoceros looks like, right? A rhinoceros is a large animal with a huge horn growing out of its nose (Fig. C-1). *Rhin-* comes from the Greek word for "nose," and *-ceros* comes from the Greek word *keras,* or "horn." Now where else might you find the Greek word *rhin-?* Well, if the mucous membranes on the inside of your nose are inflamed because you have a cold or allergies, the doctor might say that you have *rhinitis* (*rhin-,* nose + *itis,* inflammation). If a movie star has had a "nose job," then her publicist may tell the press that the celebrity has had *rhinoplasty,* the medical term for a nose job (*rhin-,* nose + *-plasty,* surgical repair).

Perhaps you have noticed a pattern here. Big words can be broken down into smaller parts, and if you know the meaning of the individual parts, you can figure out the meaning of the entire word. There are four types of word parts (Fig C-2):

- **Roots** contain the essential, basic meaning of the word. For example, *cardi-* means "heart." Common roots are listed in Table C-1, at the end of this appendix.
- **Suffixes** are attached to the end of a root to make the root more specific. For example, *carditis* is "inflammation of the heart" (*cardi-,* heart + *-itis,* inflammation). Common suffixes are listed in Table C-2, at the end of this appendix.

- **Prefixes** are attached to the beginning of a root to make the root more specific. For example, *pericarditis* is "inflammation of the sac that surrounds the heart" (*peri-,* around + *cardi-,* heart + *-itis,* inflammation). Common prefixes are listed in Table C-3, at the end of this appendix.
- **Combining vowels** are often added in between the root and the suffix to make the new word easier to pronounce. When a word has more than one root, combining vowels may also be used between the roots. For example, *cardiomyopathy* is "disease of the heart muscle" (*cardi-,* heart + *o* + *my-,* muscle + *o* + *-pathy,* disease). The combining vowel is usually "o," but "a" or "i" may also be used sometimes. The combining vowel that is used most often with each root is listed in Table C-1.

You will come across many medical terms as you study each chapter in this textbook. When you come across a term in your reading that is new to you, try using what you have learned about the different word parts to guess at the word's meaning. Then look up the word in the glossary and see how well you did!

ANATOMICAL TERMS

Anatomy is the study of the structure of the body. To describe the location of one body part in relation to another, health care professionals use specific terms. To ensure that these terms always have the same meaning to everyone, we always imagine the body to be in *normal anatomical position* when we describe it. A person who is in normal anatomical position is standing upright and facing forward, with his feet slightly spread apart, and with his arms to the sides and the palms facing forward (Fig. C-3). *Anatomical planes* are used as standard points of reference when describing the body. A *plane* is a flat surface, like a pane of glass. Health care professionals use three main imaginary planes to divide the body (Fig. C-4):

- The **sagittal plane** is a vertical plane that divides the body into right and left sides. A sagittal plane that divides the body into exact right and left halves is sometimes referred to as the *mid-sagittal plane.*
- The **transverse plane** is a horizontal plane that divides the body into upper and lower segments.
- The **frontal (coronal)** plane is a vertical plane that divides the body into front and back segments.

DIRECTIONAL TERMS

When describing the body, health care professionals often need to describe something that is above, under, to the side of, or further away from

A. Sagittal plane   **B.** Transverse plane   **C.** Frontal (coronal) plane

FIGURE C-4

The body is divided into imaginary planes, which are used as points of reference when describing the location of one body part with relation to another. (*A*) The sagittal plane is a vertical plane that divides the body into right and left segments. Shown here is the mid-sagittal plane, which divides the body into equal right and left halves. (*B*) The transverse plane is a horizontal plane that divides the body into upper and lower segments. (*C*) The frontal (coronal) plane is a vertical plane that divides the body into front and back segments.

something else. To do this, they use standard directional terms. Directional terms are used to describe the location of one body part in relation to another. When we use directional terms, we have to have a point of reference that stays the same. If not, just changing a person's body position would change a directional reference. This is where normal anatomical position and the anatomical planes come in.

Using the anatomical planes as reference points gives us the following directional terms (Fig. C-5):

- **Medial:** closer to the mid-sagittal plane of the body (toward the inner side). For example, the nose is medial to the eyes.
- **Lateral:** further away from the mid-sagittal plane of the body (toward the outer side). For example, the ears are lateral to the nose.
- **Superior:** closer to the top of the body (closer to the head). For example, the chin is superior to the breast.

FIGURE C-3

When describing the location of one part of the body in relation to another, we imagine the body to be in normal anatomical position. In normal anatomical position, the person is standing upright, facing forward, with the legs slightly apart and the arms at the sides, with the palms facing forward.

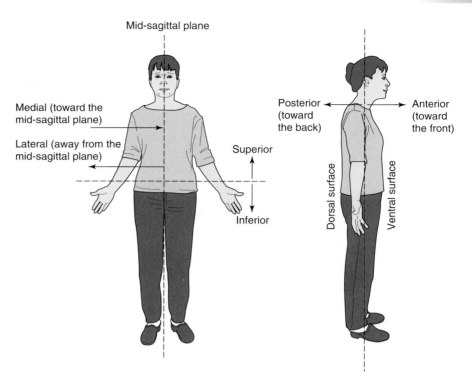

FIGURE C-5

Directional terms are used to describe the location of one body part in relation to another.

- **Inferior:** further away from the top of the body (closer to the feet). For example, the belly button is inferior to the breast.
- **Anterior:** toward the front, or *ventral surface,* of the body. For example, the abdomen is anterior to the buttocks.
- **Posterior:** toward the back, or *dorsal surface,* of the body. For example, the buttocks are posterior to the abdomen.

Two other directional terms are used to describe the location of one body part in relation to another. These terms describe the relationship between parts of the extremities (the arms and legs) and their points of attachment to the body (the shoulders and hips):

- **Proximal:** closer to the point of origin in relation to something else (for example, the elbow is proximal to the wrist)
- **Distal:** further away from the point of origin in relation to something else (for example, the wrist is distal to the elbow)

Like other terms used in the health care profession, many of these directional terms have similar meanings to words you use every day. For example, *distal* sounds like *distant,* or "further away." Similarly, *proximal* sounds like *proximity,* which means "close by." If you find the terms *ventral* and *dorsal* hard to remember, just think of a shark swimming close to the surface of the water. The shark's dorsal fin, the fin located on the shark's back, is usually visible above the water.

TERMS USED TO DESCRIBE BODY CAVITIES

A *cavity* is a hollow space. In the body, cavities contain organs. There are two major cavities inside the body. The *dorsal cavity,* which contains the brain and spinal cord, is toward the back of the body. The *ventral cavity* is toward the front of the body (Fig. C-6). The ventral cavity is divided by the diaphragm into the *thoracic (chest) cavity* and the *abdominal (belly) cavity.*

- The thoracic cavity contains the lungs, the heart, and the large blood vessels that enter and leave the heart. Most of the esophagus is also contained in the thoracic cavity.
- The upper abdominal cavity contains the stomach, liver, pancreas, spleen, large intestine, and small intestine. The lower abdominal cavity contains the urinary bladder, the rectum, and the female reproductive organs. The kidneys lie behind the abdominal cavity. Sometimes the upper and lower abdominal cavity are referred to together as the *abdominopelvic cavity.*

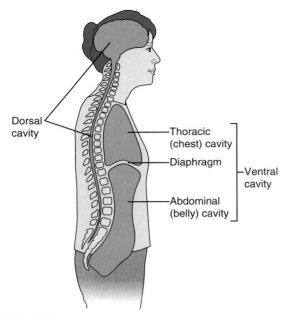

FIGURE C-6

The body has two major cavities, the dorsal cavity (*blue*) and the ventral cavity (*pink*). The diaphragm divides the ventral cavity into the thoracic (chest) cavity and the abdominopelvic (belly) cavity.

TERMS USED TO DESCRIBE THE ABDOMINAL AREA

Many patients or residents will experience pain or discomfort in the abdominal area. Often, knowing exactly where the pain or discomfort is occurring can provide clues to the source of the person's symptoms. Therefore, health care professionals use a number of different terms to describe the abdominal area. The abdominal area can be described in terms of quadrants (fourths) or regions (Fig. C-7). Quadrants are typically used to describe general information, such as where a person is experiencing pain. Regions are used when it is necessary to be very specific (for example, when describing where an incision is located).

Quadrants

Quad means "four." The simplest way to describe the abdominal area is to divide it into fourths, or quadrants. The quadrants are named according to their location: right upper quadrant (RUQ), left upper quadrant (LUQ), right lower quadrant (RLQ), and left lower quadrant (LLQ). By using these quadrants as reference, you can describe where your patient or resident is experiencing

pain by saying, "Mrs. Jones is complaining of a sharp pain in her RUQ."

Regions

The abdomen can also be divided into smaller sections, called *regions*, for the purpose of description. There are nine regions (three rows of three):

- The upper row consists of the right and left hypochondriac regions and the epigastric region. The hypochondriac regions are named for their relationship to the ribs: *hypo-* means "below" and *chondr/o-* means "cartilage" (of the ribs). The epigastric region is named for its relation to the stomach: *epi-* means "above" and *gastric* means "stomach."
- The middle row consists of the right and left lumbar regions and the umbilical region. The right and left lumbar regions are named for the region of the spinal column in that area. The umbilical region is named for the umbilicus, or belly button.
- The lower row consists of the right and left iliac regions and the hypogastric region. The iliac regions are named after the iliac crest, the bone that forms the hip bones. The iliac regions are also sometimes called the inguinal (groin) regions. The hypogastric region is named for its relation to the stomach: *hypo-* means "below" and *gastric* means "stomach."

ABBREVIATIONS

Abbreviations are shortened versions of words or phrases. Health care professionals use abbreviations to make recording more efficient. Some abbreviations come from English words. For example, you just learned that *RUQ* means "right upper quadrant." Other abbreviations come from Latin or Greek words, and therefore may seem foreign at first. For example, *bid* is the abbreviation for "twice daily," from the Latin words **bis** (twice) **in** (a) **die** (day). And *NPO*, which means "nothing by mouth," comes from the Latin words **nils** (nothing) **per** (by) **os** (mouth). As with other terms used in health care, you can often remember the meaning of a new abbreviation by relating

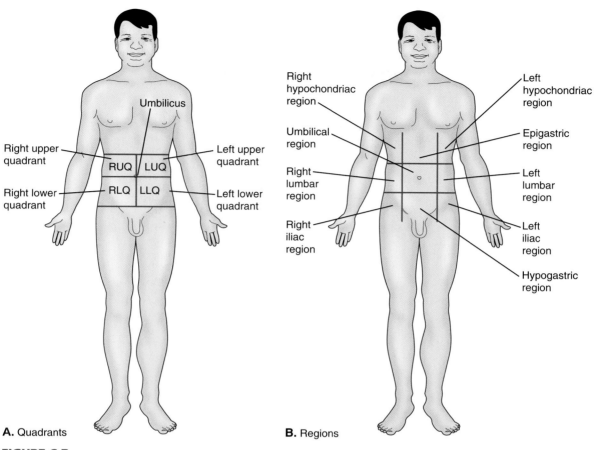

A. Quadrants   **B.** Regions

FIGURE C-7

The abdominal area can be described in terms of (*A*) quadrants or (*B*) regions. (Remember that when you are using the terms *right* and *left*, these terms are used in relation to the patient's or resident's right or left, not your right or left.)

it to an everyday word that you already know. For example, *bid, tid,* and *qid* are abbreviations that describe how many times a day an action is to be carried out. The abbreviation *bid* means "twice daily." Now think of how many wheels a *bi*cycle has: two, right? Similarly, the abbreviation *tid* means "three times daily." How many wheels does a *tri*cycle have?

Abbreviations that are commonly used in health care settings are listed in Table C-4, at the end of this appendix. Although abbreviations can help us save time and space when recording, it is very important to use only abbreviations that are approved for use in your facility. Otherwise, other members of the health care team may be confused by your meaning. In addition, if you are unsure of the meaning of an abbreviation that you read in a patient's or resident's care plan, please either look the abbreviation up or ask the nurse to explain it to you. It is important not to just guess at the meaning, because guessing could cause harm to the patient or resident.

TABLE C-1 ■ Common Roots and Their Combining Vowels

Root / Combining Vowel	Meaning	Root / Combining Vowel	Meaning
abdomin / o	abdomen	mening / o	meninges
aden / o	gland	men / o	menses, menstruation
adip / o	fat	muc / o	mucus
adren / o	adrenal glands	myel / o	spinal cord, bone marrow
angi / o	vessel (usually blood or lymph)	my / o	muscle
arteri / o	artery	myring / o	tympanic membrane (eardrum)
arthr / o	joint	nas / o	nose
blephar / o	eyelid	necr / o	death
bronchi / o	bronchus	nephr / o	kidney
calc / o	calcium	neur / o	nerve
carcin / o	cancer	noct / o	night
cardi / o	heart	odont / o	teeth
cephal / o	head	oophor / o	ovary
cerebr / o	cerebrum (brain)	ophthalm / o	eye
chol / e	bile, gall	orchi / o	testis
cholecyst / o	gallbladder	os / o	mouth
choledoch / o	bile duct	oste / o	bone
chondr / o	cartilage	ot / o	ear
col / o	colon	pancreat / o	pancreas
cost / o	ribs	pelv / i / o	pelvis
crani / o	cranium (skull)	pharyng / o	pharynx (throat)
cutane / o	skin	phleb / o	vein
cyan / o	blue	pleur / o	pleura
cyst / o	bladder	pneum / o	lung, air
dent / o	teeth	proct / o	anus, rectum
dermat / o	skin	pyel / o	renal pelvis
dipl / o	double	radi / o	x-rays, radiation
electr / o	electric	ren / o	kidney
encephal / o	brain	retin / o	retina
enter / o	intestine (usually the small intestine)	rhin / o	nose
erythr / o	red	salping / o	fallopian tube
esophag / o	esophagus	scler / o	hardening, sclera (white of the eye)
femor / o	femur (thigh bone)	sigmoid / o	sigmoid colon
gastr / o	stomach	spermat / o	sperm
gingiv / o	gum	spin / o	spine
gluc / o	sugar, glucose	spondyl / o	vertebra (backbone)
glyc / o	sugar, glucose	stern / o	sternum (breastbone)
gynec / o	woman, female	stomat / o	mouth
hemangi / o	blood vessel	tend / o	tendon
hemat / o	blood	therm / o	heat
hepat / o	liver	thorac / o	chest
hydr / o	water	thromb / o	blood clot
hyster / o	uterus	thyr / o	thyroid gland
irid / o	iris	toxic, tox / o	poison
lapar / o	abdomen	trache / o	trachea (windpipe)
laryng / o	larynx (voice box)	tympan / o	tympanic membrane (eardrum)
leuk / o	white	ureter / o	ureter
lingu / o	tongue	urethr / o	urethra
lip / o	fat	ur / o	urine
lith / o	stone, calculus	uter / o	uterus
lumb / o	lower back	vagin / o	vagina
lymphangi / o	lymph vessel	vascul / o	blood vessel
lymph / o	lymph	vas / o	vas deferens, vessel
mamm / o	breast	ven / o	vein
mast / o	breast	ventricul / o	ventricle (of brain or heart)
megal / o	enlargement	vesic / o	bladder
melan / o	black	vertebr / o	vertebra (backbone)

TABLE C-2 ■ Common Suffixes

Suffix	Meaning
-al	pertaining to
-algia	pain
-ar, -ary	pertaining to
-cele	hernia, swelling
-centesis	surgical puncture
-cyte	cell
-derma	skin
-dipsia	thirst
-ectomy	excision, removal of
-edema	swelling
-emesis	vomiting
-emia	blood
-gram	record
-graphy	process of recording
-ia	condition
-ic	pertaining to
-ism	condition
-ist	specialist
-itis	inflammation
-lith	stone, calculus
-logist	specialist in the study of
-logy	study of
-lysis	separation, destruction, loosening
-malacia	softening
-megaly	enlargement
-meter	measure, instrument for measuring
-oid	resembling
-oma	tumor
-opia	vision
-osis	abnormal condition
-pathy	disease
-pause	cessation
-penia	decrease
-pepsia	digestion
-pexy	fixation
-phagia	swallow, eat
-phasia	speech
-phobia	fear
-plasty	surgical repair
-plegia	paralysis
-pnea	breathing
-rrhaphy	suture
-rrhea	flow, discharge
-scope	instrument to view
-scopy	visual examination
-stenosis	structure, narrowing
-stomy	forming a new opening
-therapy	treatment
-tome	instrument to cut
-tomy	incision, cut into
-tripsy	crushing
-uria	urine, urination

TABLE C-3 ■ Common Prefixes

Prefix	Meaning
a-, an-	without, not, absent
ab	away from
amb-, ambi-	both, on two sides
auto-	self
bi-	two, double
brady-	slow
dys-	bad, painful, difficult
epi-	above, upon
hemi-	half, partly
hyper-	excessive
hypo-	under, below
inter-	between
intra-	within
macro-	large
micro-	small
neo-	new
para-	near, beside, around
peri-	around
poly-	many, much
post-	after, behind
pre-	before
quadri-	four
sub-	under, below
supra-	above
tachy-	rapid
tri-	three

TABLE C-4 ■ Common Medical Abbreviations

Abbreviation	Meaning	Abbreviation	Meaning
Ab	antibody	ft	foot or feet
abd	abdomen	Fx	fracture
ac	before a meal	gal	gallon
ADL	activities of daily living	GB	gallbladder
ad lib	as desired	GI	gastrointestinal
Adm (adm)	admitted or admission	GSW	gunshot wound
AFB	acid-fast bacillus (usually tuberculosis)	GU	genitourinary
		h (hr)	hour
AIDS	acquired immunodeficiency syndrome	H_2O	water
		HBV	hepatitis B virus
AKA	above-the-knee amputation	HIV	human immunodeficiency virus
AM (am)	morning	HOB	head of bed
amb	ambulate, ambulatory	HS (hs)	hour of sleep (bedtime)
AMI	acute myocardial infarction (heart attack)	ht	height
		ICU	intensive care unit
amt	amount	IDDM	insulin-dependent diabetes mellitus
ap	apical	in	inch
approx	approximately	I&O	intake and output
ASAP	as soon as possible	IV	intravenous
as tol	as tolerated	L	left, liter
ax	axillary	lab	laboratory
bid	twice a day	lb	pound
BKA	below-the-knee amputation	lg	large
BM (bm)	bowel movement	liq	liquid
BP, B/P	blood pressure	LLQ	left lower quadrant
B.R.	bed rest	LMP	last menstrual period
BRP	bathroom privileges	LPN	licensed practical nurse
BSC	bedside commode	lt	left
C	centigrade, Celsius	LVN	licensed vocational nurse
C̄	with	LUQ	left upper quadrant
CA	cancer	meds	medications
cath	catheter, catheterize	MI	myocardial infarction (heart attack)
CBC	complete blood count		
CBR	complete bed rest	mid noc	midnight
cc	cubic centimeter	min	minute
CCU	coronary care unit	ml	milliliter
CHD	coronary heart disease	NA	nursing assistant
CHF	congestive heart failure	NB	newborn
cl liq	clear liquids	neg	negative
CNA	certified nursing assistant	NIDDM	non-insulin–dependent diabetes mellitus
c/o	complains of		
COPD	chronic obstructive pulmonary disease	nil	none
		no	number
CPR	cardiopulmonary resuscitation	noc, noct	night
CVA	cerebral vascular accident (stroke)	NPO (npo)	nothing per mouth (nils per os)
dc (d/c)	discontinue	N&V	nausea and vomiting
disch	discharge	O_2	oxygen
DJD	degenerative joint disease	OB	obstetrics
DNR	do not resuscitate	OJ	orange juice
DOA	dead on arrival	OOB	out of bed
DOB	date of birth	O	oral
DON	director of nursing	OR	operating room
drsg	dressing	OT	occupational therapy
Dx	diagnosis	oz (Oz)	ounce
ECG (EKG)	electrocardiogram	PAR	post anesthesia recovery
EEG	electroencephalogram	pc	after a meal
ER	emergency room	Peds	pediatrics
F	Fahrenheit	per	by, through
FBS	fasting blood sugar	PM (pm)	afternoon or evening
FF	force fluids	po (per os)	by mouth
fl (fld)	fluid	post op	postoperative

TABLE C-4 ■ **Common Medical Abbreviations (*continued*)**

Abbreviation	Meaning	Abbreviation	Meaning
pre op	preoperative	SOB	shortness of breath
prep	preparation	Spec (spec)	specimen
prn	as necessary	SSE	soapsuds enema
Pt (pt)	patient	ST	speech therapy
PT	physical therapy	STAT, stat	at once, immediately
q	every	STD	sexually transmitted disease
qd	every day	Surg	surgery
qh	every hour	Sx	symptoms
q2h, q3h, q4h, etc.	every 2 hours, every 3 hours, every 4 hours, etc.	tbsp	tablespoon
		tid	three times a day
qhs	every night at bedtime	TIA	transient ischemic attack
qid	four times a day	TLC	tender loving care
qod	every other day	TPN	total parenteral nutrition
qs	sufficient quantity	TPR	temperature, pulse, and respirations
qt	quiet		
R	rectal	tsp	teaspoon
RBC	red blood cell, red blood cell count	Tx	treatment
rehab	rehabilitation	ty	tympanic
resp	respiration	UA (u/a)	urinalysis
RLQ	right lower quadrant	UK	unknown
RN	registered nurse	URI	upper respiratory infection
ROM	range of motion	UTI	urinary tract infection
RR	recovery room	VS (vs)	vital signs
rt (R)	right	WA	while awake
RT	respiratory therapy	WBC	white blood cell, white blood cell count
RUQ	right upper quadrant		
Rx	treatment	w/c	wheelchair
$\bar{s}$	without	WNL	within normal limits
$\bar{ss}$	half	wt	weight

Glossary

Use the CD in the back of your book to hear these terms pronounced, defined, and used in a sentence. (The number following the entry refers to the chapter in which the entry is found.)

A

Abandonment: the act of withdrawing support or help from another person, in spite of duty or responsibility (42)

Absorption: transfer of nutrients from the digestive tract into the bloodstream (19)

Abuse: intentional act that causes harm to another person (4)

Acceptance: one of the stages of grief; the person comes to terms with the reality of his or her own impending death, and is finally at peace with this knowledge (21)

Acquired immunodeficiency syndrome (AIDS): a disease caused by human immunodeficiency virus (HIV), a bloodborne virus that attacks the body's immune system; death usually results when the body becomes unable to recognize and fight off infections (8)

Activities of daily living (ADLs): routine tasks of daily life, such as bathing, eating, and grooming (17)

Acute illness: an illness with a rapid onset and a relatively short recovery time, usually unexpected (6)

Acute pain: sharp, sudden pain (29)

ADLs: see *activities of daily living*

Admission: official entry of a person into a health care setting (14)

Admission sheet: form that is completed when a person is admitted to a health care setting; gathers standard information about the person such as the person's name, address, date of birth, age, Social Security number, gender, and insurance and employment information, emergency notification information, and advance directive information (14)

Advance directive: a document that allows a person to make his wishes regarding health care known to family members and health care workers, in case the time comes when he is no longer able to make those wishes known himself; examples include living wills and durable powers of attorney for health care (21)

Aerobic: an adjective used to describe bacteria that need oxygen in order to live (compare with *anaerobic*) (7)

Afterlife: a state of being where the dead meet again with loved ones who have passed on before them (22)

Afternoon care: care that is provided before and after lunch and dinner (17)

Against medical advice (AMA): term used to describe a person's actions when a person leaves a health care facility without a doctor's order (14)

AIDS: see *acquired immunodeficiency syndrome*

Airborne pathogen: pathogens that can be transmitted through the air (8)

Airborne precautions: used when caring for people infected with pathogens that can be transmitted through the air; include placing the patient or resident in a private room with the door closed, wearing a mask when caring for the person, and minimizing the amount of time the person spends out of his or her private room (7)

Alopecia: baldness, loss of hair (18)

Alignment: good posture; the "A" in the ABCs of good body mechanics (9)

Alveoli: grape-like clusters of tiny air sacs in the lungs, where gas exchange takes place (26)

Alzheimer's disease: the most common type of dementia; characterized by the permanent and progressive loss of the ability to think and remember caused by damage to the brain (36)

Amenorrhea: absence of menstrual flow (33)

Amino acids: molecules that are the building blocks of the body's cells; found in proteins (19)

Amputation: the surgical removal of all or part of an extremity (25)

Anaerobic: an adjective used to describe bacteria that can survive without oxygen (compare with *aerobic*) (7)

Anaphylactic shock: shock caused by a serious allergic reaction to a medication, bee sting, or certain foods (12)

Anatomy: the study of what body parts look like, where they are located, how big they are, and how they connect to other body parts (23)

Anemia: a general term for a group of disorders that affect the ability of the red blood cells to carry oxygen to the cells and tissues of the body (27)

Anger: one of the stages of grief; the person realizes that she is actually going to die as a result of her illness and has feelings of rage, which may be directed toward herself or others (21)

Angina pectoris: the classic chest pain that is felt as a result of the heart muscle being deprived of oxygen (27)

Anorexia: loss of appetite (19)

Anorexia nervosa: an eating disorder characterized by an intense fear of gaining weight or becoming obese; people with this disorder cannot maintain a healthy body weight because they engage in activities such as extreme dieting, excessive exercising, or both (35)

Antepartum (prenatal) period: the period of time from conception until the baby is born (40)

Antibodies: specialized proteins produced by the immune system that help our bodies to fight off specific microbes, preventing infection (7)

Antiperspirant: a grooming product that contains ingredients to stop or slow the production of sweat (17)

Antisepsis: practices that kill microbes or stop them from growing; one of the techniques of medical asepsis (compare with *sanitization*, *disinfection*, and *sterilization*) (7)

Anuria: the state of voiding less than 100 mL of urine over the course of 24 hours (20)

Anxiety: feeling of uneasiness, dread, apprehension, or worry (35)

Aphasia: a general term for a group of disorders that affect a person's ability to communicate with others; may be expressive (an inability to form words) or receptive (an inability to understand words); often occurs following a stroke (28)

Aponeurosis: a broad, flat sheet of tendon that attaches skeletal muscles to other muscles (25)

Appetite: the desire for food (compare with *anorexia*) (19)

Arteries: vessels that carry blood away from the heart (27)

Arterioles: the smallest arteries (27)

Arteriosclerosis: "hardening of the arteries"; occurs when atherosclerotic plaques interfere with the elasticity of the arterial walls, making them brittle and prone to breaking (27)

Arthritis: inflammation of joints, usually associated with pain and stiffness (25)

Aspiration: the accidental inhalation of foreign material (such as food, liquids, vomitus) into the airway (12)

Assault: threatening or attempting to touch a person without the person's consent (4)

Assisted-living facility: type of long-term care facility that provides residents with limited assistance with tasks such as medication administration, transportation, meals, and housekeeping (1)

Assistive devices: devices that make certain tasks (such as walking, eating, or dressing) easier for a person with a disability (23)

Asthma: a condition that affects the bronchi and bronchioles of the lungs; triggers (such as cold weather, allergies, respiratory infections, stress, smoke, and exercise) cause the bronchi and bronchioles to become narrower, making breathing difficult (26)

Astigmatism: an inability to focus images properly because the cornea of the eye is not perfectly curved (29)

Atelectasis: collapse of the alveoli of the lungs; a common respiratory complication following surgery (39)

Atherosclerosis: blocking of the arteries, caused by the build-up of fatty deposits called plaques on the inside of the vessel wall (27)

Atria (singular, *atrium*): the upper chambers of the heart (27)

Atrophy: the loss of muscle size and strength (25)

Attitude: the side of ourselves that we display to the world, communicating outwardly how we feel about things (3)

Autism: a developmental disability characterized by extreme difficulty communicating and relating to other people and surroundings (34)

Autonomy: an ethical principle that requires health care workers to respect a person's rights and personal preferences (4)

Autopsy: examination of a person's organs and tissues after the person has died, done to confirm or identify the cause of the person's death (22)

Axon: a long extension from the body of a neuron that *sends* information to other neurons (compare with *dendrites*) (28)

B

Bag technique: an infection control procedure used in the home health care setting to keep the nurse's bag free from contamination (43)

Balance: necessary for good body mechanics; involves holding the body's center of gravity, or area of largest mass, close to its base of support (9)

Bargaining: one of the stages of grief; the person wants to "make a deal" with someone he or she feels has control over his or her fate, such as God or a health care provider (21)

Barium: a substance that coats the mucosa of the digestive tract, making the organs appear sharper and brighter on radiologic studies (x-rays) (31)

Basic life support (BLS): basic emergency care techniques, such as rescue breathing and cardiopulmonary resuscitation (CPR) (12)

Bath blanket: a lightweight cotton blanket used to cover a person during a bed bath or linen change to help provide modesty and warmth (15)

Battery: touching a person without his or her consent (4)

Bed board: a piece of wood that is placed under the mattress to provide extra support; helps to keep the person's body properly aligned by preventing the mattress from sagging (15)

Bed cradle: a metal frame that is placed between the bottom and top sheets to keep the top sheet, the blanket, and the bedspread away from the person's feet; used when pressure on the person's feet could result in pain or skin breakdown (15)

Bedpan: a device used for elimination when a person is unable to get out of bed; women use a bedpan for both urination and bowel movements; men use a bedpan for bowel movements only (20)

Bed protector: a square of quilted absorbent fabric backed with waterproof material that measures approximately 3 feet by 3 feet; used to prevent soiling of the bottom linens; sometimes called an *incontinence pad* (15)

Bedside commode: a device used for elimination when a person is able to get out of bed, but unable to walk to the bathroom; it consists of a chair-like frame with a toilet seat and a removable collection bucket (20)

Bell: the small, rounded surface on a stethoscope that is used to pick up faint sounds; commonly used to listen to the apical pulse in infants and small children (16)

Beneficence: an ethical principle that requires health care workers to do good for those in their care by preventing harm and promoting the health and welfare of the person above all else (4)

Benign: adjective used to describe a noncancerous tumor (that is, a tumor that does not progress or invade other tissues) (compare with *malignant*) (37)

Bile: a substance produced by the liver that helps with the digestion of fats (31)

Biological death: occurs when the tissues of the brain and heart die from lack of oxygen; biological death is not reversible (compare with *clinical death*) (12)

Biopsy: a diagnostic procedure that involves obtaining a tissue sample and examining it under a microscope for cancerous cells (37)

Bipolar disorder (manic depression): a mental health disorder characterized by mood swings; people with this disorder experience excessively "high" or happy periods, followed by excessively "low" or depressed periods (35)

Bisexual: a person who is sexually attracted to members of both sexes (6)

Bloodborne pathogen: a disease-producing microbe that is transmitted to another person through blood or other body fluids (8)

Blood pressure: the force that the blood exerts against the arterial walls; one of the vital signs (16)

BLS: see *basic life support*

Body alignment: positioning of the body so that the spine is not twisted or crooked (11)

Body fluids: liquid or semi-liquid substances produced by the body, such as blood, urine, feces, vomitus, saliva, drainage from wounds, sweat, semen, vaginal secretions, tears, cerebrospinal fluid, amniotic fluid, and breast milk (8)

Body mechanics: the efficient and safe use of the body (9)

Bony prominences: parts of the body where there is very little fat between the bone and the skin, such as the ankles, heels, hips, and elbows (24)

Body temperature: how hot the body is; one of the vital signs (16)

Bonding period: the first hour or two immediately following delivery of a baby, during which emotional and physical attachments between the parents and the infant develop (40)

Bradycardia: a heart rate that is slower than normal (less than 60 beats/min in an adult) (16)

Bradypnea: a respiratory rate that is lower than normal (less than 10 breaths/min in an adult) (16)

Braille: a system that uses letters made from combinations of raised dots that allows a blind person to read (29)

Bronchi (singular, *bronchus*): passageways that carry air from the trachea ("windpipe") to the lungs, one bronchus goes to the right lung and the other goes to the left (26)

Bronchioles: the smallest branches of the bronchi (26)

Bronchitis: inflammation of the bronchi (26)

Bulimia nervosa: an eating disorder characterized by an intense fear of gaining weight or becoming obese; people with this disorder cannot maintain a healthy body weight because they engage in activities such as binging (eating large amounts of food in one sitting) and purging (vomiting the food back up) (35)

C

Call light system: a system that allows a patient or resident to call for help; usually consists of a call light control, a light in the hall, and a panel of lights at the nurses' station or some other central location (13)

Calories: the unit of measure used to describe the energy content of food (19)

Capillary bed: the network of tiny vessels in the tissues where the oxygen and nutrients in the blood pass into the tissues, and carbon dioxide and other waste materials from the tissues pass into the blood (27)

Cardiac arrest: the condition that is said to occur when the heart stops beating (12)

Cardiac cycle: the pumping action of the heart in an organized pattern (all of the events associated with one heart beat) (27)

Cardiac rehabilitation: therapy that helps a person regain strength and adopt habits that will help the cardiovascular system become healthier (27)

Cardiogenic shock: shock that occurs when the heart is unable to pump enough blood throughout the body to meet the tissues' need for oxygen (12)

Cardiopulmonary resuscitation (CPR): a technique used to sustain breathing and circulation for a person who has gone into respiratory or cardiac arrest (12)

Carrier: a person who is infected with a virus but never develops symptoms of the disease; the virus lives in the person's body and can be transmitted to another person (8)

Cartilage: a tough, fibrous substance found in joints and other parts of the body; in slightly movable joints, the cartilage acts as a "shock absorber"; in freely movable joints, the cartilage provides a smooth surface for the bones of the joint to move against (25)

Case manager: in the home health care setting, the member of the health care team who is responsible for overseeing the client's total care, from admission through discharge (42)

Cataract: the gradual yellowing and hardening of the lens of the eye (29)

Catastrophic reaction: an extreme reaction to a situation that would normally cause minimal or no stress; often seen in people with dementia (36)

Catheter: a tube that is inserted into the body for the purpose of administering or removing fluids (20)

Catheter care: thorough cleaning of the perineal area (especially around the urethra) and the catheter tubing that extends outside of the body, to prevent infection (20)

CDC: see *Centers for Disease Control and Prevention*

Cell: the basic unit of life (23)

Cell membrane: a membrane that surrounds the cytoplasm and gives the cell its shape (23)

Centers for Disease Control and Prevention (CDC): a federal agency based in Atlanta, Georgia, that is dedicated to protecting the health and safety of people in the United States (8)

Central nervous system (CNS): the brain and spinal cord; responsible for receiving information, processing it, and issuing instructions (compare with *peripheral nervous system*) (28)

Cerebral palsy: a developmental disability caused by damage to the cerebrum, the part of the brain involved with motor control (34)

Cerebrospinal fluid (CSF): a clear fluid that circulates around the brain and spinal cord and acts as a "shock absorber" to protect these structures (28)

Cerumen: a waxy substance that helps to protect the external auditory canal by trapping dirt and other particles; commonly referred to as "earwax" (29)

Cesarean section: delivery of a baby through a surgical incision made in the mother's abdomen (40)

Chain of infection: the six key conditions that must be met for a person to get a communicable infection (pathogen, reservoir, portal of exit, method of transmission, portal of entry, and susceptible host) (7)

Chain of survival: the series of events that must take place in an emergency situation to increase the person's ability to survive the emergency without any permanent damage (12)

Charge nurse: a registered nurse (RN) or licensed practical nurse/licensed vocational nurse (LPN/LVN) who supervises the other nurses for a particular shift (2)

Chemical digestion: the process of breaking down food through the use of chemical substances such as enzymes (compare with *mechanical digestion*) (31)

Chemical restraint: any medication that alters a person's mood or behavior, such as a sedative or tranquilizer (compare with *physical restraint*) (10)

Chemotherapy: the use of medications to destroy malignant cancer cells (37)

Cheyne-Stokes respiration: very irregular, shallow breaths, in an alternating fast–slow pattern; often seen in people who are dying (22)

Chronic illness: an illness that is ongoing and often needs to be controlled through continuous medication or treatment (6)

Chronic bronchitis: a disorder caused by long-term irritation of the bronchi and bronchioles, such as that caused by inhaling tobacco smoke; one of two forms of chronic obstructive pulmonary disease (COPD) (26)

Chronic obstructive pulmonary disease (COPD): a general term used to describe two related lung disorders, emphysema and chronic bronchitis; the leading cause of COPD is smoking (26)

Chronic pain: slow, diffuse, constant pain (29)

Chyme: the liquid substance produced by the digestion of food in the stomach (20)

Circulation: the continuous movement of the blood through the blood vessels; powered by the pumping action of the heart (27)

Circumcision: a procedure involving the removal of the foreskin, the fold of loose skin that covers the head of the penis; often performed on male infants for religious or cultural reasons (17)

Civil laws: laws concerned with relationships between individuals (4)

Client: a person who is receiving the services of a home health care agency (1)

Clinical death: the state of not having a pulse or breathing; can sometimes be reversed with prompt emergency treatment that restarts the heart and breathing (compare with *biological death*) (12)

Closed bed: an empty, made bed (15)

CNS: see *central nervous system*

Coagulation: clotting of the blood (27)

Coitus: sexual intercourse (6)

Collagen: a protein that supports connective tissue, such as that found in the dermis; loss of collagen contributes to the formation of wrinkles (24)

Colonies: groups of bacteria (7)

Colostomy: an alternate way of eliminating feces from the body; done when only part of the large intestine must be removed due to disease; after removing the diseased part of a person's large intestine, an artificial opening, called a stoma, is made in the abdominal wall and the remaining portion of the large intestine is connected to it (compare with *ileostomy*) (31)

Colostrum: a thin yellowish fluid that contains extra calories and proteins as well as antibodies and is produced by the mother's breasts immediately following delivery of the baby; after 2 to 3 days, colostrum is replaced by breast milk (40)

Comatose: the state of being in a coma, a state of unconsciousness from which a person cannot be aroused (10)

Communicable disease: a disease that can be given from one person to another (7)

Communication: the exchange of information (5)

Competency evaluation: an exam consisting of a written portion and a skills portion that must be passed at the end of the nursing assistant training course to obtain certification (2)

Conception (fertilization): occurs when the male and female sex cells join, forming a cell that contains the complete number of chromosomes (33)

Condom catheter: a device used to manage urinary incontinence in men; it consists of a soft plastic or rubber sheath, tubing, and a collection bag for the urine (20)

Conduction disorders: conditions that affect the pathway that the heart uses to transmit the electrical impulses that cause contraction (27)

Conductive hearing loss: hearing loss that results when something prevents sound waves from reaching the receptors in the cochlea of the ear; compare with *sensorineural hearing loss* (29)

Confidentiality: keeping personal information that someone shares with you to yourself (4)

Conflict: discord resulting from differences between people; can occur when one person is unable to understand or accept another's ideas or beliefs (5)

Congenital: adjective used to describe a disorder that a person is born with (34)

Conjunctivitis ("pink eye"): infection and inflammation of the conjunctiva, a clear membrane that lines the inside of the eyelids and covers most of the surface of the eye; characterized by redness, swelling, itching, burning and excessive tearing (29)

Constipation: a condition that occurs when the feces remain in the intestines for too long, resulting in hard, dry feces that are difficult to pass (20)

Contact precautions: used when caring for people infected with pathogens that can be transmitted directly (by touching the person), or indirectly (by touching fomites); include using barrier methods whenever contact with the infected person or items contaminated with wound drainage or body substances is necessary (7)

Contaminated: adjective used to describe an object that is soiled by pathogens (7)

Contractures: a condition that occurs when a joint is held in the same position for too long a time; the tendons shorten and become stiff, possibly causing permanent loss of motion in the joint (11)

Coordinated body movement: necessary for good body mechanics; involves using the weight of the body to help with movement (9)

COPD: see *chronic obstructive pulmonary disease*

Coping mechanisms: conscious and deliberate ways of dealing with stress (compare with *defense mechanisms*) (35)

Coronary artery disease: a disorder that occurs when the arteries that supply the heart (the coronary arteries) narrow as a result of atherosclerosis, preventing adequate blood flow to the heart muscle (27)

CPR: see *cardiopulmonary resuscitation*

Cradle cap: see *seborrheic dermatitis*

Criminal laws: laws concerned with the relationship between the individual and society (4)

CSF: see *cerebrospinal fluid*

Culture: the beliefs (including religious or spiritual beliefs), values, and traditions that are customary to a group of people; a view of the world that is handed down from generation to generation (6)

Cyanotic: adjective used to describe skin, lips, or nail beds that have a blue or gray tinge (22)

Cyanosis: blue or gray discoloration of the skin, lips, and nail beds; develops when the skin does not receive enough oxygen and is a sign of a respiratory or circulatory disorder (24)

Cystitis: infection of the bladder (32)

Cytoplasm: the jelly-like substance within a cell within which the organelles float (23)

D

Dandruff: excessive itching and flaking of the scalp (18)

Defamation: the act of making untrue statements that hurt another person's reputation (4)

Defecate: to have a bowel movement (20)

Defense mechanisms: unconscious ways of dealing with stress (compare with *coping mechanisms*) (35)

Definitive surgery: surgery that is done when the person's medical problem is known and the best way to address it is through surgery (39)

Dehydration: too little fluid in the tissues of the body (compare with *edema*) (19)

Delegate: to authorize another person to perform a task on your behalf (2)

Delirium: a temporary state of confusion (36)

Delusions: false ideas or beliefs, especially about oneself (35)

Dementia: the permanent and progressive loss of the ability to think and remember (36)

Dendrites: short extensions from the body of a neuron that *receive* information from other neurons (compare with *axon*) (28)

Denial: one of the stages of grief; the person refuses to accept the diagnosis or feels that a mistake has been made (21)

Deodorant: a grooming product that covers or masks odor (17)

Depression: *1)* an alteration in a person's mood that causes him or her to lose pleasure or interest in all usually pleasurable activities such as eating, working, or socializing; a feeling of hopelessness (35); *2)* one of the stages of grief; the person fully realizes that death will be the end result of the illness and experiences sadness and regret (21)

Dermatitis: a general term for inflammation of the skin (24)

Dermis: the deepest layer of skin, where sensory receptors, blood vessels, nerves, glands, and hair follicles are found (24)

Depth of respiration: the quality of each breath (16)

Development: changes that occur psychologically or socially as a person passes through life (6)

Developmental disability: a permanent disability that affects a person before he or she reaches adulthood (that is, before 19 to 22 years of age) and interferes with the person's ability to achieve developmental milestones (34)

Diabetes mellitus: an endocrine disorder that results when the pancreas is unable to produce enough insulin (30)

Diabetic retinopathy: a complication of diabetes that can lead to blindness (29)

Diagnosis-related groups (DRGs): a system for controlling health care costs in which the length of a person's hospital stay, as well as payment for hospitalization, surgery, or other treatment, is specified according to the person's diagnosis (1)

Dialysis: a procedure that is done to remove waste products and fluids from the body when a person's kidneys fail and can no longer perform this task (32)

Diaphoretic: adjective used to describe a person who has a medical condition that causes him to sweat a great deal (17)

Diaphragm: *1)* the large flat surface of the stethoscope that is used to hear loud, harsh sounds (16); *2)* the strong, dome-shaped muscle that separates the chest cavity from the abdominal cavity and assists in breathing (26)

Diarrhea: the passage of liquid, unformed stool (20)

Diastole: the resting phase of the cardiac cycle; during which the myocardium relaxes, allowing the chambers to fill with blood (compare with *systole*) (27)

Diastolic pressure: the pressure that the blood exerts against the arterial walls when the heart muscle relaxes; the second blood pressure measurement that is recorded (compare with *systolic pressure*) (16)

Dietitian: a person who has a degree in nutrition (19)

Digestion: the process of breaking food down into simple elements (nutrients) (19)

Digital examination: examination that is done when a person is thought to have a fecal impaction; a finger is inserted into the person's rectum to feel for the impacted mass (20)

Director of Nursing (DON): the registered nurse who directs all of the nursing care within a facility (2)

Disability: impaired physical or emotional function (23)

Disaster: a sudden, unexpected event that causes injury to many people, major damage to property, or both (9)

Discharge: the official release of a patient or a resident from a health care facility to his or her home (14)

Discharge planning: the process used by the members of the health care team to help prepare a patient or resident to leave the facility; helps to make sure that the person continues to receive quality care, either from a home health care agency or from family members, after the discharge (14)

Disease: a condition that occurs when the structure or function of an organ or an organ system is abnormal (23)

Disinfection: the use of strong chemicals to kill pathogens on non-living objects that come in contact with body fluids or substances, such as bedpans, urinals, and over-bed tables; one of the techniques of medical asepsis (compare with *antisepsis, sanitization,* and *sterilization*) (7)

Disoriented: the state of being unable to answer basic questions about person, place, or time; a state of confusion (compare with *oriented to person, place, and time*) (12)

Diuresis: excessive urine output of urine; also called *polyuria* (20)

DNR: see *do not resuscitate order*

Do not resuscitate (DNR) order: an order written on a person's chart specifying the person's wishes that the usual efforts to save his life will not be made; also called a *no-code order* (21)

Down syndrome: a developmental disability that is the result of having 47 chromosomes instead of 46; people with this disorder have mental retardation and certain key physical features, such as almond-shaped eyes and square hands with short, stubby fingers (34)

Draw sheet: a small, flat sheet that is placed over the middle of the bottom sheet, covering the area of the bed from above the person's shoulders to below his or her buttocks; see also *lift sheet* (15)

DRGs: see *diagnosis-related groups*

Droplet precautions: used when caring for people infected with pathogens that can be transmitted by direct exposure to droplets released from the mouth or nose (for example, when the person coughs, sneezes, or talks) (7)

Durable power of attorney for health care: a type of advance directive that transfers the responsibility for handling a person's affairs and making medical decisions to a family member, friend, or other trusted individual, in the event that the person is no longer able to make these decisions on his or her own behalf (21)

Dysmenorrhea: painful menstruation (33)

Dyspnea: labored or difficult breathing (16)

Dysrhythmia: an irregular pulse rhythm (16)

Dysuria: painful or difficult urination (20)

E

Early morning care: care provided after a person wakes up to prepare him or her for breakfast or early testing or treatment (17)

Eczema: a type of chronic dermatitis that is usually accompanied by severe itching, scaling, and crusting of the surface of the skin (24)

Edema: too much fluid in the tissues of the body (compare with *dehydration*) (19)

Edentulous: without teeth (17)

EEOC: see *Equal Employment Opportunity Commission*

Egg (ovum, ova): female sex cell (33)

Egocentric: an adjective used to describe someone who places himself at the center of the world and often overestimates his importance to others; a common character trait during adolescence (41)

Ejaculation: the forceful release of semen from the body; method by which sperm cells leave the man's body through the penis (33)

Elder abuse: physical, emotional, or sexual abuse of an older person (4)

Elective: adjective used to describe a surgical procedure that is planned for and scheduled ahead of time (39)

Embolus: a blood clot in a vessel that breaks off and moves from one place to another (27)

Emergency: a condition that requires immediate medical or surgical evaluation or treatment to prevent the person from dying or having a permanent disability (12)

Emergency medical services (EMS) system: a network of resources (including people, equipment, and facilities) that is organized to respond to an emergency (12)

Emergent: adjective used to describe surgery that must be performed immediately to prevent the person from dying or becoming disabled (39)

Emphysema: a disorder caused by long-term exposure of the alveoli to toxins, such as tobacco smoke; one of two forms of chronic obstructive pulmonary disease (COPD) (26)

EMS system: see *emergency medical services system*

Endocardium: the smooth inner lining of the heart wall (27)

Endotracheal tube: a device that is inserted into a person's nose or mouth and extends to the trachea; used when a person must receive mechanical ventilation for a short time (26)

Enema: the introduction of fluid into the large intestine by way of the anus for the purpose of removing stool from the rectum (20)

Enteral nutrition: placing food directly into a person's stomach or intestines, using a nasogastric tube, nasointestinal tube, gastrostomy tube, jejunostomy tube, or percutaneous endoscopic gastrostomy (PEG) tube (19)

Enzymes: substances that have the ability to break chemical bonds (31)

Epicardium: the smooth outermost layer of the heart wall (27)

Epidermis: the outer layer of the skin (24)

Epidural block: anesthesia given through a catheter that is placed in the spinal canal (40)

Epilepsy: a disorder characterized by chronic seizure activity (28)

Episiotomy: an incision made in the perineum to enlarge the vaginal opening, making delivery of the baby's head easier (40)

Equal Employment Opportunity Commission (EEOC): a government agency that says it is illegal during the hiring process for an employer to ask a candidate questions related to age, marital status, weight, religion, sexual preference, and plans to have children at any time (3)

Erythema: redness of the skin (24)

Erythrocytes: red blood cells; responsible for carrying oxygen to all of the tissues of the body (27)

Esophageal (cardiac) sphincter: a circle of muscular tissue that surrounds the place where the esophagus enters the stomach and keeps food from going back up the esophagus after it has entered the stomach (31)

Esophagus: a long narrow tube that serves mainly as a passageway for food to get from the pharynx to the stomach (31)

Ethics: moral principles or standards that govern conduct (4)

Eupnea: a normal respiratory rate (16)

Evening (hour of sleep, hs) care: care provided in preparation for sleep (17)

Excoriation: an abrasion, or a scraping away of the surface of the skin; can be caused by trauma, chemicals, or burns (24)

Exhalation (expiration): the phase of ventilation during which carbon dioxide is transported out of the lungs [compare with *inhalation (inspiration)*] (16)

Exploratory surgery: surgery that is performed when a person has a significant medical problem but the doctors do not know exactly how bad the problem is or exactly what is causing it (39)

Exposure control plan: a plan that states what actions must be taken if an employee is exposed to blood or other body fluids while on the job (8)

F

Facemask: a device used for delivering oxygen that is made of soft, molded plastic material that fits over the nose and mouth (26)

Failure to thrive: failure of an infant to grow and develop both physically and emotionally, as a result of not being held and talked to (41)

False imprisonment: confining another person against his or her will (4)

Fanfolded: adjective used to describe the top sheet, blanket, and bedspread of a closed bed when they have been turned back (toward the foot of the bed) (15)

Fat-soluble: adjective used to describe a substance that dissolves in fat (for example, certain vitamins) (19)

Febrile: adjective used to describe the state of having a fever, or increased body temperature (16)

Fecal impaction: a condition that occurs when constipation is not relieved (20)

Fecal (bowel) incontinence: the inability to hold one's feces, or the involuntary loss of feces from the bowel (20)

Feces: the semi-solid waste product of digestion; stool (20)

Fetal alcohol syndrome: a combination of physical and mental problems that affect children whose mothers consumed alcohol during pregnancy (34)

Fiber supplement: a tablet or drink additive that is used to add bulk to the feces, causing them to hold fluid, and preventing constipation (20)

Fidelity: an ethical principle that requires health care workers to act with integrity to earn others' trust (4)

Filtrate: the liquid that forms the basis for urine (32)

First aid: the care given to an injured or sick person while waiting for more advanced help to arrive (12)

Fissure: a crack in the skin (24)

Five rights of delegation: a set of guidelines that help nurses to make good decisions about which tasks to delegate and to whom (2)

Fixation: the process of holding a broken bone in one position until the fracture heals; may be *external* (accomplished through the use of a cast) or *internal* (accomplished through the use of metal plates, screws, rods, pins, or wires attached to the bone) (25)

Flatulence: the presence of excessive amounts of flatus (gas) in the intestines, causing abdominal distension (swelling) and discomfort (20)

Flatus: gas that is formed as part of the digestion process (20)

Flow meter: a device used to set the rate at which oxygen is delivered to a patient or resident who is receiving oxygen therapy (26)

Fluid balance: a state where the amount of fluid taken into the body equals the amount of fluid that leaves the body (19)

Flushing: redness of the skin (24)

Fomite: a non-living object that has been contaminated (soiled) by pathogens (7)

Food Guide Pyramid: a guide for making daily food choices that applies for all healthy people older than 2 years; published by the United States Department of Agriculture (19)

Footboard: a padded board that is placed upright at the foot of the bed; used to keep the person's feet in proper alignment (15)

Foreskin: the fold of loose skin that covers the head of the penis (17)

Fowler's position: one of the basic positions in which the head of the bed is elevated to between 45 and 60 degrees; variations include *semi-Fowler's (low Fowler's) position* and *high Fowler's position* (11)

Fracture: a broken bone (25)

Fracture pan: a wedge-shaped bedpan that is used when a person has an injury or disability that makes it too uncomfortable or dangerous to use a regular bedpan (20)

Fragile X syndrome: an inherited type of mental retardation caused by a defect in the X chromosome (34)

Fraud: deception that could cause harm to another person (4)

Frequency: the term used to describe voiding that occurs more often than usual (20)

Friction: a term used to describe the force created when two surfaces (such as a sheet and a person's skin) rub against each other; can lead to skin breakdown (11)

Functional (modular) nursing: a model for organizing the nursing team's efforts in which each member of the nursing team carries out the same assigned task for all patients or residents (compare with *primary nursing* and *team nursing*) (2)

G

Gallbladder: a small pouch-like organ that is attached to the liver; it stores bile produced by the liver that is not secreted directly into the duodenum (31)

Gas exchange: the transfer of oxygen into the blood, and carbon dioxide out of it (26)

Gastrostomy tube: a tube used for enteral nutrition that is inserted into the stomach through a surgical incision in the abdomen (19)

Gatches: the joints at the hips and knees of the mattresses of most adjustable beds that allow the mattress to "break" so that the person's head can be elevated or his knees bent (13)

General anesthesia: a loss of consciousness brought on by the administration of a combination of inhaled and injected drugs (compare with *local anesthesia* and *regional anesthesia*) (39)

General lighting: lighting that supplies overall illumination (light), allowing a person to see and move about safely (compare with *task lighting*) (13)

Gingivitis: inflammation of the gums (17)

Glaucoma: a disorder of the eye that occurs when the pressure within the eye is increased to dangerous levels (29)

Glomerulus: part of the nephron, the functional unit of the kidney where blood is filtered to form urine (32)

Glucose: the body's most basic type of fuel; supplied by carbohydrates and sometimes referred to as "blood sugar" (19)

Goals: descriptions of what nursing interventions (nursing actions that are taken to help a patient or resident) are meant to achieve (5)

Goiter: enlargement of the thyroid gland (30)

Graduate: a measuring device used to measure fluids (19)

Grand mal seizure: a seizure characterized by generalized and violent contraction and relaxation of the body's muscles [compare with *petit mal (absence) seizure*] (12)

Grief: mental anguish, specifically associated with loss (21)

Grooming: activities related to maintaining a neat and attractive appearance, such as shampooing and styling the hair, shaving, and applying make-up (18)

Grounded: an adjective used to describe electrical equipment that has a way of returning stray electrical current to the outlet so that the risk of electrical shock is reduced (9)

Group insurance: insurance that is purchased at group rates by an employer or corporation (1)

Growth: changes that occur physically as a person passes through life (6)

H

Halitosis: bad breath that does not go away (17)

Hallucinations: episodes when a person sees, feels, hears, or tastes something that does not really exist (35)

Hangnails: broken pieces of cuticle (18)

HAV: see *hepatitis A virus*

HBV: see *hepatitis B virus*

HCV: see *hepatitis C virus*

HDV: see *hepatitis D virus*

Head nurse: a registered nurse (RN) who is in charge of a department or section (2)

Health care team: group of people with different types of knowledge and skill levels who work together to provide holistic care to the patient or resident (1)

Health Insurance Portability and Accountability Act (HIPAA): a federal privacy regulation that helps to keep personal information about patients and residents private (4)

Health maintenance organization (HMO): a managed care system that contracts with health care providers to provide health care services for a prepaid fee, and people seeking care agree to see only health care providers who are part of the HMO network (1)

Heart failure: a condition that occurs when the heart is unable to pump enough blood to meet the body's needs (27)

Heimlich maneuver: abdominal thrusts; used to clear an obstructed airway in an adult or a child older than 1 year who is choking (12)

Hematuria: blood in the urine (20)

Hemiplegia: paralysis on one side of the body (compare with *paraplegia* and *quadriplegia*) (10)

Hemoglobin: a protein found in red blood cells that combines with oxygen to carry it to the tissues of the body (27)

Hemorrhage: severe bleeding (12)

Hemorrhagic shock: shock that results from massive blood loss (12)

Hemostasis: the process of stopping blood loss from the circulatory system (27)

Hemothorax: a condition that occurs when blood builds up in the space between the lungs and the chest wall (26)

Hepatitis: inflammation of the liver (8)

Hepatitis A virus (HAV): a virus that is transmitted through the oral-fecal route and causes a form of acute hepatitis (8)

Hepatitis B virus (HBV): a bloodborne virus that causes a form of hepatitis that is acute in most people but may become chronic; a serious health threat for the health care worker (8)

Hepatitis C virus (HCV): a bloodborne virus that causes a form of chronic hepatitis that can eventually lead to end-stage cirrhosis (a fatal liver disease), liver failure, or liver cancer (8)

Hepatitis D virus (HDV): a bloodborne virus that is found only in people who are already infected with hepatitis B virus (HBV)

Hepatitis E virus (HEV): a virus that is transmitted through the oral–fecal route and causes a form of hepatitis (8)

Hernia: a disorder that occurs when an internal organ bulges through a weakness in the muscular wall of the abdominal cavity

Heterosexual: a person who is sexually attracted to members of the opposite sex (6)

HEV: see *hepatitis E virus* (8)

High Fowler's position: one of the basic positions in which the head of the bed is elevated to between 60 and 90 degrees

HIPAA: see *Health Insurance Portability and Accountability Act*

HIV: see *human immunodeficiency virus*

HIV-positive: the state of being infected with human immunodeficiency virus (HIV) (38)

HMO: see *health maintenance organization*

Holistic: an adjective used to describe care of the whole person, physically and emotionally (1)

Homebound: adjective used to describe a person who cannot leave the house without a lot of help from another person (42)

Home health aide: a nursing assistant who provides skilled care in the home (42)

Home health care agency: an agency that provides skilled care in a person's home (1)

Homeostasis: a state of balance (23)

Homosexual: a person who is attracted to members of the same sex (6)

Hope: a desire for a positive occurrence or outcome (21)

Hormones: chemicals that act on cells to produce a response (30)

Hospice organization: a health care organization that provides care for people who are dying, and their families (1)

Hospital: a health care facility that provides treatment for people with acute medical or surgical conditions (1)

Human immunodeficiency virus (HIV): a virus transmitted in blood and other body fluids (such as semen) that targets the T cells of the immune system; most people infected with HIV go on to develop acquired immunodeficiency syndrome (AIDS), a fatal illness (8)

Human resources (HR) department (personnel): the department within an organization that is concerned with matters related to employees; often responsible for hiring new employees (3)

Hydrocephalus: a condition that results from the build-up of cerebrospinal fluid (CSF); sometimes called "water on the brain" (34)

Hygiene: personal cleanliness (3)

Hyperalimentation: see *total parenteral nutrition*

Hyperglycemia: a state of having too much glucose in the bloodstream (30)

Hyperopia: farsightedness; trouble seeing objects that are close (compare with *myopia*) (29)

Hypertension: high blood pressure; a blood pressure that is consistently greater than 140 mm Hg (systolic) and/or 90 mm Hg (diastolic) (16)

Hyperthyroidism: a condition caused by the excessive secretion of thyroxine, one of the thyroid hormones; characterized by increased hunger accompanied by weight loss, an irregular heart beat, an inability to sleep, irritability, confusion, increased perspiration, and intolerance to heat (30)

Hyperventilation: increased rate and depth of breathing (16)

Hypoglycemia: a dangerous drop in blood glucose levels (30)

Hypotension: low blood pressure; a blood pressure that is consistently lower than 90 mm Hg (systolic) and/or 60 mm Hg (diastolic) (16)

Hypothyroidism: a condition caused by the low secretion of thyroxine, one of the thyroid hormones; characterized by fatigue, weakness, depression, anorexia, weight gain, constipation, and intolerance to cold (30)

Hypoventilation: decreased rate and depth of breathing (16)

Hypoxic: the state of being deficient of oxygen (26)

Hysterectomy: surgical removal of the uterus (33)

I

IDDM: see *type I diabetes mellitus*

Ileostomy: an alternative way of eliminating feces from the body; done when the entire large intestine must be removed due to disease; after removing the person's diseased large intestine, an artificial opening, called a stoma, is made in the abdominal wall and the end of the small intestine is connected to it (compare with *colostomy*) (31)

Impotence (erectile dysfunction): the inability to achieve or maintain an erection long enough to engage in sexual activity (33)

Incident (occurrence) report: a preprinted document that is completed following an accident involving a patient or resident (10)

Indwelling catheter: a urinary catheter that is left inside the bladder to provide continuous urine drainage; also known as a *retention catheter* or a *Foley catheter* (20)

Infection: disease caused by pathogenic microbes (7)

Infection control: basic practices designed to decrease the chance that an infection will spread from one person to another in a health care facility (7)

Infertility: the inability to become pregnant or to carry a pregnancy to full term (33)

Influenza: an acute respiratory infection caused by the influenza virus; characterized by a sore throat, dry cough, stuffy nose, headache, body aches, weakness, and fever; commonly known as "the flu" (26)

Informed consent: permission granted by a patient or resident to begin treatment or perform a procedure after receiving a full explanation of the treatment or procedure from the health care provider (4)

Ingestion: the intake of food or fluids (19)

Inhalation (inspiration): the phase of ventilation during which oxygen is taken into the lungs [compare with *exhalation (expiration)*] (16)

Intake and output (I&O) flow sheet: a document used for recording measurements of all of the fluids that enter and leave the body (19)

Intentional tort: a violation of civil law committed by a person with the intent to do harm (4)

Intentional wound: a wound that is the result of a planned surgical or medical intervention (compare with *unintentional wound*) (24)

Interventions: actions that are taken by the nursing team to help the patient or resident (5)

Interview: a meeting between an employer and a potential employee, during which information is exchanged regarding the organization, the job, and the potential employee's qualifications for the job (3)

Intimacy: a feeling of emotional closeness to another human being (6)

Intra-operative phase: one of three phases of care for a person who is having surgery; the phase during which the surgery is actually performed (compare with *pre-operative phase* and *post-operative phase*) (39)

Intravenous (IV) therapy: an alternative method of providing fluids and nutrition; fluids are given through a small catheter (tube) that is inserted into a vein (usually in the back of the hand) (19)

Invasion of privacy: the act of violating another person's right to keep certain information and aspects of himself away from the examination of others (4)

Ischemia: the state that occurs when the flow of oxygen-rich blood to the tissues is interrupted, leading to an oxygen deficiency in the tissues (27)

Isolation (transmission-based) precautions: guidelines, based on a pathogen's method of transmission, that health care workers follow to contain the pathogen and limit others' exposure to it as much as possible (7)

J

Jaundice: a yellow discoloration of the skin and the whites of the eyes; usually associated with liver disorders (24)

Jejunostomy tube: a tube used for enteral nutrition that is inserted into the jejunum (part of the small intestine) through a surgical incision in the abdomen (19)

Joint: the area where two bones join together (25)

Justice: an ethical principle that requires health care workers to be fair and treat people equally regardless of race, religion, culture, disability, or ability to pay (4)

K

Kardex: a card file that contains condensed versions of each patient's or resident's medical record (5)

Keratin: a substance that causes mature skin cells to thicken and become resistant to water (24)

Kidney stones (renal calculi): a painful disorder characterized by the formation of clumps of minerals ("stones") in the kidney and bladder (32)

Korotkoff sounds: sounds that are heard while taking a person's blood pressure (16)

L

Labor: the process of giving birth to a baby, during which the mother's uterus contracts to push the baby out (40)

Lactation: the process by which the glandular tissue of the female breast produces milk (33)

Larceny: the act of stealing another person's property (4)

Laryngitis: inflammation of the larynx (the "voice box") (26)

Larynx: part of the respiratory airway; also known as the "voice box" (26)

Lateral position: one of the basic positions in which the person lies on his or her side (11)

Laws: rules that are made by a controlling authority, such as the state or federal government, with the intent of preserving basic human rights (4)

Laxative: a medication that chemically stimulates the bowels to move; a treatment for constipation (20)

Lesion: a general term used to describe any break in the skin (24)

Leukemia: a general term for a group of disorders characterized by the excessive production of white blood cells that are abnormal in structure (27)

Leukocyte: white blood cell (27)

Liability: the responsibility of an individual to act within the confines of the law (4)

Libel: written statements that injure someone's reputation; a form of defamation (4)

Licensed practical nurse (LPN): a specially trained person who is licensed by a state to provide routine care for the sick under the supervision of a registered nurse (RN); completes a 1- to 2-year program in a vocational school, community college, or hospital (2)

Licensed vocational nurse (LVN): another term for *licensed practical nurse*; used in the states of Texas and California (2)

Life-sustaining treatment: treatments that will prolong life, such as mechanical ventilation, cardiopulmonary resuscitation (CPR), and the placement of a feeding tube or intravenous (IV) line for the provision of nutrition (21)

Lift sheet: a draw sheet that is used to help lift or reposition a person who needs assistance with moving in bed (15)

Ligaments: very strong bands of fibrous tissue that cross over the joint capsule, attaching one bone to another and stabilizing the joint (25)

Litigation: the lawsuit, or legal action, taken against a person who is accused of breaking a law (4)

Liver: an organ that performs several important functions in the body, including the secretion of bile (a substance needed for digestion of fats), the production of clotting factors (chemicals that help our blood to clot), and the clearance of toxins (such as alcohol and drugs) from the body (31)

Living will: a type of advance directive that states a person's wish that death not be artificially postponed (21)

Local anesthesia: a loss of sensation in only a very small part of the body brought on by the injection of drugs (compare with *general anesthesia* and *regional anesthesia*) (39)

Lochia: vaginal discharge following the birth of a baby (40)

Logrolling: a technique for turning a person in which the person's body is moved in one fluid motion to keep the spine in alignment (11)

Long-term care facility: a health care facility that provides care for people who are unable to care for themselves at home, yet do not need to be hospitalized; sometimes referred to as a "nursing home" (1)

LPN: see *licensed practical nurse*

Lungs: the primary organs for respiration, the process the body uses to obtain oxygen from the environment and remove carbon dioxide (a waste gas) from the body (26)

LVN: see *licensed vocational nurse*

Lymph: fluid in the lymph vessels (vessels that return the fluid that leaks into the tissues to the bloodstream) (27)

Lymph nodes: masses of lymphatic tissue that "clean" the lymph by removing bacteria and other large particles before returning the fluid to the bloodstream (27)

M

Macular degeneration: a vision disorder that results from the build-up of deposits in the macula (part of the retina) and eventually leads to blindness (29)

Macule: a small, flat, reddened skin lesion (24)

Magical thinking: a thought process that is common among preschoolers; the child believes that if he wishes for something hard enough, it will happen (41)

Malignant: adjective used to describe a cancerous tumor (that is, a tumor that has the ability to progress or invade other tissues) (compare with *benign*) (37)

Malpractice: negligence committed by people who hold licenses to practice their profession, such as doctors, nurses, lawyers, dentists, and pharmacists (4)

Managed care system: a system designed to control health care costs by delivering health care to people who need it by arranging contacts with various health care providers; examples include preferred provider organizations (PPOs) and health maintenance organizations (HMOs) (1)

Mastectomy: surgical removal of a breast (33)

Mastication: chewing (31)

Masturbation: stimulation of the genitals for sexual pleasure or release, by a means other than sexual intercourse (6)

Materials Safety Data Sheet (MSDS): a document that summarizes key information about a chemical, such as its composition, which exposures may be dangerous, what to do if an exposure should occur, and how to clean up spills (9)

Mechanical digestion: the process of breaking down food through the use of physical means, such as chewing (compare with *chemical* digestion) (31)

Mechanical ventilation: a life-sustaining treatment in which a machine breathes for a person who cannot breathe on his or her own (26)

Medicaid: a federally funded and state-regulated plan designed to help people with low incomes to pay for health care (1)

Medical asepsis: techniques that are used to physically remove or kill pathogens (see also *sanitization, antisepsis, disinfection,* and *sterilization*) (7)

Medical record: a legal document where information about a patient's or resident's current condition, the measures that have been taken by the medical and nursing staff to diagnose and treat the condition, and the patient's or resident's response to the treatment and care provided are recorded; also called a "medical chart" (5)

Medicare: a type of insurance plan that is federally funded by Social Security and which all people 65 years and older, and some younger disabled people, are eligible to participate in (1)

Melanin: a dark pigment that gives our skin, hair, and eyes color (24)

Menarche: the onset of the first menstrual period (6)

Meninges: the three layers of connective tissue that cover and protect the brain and spinal cord (28)

Menopause: the cessation of menstruation and fertility that women typically experience in their early 50s (6)

Menorrhagia: excessive bleeding during a menstrual period, either in terms of the amount of blood lost or the number of days that bleeding lasts (33)

Menstrual period: the monthly loss of blood through the vagina that occurs in the absence of pregnancy (33)

Mental illness: a disorder that affects a person's mind, causing the person to act in unusual ways, experience emotional difficulties, or both (35)

Mental retardation: the state of having below-average intellectual functioning (that is, a decreased ability to reason, think, and understand) and problems with adaptive skills (that is, skills needed to live and work, such as communication skills, social skills, and self-care skills) (34)

Metabolism: the word used to describe the physical and chemical changes that occur when the cells of the body change the food that we eat into energy (16)

Metastasis: the process by which cancer cells spread from their original location in the body to a new location, which may be quite distant from the first (37)

Methicillin-resistant *Staphylococcus aureus* (MRSA): a type of bacteria that has become resistant to methicillin, a powerful antibiotic (7)

Microbe (microorganism): a living thing that cannot be seen with the naked eye; examples include bacteria and viruses (7)

Micturition: the process of passing urine from the body; also known as *urination* and *voiding* (20)

Midstream ("clean catch") urine specimen: a method of collecting urine that prevents contamination of the urine by the bacteria that normally exist in and around the urethra (20)

Minimum Data Set (MDS): a report that focuses on the degree of assistance or skilled care that each resident of a long-term care facility needs (1)

Mission: the officially stated purpose of a health care facility or organization (1)

Mitered corner: a corner that is made by folding and tucking the sheet so that it lies flat and neat against the mattress (15)

Morning (A.M.) care: care provided in the morning, to ready the person for the day, such as completion of personal hygiene and grooming activities, and bedmaking (17)

Motor nerves: nerves that carry commands from the brain down the spinal cord and out to the muscles and organs of the body (28)

MRSA: see *methicillin-resistant* Staphylococcus aureus

MS: see *multiple sclerosis*

Mucous membrane: a special type of epithelial tissue that lines many of the organ systems in the body and is coated with mucus (26)

Mucus: a slippery, sticky substance that is secreted by special cells and serves to keep the surfaces of mucous membranes moist (26)

Multiple sclerosis (MS): a disorder of the nervous system in which the myelin sheaths that cover the nerves are damaged, resulting in faulty transmission of nerve impulses (28)

Munchausen syndrome by proxy: a form of physical abuse seen in children; the child's caregiver (usually the mother) deliberately does things to make the child appear ill (41)

Muscle tone: the steady contraction of the skeletal muscles that helps us to maintain an upright posture, such as sitting or standing (25)

Muscular dystrophy: a general term for a group of disorders that cause the skeletal muscles to become more and more weak over time (25)

Myelin: a fatty, white substance that protects the axon and helps to speed the conduction of nerve impulses along the axon (28)

Myocardial infarction: a "heart attack"; occurs when one or more of the coronary arteries become completely blocked, preventing blood from reaching the parts of the heart that are fed by the affected arteries (27)

Myocardium: the thick, muscular middle layer of the heart wall; responsible for the pumping action of the heart (27)

Myopia: nearsightedness; trouble seeing objects that are far away (compare with *hyperopia*) (29)

N

Nasal cannula: a device used to deliver oxygen to a patient or resident; consists of two prongs of soft plastic tubing that are inserted into the nostrils (26)

Nasal cavity: the inside of the nose (26)

Nasogastric tube: a tube used for enteral nutrition that is inserted through the nose, down the throat, and into the stomach (19)

Nasointestinal tube: a tube used for enteral nutrition that is inserted through the nose, down the throat, and into the small intestine (19)

Nasopharyngeal airway: a soft rubber tube that is inserted into a person's nose and extends back toward the throat to create an opening that air can flow through (26)

Necrosis: tissue death as a result of a lack of oxygen (24)

Need: something that is essential for a person's physical and mental health (6)

Negative-feedback system: a system that works to regulate the secretion of many hormones (30)

Negligent: adjective used to describe a person who fails to do what a "careful and reasonable" person would do in any given situation (4)

Neonate: a newborn infant, 28 days or younger (6)

Nephron: the basic functional unit of the kidney; consists of a glomerulus and a series of tubules (32)

Neuron: a cell that can send and receive information (28)

NIDDM: see *type II diabetes mellitus*

Nits: the eggs of head lice, seen on the hair, near the scalp, in people with pediculosis capitis (head lice infestation) (18)

No-code order: an order written on a person's chart specifying the person's wishes that the usual efforts to save his life will not be made; see also *do not resuscitate (DNR) order* (21)

Nocturia: the need to get up more than once or twice during the night to urinate, to the point where sleep is disrupted (20)

Nocturnal emission: the harmless involuntary discharge of semen during sleep; commonly called a "wet dream" (6)

Nonmaleficence: an ethical principle that requires health care workers to avoid harming those in their care (4)

Nonverbal communication: a way of communicating that uses facial expressions, gestures, and body language, instead of written or spoken language (5)

Normal (resident) flora: the harmless microbes that live in and on the body and help it to function properly (compare with *transient flora*) (7)

Nosocomial: an infection gotten while in a hospital or other health care setting (7)

NPO status: a doctor's order specifying that a patient or resident is to have "*nils per os*" (nothing by mouth) (19)

Nucleus: the cell's "brain"; it contains all of the information the cell needs in order to do its job, grow, and reproduce (23)

Nurse's bag: a bag used by the home health aide to transport necessary supplies and equipment to each client's home (42)

Nursing care plan: a specific plan of care for each patient or resident developed by the nursing team (5)

Nursing diagnosis: a statement that describes a problem the person is having that can be identified and treated by the nursing staff independently (5)

Nursing history: a report that is completed by the nurse when a patient or resident is admitted to a health care facility that gathers information about the person's preferences, abilities, disabilities, and habits (14)

Nursing process: a process that allows members of the nursing team to communicate with each other regarding the patient's or resident's specific needs (in regard to nursing care), what steps will be taken to meet those needs, and whether the steps were effective in meeting the person's needs; consists of five parts: assessment, diagnosis, planning, implementation, and evaluation (5)

Nutrients: substances in foods and fluids that the body uses to grow, to repair itself, and to carry out processes essential for living (19)

Nutrition: the process of taking in and using food (19)

Nutritional Labeling and Education Act: an act passed in 1990 that requires that the labels of all packaged foods include information about the food's nutritional value, approximate serving size, and any related health claims (19)

Nutritional supplement: a flavored shake or drink that is used to supply extra calories or protein; often served with meals or as a snack in between meals (19)

O

Objective data: information that is obtained directly, through measurements or by using one of the five senses (sight, smell, taste, hearing, touch) (5)

OBRA: see *Omnibus Budget Reconciliation Act*

Observation: something that you notice about the patient or resident, typically related to a change in the person's physical or mental condition (5)

Obsessive-compulsive disorder: an anxiety disorder that causes a person to suffer intensely from recurrent unwanted thoughts (obsessions) that are usually associated with rituals the person feels obligated to complete constantly (compulsions) (35)

Occult: adjective used to describe something that is hidden or cannot be seen with the naked eye; often used in reference to blood in a urine or stool sample (20)

Occupational Safety and Health Administration: an agency within the Department of Labor that establishes safety and health standards for the workplace, to protect the safety and health of employees (1)

Occupied bed: a bed with a person in it (15)

OCD: see *obsessive-compulsive disorder*

Oliguria: the state of voiding a very small amount of urine over a given period of time (20)

Omnibus Budget Reconciliation Act (OBRA): an act passed in 1987 to improve the quality of life for people who live in long-term care facilities by making sure that residents receive a certain standard of care (1)

Open bed: a bed ready to receive a patient or resident (15)

Opportunistic microbes: microbes that are considered normal (resident) flora when they are in or on one part of the body, but can cause infection if they move out of that area and into or onto another part of the body (7)

Oral–fecal route: a method of transmitting an infection; occurs when feces containing a pathogen contaminate food or water, which is then consumed by another person (8)

Organ: a group of tissues functioning together for a similar purpose (23)

Organelles: structures inside of the cell that help the cell to make the energy it needs to stay alive and to rid itself of waste products (23)

Organism: a living thing, such as an animal or a plant (23)

Organ system: a group of organs that work together to perform a specific function for the body (23)

Oriented to person, place, and time: the state of being able to answer basic questions about person, place, or time; alert (compare with *disoriented*) (12)

Oropharyngeal airway: a hard plastic device that is inserted into a person's mouth to stop the tongue from falling back into the throat; used to keep the airway open (26)

Orthostatic hypotension: a sudden decrease in blood pressure that occurs when a person stands up from a sitting or lying position (16)

OSHA: see *Occupational Safety and Health Administration*

Osteoporosis: a disorder characterized by the excessive loss of bone tissue (25)

Ostomy: a surgically created opening between an internal structure and the skin, usually located on the abdomen (see also *ileostomy* and *colostomy*) (31)

Otitis externa: an infection of the lining of the external auditory canal; commonly referred to as "swimmer's ear" (29)

Otitis media: an infection of the middle ear that is common in young children (29)

Otosclerosis: an inherited form of hearing loss (29)

Over-bed table: a table that fits over a bed or a chair and can be raised or lowered as needed (13)

Ovulation: the release of a ripe, mature egg from the female ovaries each month (33)

P

PACU: see *post-anesthesia care unit*

Palliative care: care that focuses on relieving uncomfortable symptoms, not on curing the problem that is causing the symptoms (21)

Pallor: paleness of the skin (24)

Pancreas: an organ that produces substances that aid in digestion, as well as the hormones insulin and glucagon (31)

Panic disorder: a mental health disorder in which a person experiences episodes of sudden, overpowering fright (panic) and anxiety, usually accompanied by chest or abdominal pain, a rapid heart rate, shortness of breath, and/or dizziness (35)

Papule: a small, raised, firm skin lesion that can be easily felt by passing your fingers lightly over the affected area (24)

Paraplegia: paralysis from the waist down (compare with *quadriplegia* and *hemiplegia*) (10)

Parkinson's disease: a progressive neurologic disorder that is characterized by tremor and weakness in the muscles and a shuffling gait (28)

Pathogen: a microbe that can cause illness (7)

Patient: a person who is receiving health care in a hospital, clinic, or extended-care facility (1)

Patient Self-Determination Act of 1990: an act passed to ensure that the wishes patients and patients' family members have regarding measures to be taken on their own behalf (or on the behalf of their loved one) are followed (21)

Pediculosis capitis: head lice (18)

Pelvic inflammatory disease (PID): infection of the fallopian tubes and abdominal cavity that can lead to infertility (33)

Percutaneous endoscopic gastrostomy (PEG) tube: a special type of gastrostomy tube that is inserted into the stomach with the aid of an endoscope (19)

Pericardium: a double-layered protective sac that surrounds the heart (27)

Perineal care (peri-care): cleaning the perineum and anus, as well as the vulva (in women) and the penis (in men) (17)

Perineum: the area from the bottom of the vagina to the anus (in women) or the area from the root of the penis to the anus (in men) (17)

Peri-operative period: the term used to describe all three phases of the surgical process as a whole—the pre-operative, intra-operative, and post-operative phases (39)

Peripheral nervous system (PNS): the nerves outside of the brain and spinal cord; receives information from the environment, and carries commands from the brain and spinal cord to the other organs of the body, such as the muscles (compare with *central nervous system*) (28)

Peripheral vascular disease: a disorder characterized by pain and cramping in the legs, caused by atherosclerosis of the arteries that supply the legs (27)

Peristalsis: involuntary wave-like muscular movements, such as those that occur in the digestive system to move chyme (partially digested food) through the intestines (20)

Perseveration: the inappropriate and constant repetition of a phrase or act; often seen in people with dementia (36)

Personal protective equipment (PPE): barriers that are worn to physically prevent microbes from reaching a health care provider's skin or mucous membranes, such as gloves, gowns, masks, and protective eyewear (7)

Petit mal (absence) seizure: a seizure characterized by a sudden, brief break in consciousness or activity (compare with *grand mal seizure*) (12)

Phantom pain: the feeling that a body part is still present, after it has been surgically removed (amputated) (25)

Pharyngitis: inflammation of the throat (pharynx) (26)

Pharynx: throat region (26)

Phobia: an excessive, abnormal fear of an object or situation (35)

Physical abuse: the repetitive and deliberate infliction of physical injury on another person, such as that caused by striking, biting, slapping, shaking, or failing to meet a dependent person's physical needs (for example, for food, water, and cleanliness) (compare with *psychological [emotional] abuse* and *sexual abuse*) (4)

Physical restraint: a device that is attached to or near a person's body to limit a person's freedom of movement or access to his or her body (compare with *chemical restraint*) (10)

Physiology: the study of how the body parts work (23)

Placenta: the structure that develops from the inside lining of the uterus during pregnancy and participates in the exchange of gases and nutrients between the mother and the fetus (40)

Plaques: fatty deposits that build up on the inside of the artery wall, blocking blood flow to the tissues and making the artery wall brittle and prone to breaking (27)

Plasma: the liquid part of the blood (27)

Pleura: the membrane that lines the chest cavity and covers the outside of the lungs (26)

Pleurisy: inflammation of the pleura, the membrane that lines the chest cavity and covers the lungs (26)

Pneumonia: inflammation of the lung tissue, caused by infection with a virus or a bacterium, and resulting in impaired gas exchange (26)

Pneumothorax: the build-up of air in the space between the lungs and the chest wall (26)

PNS: see *peripheral nervous system*

Podiatrist: a doctor who specializes in the care of the feet (18)

Polyuria: excessive urine output; see also *diuresis* (20)

Post-anesthesia care unit (PACU): the recovery room where patients are taken following surgery so that they can be closely monitored by the health care team to make sure that they are recovering without complications from the surgery or the anesthesia (39)

Postmenopausal bleeding: uterine bleeding after menopause (33)

Postmortem care: the care of a person's body after the person's death (22)

Post-operative phase: one of three phases of care for a person who is having surgery; the phase after the surgery is actually performed (compare with *preoperative phase* and *intra-operative phase*) (39)

Postpartum period: the 6-week period of time following the birth of a baby (40)

Post-procedure actions: steps that are routinely performed at the end of each patient or resident care procedure, called "Finishing Up" actions in this book (compare with *pre-procedure actions*) (10)

PPE: see *personal protective equipment*

PPO: see *preferred provider organization*

Precertification (preapproval) process: a system for controlling health care costs in which the health care provider must prove that a person's medical condition meets certain criteria and obtain the insurance company's go-ahead for the proposed treatment before starting treatment (1)

Preeclampsia/eclampsia: dangerously high blood pressure in a pregnant woman (40)

Preferred provider organization (PPO): a managed care system that contracts with an insurance company to accept a standard payment

as total payment for services rendered; in return for seeking care only from health care providers who are part of the PPO network, the insured person usually receives that care at a reduced cost to herself (1)

Prenatal care: the health care given to a woman in the months leading up to the birth of her baby (40)

Pre-operative phase: one of three phases of care for a person who is having surgery; the phase before the surgery is actually performed (compare with *intra-operative phase* and *post-operative phase*) (39)

Pre-operative teaching: teaching done by members of the health care team to prepare a person and his or her family members for surgery; during pre-operative teaching, the person learns about the surgical procedure, its benefits and possible risks, and what can be expected during the post-operative recovery period (39)

Pre-procedure actions: steps that are routinely performed before each patient or resident care procedure; called "Getting Ready" actions in this book (compare with *post-procedure actions*) (10)

Presbycusis: age-related hearing loss (29)

Presbyopia: age-related loss of the eye's ability to focus on objects that are close (29)

Preschooler: a person between the ages of 3 and 6 years (41)

Pressure-relieving mattress: a mattress that is placed on top of the regular mattress to help prevent skin breakdown in patients and residents who must stay in bed for long periods of time (15)

Pressure points: bony areas where pressure ulcers are most likely to form; include the heels, ankles, knees, hips, toes, elbows, shoulder blades, ears, the back of the head, and along the spine (24)

Pressure ulcer: a difficult-to-heal (and possibly even fatal) sore that forms when part of the body presses against a surface (such as a mattress or chair) for a long period of time; also known as *pressure sores* and *decubitus ulcers* (11)

Pre-term labor: labor that begins too early, before the fetus can survive on its own (40)

Primary nursing: a model for organizing the nursing team's efforts in which one nurse is assigned several patients or residents, and is responsible for planning and carrying out all aspects of care for those people [compare with *functional (modular) nursing* and *team nursing*] (2)

Procedure: a series of steps followed in a particular order when providing care to a patient or resident that helps to ensure that the care provided is safe and correct (10)

PRN (as-needed) care: personal hygiene care that is provided whenever a patient or resident needs it, throughout the day or night (17)

Professional: a person who has credentials, obtained through education and training, that enable him or her to become licensed or certified to practice a certain profession; also, a person who demonstrates a professional attitude (3)

Professionalism: the attitude of being a professional, characterized by a positive outlook and a commitment to doing one's best at all times (3)

Prognosis: a doctor's prediction of the course of a person's disease, and his or her estimation of the person's chances for recovery (37)

Prone position: one of the basic positions in which the person lies on his abdomen with his head turned to one side (11)

Prosthetic devices: artificial replacements for legs, feet, arms, or other body parts (23)

Psychiatrist: a doctor who specializes in the diagnosis and treatment of mental illness (35)

Psychological (emotional) abuse: the repetitive and deliberate infliction of emotional injury on another person, such as that caused by threatening a person with physical harm or abandonment, teasing a person in a cruel way, or preventing a person from interacting with others (compare with *physical abuse* and *sexual abuse*) (4)

Psychologist: a health care professional who is trained to provide counseling services for people with mental illness (35)

Puberty: the period during which the secondary sex characteristics appear and the reproductive organs begin to function (6)

Pulmonary circulation: the pattern of circulation that takes blood from the heart to the lungs to pick up oxygen and release carbon dioxide (compare with *systemic circulation*) (27)

Pulmonary embolism: a potentially fatal condition caused by blocking of the pulmonary artery by an embolus (a blood clot in a vessel that breaks off and moves from one place to another) (39)

Pulse: the wave of blood sent through the arteries each time the heart beats (16)

Pulse amplitude: the force or quality of the pulse (16)

Pulse deficit: the difference between the apical pulse rate (the pulse that is measured by listening over the apex of the heart with a stethoscope) and the radial pulse rate (the pulse that is measured by placing the middle two or three fingers over the radial artery, located on the inside of the wrist) (16)

Pulse points: the points where the large arteries run close enough to the surface of the skin to be felt as a pulse (12)

Pulse pressure: the difference between the systolic and diastolic pressures (16)

Pulse rate: the number of pulsations that can be felt over an artery in 1 minute; an indication of the heart rate (one of the vital signs) (16)

Pulse rhythm: the pattern of the pulsations and the pauses between them (16)

Pustule: a small, blister-like skin lesion that contains pus, a thick, yellowish fluid that is a sign of infection (24)

Pyelonephritis: a kidney infection (32)

Pyloric sphincter: a circle of muscular tissue that surrounds the place where the stomach empties into the small intestine and helps to prevent food from returning to the stomach once it enters the small intestine (31)

Pyorrhea: gum disease (17)

Pyrexia: the state of having a body temperature that is much higher than normal (16)

Q

Quadriplegia: paralysis from the neck down; compare with *paraplegia* and *hemiplegia* (10)

R

Race: a general characterization that describes skin color, body stature, facial features, and hair texture (6)

RACE fire response plan: the general actions that are taken in the event of a fire emergency (remove to safety, activate the alarm, contain the fire, extinguish or evacuate) (9)

Radiation therapy: a type of therapy that uses energy transmitted by waves to destroy cancer cells (37)

Range of motion: the complete extent of movement that a joint is normally capable of without causing pain (25)

Rash: a group of skin lesions (24)

Reciprocity: the principle by which one state recognizes the validity of a license or certification granted by another state (2)

Recording: communicating information about a patient or resident to other health care team members in written form; sometimes called *charting* (5)

Reduction: the word used to describe the process of bringing the ends of a broken bone into alignment (25)

Reference list: a list of three or four people who would be willing to talk to a potential employer about a job candidate's abilities (3)

Referred (radiating) pain: pain that is felt somewhere other than where it originated (29)

Regional anesthesia: a loss of sensation in part, but not all, of the body brought on by the injection of drugs (compare with *general anesthesia* and *local anesthesia*) (39)

Registered nurse (RN): a specially trained person who is licensed by a state to develop nursing care plans and coordinate all aspects of patient or resident care, as well as to provide that care; holds a baccalaureate degree from a liberal arts college or university (4 years) or an associate degree from a junior or community college (2 years)

Registry: an official record maintained by the state of the people who have successfully completed the nursing assistant training program (2)

Regress: to return to an earlier stage of development, as when an older child who is experiencing stress as a result of being hospitalized begins demonstrating behaviors from when she was younger, such as thumb-sucking or bedwetting (41)

Rehabilitation: the process of helping a person with a disability to return to his or her highest level of physical, emotional, or economic function (23)

Reincarnation: the idea that a person's spirit or soul will live again on Earth in the form of an animal or human being yet to be born (22)

Religion: a person's spiritual beliefs (6)

Reminiscence therapy: a technique used for interacting with people who have dementia, in which the person with dementia is encouraged to remember and share experiences from his or her past with others (36)

Renal: related to, involving, or located in the region of the kidneys (32)

Renal calculi: kidney stones (32)

Reporting: the spoken exchange of information between health care team members (5)

Reproduction: the process by which a living thing makes more living things like itself (33)

Rescue breathing: a basic life support (BLS) technique in which the rescuer blows air into the victim's mouth to perform the function of breathing for the victim until the victim begins breathing again on her own (12)

Resident: a person who is living in a long-term care facility or assisted-living facility (1)

Resident inventory sheet: a document that lists and briefly describes all of the resident's personal belongings; completed when a resident is admitted to a long-term care facility (14)

Respiration: the process the body uses to obtain oxygen from the environment and remove carbon dioxide (a waste gas) from the body (26)

Respiratory arrest: the condition where breathing has stopped (12)

Respiratory rate: the number of times a person breathes in 1 minute (one breath is both an inhalation and an exhalation); one of the vital signs (16)

Respiratory rhythm: the regularity with which a person breathes (16)

Respiratory therapy: any treatment that is used to help a person achieve satisfactory respiration (26)

Respite care: home care that gives the primary caregiver an opportunity to rest or leave the home for a short period of time (42)

Restorative care: measures that health care workers take to help a person regain health, strength, and function; the means by which rehabilitation is achieved (23)

Restraint alternatives: measures taken to avoid the use of chemical or physical restraints (10)

Résumé: a brief document that gives a possible employer general information about a job candidate's education and work experience (3)

Reverse Trendelenburg's position: one of the basic positions in which the head of the mattress is raised so the person's head is higher than her feet (compare with *Trendelenburg's position*) (13)

Rigor mortis: the stiffening of the muscles that usually develops within 2 to 4 hours of death (22)

Rugae: folds in the lining of the stomach (31)

S

Salivary glands: glands located near the mouth that produce and secrete saliva, a substance that helps with chewing and swallowing by moistening the food (31)

Sanitization: practices associated with basic cleanliness, such as handwashing, cleansing of eating utensils and other surfaces with soap and water, and providing clean linens and clothing; one of the techniques of medical asepsis (compare with *antisepsis, disinfection,* and *sterilization*) (7)

SCD: see *sequential compression device*

Schizophrenia: a mental health disorder that affects how a person thinks, feels and acts; the person has difficulty determining what is real from what is imaginary (35)

Scope of practice: the range of tasks that a nursing assistant is legally permitted to do (2)

Seborrheic dermatitis ("cradle cap"): severe scaling of the scalp with thick, yellow, crusty patches (18)

Sebum: an oily substance secreted by glands in the skin that lubricates the skin and helps to prevent it from drying out (24)

Semi-Fowler's (low Fowler's) position: one of the basic positions in which the head of the bed is elevated approximately 30 to 45 degrees (11)

Sense organs: a general term used to describe the eyes, the ears, the nose, and the taste buds (29)

Sensorineural hearing loss: hearing loss that occurs when the receptors in the ear are unable to receive stimuli or transmit nerve impulses (compare with *conductive hearing loss*) (29)

Sensory nerves: nerves that carry information from the internal organs and the outside world to the spinal cord and up into the brain so that the brain can analyze the information (28)

Sensory receptors: specialized cells or groups of cells associated with a sensory nerve (29)

Septic shock: shock caused by a severe bacterial infection that involves the entire body (12)

Sequential compression device (SCD): a device that is applied to the calves to help prevent pooling of blood in the lower legs; often used following surgery to prevent cardiovascular complications (39)

Sex: the physical activity one engages in to obtain sexual pleasure and reproduce (6)

Sexual abuse: forcing another person to engage in sexual activity [compare with *psychological (emotional) abuse* and *physical abuse*] (4)

Sex cell (gamete): special cells contributed by each parent that contain half of the normal number of chromosomes (33)

Sexuality: how a person perceives his or her maleness or femaleness (6)

Sexually transmitted disease (STD): an infection that is most commonly transmitted by sexual contact; also known as *venereal disease* (33)

Shaken baby syndrome: severe brain damage or death in an infant or toddler resulting from violent shaking that causes the child's brain to hit the inside of his skull repeatedly (41)

Shearing: a term used to describe the force created when something or someone is pulled across a surface that offers resistance; can lead to skin breakdown (11)

Shock: the condition that results when the organs and tissues of the body do not receive enough oxygen-rich blood; see also *cardiogenic shock, hemorrhagic shock, anaphylactic shock, and septic shock* (12)

Shroud: a covering used to wrap the body of a person who has died (22)

Signs: objective observations (that is, observations based on information that is obtained directly, through measurements or by using one of the five senses) (compare with *symptoms*) (5)

Sims' position: one of the basic positions in which the person lies on his side with his head turned to one side and his knee sharply bent and supported by a pillow; the corresponding arm is bent at the elbow with the hand in front of the face, palm down, resting on a pillow; the lower leg is straight and the lower arm extends out from the side with the hand down near the hips and the palm turned upward (11)

Sitz bath: a hot water soak for the perineal area (40)

Skeleton: the framework for the body formed by the bones (25)

Slander: spoken statements that injure someone's reputation; a form of defamation (4)

Sperm cell: male sex cell (33)

Sphygmomanometer: a device used to measure blood pressure (16)

Spina bifida: a congenital defect of the spinal column that occurs when the vertebrae do not close properly during development, leaving the spinal cord exposed (34)

Sputum: mucus and other respiratory secretions that are coughed up from the lungs, bronchi, and trachea; also known as *phlegm* (26)

Standard precautions: precautions that a health care worker takes with each patient or resident to prevent contact with bloodborne pathogens; include the use of barrier methods (such as gloves) as well as certain environmental control methods (8)

STD: see *sexually transmitted disease*

Sterilization: the process of completely eliminating microbes from the surface of an object using an autoclave or chemicals; one of the techniques of medical asepsis (compare with *antisepsis, disinfection, and sanitization*) (7)

Stethoscope: a device that amplifies sound and transfers it to the listener's ears (16)

Stomach: a hollow, muscular pouch for holding food (31)

Stomatitis: inflammation of the mouth, often seen in people who are receiving chemotherapy (37)

Stool: a term used to refer to fecal material after it has left the body (20)

Stool softener: a medication that helps to prevent constipation by keeping fluid in the feces (20)

Straight catheter: a urinary catheter that is inserted and then removed immediately, after the urine in the bladder has drained out (20)

Stress: a physical or emotional factor that changes the body's normal balance or equilibrium (35)

Stroke: a disorder that occurs when blood flow to a part of the brain is completely blocked, causing the tissue to die; also known as a "brain attack" or cerebrovascular accident (CVA) (28)

Stump: the end of an amputated limb that is left after surgery (25)

Sub-acute care unit (skilled nursing unit, skilled nursing facility): a unit within a hospital or a long-term care facility, or a separate facility, that provides care focused on rehabilitation and helping the patient to move from hospital care to home care (1)

Subcutaneous tissue: the layer of fat that supports the dermis (the deepest layer of the skin) (24)

Subjective data: information that cannot be objectively measured or assessed (5)

Suicide: the act of taking one's own life intentionally and voluntarily (35)

Suctioning: the process of removing fluid and mucus from a person's airway (26)

Sundowning: the worsening of behavioral symptoms in the late afternoon and evening (as the sun goes down) of a person with dementia (36)

Supine (dorsal recumbent) position: one of the basic positions in which the person lies on his back, with the bed flat and the head supported by a pillow (11)

Supportive care: treatments that will not prolong life, but will make a person more comfortable, such as oxygen therapy, nutritional supplementation, pain medication, range-of-motion exercises, grooming and hygiene, and positioning assistance (21)

Supportive devices: 1) devices used when positioning a person to help the person maintain proper body alignment, such as pillows or rolled sheets, towels, or blankets (11); 2) devices that help to stabilize a weak joint or limb; used in physical therapy to help a person with a disability regain function (23)

Suprapubic catheter: a urinary catheter that is inserted into the bladder through a surgical incision made in the abdominal wall, right above the pubic bone (20)

Surgical bed: a closed bed that has been opened to receive a patient or resident who will be arriving by stretcher; the top sheet, blanket, and bedspread are folded toward the side of the bed, leaving one side open and ready to receive the person (15)

Symptoms: subjective observations (that is, observations that are based on information that cannot be measured or observed first-hand, such as a patient's or resident's complaint of pain) (compare with *signs*) (5)

Synapse: the gap between the axon of one neuron and the dendrites of the next (28)

Syncope: fainting (12)

Systemic circulation: the pattern of circulation that takes blood from the lungs to the rest of the body to release oxygen and pick up carbon dioxide (compare with *pulmonary circulation*) (27)

Systole: the active phase of the cardiac cycle, during which the myocardium contracts, sending blood out of the heart (compare with *diastole*) (27)

Systolic pressure: the pressure that the blood exerts against the arterial walls when the heart muscle contracts; the first blood pressure measurement that is recorded (compare with *diastolic pressure*) (16)

T

Tachycardia: a heart rate that is faster than normal (more than 100 beats/min in an adult) (16)

Tachypnea: a respiratory rate that is higher than normal (more than 24 breaths/min in an adult) (16)

Tactile receptors: receptors found in the skin that are stimulated when something comes in contact with the surface of the body and presses on them, causing them to change shape (29)

Tasks: growth and development milestones that must be completed before a person can move on to the next stage of growth and development (6)

Task lighting: bright light directed toward a specific area, used for activities that require good lighting to prevent eyestrain (compare with *general lighting*) (13)

TB: see *tuberculosis*

T cells: special white blood cells (leukocytes) that play a role in the immune response to invading pathogens; the main target of the human immunodeficiency virus (HIV) (8)

Team nursing: a model for organizing the nursing team's efforts in which a team leader (a registered nurse) determines all of the nursing needs for the patients or residents assigned to the team, and assigns tasks according to each team member's skills and level of responsibility [compare with *functional (modular) nursing* and *primary nursing*] (2)

Tendons: bands of connective tissue that attach the skeletal muscles to the bones (25)

Terminal illness: an illness or condition from which recovery is not expected (6)

Tetany: a condition that occurs when the body's calcium level drops too low; characterized by cramping of the skeletal muscles and an irregular heart beat (30)

Thrombi (singular, *thrombus*): blood clots that form in the small blood vessels, blocking the flow of blood and depriving the tissues of oxygen and nutrients (27)

Thrombocytes: pinched-off pieces of larger cells that are found in the red bone marrow and are responsible for clotting of the blood; also called *platelets* (27)

Thrombophlebitis: a condition characterized by inflammation and pain in the legs, caused by a thrombus in one of the veins of the legs (39)

TIA: see *transient ischemic attack*

Tinea capitis: a fungal infection of the scalp (18)

Tinea pedis: a fungal infection of the skin and nails, commonly known as "athlete's foot" (18)

Tinnitus: ringing in the ear (29)

Tissue: a group of cells similar in structure and specialized to perform a specific function (23)

Toddler: a person between the ages of 1 and 3 years (41)

Toe pleat: loosening of the top linens over a person's feet to relieve pressure and promote comfort (15)

Tort: a violation of civil law (4)

Total parenteral nutrition (TPN, hyperalimentation): an alternative method of providing fluid and nutrition; nourishment is delivered directly into the bloodstream through a large catheter (tube) inserted into a large vein near the heart (19)

TPN: see *total parenteral nutrition*

Trachea: the passage that carries air from the larynx down into the chest toward the lungs; commonly known as the "windpipe" (26)

Tracheostomy: a surgically created opening in the neck that opens into the trachea; often used with a tracheostomy tube (instead of an endotracheal tube) when a person must be on a mechanical ventilator for more than a week or so (26)

Traction: a treatment for fracture in which the ends of the broken bone are placed in the proper alignment and then weight is applied to exert a constant pull and keep the bone in alignment (25)

Transfer: 1) to move a person from one place to another, for example, from the bed to a wheelchair (11); 2) to move a patient or resident within or between health care settings (14)

Transfer belt (gait belt): a webbed or woven belt with a buckle that is used to assist a weak or unsteady person with standing, walking, or transferring; called a *gait belt* when used to help a person walk (11)

Transient flora: microbes that are picked up by touching contaminated objects or people who have an infectious disease [compare with *normal (resident) flora*] (7)

Transient ischemic attack (TIA): a temporary (transient) episode of dysfunction caused by decreased blood flow to the brain (28)

Transsexual: a person who believes that he or she should be a member of the opposite sex (6)

Transvestite: a person who becomes sexually excited by dressing as a member of the opposite sex (6)

Trapeze bar: a device that is attached to the overhead frame of a person's bed; used to assist with movement (25)

Trendelenburg's position: one of the basic positions in which the foot of the mattress is raised so that the person's head is lower than her feet (compare with *reverse Trendelenburg's position*) (13)

Tuberculosis (TB): an airborne infection caused by a bacterium that usually infects the lungs (8)

Tumor: an abnormal growth of tissue; the cells that form the tumor may be benign or malignant (37)

Type I diabetes mellitus (insulin-dependent diabetes mellitus, IDDM): a type of diabetes caused by destruction of the insulin-producing cells of the pancreas (30)

Type II diabetes mellitus (non–insulin-dependent diabetes mellitus, NIDDM): a type of diabetes caused by the inability of the cells of the body to respond to insulin; the pancreas still produces some insulin (30)

U

Ulcer: a shallow crater on the surface of the skin that is formed when the tissue dies and is shed (24)

Umbilical cord: a cord that supplies the growing fetus with nutrients and oxygen, and removes waste (40)

Unintentional tort: a violation of civil law that occurs when someone causes harm or injury to another person or that person's property without the intent to cause harm (4)

Unintentional wound: an unexpected injury that usually results from some type of trauma (compare with *intentional wound*) (24)

Unit: a patient's or resident's room (13)

Unresponsive: adjective used to describe a person who is unconscious and cannot be aroused, or conscious but not responsive when spoken to or touched (12)

Urethritis: infection of the urethra, the passageway that carries urine from the bladder to the outside of the body (32)

Ureterostomy: an alternative way of eliminating urine from the body; a surgical procedure in which the ureters are brought through the abdominal wall by way of small incisions and sutured in place (32)

Urgency: a need to urinate immediately (20)

Urgent: adjective used to describe surgery that is planned and scheduled ahead of time, but must be done as soon as possible to prevent the person's condition from getting worse (39)

Urinal: a device used for urination when a man is unable to get out of bed (20)

Urinalysis: examination of the urine under a microscope and by chemical means (20)

Urinary incontinence: the inability to hold one's urine, or the involuntary loss of urine from the bladder (20)

Urinary retention: the inability of the bladder to empty either completely during urination, or at all (20)

Urination: the process of passing urine from the body; also known as *micturition* and *voiding* (20)

Urine: formed by the kidneys; consists of waste products that have been filtered from the bloodstream, along with excess fluid (32)

Urostomy: an alternative way of eliminating urine from the body; a surgical procedure in which the ureters are attached to a small portion of the small intestine, one end of the segment of intestine is sealed off, and the other end is brought through the abdominal wall and sutured into place to create a stoma (32)

V

Validation therapy: a technique used for interacting with people who have dementia, in which the caregiver acknowledges the person's reality; rather than correcting the person, the caregiver attempts to distract the person and redirect the conversation whenever possible (36)

Value: a cherished belief or principle (4)

Vancomycin-resistant enterococcus (VRE): a type of bacteria that has become resistant to vancomycin, a powerful antibiotic (7)

Varicose veins: a condition that results from pooling of blood in the veins just underneath the skin, causing them to become swollen and "knotty" in appearance (27)

Vascular (multi-infarct) dementia: a type of dementia caused by the loss of function in multiple areas of the brain due to tissue death caused by a lack of adequate oxygen and nutrients (36)

Vector: a living creature, such as an insect, that can transmit disease (7)

Veins: vessels that return blood to the heart (27)

Ventilation: the mechanical process of moving air in and out of the lungs (breathing) (16)

Ventilation system: a system that provides fresh air and keeps air circulating throughout a building (13)

Ventricles: the lower chambers of the heart (27)

Venules: the smallest veins (27)

Verbal communication: a way of communicating that uses written or spoken language (5)

Vernix: a protective, cheese-like substance that is present on the skin of newborns (40)

Vertigo: dizziness (29)

Vesicle: a small, blister-like skin lesion that contains fluid (24)

Villi (singular, *villus*): tiny, finger-like structures on the lining of the small intestine that increase the small intestine's ability to absorb nutrients

Virulence: the strength or disease-producing potential of a pathogen (7)

Vital signs: certain key measurements that provide essential information about a person's health (16)

Voiding: the process of passing urine from the body; also known as *urination* and *micturition* (20)

VRE: see *vancomycin-resistant enterococcus*

W

Water-soluble: adjective used to describe a substance that dissolves in water (for example, certain vitamins) (19)

Weight bearing: a term used to refer to a person's ability to stand on one or both legs (11)

Will: a legal statement that expresses a person's wishes for the management of his or her affairs after death (4)

Work ethic: a person's attitude toward his or her work (3)

Wound: an injury that results in a break in the skin (and usually the underlying tissues as well) (24)

Index

Note: A *t* following a page number indicates tabular material, an *f* indicates a figure, and a *b* indicates a boxed feature.

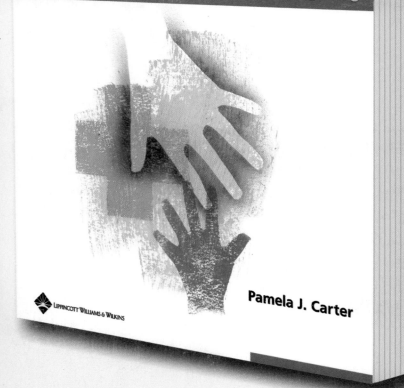